Stephanie

W9-BEO-581

# Physical Dysfunction Practice Skills for the Occupational Therapy Assistant

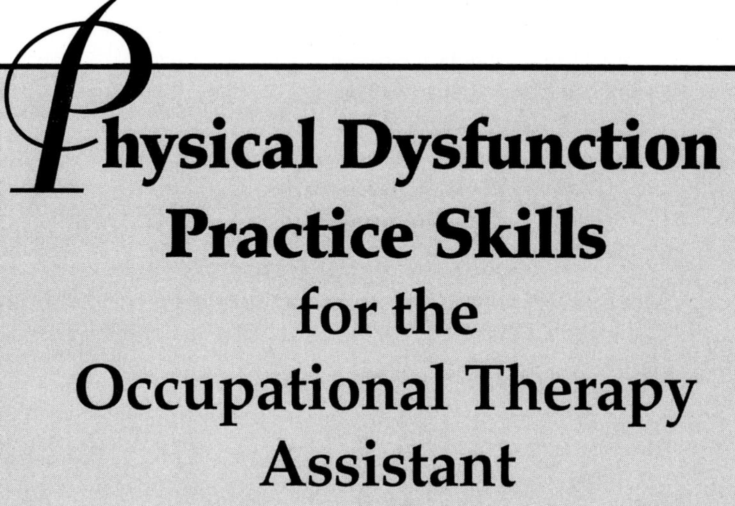

# Physical Dysfunction Practice Skills for the Occupational Therapy Assistant

*Edited by*
**MARY BETH EARLY, MS, OTR/L**

Professor
Occupational Therapy Assistant Program
F.H. LaGuardia Community College
The City University of New York
Long Island City, New York

**with editorial contributions from Lorraine Williams Pedretti, MS, OTR**

*with* 48 *contributors*
*with* 556 *illustrations*

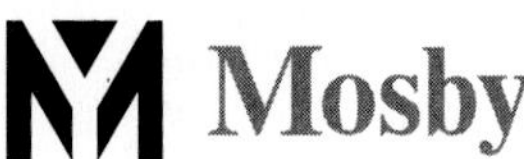

St. Louis Baltimore Boston Carlsbad Chicago Minneapolis New York Philadelphia Portland
London Milan Sydney Tokyo Toronto

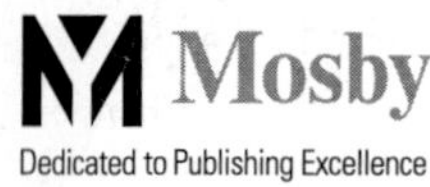

A Times Mirror Company

*Vice President and Publisher:* **Don Ladig**
*Executive Editor:* **Martha Sasser**
*Developmental Editor:* **Amy Christopher**
*Project Manager:* **Linda McKinley**
*Production Editor:* **Catherine Comer**
*Designer:* **Elizabeth Young**
*Manufacturing Supervisor:* **Don Carlisle**
*Cover Photos by:* **Randy Fader-Smith, with direction by Margit Lesser, COTA, SCLT**

Much of the text and illustrations have been revised from the fourth edition of *Occupational Therapy: Practice Skills for Physical Dysfunction* by Lorraine Williams Pedretti, editor.

**Copyright © 1998 by Mosby–Year Book, Inc.**

All rights reserved. No part of this publication may be reproduced, stored in a retrieval system, or transmitted, in any form or by any means, electronic, mechanical, photocopying, recording, or otherwise, without prior written permission from the publisher.

Permission to photocopy or reproduce solely for internal or personal use is permitted for libraries or other users registered with the Copyright Clearance Center, provided that the base fee of $4.00 per chapter plus $.10 per page is paid directly to the Copyright Clearance Center, 222 Rosewood Drive, Danvers, MA 01923. This consent does not extend to other kinds of copying, such as copying for general distribution, for advertising or promotional purposes, for creating new collected works, or for resale.

Printed in the United States of America
Composition by Graphic World, Inc.
Printing/binding by Maple-Vail Book Manufacturing Group

Mosby–Year Book, Inc.
11830 Westline Industrial Drive
St. Louis, MO 63146

**Library of Congress Cataloging in Publication Data**

Early, Mary Beth.
Physical dysfunction practice skills for the occupational therapy assistant / Mary Beth Early, with editorial contributions from Lorraine Williams Pedretti.
p. cm.
Includes bibliographical references and index.
ISBN 0-8151-3091-0
1. Occupational therapy assistants. I. Pedretti, Lorraine Williams, 1936- . II. Title.
RM735.E27 1997 97-16858
615.8′515—dc21 CIP

97 98 99 00 01 / 9 8 7 6 5 4 3 2 1

# Contributors

CAROLE ADLER, BS, OTR
Clinical Supervisor, Department of Occupational Therapy, Santa Clara Valley Medical Center, San Jose, California

PHYLLIS BER, OTR, MPA, BS
Director, Occupational Therapy, Waterview Nursing Care Center, Flushing, New York

SERENA BERGER, MA, OTR
Occupational Therapist; Teaching Assistant, Occupational Therapy Department, New York University, New York, New York;
Clinical Sales Consultant, Smith and Nephew Rolyan, Germantown, Wisconsin

ELIZABETH MARIA BIANCHI, BS, MS, OTR
Former Senior Occupational Therapist, Stanford University Hospital, Stanford, California

HELEN BOBROVE, OTR
Former Clinical Specialist, Orthopedics, Stanford University Hospital, Stanford, California

WENDY S. BUCKNER, MHE, OTR/L
Assistant Professor, Occupational Therapy Department, Medical College of Georgia, Augusta, Georgia

ANN BURKHARDT, MA, OTR/L
Assistant Director of Occupational Therapy;
Clinical Instructor of Occupational Therapy, Columbia-Presbyterian Medical Center, The Presbyterian Hospital, Columbia University, New York, New York

GORDON UMPHRED BURTON, PhD, OTR
Graduate Coordinator; Associate Professor, Occupational Therapy Department, San Jose State University, San Jose, California

SONIA COLEMAN, MEd, OTR/L
Assistant Professor, Occupational Therapy Department, Towson State University, Towson, Maryland;
Adjunct Faculty, Catonsville Community College, Catonsville, Maryland

ALBERT M. COOK, PhD, PE
Dean; Professor, Faculty of Rehabilitation Medicine, University of Alberta, Edmonton, Alberta, Canada;
Partner, Assistive Technologies 2000, Sacramento, California

JAN ZARET DAVIS, BS, OTR
NDT Occupational Therapy Instructor in Adult Hemiplegia;
President, International Clinical Educators, Inc., Port Townsend, Washington

MICHAEL K. DAVIS, MBA, OTR
Assistant Professor, Department of Occupational Therapy, Loma Linda University, Loma Linda, California

JANNA M. DREHER, MS, OTR
Program Director, Occupational Therapy Assistant Program,
Lake Superior College, Duluth, Minnesota

MARY BETH EARLY, MS, OTR/L
Professor, Occupational Therapy Assistant Program, F.H. LaGuardia Community College, The City University of New York, Long Island City, New York

FRED FEUCHTER, PhD
Associate Professor of Anatomy and Physiology, Department of Occupational Therapy, Samuel Merritt College, Oakland, California

DIANE FOTI, MS, OTR
Occupational Therapist/Lecturer, Department of Occupational Therapy, San Jose State University, San Jose, California;
Senior Occupational Therapist, Kaiser Permanente Medical Center, Redwood City, California

PATRICIA A. GENTILE, MS, OTR/L
Chief Occupational Therapist, Physical Medicine and Rehabilitation Department, The Jamaica Hospital Medical Center, Jamaica, New York

DIANE D. HARDY, BS, OTR
Senior Therapist; Spinal Cord Injury Specialist,
Loma Linda Medical Center;
Clinical Instructor and Lecturer,
Occupational Therapy Department,
Loma Linda University School of Allied Health,
Loma Linda, California

MARIANNE HEDL, MS, OTR, CHT
Private Practitioner,
Hand Therapy and Orthopaedic Rehabilitation,
Astoria, New York

SUSAN M. HUSSEY, MS, OTR
Program Coordinator, Occupational Therapy Assistant Program,
Sacramento City College;
Partner, Assistive Technologies 2000,
Sacramento, California

JANET JABRI, MBA, OTR, FAOTA
National Director of Rehabilitation,
GCI Rehabilitation Division, Pan Care, Inc.,
San Jose, California

MARY C. KASCH, OTR, CHT, FAOTA
Director, Hand Rehabilitation Center of Sacramento,
Sacramento, California

REGINA M. LEHMAN, MS, OTR/L
Assistant Director, Occupational Therapy Department,
Goldwater Memorial Hospital, New York, New York

SHERI L. LIEBERMAN, OTR
Carmel, California;
Former Clinical Coordinator of Occupational Therapy,
Department of Rehabilitation Services,
Stanford University Hospital, Stanford, California

SUSAN M. LILLIE, OTR
Senior Occupational Therapist,
Adaptive Driver Evaluation Program,
Santa Clara Valley Medical Center;
Guest Lecturer, Department of Occupational Therapy,
San Jose State University, San Jose, California;
Member, State of California Department of Motor Vehicles Medical Advisory Board

MAUREEN MICHELE MATTHEWS, BS, OTR
Clinical Supervisor, Occupational Therapy Department,
Santa Clara Valley Medical Center, San Jose, California

GUY L. McCORMACK, OTR, PhC
Chairperson; Associate Professor,
Department of Occupational Therapy,
Samuel Merritt College, Oakland, California

DEBORAH MORAWSKI, BS, OTR
Supervisor, Occupational Therapy Department,
Community Hospital and Rehabilitation Center of Los Gatos—Saratoga,
Los Gatos, California

PATRICIA ANN MORRIS, OTR, BS
Senior Occupational Therapist,
Occupational Therapy/Physical Medicine and Rehabilitation Department Unit,
Wayne State University, Detroit, Michigan

LAURIE MUHN, OTR/BS
Senior Occupational Therapist,
Upper Extremity Amputee Clinic Coordinator,
Occupational Therapy/Outpatient Department,
Eastern Michigan University, Ypsilanti, Michigan

KAREN L. NELSON, MS, OTR
Clinical Supervisor, Rehabilitation, Home Health Plus,
Santa Clara, California;
Lecturer, Department of Occupational Therapy,
San Jose State University, San Jose, California

JAN POLON NOVIC, OTR
Santa Cruz, California;
Former Clinical Coordinator of Neurological and Intensive Care Units,
Stanford University Hospital, Stanford, California

LORRAINE WILLIAMS PEDRETTI, MS, OTR
Professor Emeritus, Department of Occupational Therapy,
San Jose State University, San Jose, California

ANGELA M. PERALTA, AS, COTA
Adjunct Instructor, Occupational Therapy Assistant Program,
Touro College, New York, New York

KAREN PITBLADDO, MS, OTR
Clinical Specialist, Occupational Therapy Department,
Brigham and Women's Hospital, Boston, Massachusetts;
Former Clinical Coordinator of Occupational Therapy in Orthopedics,
Stanford University, Stanford, California

MICHAEL PIZZI, MS, OTR/L, CHES, FAOTA
Founder, Positive Images and Wellness, Inc.,
Silver Spring, Maryland

SALLY E. POOLE, MA, OTR, CHT
Clinical Assistant Professor,
Occupational Therapy Department, New York University,
New York, New York;
Private Practitioner, Hands-On Rehab,
Valhalla, New York

SARA A. POPE-DAVIS, MOT, OTR/L
Staff Occupational Therapist, Laurel Regional Hospital,
Laurel, Maryland

SHERRELL POWELL, MA, OTR
Professor, Occupational Therapy Assistant Program,
Natural and Applied Science Department,
F.H. LaGuardia Community College,
The City University of New York,
Long Island City, New York

ELIZABETH A. RIVERS, OTR, RN
Burn Rehabilitation Clinical Specialist,
The Burn Center at Ramsey;
Part-Time Clinical Instructor,
University of Minnesota, St. Paul, Minnesota

KATIE SCHLAGETER, OTR
Assistant Manager, Out Patient Rehabilitation Program,
Alta Bates Medical Center, Berkeley, California

LORI M. SHIFFMAN, MS, OTR, BCN
Adjunct Faculty, Department of Occupational Therapy,
J. Sargent Reynolds Community College,
Virginia Commonwealth University/
Medical College of Virginia; Patient Evaluator,
Defense and Veteran's Head Injury Program,
Richmond, Virginia

JEAN W. SOLOMON, MHS, OTR/L
Clinical Coordinator, Rehabilitative Services Department,
Occupational Therapy Assistant Program,
Trident Technical College, Charleston, South Carolina

MICHELLE TIPTON-BURTON, MS, OTR
Clinical Instructor;
Senior Occupational Therapist,
Santa Clara Valley Medical Center,
San Jose State University, San Jose, California

DARCY ANN UMPHRED, PhD, PT
Professor; Vice Chairperson,
Department of Physical Therapy,
University of the Pacific, Stockton, California

INGRID WADE, BSOT, OTR, CHT
Clinical Director,
R.L. Petzoldt Memorial Center for Hand Rehabilitation,
San Jose, California

MARY WARREN, MS, OTR
Director, Occupational Therapy Department,
Visual Independence Program,
The Eye Foundation of Kansas City;
Department of Ophthalmology—School of Medicine,
University of Missouri—Kansas City,
Kansas City, Missouri

CAROL J. WHEATLEY, MS, OTR/L
Assistant Supervisor of Occupational Therapy,
Maryland Rehabilitation Center,
Division of Rehabilitation Services,
Maryland State Department of Education,
Baltimore Maryland;
Instructor, Department of Occupational Therapy,
Towson State University, Towson, Maryland

BARBARA ZOLTAN, MA, OTR
Consultant in Private Practice,
Saratoga, California

# Reviewers

CAROLE ADLER, BS, OTR
Clinical Supervisor, Department of Occupational Therapy,
Santa Clara Valley Medical Center, San Jose, California

LAURA E. DUNLOP, BS, OTR/L
Clinical Specialist, Pain Management,
The Pain Center,
Hospital Joint Diseases/Orthopaedic Institute,
New York, New York

HARU HIRAMA, EdD, OTR/L, FAOTA
Director, Occupational Therapy;
Professor and Chairperson,
Occupational Therapy Department,
Alvernia College, Reading, Pennsylvania

ANNE MacKAY LAWTON, OTR/L, BA
Department Chair; Program Director,
Department of Occupational Therapy,
Delaware Technical and Community College,
Owens Campus, Georgetown, Delaware

ARLETTE LOESER, MA, OTR
Clinical Specialist in Assistive Technology,
Department of Rehabilitation Medicine,
Mount Sinai Medical Center;
Private Practitioner,
New York, New York

PATRICIA MARTIN, AAS, COTA/L
Clinical Coordinator,
Occupational Therapy Assistant Program,
School of Health Science,
Pennsylvania College of Technology,
Williamsport, Pennsylvania

MAUREEN MICHELE MATTHEWS, BS, OTR
Clinical Supervisor, Occupational Therapy Department,
Santa Clara Valley Medical Center, San Jose, California

M. TERESA MOHLER, OTR/L, MA (ACE)
Assistant Professor (Retired),
Occupational Therapy Assistant Program,
Mount Aloysius College, Cresson, Pennsylvania

KAREN L. NELSON, MS, OTR
Clinical Supervisor, Rehabilitation,
Home Health Plus, Santa Clara, California;
Lecturer, Department of Occupational Therapy,
San Jose State University, San Jose, California

LORI M. SHIFFMAN, MS, OTR, BCN
Adjunct Faculty, Department of Occupational Therapy,
J. Sargent Reynolds Community College,
Virginia Commonwealth University/
Medical College of Virginia;
Patient Evaluator,
Defense and Veteran's Head Injury Program,
Richmond, Virginia

TEEPA L. SNOW, MS, OTR/L, FAOTA
Program Director,
Occupational Therapy Assistant Program,
Health Technologies Department,
Durham Technical Community College,
Durham, North Carolina

JEAN W. SOLOMON, MHS, OTR/L
Clinical Coordinator, Rehabilitative Services Department,
Occupational Therapy Assistant Program,
Trident Technical College,
Charleston, South Carolina

# Preface

Modeled on the fourth edition of the classic text *Occupational Therapy: Practice Skills for Physical Dysfunction* by Lorraine Williams Pedretti, MS, OTR, this book was written to fill a need for a basic physical disabilities text specifically for the occupational therapy assistant student. It is designed for entry-level practice and aims to include major content required by the American Occupational Therapy Association's (AOTA's) Essentials and Guidelines for an Accredited Program for the Occupational Therapy Assistant. The text may also serve as a resource for occupational therapy practitioners at all levels seeking to understand the role of the certified occupational therapy assistant (COTA) in physical dysfunction practice. Strict attention has been given to AOTA guidelines for practice, supervision, and service competency.

This text includes significant amounts of content beyond entry level so that it may continue to serve as a resource to the COTA in the clinic. We have also recognized that individual schools and practitioners in different areas of the country may need additional material to meet the needs of their local practice environment and have tried to include this information without compromising the parameters of technical level practice or unduly enlarging the book.

Certain assumptions were made when designing this book for the technical level student. First, the student should have completed basic anatomy and physiology and foundation occupational therapy courses. Second, the student should have completed or should be taking as a corequisite a course in medical conditions or pathology. Third, the student must be willing to supplement this text with references, such as medical dictionaries and pathology texts, that will provide background information. We have made a sincere effort to write the book in such a way that it is understandable to an associate degree student, but it is not an elementary text.

The book is organized into six sections. Part I covers theory, practice models, and the history and role of the COTA in physical dysfunction practice. Part II addresses the occupational therapy process and includes documentation. Part III provides extensive information on evaluation and includes many evaluations that are beyond entry level but in which the COTA might reasonably be expected to achieve competency, at least in certain practice environments. Part IV outlines broad aspects of treatment, including infection control and safety, psychosocial aspects, sexuality, purposeful activities, therapeutic exercise, and physical agent modalities. Part V catalogs and discusses the major treatment interventions used for physical dysfunction, including activities of daily living, orthoses, assistive and adaptive devices and equipment, splinting, assistive technology, and the sensorimotor approaches to treatment. Part VI introduces specific treatment applications, including those for oncology, HIV, cardiac dysfunction and chronic obstructive pulmonary disease, older adults and multidiagnosis patients, as well as cerebrovascular accident, traumatic brain injury, degenerative diseases, amputations, lower and upper extremity orthopedics, spinal cord injury, burns, and others.

Special features include lists of key terms and objectives for each chapter, selected reading guide questions at the end of each chapter, text boxes highlighting special techniques, case studies and treatment plans, and a wealth of illustrations and photographs. A guide to selected acronyms has been included inside the cover.

To make the best use of this text, we recommend that readers begin with the objectives, key terms, and reading guide questions for the targeted chapter. Then, making use of a medical dictionary as needed, the student should read the chapter or section completely, without taking notes and with an aim to understanding what is being read. During a separate session, the student should then do a second reading, make an outline or notes from the text, and attempt to answer the reading guide questions. This level of thoroughness and repetition is critical to mastery of the material.

Certain terms in this book have been used to describe both the occupational therapy service provider and the consumer. The consumer may be referred to as *patient, client,* or *caregiver* depending on the context of the intervention.

The terms *practitioner* and *clinician* refer to providers of occupational therapy services at both levels of practice (i.e., both the registered occupational therapist [OTR] and the COTA). The words *assistant, COTA,* and *certified occupational therapy assistant* are used to designate the technical level practitioner. Conversely, the terms *therapist, OTR,* and *occupational therapist* indicate the professional level practitioner. Very occasionally the word *therapist* is used more generically to describe the provider of therapy but is intended to designate both levels of practitioners.

MARY BETH EARLY

# Acknowledgments

The first acknowledgment belongs to Lorraine Williams Pedretti and her contributors, whose pioneering efforts in their text, *Occupational Therapy: Practice Skills for Physical Dysfunction* (now in its fourth edition), inspired the present work and without whose initial contributions this book would not have been possible. A second acknowledgment is due to Maureen Michele Matthews, my sister and colleague, for her urging that I involve myself with this project and for her dedicated work on several chapters in a variety of ways.

I am indebted to the chapter authors and contributors for their dedication, professionalism, and hard work, often involving several drafts. Among the many contributors are several established writers and many new authors, quite a few of whom are occupational therapy assistant program educators. Particular thanks are due to Jeanie Solomon, for editorial advice and assistance, and to Wendy Buckner, Gina Lehman, and Michael Davis for their gracious willingness to take on more than one chapter. To provide a uniform style, I have extensively edited or rewritten many chapters; any alteration from the authors' original intent is unintentional and solely my responsibility.

Educators from occupational therapy assistant programs across the country who have contributed information, material, or advice include Johannes Kicker, Kathryn Mason, Liane Hewitt, Janet Delany, Lori Shiffman, and Brenda Smaga. In addition, educators too numerous to mention responded to a market survey that helped shape this book. Their comments and suggestions were immensely helpful.

I owe special thanks to all of the reviewers—Carole Adler, Laura Dunlop, Haru Hirama, Anne MacKay Lawton, Arlette Loeser, Patricia Martin, Maureen Matthews, M. Teresa Mohler, Karen Nelson, Angela Peralta, Lori Shiffman, Jeanie Solomon, and Teepa Snow—for their time, expertise, and advice.

All of the editors and staff at Mosby have been supportive, professional, and endlessly helpful. In particular I would like to thank Martha Sasser, Executive Editor, and Amy Christopher, Developmental Editor, for their patient and reliable guidance and assistance, and Laura MacAdam for her management of many details. Thanks are also due to Cathy Comer, Production Editor, for her careful scrutiny and stewardship of the production process.

I am grateful to the publishers, vendors, health care facilities, and in particular the individuals who permitted us to use material from their publications, as well as to the patients and models who posed for photographs.

I extend special thanks to my colleagues, friends, and students at LaGuardia Community College, whose camaraderie, support, and ability to listen have been so important.

Finally, I thank my husband, Bob, and our son, Jeffrey, whose love, flexibility, and personal sacrifice have supported and nourished me through the 2 years of work on this task.

MARY BETH EARLY

# Contents

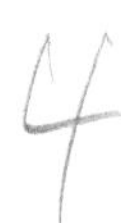

# Physical Dysfunction Practice Skills for the Occupational Therapy Assistant

Part I

# History and Theory

Chapter 1

# Brief History of Occupational Therapy and Role of the COTA in Physical Disabilities Practice

Mary Beth Early

## Chapter Objectives

*After studying this chapter, the student or practitioner will be able to:*

1. Identify the origins of occupational therapy in the Enlightenment, the concept of moral treatment, and the arts and crafts movement.
2. Recognize the effects of World War I, the Great Depression, and World War II on occupational therapy.
3. Discuss the conflicting concepts of holism and reductionism within the history of occupational therapy.
4. Trace the history of the certified occupational therapy assistant, particularly in the practice area of physical dysfunction.

## Key Terms

the Enlightenment
moral treatment
humanitarianism
arts and crafts movement
holism
reductionism
purposeful activity
physical agent modalities
*Occupational Therapy Roles*
occupational therapy practitioners
general supervision
close supervision

Imagine the certified occupational therapy assistant (COTA) practicing in a nursing home. During the day the COTA may come into contact with 20 patients, providing treatments and therapeutic activities that include dressing training, reality orientation, feeding training with adapted equipment, stacking paper cones, exercising a weak upper extremity using a small wheeled platform called a *skateboard,* weaving at an upright loom, and assembling small wood kits. How did all these tools come to be part of the COTA's practice? This question can be answered only by exploring the history of occupational therapy.

Although this text is about physical disabilities, occupational therapy took root in a broadly social foundation and first embraced the needs of the mentally ill patient, the immigrant, and the factory worker. Care of those with primarily physical problems developed later. The story begins with the treatment of mentally ill persons in Europe.

## HISTORY OF OCCUPATIONAL THERAPY IN PHYSICAL DISABILITIES PRACTICE

### Moral Treatment: Foundations in the Enlightenment

Occupational therapy is rooted in eighteenth-century Europe in the era known as **the Enlightenment.** Before the Enlightenment, popular culture was dominated by pessimism, superstition, and ignorance. People believed that the sun revolved around the earth.[20,21] Mentally ill persons were believed to be sinners or possessed by demons and were typically housed in crude stalls and treated no better than animals.[15,19]

The scientific discoveries of Isaac Newton (gravity, theory of optics), Malpighi (workings of the lung), Swammerdam (existence of red blood cells), and others stimulated an appetite among educated people for "the facts." No longer content with beliefs based on religious teachings and cultural traditions, Enlightenment philosophers argued for the use of reason and the scientific method as means of understanding the world.[20,21] It was from this atmosphere that the concept of **moral treatment** of mentally ill persons arose.

The most famous advocates of moral treatment were Philippe Pinel, a French physician, and Samuel Tuke, an Englishman and a Quaker. Their efforts in moral treatment reflected a larger social ideal of **humanitarianism,** or a regard and respect for all humans. This contrasted with the previous belief that mentally ill persons were little more than animals. Moral treatment included the following principles: a respect for the individual, a belief in the unity of the mind and the body, the importance of a regular daily routine, and the value of productive activity for even the most disabled person. Mentally ill patients were moved into residential settings, where they and the staff produced most of the goods and services provided to the patients. The patients grew their own crops, cared for animals, constructed buildings and furniture, wove cloth and made clothing, and did laundry, cleaning, and general maintenance and repairs.

The *moral* aspect of the treatment was twofold. On the one hand, it was moral to treat mentally ill patients in a more humane or humanitarian manner. On the other, it was believed that madness was often (if not generally) the result of immoral thoughts or actions. Consequently, inmates were forced into self-examination, were confronted by their physicians, and were expected to make confessions of error as an important part of the treatment. It is easy to see the beginnings of psychoanalysis in these methods.[19]

It is believed that moral treatment was introduced to the United States by Benjamin Rush, a Quaker and signer of the Declaration of Independence.[28] Moral treatment required a low patient/staff ratio, was practiced with small groups, and was more expensive than simply housing the patients in large institutions. The movement grew in popularity during the early 1800s but fell into disuse in the latter part of the century. The economic costs of the Civil War and the arrival of large numbers of non–English-speaking immigrants were two reasons for this decline.

### The Arts and Crafts Movement

Another important influence on early occupational therapy was the arts and crafts movement, which began in the late 1800s in response to the Industrial Revolution. Before industrialization, all objects used in daily life were made by hand. Most adults (except very wealthy ones) worked in agriculture, in commerce, or at some craft, such as smithing or metalwork, carpentry, or tanning or leatherwork. Women typically engaged in many different crafts needed for the operation of their homes and the needs of their families.

The rise of factories and the availability of manufactured goods caused a revolution in the way people lived and worked. No longer needed to craft objects by hand, skilled workers moved to factories, where they performed relatively low-skill, repetitious activities. Despite society's gain in more efficient production and more ready access to manufactured items, many workers lost their identity as skilled craftspersons. This immediately sparked an interest, mainly in the wealthy population, in reviving crafts and the crafts traditions. The leaders of the arts and crafts movement promoted crafts production as more aesthetically satisfying (more beautiful) than factory manufacture and as more therapeutic for the person making the craft.[25]

Among the values advanced by the arts and crafts movement were the importance of manual training for both rich and poor people, the value of good taste and an appreciation of beautiful things, and the development of physical strength and technical expertise as essential aspects of education.[25] One core idea that became fundamental to occupational therapy was that the regular schooling of children (and by extension the treatment of ill and injured persons) should include training in productive activities similar or identical to those performed by able-bodied adults.

It is important to recognize that the major traditional occupational therapy activities date from the arts and crafts movement. These activities—weaving, leathercraft, metalwork, pottery, woodworking, and needlecrafts—were ordinary tasks in preindustrial times. They were performed by many people in the course of their daily lives. Today, however, these activities are much more unusual and novel for the average person, who may perceive them as quaint, old-fashioned, or childish. The creation of tangible objects (things that can be held) with the hands is a rare experience for most people today. The relevance and place of crafts in occupational therapy practice continues to be hotly debated, as discussed later in this chapter.

### Occupational Therapy: The Beginning

Many people working with sick patients during the first years of the twentieth century tried to apply the ideas of moral treatment and the arts and crafts movement in their work. Herbert James Hall, a physician, employed needlework in the treatment of women with neurasthenia, a nervous disorder characterized by weakness, fatigue, irritability, and headaches. Beginning with short work periods, Hall gradually increased the time and demands on the patient.[28] Susan Tracy, a nurse, wrote the book *Invalid Occupations* in which she documented her work using occupations with patients in the hospital.[26] Adolph Meyer, a physician who emigrated to the United States from Switzerland in 1892, revived interest in moral treatment and specifically promoted occupation as a healing agent.[27] George Edward Barton, an architect with tuberculosis, nervous paralysis, and an amputation, realized occupation was a cure while he was recovering from these disorders. He is credited with coining the term *occupational therapy*.[28]

In 1917 Barton and five others founded the National Society for the Promotion of Occupational Therapy (N-SPOT), which in 1923 became the American Occupational Therapy Association (AOTA). The leaders included two architects, a physician, a social worker, a secretary, and an arts and crafts teacher. They shared a devotion to occupation as a means of healing and an interest in furthering the study of the relationship among the therapist, patient, and occupation. The first applications of occupation were primarily with patients with tuberculosis or psychiatric disorders. Manual training, or the use of arts and crafts to improve hand skills and dexterity, was also a common practice.

### World War I

Almost immediately after the founding of N-SPOT, the United States entered World War I, which had started in Europe in 1914. In 1918 reconstruction aides were recruited; these women were trained to occupy the hands and minds of convalescing war-injured patients. The diagnoses treated included anxiety and stress disorders (although these were not the terms used at the time), amputations, blindness, and neurological and other injuries. The reconstruction aides employed various craft activities in their work and developed specific methods for treating the various physical disabilities. Once the war ended, however, many reconstruction aides left the service, and occupational therapy practice again centered primarily on patients with psychiatric disorders. Skills and methods developed to treat physical disabilities were not properly documented and were lost.[28]

### Between the Wars

The Great Depression of the 1930s affected occupational therapy adversely. With less money available generally, budgets were cut, staff were laid off, and many schools and clinics closed. Only a small number of therapists worked with physically disabled patients. During this period, occupational therapists allied themselves with the American Medical Association, primarily as a means of enforcing educational standards.[29]

This alliance came at some cost. Occupational therapy had its roots in the holism of moral treatment. **Holism** is a philosophy that values the whole above the sum of its parts; in the case of occupational therapy, the whole was the essential unity of mind and body. In the atmosphere of the new medical era, holism was seen as sentimental and unscientific. The medical trend of the time was toward **reductionism,** or the analysis of phenomena in small measurable parts, such as range of motion or muscle strength. Occupational therapy was pushed in this direction and away from its holistic roots.[24]

### World War II and Its Aftermath: The Rise of Reductionism

World War II increased the demand for occupational therapists, but few were available. War Emergency training courses were commissioned to prepare occupational therapists for the war. The number of therapists increased by 50% over the 4 years from 1941 to 1945, and physical medicine became better established. Still by 1953 only 3% of occupational therapists were employed in physical disabilities practice. The vast majority of therapists practiced in mental health, with large numbers also in general medicine and tuberculosis treatment.[28]

Despite this trend in practice, principles of treatment for physical dysfunction were recorded and disseminated through the first edition of Willard and Spackman's *Principles of Occupational Therapy.* Clare S. Spackman listed the goals of occupational therapy in physical dysfunction as follows: "(1) to improve the motion of joints and the strength of muscles; (2) to develop co-ordination, motor skills and work tolerance; and (3) to prevent the building up of unwholesome psychologic reactions or to correct them if they are already established."[36] Spackman provided guidelines to analyze, select, adapt, and grade activities to develop specific motions. She directed the reader to pay attention to the patient's posture, the position of furniture and equipment, and the possibility of undesirable substitute motion.

Spackman's first two goals had a clearly reductionist orientation. Continued focus on these and other technical concerns through the 1950s, 60s, and 70s led to increased use of techniques (rather than occupation) in treatment. Development of splinting materials and methods and use of mechanical exercisers and physical agents such as paraffin are a few examples. These techniques had little to do with the profession's original holistic philosophy and were often unrelated to each other. A schism was developing within the field. Shannon[34] identified a split between a "technique philosophy" and the original values and beliefs on which the profession was founded. Fidler[18] associated the technique philosophy with a weak professional identity and believed that occupational therapists were borrowing the modalities of other professions to achieve credibility. In so doing, they were forgetting the most fundamental principle of occupational therapy—the patients as "doers" or creators of their own therapy. When the modalities are applied from the outside, patients never act on their own, rather they merely receive treatment.

### AOTA Adopts a Holistic Philosophy

In 1979 the Representative Assembly of AOTA voted to endorse a philosophical base, which reads in part as follows[5]:

> Man is an active being whose development is influenced by the use of purposeful activity. Human beings are able to influence their physical and mental health and their social and physical environment through purposeful activity.

In this statement the term **purposeful activity** replaces the historical term *occupation*. Adoption of this philosophical base and a companion policy[6] marks the official beginning of AOTA's efforts to promote the use of purposeful activity as the core of occupational therapy. The use of techniques and "facilitating procedures" was considered acceptable only when used to prepare the patient for purposeful activity. Despite the emphasis on purposeful activity, many therapists treating patients with physical disabilities continued to limit the use of activities in their practice. Instead they used splinting, exercise, and sensorimotor techniques that involved stimulation of the nervous system.

In 1983 AOTA further clarified the place of **physical agent modalities** in occupational therapy practice and amended and strengthened its position again in 1991 and 1992.[7] Modalities were defined as "employment of a therapeutic agent" and were to be used "only in preparation for, or as an adjunct to, purposeful activity to enhance occupational performance." In other words the use of modalities alone is not considered occupational therapy. Modalities can be used in preparation for purposeful activity, but not instead of it.

### Summary

Historically, conflicts have flared within occupational therapy regarding its philosophical base and treatment techniques. Although the national professional organization has reaffirmed its belief in the unity of mind and body and the primacy of activity within human life, we continue to apply techniques and treatments that originated in reductionist theories. How will we reconcile the use of ultrasound and other externally applied modalities with our view that the patient is the originator of purposeful activity? Numerous AOTA position papers, policies, and other documents[5-7,9] limit the use of such modalities to facilitate performance within the context of purposeful activity. However, many therapists continue to use these modalities in isolation.

Crafts, which we have used as treatment tools since the origin of the profession, are repeatedly attacked from within our own ranks and by outsiders. To what extent should we continue to use crafts with our patients? If the purposefulness of a given activity depends on the individual patient and the context or situation in which it is performed, do we give crafts only to those patients who have enjoyed them in the past and who prefer them? Or do we introduce crafts to patients as an alternative to strictly mechanical exercise, hoping that the purposefulness of the treatment goal (to increase range of motion or muscle strength) will motivate the patient long enough for him or her to find another purpose in doing the activity?

Occupational therapy is rooted in a tradition of holism, which views occupation (purposeful activity) as an essential aspect of human life and health. By engaging in activities, humans use their minds and bodies as one, develop skills and ideas, produce things that benefit themselves and others, create their own lives, and maintain their own health. Occupation is seen as a powerful tool in restoring health to injured and disabled patients.

Our profession has branched prolifically from the roots that emerged from the moral treatment era and the arts and crafts movement. Just as a tree, when cut deeply, sprouts new growth, so has occupational therapy grown despite the political, social, and economic obstacles it has encountered. From the experiences of treating wounded soldiers from two wars sprouted many creative methods that are still used today. From the reductionist era, during which occupation was almost abandoned as ridiculous and unscientific, grew many sensorimotor and exercise techniques. The challenge today is to nurture the tree around its main core of occupation so that all the branches will have a strong center from which to flourish.

## HISTORY OF THE COTA IN PHYSICAL DISABILITIES PRACTICE

As with the history of occupational therapy, the history of the certified occupational therapy assistant begins in mental health. The movement of large numbers of COTAs into physical disabilities practice occurred slowly, over decades.

### COTAs: The Beginning

During World War II, many occupational therapists were trained in war emergency courses to meet the tremendous demand. Shortages continued after the war, particularly in psychiatry, and a training program for occupational therapy assistants was proposed by AOTA in 1949. Formal standards were finally adopted in 1957.[33] The original training programs of 460 hours over 12 weeks prepared assistants to work only in psychiatry where the demand was greatest. The programs were based in the facilities where COTAs were needed to provide services. In the next few years a number of occupational therapy aides, who had been working and had received on-the-job training, were "grandfathered in" as assistants by AOTA.

### COTAs Move into General Practice and Beyond

In 1961 general practice was added to the standards for occupational therapy assistant education; training programs were specialized into the two areas of psychiatry and general practice. General practice was introduced because occupational therapy services were needed in nursing homes. By 1966 all students were required to be trained to work in both practice areas. A study at that time by Adamson and Anderson[1] showed that of those surveyed (who included uncertified assistants and aides as well as COTAs), most were planning and providing functional programs in both psychiatry and physical disabilities. Thus COTAs produced important treatment services beyond diversional activities.

The passage of Medicare legislation in 1967 increased demand for occupational therapy practitioners, particularly assistants, in nursing homes.[22] In the decade after the passage of Medicare, occupational therapy practice began to shift away from mental health and toward physical disabilities, to the point where today 89% of registered occupational therapists (OTRs) practice in physical disabilities and only 11% in mental health. COTA practice also shifted away from psychiatry to areas such as physical disabilities, school settings, and nursing homes. In 1963, 85% of COTAs were practicing in psychiatry and only 15% in general practice.[22] By 1994 these figures had almost reversed, with only 22% in mental health and 78% in physical disabilities.[10] Figures 1-1, 1-2, and 1-3 show the shift in numbers of COTAs and OTRs practicing in the two areas over the decades from 1973 to 1994.

### COTAs and OTRs: History of the Relationship

Given the tremendous shortages of personnel that motivated AOTA's decision to develop programs to train assistants, one might think that the new COTA would have been welcomed into the ranks of the occupational therapy community. Almost from the beginning, however, OTRs voiced concern about the proper role of COTAs. Some OTRs tried to limit and control the development of COTA programs, as well as the role of the COTA in the American Occupational Therapy Association.[17,22,33] The AOTA, recognizing that clarification was needed, published in 1967 *A Guide for the Supervision of the Certified Occupational Therapy Assistant*.[14] By the 1970s, however, OTRs and COTAs were engaging in open and often bitter debate about the place of the COTA in the profession. Some

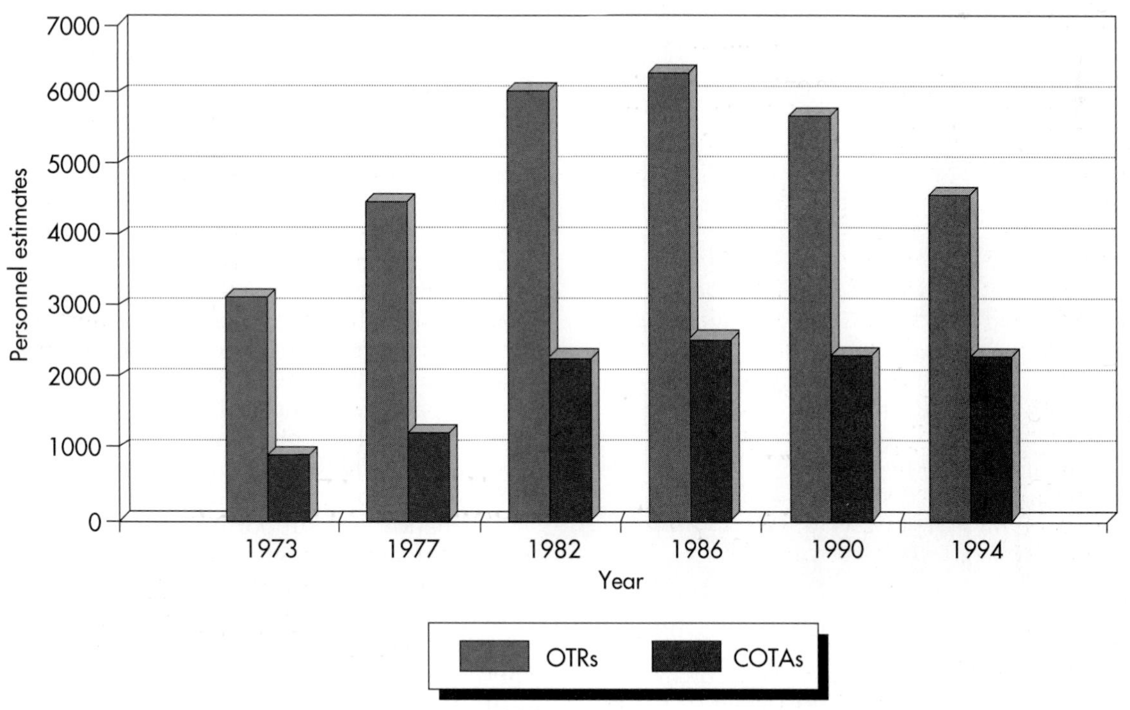


*Figure 1-1* Occupational therapy mental health personnel, 1973-1994. (Data from American Occupational Therapy Association Research Division, February 1995, private communication.)

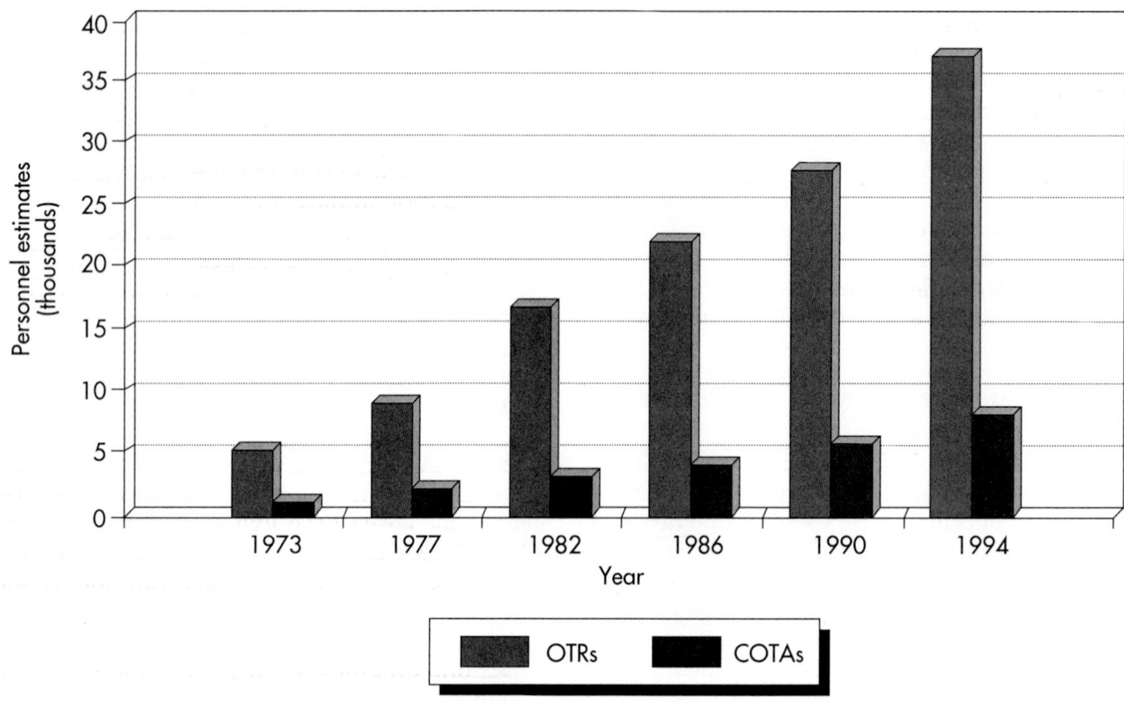


*Figure 1-2* Occupational therapy physical disabilities personnel, 1973-1994. (Data from AOTA Research Division, February 1995, private communication.)

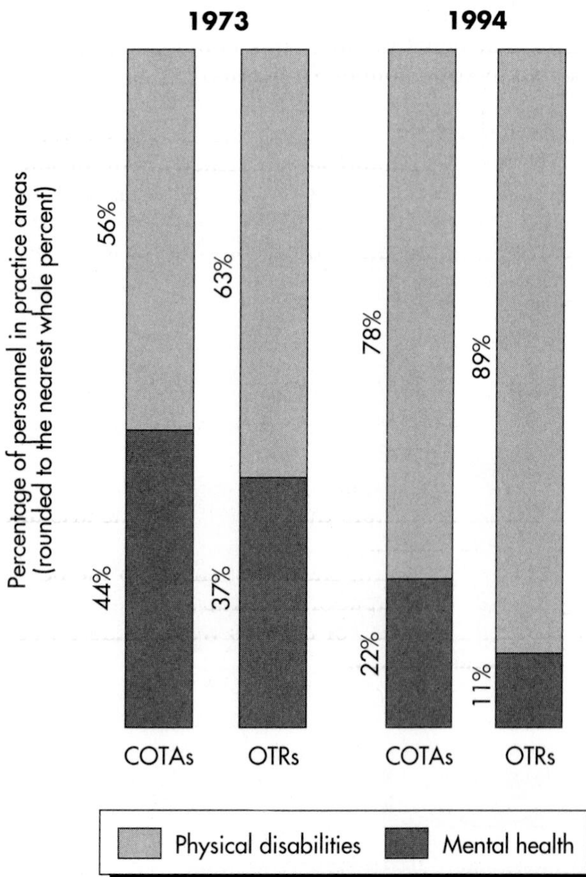


*Figure 1-3* Occupational therapy personnel practicing in mental health and physical disabilities in 1973 and 1994.

OTRs admitted they felt threatened by the possibility of being replaced by lesser trained personnel. Some COTAs responded that OTRs would feel less threatened if they pursued continuing education and kept up with advances in the field.[22]

It is helpful to understand that the OTRs and COTAs in practice at that time had come to the profession through a variety of training routes. In the 1970s some OTRs in practice had been trained in the war emergency courses of World War II, some had been grandfathered into the profession, some had graduated from 4-year degree programs, and some had completed graduate programs at the master's level. Of COTAs, some had been trained in the early 12-week psychiatry courses, some had been aides who were grandfathered in, some had graduated from 2-year college programs, and some had completed 6 months of military training in occupational therapy. Thus Carr was accurate in stating that "Therapists away from current practice should be aware that what was taught 15 years ago as functional treatment is taught to COTAs today as maintenance and supportive therapy."[16] Also, many OTRs were unaware of the qualifications and value of the COTA, because information on the COTA's role was not part of the essentials for the educational program for the registered occupational therapist at that time.

In 1976 AOTA conducted a study of practice to delineate (draw a line around) the roles of the COTA and the OTR.[35] Roles were studied at entry-level practice (the first 12 months of practice after completing AOTA certification). Of those surveyed, 48% of

COTAs worked in physical rehabilitation. Half of these were the only OT personnel at the facility, and about 14% were supervised by a non-OT administrator. Data from this study were used to develop a roles and functions statement, the purpose of which was to clarify the separate but complementary roles of the OTR and the COTA.[13]

Further attempts by AOTA to clarify the role of the COTA and the level of supervision required included various guidelines for supervision [11,12] and a requirement to include content about the COTA's role in the educational program for the OTR, beginning in 1991.[10]

More recently, ***Occupational Therapy Roles***[8] and *Career Exploration and Development: a Companion Guide to the Occupational Therapy Roles Document*[3] have provided direction for placing the COTA role within the broader context of occupational therapy practice. These two documents are meant to be used together as a guide for OTRs and COTAs in understanding and further developing their career paths within occupational therapy. *Occupational Therapy Roles* describes the COTA practitioner, listing skills for entry, intermediate, and advanced levels of practice. It also describes more independent roles to which the COTA can aspire. COTAs are specifically listed as qualified to enter the career paths of educator, fieldwork educator, fieldwork supervisor, consultant, fieldwork coordinator, faculty member, researcher, and entrepreneur.

In the opening paragraph of *Occupational Therapy Roles,* OTRs and COTAs are described together as **occupational therapy practitioners.** AOTA has clearly signaled that both levels of practice are equally valued. The two documents emphasize the need for practitioners at all levels to prepare themselves through education and skill acquisition to enter new roles. The emphasis on personal responsibility for professional development underscores that all who aspire to advance in the profession must "do their homework" and keep their information and skills current.

In 1994 AOTA published a *Guide for Supervision of Occupational Therapy Personnel.*[4] This document states that COTAs "at all levels require at least general supervision by a registered occupational therapist. The level of supervision is related to the ability of the certified occupational therapy assistant to safely and effectively provide those interventions delegated by a registered occupational therapist."[4] **General supervision** is defined as monthly (or more frequent) by direct contact (not by telephone). The document further categorizes practitioners into entry level, intermediate level, and advanced level and suggests the appropriate level of supervision for each. Entry-level COTAs should receive **close supervision,** which is defined as direct and daily supervision, at the work site.[4]

In some practice settings, however, OTR supervision is difficult to arrange. For example, the experienced COTA working in a nursing home may be supervised by a succession of OTR consultants and at times may have no consultant supervision because none can be found. The ethical and legal implications of this situation may create pressures in some states to do away with legal requirements for OTR supervision of COTAs. Is this a reasonable solution? Should it apply to all COTAs or only to those with experience? Or should COTAs be required to obtain, at their own expense, supervision from contracting OTRs? The question of who should supervise the COTA, particularly in geographical areas and practice settings where OTRs are scarce, needs to be resolved.

Despite the guidance provided by AOTA and the inclusion of information related to the COTA role in educational programs for the OTR, confusion and uncertainty still exist about the way in which the OTR and COTA should work together. Textbooks for the COTA by Ryan[30-32] and others have explicitly described how the OTR/COTA team might work together in various disability areas, but major texts for the OTR do not provide the same information.[23,37] Thus the wise COTA will anticipate that a given OTR might need more information and direction to appreciate the role and potential contributions of the COTA.

### Summary

Training programs for the occupational therapy assistant were introduced by AOTA in 1957 as a response to an increased demand for occupational therapy personnel, particularly in psychiatry. As general practice and physical disabilities were added to the content included in educational programs for the assistant and as the numbers of COTAs increased, OTRs began to clamor that their territory was being taken over by lesser trained personnel. Concerted efforts by AOTA and by COTAs and COTA educators have increased the visibility and the credibility of the COTA. COTAs in any practice area should stay informed about the latest AOTA guidelines, local legislative requirements, and developments within their practice area and should be prepared to share their understanding of their roles with OTRs in the interest of team building and professional unity.

## *Selected Reading Guide Questions*

1. Describe some of the changes that occurred as a result of the Enlightenment.
2. Discuss *moral treatment.*
3. Describe the factors that gave rise to the arts and crafts movement.
4. Relate the arts and crafts movement to the beginnings of occupational therapy.
5. Discuss the effects of the two world wars on occupational therapy.
6. Contrast holism and reductionism.
7. State the AOTA's position regarding the use of physical agent modalities.
8. Describe the content, length, and location of the first training programs for the COTA.
9. When and why did the focus of COTA training programs shift to include general practice?
10. List reasons some OTRs may be unaware of the potential and qualifications of COTAs.
11. Discuss issues surrounding COTA supervision.

## REFERENCES


1. Adamson MJ, Anderson MA: A study of the utilization of occupational therapy assistants and aides, *Am J Occup Ther* 20:75-79, 1966.
2. American Occupational Therapy Association: Member data survey information from research division, private communication, February 1995.
3. American Occupational Therapy Association: Career exploration and development: a companion guide to the occupational therapy roles document, *Am J Occup Ther* 48:844-851, 1994.
4. American Occupational Therapy Association: Guide for supervision of occupational therapy personnel, *Am J Occup Ther* 48:1045-1046, 1994.
5. American Occupational Therapy Association: Association policy 1.11: the philosophical base of occupational therapy, *Am J Occup Ther* 47:1119, 1993.
6. American Occupational Therapy Association: Association policy 1.12: occupation as the common core of occupational therapy, *Am J Occup Ther* 47:1119, 1993.
7. American Occupational Therapy Association: Association policy 1.25: registered occupational therapists and certified occupational therapy assistants and modalities, *Am J Occup Ther* 47:1118-1119, 1993.
8. American Occupational Therapy Association: Occupational therapy roles, *Am J Occup Ther* 47:1087-1099, 1993.
9. American Occupational Therapy Association: Position paper: purposeful activity, *Am J Occup Ther* 47:1081-1082, 1993.
10. American Occupational Therapy Association: Essentials and guidelines for an accredited educational program for the occupational therapist, *Am J Occup Ther* 45:1077-1084, 1991.
11. American Occupational Therapy Association: Supervision guidelines for certified occupational therapy assistants, *Am J Occup Ther* 44:1089-1090, 1990.
12. American Occupational Therapy Association: Guide for supervision of occupational therapy personnel, *Am J Occup Ther* 35:815-816, 1981.
13. American Occupational Therapy Association: *The roles and functions of occupational therapy personnel,* Rockville, Md, 1973, The Association.
14. American Occupational Therapy Association: *A guide for the supervision of the certified occupational therapy assistant,* Rockville, Md, 1967, AOTA.
15. Bockhoven JS: Legacy of moral treatment—1880's to 1910, *Am J Occup Ther* 25:223-225, 1971.
16. Carr SH: A modification of role for nursing home service, *Am J Occup Ther* 21:259-262, 1971.
17. Carr SH: The COTA heritage: proud, practical, stable, dynamic. In Ryan SE, editor: *The certified occupational therapy assistant,* ed 2, Thorofare, NJ, 1993, Slack.
18. Fidler GS: From crafts to competence, *Am J Occup Ther* 35:567, 1981.
19. Foucault M: *Madness and civilization—a history of insanity in the age of reason,* New York, 1965, Random House.
20. Gay P: *The Enlightenment: an interpretation—the rise of modern paganism,* New York, 1968, Vintage Random House.
21. Gay P, Webb RK: *Modern Europe,* New York, 1973, Harper & Row.
22. Hirama H: The COTA: a chronological review. In Ryan S, editor: *The certified occupational therapy assistant—roles and responsibilities,* Thorofare, NJ, 1986, Slack.
23. Hopkins HL, Smith HD: *Willard and Spackman's occupational therapy,* ed 8, Philadelphia, 1993, Lippincott.
24. Kielhofner G, Burke JP: A model of human occupation. I. Conceptual framework and content, *Am J Occup Ther* 34:572-581, 1980.
25. Lears J: *No place of grace—antimodernism and the transformation of American culture, 1880-1920,* New York, 1981, Pantheon.
26. Licht S: The founding and founders of the American Occupational Therapy Association, *Am J Occup Ther* 21:269-277, 1967.
27. Meyer A: The philosophy of occupational therapy, *Occup Ther Mental Health* 2(3):79-86, 1982. (Originally published in *Arch Occup Ther* 1:1, 1921.)
28. Reed KL: The beginnings of occupational therapy. In Hopkins HL, Smith HD: *Willard and Spackman's occupational therapy,* ed 8, Philadelphia, 1993, Lippincott.
29. Rerek MD: The Depression years: 1929 to 1941, *Am J Occup Ther* 25:231, 1971.
30. Ryan S, editor: *The certified occupational therapy assistant—roles and responsibilities,* Thorofare, NJ, 1986, Slack.
31. Ryan SE, editor: *The certified occupational therapy assistant,* ed 2, Thorofare, NJ, 1993, Slack.
32. Ryan SE, editor: *Practice issues in occupational therapy—intraprofessional team building,* Thorofare, NJ, 1993, Slack.
33. Ryan SE: Scope of occupational therapy: the certified occupational therapy assistant. In Hopkins HL, Smith HD: *Willard and Spackman's occupational therapy,* ed 8, Philadelphia, 1993, Lippincott.
34. Shannon PD: The derailment of occupational therapy, *Am J Occup Ther* 31:229, 1977.
35. Shapiro D, Brown D: The delineation of the role of entry-level occupational therapy personnel, *Am J Occup Ther* 35:306-311, 1981.
36. Spackman CS: Occupational therapy for patients with physical injuries. In Willard HS, Spackman CS, editors: *Principles of Occupational therapy,* ed 1, Philadelphia, 1947, Lippincott.
37. Trombly CA, editor: *Occupational therapy for physical dysfunction,* ed 4, Baltimore, 1995, Williams & Wilkins.


## RECOMMENDED READING


Breines EB: Therapeutic activities: yesterday and today. In *Occupational therapy: from clay to computers—theory and practice,* Philadelphia, 1995, Davis.

Clark EN: Certified occupational therapy assistants need a name change: a response to Hirama, *Am J Occup Ther* 49:368-369, 1995.

Friedland J: The issue is—diversional activity: does it deserve its bad name? *Am J Occup Ther* 42:603-608, 1988.

Gutman SA: Influence of the US military and occupational therapy reconstruction aides in World War I on the development of occupational therapy, *Am J Occup Ther* 49:256-262, 1995.

Hirama H: The issue is—should occupational therapy assistants provide occupational therapy services independently? *Am J Occup Ther* 48:840-843, 1994.

Peloquin SM: Moral treatment: contexts reconsidered, *Am J Occup Ther* 43:537-544, 1989.

Quiroga VAM: *Occupational therapy: the first 30 years—1900 to 1930,* Rockville, Md, 1995, American Occupational Therapy Association.

Schemm RL: Bridging conflicting ideologies: the origins of American and British occupational therapy, *Am J Occup Ther* 48:1082-1088, 1994.

West WL: Ten milestone issues in AOTA history, *Am J Occup Ther* 46:1066-1074, 1992.

Chapter 2

# Occupational Therapy's Domain of Concern

Mary Beth Early

## Chapter Objectives

*After studying this chapter, the student or practitioner will be able to:*

1. Outline the structure of *Uniform Terminology for Occupational Therapy—Third Edition.*
2. Differentiate occupational therapy's domain of concern from that of other professions.
3. Name and describe the three occupational performance areas.
4. List and describe the categories of performance components.
5. Illustrate the way in which performance context affects occupational performance.
6. Analyze the effect of physical dysfunction on occupational performance within a specific context.

## Key Terms

occupation
domain of concern
occupational performance
performance areas
activities of daily living
work and productive activities
play and leisure activities
performance components
sensorimotor
cognitive
psychosocial
psychological
performance context

The following chapter discusses some of the theories used in occupational therapy practice in physical dysfunction. First, however, the reader must be clear about the scope and interests of occupational therapy, as differentiated from other professions and scholarly disciplines. It is hoped that the material presented in this chapter is not entirely new to the reader. For many it is a review.

Review or not, it is essential in physical disabilities practice (where so many techniques and modalities address biological functions of the body) to clarify the purposes, aims, and concerns of occupational therapy. Students and new practitioners are sometimes seduced by medical jargon and fall into the role of mini-diagnosticians. They become completely sidetracked by the patient's symptoms, medical history, and test

The reader is strongly encouraged to obtain, read, understand, and if possible commit to memory the most recent edition of the *Uniform Terminology for Occupational Therapy* published by AOTA.

results or become fascinated by mechanical devices (pulleys, weights, exercise machines) and modalities (hot packs, cold packs, paraffin). In these new preoccupations, they can easily lose sight of **occupation.** Their primary concern should be the patient's *occupational functioning* in life roles that are important to the *patient.*

The American Occupational Therapy Association (AOTA), in its *Uniform Terminology for Occupational Therapy—Third Edition,*[1] outlines the domain of concern of the profession. The domain of concern delineates the issues that should be addressed by occupational therapy. The purpose of this is to make clear which topics and factors should be considered by occupational therapists and assistants in their practice. By analogy, a licensed plumber's domain of concern would be pipes and valves. The plumber is concerned with the outlets to and from the main lines (water and sewage) and with how the pipes are routed in the house. An electrician's domain of concern would be electrical circuits, wiring, and fixtures. The electrician is concerned with the main line from the power source (electrical utilities) and the routing of the electrical circuits inside the building.

We might even say that by describing our domain of concern, we lay claim to a certain territory as belonging to our profession. Certainly, in the case of plumbers and electricians, the territory is clearly marked out. However, the territories of plumbers and electricians are necessarily shared with other professionals, such as architects, engineers, and general contractors. This is also the case in our profession,

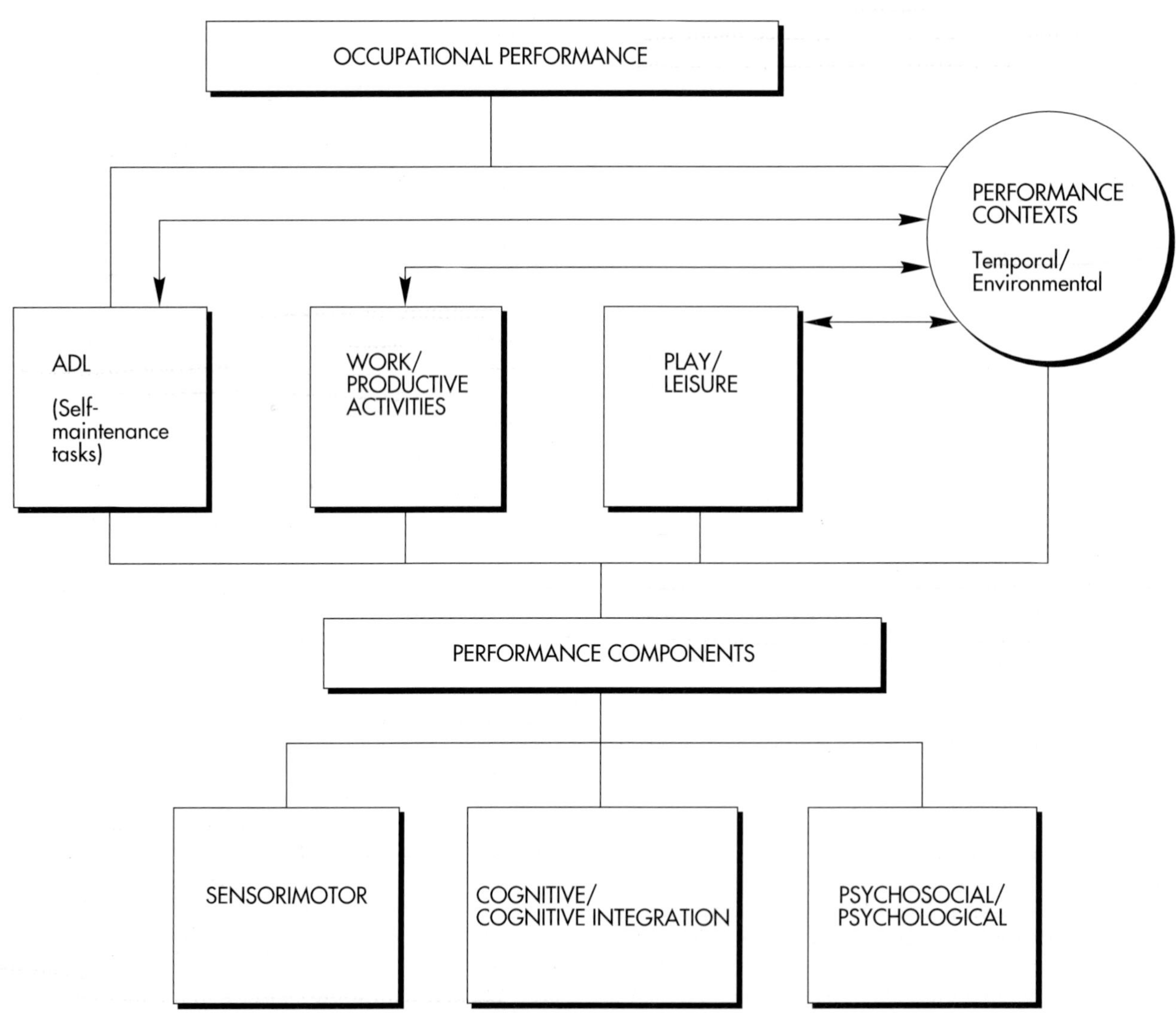


*Figure 2-1* Occupational performance model. (Modified from Uniform terminology for occupational therapy—third edition, *Am J Occup Ther* 48:1047-1054, 1994; and American Occupational Therapy Association: *A curriculum guide for occupational therapy educators,* Rockville, Md, 1974, AOTA.)

where many areas of our practice overlap with other professions (physical therapists, physicians, social workers, psychologists, etc.).

Occupational therapy's domain of concern is **occupational performance.** Occupational performance refers to the way humans carry out functional life activities (e.g., grooming, working, caring for children) and occupational roles (e.g., Little League coach, watercolorist, first grader, homemaker, lawyer, poker player). This domain of concern, which is detailed in the *Uniform Terminology,*[1] was described but did not originate with Mosey[7] and has evolved through successive AOTA documents[1-6] and years of debate and development within the occupational therapy community. It will continue to evolve as we become more knowledgeable and more focused in our theory and practice. Occupational performance incorporates ideas from the early years of our profession and includes both humanist and reductionist perspectives, as discussed later in this chapter.

Within occupational performance, three major topics or divisions exist: performance areas, performance components, and performance context. Figure 2-1 outlines the relationship among these elements of occupational performance.

## PERFORMANCE AREAS

The **performance areas** are "broad categories of human activity that are typically part of daily life."[1] Three such areas are named: activities of daily living, work and productive activities, and play and leisure activities. **Activities of daily living** are those that maintain the self, such as dressing, grooming, and being able to move about within one's home and community. **Work and productive activities** are those that contribute to society or to personal welfare, including activities that prepare a person for work, such as school. **Play and leisure activities** are those performed for enjoyment and are not necessarily productive. Despite the distinct divisions suggested by these categories, the meaning of the activity comes from the person performing it. In other words, an activity that might be seen as work by the therapist may be viewed by the patient as leisure. For example, mending a throw pillow is a homemaking task (therefore within the category of work and productive activities), but if the patient made the pillow in a creative burst of home decorating *and* views home decorating as a hobby, the activity is at least in part a leisure one to this patient. Another example is shopping for clothing, categorized as a self-maintenance activity. Some people enjoy this activity so much that for them it is clearly recreational.

For the purposes of communication within and outside the profession, however, it is recommended that the uniform terminology and its categories be used.

### Activities of Daily Living

The first area is activities of daily living, or self-maintenance tasks.[1] There are 15 categories within activities of daily living. Nine of these involve basic care of the body and the personal self: grooming, oral hygiene, bathing/showering, toilet hygiene, care of personal devices (e.g., eyeglasses, adaptive equipment), dressing, feeding and eating, medication routine, and health maintenance (e.g., physical fitness, seeking medical attention). The remaining six categories involve interactions with others or responsiveness within the community: socialization, functional communication, functional mobility (e.g., transfers), community mobility (using a car or public transportation), emergency response, and sexual expression.

### Work and Productive Activities

The second area is work and productive activities, or activities that contribute to personal livelihood or to the good of society.[1] This includes schooling, which is a preparation for work. The four major categories within this occupational performance area are as follows:

1. *Home management,* which includes the subcategories of clothing care, cleaning, meal preparation and cleanup, shopping, money management, household maintenance, and safety procedures
2. *Care of others,* such as providing for children, spouse, or parents through nurturing and physical care
3. *Educational activities,* whether through school, community, or work-sponsored activities
4. *Vocational activities,* which encompass all work-related activities (vocational exploration, job acquisition, work or job performance, retirement planning, volunteer participation)

### Play and Leisure Activities

The third performance area is play or leisure activities, or activities that are pursued for their own sake because they amuse us, help us to relax, or allow us to express ourselves.[1] Within this area are two categories: play or leisure exploration (to identify and investigate potential activities) and play or leisure performance (the actual participation in activities).

## HOW PHYSICAL DYSFUNCTION AFFECTS OCCUPATIONAL PERFORMANCE

We can easily imagine how occupational performance is affected by physical disability. A simple wrist fracture, with its resulting cast and period of immobilization, causes problems in dressing, bathing, handling money, driving a car, caring for a child, and so on.

Some activities cannot be done independently while the cast is on (e.g., bathing an infant); others can be accomplished with some changes in the methods used (e.g., donning a coat). It is not that persons with physical disabilities lack an interest in doing these activities. Rather, they cannot do the activities in the "normal" or customary way because of impairments in underlying abilities needed to perform the activities.

For example, a mother whose wrist is in a cast cannot bathe a squirming infant because she does not have the ability to hold the child with both hands; because of the cast, she lacks the tactile sensitivity, strength, range of motion, and grasp that are needed.

The occupational therapy practitioner needs to understand what these underlying abilities are and should be able to identify which ones are responsible for the patient's problems in occupational performance. These underlying abilities are called performance components.

## PERFORMANCE COMPONENTS

The **performance components** are "fundamental human abilities that—to varying degrees and in differing combinations—are required for successful engagement in performance areas."[1] The performance components support a person's ability to function in the occupational performance areas. An example of a performance component is strength, which is needed for sports, household maintenance, many types of work, and movement in the community. There are three main groupings of performance components: sensorimotor, cognitive, and psychosocial and psychological. The performance components are described briefly here by group and in more detail in Chapters 8 through 11 and 13.

### Sensorimotor Components

The first group, the **sensorimotor components**, is organized into three categories: sensory, neuromusculoskeletal, and motor. The *sensory* category includes both sensory and perceptual processes. The sensory processes are responsible for receiving and interpreting information that comes in through the senses: what we see, hear, smell, feel by touch, feel by our balance mechanisms, and feel through our muscles and joints. The senses are tactile, proprioceptive, vestibular, visual, auditory, gustatory, and olfactory.

*Perceptual* processes organize the information received through the senses into meaningful patterns.[1] Perceptual processes give us an understanding of what we are experiencing through our senses. From this understanding, we can take appropriate action. For example, as you try to get your bearings on an unfamiliar street corner, you search for a way to understand where you are. You use your eyes and see many things, too many to make sense of without being selective. Using figure-ground discrimination to pull the object (sign) from its background (everything else), you focus on a street sign, but it is partially obstructed by foliage. You can make out only a few letters. It looks like M, then maybe two more letters, then LE. Using visual closure, you mentally supply the missing letters to make up MAPLE, the street you are looking for. We use perceptual processes constantly, most of the time without being aware of them. You are using them now to read this page, applying figure-ground discrimination to read one word after the other. The perceptual processes

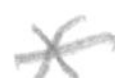

listed in the sensorimotor category are stereognosis, kinesthesia, pain response, body scheme, right-left discrimination, form constancy, position in space, visual closure, figure-ground perception, depth perception, spatial relations, and topographical orientation.

*Neuromusculoskeletal* processes concern the nerves (neuro), the muscles (musculo), and the bones and skeleton (skeletal). These processes give us a foundation from which movement can occur. The abilities to move parts of the body, to stand and sit with our bones in alignment, and to use our muscles to work against forces such as gravity are fundamental to all activities in which we use the body. For example, to ride in an elevator, we need to lift our shoulder, elbow, and hand against gravity to press the button (range of motion and strength). We also need to be able to stand for a time (endurance) and to make rapid adjustments of posture if the elevator jerks or quickly comes to a stop (reflexes). The neuromusculoskeletal processes listed in the uniform terminology are reflex(es), range of motion, muscle tone, strength, endurance, postural alignment, and soft tissue integrity.

*Motor* processes are associated with movement, particularly with the qualities of movement, or how well movement is done. The importance of these processes is readily seen in skilled activities such as playing the piano, which requires moving up and down the keyboard with both hands, sometimes crossing one over the other (bilateral integration and crossing the midline), and using the foot pedals while striking the keys with the fingers in combination and separately and with varying degrees of force (fine coordination, motor control, praxis). These processes are also needed for grooming activities such as buttoning a shirt and brushing one's teeth. As with other performance components, our motor processes are so well developed and we are so accustomed to using them that we rarely notice them unless something goes wrong or we are asked to do something new or difficult (e.g., play the piano). The motor processes are gross coordination, crossing the midline, laterality, bilateral integration, motor control, praxis, fine coordination/dexterity, visual-motor integration, and oral-motor control.

### Cognitive Components

**Cognitive** integration and cognitive components refer to the ability to use higher (cortical) brain functions to further organize and interpret information. Cortical refers to the cortex, the newest part of the brain. The cognitive components are concerned with awareness and thinking skills. We use cognitive components continuously; we are sometimes aware of doing so but often are not. For example, when studying for a test, you are conscious of trying to remember what you have learned and read (memory), you work at getting your notes and your thinking organized around the main ideas (concept formation), and you try to imagine how these ideas can be applied to case examples your instructor might pose (generalization). When you are putting away the dishes, you are still using these skills and others but are less conscious of relying on categorization, spatial operations, and memory to put the forks, spoons, and knives in the proper bins. The 14 cognitive components are level of arousal, orientation, recognition, attention span, initiation of activity, termination of activity, memory, sequencing, categorization, concept formation, spatial operations, problem solving, learning, and generalization.[1]

### Psychosocial and Psychological Components

The **psychosocial** skills and psychological components comprise the subskills that contribute to a person's ability to relate to others (psychosocial) and to deal with feelings (psychological). Three categories within this component group are psychological, social, and self-management. Students are sometimes surprised to learn that these components must also be considered in working with patients whose conditions are physical in origin. Several reasons exist for giving these components equal importance. First, people will always have an emotional or psychological reaction to something that happens to them; a physical disability gives a direct and clear message about mortality and the limitations of the physical self, a message to which people react emotionally. Second, having a disability is stressful and requires additional coping skills just to get through the day, to ask for help from others, and to manage ordinary activities. Third, the amount of independence and functional ability that people can gain from therapy depends greatly on their level of motivation, their values, and what they hope to achieve and believe they can achieve. Fourth, physical disabilities that affect the brain (at the cortical or subcortical level) generally have some damaging effect on psychological and psychosocial functioning. A common result of head injury, for example, is a problem with impulse control. Depending on the area of the brain affected, people who have experienced strokes may experience difficulty with expressing themselves and with understanding and managing time.

The **psychological** components include values, interests, and self-concept. The term *values* refers to having and being able to identify ideas and beliefs that are important. The term *interests* concerns the ability to take an interest and to identify what that interest is (e.g., activities that give pleasure or create a challenge). *Self-concept* refers to the value placed in the physical, emotional, and sexual self and includes awareness of the self, as well as positive and negative ideas about the self.

The *social* components consist of role performance, social conduct, interpersonal skills, and self-expression. *Role performance* refers to the way a person manages and engages in a variety of roles (occupational and otherwise). It includes the notion of identifying and acquiring roles as well as balancing them. *Social conduct* refers to the way a person behaves with others. Differences in social conduct between individuals are immediately noticeable and contribute significantly to acceptance by others. Norms for social conduct vary in different social and ethnic groups and different environments. Some elements of social conduct are making eye contact, using personal space (how close one person stands to another), and following manners and customs. *Interpersonal skills* refers to those skills used to interact with others, primarily to communicate. *Self-expression* is the ability to show feelings, thoughts, and needs to others in a variety of ways so that a person is understood and accepted.

The *self-management* components include coping skills, time management, and self-control.[1] *Coping skills* concerns the response to stress. The more coping skills a person has and the better developed the skills are, the better the person can respond. Examples of coping skills include analyzing the situation, identifying possible solutions, seeking support from others, changing activities, and taking a break. *Time management* refers to the ability to use time effectively to meet goals. This includes the notion of balancing work, play, and self-maintenance activities with appropriate periods of rest. *Self-control* refers to the ability to respond effectively to different situations, regardless of feelings and impulses. It assumes that a person is aware of what is going on and that the person can respond flexibly.

If you are confused after reading these definitions, you are not alone. Considerable overlap exists among these categories and between the different skills described. Future versions of the uniform terminology should clarify some of these relationships.

## PERFORMANCE CONTEXT

The word *context* comes from the Latin word, "contexere," to weave together.[8] A context is the background into which something is interwoven. This word is used in many different ways. For example, a child who is having difficulty understanding a new word encountered in reading is told to "look for context clues," such as illustrations or other words that may help the child identify the mystery word. Also, after listening to a story or anecdote, someone who knows more about the situation may remark that "you've taken that out of context," suggesting that the speaker hasn't provided enough background information to give a fair idea of what actually happened. In both these examples, we can see that context gives meaning. In the case of occupational performance, the context supplies the background and often the meaning of the activity—how and why it is performed.

**Performance contexts** are defined by AOTA as "situations or factors that influence an individual's engagement in desired and/or required performance areas."[1] The concept of performance contexts was included as a new item in the *Uniform Terminology for Occupational Therapy—Third Edition.* Historically, this concept was not new, having been termed *life space* in earlier occupational therapy documents.[4] Performance contexts provide a setting for occupational performance. For example, the activity of cutting food with a knife will have very different meanings for a 29-year-old man depending on the context. Consider the following scenarios, each with a different context:

- He has cerebral palsy and is learning this activity for the first time.
- He is recovering from Guillain-Barré syndrome and wants to feed himself.
- He is dying of AIDS and wants to maintain his ability to feed himself for as long as possible.
- He is cutting up food for his young child.
- He is a professional chef.

The performance context is considered to have both temporal (time) and environmental (space and people) aspects.

#### Temporal Aspects

The *temporal* aspects of performance contexts are chronological age (age in years), developmental age (stage of maturation), place in the life cycle (especially in relation to important life roles such as student, worker, parent), and health status (whether the condition is acute or chronic, or terminal). These temporal aspects affect expectations for performance, both by the individual and by others. In other words, differences in performance are expected in, for example, small children, mentally retarded persons, and terminally ill patients.

#### Environmental Aspects

The *environmental* aspects of performance contexts are physical considerations, social considerations, and cultural considerations. *Physical considerations* include all non-human aspects of the environment: buildings, furniture, natural terrain, objects, tools, machines, animals, and plants. Where does the patient live? What tools does the patient handle every day? *Social considerations* focus on other people who are important in the daily life of the patient, such as spouse, relatives, friends, and caregivers. What do these people expect from the patient? How available are they to help, and how capable are they of assisting? Also considered are some larger social groups (e.g., a church) that may control social routines, expected behavior, or roles. *Cultural considerations* address society at large, as well as any ethnic, political, racial, or other groups to which the individual may belong. These groups are sources of customs, beliefs, activity patterns, behavior standards, and expectations that will influence the individual. AOTA includes opportunities for education, employment, and economic support in this category.

### OCCUPATIONAL PERFORMANCE AS A PROCESS WITHIN A CONTEXT

Although it is useful to categorize and describe all the aspects just discussed, you will never understand occupational performance by looking at the sum of its parts, even with the additional perspective of performance contexts. Rather, you must travel deep within the experience of occupational performance and learn how these parts are related to each other.

First, try to remember a personal example, a time when you performed an activity for the first time, such as riding a bicycle, skiing, or cooking a meal for guests. Remember in great detail the specifics of the activity: the things you had to do, the tools you used, and the environment in which it occurred. Remember the motions involved, the sensory and physical experiences, and the thinking skills you needed to do the activity. Remember why you were doing it, why it was important to you. Remember the people who were around you, how they felt about it, and how they helped or hindered you. Remember who you are, whether a native-born American or a member of another culture, or both. How did this affect your expectations and experience of the activity?

Now, from this perspective, consider the following case study:

#### *Case Study*

Mrs. A. is a 34-year-old seamstress who completed eleventh grade in the Dominican Republic. She moved to the United States 8 years ago with her two daughters, now ages 11 and 9, after separating from her husband. A devout Catholic, Mrs. A. has been an active member of her church, making handicrafts and participating in bazaars, potluck dinners, and other activities. She understands English fairly well but speaks haltingly and is embarrassed by her accent. She is right-handed and lives with her daughters in a small fourth-floor walk-up apartment in Red Hook, Brooklyn. Two months ago she was injured at the factory where she has worked since coming to the United States. The right radial nerve was affected at elbow level, and the median nerve was damaged to a lesser extent. Partial to full recovery is expected within 10 months. Mrs. A. is able to support herself and her daughters with insurance compensation payments, but she is afraid that these will not last until she is able to recover completely. She is very worried and depressed over this.

Mrs. A. has been referred for occupational therapy for physical and functional restoration. She has weakness in the extensors of the wrist and the hand and the supinator muscle. Because the flexors and pronators are stronger than these affected muscles, her wrist drops into a flexed position, her fingers stay slightly curled, and she cannot turn her palm to face up.

Although this is a small amount of information, it is sufficient to provide some idea of the occupational performance areas affected, the performance components involved, and the performance context in Mrs. A.'s case. At this point, it would be a useful exercise for you to cover Box 2-1 and on a separate paper write down your analysis of how this patient's disability has affected her occupational performance (using the correct uniform terminology). When you are finished, check your work against Box 2-1.

Were your ideas about Mrs. A. similar to those listed? You may have identified areas, components, and aspects of the context that were not discussed. If so, congratulate yourself. The point of this exercise has been to illustrate the complexities of occupational performance and the importance of considering the context.

In the case of Mrs. A. the context would change dramatically if her injury had occurred 7 years earlier. Do you understand why? She would have been in the United States only 1 year; she would have had less time to develop her English skills; and most importantly in terms of her ability to cope with her injury, her daughters would be 2 and 4 years of age. They could not help her with the chores, and she would have the additional tasks of bathing and dressing them and perhaps also diapering the younger child.

As mentioned earlier, occupational performance incorporates ideas from the early years of our profession and includes both humanist and reductionist perspectives. The reductionist perspective is apparent in the detailed breakdown of the performance components, with each analyzed in turn as a separate element. Remember that reductionism examines phenomena in small pieces, pieces small enough for research and investigation, and that we acquired the habits and attitudes of reductionism when we allied ourselves with the medical profession. Thus, in Mrs. A.'s case, we must consider her muscle strength and coordination. From a humanist perspective, however, reaching back to the unity of mind and body that was recognized in the moral treatment era, we also consider the psychological and psychosocial components: her values, self-concept, and coping skills. Most importantly, we consider all these factors within the performance context—the unique nature of Mrs. A.'s situation at this point in her highly specific and individual human life.

## SUMMARY

Occupational therapy's domain of concern, occupational performance, focuses on the functioning of

*Box 2-1*

### Occupational Performance Summary of the Case of Mrs. A.

**Performance areas**

Because of limitations in the right hand, Mrs. A. would have difficulty with grooming, oral hygiene, bathing, toilet hygiene, dressing, applying makeup, feeding and eating, and using the telephone. She is unable to work at her job as a seamstress. Her daughters are old enough to take care of their own dressing and bathing and may be able to help Mrs. A. with the housework, which would otherwise be difficult for her. If they are interested in learning to cook, they could be taught enough to relieve her of this responsibility until she is recovered.

Mrs. A. is worried about whether she will recover enough to return to her job. If her recovery is less than complete, her job should be analyzed to see if it can be adapted to allow her to perform it. Otherwise, given her low educational level, limited job skills, and relative lack of proficiency with English, Mrs. A. may have trouble finding another job.

**Performance components**

Sensorimotor components are most obviously affected. Mrs. A. has limited strength in her right hand. Sensation may also be affected. Coordination, both fine and gross, in use of the right hand is affected by the loss of strength. It is not clear whether range of motion is affected and, if so, to what extent. There is no reason to suspect any problems with cognitive components. On the basis of Mrs. A.'s involvement with her church and her strong work history and family relationships, it appears she has good psychological and psychosocial skills. However, she is depressed over the injury, anxious about the future, and embarrassed about her limited English-speaking ability. These factors may affect her self-concept and her ability to cope with her situation.

**Performance context**

Mrs. A. is a young adult with two children in the middle years. Living on the fourth floor, Mrs. A. must carry groceries up the stairs, trash down the stairs, and laundry both down and up. Having only one useful hand is very restrictive, although her daughters can help her. Coming from a Dominican background, with its strong emphasis on family solidarity, Mrs. A.'s daughters are likely to take on these responsibilities easily. Besides Mrs. A.'s involvement with the church, it is not known if she has any relationships with neighbors or other adults. Because she is no longer going to work every day, Mrs. A. is in some danger of becoming isolated. If Mrs. A. is able to call on her relationships with fellow church members, she should be able to manage her household adequately for at least a few months. With respect to returning to work, Mrs. A.'s employer most likely has replaced her already, because many skilled garment workers reside in the area. Because her injury occurred on the job, he will be required to rehire her, but this is probably not in his economic self-interest, especially if he must make accommodations for a residual disability. Nonetheless, Mrs. A. was a valued employee, with 8 years at the same job, and this may affect his feelings about accommodating her, which he is legally required to do.

people in their daily lives and the activities and roles they have chosen. This domain is clarified by exploring the categories used by the American Occupational Therapy Association in its *Uniform Terminology—Third Edition*[1] and examining the relationships among activities, their components, and their context. These concepts can be applied to our own experiences and used to analyze case examples. The concepts described and defined in the *Uniform Terminology* have developed out of our professional history and our collective experiences with countless patients over almost 80 years.

## Selected Reading Guide Questions

1. Identify occupational therapy's domain of concern.
2. Define *performance component.*
3. Differentiate *sensory* and *perceptual.*
4. Give an example of how a perceptual skill is used in daily life.
5. Define *neuromusculoskeletal.*
6. Give an example of how neuromusculoskeletal skills are used in daily life.
7. Define *motor* as this term is used in occupational therapy.
8. Define *cognitive.*
9. Give an example of how cognitive skills are used in daily life.
10. Differentiate psychosocial skills from psychological skills.
11. Give an example of how psychosocial and psychological skills are used in daily life.
12. What is meant by *performance context,* and why is it important?
13. Give examples of the temporal and the environmental aspects of performance context.

### REFERENCES

1. American Occupational Therapy Association: Uniform terminology for occupational therapy—third edition, *Am J Occup Ther* 48:1047-1054, 1994.
2. American Occupational Therapy Association: Occupational therapy product output reporting system and uniform terminology for reporting occupational therapy services. In *Reference manual of the official documents of the American Occupational Therapy Association,* Rockville, Md, 1989, The Association.
3. American Occupational Therapy Association: Uniform terminology for occupational therapy—second edition, *Am J Occup Ther* 43:808-815, 1989.
4. American Occupational Therapy Association: *A curriculum guide for occupational therapy educators,* Rockville, Md, 1974, The Association.
5. American Occupational Therapy Association: Task force on target populations, Association report II, *Am J Occup Ther* 28:231, 1974.
6. American Occupational Therapy Association: *The roles and functions of occupational therapy personnel,* Rockville, Md, 1973, The Association.
7. Mosey AC: *Occupational therapy: configuration of a profession,* New York, 1981, Raven.
8. Oxford University Press: *The compact edition of the Oxford English dictionary,* Oxford, 1971, Oxford University Press.

### RECOMMENDED READING

American Occupational Therapy Association: Uniform terminology—third edition: application to practice, *Am J Occup Ther* 48:1055-1059, 1994.

Cynkin S: *Occupational therapy: toward health through activities,* Boston, 1979, Little, Brown.

Chapter 3

# A Frame of Reference and Practice Models for Physical Dysfunction

*Mary Beth Early*
*Lorraine Williams Pedretti*

## Chapter Objectives

*After studying this chapter, the student or practitioner will be able to:*

1. Describe the *model of human occupation* and illustrate its application to a person with a physical disability.
2. Explain the principles of occupational therapy intervention that derive from the model of human occupation.
3. Describe the *biomechanical* practice model, clarify the principles that support it, identify the conditions in which it is most effective, and establish its relationship to the model of human occupation.
4. Describe the *sensorimotor* practice model, clarify the principles that support it, identify the conditions in which it is most effective, and establish its relationship to the model of human occupation.
5. Describe the *rehabilitation* practice model, clarify the principles that support it, identify the conditions in which it is most effective, and establish its relationship to the model of human occupation.
6. Describe the *treatment continuum model* and its four stages: adjunctive methods, enabling activities, purposeful activity, and occupational performance and occupational roles.

## Key Terms

frame of reference
practice model
model of human occupation
systems model
volition
habituation
performance
biomechanical approach
kinetics
statics
sensorimotor approach
neurophysiological
reflex
rehabilitation approach
treatment continuum
adjunctive methods
enabling activities
purposeful activity
occupational roles
occupational performance

Students beginning fieldwork are typically asked about their "frame of reference" or "practice model." A supervisor may ask, "Which frames of reference are you comfortable with?" or "Which frames of reference did you learn in school?" A particular practice model may be named and the student asked to tell what she knows about it. Such questions may bring on cold sweats and sudden faintness. The purpose of this chapter is to show you that you *can* learn frames of reference or practice models well enough to explain them to others. You will see that they are useful—and that *you* will find them useful. This discussion starts with a patient situation you might face some day.

Imagine that you are working in a nursing home. On Monday morning, your first day of fieldwork, you are assigned a new admission and go to visit him in his room, having first read the chart and learned the following facts:

1. The patient is 87 years old, married, and of German-Jewish background.
2. His diagnoses are congestive heart failure, multiinfarct dementia, and Parkinson's disease.
3. He was admitted over the weekend after being discharged from a local hospital.

When you enter his room, you find him lying, fully clothed, on his back, in bed, with his knees drawn up. He seems to be staring into space and looks worried. You greet him by name, tell him your name, and ask him if he can sit up and talk with you. You assist him to sitting, although with difficulty because he seems stiff and almost uncooperative. Once up, he looks you in the eye and begins talking. You can't make any sense of what he's saying, so you ask him to speak louder. Even understanding the words, you can't tell what he's talking about. After trying some simple questions ("How are you feeling today?" "Would you like to come for a walk with me?"), you feel frustrated by his lack of response and wish you were somewhere else. After helping the patient to lie down again, you excuse yourself, promising to come back another time.

On returning to the chart area, you learn that his medical record from the hospital is now available. It's an inch and a half thick, and every page is filled with details. It's difficult to see where to start first. What is wrong with this patient? How did he come to be in this situation? What can we do to help him? How should we do it? And where should we start?

It seems practical to start with the chart. But what should you look for? This is where a frame of reference is useful. A frame of reference gives you a structure for organizing your thoughts about the patient. It identifies the most important areas in which to gather information. It provides concepts for analyzing the patient's problems and for developing broad goals. The frame of reference discussed in this chapter is the model of human occupation, which has been used across all practice areas, from psychiatry to physical medicine, and with all age groups.

The model of human occupation gives a broad perspective for organizing the occupational therapy process. In physical disabilities, however, the main focus is at times much narrower, and in this case, practice models are useful. A practice model allows the occupational therapist to focus on a selected area of the patient's problems, helps to define realistic goals, and helps in the selection of evaluation and treatment interventions that are likely to work. This chapter examines three practice models for occupational therapy: the biomechanical approach, the sensorimotor approach, and the rehabilitation approach. These models are compatible with the model of human occupation. Each focuses on one aspect of the larger picture of human occupation. The biomechanical and sensorimotor approaches are used most often with patients with physical disabilities, but the rehabilitation approach is also used in other practice areas. Each model is introduced here and elaborated in later chapters.

## PRACTICE MODEL VERSUS FRAME OF REFERENCE

Terminology can be confusing. Many scholarly authors, starting with Mosey,[11,12] have attempted to devise a structure to evaluate the theories and ideas that occupational therapists use to guide their practice. A **frame of reference,** as defined by Mosey, is based on a theory and contains specific elements, asking or answering specific questions about the patient. A frame of reference is theoretical, not necessarily practical. In other words, it may help us speculate on what is occurring with a patient. Ideally, it gives us a direction in which to look. However, it is not necessarily going to help us in our day-to-day treatment interventions.

A **practice model,** as defined by Reed,[15] has a practical focus. Its purpose is to guide the occupational therapy process to help us identify problems and technical solutions. Some practice models are derived from theories. Others have evolved from techniques that worked, although the reason why they worked was not known. The theory in these practice models was developed later to explain why these solutions or techniques were successful.

As an occupational therapy assistant, you will most likely be providing direct care to patients, performing evaluations and treatments, adapting equipment and environments, and working in a very practical world—the world of patients and their goals and problems. In the area of physical disabilities, most often you will be basing your work on one of the practice models in this book. These practice models focus on physical functions and on practical considerations of day-to-day life.

So, you might ask, why bother to learn a frame of reference if the practice models are more central to your work? The simple reason is that people are complicated, and their occupational functioning is complicated. People have needs, desires, hopes, fears, personal histories, and family and cultural backgrounds, all of which affect their beliefs in the possibilities of therapy and their willingness to try. It is not just a matter of a reflex here, some limitation in range there, or the need for a piece of adaptive equipment. Rather, the central question is how best to help each patient achieve the highest level of independent functioning possible in daily life activities. This question needs to be asked and answered from a broader perspective than any of the practice models can supply. In working with patients with physical disabilities, the patient's motivation, sense of hope, and drive to master the environment despite disability must be uppermost in the therapist's mind, even though the focus of day-to-day therapy may be on an isolated physical element such as the functioning of a muscle. For this reason, therapists guide practice from a frame of reference such as the model of human occupation.

This chapter shows how the model of human occupation provides a clear, organized system for understanding occupational performance. Occupational performance, as detailed in Chapter 2, names and defines various aspects of human activity. We can compare it to a catalog of home-building materials. The model of human occupation suggests how these aspects of human activity work together and how they are related. We can compare it to a building plan or blueprint.

## HUMAN OCCUPATION: A FRAME OF REFERENCE*

The core idea of the **model of human occupation**[9,10] is that humans have an inborn drive to explore and master their surroundings.† This activity of exploring and attempting to control the environment is called *occupation.* The model of human occupation attempts to explain how the drive toward occupation can be nurtured and developed or obstructed and crushed. In this model the individual and the environment are seen as interacting and affecting one another.

The model of human occupation is a **systems model.** The systems model is the modern equivalent of the holistic (versus reductionistic) model discussed in Chapter 1. In a systems model the whole—in this case the human individual engaged in occupation—is seen as a complex interaction of parts that cannot make sense viewed separately. In other words, therapists cannot look only at the right upper extremity or at the ability to sequence an activity without considering how this fits within the life of occupation that individuals have shaped for themselves. Persons cannot be considered separately from their environment. Their family, community, culture, and the objects they use every day are forces that shape their nature as actors in the world.

First, some terms used in the model should be defined (Box 3-1). When a person acts on the environ-

*The information in this section is modified from Early MB: *Mental health concepts and techniques for the occupational therapy assistant,* ed 2, New York, 1993, Raven.

†A second edition of *A Model of Human Occupation: Theory and Application* was released while this text was in press. The reader may wish to consult the new edition for changes in the model.

Box 3-1

### Model of Human Occupation: Definitions

**Human occupation** Process of exploring, responding to, and mastering the environment through activity.

**Environment** Human and nonhuman object world in which human occupation is carried out.

**Output** Action performed by a person.

**Intake** Information taken in from the environment.

**Feedback** Information about the effects of one's output or actions.

**Throughput** Process of attending to, evaluating, organizing, and responding to environmental intake and feedback.

**Volition** Motivation or the desire to act. The highest of the three subsystems within the model of human occupation. Personal causation, values, and interests are aspects of volition.

**Personal causation** Individual's sense of own competence and effectiveness.

**Values** Internalized images of what is good, right, and important.

**Interests** Personal preferences in activities or people.

**Habituation** Patterns or routine behavior. The second and middle of the three subsystems within the model of human occupation. Aspects of habituation include habits and internalized roles.

**Habits** Automatic routines. Actions carried out so frequently that they can be done without conscious effort.

**Internalized roles** Individual's personal interpretation and enactment of the (more general and less specific) occupational role.

**Occupational roles** Patterns for organizing productive activity, usually according to the product or service produced. Examples are grade-school student, homemaker, basketball player.

**Role change/role transition** Movement from one role to another, or movement within a role. Examples are going to work after finishing school, and moving from full-time to part-time work.

**Performance** Third or foundation level of the three subsystems within the model of human occupation. Skills and rules for using skills are aspects of performance.

**Skills** Small, simple actions that make up more complex actions.

**Rules for using skills** Principles used to adjust a skill to apply to particular situations.

**Resonance** Response of the rest of the system to a change in any part.

**Trajectory** Direction of movement of the system, which may be positive (benign cycle) or negative (vicious cycle).

**Benign cycle** Pattern of effective activity coupled with a reasonable amount of positive feedback from the environment.

**Vicious cycle** Pattern of inactivity or ineffective activity accompanied by less positive responses from the environment.

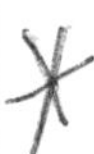

ment, the action is called *output.* Information coming from the environment about the results of this action is called *feedback.* Feedback provides a way to learn about the effects of actions. Of the available feedback, the part that the person actually takes in is called *intake.* This distinction is important; persons only use the information of which they are aware. Awareness may be unconscious, but some level of awareness must exist for intake to occur. Intake includes *all* information taken in, not just feedback from actions. This might comprise background data that can be seen, heard, or felt in some way.

By continuously taking in information (intake) and reflecting on feedback, individuals change their behavior and become more effective in controlling their environment. For example, a man sees (intake) a door that is labeled PUSH. He might push (output) on the door, but the door does not move (feedback). When he realizes (intake) that the door will not open with a push, he may try other methods, such as pulling (output) or using another door (output).

The processing of feedback and intake into new action is called *throughput.* Throughput consists of organizing, evaluating, and reorganizing information from the environment using information from within the self (e.g., memory). In the previous example, memory of other ways to open door and alternate routes to the other side would be combined with the realization that the door will not open by pushing. The process just described is depicted in Figure 3-1, which shows the relationships among intake, feedback, throughput, and output, as processed through the environment.

### Three Subsystems of Human Occupation

Besides the relatively simple output-feedback-intake-throughput-output cycle of behavior, the model of human occupation seeks to explain more complex interactions between the person and the environment. For example, people may or may not respond to the environment. Sometimes they do not want to respond. At other times, they may keep repeating an ineffective action, perhaps out of habit. Also, their actions may be limited or ineffective because they cannot organize the information they receive into any meaningful ideas or because their bodies lack the strength or coordination to act effectively. To explain these factors, the model of human occupation recognizes three levels of subsystems of human occupation: volition, habituation, and performance (Figure 3-2).

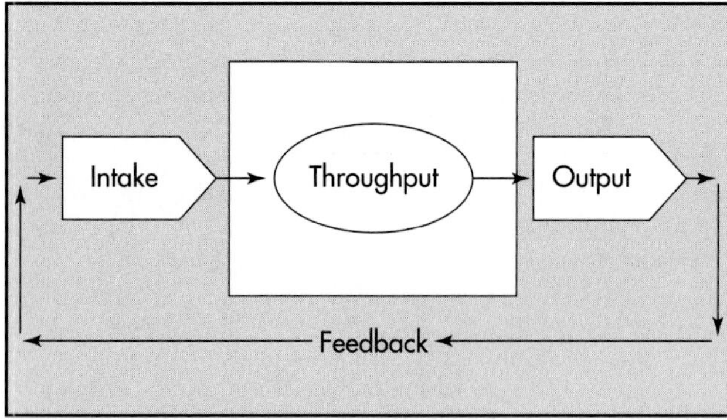


*Figure 3-1* The open system cycle: human occupation and the environment. (Modified from Kielhofner G, editor: *A model of human occupation: theory and application,* Baltimore, 1985, Williams & Wilkins.)

#### *Volition*

**Volition** is the highest level and governs the other subsystems. Another word for volition is motivation. Without motivation, there is no action, since the desire to act begins the action. Three key elements of volition are personal causation, values, and interests. *Personal causation* refers to the person's beliefs about personal effectiveness. Am I in control, or am I controlled by forces outside me? Am I good at things? Can I succeed if I try? These are questions of personal causation.

*Values* are internalized images of what is good, right, and important.[9] Values motivate behavior in many ways. For example, someone who is very ill may make a special effort to get dressed and go to church. A father may neglect professional reading to spend more time helping his child with homework because to him the child is more important.

*Interests* are "personal dispositions to find pleasure in certain objects, events, or people."[10] Interests are the things that attract people. When people are interested, they are energized, alive, and ready to attempt new things. Interests make the eyes light up and the heart beat faster and send blood coursing through the veins.

Together and separately, personal causation, values, and interests supply motivation to engage in occupation. This is the volition subsystem.

#### *Habituation*

**Habituation** is the middle-level subsystem and refers to activities that have been done often enough to become routine and customary. The two elements of the habituation subsystem are habits and internalized roles. *Habits* are automatic routines or patterns of activity that a person seems to perform almost by reflex, without much conscious awareness. An example would be folding towels or locking a door when leaving. Having habits helps conserve energy; tasks are accomplished without too much effort or concentration, and more time and attention are available for other things.

*Internalized roles* are personalized occupational roles that consist of many different habits, routines, and skills. Some typical occupational roles are homemaker, student, and retiree. Although each role carries certain socially expected behaviors, these are internalized or personalized by the individual. For example, one homemaker may pay more attention to preparing food for family and guests, whereas another is more involved in keeping the house clean and organized. The internalized role of a particular student might reflect habits established in childhood, as when the adult student sets up to study at the kitchen table immediately on returning home, just as the person was taught to do in grade school 30 years ago. Also, it may reflect values and interests, as when the student organizes study time around a favorite television program.

*Role change* or *role transition* affects the habituation subsystem. As life moves forward and the person grows, roles change. They contract, expand, are modified, and sometimes are abandoned or replaced. Former roles are rediscovered and renewed. New ones are attempted. The grade-school student becomes the high-school student. The student becomes a worker. The worker becomes a student again. The worker changes to another field. These are all examples of role change. Role change can be exciting or terrifying; occasionally it is both. Time for learning and adjustment is needed before a new role becomes internalized.

### *Performance*

**Performance** is the third and lowest level or subsystem of human occupation and consists of skills and rules for using those skills. *Skills* are small, simple actions that make up more complex actions. Touching the tip of a single finger to a surface and then lifting it is a skill. Modified and combined with other skills, it becomes part of playing a musical instrument, typing, or using a telephone, adding machine, or automated teller machine. *Rules for using skills* adjust the skill for particular situations. A manual typewriter, for example, requires much more pressure on each key than a computer key. Typing at a keyboard requires that each key be struck in turn rather than simultaneously. Playing the piano involves different chord structures and timings so that more than one key must be struck at once, and some are held when others are released.

Performance is the foundation level. Just as a building rises with strength from a sturdy foundation at the ground, so does effective human occupation arise out of a solid interlocking structure of skills. Occupational therapy for patients with physical dysfunction is most often directed at this level.

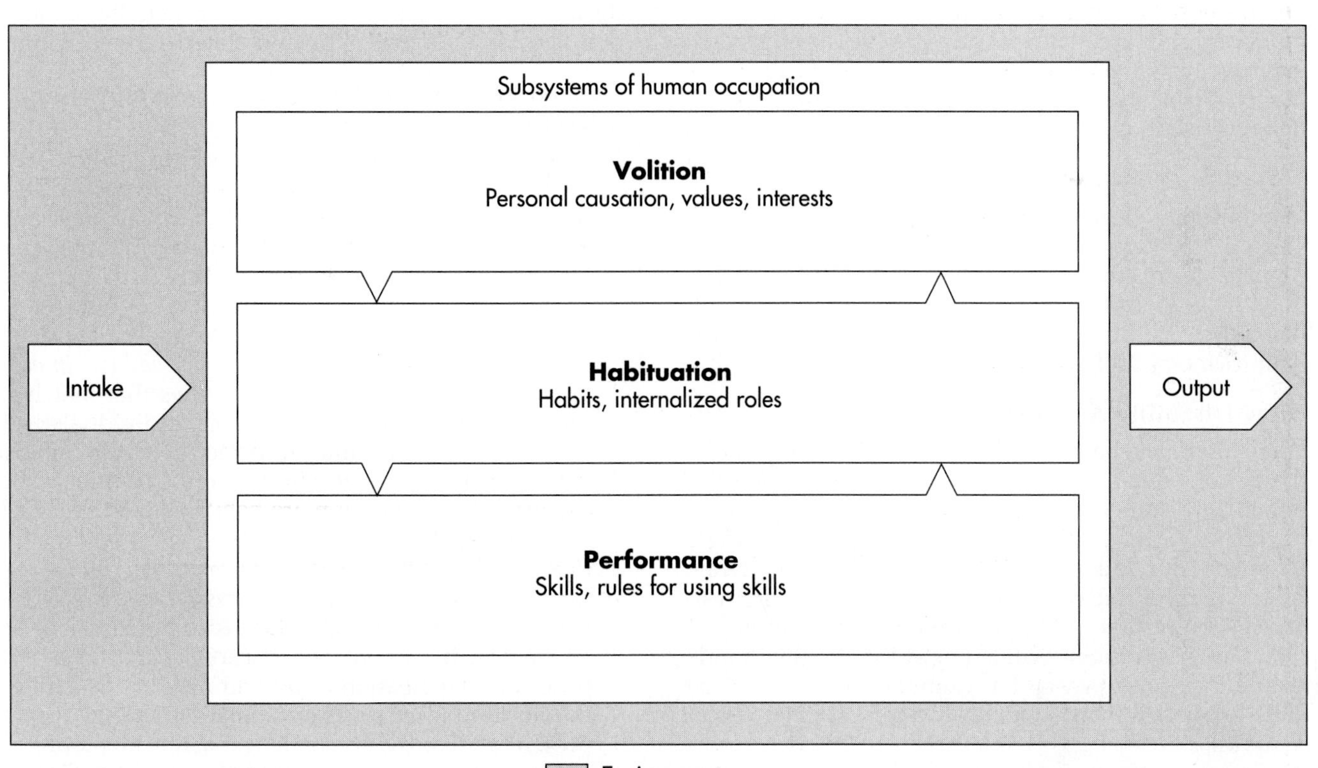


*Figure 3-2* Internal organization of the system of human occupation. (Modified from Kielhofner G: A model of human occupation. 2. The American Occupational Therapy Association: Ontogenesis from the perspective of temporal adaptation, *Am J Occup Ther* 34:657-663, 1980.)

### *Resonance Among the Subsystems*

As noted, the model of human occupation is a systems model. In a systems model a disturbance in one part affects the rest of the system. By analogy, a volcanic eruption or buildup of pollution in one country affects the weather systems for the entire planet. Similarly, in the model of human occupation, any [illegible] will resonate [illegible]

[illegible] and [illegible] challenging tasks and the perseverance to keep trying despite minor setbacks. In the opposite case, a failure can make people feel defeated and ineffective, leading to less enthusiasm for new tasks and perhaps to a loss of willingness to try. These examples illustrate two possible *trajectories* (directions of movement). A *benign cycle* consists of a pattern of effective activity coupled with a reasonable amount of positive feedback from the environment, leading to increased enthusiasm, energy, effectiveness, and optimism. A *vicious cycle* is a pattern of inactivity or ineffective activity accompanied by less positive responses from the environment, leading to diminished self-esteem, reduced activity, helplessness, and pessimism.

### How Disability Affects Human Occupation

Now that you have a general understanding of the model of human occupation, consider what happens when a person encounters the challenge of a physical disability. Consider the case of a young, healthy, single woman who falls and fractures both wrists while roller-blading. She will probably experience this physical disability first at the performance level because it takes away skills. She will not be able to use her hands while they are in casts. For example, she will not be able to operate many switches, doorknobs, and faucet handles.

Following the principle of resonance, however, this leads quickly to a change in habits and roles, since the necessary skills are not available. She cannot bathe herself, prepare her own food, or perform her job. Ultimately, personal causation is affected, with the normal feedback of success from participating in accustomed roles reduced or eliminated. She is confined to her home and begins to feel isolated. She no longer enjoys the company of co-workers or the feeling of satisfaction from doing her job. This may lead to a feeling of discouragement, helplessness, and apathy (lack of interest). She begins to feel worthless, depressed, and self-pitying. The woman may adopt a new role, that of helpless patient, in which she receives more pleasant (less demanding and less frustrating) feedback from the environment. She sees herself as less capable, more dependent on others, and more needy of support. She watches television and sleeps all day. Although such dependence may be appropriate for a time, if prolonged it might damage the volition subsystem so deeply that the patient has little motivation for anything. This is an example of a vicious cycle.

Not all persons who sustain a physical disability react in this way. Many patients respond to the challenge with inventive solutions and creative and energetic changes in behavior. Environmental supports such as family or friends can ease the adjustment so that patients feel more in control. They can look on the disability as an inconvenience, but not a serious obstacle to achieving what they want in life. Given sufficient motivation and adequate environmental support, this has the makings of a benign cycle of recovery. Patients may experience both benign and vicious cycles of varying intensity as they respond to a disability. The course of adjustment is usually not just one way or the other. Ups and downs are common.

### General Principles of Occupational Therapy Intervention

In addition to the descriptive concepts already described (Box 3-2), the model of human occupation provides guidelines for designing and carrying out occupational therapy treatment. These principles are discussed next and summarized in Box 3-3.[9,11]

1. *Through occupations designed as therapy, individuals can restore, develop, and maintain their abilities in occupation.* By participating in activities that match their needs, interests, and abilities, individuals can improve their ability to perform in daily life activities. The occupational therapy practitioner selects and designs activities to match the patient's characteristics and goals.
2. *Purposefulness, challenge, and the oppportunity for accomplishment and satisfaction are essential characteristics of occupation.* If occupation is to be effective as therapy, it must have a purpose. Typical purposes are the creation of an end product or exploration of an interest. The occupation should also present a "just right" challenge, achievable but not too easy. The careful gradation of the activity to the patient's capabilities allows for feelings of accomplishment while avoiding boredom on the one extreme or frustration on the other.
3. *Occupational therapy should present demands for performance that can result in positive feedback.* This is

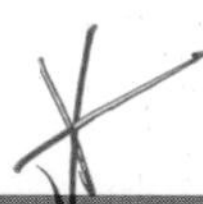

Box 3-2

### Model of Human Occupation: Concepts

1. A person is an open system. The individual affects and is affected by the environment.
2. Humans are born with a drive to explore and master their environment.
3. A person takes in information from the environment (intake).
4. A person acts on the environment (output).
5. The environment provides information about the effects of a person's actions (feedback).
6. A person evaluates, analyzes, and organizes actions using information from the environment. This process is called throughput.
7. The aspect of a person that acts in the environment is called human occupation. Human occupation is organized into three subsystems: volition, habituation, and performance.
8. Volition (motivation), the highest level, initiates action.
9. Habituation, the middle level, organizes activity into routines, which conserve energy.
10. Performance, the lowest or foundation level, includes small action patterns (skills) and the rules for using skills.
11. Changes in any of the subsystems will resonate or affect the others.
12. Occupational therapy intervention can be directed at any of the subsystems, the environment, or the interface between the environment and the individual.

y should
he patient.
the patient
een well
nance
back from
vates ongo-

*y to explore*
ve toward
volition sub-
ment of
ration.
pportunity
m. Just as
n marks
y of making
, espe-
encouraged
to explore first.

5. *Therapy should begin with the development of skills.* The foundation level of human occupation is performance. Occupational competence begins with the development of skills and the rules for

Box 3-3

### Principles of Occupational Therapy Intervention in the Model of Human Occupation

1. Through occupations designed as therapy, individuals can restore, develop, and maintain their abilities in occupation.
2. Purposefulness, challenge, and the opportunity for accomplishment and satisfaction are essential characteristics of occupation.
3. Occupational therapy should present demands for performance that can result in positive feedback.
4. Therapy should begin with an opportunity to explore rather than a demand to achieve.
5. Therapy should begin with the development of skills.

using skills. Skills should be established before organizing these into habits and occupational roles.

**Relationship of the Model of Human Occupation to Occupational Performance: The Domain of Concern**

At the beginning of this chapter, we compared occupational performance to a building materials catalog and the model of human occupation to a blueprint for a house. Examining the relationship between them in more detail reveals significant overlap, despite differences in terminology.

Both occupational performance and the model of human occupation emphasize the influence of the *environment,* part of the *context* in occupational performance. Both suggest that a change in the environment may cause a change in occupation. Equally, both give importance to occupational roles and habits; in human occupation this is the *habituation level,* and in occupational performance it is *performance areas.* Also, both identify skills as the foundation of occupational competence; in occupational performance these are called *performance components,* and in the model of human occupation they are called *skills and rules for using skills.* A key difference between occupational performance and the model of human occupation lies in the *volition subsystem,* for which no equivalent exists in occupational performance. The elements that make up this subsystem (values, interests, personal causation) fall within the *psychosocial and psychological components* section of the uniform terminology. Its components share equal status with skills such as range of motion or figure-ground perception.

Without belaboring the reasons for this difference, we must recognize that it exists. We have explored the model of human occupation as a frame of reference because it provides a direction, a point of view, and a starting point for considering how to improve the occupational experience of our patients. The volition subsystem is the highest level within human occupation and is the originator of all action. It is here that we must always start.

## THREE PRACTICE MODELS

Having described the model of human occupation and its relationship to occupational performance, we now examine the practice models most often used in physical disabilities practice: the biomechanical approach, the sensorimotor approach, and the rehabilitation approach. Each model is described, and its relationship to the model of human occupation and to occupational performance is discussed and illustrated.

### Biomechanical Approach

The **biomechanical approach** to the treatment of physical dysfunction considers the human body as a living machine. Techniques in this approach derive from **kinetics,** the science of the motions of objects and the forces acting on them.[13] To some extent, the principles of **statics,** the study of the forces acting on objects at rest, are also used in this approach. The object here is the human body, which is studied at rest and in motion. Treatment methods employ principles of physics[6] related to forces, levers, and torque (Box 3-4).

Typical evaluation and treatment techniques used in this approach are measurement of joint range of motion (ROM) and muscle strength, therapeutic exercise, and orthotics. Therapeutic activity for kinetic purposes, or the application of movement principles in the performance of activities, is also part of this approach. Sanding with a weighted sander to improve strength or weaving on an upright loom to increase shoulder ROM are examples. The goals of the biomechanical approach are to (1) evaluate specific physical limitations in ROM, strength, and endurance; (2) restore these functions; and (3) prevent or reduce deformity.

The biomechanical approach is most appropriate for patients whose central nervous system (CNS) is intact but who have lower motor neuron or orthopedic disorders. These patients can control isolated movements and specific movement patterns but may have weakness, low endurance, or joint limitation. Disabilities typically treated with this approach include orthopedic conditions (e.g., rheumatoid arthritis, osteoarthritis, fractures, amputations, hand trauma), burns, lower motor neuron disorders (e.g., peripheral nerve injuries), Guillain-Barré syndrome, spinal cord injuries, and primary muscle diseases (e.g., muscular dystrophy). Biomechanical principles are also applied in ergonomics and work hardening, with an emphasis on proper positioning and the optimum fit between the biomechanics of the individual and the work environment.

The biomechanical approach addresses the performance level of the model of human occupation and focuses on physical skills (e.g., lifting the hand) and their subskills (e.g., ROM, strength). Its principles can also be applied to the occupational performance areas and to the performance context, for example, when the height of a chair and a desk are lowered to fit a person of less than standard height. Within the context of occupational performance and uniform terminology, the biomechanical approach is primarily directed at restoration of elements of the sensorimotor component. In other words, this approach is most often employed to restore sensation, perception, strength, endurance, coordination, and so on.

How does the biomechanical approach relate to the model of human occupation and to occupational performance? Within the model of human occupation, it overlaps with the performance subsystem. Some minor overlap also occurs with the environment when the environment is adapted to fit the dimensions and biomechanical structure of the individual. Within occupational performance, the biomechanical approach overlaps with the sensorimotor components. Figure 3-3 illustrates these relationships of overlap.

*Box 3-4*

**Biomechanical Approach: Definitions**

**Kinetics** Study of the motions of objects and the forces acting on them
**Statics** Study of the forces acting on objects at rest
**Force** Measurable influence acting on a body
**Lever** Rigid structure fixed at a point called the *fulcrum* and acted on at two other points by two forces, causing movement in relation to the fulcrum; a seesaw and a crowbar are examples
**Torque** Rotary or twisting force
**Joint** Point where two bones meet and around which motion occurs
**Range of motion** Extent, measured in degrees of a circle, to which movement can occur at a joint
**Strength** Work against resistance (including the force of gravity), measured in pounds
**Endurance** Exertion or work sustained over time

### Sensorimotor (Neurophysiological) Approach

When earlier generations of occupational therapists tried to apply biomechanical principles to patients with a damaged CNS, they were frustrated by their patients' inability to carry out the desired motions. These patients could not coordinate and regulate their movements because their muscles were not receiving normal directions from the CNS. Biomechanical treatment approaches, which demand controlled voluntary movement, clearly were inappropriate for patients who lacked such control.

Methods using the **sensorimotor approach** were developed for treatment of patients who have CNS dysfunction. These methods belong to various theories

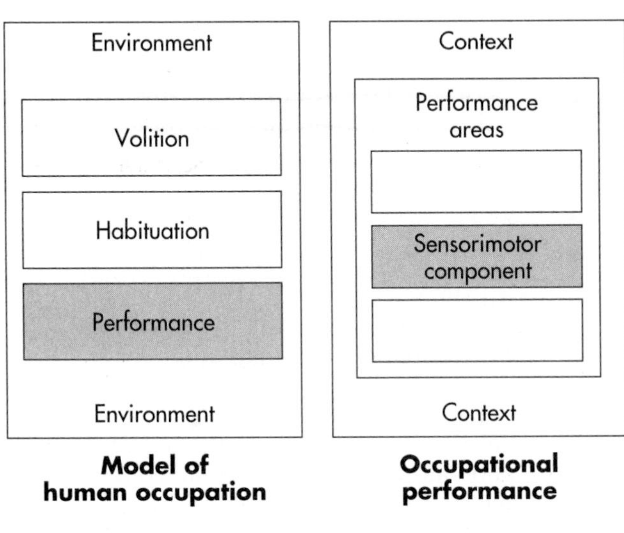


*Figure 3-3* Relationship of the biomechanical approach to the model of human occupation and to occupational performance.

of motor recovery.[7] The normal CNS functions to produce controlled, well-modulated (regular and adjusted) movement. The damaged CNS cannot coordinate and produce such movement.

All sensorimotor approaches to treatment use **neurophysiological** mechanisms to normalize muscle tone and elicit more normal motor responses.[7,19] They provide controlled input to the nervous system; this controlled input is meant to stimulate specific responses. Some approaches use **reflex** mechanisms, and the sequence of treatment may be based on the recapitulation of ontogenetic development.[17] In other words, these approaches might employ primitive reflexes such as those infants display or those that humans share with other creatures such as fish. Therapy is directed at incorporating these reflexes into purposeful activity and at integrating them so that their power is reduced and movement becomes more controlled and voluntary. Chapter 23 describes the sensorimotor approaches of Rood, Brunnstrom (movement therapy), Bobath (neurodevelopmental treatment), and Knott and Voss (proprioceptive neuromuscular facilitation). (See Box 3-5 for definitions of terms.)

The sensorimotor approach overlaps the model of human occupation and occupational performance in slightly different areas from the biomechanical approach. All the sensorimotor approaches use sensorimotor mechanisms to elicit specific motor responses. Many similarities and differences exist among the approaches, but they are all directed to motor recovery and improvement of motor performance. Within occupational performance, these are sensorimotor components.

*Box 3-5*

## Sensorimotor Approach: Definitions

**Central nervous system (CNS)** The brain and spinal cord

**Neurophysiological** Pertaining to the study of the physical and chemical nature of the nervous system

**Muscle tone** Resistance of a muscle to being stretched by an external force

**Motor response** Movement or muscle action evoked by sensory input; may be voluntary or involuntary

**Reflex mechanism** Involuntary motor response to sensory input

**Recapitulation of ontogenetic development** Theory that the organism in its development goes through the same stages as did the species in its development from lower organisms; as applied to recovery from CNS damage, also implies that recovery must go through the same stages as individual human development (i.e., from infancy)

In addition, the sensorimotor approaches intervene in some of the performance components of cognitive integration and cognitive arousal. Specifically, they address sequencing and motor learning. The sensorimotor approaches do not consider motivation, arousal, attention, or role dysfunction or the influence of these factors on motor behavior.[7] Therefore only a limited number of cognitive components are addressed. Within the model of human occupation, only the performance level is involved; the volition and habituation subsystems are not considered in these approaches (Figure 3-4).

Sensorimotor approaches have been criticized because they do not include purposeful activity or the involvement of patients as creators and actors in their own occupational world. Sensorimotor approaches are used by other health practitioners, including physical therapists, speech therapists, and physiatrists. They are not tools exclusively of occupational therapy. Although some approaches were developed by occupational therapists, others were designed or discovered by practitioners of these other disciplines.

The principles of the sensorimotor approaches can be used as an occupational therapy method when the practitioner applies them to purposeful activity, as described in Chapter 23. The American Occupational Therapy Association (AOTA) advises that the application of the techniques of an approach not associated with purposeful activity may be used "to prepare the client or patient for better performance and prevention of disability through self-participation in occupation."[4] These techniques should be a part of occupational therapy only when they are used to stimulate or condition the nervous system so that purposeful activity can be attempted, ideally during the same treatment session. When they are used in this way, the sensorimotor approaches can address the sensorimotor and cognitive/cognitive integration components and the performance areas.

## Rehabilitation Approach

The term *rehabilitation* means a restoration to a former state or to a proper state.[13] In medicine it means the return to the fullest physical, mental, social, vocational, and economic usefulness that is possible for the individual. It refers to the ability to live and work with remaining capabilities.[8] Therefore the focus in the treatment program is on abilities rather than disabilities.

Rehabilitation is concerned with the intrinsic worth and dignity of the individual and with the restoration of a satisfying and purposeful life. The **rehabilitation approach** uses measures that enable a person to live as independently as possible despite residual disability. Its goal is to help the patient learn to work around or compensate for physical limitations.[15]

The rehabilitation approach assumes that the patient is an active, involved, contributing member of the rehabilitation team. The occupational therapist must identify the patient's capabilities and assets so that these can be engaged to overcome the effects of the disability on function. To achieve this, the therapist must consider the latest scientific advances in methods and equipment (rehabilitation technology), social change, and community resources to provide the best services and opportunities for each patient.[8]

The treatment methods of the rehabilitation approach include modalities such as the following:

1. Self-care evaluation and training
2. Acquisition and training in assistive devices
3. Acquisition and training in use of adaptive clothing
4. Homemaking and child care
5. Work simplification and energy conservation
6. Work-related activities
7. Leisure activities
8. Prosthetic training
9. Wheelchair management
10. Home evaluation and adaptation
11. Community transportation
12. Architectural adaptations
13. Acquisition and training in the use of communication aids and environmental control systems.

In relation to occupational performance, the rehabilitation approach focuses on the performance areas more than on performance components. The aim of the occupational therapy program is to enable role performance and to minimize the effects of residual disability on role performance. The rehabilitation approach takes into account the influence of the environment and provides methods to adapt the environment to the individual.

The rehabilitation approach addresses most of the elements of the model of human occupation. Including the patient as a member of the rehabilitation team engages the volition subsystem. However, the patient's values, interests, and sense of personal causation are not addressed directly. The habituation subsystem is

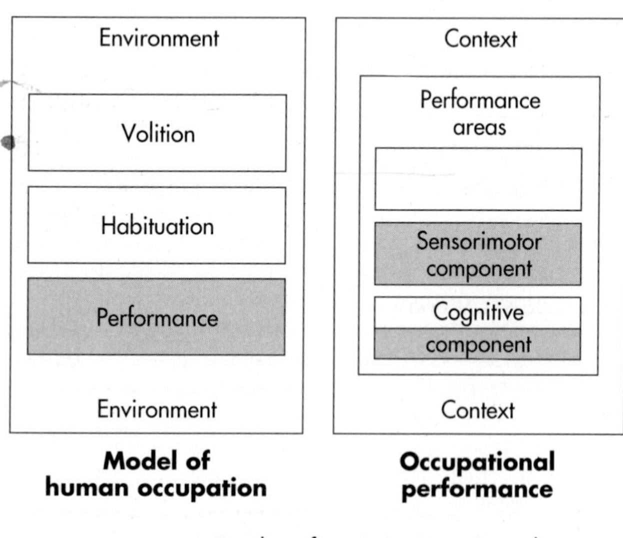


*Figure 3-4* Relationship of the sensorimotor approach to the model of human occupation and to occupational performance.

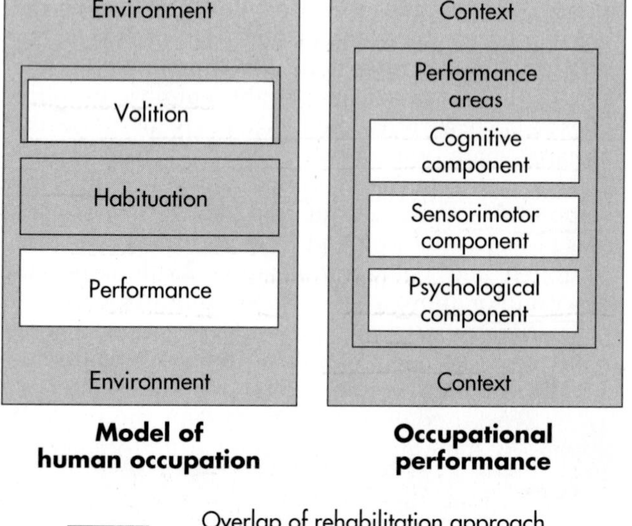


*Figure 3-5* Relationship of the rehabilitation approach to the model of human occupation and to occupational performance.

the main focus of intervention, with the emphasis on occupational role performance. As mentioned, the environment and possible changes to the environment are also considered. The performance level is emphasized less in this approach than in the biomechanical and sensorimotor approaches. Figure 3-5 illustrates these relationships.

Frequently, therapists use methods of the rehabilitation approach in combination with methods from the biomechanical or sensorimotor approaches. Biomechanical or sensorimotor principles can be applied *during* rehabilitation activities to reinforce the functioning of sensorimotor and cognitive components. An example is the use of cross-diagonal patterns (a sensorimotor approach) to normalize muscle tone and coordination during dressing. This complements and enhances the success of rehabilitation. At the same time, it ties the sensorimotor technique to purposeful activity.

### Limitations of These Practice Models

The three practice models just described have proved useful in evaluating and treating problems frequently encountered in physical disabilities practice. Used separately or together, however, they do not provide a complete view of the patient. None of the three practice models addresses the cognitive/cognitive integration performance components and psychosocial/psychological performance components explicitly. They also do not address the temporal, social, or cultural aspects of the performance context.

Di Joseph[7] urges occupational therapists to consider not only motor control but also motor behavior, that is, "a person acting purposefully within and upon his or her environment." She further states that ignoring the emotive and cognitive aspects of motor behavior is a reductionistic approach that fails to consider all factors in the production of "purposeful action." Treatment goals for patients must be based on an evaluation of mind, body, and environment. These goals should be reached through the use of activities that are compatible with the needs and values of the person and not necessarily with those of the therapist. Interaction between the person and the environment is essential to the development of functional independence.[16] The person is mind and body, not just a motor system to be evaluated and "treated."[7] Keeping this warning in mind, consider next the progress of a patient from first meeting the occupational therapist to discharge from treatment.

## THE TREATMENT CONTINUUM IN PHYSICAL DISABILITIES PRACTICE

A *continuum* is a "continuous series of elements passing into each other."[13] A **treatment continuum** begins with the onset of injury or disability and ends with the restoration of the patient to maximal independence. It is not a series of steps, but a gradual movement from disease and disability toward health and ability. The best prognosis for many conditions leaves the patient with some residual disability. For every patient the end point of the continuum is the maximal *possible* functional return.

Figure 3-6 is a model for the treatment continuum in physical disabilities practice. The stages in this treatment continuum overlap and can occur simultaneously. Although four stages are identified within it, the treatment continuum is not meant to illustrate a strict step-by-step progression. It takes the patient through a logical progression from dependence to skill development, then to purposeful activity, and finally to resumption of life roles.[14] The treatment continuum identifies the concerns of occupational therapy practice within the context of occupational performance and is compatible with the model of human occupation.

### Stage One: Adjunctive Methods

**Adjunctive methods** are used within occupational therapy to prepare the patient to engage in activity.[5] These procedures may include exercise, facilitation and inhibition techniques, positioning, sensory stimulation, selected physical agent modalities, and devices such as braces and splints.[18] Adjunctive methods are used by physical therapists and other health care providers; it is the application of these methods *as a preparation for purposeful activity* that differentiates occupational therapy from other professions.

Adjunctive methods are often used in, but are not limited to, the acute stages of illness or injury. During this stage the occupational therapist is likely to be most concerned with evaluating and remediating performance components. The occupational therapist should plan the progression of treatment so that adjunctive modalities are used to prepare the patient for purposeful activity and are directed toward the achievement of maximal independence in the performance areas. Adjunctive methods require the advanced education and training of the occupational therapist and are not appropriately performed by the entry-level occupational therapy assistant.[1]

To illustrate the treatment continuum, we use the example of a male patient who has recently suffered a stroke, or cardiovascular accident (CVA). The most obvious effect of a stroke is paralysis or weakness on one side of the body. (Other effects of this condition are addressed in Chapter 25.) In this example the patient is unable to move his arm or leg. Without normal exercise, the muscles will contract, and motion will be limited in the future. To prevent this, the therapist moves the patient's limbs passively (passive range of motion), maintaining as normal a range as possible. Passive ROM is a component needed for development of skills.

At stage one the therapist is mainly concerned with maintaining or remedying the components of skills. Within the model of human occupation, these components fall within the performance subsystem. Within occupational performance, they are performance components.

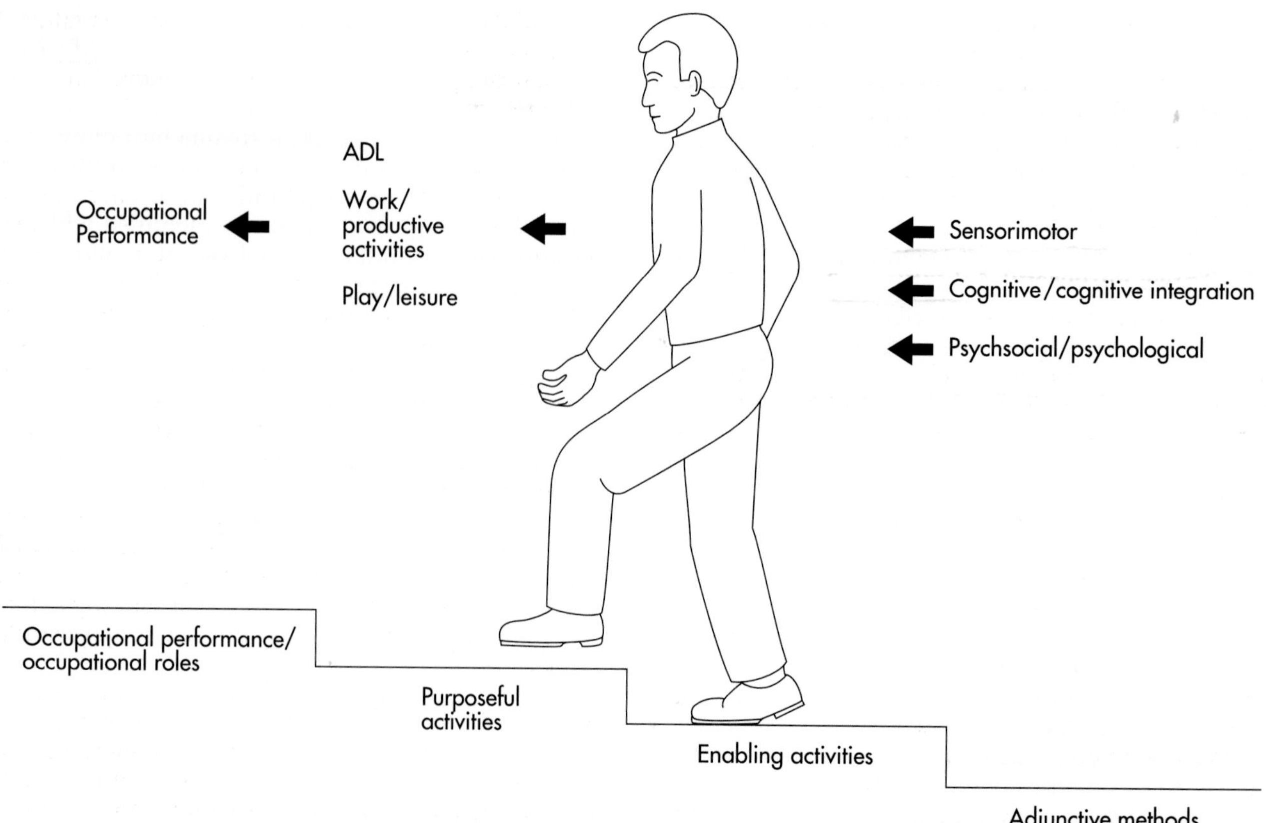


*Figure 3-6* Treatment continuum for physical disabilities practice. (Courtesy Karin Boyce.)

**Stage Two: Enabling Activities**

Occupational therapists have created many enabling methods for simulating purposeful activities. Examples are sanding boards, skateboards, stacking cones or blocks, practice boards for mastery of clothing fasteners and hardware, driving simulators, work simulators, and table-top activities such as pegboards for training perceptual-motor skills. These methods cannot be considered purposeful activity. Such activities are not likely to be as meaningful to the patient or to stimulate as much interest and motivation as purposeful activities. However, it may be necessary to use them as a preparatory or ancillary part of the treatment program to train specific sensorimotor, perceptual, or cognitive functions necessary for activities in the performance areas.

**Enabling activities** require more patient involvement than do adjunctive methods. While adjunctive methods are usually applied by the therapist to the patient who passively receives them, the enabling methods are carried out by the patient. Enabling activities meet two of the three characteristics of purposeful activity: (1) the patient participates actively, and (2) the activity requires and elicits coordination of sensorimotor, psychosocial, and cognitive systems.[5,7]

However, enabling methods fail to meet the third characteristic of purposeful activity: the presence of an autonomous or inherent goal beyond the motor function required to perform the task.[5] In other words, getting exercise should not be the *only* reason for doing the activity. Nonetheless, although enabling methods might not be considered purposeful, they are often used as a necessary step toward the ability to perform purposeful activities. Prep work

Special equipment, such as wheelchairs, ambulatory aids, assistive devices, special clothing, communication devices, and environmental control systems, may also be needed to enable independence in the performance areas and assumption of occupational roles.

Returning to our example, the patient at this stage may have some voluntary movement of his arm and leg. The movement is too weak and uncoordinated because of spasticity, however, to allow for activity performance that would satisfy the patient's self-esteem needs. In other words, the patient might be able to pick up and place very large mosaic tile pieces, but the result would be uneven and unattractive. An activity such as stacking cones or pegboard designs may be given to the patient at stage two to allow him to practice motions that later will be applied to purposeful activities.

In stage two the therapist is still concerned with evaluation and remediation of skills and the components of skills. Rules for using skills may be added at this stage, with the patient experiencing the different weights and textures of materials handled. Within the model of human occupation, stage two work is at the level of the performance subsystem. Within occupational performance, the emphasis is on performance components. The occupational therapy assistant may safely carry out most stage two enabling activities but must be careful to obtain guidance on the purpose, objectives, procedures, and precautions that apply to each patient situation.

### Stage Three: Purposeful Activity

**Purposeful activity** has been the core of occupational therapy since its inception. Purposeful activity has an inherent or autonomous goal and is relevant and meaningful to the patient.[5] It is part of the daily life routine and occurs in the context of occupational performance.[2,3] Examples are feeding, hygiene, dressing, mobility, communication, arts, crafts, games, sports, work, and educational activities.

The purposefulness of an activity is determined by the individual performing it and the context in which it is performed. Occupational therapy practitioners use purposeful activities to evaluate, facilitate, restore, or maintain a person's ability to function in life roles.[3] Purposeful activity can be carried out in a health care facility or in the patient's home.

Returning to our example, the patient at this stage has achieved more control of his arm and leg. Weakness and spasticity may remain, but significant improvement has occurred. The therapist at this point would teach the patient techniques for dressing, self-feeding, toileting, and transfer from the wheelchair. The patient might participate in crafts or games that have been adapted to improve his skills in, for example, reaching and holding and pinch and release.

In stage three the therapist is concerned with evaluating and remediating deficits in the performance of daily life activities. Within the model of human occupation, stage three work is at the level of the habituation subsystem. Within occupational performance, the emphasis is on performance areas. Again, stage one and stage two activities would overlap and continue, to reinforce the development of performance components. Some activities also may overlap with stage four. The occupational therapy assistant can expect to be prominently involved in the patient's treatment at this point, since the performance areas are the focus of the assistant's treatment skills.

### Stage Four: Occupational Performance and Occupational Roles

In the final stage of the treatment continuum, the patient resumes or assumes **occupational roles** in the living environment and in the community. Appropriate tasks in activities of daily living, work and productive activities, and play and leisure are performed to the patient's maximal level of independence. This level is defined by each patient according to personal capacities and limitations and values, interests, and goals. Residual disability may remain, but the patient has learned compensatory techniques. Formal occupational therapy intervention is decreased and ultimately discontinued.

The stroke patient at this stage has achieved as much motor return as is believed medically possible. He has learned some sensorimotor techniques to counteract the effects of abnormal spastic tone so that he can dress and feed himself. He has practiced and relearned the many skills and habits that make up his daily life. Working with the therapist, he has identified his needs in work and home life and has selected and been trained with adaptive devices appropriate to his situation. He resumes his life in the community, shaping this new occupational life with the strategies and techniques he has learned in therapy.

In stage four the therapist is concerned with assisting the patient in the transition to community life. Within the model of human occupation, stage four work is at the level of the habituation subsystem as it interfaces with the environment. Within **occupational performance,** the emphasis is on performance areas and the performance context. Both the occupational therapy assistant and the occupational therapist would be involved in this stage.

A particular occupational therapy practitioner may be responsible for only one or two phases in the continuum. In fact, the continuum may occur over two or more treatment settings, such as an acute care hospital and an intermediate care facility, and finally in the community.

## SUMMARY

The model of human occupation is a frame of reference for occupational performance. This model has three subsystems, of which volition (motivation) is the highest or governing level. The other levels are habituation, a main focus of the occupational therapy assistant's expertise, and performance, in which patients with physical dysfunction experience the most direct and visible disruption of their occupational lives.

The three treatment approaches usually applied in physical disabilities practice are the biomechanical, sensorimotor, and rehabilitation approaches. These approaches apply to specific types of patient situations and overlap with some aspects of occupational performance and the model of human occupation.

The treatment continuum in physical disabilities practice is a process of four stages through which the patient gradually acquires the abilities to resume occupational life after disability. The occupational therapy assistant is most involved in the final two stages of purposeful activity and resumption of occupational roles.

The goal of occupational therapy intervention is to facilitate the development of maximal functioning in occupational roles, which is defined for each individual according to that person's capacities and limitations. Recognizing that the patient is the starting point, we consider this individual's goals, values, and interests throughout the occupational therapy process.

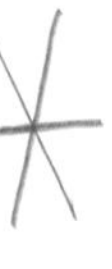

## Selected Reading Guide Questions

1. Explain the difference between a frame of reference and a practice model.
2. Explain how a systems model works.
3. Define the following terms: output, intake, throughput, feedback, environment.
4. List and describe the three levels or subsystems of the model of human occupation.
5. Relate *role change* or *role transition* to the model of human occupation.
6. Discuss what is meant by *benign and vicious cycles* in the model of human occupation.
7. How does the model of human occupation fit within occupational performance, occupational therapy's domain of concern?
8. List the typical evaluation and treatment methods used in the biomechanical approach.
9. Identify the conditions for which the biomechanical approach is most appropriate.
10. How does the biomechanical approach relate to the model of human occupation?
11. Identify the conditions for which the sensorimotor approach is most appropriate, and explain why this approach is preferred.
12. List some of the theorists whose work is used in the sensorimotor approach.
13. Discuss the relationship between the sensorimotor approach and purposeful activity.
14. How does the sensorimotor approach relate to the model of human occupation?
15. Define *rehabilitation.*
16. State the goal of the rehabilitation approach.
17. List some of the treatment methods of the rehabilitation approach.
18. How does the rehabilitation approach relate to the model of human occupation?
19. Explain why the three practice models used in physical disabilities practice have been criticized for providing an incomplete view of the patient.
20. Discuss why each of the four stages in the occupational therapy treatment continuum requires a different level of patient involvement.

## REFERENCES


1. American Occupational Therapy Association: Association policy 1.25: registered occupational therapists and certified occupational therapy assistants and modalities, *Am J Occup Ther* 47:1118-1119, 1993.
2. American Occupational Therapy Association: Position paper: purposeful activity, *Am J Occup Ther* 47:1081-1082, 1993.
3. American Occupational Therapy Association: Purposeful activities, a position paper, *Am J Occup Ther* 37:805, 1983.
4. American Occupational Therapy Association: Resolution 532-79 (1979): occupation as the common core of occupational therapy, Representative Assembly minutes, Detroit, April 1979, *Am J Occup Ther* 33:785, 1979.
5. Ayres AJ: Basic concepts of clinical practice in physical disabilities, *Am J Occup Ther* 12:300, 1958.
6. Brunnstrom S: *Clinical kinesiology,* ed 3, Philadelphia, 1972, Davis.
7. Di Joseph LM: Independence through activity: mind, body, and environment interaction in therapy, *Am J Occup Ther* 36:740, 1982.
8. Hopkins HL, Smith HD, Tiffany EG: Rehabilitation. In Hopkins HL, Smith HD, editors: *Willard and Spackman's occupational therapy,* ed 6, Philadelphia, 1983, Lippincott.
9. Kielhofner G, editor: *A model of human occupation: theory and application,* Baltimore, 1985, Williams & Wilkins.
10. Kielhofner G, Burke JP: A model of human occupation. 1. Conceptual framework and content, *Am J Occup Ther* 34:572-581, 1980.
11. Mosey AC: *Occupational therapy: configuration of a profession,* New York 1981, Raven.
12. Mosey AC: *Three frames of reference for mental health,* Thorofare, NJ, 1970, Slack.
13. Oxford University Press: *The compact edition of the Oxford English dictionary,* Oxford, 1971, Oxford University Press.
14. Pedretti LW: The compatibility of treatment methods in physical disabilities with the philosophical base of occupational therapy. Paper presented at the American Occupational Therapy Association National Conference, Philadelphia, May 1982.
15. Reed KL: *Models for practice in occupational therapy,* Baltimore, 1984, Williams & Wilkins.
16. Rogers JC: The spirit of independence: the evolution of a philosophy, *Am J Occup Ther* 36:709, 1982.
17. Stockmeyer SA: An interpretation of the approach of Rood to the treatment of neuromuscular dysfunction, *Am J Phys Med* 46:900, 1967.
18. Trombly CA: Include exercise in purposeful activity, *Am J Occup Ther* 36:467, 1982 (letter to the editor).
19. Willard HL, Spackman CS, editors: *Occupational therapy,* ed 4, Philadelphia, 1971, Lippincott.


## RECOMMENDED READING


Clark F: Occupation embedded in a real life: interweaving occupational science and occupational therapy, *Am J Occup Ther* 47(12):1067-1078, 1993.

Dunn W, Brown C, McGuigan A: The ecology of human performance: a framework for considering the effect of context, *Am J Occup Ther* 48(7):595-607, 1994.

Early MB: *Mental health concepts and techniques for the occupational therapy assistant,* New York, 1993, Raven.

Sharrott GW, Cooper-Fraps C: Theories of motivation in occupational therapy: an overview, *Am J Occup Ther* 40(4):249-257, 1986.

Part II

# Occupational Therapy Process

Chapter 4

# Overview of Occupational Therapy Process

Mary Beth Early

## Chapter Objectives

*After studying this chapter, the student or practitioner will be able to:*

1. Identify and describe the major stages in the occupational therapy process.
2. Describe the "flow" of the occupational therapy process, and give examples to illustrate this.
3. Identify and contrast the roles of the OTR and the COTA in the occupational therapy process.
4. Discuss ways in which the COTA can achieve greater responsibility in the occupational therapy process.

## Key Terms

referral
screening
evaluation
treatment planning
treatment implementation
reevaluation
discharge planning
termination of treatment
occupational therapy practitioner
transition services

The patient with a physical disability may never have heard of occupational therapy before the first encounter with the OTR or COTA in the clinic. For many patients, however, occupational therapy will be an important bridge back to life, to the ability to function with maximal independence in occupational roles and daily life activities. Every encounter with the patient, from the first referral or screening meeting to the final discharge, is directed toward this end.

The purpose of this chapter is to give an overview of the occupational therapy process, with particular emphasis on the role of the COTA and the relationship between the COTA and OTR and the patient. Chapters 5 and 6 focus more specifically on evaluation and treatment, two important stages in the occupational therapy process.

## STEPS OR STAGES IN THE OCCUPATIONAL THERAPY PROCESS

Traditionally, the occupational therapy process has been seen as a series of separate stages or steps, as follows:

1. **Referral.** The physician or other legally qualified professional requests occupational therapy services for the patient. Referral may be oral, but a

written record is also necessary.
2. **Screening.** The registered occupational therapist performs a quick assessment to determine whether occupational therapy services would be helpful to this patient.
3. **Evaluation.** The registered occupational therapist identifies the information to be collected and the areas to be evaluated and selects the evaluation and assessment instruments. Areas of the evaluation may be carried out by the COTA. The data are then analyzed to determine the patient's specific strengths and deficits.
4. **Treatment planning.** Working with the patient, the occupational therapy practitioners develop a plan for restoring, improving, or maintaining the patient's ability to function in daily life roles and activities. The treatment plan includes goals and methods for reaching them. It recognizes the patient's values and goals and considers the cultural, social, and environmental situation.
5. **Treatment implementation.** The occupational therapy team carries out the treatment plan. The certified occupational therapy assistant may have significant responsibilities for this part of the process.
6. **Reevaluation.** With the same instruments used in the evaluation, the occupational therapy team again evaluates the patient to determine what changes have occurred since the previous evaluation. This measurement of the outcomes of treatment is critical in showing the effectiveness of the therapy. The treatment plan may be changed or continued based on the results of the reevaluation.
7. **Discharge planning.** Working with the patient, the patient's family, and the treatment team, the occupational therapist and assistant develop a plan for the patient once discharge occurs. The discharge may be to the patient's home or to an intermediate care or long-term care facility.
8. **Termination of treatment.** The patient is discharged from the treatment program. Final outcomes are analyzed and documented. Follow-up information is given to the patient should problems arise in the future.

## PROCESS AND FLOW

Despite the discrete stages just listed, the occupational therapy process more closely resembles a flowing or fluid current (like a river) than a stepwise progression (like climbing a mountain). Although referral generally comes first, in some cases the occupational therapy practitioner (therapist or assistant) may initiate the referral and actually perform a cursory screening before the physician becomes involved. Some physicians rely on occupational therapy staff to identify those patients who are most likely to benefit, and issue referrals at their suggestion.

Similarly, evaluation and treatment may be interwoven throughout the process. In a patient with a biomechanical problem, range of motion (ROM) and muscle strength may be evaluated and treated first; evaluation (and treatment planning) of other areas would be deferred until pain is diminished and ROM is within a functional range.

Significantly, most occupational therapists consider discharge planning almost immediately on meeting the patient. This is partly a result of demands for quick discharge because of restrictions on reimbursement. However, occupational therapists have historically viewed their patients in the context of their occupational lives; by envisioning the patient's future, the therapist creates a scenario of hope toward which the patient and staff can direct their energies.

Novices at clinical practice may find it difficult to immerse themselves in the flowing of the occupational therapy process, preferring the structure and comfort of readily identified steps and stages. Good supervision is essential if beginners are to acquire this important clinical habit.

## ROLE OF THE REGISTERED OCCUPATIONAL THERAPIST

In keeping with the most recent *Standards of Practice for Occupational Therapy* issued by the American Occupational Therapy Association (AOTA),[2] we recognize the leadership role of the registered therapist in the occupational therapy process. The OTR is responsible for accepting and acting on referrals and for designing and supervising individual or group screenings.

The OTR is the manager, director, analyst, and documenter of occupational therapy evaluation. The OTR selects the areas to be evaluated and chooses appropriate evaluation instruments. The OTR may delegate administration of parts of the evaluation to the COTA, who may also be asked to document these areas.

The OTR is the designer, developer, and documenter of the treatment plan. Planning should include the following[2]:

1. Formulating a list of strengths and weaknesses
2. Estimating rehabilitation potential
3. Identifying measurable short-term and long-term goals
4. Collaborating with the individual, family members, other caregivers, professionals, and community resources
5. Selecting the media, methods, environment, and personnel needed to accomplish the intervention goals
6. Determining the frequency and duration of occupational therapy services
7. Identifying a plan for reevaluation
8. Planning for discharge

The OTR may delegate some aspects of treatment planning to the COTA. However, the OTR retains legal and supervisory responsibility for the plan and its implementation.

The OTR is the manager and documenter of treatment implementation and reevaluation. Major portions of implementation may be delegated to the COTA. Nevertheless, the OTR is responsible for overseeing and supervising treatment and reevaluating and documenting progress.

The OTR determines when service should be discontinued and develops a discharge plan. Parts of the planning for discharge may be delegated to the COTA. The OTR is responsible to document all outcomes and recommendations for follow-up in the final report.

## ROLE OF THE CERTIFIED OCCUPATIONAL THERAPY ASSISTANT

The COTA is a co-participant in the entire occupational therapy process, at the discretion of the supervising OTR and depending on the experience and service competencies of the particular COTA. The 1994 *Standards of Practice* employs the term **occupational therapy practitioner,** referring to both the OTR and the COTA.[2] Thus the training and qualifications of the COTA are recognized to be consistent with significant responsibilities in the occupational therapy process.

With regard to referral, the COTA can educate physicians and other potential referral sources about how to initiate occupational therapy referrals. The COTA may carry out parts of the screening under OTR supervision.[2]

Once appropriate evaluation instruments have been selected by the OTR, the COTA may administer some of these.[2] As a general rule, the more standardized and structured the instrument, the more quickly the COTA can acquire adequate service competency for administration. The COTA must be able to communicate results, both orally and in writing, of evaluation instruments he or she administers. The COTA may be given responsibility for educating the patient and family about the purposes of the evaluation.

The COTA can contribute to the treatment plan.[2] This is especially true in the occupational performance areas of daily living activities, work and productive activities, and play and leisure. The COTA with sufficient experience and expertise may work fairly independently in these areas. Generally, treatment of performance components (e.g., motor skills, cognitive skills) is planned by the OTR.

According to the 1994 *Standards of Practice,* the COTA may implement the treatment plan under OTR supervision.[2] This might include carrying out treatment activities, educating the patient and family about treatment, and documenting the services provided. The COTA may also contribute to reevaluation, as directed.

The COTA may have responsibility for **transition services,** which help the patient change from one level or one environment to another.[2] For example, the patient with a head injury may need to move toward independent community living. This type of transition might require the services of a community agency. Depending on the practice area and personal expertise, the COTA may coordinate or carry out a plan for moving the patient through such a transition. Generally the OTR designs the transition plan.

## EXPERIENCE, EXPERTISE, AND SERVICE COMPETENCY

The occupational therapy assistant student or recent graduate, as a matter of personal responsibility and professional prudence, should follow the guidelines set forth in the 1994 *Standards of Practice.* New practitioners need and benefit from close supervision and direction in all stages of the occupational therapy process. They should undertake independent service provision in evaluation and treatment planning only when service competency is assured after careful training.

The more experienced COTA may function fairly autonomously in designated areas of evaluation and treatment planning with only general supervision from the OTR.[1,3] Years of experience are not sufficient by themselves. COTAs wanting more autonomy and responsibility must study, learn, and practice the service tasks they want to provide. The more experienced and expert COTA may find opportunities for greater independence and responsibility both within the occupational therapy team and in related fields.

The experienced COTA might assume leadership or specialty positions within the OT department, perhaps within an area of practice or administration.[1] Examples might include technology specialist, pain management specialist, or director of student training. Each of these roles requires certain skills and competencies that can be achieved by COTAs. Alternative roles exist outside the occupational therapy field, such as director of durable medical equipment or director of adult day care.

## SUMMARY

The occupational therapy process begins with referral and ends with termination of treatment. Although the process includes discrete stages that can be named and described, the process is not stepwise but rather is fluid, with the stages intermingled at times. To the novice this may appear confusing, but it is a hallmark of good clinical reasoning.

The registered occupational therapist and certified occupational therapy assistant have specific responsibilities and areas of emphasis within the occupational therapy process. The OTR is the manager and director of the process and delegates specific tasks and steps to the qualified COTA. With time, study, and experience, COTAs can develop sufficient service competency that allows them to take on additional responsibilities and specialty roles.

## Selected Reading Guide Questions

1. List and describe the eight stages or steps in the occupational therapy process.
2. Describe and contrast the roles of the OTR and the COTA with regard to each stage of the occupational therapy process.
3. Give at least one example that shows the "flow" of the occupational therapy process.
4. Summarize what the COTA must do to achieve greater responsibility for the occupational therapy process.

### REFERENCES

1. American Occupational Therapy Association: Career exploration and development: a companion guide to the occupational therapy roles document, *Am J Occup Ther* 48:844-851, 1994.
2. American Occupational Therapy Association, Commission on Practice: Standards of practice for occupational therapy, *Am J Occup Ther* 48:1039-1043, 1994.
3. American Occupational Therapy Association: Occupational therapy roles, *Am J Occup Ther* 47:1087-1099, 1993.

### RECOMMENDED READING

Greenberg NS: *Occupational therapy assistant career profile,* St Louis, 1990, Green.

Chapter 5

# Occupational Therapy Evaluation of Physical Dysfunction

*Lorraine Williams Pedretti*
*Mary Beth Early*

## Chapter Objectives

*After studying this chapter, the student or practitioner will be able to:*

1. Differentiate among evaluation, evaluation procedure, and assessment.
2. Contrast the roles of the OTR and the COTA in the evaluation process.
3. Define clinical reasoning and discuss its role in the evaluation process.
4. Describe the typical content of the initial evaluation.
5. Explain how the medical record can assist the practitioner in preparing to evaluate the patient.
6. Describe the skills and behavior of an effective interviewer.
7. Describe the daily schedule interview and discuss its purpose.
8. Contrast standardized and nonstandardized tests.
9. Discuss the general guidelines for administering standardized tests.
10. Discuss some reasons why nonstandardized tests continue to be used in occupational therapy.

## Key Terms

evaluation
assessment
evaluation procedure
clinical reasoning
active listening
daily schedule interview
standardized test
norms
reliability
validity
nonstandardized test

Before treating the patient, the occupational therapy team must gather information about the patient's problems, strengths, goals, life situation, and occupational roles. The process of gathering and analyzing this information is called *evaluation*.[3] The registered occupational therapist (OTR) is responsible for the evaluation process, in which the certified occupational therapy assistant (COTA) may assist. Evaluation may involve formal and informal screening and evaluation methods, including review of the medical record, interview, observation, standardized tests, and nonstandardized tests. Occupational therapy evaluation focuses on the occupational performance areas and performance components. Problems identified through evaluation become the basis for developing treatment objectives and strategies to remediate or compensate for these problems.

## EVALUATION AND ASSESSMENT

The terms *assessment* and *evaluation* have been used interchangeably. The American Occupational Therapy Association (AOTA)[3] in 1995 clarified the meaning of evaluation and assessment as follows:

> **Evaluation** shall be used to refer to the process of obtaining and interpreting data necessary for intervention. This includes planning for and documenting the evaluation process and results.
>
> **Assessment** shall be used to refer to specific tools or instruments used during the evaluation process.

Before this, AOTA documents had used these terms to mean exactly the reverse. The change in definitions was made to conform to patterns within the health care industry and to bring occupational therapy language in line with the language of other disciplines. This text follows the AOTA guidelines with regard to the term *evaluation*. Thus evaluation includes both the battery of specific tests of measurable deficits (i.e., a set of tests identified by the OTR as appropriate for measuring this patient's problems) *and* the clinical reasoning process used by the OTR to organize and interpret the results of these tests. In this text, **evaluation procedure** or *assessment procedure* refers to one specific method, such as a test or structured observation (e.g., range of motion), used in the evaluation. The COTA may carry out selected evaluation and assessment procedures.

The evaluation ideally will provide a composite picture of the person's functioning based on the results of the evaluation procedures and assessments. Evaluation represents the product of the therapist's thinking and analysis, using all the data gathered, which the therapist considers in light of previous learning, both academic and clinical, and past cases. By sifting through a variety of facts, memories, and ideas, the therapist arrives at an understanding or interpretation of the nature and causes of the patient's problems. The therapist identifies deficits in performance components, performance areas, and occupational role performance. The evaluation is used for planning treatment and selecting treatment objectives and methods.

An initial evaluation is performed before treatment; reevaluation occurs periodically during the course of occupational therapy intervention.[21] The results of the initial evaluation are used to make the initial treatment plan. Reevaluation is essential to determine the effectiveness of treatment, to modify treatment to suit the patient's current needs, and to revise the evaluation. This may involve eliminating unattainable goals, modifying goals that were partially or completely achieved, and adding new goals as additional problems are identified or progress is made.

### Role of the Registered Occupational Therapist

The OTR is the planner, coordinator, and manager of evaluation, which forms the scientific foundation for the decisions in the treatment plan.[22] The OTR determines the evaluation procedures to be used and administers those evaluations or delegates their administration to another therapist or qualified occupational therapy assistant. The therapist must be knowledgeable about the dysfunction and its causes, course, and prognosis; be familiar with a variety of evaluation procedures, their uses, and proper administration; and be able to select evaluation procedures that are suitable to the patient and the dysfunction.

Evaluation provides specific information that can be communicated to other members of the rehabilitation team. In addition, researchers may use carefully collected evaluation data to develop more standardized evaluation instruments. Finally, evaluation data demonstrate the outcome of treatment and may indicate which techniques are most suitable and effective in occupational therapy practice.

### Role of the Certified Occupational Therapy Assistant

COTAs may administer evaluation procedures for which they have achieved service competency. Such evaluations are performed with the guidance and supervision of the OTR. COTAs can perform these procedures with only general supervision once they have demonstrated consistent and reliable administration techniques. When performing evaluation procedures, the assistant must approach the patient with openness and without preconceived ideas about the patient's limitations or personality. The assistant must have good observation skills and be able to enlist the trust of the patient in a short time.[25]

Occasionally, COTAs may encounter pressure to administer evaluation procedures for which they are not qualified. Administrators or other staff may even ask the COTA to conduct an entire evaluation. To do so would be inappropriate, exceeding the scope of practice and expertise of the COTA role. The COTA who encounters such pressure may take several courses of action. The first is to explain as clearly as possible the difference between the OTR and COTA roles. The COTA also must contact the OTR supervisor for guidance. If pressure continues or if the COTA is threatened with loss of a job or other penalties by the employer, the COTA should contact the local and state practice associations and the AOTA. Under no circumstance should COTAs ever attempt any procedure for which they do not have service competency.

## THE EVALUATION PROCESS

The evaluation process (Figure 5-1) begins with screening. Screening most often requires reviewing the patient's record to determine the need for further evaluation and occupational therapy intervention.[8] This is performed by the OTR. Quick tests or evaluations may be conducted to determine whether occupational therapy services are needed and the types of services required.[21] The occupational therapist may also interview the patient, make observations, and estimate time of treatment and the need to coordinate treatment with other services.[8]

After the screening the OTR selects an appropriate practice model for treatment. The selection of the practice model determines the range of evaluation procedures that might be used to yield the information needed for planning treatment. The therapist selects and administers (or directs the COTA to administer) specific tests, clinical observations, structured interviews, standardized tests, performance checklists, and activities and tasks. These are used to evaluate specific performance abilities and deficits.

The therapist gathers, interprets, and analyzes the information from the evaluation procedures.[8] The therapist then considers the individual's occupational roles and role dysfunction and generates a list of problems and assets to be used in planning occupational therapy intervention.[21] A treatment plan is developed, with the selection of treatment objectives and treatment methods. The certified occupational therapy assistant may contribute to planning treatment, particularly in the occupational performance areas. It is important that the patient be involved, to the extent possible, throughout the evaluation process.

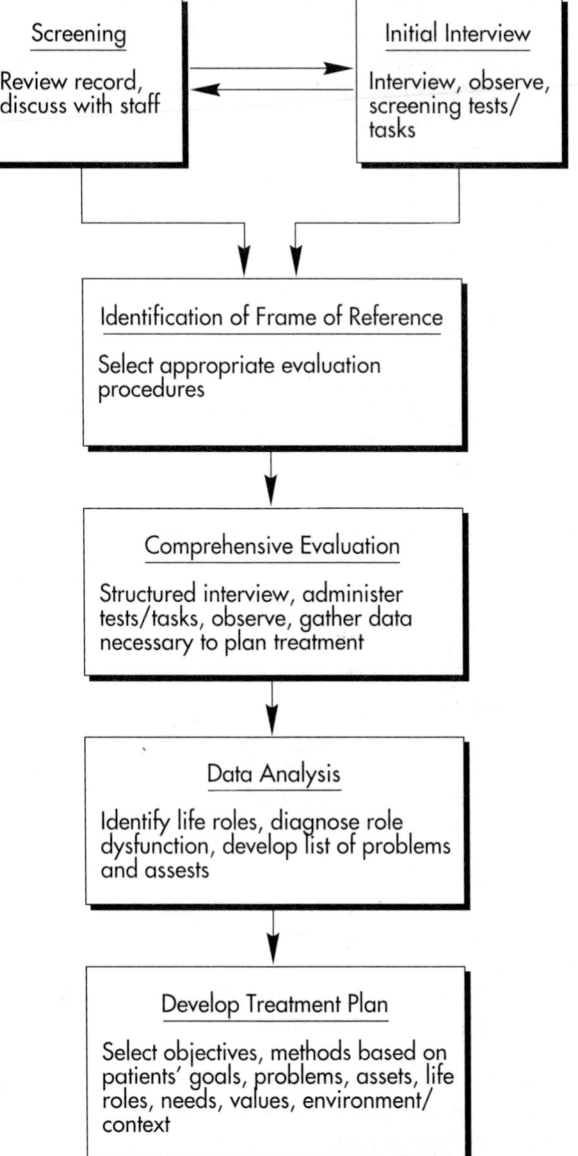


*Figure 5-1* Diagram of the evaluation process.

### Clinical Reasoning

Given the various practice models and many tests and procedures that might be used in evaluation, it may seem incredible that the therapist "knows" which ones to select and can remember and put together all the information to determine an effective analysis and treatment plan. In fact, the therapist does not "know" in a conscious and preordained way, but rather works through a series of of decisions in a process known as **clinical reasoning.** Fleming[14] defined clinical reasoning as "the many types of inquiry that an occupational therapist uses to understand patients and their difficulties." Further, she stated that it includes, but is not limited to, hypothetical reasoning and problem solving. Clinical reasoning refers to the complex processes used when the occupational therapist thinks about the patient, the disability, the circumstance, and the meaning of the disability to the patient.

Clinical reasoning has been the focus of much study in the past several years.[2,14] Clinical reasoning results in the development of professional expertise, a form of knowing that comes from doing or action. Such knowledge is difficult to articulate and in a sense is greater than the knowledge that can be expressed verbally.[19] Clinical reasoning includes the ability to express theoretical reasons for clinical decisions, but it is more than that. It embodies the tacit knowledge and habitual ways of seeing and doing things and dealing with patients that are based on expertise gained from experience. It is directed toward determining appropriate action for the particular patient at a particular time in a specific circumstance. It is not merely the response to a technical question or theoretical hypothesis. In essence, clinical reasoning is a process of deciding how to act and what to do in a specific circumstance involving the patient's well-being.[19]

Occupational therapy theory can provide a starting

place for clinical reasoning but cannot provide all the answers for the course of action in a particular case. Since each patient is unique and complex, treatment must be individualized, and this requires judgment, creativity, and improvisation. Mattingly[19] proposed that clinical reasoning in occupational therapy be primarily directed to the "human world of motives and values and beliefs—a world of human meaning," rather than to a biological world of disease. "Occupational therapists' fundamental task is treating . . . the illness experience," that is, what the disability means to the individual person.[19]

Occupational therapy practitioners teach everyday activities, such as dressing skills and toilet transfers, to increase self-care independence. In the teaching process they are confronted with the patient's experiences of profound life changes resulting from the disability—the loss of capacities taken for granted and the necessity to reorient to the world as a person with physical and functional limitations. The practitioner treats not only the physical dysfunction but also the person who has the dysfunction. The therapist and assistant must help the patient confront the limitations, "claim the disability," reclaim a changed body and functioning, and develop a new sense of self with meaning, purpose, and value. Thus the simple application of theoretical constructs to arrive at answers to questions about appropriate intervention strategies is only a part of the clinical reasoning process. Practitioners must plan treatment based on the unique meaning of the disability to the patient, not only on the physical impairments resulting from the disability.[19]

A pilot study of clinical reasoning found that registered occupational therapists in physical disabilities practice used six stages of clinical reasoning during the initial evaluation, as follows[23]:

1. Obtaining available information from the medical record, referral statement, and reports before meeting the patient
2. Selecting evaluation procedures based on medical diagnosis, prognosis, and the patient's ability to cooperate and participate in the evaluation
3. Implementing the evaluation plan by interacting with the patient and carrying out selected evaluation procedures
4. Defining problems and possible causes
5. Defining treatment objectives based on the problem list with the patient's involvement and selecting some treatment tasks and plans to carry out additional evaluation
6. Evaluating the effectiveness of the evaluation plan and the reliability of evaluation results

In this study, therapists used the medical diagnosis to select evaluation procedures, to recall standard problem lists for the diagnoses, and to select objectives and methods of treatment.[23] This reflects a medical model of clinical reasoning that focuses on the diagnosis.[15] It is a formula approach that bypasses important considerations about the patient as a person, which are critical factors in effective treatment planning and treatment outcomes.[19,23] This approach has value as an element of clinical reasoning, but it omits the complex needs, unique situation, and meaning of the disability in the patient's life—all important considerations for treatment planning. The occupational therapist may use a medical model of reasoning when considering the physical disability. However, this model is inadequate for individualizing treatment, facilitating independence, and creating a new future.[15,16]

Fleming[16] proposed that three types of reasoning are used by occupational therapists. The first is *procedural reasoning,* used to consider physical problems; an example is evaluating and analyzing the extent and possible causes of limited range of motion. *Interactive reasoning* is used to guide interactions with the patient, for example, when trying to obtain information, elicit cooperation, or develop rapport. Finally, *conditional reasoning* is used to consider patients within their personal and social context and future.[14,16] Conditional reasoning uses a "what if" approach. The therapist considers what might happen if different treatment methods, approaches, techniques, and goals were applied. Clinical reasoning is a complex, changing process for meeting the individual's unique needs for reclaiming a valued sense of self and a meaningful life.[19]

### Content of the Evaluation

The initial occupational therapy evaluation generally includes an evaluation of the patient's goals, functional abilities, and deficits in occupational performance areas.[4,6,7] Performance components may also be evaluated, with particular attention to the sensorimotor component and cognitive integration/cognitive components. Psychosocial skills and psychological components[7] are also evaluated or observed during the initial patient visits. The occupational therapist may need to plan remediation for these latter components and for the more obvious sensorimotor deficits or to refer the patient to the appropriate service for remediation, depending on the severity of the problems.

Additional information needed includes the patient's medical, educational, and work histories and family and cultural background.[6] The patient's environment (social, cultural, physical) should also be evaluated as a determinant of occupational performance. The patient's environments and person-environment relationships may harbor disabling and enabling factors that require evaluation and consideration.[6,18] A perspective of patients from their own environmental and sociocultural context should guide the therapist in selecting appropriate and meaningful treatment objectives and methods that will elicit full participation in the treatment process.

### Methods of Evaluation

#### *Review of Medical Records*

The medical record can provide information on the diagnosis, prognosis, medical history, precautions, current treatment regimen, social data, psychological data, and other rehabilitation therapies. Daily notes from nurses and physicians list current medications and the patient's reactions and responses to the facility, treatment regimen, staff, and other patients.[24] The information from the medical record serves as a good basis for selecting evaluation procedures and possibly an approach to the patient. It indicates problem areas and helps the therapist focus attention on the relevant factors of the case.[25] Ideally, the occupational therapy practitioner had the opportunity to study the medical record before seeing the patient to begin specific evaluation. This is not always possible, however, and the practitioner may have to begin the evaluation with an interview and some simple screening tests, without benefit of the medical information. Generally, COTAs should not begin evaluation without seeing the medical record. To do so without this information requires considerable experience and expertise and specific direction from supervising OTRs.

### Interview

The initial interview is a valuable step in the evaluation process. At this time the occupational therapist gathers information on how patients perceive their roles, dysfunction, needs, and goals. Simultaneously, patients can learn about the role of the occupational therapist and occupational therapy in the rehabilitation program.[25] The rapport and trust that develop between therapist and patient are important outcomes of the initial interview. In certain settings and situations (e.g., when working with occasional consultation) the COTA may be required to conduct the initial interview.

The initial interview should take place in a quiet environment that ensures privacy. The practitioner should plan the interview in advance to know what information must be obtained and to have some specific questions prepared. A specified period of time, known to interviewer and patient before the interview, should be set aside. The first few minutes of the interview may be devoted to getting acquainted and orienting the patient to the occupational therapy clinic or service and to the role and goals of occupational therapy.

The two essential characteristics of the successful interviewer are a solid knowledge base and active listening skills. These qualities require study, practice, and preparation. The clinician's knowledge will influence the selection of questions or topics to be covered in the interview. Although the COTA follows a structured format in any interview, a knowledge base is still helpful for deciding which questions to skip and which to repeat, expand, or rephrase.

The interviewer who actively listens demonstrates respect for and interest in the patients.[1] In **active listening** the receiver (interviewer) tries to understand what the sender (patient) is feeling or the meaning of the message. Interviewers then put that understanding into their own words and feed it back for verification by saying, for example, "This is what I believe you mean. . . . Have I understood you correctly?" While listening actively, the interview does not send a new message, such as an opinion, judgment, advice, or analysis. Rather, interviewers send back only what they think the patient meant.[17]

Throughout the interview the practitioner should listen to ascertain the patient's attitude toward the dysfunction. Patients should have an opportunity to express what they see as the primary problems and goals for rehabilitation. These may differ substantially from what the practitioner believes but must be given careful consideration when the occupational therapy team and patient reach the point of setting treatment objectives together. As the interview progresses, the patient should have an opportunity to ask questions as well. The occupational therapy practitioner must have good listening and observation skills to gather maximum information from the interview.

The rapport and trust that develop between the patient and the occupational therapy practitioner are based on their communication. The communication in the interview and observation phases of the evaluation are critical to all subsequent interactions and thus to the effectiveness of treatment. Patients need to sense that they have been heard and understood by someone who is empathetic and has the necessary knowledge and skills to facilitate rehabilitation. The practitioner needs to project self-confidence and confidence in the profession. This will set the tone for all future patient interaction. It will enhance the development of the patient's trust in the practitioner and in the potential effectiveness of occupational therapy.[25]

The practitioner usually needs to take notes or record the initial interview. The patient should be advised of this in advance and told how the material will be used. If requested, the patient should be allowed to view or listen to the record.[24,25]

During the initial phase of the interview, the occupational therapy practitioner should explain the role of occupational therapy, the respective roles of the therapist and the therapy assistant, the purpose of the interview, and how the information is to be used. As the interview progresses, the interviewer may seek the desired information by asking appropriate questions and guiding the responses and ensuing discussion so that relevant topics are addressed. (In general, this sort of unstructured or semistructured interview is conducted by the registered therapist; the COTA follows a structured interview protocol with specific questions to be asked.) The interview can be concluded with a summary of the major points covered, information gained, estimate of problems and assets, and plans for further occupational therapy evaluation.

The occupational therapist may want information about the patient's family and friends, community and work roles, educational and work histories, leisure and social interests and activities, and living situation. Information about how the patient spends and manages time is important. This can be determined by using a tool such as the daily schedule interview, the Activities Configuration described by Watanabe,[26] or the Activities Health Assessment described by Cynkin and Robinson.[13] All three instruments are structured and can be administered by the COTA.

*Daily schedule* The therapist or assistant should interview the patient to obtain a detailed account of his or her activities for a typical day (or week) before the onset of physical dysfunction. Information that should be elicited in the **daily schedule interview** is outlined as follows:

Rising hour
Morning activities with hours
Hygiene
Dressing
Breakfast
Work/leisure/home management
Child care
Luncheon
Afternoon activities with hours
Work/leisure/home management
Child care
Rest
Social activities
Dinner
Evening activities with hours
Leisure and social activities
Preparation for retiring
Bedtime

The amount of time spent on each activity should be recorded carefully. During the interview the occupational therapy practitioner should cue with appropriate questions so that the patient will not gloss over or omit any of the daily activities. The interviewer might ask, "What time did you get up?" "What was the first thing that you did?" "When did you eat lunch?" and "Who fixed it for you?"

The therapist or assistant helps the patient review the daily schedule as it was before the disability. The patient may share information freely, giving many recollections of social, community, vocational, and leisure activities. At times this digression from the schedule itself is desirable to elicit a well-rounded picture of the patient's roles and relationships. The patient's needs, values, and personal goals may be revealed. However, digressions that are tangential and contribute no new information should be limited or discouraged. Instead, the interviewer should focus the patient's attention on the specific daily schedule. If the patient is unable to remember or communicate the schedule, the occupational therapy practitioner should seek information from friends or family members to reconstruct the patient's activities pattern.

The practitioner then helps the patient to construct a second daily schedule of activities pattern, focusing on the present situation in the treatment facility (or at home if the patient is an outpatient or is treated at home). It is important during this interview to ask the patient who helps with each activity and how much assistance is needed and received. The practitioner and patient can discuss and compare the two schedules. This process should yield valuable information about the patient's needs, values, satisfaction/dissatisfaction with the activities pattern, primary and secondary goals for change, interests, motivation, interpersonal relationships, and fears. This information gives a basis for treatment objectives according to the patient's needs and values. Activities can be identified that are appropriate for use in the intervention plan and that will be meaningful to the patient as an individual in a particular environment and social group.

The daily schedule reveals how patients' view themselves in their occupational and life roles. The practitioner can see the patient as a functioning human rather than merely a diagnosis or disability. The patient's individual needs become the basis for treatment (rather than standard evaluation and treatment regimens established for a given disability). Knowing the patient's roles, interests, and activities is most helpful for diagnosing role dysfunction. It is valuable for determining the patient's values and establishing realistic possibilities for resuming former roles or structuring new ones.

### Observation

The skillful clinician relies heavily on observations of the patient during the interview, evaluation, and treatment. By carefully watching, looking, and seeing, the practitioner learns much about the patient's functioning under different circumstances. Consider what may be learned by observing patients as they approach or are approached. What is the posture, mode of ambulation, and gait pattern? How is the patient dressed? Is there obvious motor dysfunction? Are there apparent musculoskeletal deformities? What is the facial expression, tone of voice, and manner of speech? How are the hands held and used? Are there pain mannerisms, such as protection of an injured part or grimaces and groans?

In addition to these informal observations, which can be made during the first few minutes of the initial contact with the patient, occupational therapy practitioners use structured observation to evaluate performance of self-care, home management, mobility, and transferring. These structured observations, which may be performed by the COTA, are usually carried out by observing the patient perform real tasks in real or simulated environments. Data from these observations yield information about the patient's level of independence, speed, skill, and need for special equipment and the feasibility for further training.

### Formal Evaluation Procedures

Along with the informal evaluation procedures already discussed, occupational therapists rely on formal evaluation and assessment, including tests and measurements. The occupational therapist's interpretations, derived from the results of evaluation, can be the basis for critical decisions about the patient's treatment, school and community living placement, admission and discharge to clinical programs, and other dispositions. Therefore it is essential that the information be supported by accurate testing.[10]

Occupational therapists use both standardized and nonstandardized tests, as discussed next.

*Standardized tests* Standardized tests generally follow a strict protocol or set of administration procedures. A **standardized test** usually has been normed, or tested against a sample population, to demonstrate the normal ranges **(norms)** and abnormal ranges. This allows the score of the person being evaluated to be compared with those of a norm group.[9,10]

Standardized tests also have known reliability and validity. **Reliability** refers to the consistency of results. In other words, two different evaluators should be able to obtain very similar results on the same patient. Also, the same evaluator should be able to administer the test in the same way to each person. **Validity** is concerned with the degree to which the test measures what it is supposed to measure. For example, a test of cognitive skills should be measuring just those skills, uncontaminated by psychosocial factors or motor skill factors.

Occupational therapists have been encouraged to use standardized tests to record information obtained from patients. Because such assessments yield quantitative (numerical) results, they are useful in showing outcomes of treatment. Results of the initial evaluation and follow-up evaluations can be reported in a consistent, objective, and reliable manner.[27]

Standardized tests are considered superior to nonstandardized tests, and most clinicians apparently would prefer to use standardized tests.[2] However, relatively few standardized evaluation procedures are available in occupational therapy.[21] Many evaluation procedures in use have unknown reliability and validity. Many are informal instruments developed by occupational therapists to suit the needs of their own practice settings. Still others are adaptations of existing evaluation instruments and are used with patients other than those for whom they were designed.

Occupational therapists use many standardized tests that were designed by professionals in other disciplines.[11,28] These include tests for measuring achievement, development, intelligence, manual dexterity, motor skills, personality, sensorimotor function, and vocational skills.[9,11] Several excellent sources of information about standardized tests are available.[9,12,20,24] Current health care journals and psychological abstracts are other sources of information about standardized evaluations that may be relevant to occupational therapy.[10] Although having standardized and objective measures is desired, professional judgment and interpretation are also essential to the evaluation process.[21]

To participate in the administration of standardized tests, the occupational therapy assistant needs certain skills. The assistant should understand the theoretical reason for using the tests; be able to follow directions, administer, and score the standardized tests; and be able to communicate and document the information for the OTR to interpret. While administering a standardized test, the COTA must scrupulously follow the procedures outlined in the directions. Varying from the standard procedure will yield unreliable results. The OTR selects appropriate tests and interprets the results.[5]

*Nonstandardized tests* In contrast to a standardized test, a **nonstandardized test** is subjective and often has no specific stated instructions for administration, no criteria for scoring, and no information on interpreting results of the evaluation.[21] Nonstandardized tests are valued and continue to be used because they provide information that is subtle and not necessarily quantifiable, but very meaningful for planning treatment. The quality of the information from such a test depends on the clinical skill, experience, judgment, and bias of the evaluator.[10] Some nonstandardized evaluation procedures provide broad criteria for scoring and interpretation but still require the use of considerable subjective professional judgment.[21] The manual muscle test, described in Chapter 9, is an example of such a test.

## SUMMARY

The occupational therapy process begins with evaluation, in which information about the patient is gathered and analyzed to identify problems and assets in the patient's life and to plan appropriate treatment strategies. Evaluation of the patient with physical dysfunction includes an examination of medical records, one or more interviews, observations, and the administration of specific formal and informal evaluation procedures.

The registered occupational therapist selects appropriate evaluation procedures depending on the patient's diagnosis, medical history, lifestyle, interests, living situation, needs, values, and environment. The occupational therapy assistant contributes to the evaluation process by performing structured interviews, observations, and tests as directed by the supervising OTR.

Throughout the evaluation process, the assistant must demonstrate good observation skills and the ability to listen actively. Clinical reasoning, or the ability to "think on one's feet" while gathering data from the patient, is a skill worth developing. The assistant must learn to obtain the requested information while simultaneously establishing a comfortable relationship with the patient.

Occupational therapists have developed many informal evaluation procedures that are useful in particular treatment facilities, including tests, checklists, and rating scales. Some of these have been developed into standardized tests. The need for reliable standardized tests pertinent to occupational therapy continues, however, as occupational therapists have recognized the need to identify and employ discipline-specific evaluation procedures to help establish the scientific basis of the profession.

## Selected Reading Guide Questions

1. Define *evaluation.*
2. Differentiate *evaluation* and *assessment.*
3. Discuss the purposes of occupational therapy evaluation.
4. Describe the role of the registered occupational therapist in evaluation.
5. Describe the role of the certified occupational therapy assistant in evaluation.
6. What skills must the occupational therapist possess to be an effective evaluator?
7. List and describe the steps in the evaluation process.
8. Define and discuss *clinical reasoning.*
9. List and differentiate three types of clinical reasoning.
10. Which specific occupational performance areas and performance components are generally evaluated by the occupational therapist when treating patients with physical dysfunction?
11. Describe four methods of evaluation that the occupational therapist may use in the evaluation process.
12. Describe the daily schedule interview, including the information to be covered and the recommended ways of obtaining this information.
13. Along with diagnosis and medical data, which other important factors about the patient should be considered by the occupational therapist during the evaluation and later in treatment planning?
14. Compare standardized and nonstandardized tests. What are some advantages and disadvantages of each?
15. To administer standardized tests, the certified occupational therapy assistant should have certain skills. List at least three that are identified in this chapter.

### REFERENCES


1. Allen C: The performance status examination. Paper presented at the American Occupational Therapy Association Annual Conference, San Francisco, October 1976. Cited in Smith HD, Tiffany EG: Assessment and evaluation: an overview. In Hopkins HL, Smith HD: *Willard and Spackman's occupational therapy,* ed 6, Philadelphia, 1983, Lippincott.
2. *American Journal of Occupational Therapy:* Special issue on clinical reasoning, 45(11), 1991.
3. American Occupational Therapy Association: The Association: clarification for the use of the terms *assessment* and *evaluation, Am J Occup Ther* 49(10):1072-1073, 1995.
4. American Occupational Therapy Association: Uniform terminology for occupational therapy—third edition, *Am J Occup Ther* 48(11):1047-1054, 1994.
5. American Occupational Therapy Association: Hierarchy of competencies relating to the use of standardized instruments and evaluation techniques by occupational therapists. In *Reference manual of the official documents of the American Occupational Therapy Association,* Rockville, Md, 1989, AOTA.
6. American Occupational Therapy Association: Standards of practice for occupational therapy services for clients with physical disabilities. In *Reference manual of the official documents of the American Occupational Therapy Association, Inc,* Rockville, Md, 1986, AOTA.
7. American Occupational Therapy Association: Uniform occupational therapy evaluation checklist. In *Reference manual of the official documents of the American Occupational Therapy Association, Inc,* Rockville, Md, 1986, AOTA.
8. American Occupational Therapy Association: Uniform terminology system for reporting occupational therapy services. In *Reference manual of the official documents of the American Occupational Therapy Association, Inc,* Rockville, Md, 1986, AOTA.
9. Asher IE: *An annotated index of occupational therapy evaluation tools,* Rockville, Md, 1989, American Occupational Therapy Association.
10. Atchison B: Selecting appropriate assessments, *Phys Disabil Special Interest Sect Newslett* 10:2, 1987, AOTA.
11. Bowker A: Standardized tests utilized by therapists in the field of physical disabilities, *Phys Disabil Special Interest Sect Newslett* 6:4, 1983, AOTA.
12. Christiansen C: Occupational performance assessment. In Christiansen C, Baum C, editors: *Occupational therapy: overcoming human performance deficits,* Thorofare, NJ, 1991, Slack.
13. Cynkin S, Robinson AM: *Occupational therapy and activities health: toward health through activities,* Boston, 1990, Little, Brown.
14. Fleming MH: Aspects of clinical reasoning in occupational therapy. In Hopkins HL, Smith HD: *Willard and Spackman's occupational therapy,* ed 8, Philadelphia, 1993, Lippincott.
15. Fleming MH: Clinical reasoning in medicine compared with clinical reasoning in occupational therapy, *Am J Occup Ther* 45(11):988, 1991.
16. Fleming MH: The therapist with the three-track mind, *Am J Occup Ther* 45(11):1007, 1991.
17. Gordon T: *PET: parent effectiveness training,* New York, 1970, New American Library.
18. Letts L et al: Person-environment assessment in occupational therapy, *Am J Occup Ther* 48(7):608, 1994.
19. Mattingly C: What is clinical reasoning? *Am J Occup Ther* 45(11):979, 1991.
20. Mitchell JV, editor: *Mental measurements yearbook,* ed 11, Highland Park, NJ, 1992, Rutgers University.
21. Mosey AC: *Occupational therapy: configuration of a profession,* New York, 1981, Raven.
22. Opacich KJ: Assessment and informed decision-making. In Christiansen C, Baum C, editors: *Occupational therapy: overcoming human performance deficits,* Thorofare, NJ, 1991, Slack.
23. Rogers JC, Masagatani G: Clinical reasoning of occupational therapists during the initial assessment of physically disabled patients, *Occup Ther J Res* 4:195, 1982.
24. Smith HD: Assessment and evaluation: an overview. In Hopkins HL, Smith HD: *Willard and Spackman's occupational therapy,* ed 8, Philadelphia, 1993, Lippincott.
25. Smith HD, Tiffany EG: Assessment and evaluation: an overview. In Hopkins HL, Smith HD: *Willard and Spackman's occupational therapy,* ed 6, Philadelphia, 1983, Lippincott.
26. Watanabe S: *Activities configuration,* 1968 Regional Institute on the Evaluation Process, Final report RSA-123-T-68, New York, 1968, American Occupational Therapy Association.
27. Watson M: Analysis: standardized testing objective, *Phys Disabil Special Interest Sect Newslett* 6:4, 1983, American Occupational Therapy Association.
28. Watts JH et al: The assessment of occupational functioning: a screening tool for use in long-term care, *Am J Occup Ther* 40:231, 1986.

Chapter 6

# Occupational Therapy Treatment Planning

*Lorraine Williams Pedretti*
*Mary Beth Early*

## Chapter Objectives

*After studying this chapter, the student or practitioner will be able to:*

1. Define treatment planning and describe its process.
2. Contrast the roles of the registered occupational therapist and the certified occupational therapy assistant in treatment planning.
3. Identify and describe the elements of a comprehensive treatment objective.
4. Write clear, measurable, relevent treatment objectives.
5. Discuss the process by which treatment methods are selected.
6. Describe the steps of reevaluation, discharge planning, and termination of treatment.

## Key Terms

goals
objectives
terminal behavior
conditions
criterion
treatment method

A treatment plan is a design or proposal for a therapeutic program. Pelland described it as "the core of occupational therapy practice."[8] The treatment plan is based on the therapist's analysis of performance deficits and the unique circumstances of the individual patient. Treatment planning presents a challenge because of the complexity and variety of circumstances, goals, and problems seen in patients.

The registered occupational therapist is responsible for the treatment plan, to which the occupational therapy assistant can contribute. Treatment planning for the occupational performance areas of daily living activities, work and productive activities, and play and leisure is a particular emphasis for the COTA. Although the COTA may become more practiced, expert, and independent with experience, the final responsibility for planning treatment rests with the OTR.

To plan treatment effectively, the therapist must (1) make a thorough and careful evaluation; (2) review, analyze and summarize the data; (3) identify treatment goals and objectives; and (4) select appropriate treatment methods. The treatment plan should include ongoing reevaluation and data collection and the development of treatment priorities.[2]

The importance of having a written treatment plan cannot be overstated. Specific objectives must be outlined in an orderly and sequential manner so that these will be clear to the therapist, therapy assistant, patient, and other concerned personnel. The treatment plan helps occupational therapy practitioners know how to proceed efficiently and provides a standard for measuring the patient's progress and the plan's effectiveness. For the occupational therapy assistant, a written treatment plan is essential to provide a clear structure and sequence for treatment interventions. Without a written plan, the COTA may feel hesitant, uncertain, and unclear about what to do with the patient. The patient will sense this insecurity as reduced confidence in the occupational therapy process.

In writing the treatment plan, the therapist formally plans and analyzes the proposed course of action. Some questions considered in the planning process include the following:

1. What is the most appropriate frame of reference or practice model on which to base the treatment plan?
2. What are the patient's capabilities and assets?
3. What are the patient's limitations and deficits?
4. What does occupational therapy have to offer this patient?
5. What are the goals of treatment?
6. What are specific long-term and short-term objectives?
7. Are the treatment objectives consistent with the patient's needs and personal aspirations?
8. If objectives are not compatible, how do they need to be modified?
9. Which treatment methods are available to meet these objectives?
10. When should the patient have met the objectives?
11. What standards will be used to determine when the patient has reached an objective?
12. How will the effectiveness of the treatment plan be evaluated?
13. What is the estimated length of treatment?

The written treatment plan affirms the professionalism of occupational therapy. It documents the purposes and effectiveness of occupational therapy services and can provide a systematic method for gathering research data. Most importantly, it guides the COTA and OTR in implementing treatment.

## THE TREATMENT PLANNING PROCESS

The occupational therapy treatment planning process (Figure 6-1) requires identifying problems and finding their solutions. The goal is to promote health, well-being, and optimal functioning in persons who are ill or disabled. Treatment planning is a problem-solving process that has a logical progression.[4] The first step is evaluation and analysis and identification of problems. This is followed by exploration of prospective solutions and development of treatment objectives. From these, the therapist designs and implements a plan of action, the treatment plan. After some time the therapist assesses the outcomes of the plan and modifies it if necessary. The therapist terminates treatment when the plan has been achieved or treatment is no longer feasible.[4]

### Data Gathering

As discussed in Chapter 5, the therapist must gather data to develop an appropriate treatment plan. Sources for these data are the referral form; the medical record; social, educational, vocational, and play histories; the interview with the patient or family and friends; and the results of evaluation procedures completed by occupational therapy and other services.

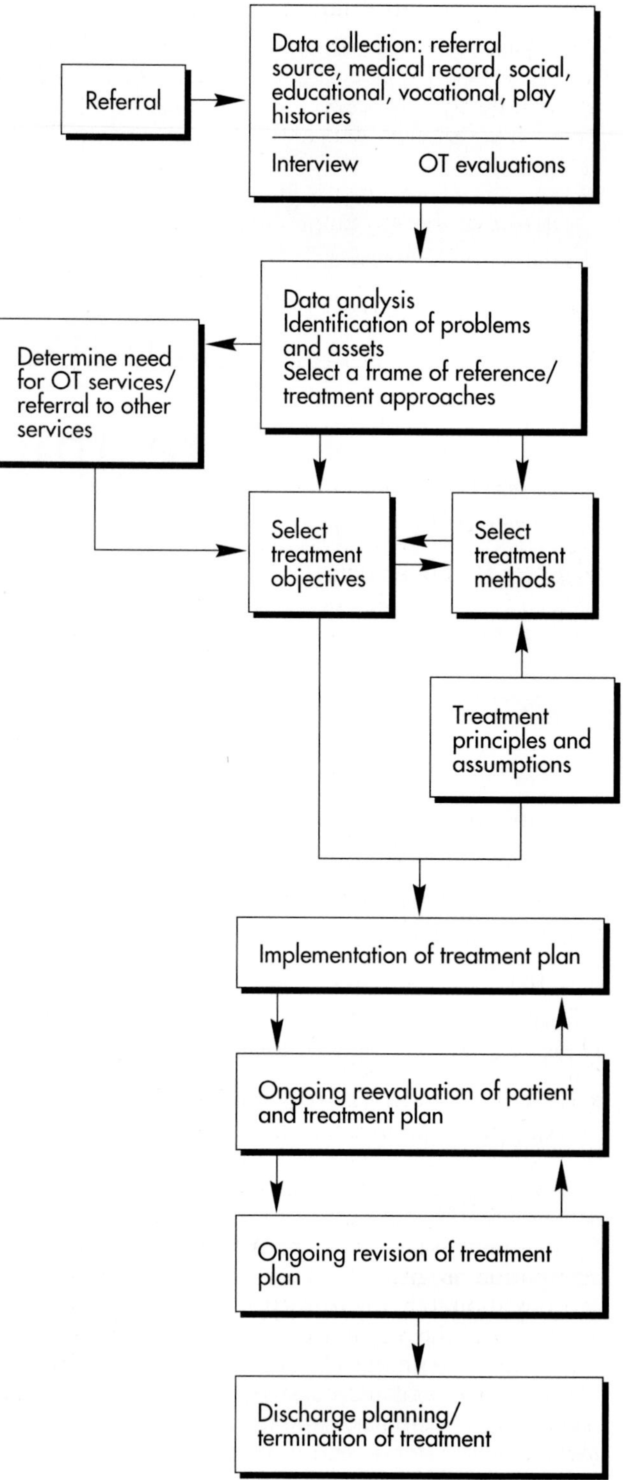


*Figure 6-1* Schematic of the treatment planning process.

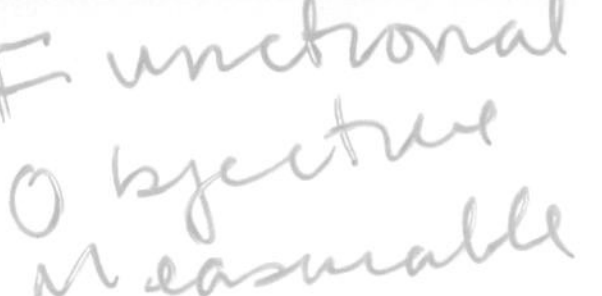



### Data Analysis and Problem Identification

Once gathered, data are analyzed to identify functions and dysfunctions. The therapist determines if occupational therapy is appropriate for the patient's problems.[9] A list of problems and assets is developed. The therapist notes deficits in the performance areas and performance components that may be amenable to occupational therapy intervention. The therapist considers how the patient's assets might enhance progress toward independence. This analysis of problems and assets becomes the basis of the treatment plan.

### Selecting a Frame of Reference or Practice Model

A treatment plan should be based on an occupational therapy frame of reference or a specific practice model. The model or frame of reference determines which evaluation procedures, objectives, and methods will be most appropriate for the patient.[8,9] The problem-solving process is influenced by the frame of reference or practice model being used. Each model has its particular philosophy, body of knowledge, and methods of evaluation and treatment, although some overlap exists. Each provides some guidelines for the clinical reasoning process in treatment planning.[4]

For example, if the therapist is treating a patient with a fractured arm resulting in limited joint motion and muscle weakness from disuse, the biomechanical practice model might be selected. Evaluation procedures in this model focus on joint range of motion measurement and muscle strength testing. Treatment might involve therapeutic exercise and activities. On the other hand, if the patient has hemiplegia, the therapist might choose the sensorimotor practice model and the neurodevelopmental (Bobath) approach and would evaluate muscle tone and postural mechanisms. Treatment would be directed toward normalizing tone through positioning, handling techniques and special movement patterns, and facilitating a more normal postural mechanism through activities that demand weight shifts and weight bearing.

The patient's motivation and goals must also be considered in planning treatment. For this reason, a frame of reference such as the model of human occupation is helpful. As explained in Chapter 3, the three practice models typically used in physical dysfunction practice neglect this important element of the treatment process. (See Chapter 3 for discussions of the model of human occupation and the biomechanical, rehabilitation, and sensorimotor practice models.)

### Selecting and Writing Treatment Goals and Objectives

The therapist writes treatment goals and objectives to address the problems identified in the occupational therapy evaluation. At the same time the therapist considers which treatment methods to use. Writing objectives and selecting treatment methods are mutually dependent elements of the treatment planning process.

Beginners may be confused by the terms *goal* and *objective*. These are explained as follows:

> **Goals** are general statements that describe global or general changes in function at some time in the future. Goals might also be viewed as long-term objectives. For example, a goal might be: *The patient will be independent in self-care.* Since self-care encompasses many activities, it is not possible to achieve this goal without many intervening objectives. Objectives therefore are more short term than are goals.
>
> **Objectives** are steps in the process of achieving goals. An example of an objective related to the goal just stated is: *The patient will transfer to and from the toilet without assistance.*

#### *Thinking about Objectives*

A treatment objective states a proposed change in the patient that will occur as a result of occupational therapy intervention. The objective should clearly convey the change in function, performance, or behavior that the patient will demonstrate when the treatment procedure or program has been successfully completed. Whenever possible, the therapist (and assistant) should involve the patient in selecting objectives and planning the treatment program. All involved must consider whether objectives are attainable within the time limits of the treatment program. Objectives should reflect the patient's needs and should be consistent with the general goals stated on the referral and determined by the evaluation. The occupational therapy objectives should complement those of other rehabilitation services.

When clearly defined objectives have *not* been stated, no sound basis exists for selecting appropriate treatment methods, and it is impossible to evaluate the effectiveness of the treatment program. It is important to state objectives clearly and in quantifiable terms if possible. Clear objectives permit the therapist to measure the degree to which the patient has achieved them.

### Writing Treatment Objectives

It is not difficult to write clear treatment objectives. However, it does require time, thoughtfulness, and thoroughness. It is helpful to have a method or structure to guide the process. One method for writing treatment objectives, described next, is based on models for writing competency-based educational objectives described by Mager[7] and Kemp.[6]

The objective should convey the patient's future functioning and performance once the objective has been achieved. It should do so in simple language and should be understandable to anyone who reads it. A comprehensive treatment objective has the following three elements (Box 6-1):

1. **Statement of terminal behavior.** Terminal behavior specifies the physical changes, type of behavior, or performance skill that the patient is expected to display.[7] The terminal behavior is

Box 6-1

## Elements of a Comprehensive Treatment Objective

**Statement of terminal behavior** Specifies the physical changes, type of behavior, or performance skill that the patient is expected to display. The terminal behavior consists of an action verb and the object being acted on. Example: The patient will *don* (action verb) a *shirt* (object).
**Conditions** States the circumstances required for the performance of the terminal behavior. Example: *Given verbal prompts* (condition), the patient will don a shirt.
**Criterion** States the degree of competence or the performance standard by which the patient's behavior is to be measured. Example: Given verbal prompts, the patient will don a shirt *in 5 minutes with no errors* (Criterion).

composed of an action verb and the object being acted on. Consider, for example, *To remove the blouse. Remove* is the action verb, and the *blouse* is the object of the action.

2. **Conditions.** These are the circumstances required for the performance of the terminal behavior. The conditions answer questions such as "Is special equipment needed?" "Are assistive devices necessary?" "Is supervision or assistance necessary?" "Are special cues necessary?"[6,7] Here is an example: "If given verbal cues, the patient will remove the blouse." This indicates that the patient will only be able to remove the blouse when someone is present to provide verbal cues. The phrase *if given verbal cues* represents a special circumstance or condition that enables adequate performance of the terminal behavior.

   Many treatment objectives are achieved by patients without any special devices, equipment, environmental modification, or human assistance. Therefore the statement of conditions is not always necessary. Conditions should be used only when some special circumstance is required to enable the performance of the terminal behavior. The treatment methodology and the treatment program's time frame are *not* considered conditions.
3. **Criterion.** The criterion is the performance standard or degree of competence the patient is expected to achieve, stated in measurable or observable terms.[6,7] The criterion answers questions such as "How much?" "How often?" "How well?" "How accurately?" "How completely?" and "How quickly?"[6] It is important to include a criterion or performance standard that estimates the patient's potential level of competence. This is the only way the therapist can determine achievement of the stated terminal behavior with certainty. As with conditions, the criterion is an optional element in the treatment objective.

   Here is an objective that contains a criterion: "If given verbal cues, the patient will remove the blouse within 1 minute." The criterion or performance standard indicates that the task will be completed *within 1 minute.* This might be a necessary criterion in a long-term care facility in which an aide supervises the patient's dressing; speed of performance is important so that the aide can attend to other tasks and patients.

   Although stating a performance standard is desired, it is not always necessary or possible. For example, in the objective *With minimal assistance the patient will transfer to the toilet,* a performance standard is not necessary, since the accomplishment of the transfer is evidence of achievement of the desired skill. In this example, *with minimal assistance* is the condition.

   Muscle grades, increases in range of joint motion, degree of competence in task performance, and speed of performance are possible measures for criteria. Although it is sometimes necessary to state the length of the treatment program in an objective to satisfy requirements of insurers, length of treatment is *not* a criterion.

### Critiquing Sample Objectives

Studying sample objectives and analyzing their elements can help the beginner refine skills in writing clear objectives. Consider the following examples:

1. *Given assistive devices, the patient will eat independently in 30 minutes.* In this objective the terminal behavior is the statement *the patient will eat,* and *eat* is the action verb. No object needs to be named, since the object (food) of the action is implicit. The condition is *given assistive devices.* This statement indicates the special circumstances, in this case devices, that will make eating possible. The performance standards are *independently in 30 minutes.* This statement reflects that the patient will be able to eat without human assistance and will complete eating a meal within 30 minutes, a reasonable amount of time for this activity.
2. *The joint range of motion (ROM) of the left elbow will increase.* As written, this objective is a good statement of terminal behavior. It indicates the type of change in physical function that is expected as a result of the treatment program. Conditions are not necessary, since no special circumstances are needed for the patient to demonstrate or perform the increased ROM. However, the objective does need a criterion because the amount of increase in ROM is not indicated, making it difficult to measure progress. The objective can be improved as follows: *The joint ROM of the left elbow will increase from 0-120 to 0-135 degrees.* This adds the criterion of a 15-degree increase in ROM, which is measurable.
3. *The patient will operate the control systems of the left*

*above-elbow prosthesis without hesitation.* In this objective, *operate the control systems* is the terminal behavior. *Operate* is the action verb, and *control systems* is the object of the action. This is the skill (behavior) that is expected as a result of the prosthetic training program. Conditions are not necessary, since the desired goal is for the patient to be able to perform this skill under any circumstances. *Without hesitation* is the criterion. It is an observable level of skill indicative of automaticity of performance.

4. *Given assistive devices, the patient will dress herself in less than 20 minutes. Dress* is the action verb that indicates the terminal behavior. The indirect object of the action (herself) is stated; the direct object (in clothes) does not need to be stated because it is implied in the action verb. The availability of assistive devices is a necessary condition for this patient to perform this task; thus the statement of conditions, *given assistive devices,* is needed. The criterion or performance standard is stated in terms of speed and indicates that dressing within 20 minutes is a reasonable expectation for this patient and for this task. Other standards could be added if formal neatness or appropriateness for a given occasion were important for the patient's life roles.
5. *Given equipment setup and assistive devices, the patient will use mobile arm supports to feed himself independently.* The equipment setup and the availability of assistive devices constitute the conditions for this objective. The criterion for performance under these circumstances is *independently,* which indicates that once the equipment and devices are provided, the task of eating can be performed without further human assistance.

Many variables and unknown factors exist in the performance and functions of persons with physical dysfunction. Therefore the degree to which they can benefit from, participate in, or succeed at rehabilitation programs cannot be predicted with certainty. This often makes it difficult for occupational therapy practitioners to write comprehensive treatment objectives. However, the therapist and assistant should attempt to write such objectives, using past experience with similar patients and knowledge gained during the evaluation process to describe desired terminal behavior, conditions, and criteria for each treatment objective. If the conditions and criteria cannot be predicted, practitioners should use a specific statement of terminal behavior until applicable conditions and criteria become apparent. The stated terminal behaviors can then be modified, as treatment progresses, to become comprehensive objectives.

### Selecting Treatment Methods

Once the objectives have been selected, the treatment method to help the patient achieve them are chosen. This is probably one of the most difficult steps in the treatment planning process. Therapists should select a **treatment method** based on a principle or theory related to the problem being treated and its cause. This underlying principle may come from a frame of reference or a practice model.[3] For example, nerves regenerate after peripheral nerve injury and repair. Use of reinnervated muscles helps to maintain or increase their tone and strength. Improvement of function through use is a principle of the biomechanical model. This principle guides the therapist to select graded therapeutic activity or exercise as the method of choice to effect the desired goals.

Many other factors influence the selection of treatment methods. Some of those that should be considered include the following:

1. What is the goal for the patient?
2. What are the precautions or contraindications that affect the occupational therapy program?
3. What is the prognosis for recovery?
4. What were the results of evaluations in occupational therapy and other services?
5. What other treatment is the patient receiving?
6. What are the goals of other treatment programs, and are the occupational therapy goals compatible with these?
7. How much energy does the patient expend in other therapies?
8. What is the state of the patient's general health?
9. What are the patient's interests, vocational skills, and psychological needs?
10. What is the patient's physical and sociocultural environment?
11. What roles will the patient assume in the community?
12. What kinds of activities or exercises will be most useful and meaningful to the patient?[5]
13. How can treatment be graded to meet the patient's changing needs as progression or regression occurs?
14. What special equipment or adaptations of therapeutic equipment are needed for the patient to perform maximally?

When treatment methods are selected, others reading the treatment plan should understand exactly how the methods will be used to reach specific objectives. Sometimes several methods may be needed to achieve one objective, or the same methods may be used to reach several objectives.

### Implementing the Treatment Plan

The treatment plan can be implemented once at least one objective and one or more treatment methods have been selected. During implementation the therapist and assistant guide the patient as he or she engages in the procedures that have been designed. The comprehensive treatment plan may evolve over time. For example, while a lengthy evaluation procedure is in progress, such as activities of daily living (ADLs), the patient may begin a program of therapeutic activity to strengthen specific muscle groups. Therefore, as the evaluation is being completed, an increasing number of problems may be identified, and additional objectives and methods may be added to the treatment plan. Thus the occupational therapy assistant should not be surprised by continual changes in the treatment plan.

### Reevaluating the Patient and Initial Treatment Plan

Once the treatment plan is implemented, its effectiveness is evaluated on an ongoing basis through continuous observation and reevaluation. The therapist and assistant must be alert observers and ask the following:

1. Are the objectives suitable to the patient's needs and capabilities?
2. Are the methods most appropriate for fulfilling the treatment objectives?
3. Does the patient relate to the treatment methods and see them as worthwhile and meaningful?
4. Are the treatment objectives realistic, and are they consistent with the patient's personal objectives?

The therapist may choose to reevaluate physical functions and performance skills with the same evaluation procedures used in the initial evaluation. Gains or losses may then be compared with baseline functions recorded at the outset. Such comparisons validate the treatment plan and provide the objective evidence of change required for reimbursement. Scrutinizing the treatment plan in this way enables the therapist to modify the plan as the need arises. The patient's progress toward the stated objectives is the criterion for determining the plan's effectiveness.

### Revising the Treatment Plan

The therapist may recognize a need to revise or modify the initial treatment plan, based on information gained from observations and reevaluation of the patient, as just outlined. For example, the patient's progress may be significant enough that it is beneficial to increase the duration, complexity, or resistance of the activity. Conversely, the gradual decline of physical resources may necessitate a decrease in resistance, duration, and complexity of activity. This situation applies in degenerative diseases, in which a primary objective is to maintain optimal function despite declining strength and coordination.

If the patient is unable to see the therapeutic program as helpful or meaningful, a change in treatment approaches and methods may be necessary. On the other hand, if the patient is highly motivated, the plan can be accelerated. The initial plan is continually revised according to the patient's needs and progress. This process of reevaluation, revision, and reimplementation of the treatment plan continues throughout the course of the therapeutic program.[8,9]

### Discharge Planning and Terminating Treatment

Ultimately, the whole treatment program is directed to preparing the patient to return home or to another suitable living arrangement. As discussed in Chapter 5, discharge planning is actually a continual process that occurs throughout the treatment program. It may be considered as early as the first meeting with the patient. All treatment is directed to preparing the patient to return to the community. Therapy often will continue on a less intensive basis at home or in another living environment.

#### *Discharge Planning*

Discharge planning should be initiated as the treatment program in the primary health care facility is progressing. Discharge planning is a team effort that involves the patient, the family, and all the rehabilitation specialists concerned with the patient's care. Preparation for discharge includes discussing medical considerations, providing assistive devices and mobility equipment, planning a home activity or exercise program, and making a home visit to assess architectural barriers in the environment. Discharge planning should include education and training of patient and caregivers for a smooth transition. Arrangements for home care therapies and referral to appropriate community agencies are also important.[10]

The patient and family must be prepared psychologically for discharge. Therapy staff should not assume that patients are emotionally prepared for (or functionally capable of) managing the transition to the new environment. Generalization (transfer) of learning from the health care facility to the home may be difficult for the patient. The family may not know the patient's capabilities or how best to give assistance. Emotional support, education, training, counseling, and information about resources are helpful measures in easing the transition. The family needs information about the patient's ADL status and performance expectations; solutions to accessibility problems in the home, workplace, and community; information on home modification; how to obtain, use, and care for assistive devices or mobility equipment; and availability of community resources such as emergency care, self-help groups, respite care, and independent living centers.[11] Maintaining contact with the primary care facility as a resource for information or further treatment can be reassuring and helpful.[1]

### *Termination of Treatment*

Termination of treatment requires a final evaluation of the patient. The clinician should clearly indicate objectives achieved, partially achieved, or not achieved in the treatment program. The assistant may be directed to perform parts of this evaluation. The therapist writes a discharge summary on the basis of these data. The summary should indicate expected future performance of the patient. Termination can affirm the success of the treatment program. In reality, however, termination is not always achieved, since patients may be discharged before objectives of treatment are met and treatment is concluded.[4] The patient may be referred to another facility or to home care, with another therapist continuing the treatment program. Careful communication between therapists and agencies is necessary to ensure a smooth transition and continuity of care.

## A TREATMENT PLAN MODEL

The treatment plan model is useful for learning treatment planning during academic preparation, and it may be modified for clinical use. Figure 6-2 shows one such model. The areas of the treatment plan that might be completed by the COTA are indicated in boldface. A more extensive *treatment planning guide* similar to one that would be completed by an OTR is shown in Figure 6-3.

An example of a sample treatment plan is also shown on the following pages. Only a portion of the treatment plan is shown. The occupational therapy assistant student should focus on the occupational performance areas in evaluation and treatment planning. Other areas can be added as service competency increases.

**Case #**
**Personal Data**
- **Name**
- **Age**
- **Diagnosis**
- **Disability**
- **Treatment goals stated in the referral**

Other Services
Frame of Reference/Practice Model
**O.T. Evaluation**
- Performance components
  1. sensorimotor
  2. cognitive integration and cognitive
  3. psychosocial skills and psychological
- **Performance areas**
  1. **activities of daily living**
  2. **work and productive activities**
  3. **play or leisure activities**

Evaluation Summary
Assets
Problem list
**Outline treatment plan (COTA focuses on performance areas)**
1. **Problem**
2. **Objective**
3. **Methods**
4. **Grading**

*Figure 6-2* Treatment plan model. Sections appropriate for the entry-level COTA are shown in **boldface.**

## TREATMENT PLANNING GUIDE

### PERSONAL DATA

Fill in the requested information from the medical record or case study.

- Name
- Age
- Diagnosis
- Disability
- Treatment aims stated in the referral

### OTHER SERVICES

List and describe briefly other services the patient is using.

- Physician
- Nursing
- Respiratory therapy
- Social service
- Speech pathology
- Physical therapy
- Vocational counseling
- Psychology/psychiatry
- Educational services
- Spiritual counseling
- Community social groups/day care
- Home health care services
- Sheltered employment

### FRAME OF REFERENCE/ TREATMENT APPROACH

State the frame of reference and treatment approach on which the treatment plan is based. More than one may be necessary.

### OT EVALUATION

From the list below, select the performance components and performance areas that should be evaluated. Indicate whether evaluation will be determined by testing or by observation.

**Performance components**

Sensorimotor

- Muscle strength
- ROM
- Physical endurance
- Standing tolerance
- Walking tolerance
- Sitting balance
- Involuntary movement
- Movement speed
- Level of motor development
- Equilibrium/protective responses
- Coordination/muscle control
- Spasms
- Spasticity
- Stage of motor recovery (stroke patient only)
- Postural reflex mechanism
- Functional movement patterns
- Hand function
- Swallowing/cranial nerve functions
- Sensation—touch, pain, temperature, proprioception, taste, smell
- Body schema
- Motor planning
- Stereognosis
- Visual perception
    - Visual fields
    - Spatial relations
    - Position in space
    - Figure/background
    - Perceptual constancy
    - Visual-motor coordination
    - Depth perception
    - Perception of vertical/horizontal elements
    - Eye movements
- Functional auditory perception

Cognitive/cognitive integration

- Memory
- Judgment
- Safety awareness
- Problem-solving ability
- Motivation
- Sequencing
- Rigidity

*Figure 6-3* Treatment planning guide.

## TREATMENT PLANNING GUIDE

- Abstract thinking
- Functional language skills
  - Comprehension of speech/writing
  - Ability to express ideas
  - Reading
  - Writing
- Functional mathematical skills
  - Mental calculations
  - Written calculations

Psychosocial/psychological skills
- Self-identity
- Self-concept
- Coping skills
- Maturity (developmental level)
- Adjustment to disability
- Reality functioning
- Interpersonal skills—dyadic and group interactions

**Performance areas**

Self-care
- Feeding
- Dressing
- Hygiene
- Transferring
- Community mobility

Work and productive activities
- Work habits and attitudes
- Potential work skills
- Work tolerance
- Home management
- Child care

Play/leisure
- Past and present leisure interests/play activities
- Modes of relaxation

### EVALUATION SUMMARY
Summarize findings from tests and observations.

### ASSETS
List the assets of the patient and his or her situation that can be used to enhance progress toward maximum independence.

### PROBLEM LIST
Identify and list the problems that require occupational therapy intervention.

### OBJECTIVES
Write specific treatment objectives in comprehensive form. Each should relate to a specific problem in the problem list and be identified by the corresponding number.

### METHODS OF TREATMENT
Describe in detail appropriate treatment methods for the patient.

### GRADATION OF TREATMENT
Briefly state how treatment methods will be graded to enhance the patient's progress.

*Figure 6-3, cont'd.* Treatment planning guide.

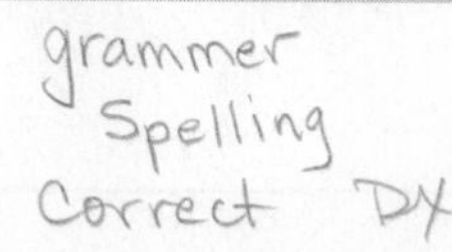

# Sample Treatment Plan

The following treatment plan is not a comprehensive plan for the hypothetical patient. Rather, it presents a sampling of parts of a proposed treatment program. The reader is encouraged to add objectives and methods to address additional problems and make the plan a more comprehensive one.

### Case study

Mrs. R. is 49 years old. She has two sons; one is age 26 and married, and the other is age 17. Mrs. R. is divorced. She and her younger son live with her married son, his wife, and their 4-year-old boy. Before the onset of her illness, Mrs. R. lived in an apartment with her younger son.

Mrs. R. had Guillain-Barré syndrome. She has been left with residual weakness of all four extremities. Mrs. R. uses a standard wheelchair for mobility.

Mrs. R. appears thin and frail. She speaks in a weak voice and appears to be passive and discouraged. She feels she cannot accomplish anything. The home situation is poor. Mrs. R. does not communicate with her daughter-in-law, and there are conflicts between the couple and Mrs. R. concerning the management of the teenage son. Mrs. R. feels unable to assert her authority as his mother or to express her needs and feelings. The disability has brought about the loss of her independence and has changed her role in relation to her younger son.

Her daughter-in-law reported that Mrs. R. is dependent for self-care, never attempts to help with homemaking, and isolates herself in her room much of the time. She believes that her mother-in-law is capable of more activity "if only she would try." She says she is willing to allow Mrs. R. to do some of the household work.

Mrs. R. was referred for occupational therapy services as an outpatient for restoration or maintenance of motor functioning and increased independence in ADL.

### Treatment plan

*Personal data*

Name: Mrs. R.
Age: 49
Diagnosis: Guillain-Barré syndrome
Disability: Residual weakness, upper and lower extremities
Treatment aims stated in referral: Restoration or maintenance of motor functioning; increased independence in ADL

### Other services

Physician: prescription of medication, maintenance of general health, supervision of rehabilitation program
Physical therapy: muscle strengthening, ambulation and transfer training
Social service: individual and family counseling
Community social group: socialization

### Frame of reference

Model of human occupation

### Treatment approaches

Biomechanical and rehabilitative

### OT evaluation

*Performance components*

Sensorimotor
- Muscle strength: test
- Passive ROM: test
- Physical endurance: observe, interview
- Walking tolerance: observe, interview
- Movement speed: observe
- Coordination: test, observe
- Functional movement: test, observe
- Sensation (touch, pain, thermal, proprioception): test

Cognitive/cognitive integration
- Judgment: observe
- Safety awareness: observe
- Motivation: observe, interview

Psychosocial/psychological skills
- Coping skills: observe
- Adjustment to disability: observe, interview
- Social skills
- Interpersonal relationships: observe

*Performance areas*

Self care: observe, interview
Home management: observe, interview

### Evaluation summary

Muscle testing revealed that all muscles are the same grades bilaterally: scapula and shoulder muscles are F + to G (3+ to 4), elbow and forearm muscles are F + to G (3+ to 4), and wrist and hand musculature is graded F+ (3 +). Trunk muscles are G (4); all muscles of the hip are G (4) except adductors and external rotators, which are F + (3 +). Knee flexors and extensors are G (4). Ankle plantar flexors and dorsiflexors are F (3), and all foot muscles are F – (3 –) to P (2).

All joint motions within normal to functional range. Physical endurance limited to 1 hour of light activity of upper extremities, with some ambulation, before rest. Mrs. R. uses a wheelchair for energy conservation and propels it using both arms and legs. Slight incoordination, evident on fine hand function, caused by muscle weakness.

Sensory modalities of touch, pain, temperature, and proprioception are intact. No cognitive deficits were observed. Mrs. R. is passive and discouraged about her disability. She feels she cannot accomplish anything and tends to stay in her room alone.

Before onset of illness, Mrs. R. lived independently with her 17-year-old son. Since her illness, she and her son have moved in with her 26-year-old son, his wife, and their 4-year-old son. This arrangement has proved less than ideal. There is little communication between Mrs. R. and her daughter-in-law. There are conflicts between the couple and Mrs. R. about the management of her teenage son.

## Sample Treatment Plan—cont'd

**Evaluation summary—cont'd**

The disability has brought about the loss of Mrs. R.'s independence and has changed her roles as homemaker and mother. She feels unable to assert her authority as mother of her 17-year-old or to express her needs and feelings.

Mrs. R. manages some personal care such as facewashing and hair and teeth care. She needs some assistance with dressing and has difficulty with buttons and zippers. She requires an adaptive toothbrush and needs assistance in toilet transferring and showering. Mrs. R. does not perform any home management tasks but is potentially capable of light activities such as table setting, dusting, and folding clothes. Mrs. R.'s daughter-in-law is willing to allow her mother-in-law some household activities if understanding about their respective roles can be established.

**Assets**

Some functional muscle strength
Good joint mobility
Potential for good living situation
Presence of able-bodied adults who can assist
Potential for some further recovery
Good sensation

**Problem list**

1. Muscle weakness
2. Low physical endurance
3. Limited walking tolerance
4. Mild incoordination
5. Self-care dependence
6. Homemaking dependence
7. Dependent transferring
8. Isolation, apparent depression
9. Reduced social interaction
10. Lack of assertiveness

**Problem 1**

Muscle weakness

*Objective*

Muscle strength of shoulder flexors will increase from F+ (3+) to G (4).

*Method*

Light progressive resistive exercise to shoulder flexion: patient is seated in a regular chair, wearing a weighted cuff one half the weight of her maximum resistance above each elbow. Lifts arms alternately through 10 repetitions and then rests. Repeated using three quarters maximum resistance, then full resistance. Activities: reaching for glasses in overhead cupboard and placing them on the table, replacing glasses in cupboard when dry; rolling out pastry dough on a slightly inclined pastry board; wiping table, counter, and cupboard doors, using a forward push-pull motion; Turkish knotting project with weaving frame set vertically in front of her and tufts of yarn on right and left sides, at hip level.

*Gradation*

Increase resistance, number of repetitions, and length of time as strength improves.

**Problem 1**

Muscle weakness

*Objective*

Strength of wrist flexors and extensors and finger flexors will increase from F+ (3+) to G (4).

*Method*

Light progressive resistive exercises for wrist flexors and extensors: patient is seated, side to table, with pronated forearm resting on the table and hand extended over edge of table; a hand cuff, with small weights equal to one half of her maximum resistance attached to the palmar surface, is worn on the hand; patient extends the wrist through full range of motion against gravity for 10 repetitions, then rests. Exercise is repeated, using three quarters maximum resistance and then full resistance. The same procedure is used to exercise wrist flexors, except that the forearm is supinated on the table, and the weights are suspended from the dorsal side of the hand cuff. Activities to improve finger flexors: tearing lettuce to make a salad; handwashing panties and hosiery. Progress to kneading soft clay or bread dough.

*Gradation*

Increase resistance, repetitions, and time.

**Problem 5**

Self-care dependence

*Objective*

Given assistive devices, Mrs. R. will be able to dress herself independently within 20 minutes.

*Method*

Putting on bra: using a back-opening stretch bra, pass bra around waist so that opening is in front and straps are facing up; fasten bra in front at waist level; slide fastened bra around at waist level so that cups are in front; slip arms through straps and work straps up over shoulders; adjust cups and straps. Putting on shirt: place loose-fitting blouse on lap with back facing up and neck toward knees; place arms under back of blouse and into arm holes; push sleeves up onto arms past elbows; gather back material up from neck to hem with hands and duck head forward and pass garment over head; work blouse down by shrugging shoulders and pulling into place with hands; use button hook to fasten front opening. Putting on underpants and slacks: sitting on bed or in wheelchair, cross legs, reach down, and place one opening over foot; cross opposite leg, place other opening over foot; uncross legs, work pants up over feet and up under thighs (a dressing stick may be used to pull pants up if leaning forward is difficult); shift hips from side to side and work pants up as far as possible over buttocks; stand, if possible, and pull pants to waist level, then sit and pull zipper up with prefastened zipper pull; use Velcro at waist closure on slacks. Putting on socks: using stretch socks and seated, cross one leg, place sock over toes and work sock up onto foot and over heel; cross other leg and repeat. Putting on shoes: using slip-on shoe with Velcro fasteners, use procedure for socks.

*Continued.*

## Sample Treatment Plan—cont'd

**Problem 5—cont'd**

*Gradation*

Progress to more difficult tasks such as pantyhose, tie shoes, dresses, pullover garments.

**Problem 6**

Homemaking dependence

*Objective*

Given assistive devices, Mrs. R. will perform homemaking activities.

*Methods*

Using a dust mitt, patient dusts furniture surfaces easily reached from wheelchair such as lamp tables and coffee table; sits at sink to wash dishes; practices folding small items of clothing such as panties, nylons, children's underwear, while sitting at kitchen table; have Mrs. R.'s daughter-in-law observe activities at treatment facility; work out an acceptable list of activities and a schedule with both women. Discuss how Mrs. R. could make some contributions to home management routines; ask Mrs. R. to keep activity diary, noting any performance difficulties and successes for review at next visit.

*Gradation*

Increase number of household responsibilities. Increase time spent on household activities.

**Problem 8**

Isolation, depression

*Objective*

Mrs. R. will reduce time spent alone from 6 waking hours to 3 waking hours.

*Method*

Establish acceptable graded activity schedule between Mrs. R. and son and daughter-in-law; include homemaking tasks and socialization with family through playing games, watching TV, preparing and eating meals, and conversing; family members encourage Mrs. R. to be with them but to be accepting if she refuses; have Mrs. R. keep activities diary for review; determine how time is spent and discuss how it could be more productive and enjoyable. Initiate avocational activity, such as needlework or tile mosaics, to complete at home; set goals for where and how much activity will be performed.

*Gradation*

Increase time spent out of own room; include friends, neighbors, family, in household social activities; plan a community outing for shopping or lunch.

## SUMMARY

Treatment planning involves the identification of goals, objectives, and methods. These are directed toward resolving the problems noted in the evaluation stage. The registered occupational therapist is responsible for the treatment plan, to which the certified occupational therapy assistant can contribute significantly, especially in the occupational performance areas. Treatment plans should be written so that staff members have a clear procedure to follow and effectiveness can be measured.

The patient's motivation cannot be underestimated as a factor in treatment success. Treatment goals should coincide with the patient's own goals. Goals are broad descriptive statements of how the patient might function at some future time (e.g., "The patient will be independent in activities of daily living"). Goals may be broken down into component objectives, each of which is a step toward the ultimate goal (e.g., "The patient will transfer from the wheelchair to the toilet without assistance"). A comprehensive treatment goal contains a terminal behavior, a statement of conditions, and a criterion (or set of criteria) for measuring accomplishment. Methods are chosen based on the objectives, the practice model or frame of reference, the patient's values and motivations, and the performance context.

The certified occupational therapy assistant is encouraged to study and practice writing clear and comprehensive treatment objectives. Such study will yield great rewards: clinical clarity, effective communication, and professional self-confidence.

## Selected Reading Guide Questions

1. Define *treatment plan.*
2. Describe the roles of the OTR and the COTA in treatment planning.
3. Why should a treatment plan be written down?
4. Why should a treatment plan be based on a specific frame of reference or treatment approach?
5. List the steps in developing a treatment plan.
6. List, define, and give examples of the three elements of a comprehensive treatment objective.
7. If a comprehensive objective cannot be written, which one element would be *most* important to identify first?
8. List six factors to consider when selecting treatment methods.
9. Is it necessary to develop a comprehensive treatment plan before treatment can begin? Explain.
10. Is it ever necessary to change the initial treatment plan? Why?
11. What criterion is used to evaluate the effectiveness of a treatment plan?
12. How does the therapist know when to modify or change the plan?
13. What are some of the concerns and preparations involved in termination of treatment?

## REFERENCES


1. Baum C: Identification and use of environmental resources. In Christiansen C, Baum C: *Occupational therapy: overcoming human performance deficits,* Thorofare, NJ, 1991, Slack.
2. Christiansen C: Occupational therapy: intervention for life performance. In Christiansen C, Baum C: *Occupational therapy: overcoming human performance deficits,* Thorofare, NJ, 1991, Slack.
3. Day D: A systems diagram for teaching treatment planning, *Am J Occup Ther* 27:239, 1973.
4. Hopkins HL: Problem solving. In Hopkins HL, Smith HD: *Willard and Spackman's occupational therapy,* ed 8, Philadelphia, 1993, Lippincott.
5. Hopkins HL et al: Therapeutic application of activity. In Hopkins HL, Smith HD: *Willard and Spackman's occupational therapy,* ed 6, Philadelphia, 1983, Lippincott.
6. Kemp JE: *The instructional design process,* New York, 1985, Harper & Row.
7. Mager RF: *Preparing instructional objectives,* ed 2, (revised), Belmont, Calif, 1984, Lake.
8. Pelland MJ: A conceptual model for the instruction and supervision of treatment planning, *Am J Occup Ther* 41:351, 1987.
9. Smith HD: Assessment and evaluation: an overview. In Hopkins HL, Smith HD, editors: *Willard and Spackman's occupational therapy,* ed 8, Philadelphia, 1993, Lippincott.
10. Spencer EA: Functional restoration: preliminary concepts and planning. In Hopkins HL, Smith HD, editors: *Willard and Spackman's occupational therapy,* ed 8, Philadelphia, 1993, Lippincott.
11. Versluys HP: Family influences. In Hopkins HL, Smith HD: *Willard and Spackman's occupational therapy,* ed 8, Philadelphia, 1993, Lippincott.

Chapter 7

# Documentation of Occupational Therapy Services

*Janet Jabri*
*Janna M. Dreher*

## Chapter Objectives

*After studying this chapter, the student or practitioner will be able to:*

1. Describe the purposes of documentation for occupational therapy services.
2. Describe the legal implications for complete and accurate documentation.
3. List fundamental elements of documentation.
4. Differentiate COTA and OTR documentation responsibilities.
5. Describe various types of records and reports.
6. List the sequential steps in the clinical reasoning process for documentation.
7. Describe the reporting process, including initial evaluation reports, treatment plans, progress reports, and discharge summaries.

## Key Terms

problem-oriented medical record
SOAP note
*Uniform Terminology*
classification codes
clinical reasoning
referral
treatment plan
critical pathway
behavioral objective
functional outcome
RUMBA
initial evaluation report
progress notes
discharge summary

Documenting patient care is essential to occupational therapy. Although most practitioners choose this profession in order to work with people and assist in improving their quality of life, the documentation of treatment justifies the therapy. The certified occupational therapy assistant (COTA) plays a valuable role in the documentation process.

Documentation of occupational therapy services refers to the written record of all information relevant to the patient from admission to discharge. The documentation process begins immediately on receipt of the initial referral. The written record should include confirmation of the referral, initial evaluation results, and ongoing daily and/or weekly progress notes. These notes include treatment goals, methods and modalities used, response to treatment, and functional outcomes.[13] Any periodic reevaluation reports and a discharge summary are also included. The complete medical record contains pertinent information about the patient's history, status, progress, and performance, as described by all health care practitioners involved in the patient's care.

No standard or single method exists for documenting occupational therapy services within the profession. The types of records and reports to be written may be determined by the individual treatment facility and the funding agencies. All entries should be clear, concise, objective, accurate, complete, and timely, regardless of the method used. Since the documentation is part of a legal record, omissions or errors in the record may raise doubts about the accuracy of the entire record.[7]

## PURPOSES OF DOCUMENTATION

The purposes of documentation are as follows:[16]

1. Provide a sequential and legal record of the patient's status and the course of treatment.
2. Provide information about the patient's care.
3. Facilitate communication among health care practitioners involved in the patient's care.
4. Reflect the practitioner's reasoning.
5. Justify the need for continuing treatment.
6. Provide data for use in treatment, reimbursement, education, and research.

## DOCUMENTATION AND ETHICS

Occupational therapy practitioners are required to examine the quality of their practice and the documentation of that practice through the American Occupational Therapy Association's (AOTA's) Code of Ethics.[12] Unethical, incompetent, or fraudulent documentation places the COTA at risk for legal repercussions and jeopardizes the credibility of the entire profession. Conversely, competent documentation effectively communicates a patient's response to therapy and also educates other health care providers and fiscal intermediaries about the value of occupational therapy. Recently, financial constraints have motivated reimbursement intermediaries to scrutinize the need for occupational therapy services. To pass scrutiny, OT practitioners must provide a clear rationale for service through competent, ethical, and truthful documentation.

## LEGAL ASPECTS OF DOCUMENTATION

Numerous state and federal laws govern documentation, including Medicare, Medicaid, licensure laws, privacy acts, and state laws governing medical records.[15] Practitioners must know the laws that affect their practice and must meet the requirements of these laws in their documentation.

Health records may be used in litigation to settle insurance claims and may be examined by third-party payers, fiscal intermediaries, and other utilization review boards.[15,17] The review of the records is governed by principles of ethical practice in relation to confidentiality, and the records are under strict control of the physician or health care agency. No privileged information, verbal or written, can be released without the patient's written consent. [7] In addition, the patient has the right to know what is in the record and can ask for this information. The physician is responsible to provide the information in the appropriate manner.

Because documentation is part of the legal record and may be used in court, the services documented by the occupational therapy practitioner must accurately reflect the treatment given. The legal written record is the only acceptable proof of the treatment intervention. A standard phrase among outside reviewers, whether a third-party payer or a jury, is, "If it was not written, it did not happen." Therefore, completeness and accuracy of the record are essential.

Some documentation guidelines that may be used to ensure meeting the therapist's legal and ethical obligations include the following[15]:

1. Date all entries for accurate sequencing of the treatment.
2. Document missed treatments.
3. Document at the time of treatment so that the entry will completely and accurately reflect the treatment session.
4. Document using specific facts rather than general terms.
5. Do not criticize another health care provider in the written record.
6. Do not change a legal record after the fact without clarifying the time and nature of the change.

To promote uniformity in occupational therapy documentation and to improve continuity of legal records, AOTA has provided a guideline that includes the content of various types and fundamental elements of documentation.[16] This guideline is helpful regardless of the method used to document the occupational therapy intervention. Box 7-1 lists the 10 elements of the documented record.

Although the registered occupational therapist (OTR) has ultimate responsibility for all documentation, the COTA has complete responsibility for preparation of certain reports.[5] The COTA contributes to evaluation data and may perform certain screenings and standardized assessments. The COTA may also prepare the treatment plan, document progress, report any necessary revisions in the treatment plan based on reevaluation, and complete the discharge summary in collaboration with the OTR.

In many instances, co-signature of the COTA's documentation by the OTR may be required by the facility's accrediting bodies.[4] Accrediting bodies may include the Joint Commission on Accreditation of Healthcare

Box 7-1

**Fundamental Elements of Documentation**

1. Patient's full name and case number on each page of documentation
2. Date stated as month, day, and year for each entry; time of intervention; and length of session
3. Identification of type of documentation and department name
4. Practitioner's signature with a minimum of first name or initial, last name, and professional designation
5. Signature of the recorder directly at the end of the note, without space left between the body of the note and the signature
6. Co-signature by a registered occupational therapist (OTR) on documentation written by students and certified occupational therapy assistants (COTAs) when required by law or the facility
7. Compliance with confidentiality standards
8. Acceptable terminology as defined by the facility
9. Facility-approved abbreviations
10. Errors corrected by drawing a single line through an error, liquid correction fluid and erasures are not acceptable, and the correction initialed; or facility requirements followed

Modified from Thomson LK, Foto M: Elements of clinical documentation, *Am J Occup Ther* 49 (10):1032, 1995.

Organizations (JCAHO), the Commission on the Accreditation of Rehabilitation Facilities (CARF), and the Comprehensive Outpatient Rehabilitation Facilities (CORF). Medicare, Medicaid, and other third-party payers also have documentation requirements. In addition, state laws related to licensure, registration, and certification may require co-signature of documentation. The COTA must be familiar with the documentation requirements of the facility, third-party payers, and the state.

## QUALITY OF DOCUMENTATION CONTENT

The quality of the documentation content is significant. Documentation must be well organized, contain only pertinent information, and be objective and accurate. Conciseness and brevity are also critical because both the writer and the reader have other demands on their time. When writing a report, the occupational therapy practitioner must consider who will read it.[6] This may influence what needs to be reported and how the report will be written. An audience of clinicians, insurance payers, or lay persons may determine the type of medical terminology or accepted medical abbreviations used and the amount of detail needed for accurate understanding of the report.

## PERMANENT LEGAL RECORD

The documents contained in the permanent record are considered the only official records related to that patient. Each facility determines the official contents of this record. This may be based on requirements set by internal systems, licensing agencies, accrediting bodies, and third-party payers. This record will be used internally by the treatment team to understand the total patient treatment plan, by utilization reviewers to determine justification for continued treatment, and by quality assurance teams to assess overall patient outcomes and services. These records may be used externally by third-party payers to determine payment for services, by the court system for legal litigation, and by outside agencies for continued treatment or services after discharge from the facility.

## OCCUPATIONAL THERAPY RECORD

The occupational therapy documents contained in the permanent legal record consist of the physician's referral, initial evaluation, ongoing progress notes, reevaluation reports, and discharge summary. These records identify all tests and observations, treatment goals, treatment plans, and progress toward the established goals. The practitioner may also be required to provide entries in other sections of the permanent record, such as the interdisciplinary care plan or the patient care conference note.

In some facilities the occupational therapy service will maintain separate departmental files. This file includes supporting records, notes, and worksheets as well as copies of the reports prepared for the permanent legal record. The supporting data may include test results (e.g., muscle test form), treatment observations (e.g., activities of daily living checklist), informal therapy team conference notes, or treatment plan approaches. The supporting data form the basis for the reports that become part of the permanent legal record.

## PROBLEM-ORIENTED MEDICAL RECORD

The **problem-oriented medical record** (POMR) is one format often used to structure documentation.[8] The POMR encourages an interdisciplinary model in which all health care services integrate information into one document. The POMR allows for adequate documentation required for quality assurance and third-party payers. It consists of four sections: a data base, a problem list, treatment plan, and SOAP or progress notes.[6] SOAP notes are often used for communicating daily or weekly information within facilities. The data base is composed of physical, social, and demographic information and is contained in one report. From this data base a problem list is formulated and kept at the front of the record. It serves as an index to all problems and may include anticipated problems. Each problem is numbered and named, and these designations remain the same for each hospitalization of the patient. All the treatment plans must be titled and numbered according to the problem list, dated, and signed.

Each section of the **SOAP note** includes specific information, as follows:

*Subjective:* what has been said subjectively by the patient or what has been reported by significant others

*Objective:* observable and measurable data derived from evaluation and treatment results

*Assessment:* the opinion, interpretation, or assessment of the results of the patient's functional performance and anticipated outcomes

*Plan:* the treatment plan, including long-term and short-term goals and the frequency and length of treatment

The value of SOAP note charting is that the reader can easily review information. The original format has been adapted by many professionals in medical and allied health fields.[9] COTAs encounter many variations of the note in professional practice.

## AUTOMATED DOCUMENTATION SYSTEMS

With the development of computer technology, therapy documentation software systems have become increasingly available. These systems range from primary documentation formats to integrated systems that not only accomplish the basic documentation but also complete billing processes, provide administrative tracking information, and collate outcome data.

The ultimate advantage in using an automated system is the time saved in completing the documentation and collating the data for outcome studies and other required administrative reports. In addition, the sophistication of the data collected is much more advanced and accurate than can be provided by manual systems. The primary disadvantages of automated systems are difficulty in designing a system that meets all the needs of the particular program or the specific requests from various outside agencies; the cost of sufficient hardware to meet the needs of the facility; the cost of staff training; and the need for staff to accept and use the system.[13] The occupational therapy practitioner who possesses basic keyboarding and word-processing skills is well prepared for the increasing use of automated documentation systems.

## CLASSIFICATION CODES FOR BILLING OF SERVICES

Occupational therapy practitioners who work in facilities where Medicare, Medicaid, other major insurance plans such as Blue Cross/Blue Shield, and managed care organizations are billed for services must be familiar with **classification codes** known as the *Health Care Financing Administration* (HCFA) *Common Procedure Coding System* (HCPCS).[14] These codes are used in reimbursement programs to classify the various types of services rendered. As part of this coding system, the Physician's Current Procedural Terminology (CPT) lists descriptive terms and identifying codes for reporting medical services and procedures performed by physicians and nonphysician practitioners. The terminology provides a uniform language that designates medical, surgical, and diagnostic services and accurately and effectively provides a means of reliable, nationwide communication among health care practitioners, patients, and third parties.

Occupational therapy practitioners must classify the services rendered according to the terminology used in the coding system. These codes provide uniform language related to occupational therapy and aid in the reimbursement process. Recently, occupational therapy practitioners have been instrumental in collaboratively revising the physical medicine section of the CPT to reflect better the type of procedures performed in practice.

## UNIFORM TERMINOLOGY FOR OCCUPATIONAL THERAPY

Occupational therapy practitioners must also become familiar with the document *Uniform Terminology for Occupational Therapy*.[3] An official document of AOTA, it provides a generic outline of the scope of practice within the profession and creates a common terminology for explaining the practice to others. Essentially, the ***Uniform Terminology*** outlines three interrelated sections: performance areas, performance components, and performance contexts. We recommend that the occupational therapy practitioner refer to the document, available from the American Occupational Therapy Association, for further understanding. (See Chapter 2.)

## OVERVIEW OF THE REPORTING PROCESS

### Documentation and Clinical Reasoning

Creating documentation that is accurate and reflects effective occupational therapy intervention requires a step-by-step process of **clinical reasoning**.[1] The process provides useful information for treatment planning and note writing. The COTA completes an eight-step process collaboratively with the OTR (Box 7-2).

### The Referral

Occupational therapy evaluation and treatment is usually initiated by receipt of a patient referral. This **referral** is generally (but not always) received from the physician and may specify the reason for requesting the referral. It is sometimes called a *prescription* or *physician's orders for occupational therapy*. When a physician's referral is required, it should include the oc-

Box 7-2

## Eight-Step Process of Clinical Reasoning for Documentation

1. After referral to occupational therapy and evaluation, predict functional outcomes based on groups of people with similar problems.
2. Consider the patient, present and past functional abilities, and occupational history.
   a. Collaborate with the patient on activities that are meaningful and achievable.
   b. Set long-term goals.
3. Observe performance.
4. Establish a sequence for short-term goals.
5. Consider the timing of long-term and short-term goals, and prioritize and sequence treatment methods.
6. Reassess performance and complete daily and/or weekly notes.
7. Reexamine long-term and short-term goals, and complete the monthly summary.
8. Complete the discharge summary.

Modified from Allen C: Clinical reasoning for documentation. In Acquaviva J, editor: *Effective documentation for occupational therapy,* Rockville, Md, 1992, American Occupational Therapy Association.

cupational therapy treatment diagnosis, the onset date of the treatment diagnosis, a request for evaluation and other specific treatment orders, the date, and physician's signature.[2] Figure 7-1 provides an example of a physician's orders form that includes the entire treatment team.

The first entry into the patient's permanent record may be to document receipt of the referral and the initial plan of action, for example, "11/5/97 Occupational Therapy referral received and full evaluation initiated this date." The response time is established by each facility but is usually within 24 to 48 hours after the referral is received.

### Initial Evaluation Process

The initial evaluation process requires the OTR to gather and establish a base of general information about the patient, complete the evaluation, and establish a baseline of patient performance. Through the clinical reasoning process, the information obtained during the initial evaluation is used to make valid conclusions and establish the treatment goals and plans.

#### *General Information Data Base*

The general information data base includes the patient's name and address; important phone numbers; family members; third-party payers; family history; educational and work history; pertinent medical, physical, and mental status information related to specific primary and secondary diagnoses; and other information related to the patient's prior level of functioning. Information regarding expected treatment outcomes and discharge plans is also pertinent. The initial evaluation process begins by reviewing available data obtained from the existing permanent record; by interviewing referring sources, the patient, and family members; and by observing patient performance and behavior during the evaluation process.

This information provides a baseline, and the appropriate data are integrated into the initial evaluation report. Extraneous information may be kept in the occupational therapy record for reference during the treatment process.

#### *Evaluation Process*

The initial evaluation is a process for establishing the patient's baseline status by administering and interpreting assessment instruments and tests. Accuracy in administering and recording evaluation results is critical. All future evaluation reports will compare progress to this initial baseline status, and the degree of improvement may determine the course and amount of treatment approved by physicians and third-party payers.

Many facilities and third-party payers require the OTR to perform the initial evaluation. However, after demonstrating service competency, the COTA, working under the supervision of an OTR, may contribute to the initial evaluation by administering certain structured or standardized tests.[4] The COTA may also complete interviews, general observations, and behavioral checklists; score test protocols; and report these findings orally and in writing.

The occupational therapy file should contain the detailed results of all completed assessments. These may include range of motion (ROM) measurements; manual muscle testing, sensory testing, and perceptual/cognitive assessment results; and activities of daily living (ADLs), functional mobility, home management, vocational, and avocational assessment findings.

#### *Establishing the Treatment Plan*

The **treatment plan** involves organizing and interpreting the data gathered previously to establish a clear plan of action. This process identifies the problems impeding function and then applies clinical reasoning skills to specify predictable functional outcomes. The result is a clear set of goals with an established plan of treatment to accomplish those goals.

It is important to involve the patient (or, when necessary, a patient advocate) in treatment planning. Goals that the patient finds personally meaningful, valuable, and culturally relevant must be considered. Involvement in goal setting increases patient motivation and improves rehabilitation potential.

Many examples or types of treatment plans are available. Occupational therapy practitioners may select a form that is most suitable for the patient

MEDICAL REC. # ____________

IDENTIFICATION INFORMATION

☐ ADULT REHABILITATION ☐ PEDIATRIC SERVICES ☐ LONG TERM CARE ☐ CENTER THERAPY

**PATIENT'S NAME** ____________ BIRTHDATE ____________

ADDRESS ____________ PHONE (HOME) ____________ (WORK) ____________

PARENT/GUARDIAN ____________ DOCTOR ____________ PHONE ____________

INSURANCE TYPE: ☐ MEDICARE ☐ MEDICAL ASSISTANCE ☐ OTHER (Specify): ____________

**DIAGNOSIS** ____________

TREATMENT DIAGNOSIS ____________ ONSET DATE ____________

**PRECAUTIONS/CONTRAINDICATIONS:** ____________

PHYSICIAN RE-CHECK DATE ____________ NATURE OF INJURY: ☐ ATHLETICS ☐ EXERCISE ☐ WORK ☐ OTHER ____________

QRC ____________ SURGICAL PROCEDURE ____________ SURGICAL/INJURY DATE ____________

| | PT | OT | SPEECH | PSYCH | SOC. SVS. | OCC. MED. | BLADDER | THER. REC. |
|---|---|---|---|---|---|---|---|---|
| DATE | | | | | | | | |
| TIME | | | | | | | | |
| THER. | | | | | | | | |

PHYSICIAN'S ORDERS

**SPECIAL PROGRAMS**

___ BACK IN BALANCE (BIB) (PT, OT)
___ DRIVERS POTENTIAL ASSESS. (OT, PT)
___ RA PROTOCOL (PT, OT)
___ TMJ AND CRANIOFACIAL PAIN CLINIC (PT, Psych, Dental)
___ THERAPEUTIC HORSEBACK RIDING
___ POST MASTECTOMY PGM.
___ THERAPEUTIC EXER. GRP. (LTC)
___ FIBROMYALGIA PGM (PT, OT, Psych)
___ CHRONIC PAIN PGM (PT, OT, Psych)

**OCCUPATIONAL MEDICINE** ___ Eval. ___ Eval. and treat Frequency ___ X/Week ___ X/Day Duration ___ Weeks

___ Functional capacities assessment (FCA) ___ Modified FCA ___ Upper extremity functional eval. ___ Work hardening (includes back in balance and back on track)

**UPPER EXTREMITY REHAB.** ___ Eval. ___ Eval. and treat ___ Splint Frequency ___ X/Week ___ X/Day Duration ___ Weeks

**PHYSICAL THERAPY** ___ Eval. ___ Eval. and treat ___ Treat Frequency ___ X/Week ___ X/Day Duration ___ Weeks

☐ ELECTROTHERAPY
___ HVGS
___ Interferential
___ Iontopharesis
___ Muscle Re-ed.
___ TENS
☐ HYDROTHERAPY
___ Contrast baths
___ Pool therapy
___ Whirlpool

☐ GAIT TRAINING
☐ HOME EXERCISE PROGRAM
☐ FUNCTIONAL ACTIVITIES
___ Body mechanics
___ Endurance
___ Mobility
___ Postural training
___ Transfers
☐ ADAPTIVE EQUIPMENT
☐ TRACTION ☐ Mechanical ☐ Manual
___ Cervical ___ Pelvic

☐ MODALITIES
___ Cold packs (Ice) ___ Hot packs
___ Diathermy ___ Ultrasound
☐ MUSCLE REEDUCATION
___ ROM ____________
___ Strengthening ____________
☐ PROCEDURES
___ Massage ☐ Regular ☐ Ice
___ Spray and stretch
___ Paraffin bath
☐ SPLINTS

☐ THERAPEUTIC EXERCISE
___ BTE
___ Cybex
___ Circuit training
___ CPM
___ Functional training
___ Stretching
___ Joint mobilization
___ Myofascial release
___ Pelvic stabilization
___ Relaxation

**OCCUPATIONAL THERAPY** ___ Eval. ___ Eval. and treat ___ Treat Frequency ___ X/Week ___ X/Day Duration ___ Weeks

___ ADL
___ Adaptive equipment
___ Cognition
___ Feeding
___ Pool therapy
___ Sensory
___ Splint
___ Visual percept. ____________
☐ UPPER EXTREMITY-NEURO
___ Coordination ____________
___ Neuromuscular re-ed.
___ ROM
___ Strengthening

**SPEECH THERAPY** ___ Eval. ___ Eval. and treat ___ Treat Frequency ___ X/Week ___ X/Day Duration ___ Weeks

___ Feeding ___ Speech language ___ Swallowing ___ Other ____________

**PSYCHOLOGY** ___ Eval. ___ Eval. and treat ___ Treat Frequency ___ X/Week ___ X/Day Duration ___ Weeks

___ Adjustment counseling
___ BACK ON TRACK (BOT) (Psych)
___ Biofeedback/relaxation
___ Cognitive Eval/retraining
___ MMPI ____________
___ Vocational ____________

**SOCIAL SERVICES** Frequency ___ X/Week ___ X/Day Duration ___ Weeks

___ Assess. ___ Counsel ___ Case mgmt./DC planning ___ Adj. group ___ Financial resource/needs assess. ___ Info and referral

**THERAPEUTIC REC.** ___ Eval. ___ Eval. and treat ___ Treat Frequency ___ X/Week ___ X/Day Duration ___ Weeks

**BLADDER THERAPY** ___ Eval. ___ Eval. and treat ___ Treat ___ PRN per patient progress and M.D. instruction

**OTHER (Please specify)** ____________

Inpatient treatment may include therapeutic group sessions.
Pertinent History, Rehab Problem(s), Goal(s) and Precaution Information available in therapist's documentation.

Verbal order taken by ____________ Date ____________

Except as listed above, this patient has no infections and there are no contraindications/precautions to the above ordered treatment.
Except as listed above, all referrals for musculoskeletal disorders include education and exercise.

Physician's signature ____________ Date ____________

No. 0151-014 BLACK-Medical record BROWN-Medical records copy BLUE-Therapist GREEN-Scheduler

**PHYSICIAN'S ORDERS**

*Figure 7-1* Physician's orders form. (Courtesy Regional Rehabilitation Center of Duluth, Duluth, Minn.)

Name: John Doe
Doctor: Dr. J. Smith
Therapist: J. Gomez, OTR S. Johnson, COTA
Referred for: OT THA protocol including eval + tx for ADLs

DOB: 12/30/27 Date: 7/2/97
Diagnosis: THA arthroplasty
Precautions: THA precautions
Frequency: 3x/ week
Duration: 1 week
Rehab potential: Good

| PROBLEMS: | SHORT-TERM GOALS: | LONG-TERM GOALS: | APPROACHES: |
|---|---|---|---|
| ↓ ADL:<br><br>dressing<br><br>hygiene<br><br>bathing<br><br>functional mobility | • Provided assistive devices & instructions & following THA precautions, patient will dress L/E c̄ min. assist in 3 days.<br>• Provided raised toilet seat, patient will transfer from standing ↔ toilet c̄ min. assist following THA precautions within 3 days.<br>• Provided tub chair and grab bars, patient will transfer from standing ↔ tub chair c̄ min. assist following THA precautions within 3 days. | • Patient will perform ADLs independently in order to return to ADL activities at home by D/C. | • Instruct and demo THA precautions.<br>• Train in use of assistive devices including: reacher, dressing sticks, sock aid, long-handled shoe horn, elastic shoe laces, raised toilet seat, tub chair, grab bars.<br>• Instruct in tub/shower, toilet and car transfers.<br>• Provide options for work simplification, meal preparation, & item transport.<br>• Assist in obtaining equipment as needed. |

*Figure 7-2* Occupational therapy treatment plan form.

diagnoses seen by their department. Alternatively, facilities may require a certain type of treatment plan format. Figure 7-2 provides an example of an OT treatment plan.

*Critical Pathways* Another type of treatment plan is the critical pathway (Figure 7-3). A **critical pathway** is a care plan or treatment plan based on predetermined expected outcomes and length of treatment for a specific diagnosis. Critical pathways identify what treatment is to be provided on each treatment day and include the services of the entire treatment team. Critical pathways are mutually decided by team members based on previous quantitative data related to that diagnosis.

Critical pathways are useful in managed care or prepaid health care programs. With the growth of managed care, employers are seeking employee health care services that provide quantitative measures, cost-effectiveness, quality clinical outcomes, and responsiveness to customers. Often these plans identify fixed, preset reimbursement schedules for qualifying services.

*Behavioral Objectives* Treatment plan goals often are written in the form of behavioral objectives. A **behavioral objective** is an objective or goal written in clear, specific, and measurable terms and has three basic components: an outcome statement, a condition statement, and a criterion. The easiest way to write a behavioral objective is first to consider under what

Critical Pathway

Physician: Dr. J. Smith
Nurse case manager: M. Ryan, RN
PT: R. O'Hearn, RPT; B. Crowell, PTA
OT: J. Gomez, OTR; S. Johnson, COTA
Speech: M. Swor, SLP
Psych: G. Stallig, MALP
Ther. rec.: T. Chang, TRS
Social worker: B. Kucinski, MSW
Dietician: F. Wood, RD
Additional team members:

Diagnosis: Right CVA Left Hemiplegia
Admission date: 7/6/97
Discharge date: 8/2/97
Length of stay: 1 month

*Figure 7-3* Critical pathway form for moderate to severe right cerebrovascular accident (CVA) and left hemiplegia. (Courtesy Regional Rehabilitation Center of Duluth, Duluth, Minn.)

Moderate-Severe
(Right CVA Left Hemi)

Admission date: 7/6/97

| 1 | 2 | 3 | 4 | 5 | 6 | 7 |
|---|---|---|---|---|---|---|
| Establish bowel and bladder program<br>Establish skin program<br>Begin eval<br>Oriented to unit/room<br>Oriented to rehab program<br>Bedside dysphagia screen<br>Swallow risk ID band<br>DNR/DNI status | W/C fitted<br>Assess for positioning equipment<br>Assess need for referral to DRS and/or CIL | Evaluations complete<br>Assess transfers w/team<br>Assess for dining grp<br>Assess need for psych eval<br>Conference | Assess need for CD referral<br>Assess need for TR<br>Foley out | Assess self-transport<br>Stroke films<br>Referral to Stroke Club | | Family Day<br>Members attended ____<br>____<br>____<br>____<br>Review patient goals with patient and family |
| **8** | **9** | **10** | **11** | **12** | **13** | **14** |
| Assess need for adaptive equipment<br>Reassess dysphagia<br>Re-evaluate bowel and bladder program<br>Re-evaluate skin program | | | Assess phone skills, check writing, money skills<br>Dry run | Assess simple meal prep<br>Assess appropriateness for self-meds | Assess need for positioning equipment/ splints | Family Day<br>Members attended ____<br>____<br>____<br>____<br>Assess car transfer<br>Assess light housekeeping skills<br>W/E pass |
| **15** | **16** | **17** | **18** | **19** | **20** | **21** |
| Community re-entry activity<br>Reassess dysphagia<br>Re-evaluate bowel and bladder program<br>Re-evaluate skin integrity | | Assess anticipated equipment needs<br>Assess home adaptation needs | Equipment ordered<br>Wet run | | | Family Day<br>Members attended ____<br>____<br>____<br>____<br>Begin instruction in home program<br>Assess need for DPA<br>W/E pass |
| **22** | **23** | **24** | **25** | **26** | **27** | **28** |
| | D/C FIM complete<br>Referral call to O.P. therapist | | | | | |

*Figure 7-3, cont'd* See opposite page for legend.

conditions or circumstances the goal is to occur. This statement reflects the who, what, when, where, and the occupational therapy intervention. Then the statement that describes the **functional outcome** or expected performance after treatment (the goal) is determined. The third statement indicates how well the task must be performed in order for the goal or objective to be accomplished. Consider this example: "Provided with ADL training in use of adaptive dressing aids, the patient will dress lower extremities independently, following total hip arthroplasty precautions, within 1 week." The behavioral objective is divided into the following components:

*Condition:* Provided ADL training in use of adaptive dressing aids
*Outcome:* Dress lower extremities
*Criterion:* Independently, following total hip arthroplasty precautions, within 1 week

Behavioral objectives can be written either as short-term goals or long-term results of treatment. In either case, objectives must be measurable and must describe functional outcomes.[11] Third-party payers look for documentation that indicates changes in function based on the treatment provided. For example, although treatment may be to increase ROM in the shoulder, a functional outcome is that the patient is then able to bathe independently as a result of the increased range.

A helpful tool to evaluate a behavioral objective is to use the mnemonic **RUMBA.**[5] RUMBA stands for *r*elevant, *u*nderstandable, *m*easurable, *b*ehavioral, and *a*chievable. A *relevant* goal is meaningful to the patient and reflects the patient's potential. An *understandable* goal is stated clearly and in language understood by the patient and treatment team. A *measurable* goal contains a criterion for success, stated in quantitative terms whenever possible, and an expected date for achieving the goal. A *behavioral* goal describes what the patient must do to accomplish the goal. An *achievable* goal is one the patient can accomplish within a reasonable time. (See Chapter 6 for more information on writing objectives.)

## Initial Evaluation Report

The OTR has primary responsibility to complete the initial evaluation. The **initial evaluation report,** whether it is a form (Figure 7-4) or a narrative format, can be divided into four distinct sections as follows:

1. General information, which includes patient identifying information, medical history, and prior level of functioning
2. Clinical evaluation and interpretation
3. Functional status evaluation
4. Evaluation summary, which includes problem identification, short-term and long-term goals, and the treatment plan

### *General Information Section*

Basic patient identifying information includes the patient's name, medical record or account number, the referring physician's name, the referral, and evaluation dates. This first section details pertinent medical history, including the primary treatment diagnosis and any related secondary diagnoses with their onset dates. This section should list any precautions or contraindications that need to be observed during treatment. The patient's prior level of functioning, previous living situation, and prior vocational and avocational status are also noted.

### *Clinical Evaluation Section*

This section summarizes the results of each patient assessment. The OTR selects specific assessments depending on the diagnosis and the individual patient. For example, a brain-injured patient may require a physical assessment (ROM, motor and sensory function) and perceptual and cognitive testing. The COTA completes certain aspects of the evaluation as identified by the OTR. It is helpful to use standardized results or standardized rating scales for easy interpretation by others. Standardized scales also permit reliable replication of the evaluation process at reevaluation and discharge times.

### *Functional Status Evaluation Section*

This section evaluates the patient's functional performance, or how well the patient performs in essential activities. A standardized scale (Table 7-1) is used to ensure reliability of results. The focus and scope of the OT evaluation depends on the defined roles of the various professional departments in the facility. In the sample form (see Figure 7-4), bed mobility, transfers, wheelchair mobility, and daily living skills are assessed.

### *Evaluation Summary Section*

The evaluation summary is the most important section of the report. The OTR completes the evaluation summary, and the COTA contributes to it as directed by the OTR. In this section the previously recorded information is analyzed and a problem list developed. The problems listed are those factors that will impede the patient from obtaining maximal independence. This list may include problems that occupational therapy intervention may or may not directly impact; these problems will influence the OT practitioner's treatment approach. Using this problem list, the OTR and COTA set realistic and functional therapy goals.

The goals can be divided into two sections: long term and short term. Long-term goals are the maximal predicted outcomes expected for the patient after completing the full treatment program. Short-term goals are the level of function expected after a predesignated period of treatment intervention, perhaps as short as 1 week. Each goal must reflect a measurable, realistic, and functional outcome. For example, a long-term goal

SANTA CLARA VALLEY

**SANTA CLARA VALLEY MEDICAL CENTER**
OCCUPATIONAL THERAPY DEPARTMENT
Page 1 of 2

Service ______________ ☐ Inpatient ☐ Outpatient

☐ Initial ☐ Interim ☐ Discharge
(Rating scales on back of form)

**OCCUPATIONAL THERAPY**

**INFORMATION**

Onset Date: ______________ Referral Date: ______________ Sex: M F Language: ______________

Diagnosis

Medical History:

Precautions/Diet:

Living Situation:

A/Vocational History:

**UPPER EXTREMITY**

**Range of Motion**

☐ Refer to range of motion form

**Muscle Picture**

☐ Refer to muscle test form

**Sensation**

(Light touch, pain, kinesthesia, other)

**Hand Function**

Dominance: ☐ Right ☐ Left

Splinting:

| | Right | | | Left | | |
|---|---|---|---|---|---|---|
| | Grip | 3 point | Lateral | Grip | 3 point | Lateral |
| Initial | | | | | | |
| Interim/DC | | | | | | |
| Norm | | | | | | |

**OTHER MOTOR**

(Endurance, head/trunk posture and control, sitting/standing balance, reflexes, LE picture, functional ambulation)

**VISUAL PERCEPTUAL SKILLS**

| VISUAL | Initial | Interim/DC | PERCEPTUAL | Initial | Interim/DC |
|---|---|---|---|---|---|
| Visual Attention | | | Motor planning | | |
| Near Acuity | | | Graphic praxis | | |
| Distance Acuity | | | Body scheme | | |
| Pursuits | | | R/L discrimination | | |
| Saccades | | | Form | | |
| Ocular Alignment | | | Size | | |
| Stereopsis | | | Part/whole | | |
| Visual Fields | | | Figure ground | | |
| Visual Neglect | | | Position in space | | |

SCALE: 0 = intact; 1 = impaired; 2 = severely impaired; 3 = unable to perform

COMMENTS:

Wears corrective lenses ☐Y ☐N Testing not indicated ☐

**COGNITION AND BEHAVIOR**

(Orientation, initiation, direction following, memory, judgement, organization, problem solving, impulsivity, attention span )

**DISPOSITION - White - MEDICAL RECORD Yellow - O.T. Chart**

Therapist's Signature: ______________

9502 SCVMC 6628-17

*Figure 7-4* Occupational therapy evaluation form. (Courtesy of Occupational Therapy Department, Santa Clara Valley Medical Center, San Jose, Calif.)

**SANTA CLARA VALLEY MEDICAL CENTER**
OCCUPATIONAL THERAPY EVALUATION
Page 2 of 2

SANTA CLARA VALLEY MEDICAL CENTER

Service ______________________ ☐ Inpatient ☐ Outpatient
☐ Initial ☐ Interim ☐ Discharge
(Rating scale on back of form)

OCCUPATIONAL THERAPY

| | ACTIVITY | Initial | Interim D/C | Goal | |
|---|---|---|---|---|---|
| BED MOBILITY | Rolling R | | | | Bed: Positioning: |
| | Rolling L | | | | Caregiver Training: |
| | Bridging | | | | |
| | Scooting | | | | Comments: |
| | Long Sit | | | | |
| | Sidelying to Sit | | | | |
| TRANSFERS | Bed | | | | Type: Equipment: |
| | Toilet | | | | Caregiver Training: |
| | Tub/Shower | | | | |
| | Car/Van Seat | | | | Comments: |
| | Furniture | | | | |
| WHEELCHAIR | Management | | | | Type: Weight Shift Type: |
| | Weight Shift | | | | Positioning/Cushion: |
| | Home | | | | Caregiver Training: |
| | Community | | | | Comments: |
| | In/Out of Car | | | | |
| DAILY LIVING SKILLS | Eating | | | | Equipment: |
| | Upper Body Dressing | | | | Home Environment: |
| | Lower Body Dressing | | | | |
| | Hygiene/ Grooming | | | | A/Vocational/Driving Skills: |
| | Bathing | | | | |
| | Toileting | | | | |
| | Kitchen | | | | Caregiver Training: |
| | Homemaking | | | | Comments: |
| | Community | | | | |
| | Communication Tasks | | | | |

| Problems: | Goals/Recommendation: ☐ Patient/Caregiver participated in goal setting |
|---|---|
| ____X____ / ________ / ________<br>Frequency / Session Length / Duration of Treatment | Therapist's Signature ______ Date ______ Physician's Signature ______ |

**DISPOSITION - White - MEDICAL RECORD Yellow - O.T. Chart** 9502 PAGE 2 of 2 SCVMC 6628-17

*Figure 7-4, cont'd* See previous page for legend.

Table 7-1

## Definitions of Levels of Assistance

| Level of assistance | Abbreviation | Definition |
|---|---|---|
| Independent | Ind. | • Patient requires no assistance or cuing in any situation and is trusted in all situations 100% of the time to do the task safely. |
| Supervision | Sup. | • Caregiver is not required to provide any hands-on guarding but may need to give verbal cues for safety. |
| Contact guard/standby | Con. Gd./Stby | • Caregiver must provide hands-on contact guard to be within arms length for patient's safety. |
| Minimum assistance | Min. | • Caregiver provides 25% physical and/or cuing assistance. |
| Moderate assistance | Mod. | • Caregiver assists patient with 50% of the task. Assistance can be physical and/or cuing. |
| Maximum assistance | Max. | • Caregiver assists patient with 75% of the task. Assistance can be physical and/or cuing. |
| Dependent | Dep. | • Patient is unable to assist in any part of the task. Caregiver performs 100% of the task for patient physically and/or cognitively. |

Courtesy Occupational Therapy Department, Santa Clara Valley Medical Center, San Jose, Calif.

Fims

for a patient currently requiring maximum assistance for eating might read, "Using an adapted utensil, the patient will eat independently by discharge to home." The short-term goal for the week might read, "Using an adapted utensil, the patient will eat with moderate assistance within 1 week."

Once goals have been established, a treatment plan is completed. Using the goal just listed, daily eating retraining and upper extremity functional strengthening for 2 weeks may be identified as treatment methods to achieve improved independence in eating.

Other critical entries in this summary section may include a discharge plan once therapy has been completed and a section noting that the stated goals have been discussed with and reflect the goals of the patient and family. Finally, if the initial physician's order was for an evaluation only or was not specific for the treatment intervention now planned, a physician's review of the plan and verifying signature may be necessary.

### Progress Notes

**Progress notes** may be required on a per treatment, daily, or weekly basis. Generally, daily notes are very brief and reflect the patient's response to treatment, treatment provided, and progress noted. Revision of the treatment plan and goals is not always necessary.

Weekly progress notes are more thorough and should summarize the treatment provided, the treatment frequency, the patient's response to treatment and progress toward goals (or lack of progress, with justification). The goals should be updated and the treatment plan revised. The new goals and treatment plan are usually considered short-term goals and reflect the expected outcome for the following week's treatment regimen.

give examples

Various styles or formats for progress notes are used to ensure consistency of the notes' content. SOAP notes are one format frequently used. Figure 7-5 shows a form for a narrative style. Another format for short daily notes states the problem, progress, description of the treatment program, and future plans. Another approach is to record the treatment frequency, goal, method, patient's response and progress, and future treatment plan. Boxes 7-3 to 7-6 provide some examples of progress notes.

### Reevaluation Report

If treatment occurs over an extended period, the OTR may need to complete a full reevaluation. Again, the COTA contributes to this process. The format is often the same as the initial evaluation. The primary difference is that this report reflects the differences between the initial baseline of evaluation results and the patient's present clinical status. The reevaluation report reflects progress made toward the predicted goals and is a measure of success of the treatment intervention. Based on the new evaluation results, initial goals and treatment timelines can be revised. The reevaluation is an important tool for the ongoing utilization review process. It allows the occupational therapy practitioner to justify continued intervention by clearly quantifying the effectiveness and efficiency of the treatment.

**PROGRESS NOTE**

**GOALS:**

| **DATE** | **NARRATIVE** |
|---|---|

**Assessment:**

**NOTE: Please refer to Initial Evaluation for long-term goals and critical pathway for short-term goals.**

| **DATE** | AM | PM | AM | PM | AM | PM | AM | PM | AM | PM | AM | PM |
|---|---|---|---|---|---|---|---|---|---|---|---|---|
| Therapeutic Ex. | | | | | | | | | | | | |
| Neuromuscular Re-ed | | | | | | | | | | | | |
| Functional Activity | | | | | | | | | | | | |
| Kinetic Activity | | | | | | | | | | | | |
| ADL | | | | | | | | | | | | |
| Perception | | | | | | | | | | | | |
| Other | | | | | | | | | | | | |
| | | | | | | | | | | | | |
| | | | | | | | | | | | | |

1 Unit = 15 minutes

Signatures: Therapist(s) (and initials)

**OCCUPATIONAL THERAPY**
**Service Documentation and Progress Notes**
**Form # 6/93**

*Figure 7-5* Progress note form. (Courtesy Occupational Therapy Department, Regional Rehabilitation Center of Duluth, Duluth, Minn.)

*Box 7-3*

### Brief Daily Note Sample

Patient actively participated in eating retraining and RUE strengthening program. Patient ate 75% of meal with adapted utensils and required minimal assistance for cutting meat. Established treatment plan to continue.

*Box 7-4*

### Weekly Progress Note Sample

Patient has been seen daily for eating retraining and RUE functional strengthening program. Using adapted utensils, patient ate 75% of meal with minimal assistance for cutting meat. Previously, patient ate 50% of meal and required moderate assistance for cutting meat. Patient will eat independently with no assistive devices in 1 week.

*Box 7-5*

### SOAP Note Sample

**S:** Patient stated satisfaction with feeding self.
**O:** Using adapted utensils, patient ate 75% of meal with minimal assistance for cutting meat. Previously, patient ate 50% of meal and required moderate assistance for cutting meat. Presently, OTR evaluates fair to fair minus strength in elbow flexors compared with poor strength previous week.
**A:** Patient continues to exhibit low endurance for maintaining handgrip and weakness in elbow flexors.
**P:** Provided with eating retraining and RUE functional strengthening program, patient will eat independently with no assistive devices in 1 week.

*Box 7-6*

### Problem-Focused Progress Note Sample

**Problem:** Assisted eating.
**Progress:** Using adapted utensils, patient ate 75% of meal with minimal assistance for cutting meat. Previously, patient ate 50% of meal and required moderate assistance for cutting meat.
**Program:** Eating retraining and RUE functional strengthening.
**Plan:** Achieve independent eating with no assistive devices in 1 week.

### Discharge Summary Report

At completion of the treatment regimen, the patient's status must be documented. Insurance or facility requirements may stipulate that the OTR complete the discharge summary. Again, the format can be the same as that used for the initial evaluation and reevaluation. The **discharge summary** is a description of the patient's final status on discharge from the facility. The progress made from the initial evaluation to discharge must be accurately outlined. Some key elements may be added, including a statement of which goals were and were not achieved, with a reason why for those not achieved. Discharge recommendations are provided, clearly indicating the additional interventions and follow-up that may be required to ensure continued functional improvement or maintenance of the functional gains made. Any home program plans or referral plans are described.

The discharge summary is the key document that reflects the patient's total progress and all the accomplishments achieved. The data can be used for many purposes. Quality assurance committees may use the data to evaluate the effectiveness of treatment. The data may also be used for outcome studies to prove overall effectiveness of treatment within certain diagnostic categories. Insurance payers may use the report to determine payment for the service. Other service agencies, such as outpatient clinics, will use the data to help establish continued goals and treatment plans in the new treatment setting. Figure 7-6 provides a sample form for the discharge summary.

## TREATMENT RECORD

In addition to documenting the patient's performance, OT practitioners must complete daily records on patient attendance and the treatment provided. These records are provided to insurance payers to verify that charges and treatment interventions are consistent. Various formats are available to record this information.[10] Figures 7-7 and 7-8 provide examples of treatment records.

## MEDICARE REPORTS

Medicare is the largest single payer for occupational therapy services.[14] For this reason, occupational therapy practitioners are often required to complete reports for Medicare, Part A: Hospital Insurance Program, which pays for hospital inpatient, skilled nursing facility, home, and hospice care, and Part B: Supplemental Medical Insurance Program, which covers hospital outpatient, physician, and other professional services. Certain requirements apply to Medicare, so records may include prior authorizations, certifications, and recertifications. The occupational therapy practitioner must become familiar with Medicare regulations as they pertain to documentation. Figure 7-9 provides an example of a Medicare B form.

*Text continued on p. 74.*

| DATE DISCONTINUED: | REASON: | REFERRAL OBJECTIVES: | LENGTH OF TIME PT WAS SEEN: |
|---|---|---|---|
| DIAGNOSIS: | | | |

| GOALS | MET | NOT MET | REASON |
|---|---|---|---|
| STG: | | | |
| | | | |
| | | | |
| Pt/family will make DC plans based on level of independence at time of DC. | | | |
| LTG: | | | |
| | | | |

| PATIENT'S HOME SITUATION PRIOR TO ADMIT: | PATIENT DISCHARGED TO: ☐ Home ☐ Rehab ctr ☐ NH ☐ Other ______ | LIST HELP AVAILABLE IF DC HOME: |
|---|---|---|

**PATIENT'S ADL STATUS AT THE TIME OF DISCHARGE**

| | INDEP. | ASSIST | COMMENTS |
|---|---|---|---|
| TRANSFERS | | | |
| SELF CARE | | | |
| DRESSING | | | |
| EATING | | | |
| COOKING | | | |

**ADAPTIVE EQUIPMENT (RECOMMENDED FOR) WITH PATIENT**

☐ Long handled reacher ☐ Bath sponge ☐ Sock aide ☐ Dressing stick ☐ Elastic shoe laces ☐ Walker bag

☐ Elevated toilet seat ☐ Leg lift device ☐ Tub grab bar ☐ Other ______

**WRITTEN MATERIAL SENT WITH PATIENT**

☐ Ortho restrictions & transfer instructions
☐ Crutch/walker safety instructions
☐ Dressing equipment instructions
☐ Adaptive equipment list & purchase information
☐ Joint protection/arthritis exercises
☐ Brain trauma information
☐ One handed ADL techniques
☐ Back saving ADL techniques
☐ Low vision adaptation/safety techniques
☐ Carpal tunnel prevention
☐ U/E strengthening instructions
☐ U/E coordination instructions
☐ Adaptive dressing techniques
☐ Cognitive worksheets/instructions
☐ Range of motion instructions
☐ Other ______

**COMMENTS:** ______

**RECOMMENDATIONS FOR FURTHER TREATMENT OR SUPERVISION**

☐ None needed ☐ Outpatient OT is recommended ☐ OT at new facility ☐ Other: ______

**AREAS OF CONCERN:** ______

Occupational therapist signature ______ Date ______

61-00206 REV. 7/93

**OCCUPATIONAL THERAPY DISCHARGE SUMMARY**

OCCUPATIONAL THERAPY DISCHARGE SUMMARY

*Figure 7-6* Discharge summary form. (Courtesy Occupational Therapy Department, Unity Hospital, Fridley, Minn.)

**PRESCRIPTION AND TREATMENT RECORD**
**OCCUPATIONAL THERAPY**

Principal diagnosis ____________________________________________

____________________________________________

Diagnosis for which treatment is requested ____________________________

Treatment objective ____________________________________________

Precautions or special instructions ______________________ Rehab potential ________

Frequency of treatment: Daily ❑ BID ❑ Other ______________________ Duration ________

Date ________________ Signature of physician

| MONTH | Rx Ord. | 1 | 2 | 3 | 4 | 5 | 6 | 7 | 8 | 9 | 10 | 11 | 12 | 13 | 14 | 15 | 16 | 17 | 18 | 19 | 20 | 21 | 22 | 23 | 24 | 25 | 26 | 27 | 28 | 29 | 30 | 31 | |
|---|---|---|---|---|---|---|---|---|---|---|---|---|---|---|---|---|---|---|---|---|---|---|---|---|---|---|---|---|---|---|---|---|---|
| Evaluation | | | | | | | | | | | | | | | | | | | | | | | | | | | | | | | | | |
| Motor skills | | | | | | | | | | | | | | | | | | | | | | | | | | | | | | | | | |
| Sensory integrative skills | | | | | | | | | | | | | | | | | | | | | | | | | | | | | | | | | |
| Cognitive skills | | | | | | | | | | | | | | | | | | | | | | | | | | | | | | | | | |
| Activities of daily living | | | | | | | | | | | | | | | | | | | | | | | | | | | | | | | | | |
| Preventive skills | | | | | | | | | | | | | | | | | | | | | | | | | | | | | | | | | |
| Therapeutic adaptations | | | | | | | | | | | | | | | | | | | | | | | | | | | | | | | | | |
| Splint/follow-up | | | | | | | | | | | | | | | | | | | | | | | | | | | | | | | | | |

**Occupational Therapy Department**
**PRESCRIPTION AND TREATMENT RECORD**

Name ______________________ Room # ______
M.R. ______________________
D.O.B. ____________________ Age ______
Doctor ______________________
Admit date ______________________

*Figure 7-7* Occupational therapy prescription and treatment record form. (Courtesy Lora Taylor, OTR.)

**OCCUPATIONAL THERAPY**

IP/OP Room ________

| Month | | | | | | | | | | | | | | | |
|---|---|---|---|---|---|---|---|---|---|---|---|---|---|---|---|
| **Date** | | | | | | | | | | | | | | | |
| | | | | | | | | | | | | | | | |
| 9705 OT eval/re-eval 1-15 | | | | | | | | | | | | | | | |
| 0959 ADL training 1-15 | | | | | | | | | | | | | | | |
| 0977 OT consult/care conf 1-15 | | | | | | | | | | | | | | | |
| 9707 Cognitive treatment 1-15 | | | | | | | | | | | | | | | |
| 973 Develop treatment 1-15 | | | | | | | | | | | | | | | |
| 9877 Environmental stim 1-15 | | | | | | | | | | | | | | | |
| 0970 Motor skills 1-15 | | | | | | | | | | | | | | | |
| 0972 Preventive skills 1-15 | | | | | | | | | | | | | | | |
| 0971 Sensory integration 1-15 | | | | | | | | | | | | | | | |
| 9785 Therapeutic adapt 1-15 | | | | | | | | | | | | | | | |
| 9712 Initial out/pt ADL 30 | | | | | | | | | | | | | | | |
| 0967 Out/Pt no show 1-15 | | | | | | | | | | | | | | | |
| | | | | | | | | | | | | | | | |
| 0968 OT eval/hand 1-15 | | | | | | | | | | | | | | | |
| 0969 Motor skills/hand 1-15 | | | | | | | | | | | | | | | |
| 0963 Preventive skills/hand 1-15 | | | | | | | | | | | | | | | |
| 0960 Therap adapt/hand 1-15 | | | | | | | | | | | | | | | |
| 0962 Splint (prefab-hand) | | | | | | | | | | | | | | | |
| 0965 Splint (fabricated-H) | | | | | | | | | | | | | | | |
| | | | | | | | | | | | | | | | |
| 97832 Splint-prefab | | | | | | | | | | | | | | | |
| 609610 Splint-fabricated | | | | | | | | | | | | | | | |
| 610063 2/Piece formfit TLSO | | | | | | | | | | | | | | | |
| | | | | | | | | | | | | | | | |
| 9798 In/Pt OT adapt equip | | | | | | | | | | | | | | | |
| 0964 O/P hand equip | | | | | | | | | | | | | | | |
| 1008 O/P occ therapy supply | | | | | | | | | | | | | | | |

**OCCUPATIONAL THERAPY TREATMENT RECORD**

B, Bedside; C, clinic; H, hold treatment; S, surgery; DC, discontinued; D, discharged.

Therapist's signature ________________________________

*Figure 7-8* Occupational therapy treatment record form. (Courtesy Occupational Therapy Department, Unity Hospital, Fridley, Minn.)

Form Approved
OMB No. 0938-0227

# OCCUPATIONAL THERAPY INFORMATION AND PLAN OF TREATMENT

Attach to Medicare Billing Form. Continued reimbursement of the treatment program will be based upon the documentation of significant functional improvement of the patient's problem or problems.

1 COVERED ☐ NONCOVERED ☐ | 2 CERTIFICATION ☐ RECERTIFICATION ☐

3 Patient's name Last First Middle | 4 Date of birth | 5 Health insurance claim no.

6 Provider name and address (city and state) | 7 Provider number | 8 Attending physician

9 Admitting diagnosis | 10 Prior therapy history DATES From To | 11 Onset/exac. date | 12 Date treatment started

13 Rx diagnosis | 14 Rehab. potential | 15 Long range plan

16 Treatment precautions | 17 Functional status prior to current treatment episode

18 Functional level: ☐ - initial 0 - current ■ - last recent X - functional goal
Place appropriate symbol on bar(s).

**Assistance Level**

| **ACTIVITIES OF DAILY LIVING** | Total | Maximum | Moderate | Minimum | Standby | Independent |
|---|---|---|---|---|---|---|
| Feeding/Eating | | | | | | |
| Hygiene/Grooming | | | | | | |
| Dressing | | | | | | |
| Homemaking | | | | | | |
| Functional comm. | | | | | | |
| Functional mobility | | | | | | |
| Other | | | | | | |
| ______ | | | | | | |
| ______ | | | | | | |
| ______ | | | | | | |
| ______ | | | | | | |

THERAPEUTIC ADAPTATIONS:
(orthotics, prosthetics, assistive devices/equipment)

19 Complicating factors
Spasticity ______
Pain ______
Contracture ______
Weakness ______
Balance ______
Motivation ______
Cognition ______
Vision/hearing ______
Pt. compliance ______
Psychosocial ______
______ ______
______ ______

20 Plans for continued therapy:
Yes______ No______

21 Total no. of treatments to date:

22 Treatment plan:

Frequency Duration

23 Remarks:

24 Reason for terminating therapy:

25 Certification: The above plan of treatment is medically necessary and will reasonably treat or diagnose an illness or injury or improve the functioning of a malformed body member. The patient is under the care of a physician. This patient was examined by a physician within the past 30 days. Date of this examination was ______________. The above plan of treatment was reviewed by me in consultation with the occupational therapist on ______________ (date).

26 Physician signature Date | 27 O.T. signature Date | 28 Therapy denial or discharge date

*Figure 7-9* Occupational therapy information and plan of treatment form. (Courtesy Blue Cross/Blue Shield of Minnesota, St Paul, Minn.)

## SUMMARY

Documentation of occupational therapy services produces written records and reports that contain pertinent information about the patient's status, progress, and performance. The OT practitioner is responsible for keeping accurate records to document the patient's evaluation results, the identified problems, the treatment goals and plan, and the patient's progress toward the established plan.

Occupational therapy documentation includes the referral, evaluation data, initial evaluation, progress notes, reevaluation, and discharge summary. Records and reports should reflect clear, concise, accurate, and objective information about the patient. Documentation should be well organized and developed according to an agreed-on system for internal consistency of the record.

## *Selected Reading Guide Questions*

1. What are the role and responsibilities of the COTA in the documentation process?
2. What are four major components of a treatment plan?
3. Describe the reporting process from initial evaluation to progress reports and discharge summaries.
4. What is the purpose of the treatment record?

### *REFERENCES*

1. Allen C: Clinical reasoning for documentation. In Acquaviva J, editor: *Effective documentation for occupational therapy,* Rockville, Md, 1992, American Occupational Therapy Association.
2. Allen C, et al: A payer's review of documentation. In Acquaviva J, editor: *Effective documentation for occupational therapy,* Rockville, Md, 1992, American Occupational Therapy Association.
3. American Occupational Therapy Association: *Uniform terminology for occupational therapy,* ed 3, Rockville, Md, 1994, The Association.
4. Backhaus H: Documentation. In Ryan S, editor: *Practice issues in occupational therapy,* Thorofare, NJ, 1993, Slack.
5. Early MB: *Mental health concepts and techniques for the occupational therapy assistant,* ed 2, New York, 1993, Raven.
6. Foto M et al: Reports that work. In Acquaviva J, editor: *Effective documentation for occupational therapy,* Rockville, Md, 1992, American Occupational Therapy Association.
7. Gleave GJ: Medical records and reports. In Willard HS, Spackman CS, editors: *Occupational therapy,* ed 4, Philadelphia, 1971, Lippincott.
8. Jones RA: Service management. In Ryan S, editor: *The certified occupational therapy assistant: roles and responsibilities,* Thorofare, NJ, 1986, Slack.
9. Kettenbach G: *Writing SOAP notes,* ed 2, Philadelphia, 1995, Davis.
10. Llorens LA: *Occupational therapy sequential client care record manual,* Laurel, Md, 1982, Ramsco.
11. Mahoney P, Kannenberg K: Writing functional goals. In Acquaviva J, editor: *Effective documentation for occupational therapy,* Rockville, Md, 1992, American Occupational Therapy Association.
12. Reitz S: Ethical issues in documentation. In Acquaviva J, editor: *Effective documentation for occupational therapy,* Rockville, Md, 1992, American Occupational Therapy Association.
13. Robertson SC: Why we document. In Acquaviva J, editor: *Effective documentation for occupational therapy,* Rockville, Md, 1992, American Occupational Therapy Association.
14. Scott SJ, Somers FP: Orientation to payment. In Acquaviva J, editor: *Effective documentation for occupational therapy,* Rockville, Md, 1992, American Occupational Therapy Association.
15. Steich T: Legal implications in documentation: fraud, abuse and confidentiality. In Acquaviva J, editor: *Effective documentation for occupational therapy,* Rockville, Md, 1992, American Occupational Therapy Association.
16. Thomson LK, Foto M: Elements of clinical documentation, *Am J Occup Ther* 49(10):1032, 1995.
17. Welles C: The implications of liability: guidelines for professional practice, *Am J Occup Ther* 23:1, 1969.

### *RECOMMENDED READING*

Acquaviva J, editor: *Effective documentation for occupational therapy,* Rockville, Md, 1992, American Occupational Therapy Association.

Part III

# Occupational Therapy Evaluation Methods

Chapter 8

# Evaluation of Joint Range of Motion

*Lorraine Williams Pedretti*
*Michael K. Davis*

## Chapter Objectives

*After studying this chapter, the student or practitioner will be able to:*

1. Define goniometry as it relates to range of motion.
2. Describe functional range of motion as it relates to activities of daily living.
3. State eleven basic principles for joint measurement.
4. Determine range of motion measurements of the major upper extremity joints.
5. Contrast active and passive range of motion.
6. Describe basic goniometry testing positions of the upper extremity.
7. Recommend a therapeutic exercise program based on goniometric measurements.
8. Describe the three cardinal planes of movement.

## Key Terms

range of motion
joint movement
active range of motion
passive range of motion
functional range of motion
planes of movement
joint movement
goniometer
stationary bar
movable bar

**Range of motion (ROM)** is the extent of movement that occurs at a joint. The human body is composed of several types of joints, muscle tissue, tendons, and other supporting structures that allow for a high degree of joint mobility. Many factors (disease processes, trauma, periarticular changes, etc.) can adversely affect joint movement. Development and maintenance of the greatest ROM maximize function. The study of joint range is the foundation for understanding how movement or the lack of movement affects occupational performance. From an anatomical standpoint, normal joint movement and muscular strength provide the ability to carry out effortless movement in life activities, from simple to very complex. Joint measurement is an important tool in the assessment of physical dysfunction in conditions such as cerebrovascular accident (CVA, stroke), arthritis, fractures, and general debility.

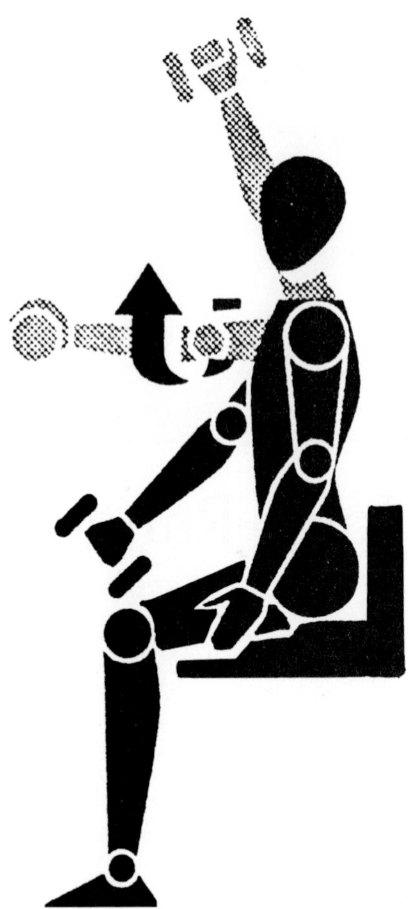

*Figure 8-1* Schematic representation of range of motion (ROM) occurring around the axis of the glenohumeral joint in shoulder flexion. (Courtesy Jerry L. Pettis VA Medical Center, Los Angeles, Calif.)

Joint measurement data assist the occupational therapy practitioner in evaluating progress or lack of progress toward the treatment goals. Many patients are motivated by seeing concrete improvement based on recorded range of motion (ROM) measures. ROM data are important to establish a baseline data base, but this information must be linked to function. Increases in motion are not significant unless the person has gained in function, such as in the ability to dress independently as a result of increased ROM.[3] Simply put, ROM is **joint movement:** active, passive, or a combination of both. Motion occurs in an arc; the joint acts as the axis or pivot of the arc (Figure 8-1). **Active range of motion** (AROM) is the arc of motion through which the joint passes when voluntarily moved by muscles acting on the joint. **Passive range of motion** (PROM) is the arc of motion through which the joint passes when moved by an outside force. Normally, PROM is slightly greater than AROM.[9] ROM is measured by an instrument or tool known as a *goniometer.*

## ROLE OF THE OCCUPATIONAL THERAPY ASSISTANT IN JOINT MEASUREMENT

The extent of the certified occupational therapy assistant's (COTA's) involvement in ROM evaluations is determined by the supervising registered occupational therapist (OTR) in agreement with the applicable laws and professional practice standards of the particular state. In many clinical practices the COTA performs basic goniometry of the upper extremity.[4] The role of the COTA in this area should be based on competency level and must consider legislation and restrictions governing the practice setting.

## GENERAL PRINCIPLES OF JOINT MEASUREMENT

The occupational therapy practitioner must have complete understanding of (1) the degree and type of motion that will occur at a specific joint,[5] (2) average normal ROM,[1] and (3) how to position self and patient during measurement.[10] It is important to establish good habits early when approaching the patient for assessment. That is, you should take a few minutes to establish rapport and to instruct the patient about the nature and purpose of the particular assessment.[2] Before measuring, ask the patient to move the extremity through a comfortable ROM. After aligning the goniometer, note any discomfort, unusual restriction or freedom of movement, or audible noise *(crepitation)* from the joint.

Formal joint measurement is not necessary with all patients. The OT practitioner can informally measure joint movement by asking the patient to position the affected extremity in a variety of normal positions. Comparing the movement of the affected extremity to that of the opposite extremity allows the examiner to detect any gross limitations. The practitioner should always check the medical record for any causes that may predispose the patient to joint limitations (e.g., fused joints, previous injuries, arthritis). Pain may limit ROM, and crepitation may be heard on movement in some conditions. Joints should not be forced when resistance is met on PROM.

Clinicians are generally concerned with **functional range of motion.** This term is typically used to describe the minimum range of motion needed to perform essential activities of daily living (ADLs) without the use of special equipment.[6] Function in ADLs is a primary goal of occupational therapy. If the patient is completely independent with all ADLs and has adequate ROM to perform these functions, treatment to increase ROM is generally not indicated, even though the patient may have less than "normal" ROM. Range of motion for any individual is affected by age, gender, and other factors, including lifestyle and occupation.[9]

## METHOD OF JOINT MEASUREMENT

Joint ROM is measured using a goniometer that is calibrated from 0° to 180°. Using this system, 0° is the

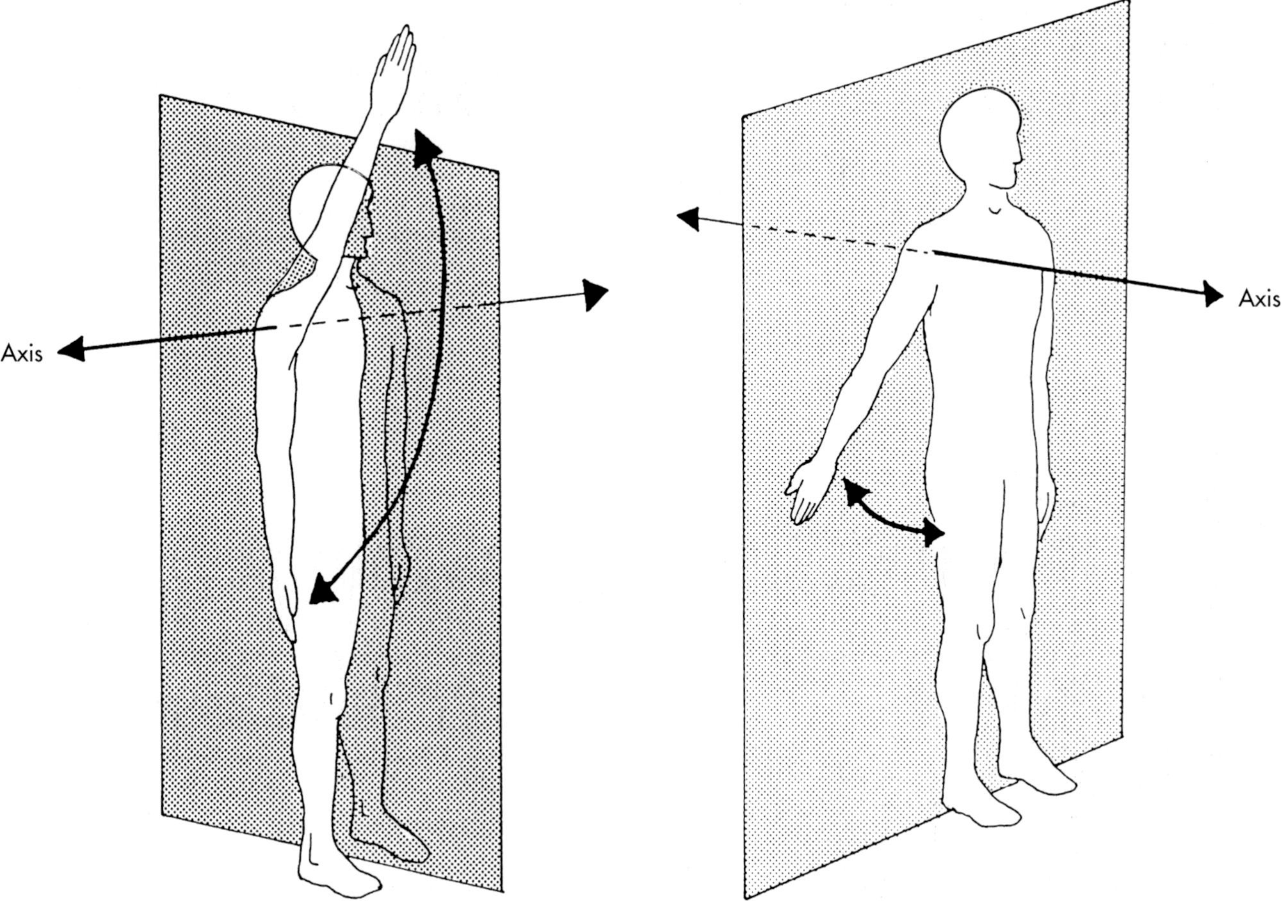


*Figure 8-2* Sagittal plane. Flexion and extension occurs in this anatomical plane around the coronal axis. (Courtesy Jerry L. Pettis VA Medical Center, Los Angeles, Calif.)

*Figure 8-3* Frontal plane. Abduction and adduction occur in this anatomical plane around the anteroposterior axis. (Courtesy Jerry L. Pettis VA Medical Center, Los Angeles, Calif.)

starting position and increases toward 180° for almost all joint motions. In general, measurements are performed with the patient in the anatomical position.

Measurement of rotation is an exception to this rule. Basically, motions of the body occur in three cardinal **planes of movement**: sagittal, frontal, and horizontal (Figures 8-2, 8-3, and 8-4, respectively). A semicircle of 180° is superimposed on the body in the plane, with degrees increasing in the direction in which movement will occur. The axis of the joint is the axis of the semicircle, or arc of motion.

## THE GONIOMETER

The universal **goniometer** is the tool most widely used to measure joint ROM in the clinical environment. The word *goniometer* is derived from the Greek *gonio,* which means angle, and *metron,* which means a measure.[7] Made of either plastic or metal, goniometers come in a variety of sizes and shapes. They can be purchased from medical supply houses or through medically oriented catalogs.

The goniometer consists of a stationary (proximal) bar and a movable (distal) bar. The body of the **stationary bar** includes a small protractor (half circle) of 0° to 180° or a full circle printed with a scale from 0° to 360°. The **movable bar** is attached at the center or axis of the protractor and acts as a dial. As the dial rotates around the protractor, the number of degrees is indicated on the scale (Figure 8-5).

One important feature of the goniometer is the *axis,* or *fulcrum.* The rivet that acts as the fulcrum must move freely but hold tightly enough to keep the arms at the measured position when the goniometer is removed from the body.

Two scales of figures are printed on the half circle. Each starts at 0° and progresses toward 180°, but in opposite directions. The key point to reading the goniometer is to use common sense. Once the movement of the body part has exceeded 90°, the larger numbers are read. A common error for beginners is to position the patient and goniometer correctly and then *misread* the actual measurement. Many practitioners find it easiest to align the two arms first and then center the axis point over the exact anatomical landmark.[8]

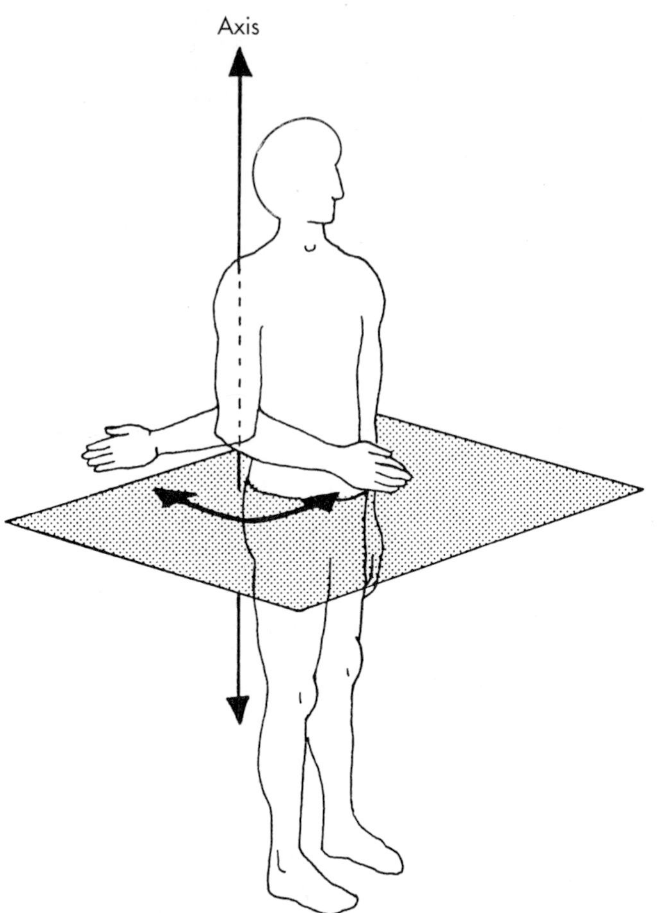


*Figure 8-4* Horizontal plane. Shoulder internal rotation and external rotation occur in this anatomical plane. (Courtesy Jerry L. Pettis VA Medical Center, Los Angeles, Calif.)

Figure 8-6 shows five styles of goniometers. The first (Figure 8-6, *A*) is a full-circle goniometer. Its longer arms are for use on the long bones or large joints of the body. The goniometer in Figure 8-6, *B*, is radiopaque and can be used during x-ray examinations. The notched dial allows an accurate reading of the motion regardless of whether the convexity of the half circle is directed toward or away from the direction of motion. The finger goniometer in Figure 8-6, *D*, has short, flattened arms designed to be used over the finger joint surfaces rather than along their sides. Small plastic goniometers are shown in Figure 8-6, *C* and *E*. These are inexpensive and easy to carry. The longer one can be used with both large and small joints. The dials of both goniometers are transparent and are marked and notched in two places similar to the goniometer in *B*. The smaller of these two goniometers is simply a larger one that has been cut to be adapted as a finger goniometer.

Other goniometers use fluid with a free-floating bubble that provides the reading after the motion is

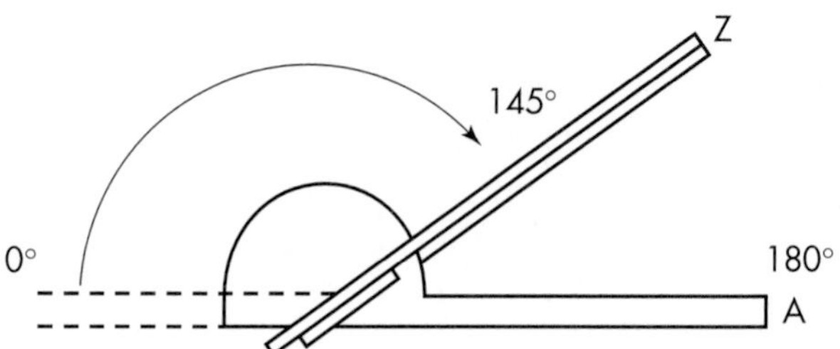


*Figure 8-5* Universal goniometer measuring 145°, using the 180° joint measurement system. Point *A* represents the stationary bar and *Z* the movable bar.

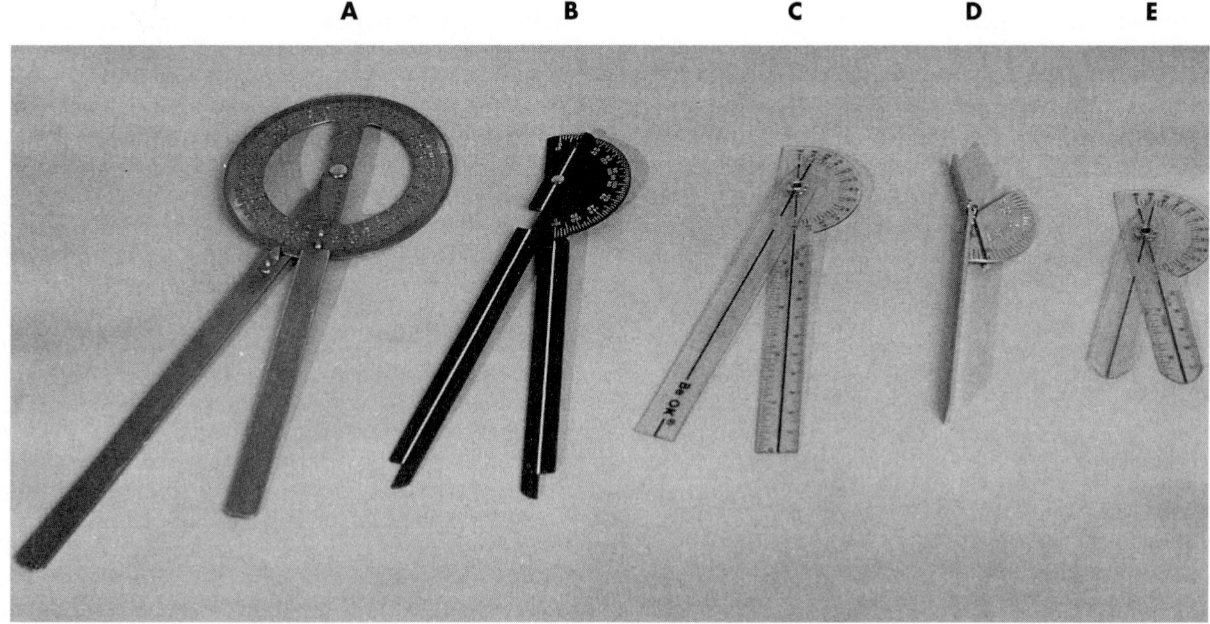


*Figure 8-6* Types of goniometers.

completed. Digital types have an LCD readout. Others can be attached to a body segment and have dials that register rotary motions, such as pronation and supination.

## RECORDING MEASUREMENT RESULTS

The occupational therapy practitioner records ROM testing results using a form similar to that shown in Figure 8-7. Table 8-1 lists average normal ranges of motion using the 180° method. The practitioner must remember that these ranges are only representative. Often the patient's unaffected extremity provides the closest approximation of what is normal for that individual. The following simple rules of thumb should clarify situations that arise during measurement:

1. Alternate methods of recording ROM are possible, and the OT practitioner should adapt to the method required by the facility.[4]

*Table 8-1*

### Average Normal Range of Motion (ROM) (180° Method)

| *Joint* | *ROM* | *Associated girdle motion* |
|---|---|---|
| **Cervical spine** | | |
| Flexion | 0° to 45° | — |
| Extension | 0° to 45° | — |
| Lateral flexion | 0° to 45° | — |
| Rotation | 0° to 60° | — |
| **Thoracic and lumbar spine** | | |
| Flexion | 0° to 80° | — |
| Extension | 0° to 30° | — |
| Lateral flexion | 0° to 40° | — |
| Rotation | 0° to 45° | — |
| **Shoulder** | | |
| Flexion | 0° to 170° | Abduction, lateral tilt, slight elevation, slight upward rotation |
| Extension | 0° to 60° | Depression, adduction, upward tilt |
| Abduction | 0° to 170° | Upward rotation, elevation |
| Adduction | 0° | Depression, adduction, downward rotation |
| Horizontal abduction | 0° to 40° | Adduction, reduction of lateral tilt |
| Horizontal adduction | 0° to 130° | Abduction, lateral tilt |
| Internal rotation | | Abduction, lateral tilt |
| Arm in abduction | 0° to 70° | — |
| Arm in adduction | 0° to 60° | — |
| External rotation | | |
| Arm in abduction | 0° to 90° | — |
| Arm in adduction | 0° to 80° | — |
| **Elbow** | | |
| Flexion | 0° to 135°-150° | — |
| Extension | 0° | — |
| **Forearm** | | |
| Pronation | 0° to 80°-90° | — |
| Supination | 0° to 80°-90° | — |

| *Joint* | *ROM* |
|---|---|
| **Wrist** | |
| Flexion | 0° to 80° |
| Extension | 0° to 70° |
| Ulnar deviation (adduction) | 0° to 30° |
| Radial deviation (abduction) | 0° to 20° |
| **Thumb*** | |
| DIP flexion | 0° to 80°-90° |
| MP flexion | 0° to 50° |
| Adduction, radial and palmar | 0° |
| Palmar abduction | 0° to 50° |
| Radial abduction | 0° to 50° |
| Opposition | |
| **Fingers*** | |
| MP flexion | 0° to 90° |
| MP hyperextension | 0° to 15°-45° |
| PIP flexion | 0° to 110° |
| DIP flexion | 0° to 80° |
| Abduction | 0° to 25° |
| **Hip** | |
| Flexion | 0° to 120° (bent knee) |
| Extension | 0° to 30° |
| Abduction | 0° to 40° |
| Adduction | 0° to 35° |
| Internal rotation | 0° to 45° |
| External rotation | 0° to 45° |
| **Knee** | |
| Flexion | 0° to 135° |
| **Ankle and foot** | |
| Plantar flexion | 0° to 50° |
| Dorsiflexion | 0° to 15° |
| Inversion | 0° to 35° |
| Eversion | 0° to 20° |

Data from American Academy of Orthopaedic Surgeons: *Joint motion: method of measuring and recording,* Chicago, 1965, The Academy; and Esch D, Lepley M: *Evaluation of joint motion: methods of measurement and recording,* Minneapolis, 1974, University of Minnesota Press.
**DIP,* Distal interphalangeal; *MP,* metacarpophalangeal; *PIP,* proximal interphalangeal.

JOINT RANGE MEASUREMENTS

Patient's name ______________________ Chart no. __________

Date of birth ______________________ Age __________ Sex __________

Diagnosis ______________________ Date of onset __________

Disability ______________________

| LEFT | | | | | RIGHT | | |
|---|---|---|---|---|---|---|---|
| 3 | 2 | 1 | SPINE | | 1 | 2 | 3 |
| | | | Cervical spine | | | | |
| | | | Flexion | 0 to 45 | | | |
| | | | Extension | 0 to 45 | | | |
| | | | Lateral flexion | 0 to 45 | | | |
| | | | Rotation | 0 to 60 | | | |
| | | | Thoracic and lumbar spine | | | | |
| | | | Flexion | 0 to 80 | | | |
| | | | Extension | 0 to 30 | | | |
| | | | Lateral flexion | 0 to 40 | | | |
| | | | Rotation | 0 to 45 | | | |
| | | | SHOULDER | | | | |
| | | | Flexion | 0 to 170 | | | |
| | | | Extension | 0 to 60 | | | |
| | | | Abduction | 0 to 170 | | | |
| | | | Horizontal abduction | 0 to 40 | | | |
| | | | Horizontal adduction | 0 to 130 | | | |
| | | | Internal rotation | 0 to 70 | | | |
| | | | External rotation | 0 to 90 | | | |
| | | | ELBOW AND FOREARM | | | | |
| | | | Flexion | 0 to 135-150 | | | |
| | | | Supination | 0 to 80-90 | | | |
| | | | Pronation | 0 to 80-90 | | | |
| | | | WRIST | | | | |
| | | | Flexion | 0 to 80 | | | |
| | | | Extension | 0 to 70 | | | |
| | | | Ulnar deviation | 0 to 30 | | | |
| | | | Radial deviation | 0 to 20 | | | |
| | | | THUMB | | | | |
| | | | MP flexion | 0 to 50 | | | |
| | | | IP flexion | 0 to 80-90 | | | |
| | | | Abduction | 0 to 50 | | | |
| | | | FINGERS | | | | |
| | | | MP flexion | 0 to 90 | | | |
| | | | MP hyperextension | 0 to 15-45 | | | |
| | | | PIP flexion | 0 to 110 | | | |
| | | | DIP flexion | 0 to 80 | | | |
| | | | Abduction | 0 to 25 | | | |
| | | | HIP | | | | |
| | | | Flexion | 0 to 120 | | | |
| | | | Extension | 0 to 30 | | | |
| | | | Abduction | 0 to 40 | | | |
| | | | Adduction | 0 to 35 | | | |
| | | | Internal rotation | 0 to 45 | | | |
| | | | External rotation | 0 to 45 | | | |
| | | | KNEE | | | | |
| | | | Flexion | 0 to 135 | | | |
| | | | ANKLE AND FOOT | | | | |
| | | | Plantar flexion | 0 to 50 | | | |
| | | | Dorsiflexion | 0 to 15 | | | |
| | | | Inversion | 0 to 35 | | | |
| | | | Eversion | 0 to 20 | | | |

*Figure 8-7* Form for recording joint ROM measurements.

2. A limitation in ROM is indicated when the start position is not 0°. Examples are (1) extension limitation at elbow joint 15° to 140° and (2) abnormal hyperextension of elbow joint –20° to 140°.
3. Glenohumeral mobility depends greatly on scapular mobility. If the scapular musculature is spastic, contracted, or orthopedically restricted, glenohumeral ROM will be affected.
4. When joint measurements may be performed in more than one position (e.g., shoulder internal and external rotation), the practitioner should note the position used on the ROM form.
5. The practitioner should observe and proceed with caution when spasticity, pain, or abnormal pathology is present.
6. Range of motion measurements are usually indicated in 5° increments. For example, if elbow flexion measures 0° to 128°, it would be recorded as 0° to 130°. Similarly, if elbow flexion is 0° to 122°, it would be recorded as 0° to 120°.

## JOINT LIMITATION AND DISEASE PROCESSES

An individual may develop joint limitations for a variety of reasons. A person with CVA might have spasticity that restricts range of motion. Individuals with significant burn injuries often develop skin adhesions and scar formation that decrease joint movement. Trauma and disease processes such as rheumatoid arthritis mechanically restrict ROM.

Future loss of ROM is expected in the course of many disease processes. Treatment planning must incorporate measures to maintain ROM for as long as possible. For example, arthritis can lead to joint stiffness and deformity. A primary therapeutic objective would be to preserve function through the use of splints, positioning, exercise, joint protection principles, and use of assistive devices.

A variety of exercises and activities can be incorporated into a therapy program to increase ROM. Active and passive stretching, resistive exercise, and exercises using equipment such as pulleys can play a significant part. Functional activities such as reaching, catching a ball, table-top activities, and throwing a bean bag can be incorporated into the therapy program. Whatever the approach, the OT practitioner should be creative and ingenious in developing enjoyable activities that increase ROM to increase function.

## PROCEDURE FOR JOINT MEASUREMENT

The illustrations that accompany the directions for measurement of each motion in the next section show both goniometer placement and general orientation of the examiner in relationship to the patient. In most cases the examiner is squared off directly with the patient so that the examiner can position the goniometer and read the result.

The way the examiner holds the goniometer and supports the part being measured is determined by factors such as degree of muscle weakness, presence or absence of joint pain, and whether passive or active range of motion is being measured. The examiner and patient should be positioned to ensure the greatest degree of comfort, correct placement of the goniometer, and adequate stabilization of the part being measured in correct anatomical plane of movement.

Box 8-1 lists principles for practitioners performing ROM testing that can be applied to the following section on measurement of upper extremity motions. The measurement section indicates the starting position and "normal" final position. Practitioners should record the *patient's* final position on the form.

## PROCEDURES FOR GONIOMETRIC MEASUREMENT AND TESTING OF SELECTED UPPER EXTREMITY MOTIONS

### Shoulder

***Flexion: 0° to 170° (Figure 8-8)***

*Position of subject:* Seated or supine with humerus in neutral position.

*Position of goniometer:* Axis is center of humerus just distal to acromion process on lateral aspect of hu-

*Box 8-1*

**Basic Principles for Range of Motion (ROM) Testing**

1. Have the patient comfortable and relaxed in testing position.
2. Explain and demonstrate the what, why, and how of goniometry to the patient.
3. Establish body landmarks for the measurement.
4. Stabilize joints proximal to the joint being measured.
5. Move the part passively through ROM to estimate available ROM and "get a feel" for joint mobility.
6. Return the part to the starting position.
7. At the starting position, place the axis of the goniometer over the axis of the joint. Place the stationary bar on the proximal or stationary bone and the movable bar on the distal or moving bone.
8. Record the number of degrees at the starting position.
9. Depending on what type of measurement is being taken (AROM or PROM), move or have the patient move the part to obtain the measurement desired (e.g., shoulder flexion).
10. Reposition the movable arm of the goniometer, checking that the axis is still accurately placed, and note the number of degrees at final position.
11. Record the reading to the nearest 5°, and make any other appropriate notations on the form (e.g., pain, crepitation).

merus. Stationary bar is parallel to trunk, and movable bar is parallel to humerus.

*Direction of movement:* Patient's arm is raised in front of body in a sagittal plane of movement.

### Extension: 0° to 60° (Figure 8-9)

*Position of subject:* Seated or prone, with no obstruction behind humerus. Humerus is in neutral position.

*Position of goniometer:* Same as for shoulder flexion.

*Direction of movement:* Patient's arm is to be brought in back of the body in a sagittal plane of movement. Excessive scapular motion should be avoided.

### Abduction: 0° to 170° (Figure 8-10)

*Position of subject:* Seated or prone with humerus in adduction and external rotation.

*Position of goniometer:* Axis is on acromion process on posterior surface of shoulder. Stationary bar is parallel to trunk, and movable bar is parallel to humerus.

*Direction of movement:* Patient's arm is raised to side of body in a frontal plane of movement.

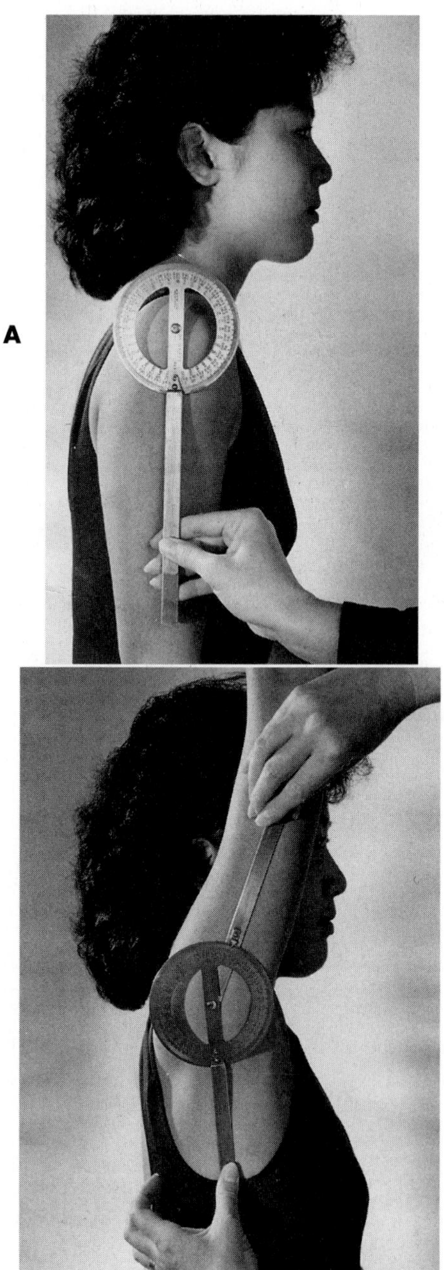


*Figure 8-8* Shoulder flexion. **A,** Starting position. **B,** Final position.

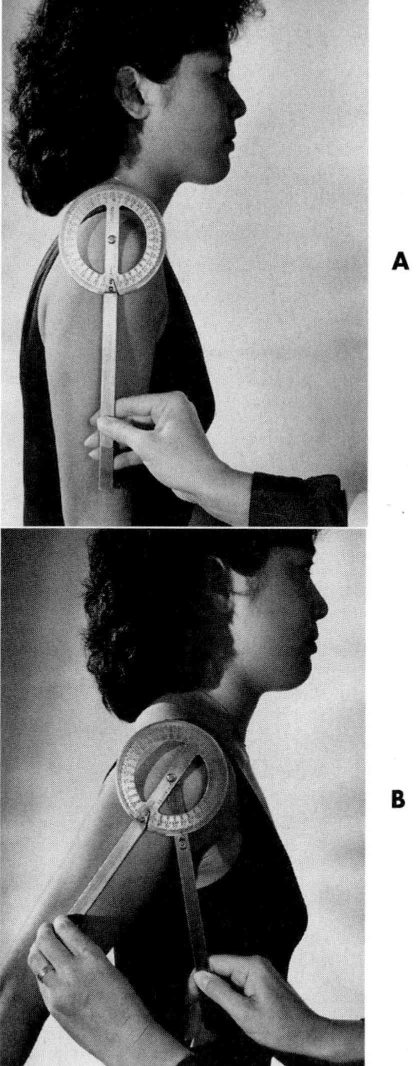


*Figure 8-9* Shoulder extension. **A,** Starting position. **B,** Final position.

***Internal Rotation: 0° to 60° (Figure 8-11)***

*Position of subject:* Seated with humerus adducted against trunk, elbow at 90°, and forearm in midposition and perpendicular to body.

*Position of goniometer:* Axis is on olecranon process of elbow, and stationary bar and movable bar are parallel to forearm.

*Direction of movement:* Patient's forearm is swung toward body through a horizontal plane of movement. Humerus must remain adducted.

***Internal Rotation: 0° to 70° (Figure 8-12)***

(Alternate position: Used in some practice settings or as preference of supervising occupational therapist.)

*Position of subject:* Seated or supine with humerus abducted to 90° and elbow flexed to 90°.

*Position of goniometer:* Axis is on olecranon process of elbow, and stationary bar and movable bar are parallel to forearm.

*Direction of movement:* Patient's forearm is swung down gently, keeping humerus parallel to floor.

***External Rotation: 0° to 80° (Figure 8-13)***

*Position of subject:* Humerus adducted, elbow at 90°, and forearm in midposition, perpendicular to body.

*Position of goniometer:* Axis is on olecranon of elbow, and stationary bar and movable bar are parallel to forearm.

*Direction of movement:* Patient's forearm is swung out from body through a horizontal plane of movement. Humerus must remain adducted.

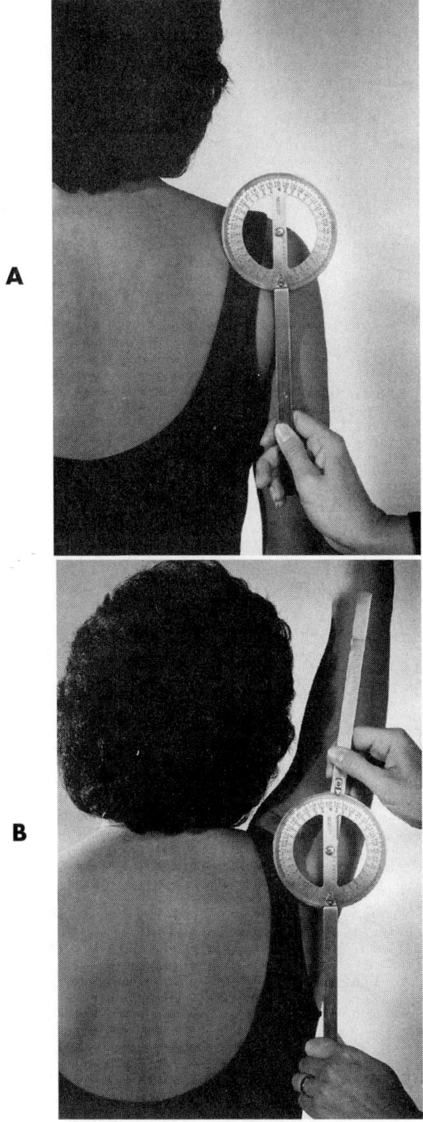


*Figure 8-10* Shoulder abduction. **A,** Starting position. **B,** Final position.

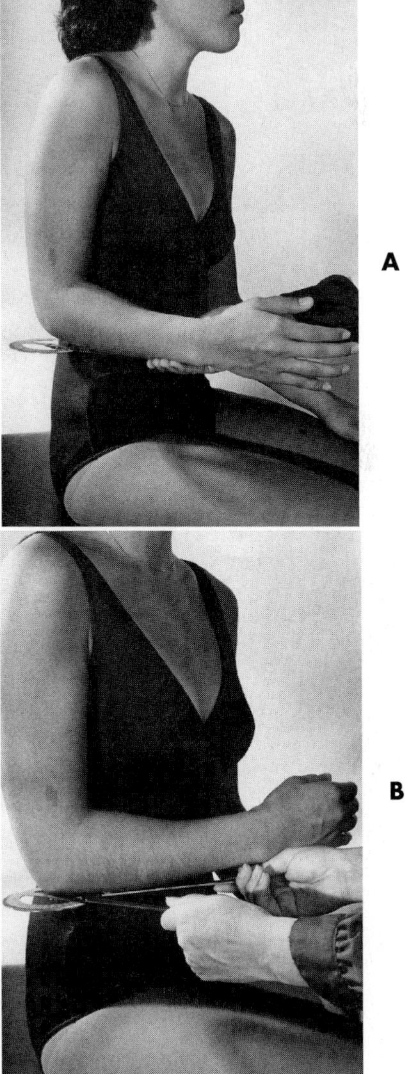


*Figure 8-11* Shoulder internal rotation. **A,** Starting position. **B,** Final position.

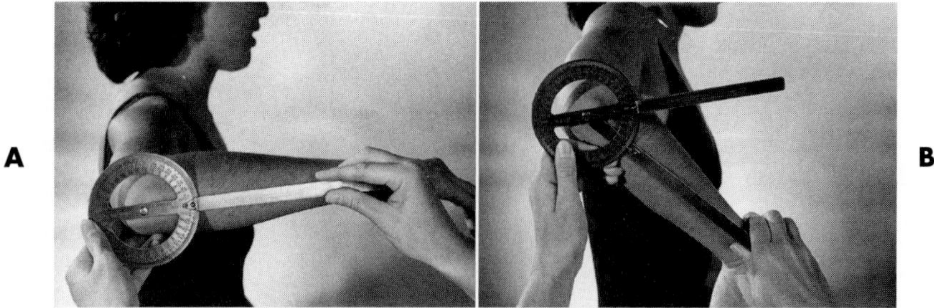

*Figure 8-12* Shoulder internal rotation, alternate position. **A,** Starting position. **B,** Final position.

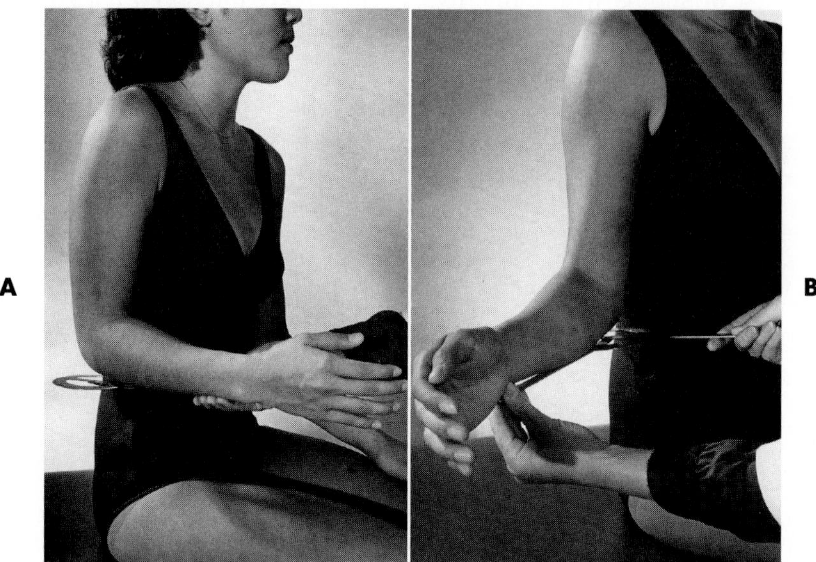

*Figure 8-13* Shoulder external rotation. **A,** Starting position. **B,** Final position.

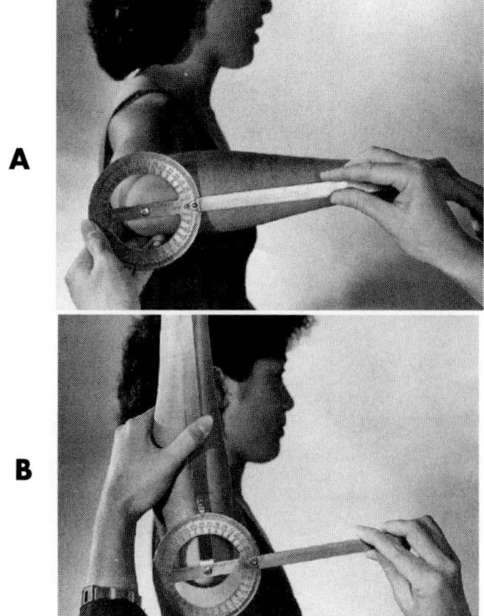

*Figure 8-14* Shoulder external rotation, alternate position. **A,** Starting position. **B,** Final position.

***External Rotation: 0° to 90° (Figure 8-14)***

(Alternate position: Used in some practice settings or as preference of supervising occupational therapist.)

*Position of subject:* Seated or supine with humerus abducted to 90°, elbow flexed to 90°, and forearm pronated.

*Position of goniometer:* Axis is on olecranon process of elbow, and stationary bar and movable bar are parallel to forearm.

*Direction of movement:* Patient's forearm is swung up gently, keeping humerus parallel to floor.

### Elbow

***Extension to Flexion: 0° to 135°-150° (Figure 8-15)***

*Position of subject:* Standing, sitting, or supine with humerus adducted and externally rotated and forearm supinated.

*Position of goniometer:* Axis is placed over lateral epicondyle of humerus at end of elbow crease. Stationary bar is parallel to midline of humerus, and movable bar is parallel to radius.

*Direction of movement:* Patient's forearm begins in

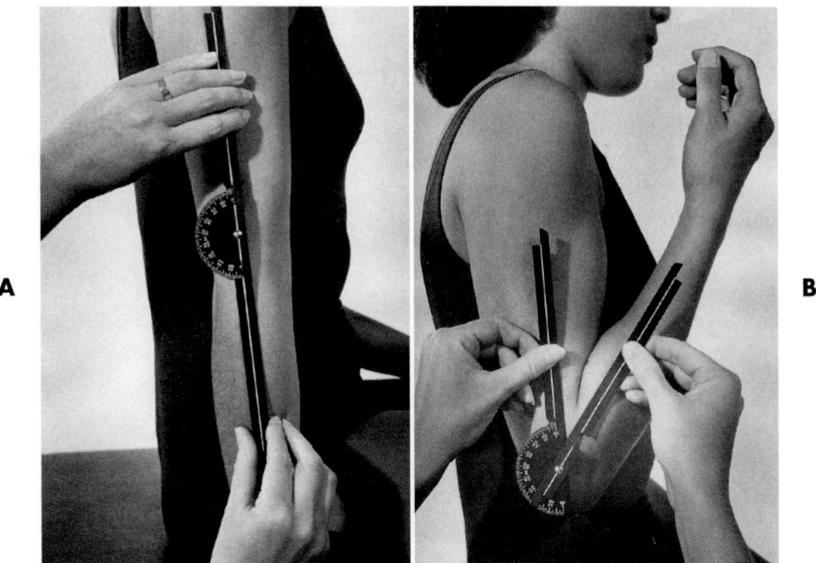


*Figure 8-15* Elbow flexion. **A,** Starting position. **B,** Final position.

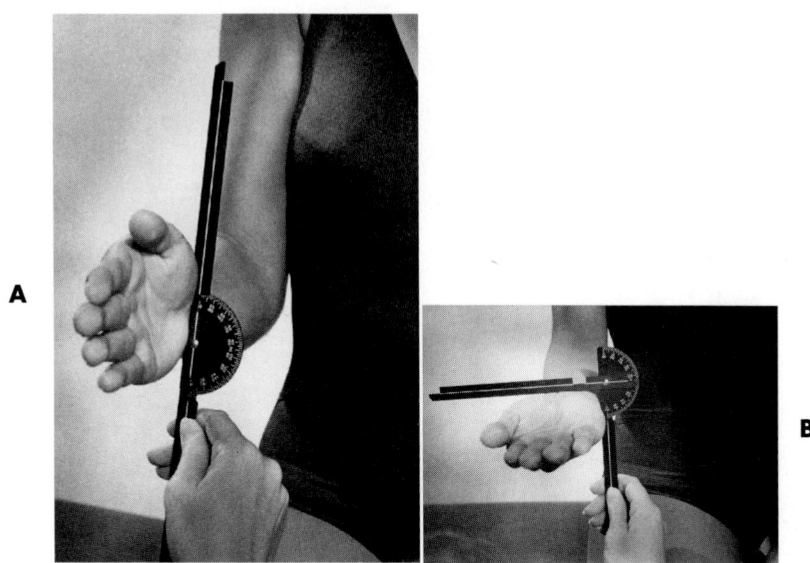


*Figure 8-16* Forearm supination. **A,** Starting position. **B,** Final position.

extended position and is raised in a sagittal plane of movement.

### Forearm

***Supination: 0° to 80°-90° (Figure 8-16)***

*Position of subject:* Seated or standing with humerus adducted, elbow at 90°, and forearm in midposition.

*Position of goniometer:* Axis is at ulnar border of volar aspect of wrist, just proximal to ulna styloid. Stationary bar is perpendicular to the floor, and movable bar is resting against volar aspect of wrist.

*Direction of movement:* Patient's forearm is rotated laterally around ulna.

***Supination: 0° to 80°-90° (Figure 8-17)***

(Alternate position: Used in some practice settings or as preference of supervising occupational therapist.)

*Position of subject:* Seated or standing with humerus adducted, elbow at 90°, and forearm in midposition. A pencil is placed in subject's hand so that it is held perpendicular to floor.

*Position of goniometer:* Axis is over midshaft of third

proximal phalanx. Stationary bar is perpendicular to floor, and movable bar overlays shaft of pencil.

*Direction of movement:* Patient's forearm is rotated laterally around the ulna.

***Pronation: 0° to 80°-90° (Figure 8-18)***

*Position of subject:* Seated or standing with humerus adducted, elbow at 90°, and forearm in midposition.

*Position of goniometer:* Axis is at ulnar border of dorsal aspect of wrist, just proximal to ulna styloid. Stationary bar is perpendicular to floor, and movable bar is resting against dorsal aspect of wrist.

*Direction of movement:* Patient's forearm is rotated medially around ulna.

***Pronation: 0° to 80°-90° (Figure 8-19)***

(Alternate position: Used in some practice settings or as preference of supervising occupational therapist.)

*Position of subject:* Seated or standing with humerus adducted, elbow at 90°, and forearm in midposition. A

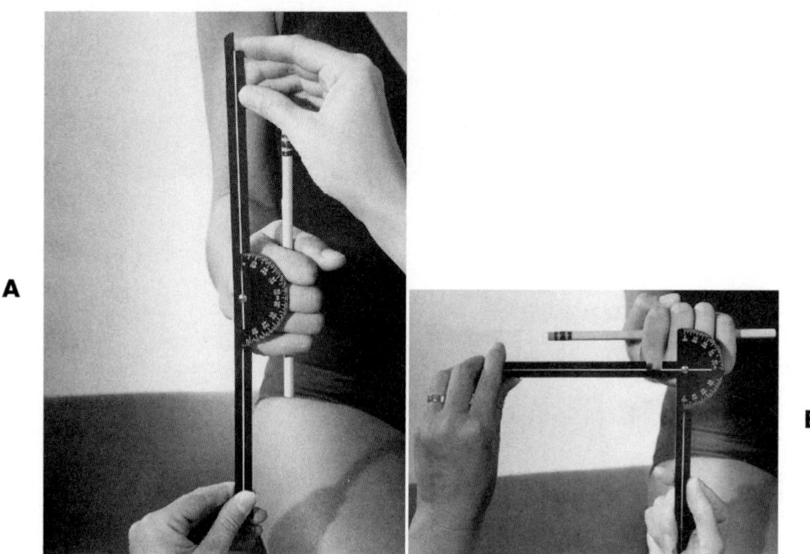


*Figure 8-17* Forearm supination, alternate position. **A,** Starting position. **B,** Final position.

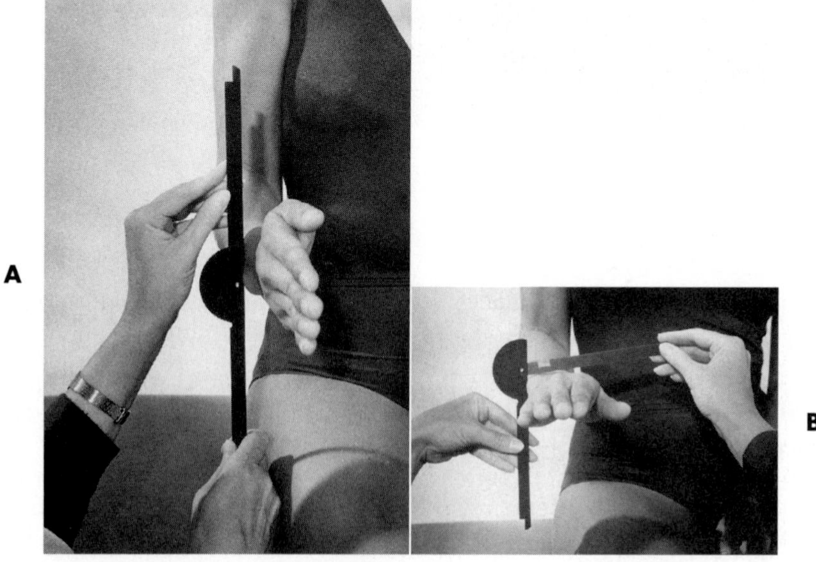


*Figure 8-18* Forearm pronation. **A,** Starting position. **B,** Final position.

pencil is placed in subject's hand so that it is held perpendicular to floor.

*Position of goniometer:* Axis is over third proximal phalanx. Stationary bar is perpendicular to floor, and movable bar overlays shaft of pencil.

*Direction of movement:* Patient's forearm is rotated medially around ulna.

### Wrist

***Flexion: 0° to 80° (Figure 8-20)***

*Position of subject:* Seated with forearm in midposition and hand and forearm resting on table on ulnar border.

*Position of goniometer:* Axis is on lateral aspect of wrist just distal to radial styloid in anatomical snuffbox. Stationary bar is parallel to radius, and movable bar is parallel to metacarpal of index finger.

*Direction of movement:* Patient's hand is flexed down so that palm moves closer to volar aspect of forearm.

***Extension: 0° to 70° (Figure 8-21)***

*Position of subject:* Same as for wrist flexion except fingers should be flexed.

*Position of goniometer:* Same as for wrist flexion.

*Direction of movement:* Patient's hand is raised up so that back of hand moves closer to dorsal aspect of forearm.

***Ulnar Deviation: 0° to 30° (Figure 8-22)***

*Position of subject:* Seated with forearm pronated and palm of hand resting flat on table surface. Goniometer is positioned so that the third finger lines up with center of forearm.

*Position of goniometer:* Axis is on dorsum of wrist at base of third metacarpal. Stationary bar is positioned in center of forearm, and movable bar is parallel to third metacarpal.

*Direction of movement:* Patient's hand is laterally extended in a horizontal plane of movement.

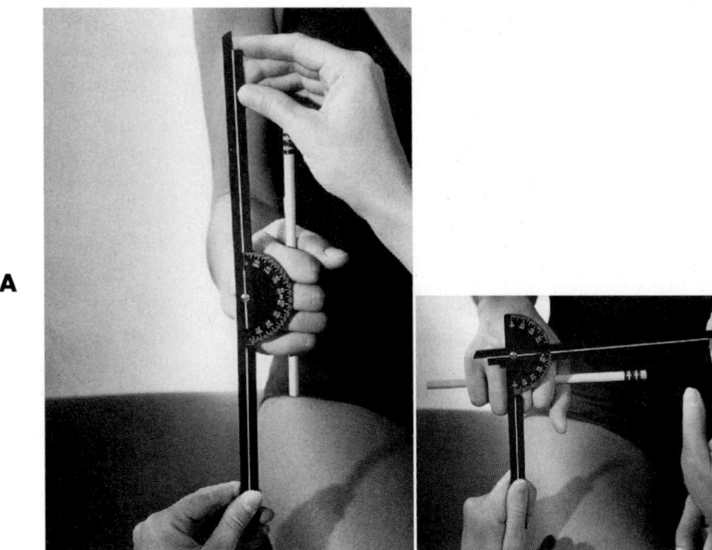


*Figure 8-19* Forearm pronation, alternate position. **A,** Starting position. **B,** Final position.

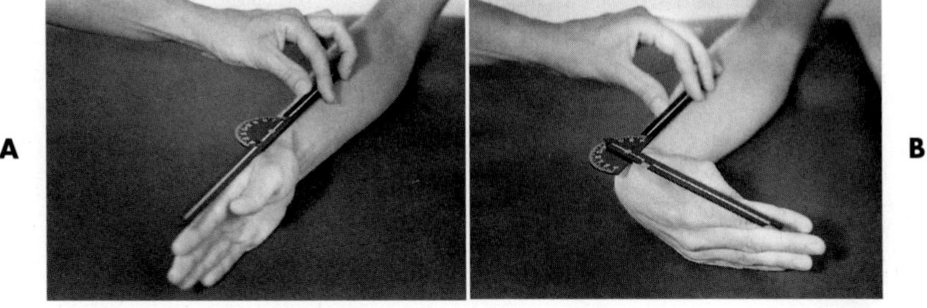


*Figure 8-20* Wrist flexion. **A,** Starting position. **B,** Final position.

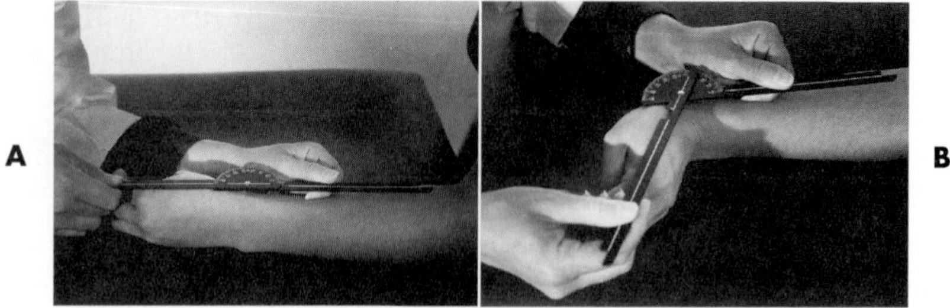


*Figure 8-21* Wrist extension. **A,** Starting position. **B,** Final position.

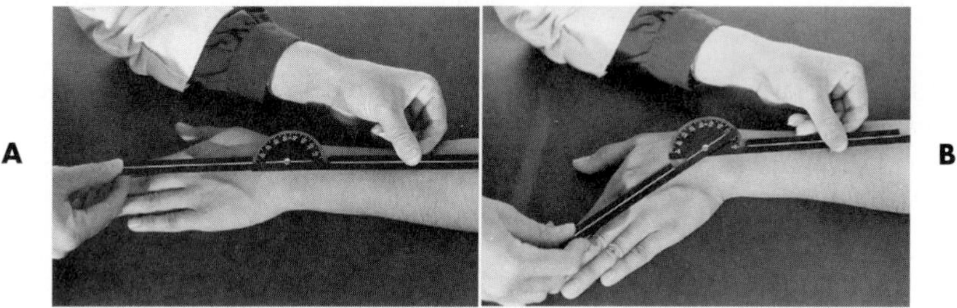


*Figure 8-22* Wrist ulnar deviation. **A,** Starting position. **B,** Final position.

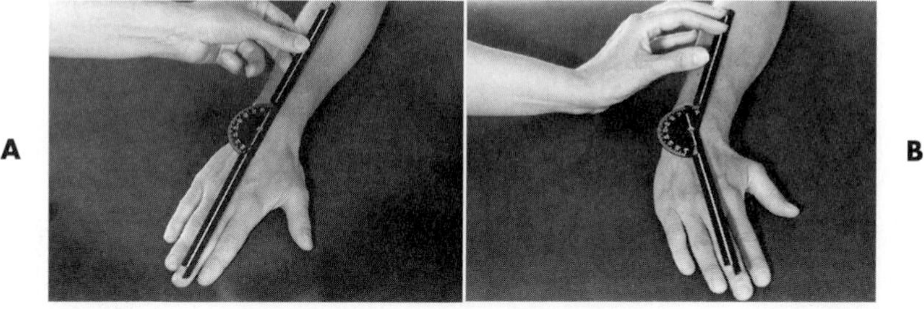


*Figure 8-23* Wrist radial deviation. **A,** Starting position. **B,** Final position.

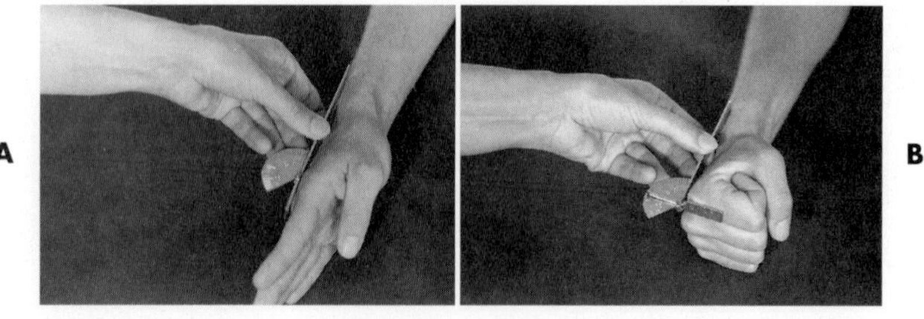


*Figure 8-24* MP flexion. **A,** Starting position. **B,** Final position.

### *Radial Deviation: 0° to 20° (Figure 8-23)*

*Position of subject and goniometer:* Same as for ulnar deviation.

*Direction of movement:* Patient's hand is medially extended in a horizontal plane of movement.

## Fingers

### *Metacarpophalangeal (MP) Flexion: 0° to 90° (Figure 8-24)*

*Position of subject:* Seated with forearm in midposition, wrist at 0° neutral, and forearm and hand supported on a firm surface on ulnar border.

*Position of goniometer:* Axis is centered on top of middle of MP joint. Stationary bar is on top of metacarpal, and movable bar is on top of proximal phalanx.

*Direction of movement:* Patient's finger distal of MP joint is flexed down in a sagittal plane.

### *MP Hyperextension: 0° to 15°-45° (Figure 8-25)*

*Position of subject:* Seated with forearm in midposition, wrist at 0° neutral, and forearm and hand supported on a firm surface on ulnar border.

*Position of goniometer:* Axis is over lateral aspect of MP joint of index finger. Stationary bar is parallel to metacarpal, and movable bar is parallel to proximal phalanx. MP joint of fifth finger may be measured similarly. ROM of third and fourth fingers can be estimated by comparison.

*Direction of movement:* Patient's finger distal of MP joint is extended up in a sagittal plane of movement.

### *Proximal Interphalangeal (PIP) Flexion: 0° to 110° (Figure 8-26)*

*Position of subject:* Seated with forearm in midposition, wrist at 0° neutral, and forearm and hand supported on a firm surface on ulnar border.

*Position of goniometer:* Axis is centered on dorsal surface of PIP joint being measured. Stationary bar is placed over proximal phalanx, and movable bar is over middle phalanx.

*Direction of movement:* Patient's finger distal of PIP joint is flexed down in a sagittal plane of movement.

### *Distal Interphalangeal (DIP) Flexion: 0° to 80° (Figure 8-27)*

*Position of subject:* Seated with forearm in midposition, wrist at 0° neutral, and forearm and hand supported on a firm surface on ulnar border.

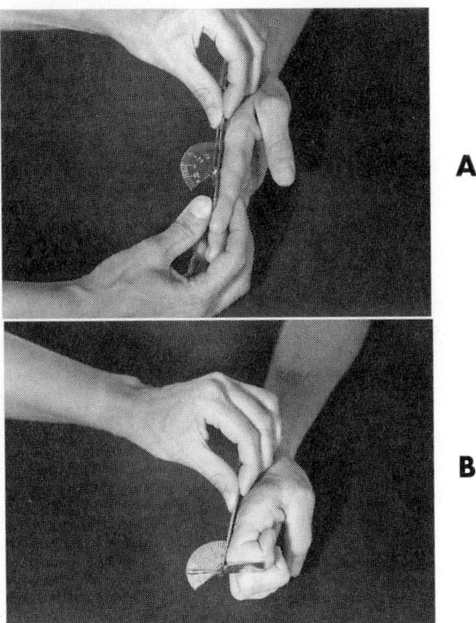


*Figure 8-26* PIP flexion. **A,** Starting position. **B,** Final position.

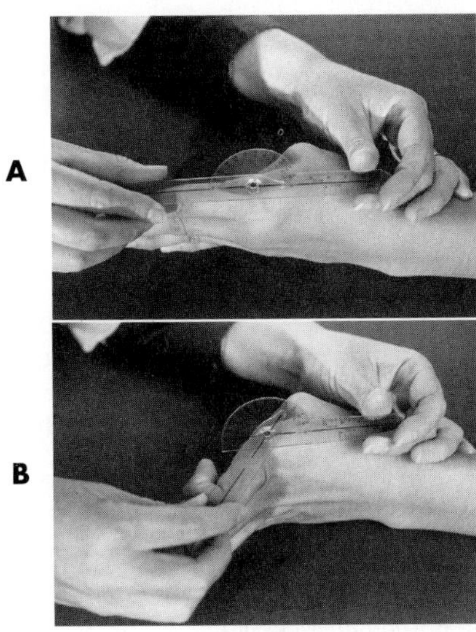


*Figure 8-25* MP hyperextension. **A,** Starting position. **B,** Final position.

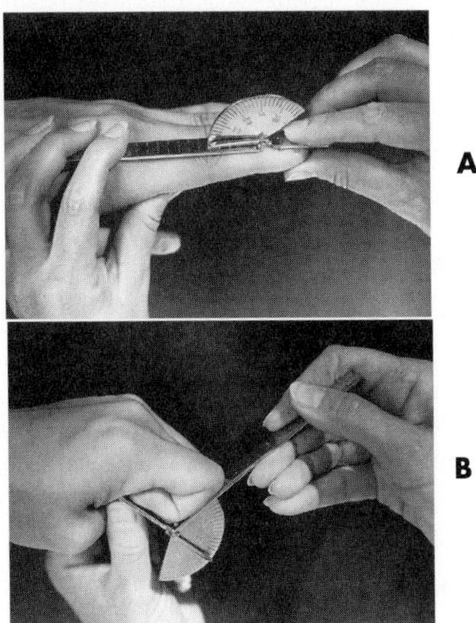


*Figure 8-27* DIP flexion. **A,** Starting position. **B,** Final position.

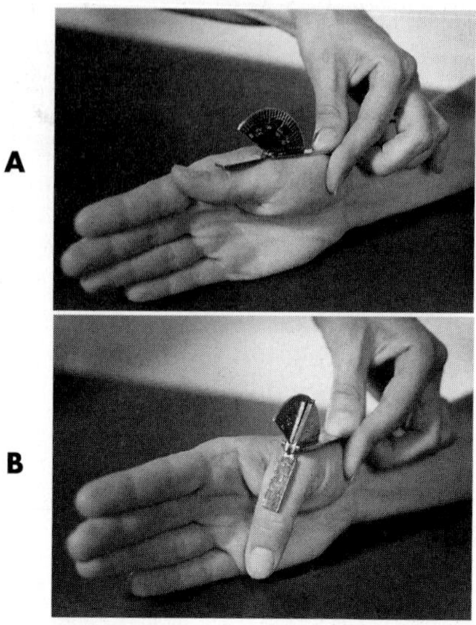


*Figure 8-28* Thumb MP flexion. **A,** Starting position. **B,** Final position.

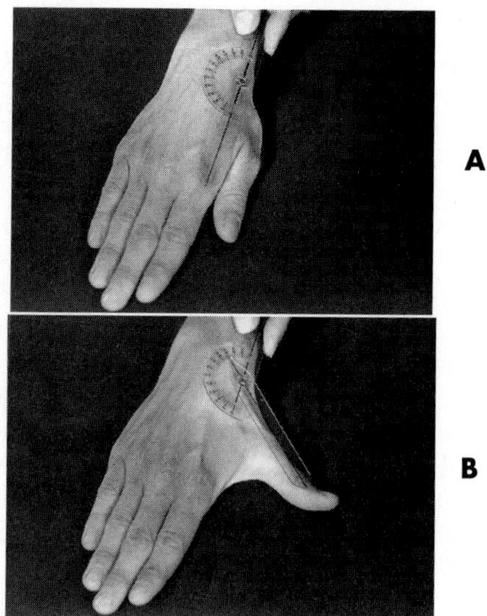


*Figure 8-30* Thumb radial abduction. **A,** Starting position. **B,** Final position.

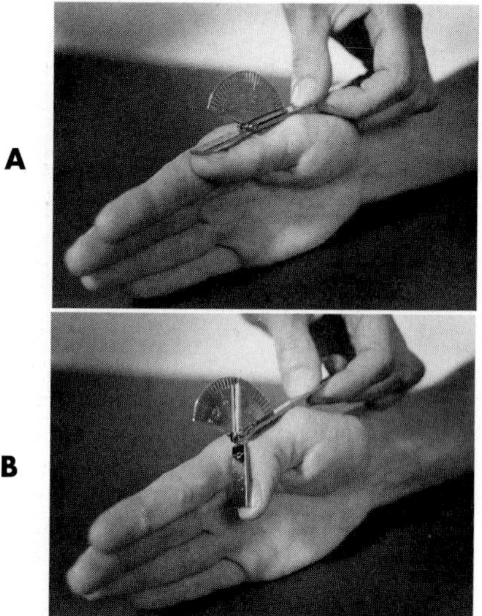


*Figure 8-29* Thumb IP flexion. **A,** Starting position. **B,** Final position.

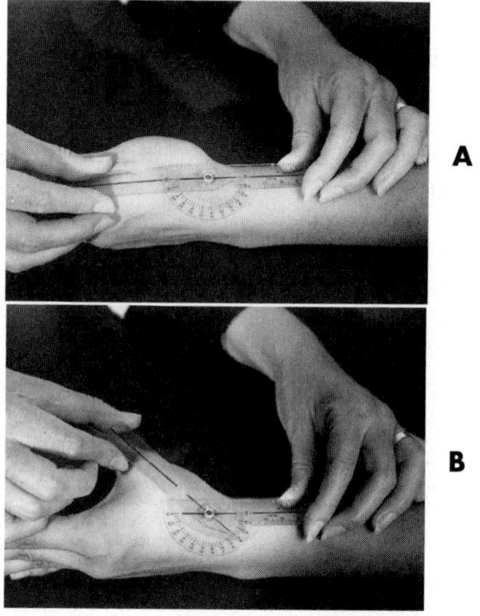


*Figure 8-31* Thumb palmar abduction. **A,** Starting position. **B,** Final position.

*Position of goniometer:* Axis is on dorsal surface of DIP joint. Stationary bar is over middle phalanx, and movable bar is over distal phalanx.

*Direction of movement:* Patient's finger distal of DIP joint is flexed down in a sagittal plane of movement.

## Thumb

### *MP Flexion: 0° to 50° (Figure 8-28)*

*Position of subject:* Seated with forearm in 45° of supination, wrist at 0° neutral, and forearm and hand supported on a firm surface.

*Position of goniometer:* Axis is on dorsal surface of MP joint. Stationary bar is over thumb metacarpal, and movable bar is over proximal phalanx.

*Direction of movement:* Patient's thumb distal of MP joint is flexed down.

### *Interphalangeal (IP) Flexion: 0° to 80°-90° (Figure 8-29)*

*Position of subject:* Same as for PIP/DIP finger flexion.

*Position of goniometer:* Axis is on dorsal surface of IP joint. Stationary bar is over proximal phalanx, and movable bar is over distal phalanx.

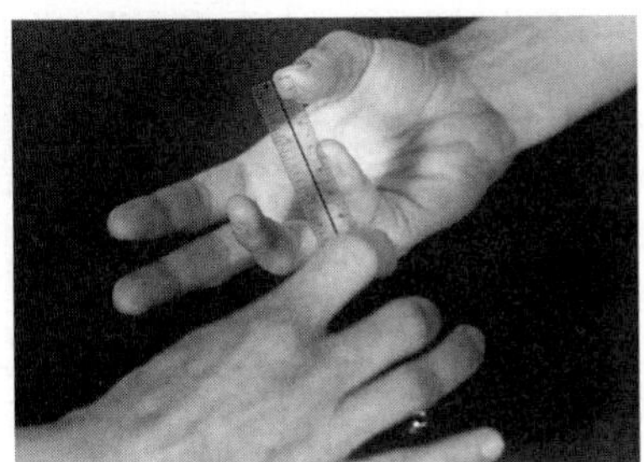

Figure 8-32 Thumb opposition to fifth finger.

*Direction of movement:* Patient's thumb distal of IP joint is flexed down.

### *Radial Abduction (Carpometacarpal [CMC] Extension): 0° to 50° (Figure 8-30)*

*Position of subject:* Seated with forearm pronated and hand palm down, resting flat on a firm surface.

*Position of goniometer:* Axis is over CMC joint at base of thumb metacarpal. Stationary bar is parallel to radius, and movable bar is parallel to thumb metacarpal.

*Direction of movement:* Patient's thumb is abducted in a horizontal plane of movement.

### *Palmar Abduction (CMC Flexion): 0° to 50° (Figure 8-31)*

*Position of subject:* Seated with forearm at 0° midposition, wrist at 0°, and forearm and hand resting on ulnar border. Thumb is rotated so that it is at right angles to palm of hand.

*Position of goniometer:* Axis is over CMC joint at base of thumb metacarpal. Stationary bar is over radius, and movable bar is over thumb metacarpal.

*Direction of movement:* Patient's thumb is abducted in a horizontal plane of movement while forearm is in midposition.

### *Thumb Opposition: (Figure 8-32)*

*Position of subject:* Seated with palmar aspect of hand exposed.

*Position of goniometer:* Distance between thumb and fifth finger pads is measured with a centimeter ruler.

*Direction of movement:* Patient's thumb and fifth digit are opposed to one another.

## SCREENING FOR FUNCTIONAL RANGE OF MOTION

**Functional range of motion** refers to the range needed to accomplish typical and ordinary daily life activities such as self-feeding, hygiene, dressing and grooming. This functional range is always less than the "normal" range given for standard measurements with a goniometer. There are many situations in which it is desirable to briefly screen a patient for functional ROM. If deficits are noted in the functional range then the standard evaluation of ROM can be used to obtain more information.

The procedure for testing functional ROM is generally demonstrated by the experienced clinician to the novice or the student on fieldwork (Box 8-2). The sequence and positioning may vary. For example, testing of forearm, wrist, and finger motions of subjects who do not have the strength to maintain shoulder abduction may be done with the forearms resting on a table top or the arms of a chair.

Box 8-2

### Brief Screening for Functional Range of Motion

S is generally seated, preferably in a chair without arms. For each of the bold-faced motions, E gives directions (in quotes) and should also demonstrate. Alternately, E may demonstrate, saying at the same time, "Do this."

**Trunk forward flexion and trunk extension:** "Reach down to your toes. Come back up."

**Trunk lateral flexion:** "Reach down to the floor on the left with your left hand. Come back up. Reach down to the floor on the right with your right hand. Come back up."

**Shoulder flexion:** "Raise your arms straight up in front of you as far as you can."

**Shoulder external rotation:** "Place your hands behind your neck."

**Shoulder internal rotation:** "Reach behind your back."

**Shoulder abduction:** "Raise your arms out to the side."

**Pronation and supination:** S keeps arms in shoulder abduction position and is instructed: "Turn your palms up. Now turn your palms down."

**Elbow flexion and extension:** S keeps arms in shoulder abduction position and is instructed: "Bend and straighten your elbows."

**Finger flexion and extension:** S keeps arms in shoulder abduction position and is instructed: "Make a fist and then straighten your fingers."

**Thumb opposition:** S keeps arms in shoulder abduction position and is instructed: "Touch the tip of your thumb to the tips of each of the other fingers."

**Wrist flexion and extension:** S keeps arms in shoulder abduction position and is instructed: "Bend your wrist up. Bend your wrist down."

**Wrist radial and ulnar deviation:** S places hands and forearms on lap or table top and is instructed: "Turn your hands out. Turn your hands in."

## Case Study

Mr. R., a retired automobile industry executive, recently fractured his right shoulder during a fall. Mr. R. was evaluated at an urgent care center. X-ray films revealed a nondisplaced fracture of the right proximal humerus. The physician ordered fabrication of a full cast, medications for pain, and a follow-up visit to the center. After 6 weeks, Mr. R. lacked independence in dressing his upper body and complained of pain around the elbow joint. The physician removed the cast and noted the following information in the medical record using the SOAP format (see Chapter 7):

**S/O:**

62 y/o, male, SP (R)Humeral fracture. Pt. c/o pain at elbow joint with generalized stiffness. Elbow ROM measurements show AROM 45°-135°, PROM 30°-150°. Strength is graded 4/5.

**A:**

Limited ROM and strength noted in right upper extremity ([R]UE) along with decreased ADLs (dressing).

**P:**

Occupational therapy 2 times per week × 2 weeks for assessment and treatment of (R)UE dysfunction.

Mr. R. was scheduled at a local occupational therapy clinic. After careful assessment, the OTR and COTA collaborated in developing the following course of treatment:

- PROM and AROM and progressive strength exercises for elbow extension
- Adaptive equipment (reacher and dressing stick)
- Functional activities such as bilateral reaching, balloon volleyball, and table-top activities
- Dynamic elbow extension splint for night use and overhead pulleys for clinic and home use.

After a 2-week course of therapy, Mr. R. had regained normal motion of his (R)UE, became independent in dressing, and was continuing a home program of general conditioning.

## SUMMARY

The medical profession has evolved to a point where positive *functional outcomes* are becoming the benchmark of sound clinical practice. The assessment process is the foundation that enables the occupational therapy practitioner to target the type and scope of therapy services specific to each patient's needs. The assessment of range of motion (ROM) cannot be based on "hunches" relative to the patient's deficits.

The measurement of ROM is an essential aspect of the assessment process. It documents objectively the biomechanical changes in joint mobility that result from trauma, disease, or aging. ROM measurement lays the foundation for documenting increases in function proportional to increases in joint ROM.

## Selected Reading Guide Questions

1. Describe upper extremity joint motions of the shoulder flexion, extension, external rotation, and internal rotation.
2. Identify major anatomical landmarks associated with joint measurements of elbow flexion and wrist flexion and extension.
3. Describe three types of functional activities that can increase range of motion in shoulder flexion.
4. List two medical conditions that can negatively influence range of motion in the upper extremity.
5. Describe why the evaluation of joint range of motion is an important assessment tool.
6. Describe how crepitation and discomfort can influence range of motion.
7. Describe the concept of *functional range of motion* as it relates to activities of daily living.
8. Contrast active and passive range of motion.
9. List the four components of a goniometer.
10. Explain why the occupational therapy practitioner records goniometric data in 5° increments. (HINT: Interrater reliability.)

### REFERENCES


1. American Academy of Orthopaedic Surgeons: *Joint motion: method of measuring and recording,* Chicago, 1965, The Academy.
2. American Occupational Therapy Association: The Association: clarification of the use of the terms assessment and evaluation, *Am J Occup Ther* 1072-1073, 1995.
3. American Occupational Therapy Association: *Effective documentation for occupational therapy,* Rockville, Md, 1992, The Association.
4. Asher IE: *An annotated index of occupational therapy evaluation tools,* Rockville, Md, 1989, The Association.
5. Cole T, Tobis J: Measurement of musculoskeletal function: goniometry. In Kottke FJ, Lehmann JF: *Krusen's handbook of physical medicine and rehabilitation,* ed 4, Philadelphia, 1990, Saunders.
6. Killingworth A: *Basic physical disability procedures,* San Jose, Calif, 1987, Maple.
7. McDonough JT, editor: *Stedman's concise medical dictionary,* ed 2, Williams & Wilkins.
8. Moore ML: Clinical assessment of joint motion. In Basmajian JV, editor: *Therapeutic exercise,* ed 3, 1978, Baltimore, Williams & Wilkins.
9. Norkin CC, White DJ: *Measurement of joint motion: a guide to goniometry,* ed 2, Philadelphia, 1995, Davis.
10. Pedretti LW: *Occupational therapy: practice skills for physical dysfunction,* ed 4, St Louis, 1995, Mosby.

Chapter 9

# Evaluation of Muscle Strength

*Lorraine Williams Pedretti*
*Michael K. Davis*

## Chapter Objectives

*After studying this chapter, the student or practitioner will be able to:*

1. Identify the six general purposes of muscle strength measurement.
2. Identify the three methods of evaluating muscle strength.
3. Discuss the relationship between joint range of motion and muscle strength measurement.
4. Define manual muscle testing.
5. Identify the four primary limitations of the manual muscle test.
6. Identify and describe the two primary factors influencing muscle function.
7. Identify and define the muscle grades.
8. Describe the six steps of the standard procedure for manual muscle testing.
9. Describe the *break test.*
10. Demonstrate muscle testing procedures for each of the upper extremity muscle groups, including positioning, stabilization, palpation, observation, and application of resistance.

## Key Terms

range of motion
passive range of motion
manual muscle test
muscle endurance
muscle coordination
palpation
hypertrophy
atrophy
resistance
gravity eliminated
substitution
muscle grades
break test

The human body is capable of infinitely complex and varied movements. Muscle strength is critical for these movements. The power for the human body comes from muscles as tiny as those that surround the eyes and others as massive as those in the legs.

Muscle function is the product of strength, endurance, and coordination. The manual muscle test allows the occupational therapy practitioner to assess, plan treatment, and perhaps predict functional changes in the musculoskeletal system.

Manual muscle testing can be approached in several ways. Simple observation of the patient interacting in the immediate environment allows the practitioner to note any obvious difficulties. However, a more precise assessment of muscle strength is often undertaken to assess primary conditions such as general debility, spinal cord injuries, Guillain-Barré syndrome, primary muscle and neurological disease processes, and traumatic conditions resulting from contractures, burns, amputation, arthritis, and fractures, as well as a variety of other orthopedic conditions.

Chapter 8 examined the movement aspect of the body. This chapter discusses the muscles, especially in relation to movement, and how muscle function affects the ability to perform activities of daily living (ADLs).

## ROLE OF THE OCCUPATIONAL THERAPY ASSISTANT IN EVALUATING MUSCLE STRENGTH

The extent of the certified occupational therapy assistant's (COTA's) involvement in data collection and measurement for muscle testing is determined by the supervising registered occupational therapist (OTR), with consideration of the applicable laws and professional practice standards of the particular state. In many clinical practices the COTA performs basic gross muscle testing of the upper extremity. The role of the COTA in this area should be based on demonstrated service competency and must be within the legislation and restrictions governing the practice setting. The American Occupational Therapy Association (AOTA) has defined *service competency* as whether the OTR and COTA can perform the same assessments or tests in the same manner and achieve the same results.

## LIMITATIONS RESULTING FROM MUSCLE WEAKNESS

Muscle weakness can restrict performance in self-care, vocational, leisure, and social activities. Documentation of strength limitations must be linked to function. The occupational therapy practitioner must assess and monitor the degree of improvement in strength as it relates to function, for example, in different aspects of ADLs, such as the ability to carry an object and sustain an activity over time.

Given good to normal endurance, the patient with good (G) to normal (N) muscle strength is able to perform all ordinary ADLs without undue fatigue.[7] The patient with fair plus (F+) muscle strength usually has low endurance and fatigues more easily than one with G or N strength. The patient is able to perform many ordinary ADLs independently but may require frequent rest periods. The patient with the muscle grade of fair (F) is able to move parts against gravity and perform light tasks that present little or no resistance.[4,7]

Low endurance is a significant problem and limits the amount of activity. It is generally accepted that for every day of hospitalization, 3 days are needed to recondition back to prehospitalization status. The patient with low endurance can probably feed finger foods and perform light self-hygiene but may do so slowly, requiring rest periods to reach the goals.[7] If muscle strength in the lower extremities is only F, ambulation is not possible.[4] Poor (P) strength is considered below functional range, but the patient can perform some ADLs with mechanical assistance, and **range of motion** (ROM) can be maintained independently.[4] Patients with muscle grades of trace (T) and zero (0) are completely dependent and can perform ADLs only with the aid of externally powered devices. Some activities are possible with special controls on equipment, such as electric wheelchairs, communication devices, and hand splints.[7]

## GENERAL PURPOSES OF MUSCLE STRENGTH MEASUREMENT

The evaluation of muscle strength helps the examiner to assess the strength of a given movement. The purposes for evaluating muscle strength are as follows[7]:

1. Determine the amount of muscle power available and thus establish a baseline for treatment.
2. Assess how muscle weakness is limiting performance of ADLs.
3. Prevent deformities that can result from imbalances of strength of agonist and antagonist muscles.
4. Determine the need for assistive devices to compensate for reduced strength.
5. Aid in the selection of activities within the patient's capabilities.
6. Evaluate the effectiveness of treatment.

## METHODS OF EVALUATION

As mentioned earlier, muscle strength can be evaluated in several ways. The most precise method is a test of individual muscles, as much as this is possible. In this procedure the muscle is carefully isolated through proper positioning, stabilization, and careful control of the movement pattern. This type of muscle testing, as described by Kendall and McCreary,[6] is not expected of COTAs.

A second and more practical means of measuring function is to assess the strength of groups of muscles that perform specific functions at individual joints, as initially described by Daniels and Worthingham.[4] A third way to evaluate muscle strength is by observing the performance of ordinary activities.[4] During an ADL performance evaluation, for example, the OT practitioner can note difficulties and movement patterns that may signal weakness, muscle imbalance, poor endurance for activity, or substitute motions. The ADL evaluation can be used together with muscle strength evaluation. The functional muscle test is often used to screen for general muscle strength.[9] The occupational therapy practitioner performs this screening and can assess effectiveness of treatment interventions based on the patient's gross improvements. *Functional muscle testing* is presented at the end of the chapter.

## RELATIONSHIP BETWEEN JOINT RANGE OF MOTION AND MUSCLE TESTING

One measure of muscle strength is the movement of the joint on which the muscle acts; that is, did the muscle move the joint through complete, partial, or no ROM? Another criterion is the amount of resistance that can be applied to the part once the muscle has moved the joint through available ROM. Available ROM is not necessarily the full average normal ROM for the given joint. Rather, it is the ROM available to the individual patient. When measuring joint motion (see Chapter 8) the **passive range of motion** (PROM) is the measure of the range available to the patient. PROM, however, is no indication of muscle strength.

The occupational therapy practitioner must know the patient's available PROM to assign muscle grades correctly. PROM may be limited or less than the average for a particular joint motion, but the muscle strength may be normal. For example, the patient's PROM for elbow flexion may be limited to 0° to 110° because of a previous fracture. If the patient can flex the elbow joint to 110° and hold against moderate resistance during the muscle test, the grade would be good (G). In such cases the examiner should record the limitation with the muscle grade, for example, 0° to 110°/G. If the patient's available ROM for elbow flexion is 0° to 140° and the patient can flex the elbow against gravity through 110°, the muscle would be graded fair minus (F–), since the part moved through only partial ROM against gravity.

## MANUAL MUSCLE TESTING

The **manual muscle test** is a means of measuring the maximal contraction of a muscle or muscle group. It is used to determine the amount of muscle power and to record gains and losses in strength. The muscle test is a primary evaluation tool for patients with lower motor neuron disorders, primary muscle diseases, and orthopedic dysfunction. The criteria used to measure strength are (1) evidence of muscle contraction, (2) amount of ROM through which the joint passes, and (3) amount of resistance against which the muscle can contract, including gravity as a form of resistance.[4]

### Limitations

The limitations of the manual muscle test are that it cannot measure **muscle endurance** (number of times the muscle can contract at its maximum level), **muscle coordination** (smooth, rhythmic interactions of muscle function), or motor performance capabilities of the patient (use of the muscles for functional activities).

The manual muscle test cannot be used accurately with patients who have spasticity caused by upper motor neuron disorders, such as cerebrovascular accident (CVA, stroke) and cerebral palsy, for the following reasons[3,5,8]:

1. In these disorders, muscles are often hypertonic.
2. Muscle tone and ability to perform movements are influenced by primitive reflexes and the position of the head and body in space.
3. Movements tend to occur in gross synergistic patterns (several muscles working together), which makes it impossible for the patient to isolate joint motion as demanded in manual muscle testing procedures.

### Examiner's Knowledge and Skill

Validity of the manual muscle test depends on the examiner's knowledge and skill in using the correct testing procedure. Careful observation of movement, careful and accurate **palpation** (detecting muscle activity by placing the fingers over the muscle), correct positioning, consistency of procedure, and the examiner's experience are critical factors in accurate testing.[4,6]

To be proficient in manual muscle testing, the examiner must have detailed knowledge about all aspects of muscle function. Joints and joint motions, muscle innervation, origin and insertion of muscles, action of muscles, direction of muscle fibers, angle of pull on the joints, and the role of muscles in fixation and substitution are important considerations. The examiner must be able to locate and palpate the muscles; recognize whether the contour of the muscle is normal, atrophied, or hypertrophied; and detect abnormal movements and positions. Knowledge and experience are necessary to detect substitutions and to interpret strength grades accurately.[6]

The examiner must acquire skill and experience in testing and grading muscles of normal persons of both genders and all ages. Some muscles in normal individuals may seem to be weak, but this may be normal for the particular person. Experience can help the examiner differentiate normal strength from slight muscle weakness if the subject's age, gender, body build, and lifestyle are taken into account.[9]

### General Principles

#### *Preparation*

The examiner should always perform a visual check to assess the general contour, comparative symmetry, and any apparent **hypertrophy** (overdevelopment) or **atrophy** (wasting away) of the muscle(s). When assessing the passive ROM, the examiner can estimate the muscle tone and determine resistance to that motion. During the active ROM the examiner can observe the quality of movement (speed, smoothness, rhythm, abnormal movements such as tremors).

#### *Positioning*

Correct positioning of the subject and body part is essential to effective and correct muscle evaluation. The subject should be positioned comfortably on a firm surface. It is common practice to test muscles with the subject seated or in a wheelchair. Clothing should be arranged or removed so that the examiner can see the muscle or muscle groups being tested. If this is not possible, the examiner must exercise clinical judgment in approximating muscle grades.[9] In addition, correct positioning, careful stabilization, and palpation of the muscle(s) and observation of movement are essential to test validity.[4]

## FACTORS INFLUENCING MUSCLE FUNCTION

### Gravity

Gravity provides **resistance** to muscle power.[6] It is used as a grading criterion in tests of the neck, trunk, and extremities. Therefore muscle grade must consider whether a muscle can move the part against gravity.[6]

Movements against gravity and applied resistance are performed in a vertical plane (i.e., moving up). Graded manual resistance is used with fair plus (F+) to normal (N) grades. Tests for weaker muscles (0, T, P, and P+ grades; see Table 9-1) are often performed in a horizontal plane (i.e., moving sideways). The term **gravity eliminated** is often used to describe this position of testing, which reduces the resistance to muscle power by eliminating the effect of gravity.

### Substitution

The brain "thinks" in terms of movement and not contraction of individual muscles.[4] Thus a muscle or muscle group may attempt to compensate for the function of a weaker muscle to accomplish the desired movement. This act of compensation is termed **substitution.**[6] To test the muscle or muscle group accurately, the examiner must eliminate substitutions in the testing procedure by correct positioning, stabilization, and palpation of the muscle being tested and careful performance of the test motion without extraneous movements. The correct body position should be maintained and movement of the part performed without shifting the body or turning the part to allow substitutions.[6] The examiner must palpate contractile tissue (muscle fibers or tendons) to detect subtle tension in the muscle group under examination. Only through correct palpation can the examiner be certain that the motion observed is being performed by the target muscle and not by substitution.[4] Detecting substitutions is a skill gained with experience.

Positioning for movement in the correct plane may not be possible with some patients because of confinement to bed, generalized weakness, trunk instability, immobilization devices, and medical precautions. Also, positioning in a gravity-eliminated position for forearm and fingers is seldom done because the weight of the part lifted against gravity is insignificant.[4,6]

## MUSCLE GRADES

Although the definitions of the **muscle grades** are standard, the assignment of muscle grades during the manual muscle test depends on the examiner's clinical judgment, knowledge, and experience.[4] This is especially true when determining slight, moderate, or full resistance. The patient's age, gender, body type, occupation, and avocations all influence the amount of resistance that the examiner perceives to be appropriate.

The amount of resistance that can be given also varies from one muscle group to another.[4] For example, the flexors of the wrist take much more resistance than the abductors of the fingers. The examiner must consider the size and relative power of the muscle(s) or muscle group and accordingly adjust the leverage used when giving resistance.[7] It is common practice to use patients as their own control standard when assessing dysfunction in a given part of the body, comparing the affected side with the unaffected side when possible.

Because weak muscles fatigue easily, results of muscle testing may not be accurate if the subject is tired. Pain, swelling, or muscle spasm in the area being tested may also interfere with the testing procedure. The examiner should note such problems on the assessment form. Psychological factors must also be considered. The examiner must assess the subject's motivation, cooperation, cognitive ability, and effort when interpreting strength.[4]

In manual muscle testing, muscles are graded according to the criteria in Table 9-1.[4,11]

The purpose of using plus and minus designations with muscle grades is to "fine-grade" the muscle strength grades. The experienced examiner will probably use these designations. It is accepted that two examiners testing the same subject may vary up to a half grade in their results, but they should not disagree by a whole grade.[9]

## PROCEDURE FOR MANUAL MUSCLE TESTING

Testing should be performed according to a standard procedure to ensure accuracy and consistency. Each test is conducted following the same basic steps: (1) position, (2) stabilize, (3) palpate, (4) observe, (5) resist, and (6) grade.

First, the subject (S) should be positioned for the specific muscle test. The examiner (E) should *position* in relation to S. Then E *stabilizes* the part proximal to the part being tested to eliminate extraneous movements, isolate the muscle group, ensure the correct test motion, and eliminate the chance of substitution. E demonstrates or describes the test motion to S and asks S to perform the desired test motion. E makes a general observation of the form and quality of movement, checking for substitutions or difficulties that may require adjustments in positioning and stabilization. E then places fingers to *palpate* one or more of the prime movers, or the tendinous insertion(s), in the muscle group being tested and asks S to repeat the test motion. E again *observes* the movement for possible substitution and the amount of range completed. When S has moved the part through the available ROM, S is asked to hold the position at the end of the available ROM. E removes the palpating fingers and uses this hand to

Table 9-1

**Muscle Grades in Manual Muscle Testing**

| Number grade | Word (letter) grade | Definition |
|---|---|---|
| 0 | Zero (0) | No muscle contraction can bè seen or felt. |
| 1 | Trace (T) | Contraction can be felt, but there is no motion. |
| 2– | Poor minus (P–) | Part moves through incomplete ROM with gravity decreased. |
| 2 | Poor (P) | Part moves through complete ROM with gravity decreased. |
| 2+ | Poor plus (P+) | Part moves through incomplete ROM (less than 50%) against gravity or through complete ROM with gravity decreased against slight resistance.[4] |
| 3– | Fair minus (F–) | Part moves through incomplete ROM (more than 50%) against gravity.[4] |
| 3 | Fair (F) | Part moves through complete ROM against gravity. |
| 3+ | Fair (F+) | Part moves through complete ROM against gravity and slight resistance. |
| 4 | Good (G) | Part moves through complete ROM against gravity and moderate resistance. |
| 5 | Normal (N) | Part moves through complete ROM against gravity and full resistance. |

*resist* in the opposite direction of the test movement. E usually must maintain stabilization when resistance is given. These muscle tests use the **break test;** that is, the resistance is applied *after* S has reached the end of the available ROM and attempts to break the contraction.

S should be allowed to establish a maximal contraction (set the muscles) before the resistance is applied.[4,7] E applies the resistance after preparing S by giving the command "hold." Resistance should be applied gradually in the direction opposite to the line of pull of the muscle or muscle group being tested.

The break test should not evoke pain, and resistance should be released immediately if pain or discomfort occurs.[4] Finally, E *grades* the muscle strength according to standard definitions of muscle grades (see Table 9-1). This procedure is used for the tests of strength of grades F and above. Resistance is *not* applied for tests of muscles from P to 0. Slight resistance is sometimes applied to a muscle that has completed the full available ROM in a gravity-decreased plane to determine if the grade is P+. Figure 9-1 is a sample form for recording muscle grades.

### General Instructions and Limitations for Testing Positions

The purpose of this chapter is to familiarize the OTA student or COTA with practical knowledge in the area of muscle testing. Therefore *only* gross muscle group evaluation in the fair (F) to normal (N) range is described in the next section. The occupational therapy practitioner can explore other sources (see References) to master muscle testing for all grade and position levels.

The following protocol does *not* include tests for the face, neck, trunk, and lower extremities and does *not* consider muscle grades below fair (F). Refer to Kendall and McCreary[6] or Daniels and Worthingham[4] for these tests.[4,6]

## MANUAL MUSCLE TESTING OF THE UPPER EXTREMITY

Again, note that *all* the following procedures apply to testing *only* muscle grades fair (F) to normal (N).

### Motion: Shoulder Flexion

| Muscles[4] | Innervation[4] |
|---|---|
| Anterior deltoid | Axillary nerve (n.), fifth and sixth cervical nerves (C5, C6) |
| Coracobrachialis | Musculocutaneous n., C6, C7 |

**Position:** S seated with arm relaxed at side of body with hand facing backward. A straight-back chair may be used to offer maximum trunk support. E stands on side being tested and slightly behind S.[4,11]

**Stabilize:** Over shoulder being tested, but allow normal abduction and upward rotation of scapula that naturally occurs with this movement.[4]

**Palpate:** Anterior deltoid just below clavicle on anterior aspect of humeral head.

**Observe:** S flexes shoulder joint by raising arm horizontally to 90° of flexion (parallel to floor) (Figure 9-2, *A*).[4]

**Resist:** At distal end of humerus downward toward shoulder extension (Figure 9-2, *B*).

### Motion: Shoulder Extension

| Muscle[2,4,6] | Innervation[4] |
|---|---|
| Latissimus dorsi | Thoracodorsal n., C6, C7, or C6 to C8 |
| Teres major | Inferior subscapular n., C5, C6 Axillary n., C5, C6 |
| Posterior deltoid | Axillary n., C5, C6 |

**Position:** S prone lying with shoulder joint adducted and internally rotated so that palm of hand is facing up. E stands on opposite side.

**Stabilize:** Over scapula on side being tested.

BRIEF FUNCTIONAL MUSCLE EXAMINATION OF THE UPPER EXTREMITY

Patient's name ______________________ Chart no.

Date of birth ______________ Name of institution ______________

Date of onset ______________ Attending physician ______________ MD

Diagnosis:

KEY

| | | | |
|---|---|---|---|
| 5 | N | Normal | Complete range of motion against gravity with full resistance. |
| 4 | G | Good* | Complete range of motion against gravity with some resistance. |
| 3 | F | Fair* | Complete range of motion against gravity. |
| 2 | P | Poor* | Complete range of motion with gravity eliminated. |
| 1 | T | Trace | Evidence of slight contractility. No joint motion. |
| 0 | 0 | Zero | No evidence of contractility. |
| S or SS | | | Spasm or severe spasm. |
| C or CC | | | Contracture or severe contracture. |

*Muscle spasm or contracture may limit range of motion. A question mark should be placed after the grading of a movement that is incomplete from this cause.

| LEFT | | | | | | | RIGHT | | | |
|---|---|---|---|---|---|---|---|---|---|---|
| | | | | Examiner's initials | | | | | | |
| | | | | Date | | | | | | |
| | | | | SHOULDER | Flexor | Anterior deltoid | | | | |
| | | | | | Extensors | Latissimus dorsi<br>Teres major | | | | |
| | | | | | Abductor | Middle deltoid | | | | |
| | | | | | Horiz. abd. | Posterior deltoid | | | | |
| | | | | | Horiz. add. | Pectoralis major | | | | |
| | | | | | External rotator group | | | | | |
| | | | | | Internal rotator group | | | | | |
| | | | | ELBOW | Flexors | Biceps brachii<br>Brachioradialis | | | | |
| | | | | | Extensor | Triceps | | | | |
| | | | | FOREARM | Supinator group | | | | | |
| | | | | | Pronator group | | | | | |
| | | | | WRIST | Flexors | Flex. carpi rad.<br>Flex. carpi uln. | | | | |
| | | | | | Extensors | Ext. carpi rad. l. & br.<br>Ext. carpi uln. | | | | |
| | | | | FINGERS | MP flexors | Lumbricales | | | | |
| | | | | | IP flexors (first) | Flex. digit. sub. | | | | |
| | | | | | IP flexors (second) | Flex. digit. prof. | | | | |
| | | | | | MP extensor | Ext. digit. com. | | | | |
| | | | | | Adductors | Palmar interossei | | | | |
| | | | | | Abductors | Dorsal interossei | | | | |
| | | | | | Abductor digiti quinti | | | | | |
| | | | | | Opponens digiti quinti | | | | | |
| | | | | THUMB | MP flexor | Flex. poll. br. | | | | |
| | | | | | IP flexor | Flex. poll. l. | | | | |
| | | | | | MP extensor | Ext. poll. br. | | | | |
| | | | | | IP extensor | Ext. poll. l. | | | | |
| | | | | | Abductors | Abd. poll. br.<br>Abd. poll. l. | | | | |
| | | | | | Adductor pollicis | | | | | |
| | | | | | Opponens pollicis | | | | | |

Additional data:

*Figure 9-1* Sample form for brief functional muscle examination of the upper extremity. (Modified from March of Dimes—Birth Defects Foundation.)

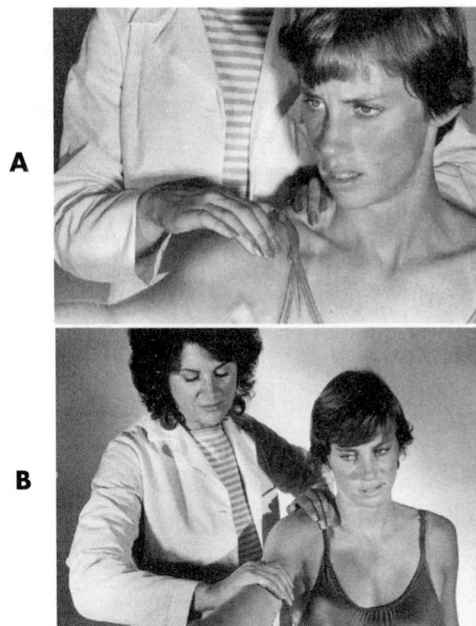

*Figure 9-2* Shoulder flexion. **A,** Palpate and observe. **B,** Resist.

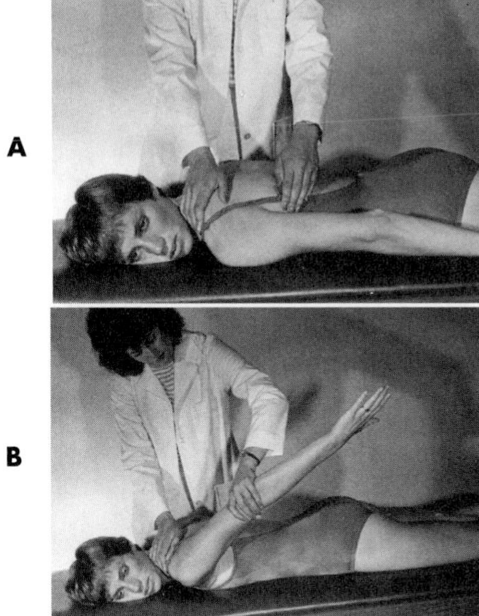

*Figure 9-3* Shoulder extension. **A,** Palpate and observe. **B,** Resist.

**Palpate:** Teres major along axillary border of scapula. Latissimus dorsi may be palpated slightly below this point or closer to its origin parallel to thoracic and lumbar vertebrae.[4] Posterior deltoid may be found over posterior aspect of humeral head (Figure 9-3, *A*).

**Observe:** S lifts up arm off table, extending shoulder joint.

**Resist:** At distal end of humerus in a downward and outward direction, toward flexion and slight abduction (Figure 9-3, *B*).[4,6]

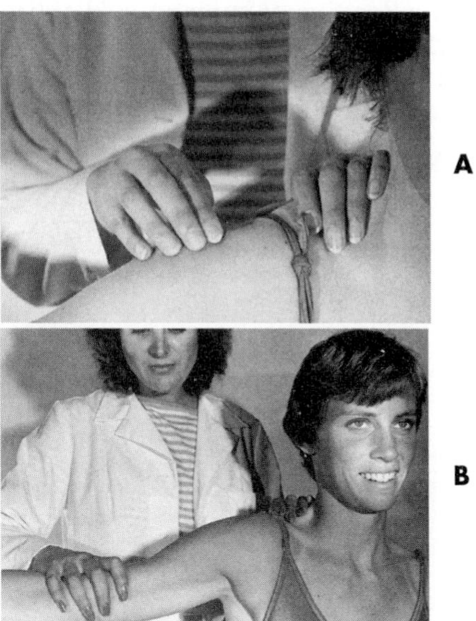

*Figure 9-4* Shoulder abduction. **A,** Palpate and observe. **B,** Resist.

### Motion: Shoulder Abduction

| Muscle[4,6] | *Innervation*[4] |
|---|---|
| Middle deltoid | Axillary n., C5 to C8 |
| Supraspinatus | Suprascapular n., C5 |

**Position:** S seated with arms relaxed at sides of body. Elbow on side to be tested should be slightly flexed with palms facing body. E stands behind S.

**Stabilize:** Over scapula on side being tested.[4,6]

**Palpate:** Middle deltoid over middle of shoulder joint from acromion to deltoid tuberosity.[4,6,7]

**Observe:** S abducts shoulder to 90°. During movement, S's palm should remain down, and E should observe that no external rotation of shoulder or elevation of scapula occurs.[4,6,7] Supraspinatus may be difficult to palpate because it lies under trapezius muscle, but it may be palpated in supraspinatus fossa (Figure 9-4, *A*).[4]

**Resist:** At distal end of humerus as if pushing arm down toward adduction (Figure 9-4, *B*).

### Motion: Shoulder External Rotation

| Muscle[2,4,6,7] | Innervation[2,4,6] |
|---|---|
| Infraspinatus | Axillary n., C5, C6 |
| Teres minor | Axillary n., C5, C6 |

**Position:** S lying prone with shoulder abducted to 90°, humerus in neutral (0°) rotation, and elbow flexed to 90°. Forearm is in neutral rotation, hanging over edge of table, perpendicular to the floor. E stands in front of supported surface toward side being tested.

**Stabilize:** At distal end of humerus by placing hand under arm on supporting surface.[6]

**Palpate:** Infraspinatus muscle just below spine of scapula, on body of scapula, or teres minor along axillary border of scapula.[4]

**Observe:** Rotation of humerus so that back of hand is moving toward ceiling (Figure 9-5, *A*).[4,6]

**Resist:** On distal end of forearm toward floor in direction of internal rotation (Figure 9-5, *B*).[4,6]

### Motion: Shoulder Internal Rotation

| Muscle[4,6,7] | Innervation[2,4,10] |
|---|---|
| Subscapularis | Subscapular n., C5, C6 |
| Pectoralis major | Anterior thoracic n., C5 through first thoracic nerve (T1) |
| Latissimus dorsi | Thoracodorsal n., C6 to C8 |
| Teres major | Subscapular n., C5, C6 |

**Position:** S lying prone with shoulder abducted to 90° and humerus in neutral (0°) rotation and elbow flexed to 90°. Forearm is perpendicular to floor. E stands on side being tested just in front of S's arm.

**Stabilize:** At distal end of humerus by placing hand under arm and on supporting surface, as for external rotation.[4,6]

**Palpate:** Teres major and latissimus dorsi along axillary border of scapula toward inferior angle.

**Observe:** Movement of palm of hand upward toward ceiling, internally rotating humerus (Figure 9-6, *A*).[4]

**Resist:** At distal end of volar surface of forearm anteriorly toward external rotation (Figure 9-6, *B*).[4,6]

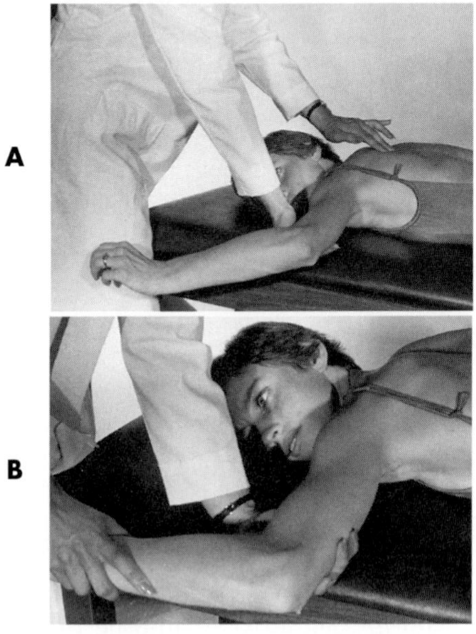


*Figure 9-5* Shoulder external rotation. **A,** Palpate and observe. **B,** Resist.

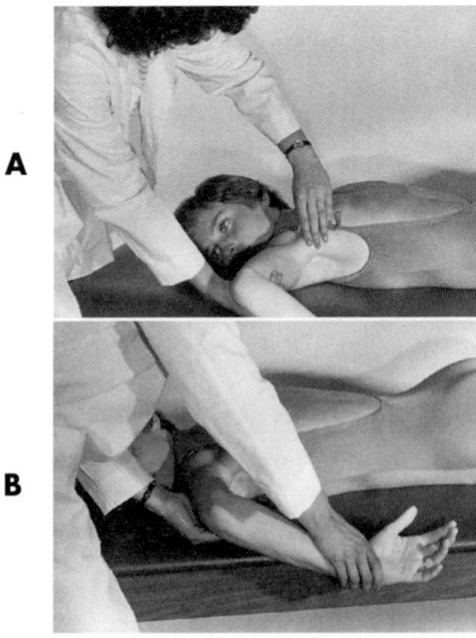


*Figure 9-6* Shoulder internal rotation. **A,** Palpate and observe. **B,** Resist.

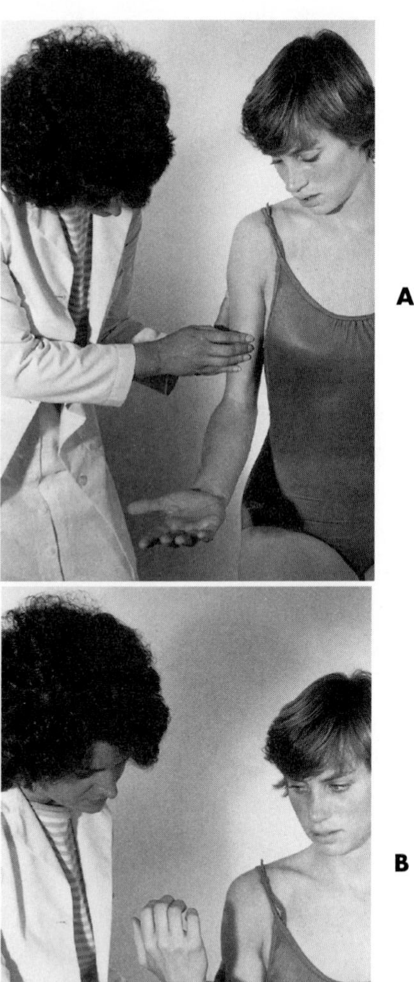


*Figure 9-7* Elbow flexion. **A,** Palpate and observe. **B,** Resist.

### Motion: Elbow Flexion

| Muscle[4,6,7] | Innervation[6] |
|---|---|
| Biceps brachii | Musculocutaneous n., C5, C6 |
| Brachialis | Musculocutaneous n., C5, C6 |
| Brachioradialis | Radial n., C5, C6 |

**Position:** S sitting with arm adducted at shoulder and extended at elbow, held against side of trunk. Forearm is supinated to test primarily for biceps. E stands next to S on side being tested or directly in front of S.

**Stabilize:** Humerus in adduction.

**Palpate:** Biceps brachii over muscle belly on middle of anterior aspect of humerus. Its tendon may be palpated in middle of antecubital space.[4] Brachioradialis is palpated over upper third of radius on lateral aspect of forearm just below elbow. Brachialis may be palpated lateral to lower portion of biceps brachii, if elbow is flexed and in pronated position.[7]

**Observe:** Elbow flexion and movement of hand toward face. E should observe for maintenance of forearm in supination (Figure 9-7, *A*).[7]

**Resist:** At distal end of volar aspect of forearm, pulling downward toward elbow extension (Figure 9-7, *B*).[4,6]

### Motion: Elbow Extension

| Muscle[4,6] | Innervation[4,6] |
|---|---|
| Triceps | Radial n., C7, C8 |
| Anconeus | Radial n., C7 |

**Position:** S prone with humerus abducted to 90° and in neutral rotation, elbow flexed to 90°, and forearm in neutral position perpendicular to floor. E stands next to S just behind arm being tested.[6,11]

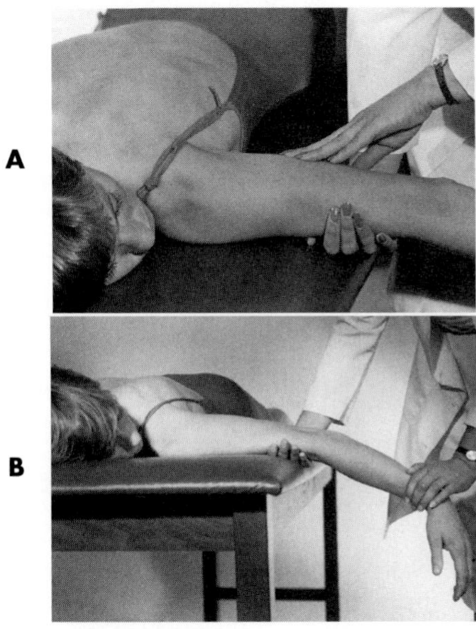

*Figure 9-8* Elbow extension. **A,** Palpate and observe. **B,** Resist.

**Stabilize:** Humerus by placing one hand for support under it, between S's arm and table.[6]

**Palpate:** Triceps over middle of posterior aspect of humerus or triceps tendon just proximal to elbow joint on dorsal surface of arm.[4,7]

**Observe:** Extension of elbow to just less than maximum range. Wrist and fingers remain relaxed (Figure 9-8, *A*).

**Resist:** In same plane as forearm motion at distal end of forearm, pushing toward floor or elbow flexion. Before resistance is given, E ensures elbow is not locked. Resistance to a locked elbow can cause joint injury (Figure 9-8, *B*).[4]

### Motion: Forearm Supination

| Muscle[2,4,7] | Innervation[4] |
|---|---|
| Biceps brachii | Musculocutaneous n., C5, C6 |
| Supinator | Radial n., C6 |

**Position:** S seated with humerus adducted, elbow flexed to 90°, and forearm in full pronation. E stands next to S on side being tested.[4]

**Stabilize:** Humerus just proximal to elbow.

**Palpate:** Over supinator on dorsolateral aspect of forearm, below head of radius. Muscle can be best felt when radial muscle group (extensor carpi radialis and brachioradialis) is pushed up and out of the way.[2] E may also palpate biceps on middle of anterior surface of humerus.

**Observe:** Supination, turning hand up. Gravity may assist the movement after the 0° neutral position is passed (Figure 9-9, *A*).

**Resist:** By grasping around dorsal aspect of distal forearm with fingers and heel of hand, turning arm toward pronation (Figure 9-9, *B*).

### Motion: Forearm Pronation

| Muscle[2,7] | Innervation[6] |
|---|---|
| Pronator teres | Median n., C6 |
| Pronator quadratus | Median n., C8, T1 |

**Position:** S seated with humerus adducted, elbow flexed to 90°, and forearm in full supination. E stands beside S on side being tested.[4]

**Stabilize:** Humerus just proximal to elbow to prevent shoulder abduction.[4,6]

**Palpate:** Pronator teres on upper part of volar surface of forearm, medial to biceps tendon and diagonally from medial condyle of humerus to lateral border of radius.[4,6,7]

**Observe:** Pronation, turning hand palm down (Figure 9-10, *A*).

**Resist:** By grasping around dorsal aspect of distal forearm with fingers and heel of hand, turning arm toward supination (Figure 9-10, *B*).[4]

### Motion: Wrist Extension with Radial Deviation

| Muscle[4,6,7] | Innervation[7] |
|---|---|
| Extensor carpi radialis longus | Radial n., C5 to C8 |
| Extensor carpi radialis brevis | Radial n., C5 to C8 |
| Extensor carpi ulnaris | Radial n., C6 to C8 |

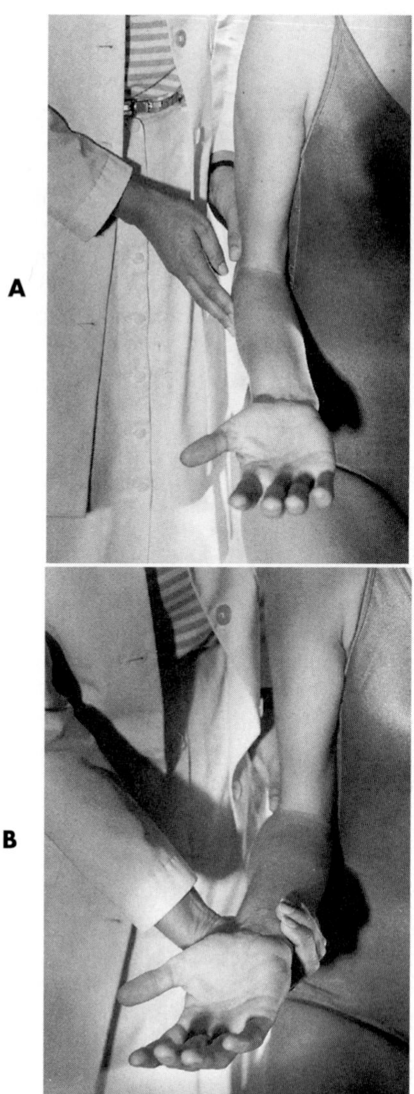

*Figure 9-9* Forearm supination. **A,** Palpate and observe. **B,** Resist.

**Position:** S seated or supine with forearm resting on supporting surface in pronation, wrist in neutral position, and fingers and thumb relaxed. E sits opposite S or next to S on side being tested.[7,8]

**Stabilize:** Over volar aspect of middle to distal forearm (Figure 9-11, *B*).[7,8]

**Palpate:** Extensor carpi radialis longus and brevis tendons on dorsal aspect of wrist at bases of second and third metacarpals, respectively.[4,7] Tendon of extensor carpi ulnaris may be palpated at base of fifth metacarpal, just distal to head of ulna (Figure 9-11, *A*).[2,4,7]

**Observe:** Wrist extension and radial deviation, lifting hand up from supporting surface and moving it medially (to radial side) simultaneously. Movement should be performed without finger extension, which could substitute for wrist motion (Figure 9-11, *B*).[4,7]

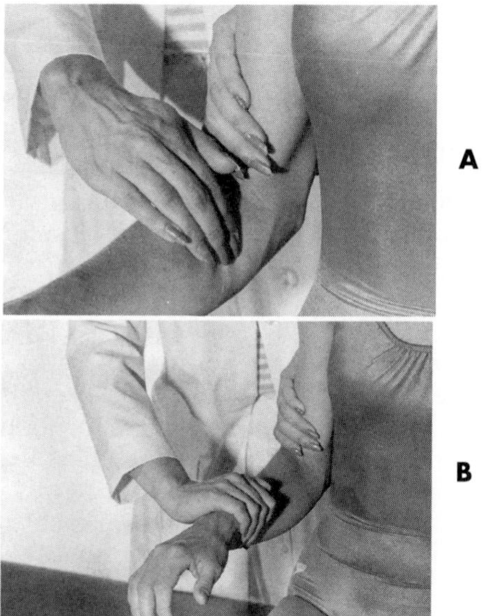

*Figure 9-10* Forearm pronation. **A,** Palpate and observe. **B,** Resist.

**Resist:** Over dorsum of second and third metacarpals toward flexion and ulnar deviation (Figure 9-11, *C*).

### Motion: Wrist Extension with Ulnar Deviation

| Muscle[4,6,7] | Innervation[6] |
|---|---|
| Extensor carpi ulnaris | Radial n., C6 to C8 |
| Extensor carpi radialis longus | Radial n., C5 to C8 |
| Extensor carpi radialis brevis | Radial n., C5 to C8 |

**Position:** S seated with forearm in pronation, wrist in neutral position, and fingers and thumb relaxed. E sits opposite or next to S on side being tested.

**Stabilize:** Over volar aspect of middle to distal forearm.[4,6]

**Palpate:** Extensor carpi ulnaris tendon at base of fifth metacarpal, just distal to head of ulna, and extensor carpi radialis longus and brevis tendons at bases of second and third metacarpals.

**Observe:** S brings hand up from supporting surface and moves it laterally (to ulnar side) simultaneously. E should observe that movement is not preceded by thumb or finger extension (Figure 9-12, *A*).[4,7]

**Resist:** Over dorsolateral aspect of fifth metacarpal toward flexion and radial deviation (Figure 9-12, *B*).[4,6]

### Motion: Wrist Flexion with Radial Deviation

| Muscle[6] | Innervation[4,6,10] |
|---|---|
| Flexor carpi radialis | Median n., C6 to C8 |
| Flexor carpi ulnaris | Ulnar n., C8, T1 |
| Palmaris longus | Median n., C7, C8, T1 |

**Position:** S seated or supine with forearm resting in almost full supination on supporting surface and fingers and thumb relaxed. E sits next to S on side being tested.

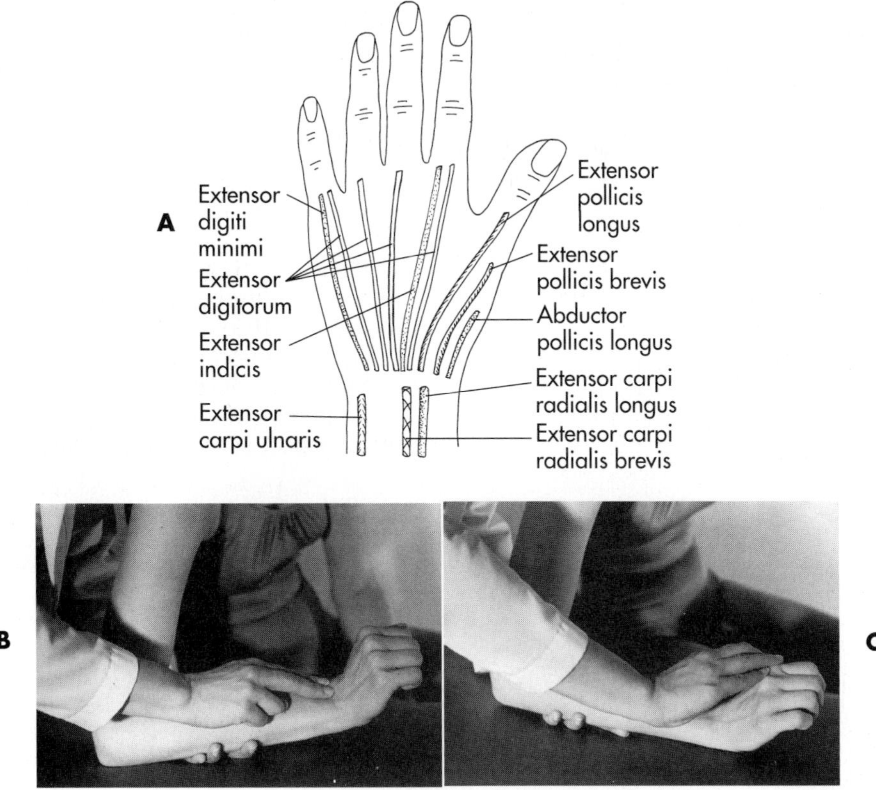


*Figure 9-11* **A,** Arrangement of extensor tendons at wrist. **B,** Wrist extension with radial deviation. Palpate and observe. **C,** Resist.

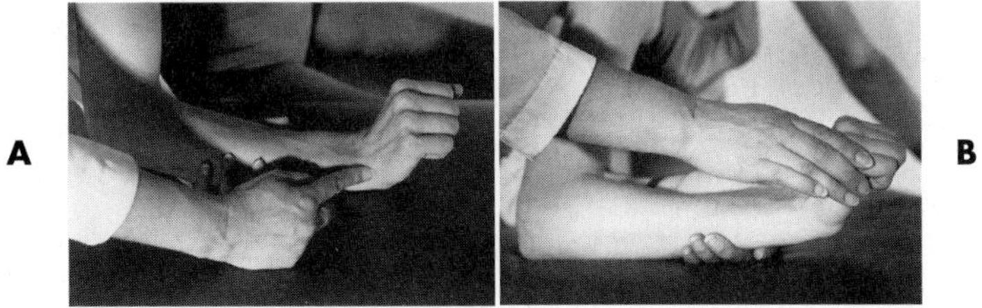


*Figure 9-12* Wrist extension with ulnar deviation. **A,** Palpate and observe. **B,** Resist.

**Stabilize:** Over volar aspect of midforearm.[4,6]

**Palpate:** Muscle tendons. Flexor carpi radialis tendon can be palpated over wrist at base of second metacarpal bone. Palmaris longus tendon is at center of wrist at base of third metacarpal, and flexor carpi ulnaris tendon can be palpated at ulnar side of volar aspect of wrist at base of fifth metacarpal (Figure 9-13, *A*).[2]

**Observe:** S brings hand up from supporting surface toward face, deviating hand toward radial side simultaneously. E should observe that fingers remain relaxed during movement (Figure 9-13, *B*).

**Resist:** In palm at radial side of hand over second and third metacarpals toward extension and ulnar deviation (Figure 9-13, *C*).

### Motion: Wrist Flexion with Ulnar Deviation

| Muscle[4] | Innervations[4,6,10] |
|---|---|
| Flexor carpi ulnaris | Median n., C8, T1 |
| Flexor carpi radialis | Median n., C6 to C8 |
| Palmaris longus | Median n., C7, C8, T1 |

**Position:** S seated or supine with forearm resting in almost full supination on supporting surface and fingers and thumb relaxed. E sits opposite or next to S on side being tested.[4,6]

**Stabilize:** Over volar aspect of middle of forearm.[4,6]

**Palpate:** Flexor tendons on volar aspect of wrist, flexor carpi ulnaris at base of fifth metacarpal, flexor carpi radialis at base of second metacarpal, and palmaris longus at base of third metacarpal.[2] Flexor carpi radialis tendon can be palpated over wrist at base of second metacarpal bone. Palmaris longus tendon is at center of wrist at base of third metacarpal.

**Observe:** S brings hand up from supporting surface, simultaneously flexing wrist and deviating it to the ulnar side (Figure 9-14, *A*).

**Resist:** In palm of hand over hypothenar eminence toward extension and radial deviation (Figure 9-14, *B*).[6]

### Motion: Metacarpophalangeal (MP) Flexion with Interphalangeal (IP) Extension

| Muscle[1,2] | Innervation[4] |
|---|---|
| Lumbricales manus 1 and 2 | Median n., C6, C7 |
| Lumbricales manus 3 and 4 | Ulnar n., C8, T1 |
| Interossei dorsales manus | Ulnar n., C8, T1 |
| Interossei palmares | Ulnar n., C8, T1 |

**Position:** S seated with forearm in supination resting on supporting surface and wrist in neutral position.[4] MP joints are extended and IP joints flexed.[11] E sits next to S on side being tested.

**Stabilize:** Over palm to prevent wrist motion.

**Palpate:** First interosseus dorsales just medial to distal aspect of second metacarpal on dorsum of hand.

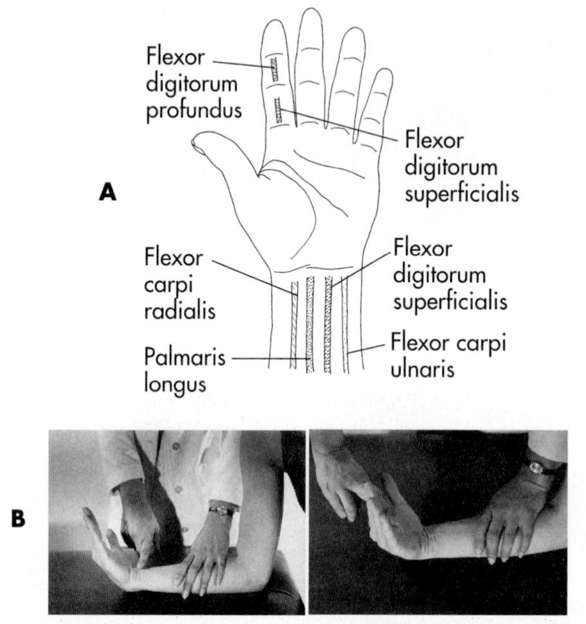


*Figure 9-13* **A,** Arrangement of flexor tendons at wrist. **B,** Wrist flexion with radial deviation. Palpate and observe. **C,** Resist.

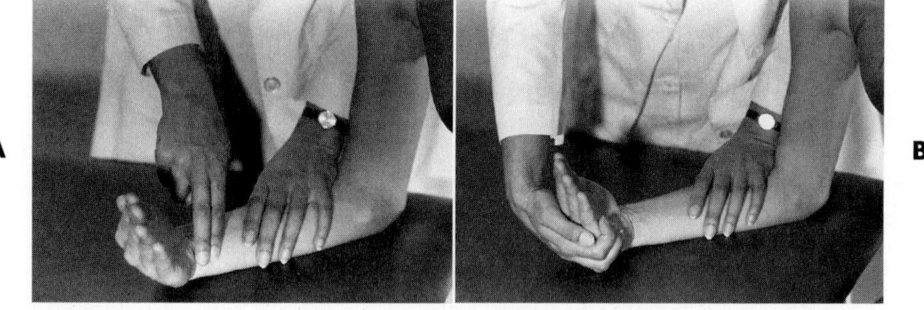


*Figure 9-14* Wrist flexion with ulnar deviation. **A,** Palpate and observe. **B,** Resist.

Remainder of these muscles are not easily palpable because of their size and deep location in hand.

**Observe:** S flexes MP joints and extends IP joints simultaneously (Figure 9-15, *A*).[6]

**Resist:** Each finger separately by grasping distal phalanx and pushing downward on finger into supporting surface toward MP extension and IP flexion, or pressure applied first against dorsal surface of middle and distal phalanges toward flexion, followed by pressure to volar surface of proximal phalanges toward extension (Figure 9-15, *B*).[6]

### Motion: MP Extension

| Muscle[4,6,7] | Innervation[4] |
|---|---|
| Extensor digitorum | Radial n., C6 to C8 |
| Extensor indicis | Radial n., C6 to C8 |
| Extensor digiti minimi | Radial n., C6 to C8 |

**Position:** S seated with forearm pronated and wrist in neutral position, with MP and IP joints partially flexed.[4] E sits opposite or next to S on side being tested.

**Stabilize:** Wrist and metacarpals slightly above supporting surface.[4,6]

**Palpate:** Extensor digitorum tendons where they course over dorsum of hand.[4] In some individuals, extensor digiti minimi tendon can be palpated or visualized just lateral to extensor digitorum tendon to fifth finger. Extensor indicis tendon can be palpated or visualized just medial to extensor digitorum tendon to first finger.

**Observe:** S raises fingers away from supporting surface, extending MP joints but maintaining IP joints in some flexion (Figure 9-16, *A*).

**Resist:** Each finger individually over dorsal aspect of proximal phalanx toward MP flexion (Figure 9-16, *B*).[4,6]

### Motion: Proximal Interphalangeal (PIP) Flexion, Second Through Fifth Fingers

| Muscle[4,6] | Innervation[4,6] |
|---|---|
| Flexor digitorum superficialis | Median n., C7, C8, T1 |

**Position:** S seated with forearm in supination, wrist in neutral position, fingers extended, and hand and forearm resting on dorsal surface.[4] E sits opposite or next to S on side being tested.

**Stabilize:** MP joint and proximal phalanx of finger being tested.[4,6]

**Palpate:** Flexor digitorum superficialis tendon on volar surface of proximal phalanx. A stabilizing finger may be used to palpate in this procedure.[7] Tendon supplying fourth finger may be palpated over volar aspect of wrist between flexor carpi ulnaris and palmaris longus tendons, if desired.[2]

**Observe:** S flexes PIP joint while maintaining distal interphalangeal (DIP) joint in extension (Figure 9-17, *A*). If isolating PIP flexion is difficult, all fingers not being tested are held in MP hyperextension and PIP extension by pulling back over IP joints. This maneuver inactivates flexor digitorum profundus (FDP) so

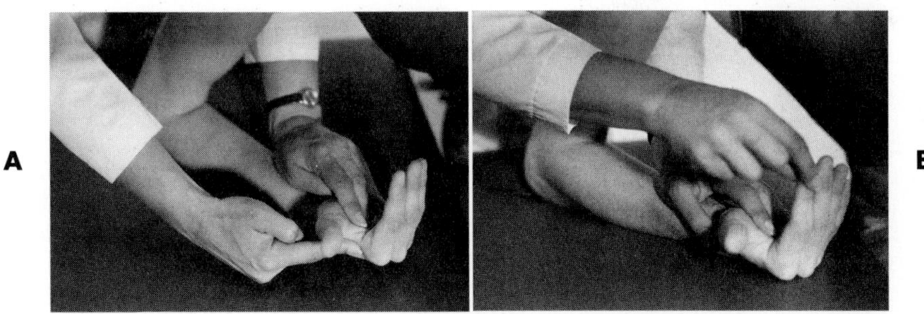


*Figure 9-15* MP flexion with IP extension. **A,** Palpate and observe. **B,** Resist.

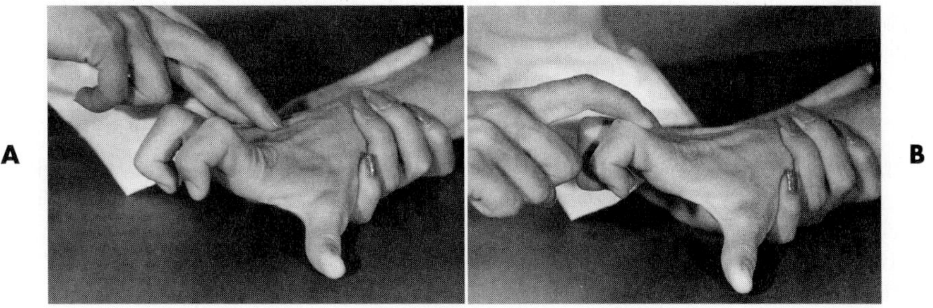


*Figure 9-16* MP extension. **A,** Palpate and observe. **B,** Resist.

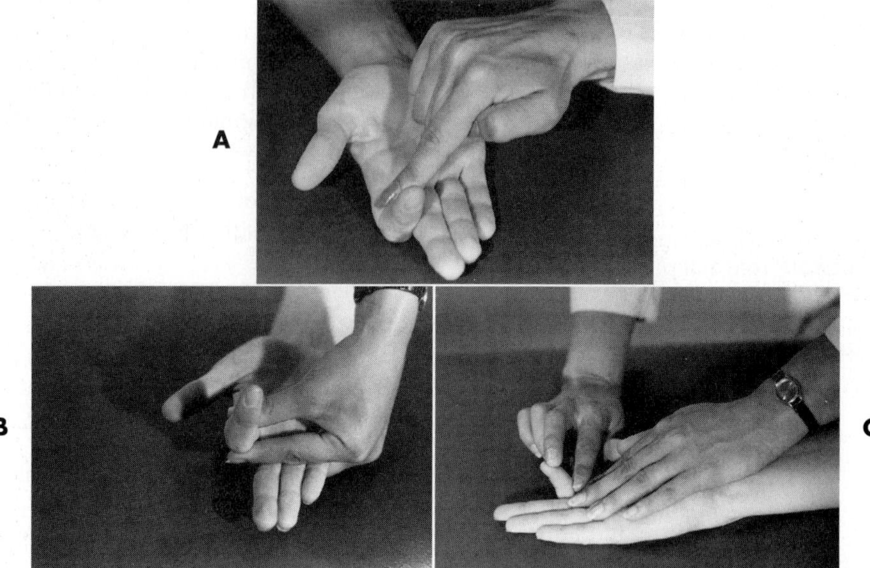


*Figure 9-17* PIP flexion. **A,** Palpate and observe. **B,** Position to assist with isolation of PIP joint flexion. **C,** Resist. Examiner checks for substitution by flexor digitorum profundus.

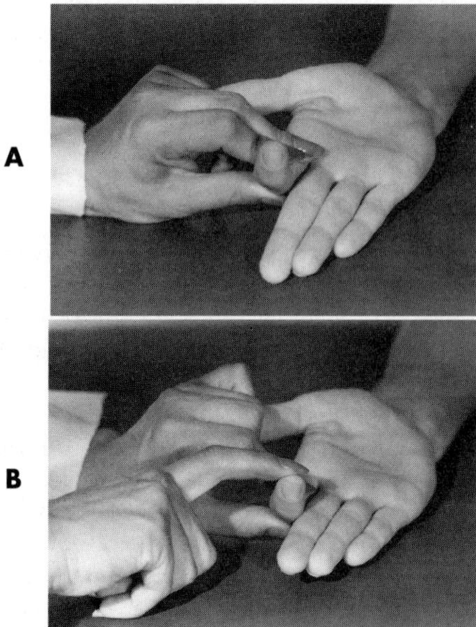


*Figure 9-18* DIP flexion. **A,** Palpate and observe. **B,** Resist.

that S cannot flex distal joint (Figure 9-17, *B*).[2,11] Most individuals cannot perform isolated action of PIP joint of fifth finger even with assistance.

**Resist:** With one finger at volar aspect of middle phalanx toward extension.[4,6] If index finger is used to apply resistance, middle finger may be used to move DIP joint back and forth to verify that FDP is not substituting (Figure 9-17, *C*).

### Motion: Distal Interphalangeal (DIP) Flexion, Second through Fifth Fingers

| Muscle[4] | Innervation[4] |
|---|---|
| Flexor digitorum profundus | Median n., ulnar n., C8, T1 |

**Position:** S seated with forearm in supination, wrist in neutral position, and fingers extended. E sits opposite or next to S on side being tested.[4]

**Stabilize:** Wrist at neutral position and PIP joint and middle phalanx of finger being tested.[11]

**Palpate:** Finger stabilizing middle phalanx used to simultaneously palpate FDP tendon over volar surface of middle phalanx.[4,7]

**Observe:** S brings fingertip up and away from supporting surface, flexing DIP joint (Figure 9-18, *A*).

**Resist:** With one finger at volar aspect of distal phalanx toward extension (Figure 9-18, *B*).[4,6]

### Motion: Finger Abduction

| Muscle[4] | Innervation[4] |
|---|---|
| Interossei dorsales | Ulnar n., C8, T1 |
| Abductor digiti minimi manus | Ulnar n., C8, T1 |

**Position:** S seated or supine with forearm pronated, wrist in neutral position, and fingers extended and adducted. E sits opposite or next to S on side being tested.[4]

**Stabilize:** Wrist and metacarpals slightly above supporting surface.

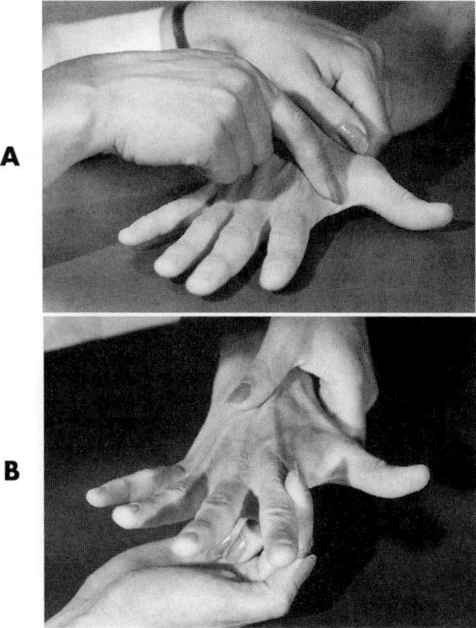


*Figure 9-19* Finger abduction. **A,** Palpate and observe. **B,** Resist.

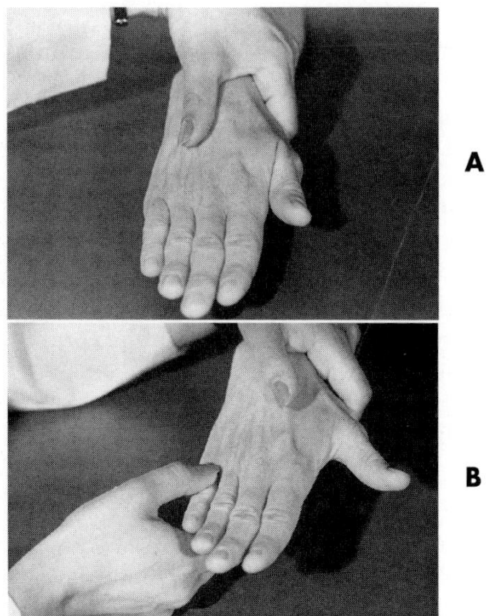


*Figure 9-20* Finger adduction. **A,** Examiner observes movement of fingers into adduction. Palpation of these muscles is not possible. **B,** Resist.

**Palpate:** First interosseus dorsales on lateral aspect of second metacarpal or of abductor digiti minimi manus on ulnar border of fifth metacarpal.[4] Remaining interossei are not palpable.

**Observe:** S spreads fingers apart, abducting them at MP joints (Figure 9-19, *A*).

**Resist:** First interosseus dorsales by applying pressure on radial side of distal end of proximal phalanx of second finger in an ulnar direction (Figure 9-19, *B*); second interosseus dorsales on radial side of proximal phalanx of middle finger in an ulnar direction; third interosseus dorsales on ulnar side of proximal phalanx of middle finger in a radial direction; fourth interosseus dorsales on ulnar side of proximal phalanx of ring finger in a radial direction; abductor digiti minimi manus on ulnar side of proximal phalanx of little finger in a radial direction.[6]

### Motion: Finger Adduction

| Muscles[4,6] | Innervation[4] |
|---|---|
| Interossei palmares | Ulnar n., C8, T1 |

**Position:** S seated with forearm pronated, wrist in neutral position, and fingers extended and abducted.[4]

**Stabilize:** Wrist and metacarpals slightly above supporting surface.

**Palpate:** Not palpable.

**Observe:** S adducts first, fourth, and fifth fingers toward middle finger (Figure 9-20, *A*).

**Resist:** Index finger at proximal phalanx by pulling it in a radial direction, ring finger at proximal phalanx in an ulnar direction, and little finger likewise (Figure 9-20, *B*).[6] These muscles are very small, and resistance must be modified to accommodate to their comparatively limited power.

### Motion: Thumb MP Extension

| Muscle[4,6] | Innervation[4,6] |
|---|---|
| Extensor pollicis brevis | Radial n., C6 to C8 |

**Position:** S seated or supine, forearm in midposition, wrist in neutral position, and hand and forearm resting on ulnar border.[4] Thumb is flexed into palm at MP joint, and IP joint is extended but relaxed. E sits opposite or next to S on side being tested.

**Stabilize:** Wrist and thumb metacarpal.

**Palpate:** Extensor pollicis brevis (EPB) tendon at base of first metacarpal on dorsoradial aspect. It lies just medial to abductor pollicis dorsoradial longus tendon on radial side of anatomical snuffbox, which is hollow space between extensor pollicis longus (EPL) and EPB tendons when thumb is fully extended and radially abducted.[2]

**Observe:** S extends MP joint. IP joint remains relaxed (Figure 9-21, *A*). It is difficult for many individuals to isolate this motion.

**Resist:** On dorsal surface of proximal phalanx toward MP flexion (Figure 9-21, *B*).[4,6]

### Motion: Thumb IP Extension

| Muscle[4,6,7] | Innervation[4,6] |
|---|---|
| Extensor pollicis longus | Radial n., C6 to C8 |

**Position:** S seated or supine, forearm in midposition, wrist in neutral position, and hand and forearm resting on ulnar border.[4] MP joint of thumb is extended or slightly flexed, and IP joint is flexed fully into palm. E sits opposite or next to S on side being tested.

**Stabilize:** Wrist in neutral position, first metacarpal, and proximal phalanx of thumb.

**Palpate:** EPL tendon on dorsal surface of hand medial to EPB tendon, between head of first metacarpal and base of second metacarpal on ulnar side of anatomical snuffbox.[2,4]

**Observe:** S brings tip of thumb up and out of palm, extending IP joint (Figure 9-22, *A*).

**Resist:** On dorsal surface of distal phalanx, down toward IP flexion (Figure 9-22, *B*).[4,6]

### Motion: Thumb MP Flexion

| Muscle[4,6] | Innervation[4,6] |
|---|---|
| Flexor pollicis brevis | Median n., ulnar n., C6 to C8, T1 |

**Position:** S seated or supine, forearm fully supinated, wrist in neutral position, and thumb in extension and adduction. E sits next or opposite to S.[4,6]

**Stabilize:** First metacarpal and wrist.

**Palpate:** Over middle of palmar surface of thenar eminence just medial to abductor pollicis brevis.[4] Hand used to stabilize may also be used for palpation.

**Observe:** S flexes MP joint while maintaining extension of IP joint (Figure 9-23, *A*). Some individuals may be unable to isolate flexion to MP joint. In this case, both MP and IP flexion may be tested together as a gross test for thumb flexion strength and graded according to E's judgment.

**Resist:** On palmar surface of first phalanx toward MP extension (Figure 9-23, *B*).[4,6]

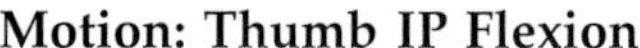

### Motion: Thumb IP Flexion

| Muscle[4,6,7] | Innervation[6] |
|---|---|
| Flexor pollicis longus | Median n., C7, C8, T1 |

**Position:** S seated with forearm fully supinated, wrist in neutral position, and thumb in extension and adduction.[4] E sits next or opposite to S.

**Stabilize:** First metacarpal and proximal phalanx of thumb in extension.[4,6]

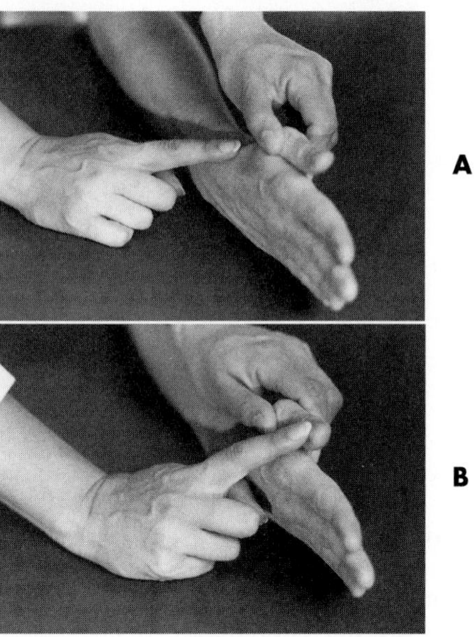


*Figure 9-22* Thumb IP extension. **A,** Palpate and observe. **B,** Resist.

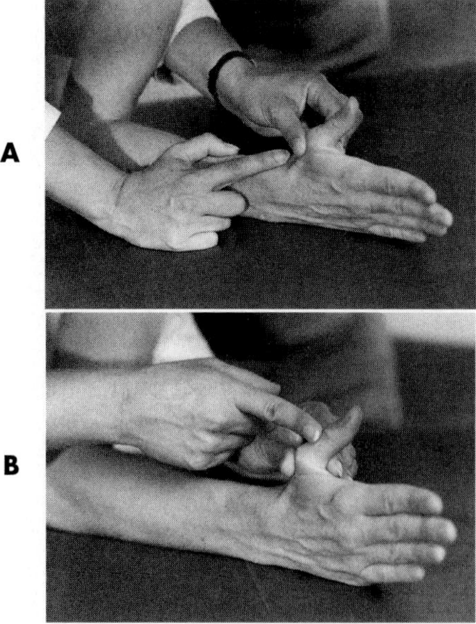


*Figure 9-21* Thumb MP extension. **A,** Palpate and observe. **B,** Resist.

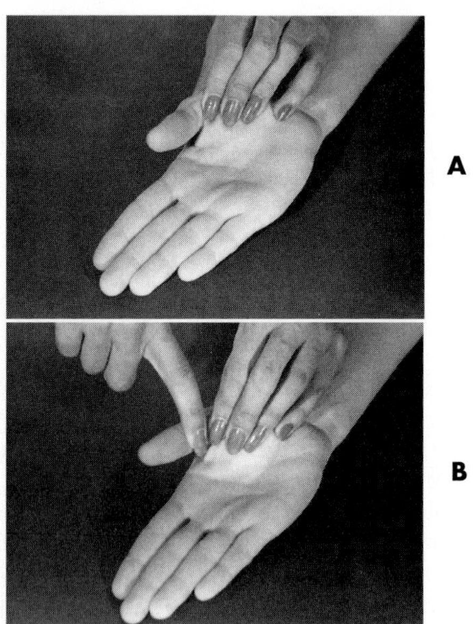


*Figure 9-23* Thumb MP flexion. **A,** Palpate and observe. **B,** Resist.

**Palpate:** Flexor pollicis longus tendon on palmar surface of proximal phalanx. In this case, palpating finger may be the same one used for stabilizing proximal phalanx.

**Observe:** S flexes IP joint in plane of palm (Figure 9-24, *A*).[4]

**Resist:** On palmar surface of distal phalanx toward IP extension (Figure 9-24, *B*).[4,6]

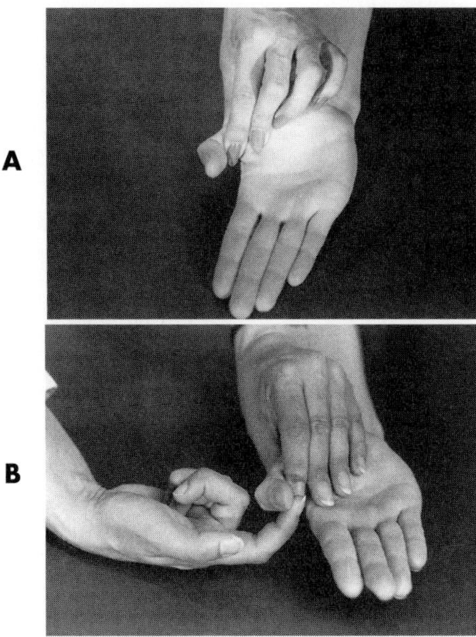

*Figure 9-24* Thumb IP flexion. **A,** Palpate and observe. **B,** Resist.

### Motion: Thumb Palmar Abduction

| Muscle[6,7] | Innervation[6] |
|---|---|
| Abductor pollicis brevis | Median n., C6 to C8, T1 |

**Position:** S seated or supine, forearm in supination, wrist in neutral position, thumb extended and adducted, and carpometacarpal (CMC) joint rotated so that thumb is resting in a plane perpendicular to palm. E sits opposite or next to S on side being tested.[4,6]

**Stabilize:** Metacarpals and wrist.

**Palpate:** Abductor pollicis brevis on lateral aspect of thenar eminence, lateral to flexor pollicis brevis.[4]

**Observe:** S raises thumb away from palm in a plane perpendicular to palm (Figure 9-25, *A*).[6]

**Resist:** At lateral aspect of proximal phalanx, downward toward adduction (Figure 9-25, *B*).[6]

### Motion: Thumb Radial Abduction

| Muscle[6] | Innervation[6] |
|---|---|
| Abductor pollicis longus | Radial n., C6 to C8 |

**Position:** S seated or supine, forearm in neutral rotation, wrist in neutral position, and thumb adducted and slightly flexed across palm. Hand and forearm are resting on ulnar border.[6] E sits opposite or next to S on side being tested.

**Stabilize:** Wrist and metacarpals of fingers.[4,6]

**Palpate:** Abductor pollicis longus tendon on lateral aspect of base of first metacarpal. It is the tendon immediately lateral (radial) to extensor pollicis brevis tendon.[2,4]

**Observe:** S moves thumb out of palm of hand, abducting it in plane of palm (Figure 9-26, *A*).

**Resist:** At lateral aspect of distal end of first metacarpal toward adduction (Figure 9-26, *B*).[4,6]

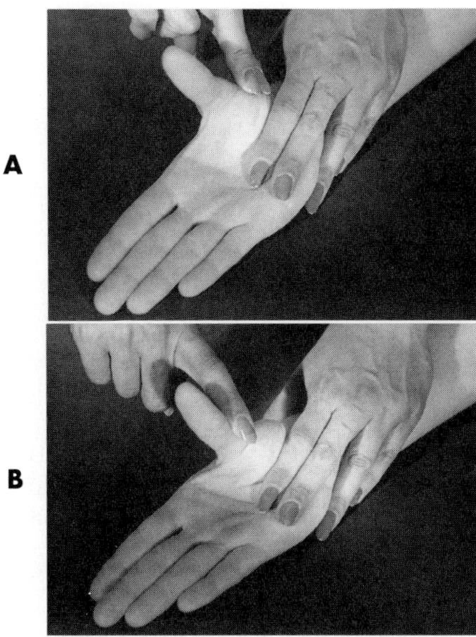

*Figure 9-25* Thumb palmar abduction. **A,** Palpate and observe. **B,** Resist.

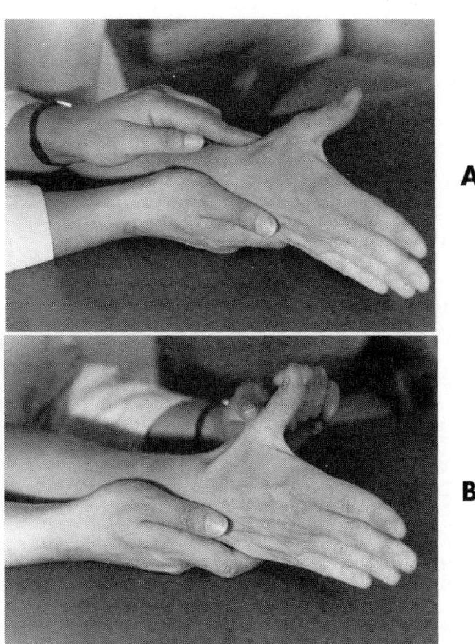

*Figure 9-26* Thumb radial abduction. **A,** Palpate and observe. **B,** Resist.

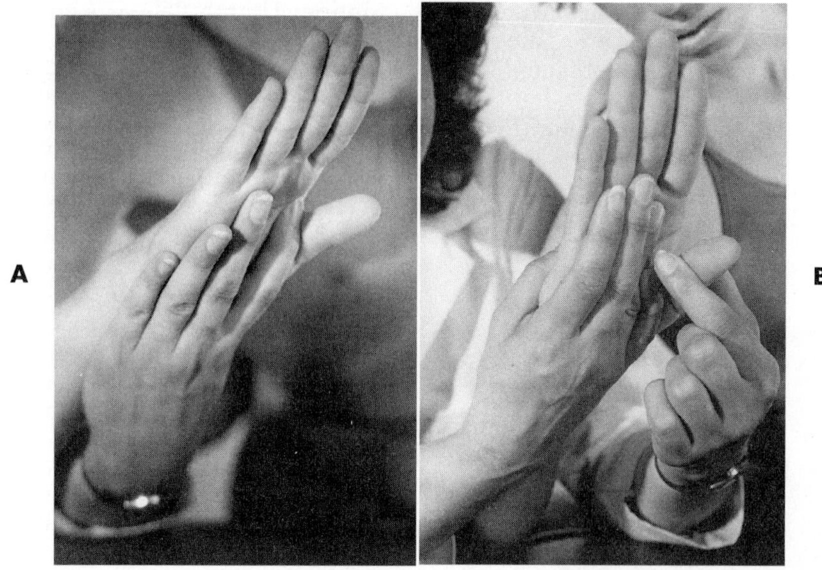


*Figure 9-27* Thumb adduction. **A,** Palpate and observe. **B,** Resist.

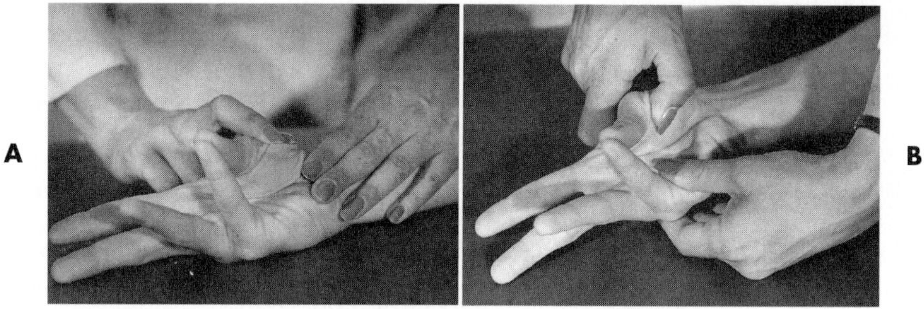


*Figure 9-28* Thumb opposition. **A,** Palpate and observe. **B,** Resist.

### Motion: Thumb Adduction

| Muscle[4,6] | Innervation[4,6] |
|---|---|
| Adductor pollicis | Ulnar n., C8, T1 |

**Position:** S seated or supine, forearm pronated, wrist in neutral position, and thumb opposed and abducted.[4,11] E sits opposite or next to S on side being tested.

**Stabilize:** Wrist and metacarpals, supporting hand slightly above resting surface.[4]

**Palpate:** Adductor pollicis on palmar side of thumb web space.[7]

**Observe:** S brings thumb up to touch palm (Figure 9-27, *A*).[4] (Thumb is turned up in Figure 9-27 to show palpation point.)

**Resist:** By grasping proximal phalanx of thumb near metacarpal head, and pulling downward, toward abduction (Figure 9-27, *B*).[4]

### Motion: Opposition of Thumb to Fifth Finger

| Muscles[4,6] | Innervation[4,6] |
|---|---|
| Opponens pollicis | Median n., C6 to C8, T1 |
| Opponens digiti minimi | Ulnar n., C8, T1 |

**Position:** S seated or supine, forearm in full supination, wrist in neutral position, and thumb and fifth finger extended and adducted.[4,6] E sits on side being tested.

**Stabilize:** Forearm and wrist.

**Palpate:** Opponens pollicis along radial side of shaft of first metacarpal, lateral to abductor pollicis brevis. Opponens digiti minimi cannot be easily palpated.[4,7]

**Observe:** S brings thumb out across palm to touch thumb pad to pad of fifth finger (Figure 9-28, *A*).

**Resist:** At distal ends of first and fifth metacarpals, exerting pressure toward, separating, and rolling away these bones and flattening palm of hand (Figure 9-28, *B*).[4]

## FUNCTIONAL MUSCLE TESTING

The functional muscle test is a useful tool when screening muscles for normal strength.[4,9] It is used by occupational therapy practitioners in some health care facilities where specific muscle testing is the responsibility of the physical therapy service. The functional muscle test assesses the general strength and motion capabilities of the patient.

The following functional muscle test should be performed while the subject is comfortably seated in a sturdy chair or wheelchair.

The subject is asked to perform the test motion against gravity. The subject may perform the motion in the gravity-decreased position, if the former is not feasible.

In all of the tests the subject is allowed to complete the test motion before the examiner applies resistance. The resistance is applied at the end of the ROM while the subject maintains the position and resists the force applied by the examiner. The examiner may make modifications in positioning to suit individual needs. As in the manual muscle tests, the examiner should stabilize proximal parts and attempt to rule out substitutions. The reader should be familiar with joint motions, their prime movers, manual muscle testing, and muscle grades before performing this test. The COTA must establish service competency to assure accuracy and safety in testing.

### Functional Muscle Test

#### *Shoulder Flexion (Anterior Deltoid and Coracobrachialis)*

With S's shoulder flexed to 90° and elbow flexed or extended, E pushes down on arm proximal to elbow into extension.

#### *Shoulder Extension (Latissimus Dorsi and Teres Major)*

S moves shoulder into full extension. E pushes from behind at a point proximal to elbow into flexion.

#### *Shoulder Abduction (Middle Deltoid and Supraspinatus)*

S abducts shoulder to 90° with elbow flexed or extended. E pushes down on arm just proximal to elbow into adduction.

#### *Shoulder Horizontal Adduction (Pectoralis Major, Anterior Deltoid)*

S crosses arms in front of chest. E reaches from behind and attempts to pull arms back into horizontal abduction at a point just proximal to elbow.

#### *Shoulder Horizontal Abduction (Posterior Deltoid, Teres Minor, Infraspinatus)*

S moves arms from full horizontal adduction as just described to full horizontal abduction. E pushes forward on arms just proximal to elbow into horizontal adduction.

#### *Shoulder External Rotation (Infraspinatus and Teres Minor)*

S holds arm in 90° of shoulder abduction and 90° of elbow flexion, then externally rotates shoulder through available ROM. E supports or stabilizes upper arm proximal to elbow; at the same time, E pushes from behind at dorsal aspect of wrist into internal rotation.

#### *Shoulder Internal Rotation (Subscapularis, Teres Major, Latissimus Dorsi, Pectoralis Major)*

S begins with arm as described for external rotation (90° of shoulder abduction and 90° of elbow flexion) but performs internal rotation. E supports or stabilizes upper arm as before and pulls up into external rotation at volar aspect of wrist.

#### *Elbow Flexion (Biceps, Brachialis)*

With forearm supinated, S flexes elbow from full extension. E sits opposite subject and stabilizes upper arm against trunk while attempting to pull forearm into extension at volar aspect of wrist.

#### *Elbow Extension (Triceps)*

With S's upper arm supported in 90° of abduction (gravity-decreased position) or 160° shoulder flexion (against-gravity position), elbow is extended from full flexion. E pushes forearm into flexion at dorsal aspect of wrist.

#### *Forearm Supination (Biceps, Supinator)*

Upper arm is stabilized against trunk by S or E. Elbow is flexed to 90°, and forearm is in full pronation. S supinates forearm. E grasps distal forearm and attempts to rotate it into pronation.

#### *Forearm Pronation (Pronator Teres, Pronator Quadratus)*

S is positioned as described for forearm supination except that forearm is in full supination. S pronates forearm. E grasps distal forearm and attempts to rotate it into supination.

#### *Wrist Flexion (Flexor Carpi Radialis, Flexor Carpi Ulnaris, Palmaris Longus)*

S's forearm is supported on its dorsal surface on a tabletop or armrest. Hand is moved up from tabletop, using wrist flexion. E is seated next to or opposite S and pushes on palm of hand, giving equal pressure on radial and ulnar sides into wrist extension or down toward tabletop.

#### *Wrist Extension (Extensor Carpi Radialis Longus and Brevis, Extensor Carpi Ulnaris)*

S's forearm is supported on a tabletop or armrest, resting on its volar surface. Hand is lifted from tabletop, using wrist extension. E sits next to or opposite S and pushes on dorsal aspect of palm, giving equal pressure at radial and ulnar sides into wrist flexion or down toward tabletop.

*Finger MP Flexion and IP Extension (Lumbricales and Interossei)*

With forearm and hand supported on tabletop on dorsal surface, E stabilizes palm and S flexes MP joints while maintaining extension of IP joints. E pushes into extension with index finger across proximal phalanges or pushes on tip of each finger into IP flexion and MP extension.

*Finger IP Flexion (Flexors Digitorum Profundus and Sublimis)*

S is positioned as described for MP flexion. IP joints are flexed while maintaining extension of MP joints. E attempts to pull fingers back into extension by hooking fingertips with those of S.

*Finger MP Extension (IP Joints Flexed) (Extensor Digitorum Communis, Extensor Indicis Proprius, Extensor Digiti Minimi)*

S's forearm and hand are supported on a table surface, resting on ulnar border. Wrist is stabilized by E in 0° neutral position. S moves MP joints from flexion to full extension (hyperextension) while keeping IP joints flexed. E pushes fingers at PIP joints simultaneously into flexion.

*Finger Abduction (Dorsal Interossei, Abductor Digiti Minimi)*

S's forearm is resting on volar surface on a table. E may stabilize wrist in slight extension so that hand is raised slightly off supporting surface. S abducts fingers. E pushes two fingers at a time together at the proximal phalanges into adduction. First, index finger and middle fingers are pushed together, then ring finger and middle fingers, and finally little finger and ring fingers. Resistance is modified to accommodate small muscles.

*Finger Adduction (Palmar Interossei)*

S is positioned as described for finger abduction. Fingers are adducted tightly. E attempts to pull fingers apart one at a time at the proximal phalanges. First, index finger is pulled away from middle finger then ring finger is pulled away from middle finger, and finally little finger is pulled away from ring finger. In normal hand, adducted finger 'snaps' back into adducted position when E pulls it into abduction and lets go quickly. An alternate method is for examiner to place index finger between two of S's fingers. S should adduct against it, thus estimating amount of force or pressure that S is exerting.

*Thumb MP and IP Flexion (Flexor Pollicis Brevis and Flexor Pollicis Longus)*

S's forearm should be supported on a firm surface, with elbow flexed at 90° and forearm in 45° supination. Thumb is flexed across palm. E pulls on tip of thumb into extension.

*Thumb MP and IP Extension (Extensor Pollicis Brevis and Extensor Pollicis Longus)*

S is positioned as for thumb MP and IP flexion. Thumb is extended away from palm. E pushes on tip of thumb into flexion.

*Thumb Palmar Abduction (Abductor Pollicis Longus and Abductor Pollicis Brevis)*

S is positioned as described for thumb flexion and extension. Thumb is abducted away from palm in a plane perpendicular to palm. S resists movement at metacarpal head into adduction.

*Thumb Adduction (Adductor Pollicis)*

S is positioned as for all other thumb movements. Thumb is adducted to palm. E attempts to pull thumb into abduction at metacarpal head or proximal phalanx.

*Opposition of Thumb to Fifth Finger (Opponens Pollicis, Opponens Digiti Minimi)*

S is positioned with elbow flexed to 90° and dorsal surface of forearm and hand resting on a flat surface such as a tabletop or armrest. Thumb is opposed to fifth finger, making pad-to-pad contact. E attempts to pull fingers apart, applying force at metacarpal heads of both fingers.

## SUMMARY

Evaluation of muscle strength contributes to the functional assessment of patients with many different physical disorders. Muscle strength is needed to maintain body posture and to perform activities when gravity or other resistance is a factor. Evaluation of muscle strength documents objectively the physiological and functional changes in the musculoskeletal system. It is an important evaluation tool for patients with lower motor neuron dysfunction, orthopedic conditions, and muscle diseases. The role of the COTA in evaluating muscle strength must start with proven service competency and is determined by the supervising OTR, in accordance with practice regulations of the state and the treatment setting.

## Selected Reading Guide Questions

1. List two medical conditions in which testing of muscle strength would be appropriate.
2. Define *endurance,* and discuss its relationship to muscle testing.
3. What is the difference between spasticity and normal muscle strength?
4. What are the purposes of functional muscle testing?
5. Explain why specific positioning is used for testing of specific muscle groups.
6. How does gravity affect the tested strength of a muscle?
7. If joint range is limited, how can strength be tested, and how would this be recorded?
8. Define each of these muscle grades: N (5), G (4), F (3), P (2), T (1), and zero (0).
9. Describe how muscle fatigue, pain, and muscle spasm may affect testing of muscle strength.
10. Why is it important to know the patient's passive ROM before muscle testing?

## Exercise

1. Demonstrate the muscle testing procedures for the following muscle groups: shoulder flexion, extension, abduction, external rotation, and internal rotation; elbow flexion and extension; forearm supination and pronation; and wrist flexion and extension.

### REFERENCES

1. Basmajian JF: *Muscles alive,* ed 4, Baltimore, 1978, Williams & Wilkins.
2. Brunstrum S: *Clinical kinesiology,* ed 5, Philadelphia, 1996, Davis.
3. Brunnstrom S: *Movement therapy in hemiplegia,* New York, 1970, Harper & Row.
4. Daniels L, Worthingham C: *Muscle testing,* ed 5, Philadelphia, 1986, Saunders.
5. Davis PM: *Steps to follow: a guide to the treatment of adult hemiplegia,* Berlin, 1985, Springer-Verlag.
6. Kendall FP, McCreary EK: *Muscles: testing and function,* ed 4, Baltimore, 1993, Williams & Wilkins.
7. Killingsworth A: *Basic physical disability procedures,* San Jose, Calif, 1987, Maple.
8. Landen B, Amizich A: Functional muscle examination and gait analysis, *J Am Phys Ther Assoc* 43:39, 1963.
9. Pact V, Sirotkin-Roses M, Beatus J: *The muscle testing handbook,* Boston, 1984, Little, Brown.
10. Pedretti LW: *Occupational therapy: practice skills for physical dysfunction,* ed 4, St Louis, 1995, Mosby.
11. Rancho Los Amigos Hospital, Department of Occupational Therapy: *Guide for muscle testing of the upper extremity,* Downey, Calif, 1978, Professional Staff Association of Rancho Los Amigos Hospital.

Chapter 10

# Evaluation of Motor Control

*Jean W. Solomon*

## Chapter Objectives

*After studying this chapter, the student or practitioner will be able to:*

1. Delineate COTA/OTR roles with regard to motor control evaluation and intervention.
2. Define *normal* and *abnormal* muscle tone.
3. Describe specific primitive reflexes and how to assess for the presence of such reflexes. Describe the impact on function when primitive reflexes persist after neurological damage in the adult patient.
4. Define protective extension, righting, and equilibrium responses and how to assess for the presence of these responses. Describe the functional significance of these responses while a patient is engaged in occupational performance activities.
5. Describe expected motor recovery patterns in the adult with central nervous system (CNS) dysfunction.
6. Define levels of assistance, and give examples of functional use of an involved extremity in the adult with CNS dysfunction.
7. Define *upper extremity coordination.*
8. List and describe three simple structured tests used by the occupational therapy practitioner to evaluate fine coordination and dexterity.
9. Define the occurrences and types of incoordination that might affect the adult with CNS dysfunction.
10. Identify how incoordination affects a patient's handling of occupational performance tasks.

## Key Terms

postural tone
muscle tone
hypotonicity
hypertonicity
spasticity
rigidity
primitive reflexes
protective extension reactions
righting reactions
equilibrium reactions
selective movement
coordination
ataxia
adiadochokinesia
dysmetria
dyssynergia
tremor
rebound phenomenon of Holmes
nystagmus
dysarthria
choreiform movements
athetoid movements
spasms
dystonia
ballism
occurrence of incoordination

Motor control is necessary for a person to be able to function independently during occupational performance tasks. When motor control is impaired, a person has difficulty performing basic self-care activities. For example, a 62-year-old male had a cerebrovascular accident (CVA, stroke) on the left side of his cerebral cortex, or brain. Four weeks after the stroke, he is unable to use his preferred right arm for self-feeding or simple oral hygiene activities because of the loss of motor control on the right side of his body.

Motor control is the unconscious ability to make continuous postural adjustments and to regulate trunk and extremity movements.[31] Complex neurological systems work together to make motor control possible. When an insult to the central nervous system (CNS) occurs (e.g., stroke) or a progressive, neurological disease exists (e.g., multiple sclerosis), motor control is affected. Functional recovery depends on the extent of the damage to the CNS and the expected neurological recovery for a particular diagnosis.

Motor control is evaluated in regard to both its components and its effect on function. The occupational therapy practitioner evaluates the components of motor control and the influence of the component parts on the patient's ability to carry out occupational performance tasks such as feeding, dressing, and personal hygiene activities. Performance components considered necessary for motor control include normal postural tone and postural mechanism, normal muscle tone, selective movement, and coordination. The registered occupational therapist (OTR) evaluates postural tone and muscle tone. On the establishment of service competency, the certified occupational therapy assistant (COTA) may contribute to the evaluation of the status of the postural mechanism (and selective movement and coordination) using simple structured tests or checklists to guide in the clinical observations. Both the OTR and the COTA observe how impaired motor control affects the patient's functional abilities and independence during activities.

## POSTURAL MECHANISM

Normal postural mechanisms are automatic, involuntary (nonintentional) movements that together provide stability and mobility during activity.[10] These automatic reactions develop in the early years of life. The normal postural mechanisms allow for the development of head control (stability) and mobility, trunk control and mobility, midline orientation of self and symmetry, weight bearing and weight shifting in all directions, balance during transitional movements, controlled voluntary limb movement, and coordination.[6,10]

The components of the normal postural mechanism include normal postural tone, normal muscle tone, integration of the primitive reflexes and mass patterns of movement, righting reactions, equilibrium reactions, protective extension reactions, and selective voluntary or intentional movement.[6,10]

In patients who have sustained CNS damage secondary to a CVA or traumatic brain injury, the normal postural mechanism is disrupted. The patient's movements are dominated by abnormal muscle tone and mass patterns. Movements may be slow and uncoordinated. Occupational therapy practitioners must evaluate the degree of damage to the postural mechanism in patients with CNS trauma or disease. The OT practitioner must also assess how the abnormal postural mechanism affects the patient's ability to engage in occupational performance activities such as dressing and feeding.

**Postural tone** refers to *tonus* (muscle tension) in the neck, trunk, and limb girdles. Normal postural tone is high enough to resist gravity, enabling persons to be upright against gravity yet low enough to allow movement.[6] It allows persons to adjust automatically and continuously to their movements or to movements imposed on them externally. Postural tone provides the necessary stability proximally (close to the body center) to enable distal (away from the body center), voluntary, selective movements. Abnormal muscle tone may be too low, which is unstable, or too high, which is rigid. High or low tone interferes with normal selective movement.

### Normal Muscle Tone

Normal **muscle tone,** a component of the normal postural mechanism, is a continuous state of mild contraction, or state of readiness of a specific muscle.[36] Muscle tone is the resting state of a muscle in response to gravity and emotion. It depends on the integrity of the peripheral nervous system (PNS) and the CNS mechanisms and the properties of muscles. Tension exists between the origin and insertion of the muscle such that resistance is felt by the therapist when passively manipulating the head, trunk, or limbs. In other words, when passively stretched, muscles offer a small amount of involuntary resistance.

Normal muscle tone varies from one individual to another and depends on factors such as age, gender, occupation, and exercise regimen. A range exists that is considered normal (Figure 10-1). Normal muscle tone is characterized by the following:

1. Effective coactivation (stabilization) at axial (neck and trunk) and proximal shoulder and pelvic girdle joints
2. Ability of a limb to move against gravity and resistance
3. Ability to maintain the limb's position if it is placed passively by the therapist and then released
4. Equal amount of resistance to passive stretch between the *agonist* (muscle that contracts to create movement at a joint) and the *antagonist* (muscle that relaxes, or elongates, to allow movement at a joint), for example, equal amount of resistance in the biceps and triceps muscles or in the wrist flexors and extensors

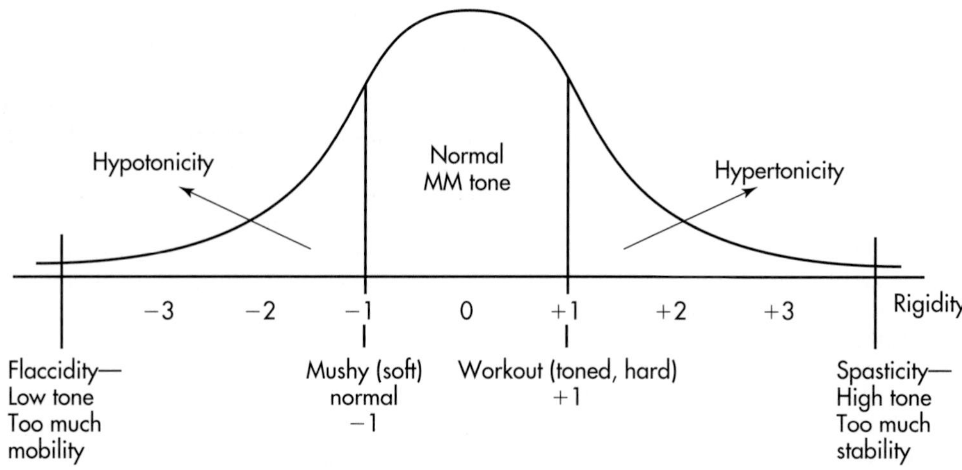


*Figure 10-1* Visual representation of the continuum of muscle tone. (Courtesy Jean W. Solomon, 1995.)

5. Ease of ability to shift from stability to mobility, and vice versa, as needed, for example, ability to raise arm above head and then to maintain that position while reaching for a glass in a high cabinet
6. Ability to use muscles in groups or selectively, if necessary,[16] for example, opening the hand to release an item versus pointing the index finger while keeping the other digits flexed
7. Slight resistance to passive movement[14]

### Evaluating Muscle Tone

Normal muscle tone is dynamic. Objective evaluation of muscle tone in the patient with CNS dysfunction is difficult because of its continuous fluctuation and its relationship to the postural mechanism.[6,20] For example, when lying supine, a patient's level of tone is lower than when the patient is sitting or standing erect against gravity. The level and distribution of muscle tone change as the position of the patient's head in space changes.[6] The emergence of primitive reflexes and associated reactions will alter muscle tone. Therefore muscle tone must be evaluated with regard to the postural mechanism, synergies present, the specific task, and other factors related to motor control. The OTR is responsible for evaluating muscle tone and its distribution. The COTA and OTR observe how abnormal muscle tone interferes with the performance of functional activities.

Abnormal muscle tone is usually described using the following terms: hypotonicity, hypertonicity, and rigidity. The occupational therapy practitioner needs to differentiate these tonic states. Clinically the therapist must be able to identify the type and distribution of abnormal muscle tone to select appropriate treatment techniques.

The OTR follows general guidelines while assessing muscle tone in the patient with CNS damage. The preferred position of the patient for assessment of muscle tone is upright, either sitting or standing, because these are the positions in which a person performs most occupational performance tasks. The therapist grasps the patient's arm proximally and distally to the joint on which the muscle acts. The joint is moved slowly through the full range of motion (ROM). The OTR notes how freely and readily the limb passively moves through ROM. The type and distribution of muscle tone are recorded for various muscle groups or movements, which provides a framework for formal assessment.

### Abnormal Muscle Tone

#### *Hypotonicity*

**Hypotonicity,** also called *flaccidity,* is a decrease in muscle tone. Hypotonicity is usually the result of a peripheral nerve injury, cerebellar disease, or frontal lobe damage and is seen temporarily in the shock phase after a stroke or spinal cord injury. The muscles feel soft and offer no resistance to passive movement. Usually a wide or excessive ROM is present.[42] When the flaccid limb is moved passively, it feels heavy. The patient is unable to hold a position once the limb is placed and released by the therapist. The hypotonic limb is unable to resist the pull of gravity and therefore drops.[4] Deep tendon reflexes (reflexive contraction of muscles when their tendons are tapped) are diminished or absent.[13,18] In CVA and spinal cord injuries, flaccidity is usually present initially but is soon replaced by hypertonicity.

#### *Hypertonicity*

Hypertonicity, also called *spasticity,* is an increase in muscle tone. Hypertonicity is defined in a variety of ways. One of the most common definitions is an increased resistance to passive stretch caused by an increased or hyperactive stretch reflex.[36,40] Any neurological condition that alters upper motor neuron pathways may result in hypertonicity.[20]

Hypertonicity is characterized by hyperactive deep tendon reflexes and *clonus* (quick, repetitive, alternate contraction of the agonist and antagonist muscles).[32] Hypertonic muscles offer greater than normal resistance to passive ROM. Hypertonicity usually occurs in patterns of flexion or extension.[6,24,32] Typically the patterns of hypertonicity occur in the antigravity muscles of the limbs. Flexor hypertonicity is more frequently apparent in the upper extremity and extensor hypertonicity in the lower extremity.

Hypertonicity varies with the site of the insult to the nervous system. Hypertonicity associated with cerebral damage, as occurs with stroke or head injury, is often seen in combination with other motor deficits, such as rigidity or ataxia. Such hypertonicity is influenced by the patient's position and the components of the postural mechanism.[20] Spinal cord hypertonicity is often violent in nature, with severe episodic muscle spasms in muscle groups normally innervated below the level of the lesion.[20,37]

*Occurrence* Hypertonicity is frequently seen in patients with upper motor neuron disorders such as multiple sclerosis, CVA, head injury, brain tumors or infections, and spinal cord injury or disease.

*Influencing factors* The postural mechanism influences the degree and patterns of hypertonicity. Therefore the positions of the body and head in space and the head in relation to the body influence the degree and distribution of abnormal muscle tone.[6] Extrinsic factors that influence the degree of hypertonicity include environmental temperature extremes, pain, infection, and emotional stress.[17,20] Therapeutic intervention focuses on empowering the patient to reduce, eliminate, or cope with these extrinsic factors.

*Method of evaluation* Hypertonicity fluctuates, making accurate measurement difficult. Several authors have documented methods of evaluating hypertonicity.[6-8] The OTR can clinically judge the degree and distribution of hypertonicity while assessing a patient with CNS dysfunction. The occupational therapist must remember the dynamic aspect of muscle tone and the factors that might influence a patient's muscle tone. While observing a patient performing occupational tasks such as feeding or dressing, the OTR or COTA must note the impact of abnormal muscle tone. The ultimate purpose of evaluating hypertonicity is to determine how function is impaired as a result of the abnormal muscle tone.

*Measurement of degree* Following the general guidelines for muscle tone assessment, the occupational therapist can determine if hypotonicity, hypertonicity, or rigidity is present. With hypertonicity the OTR determines the degree of increased muscle tone, which may be mild, moderate, or severe. In a patient with mild or minimal hypertonicity, resistance during passive movement of a joint through full ROM may be felt; however, full ROM is readily attainable. The patient with mild hypertonicity may have difficulty performing functional activities at a normal speed. A patient with moderate hypertonicity demonstrates consistent resistance during passive movement of a joint through full ROM; however, full ROM is attainable. Actively, the patient demonstrates observable deviations while performing occupational performance tasks. For example, the patient may be unable to incorporate forearm supination (palm up) and wrist extension (wrist in upward position) during self-feeding because of hypertonicity in the forearm pronator and wrist flexor muscles. The patient with severe hypertonicity demonstrates strong resistance during passive movement of a joint through full ROM. Actively, a patient with severe hypertonicity is significantly limited in the ability to control the involved extremities.

Manual muscle testing is not appropriate for patients who demonstrate abnormal muscle tone. Hypotonic patients are at risk of subluxation or dislocation of joints during manual testing. Hypertonic and rigid muscles may appear "strong" because of resistance during movement. The increased resistance to movement is not controlled by the patient and is involuntary. With severe hypertonicity the application of resistance in an effort to stretch the hypertonic muscle may cause tearing or other injuries to the muscle.[6]

### *Rigidity*

**Rigidity** is an increase in muscle tone in the agonist and antagonist muscles simultaneously. Both muscle groups contract continually, resulting in increased resistance to passive movement in any direction and throughout the joint ROM.[15,28] *Lead-pipe rigidity* is identified in patients who demonstrate a constant resistance throughout the joint ROM when a limb is passively moved in any direction. With *cogwheel rigidity* a rhythmic "give" occurs in the resistance throughout the ROM, similar to the feeling of turning a cogwheel. In rigidity the deep tendon reflexes are normal or only moderately increased.[15,28]

*Occurrence* Rigidity occurs as a result of lesions of the extrapyramidal system, such as in Parkinson's disease, certain degenerative diseases, encephalitis, tumors,[14] and traumatic brain injury. Cogwheel rigidity occurs in some types of parkinsonism and in some cases of carbon monoxide poisoning. Rigid *decerebrate posturing* (full body extension) and *decorticate posturing* (full body flexion) may occur with diffuse brain injury or anoxia. Frequently, rigidity and hypertonicity of muscles occur simultaneously in a patient with CNS dysfunction.

Muscle tone is only one component of the postural mechanism. The occupational therapist must also assess for the presence of primitive reflexes and automatic reactions.

### Reflexes

Reflexes are innate motor responses elicited by specific sensory stimuli. In normal development, **primitive reflexes** are observed in the infant and are involuntary. The primitive reflexes help to elongate muscle groups in preparation for voluntary control. In normal development the reflexes occur only under stress (e.g.,

(Pictures)

infant is hungry or tired) and are never seen in the total complement or pattern. The primitive reflexes become integrated as the infant gains voluntary motor control. The OTR, and in certain situations the COTA on the establishment of service competency, may assess for the presence of primitive reflexes. Formal reflex testing is typically performed with the patient in the sitting or supine position. The specific sensory stimulus is provided by the therapist, and the clinician observes for the expected motor response, as described in Table 10-1. The emergence or persistence of primitive reflexes in an adult will interfere with the recovery of the automatic protective extension, righting, and equilibrium reactions. The functional significance of the presence of specific reflexes is described next.

*Suck/Swallow Reflex*

The patient with a suck/swallow reflex has difficulty eating. The involuntary protrusion and retraction of the tongue makes it difficult to keep food and liquids in the oral cavity. The patient will not be able to suck from a straw.

*Asymmetrical Tonic Neck Reflex (ATNR)*

The patient with a persistent ATNR may have difficulty maintaining the head in midline while moving the eyes toward or past midline.[5] The patient may be unable to extend or flex an arm without turning the head.[5,13] The patient also may be unable to bring the hands to midline. Thus the presence of the ATNR makes it difficult to bring an object to the mouth, hold an object in both hands, or grasp an object in front of the body while looking at it.

*Symmetrical Tonic Neck Reflex (STNR)*

The patient with a persistent STNR is unable to support the body weight on hands and knees, maintain balance in quadruped, and creep normally.[6] The patient has difficulty moving from supine to sitting position because bending the head forward (flexed) to initiate the task increases extension in the legs. The patient is unable to bend at the hips to sit upright. The patient has difficulty with moving from sitting to standing. Because the arms and head are extended to initiate the movement, one or both legs may flex. Also, the patient who has had a CVA may demonstrate total flexion of the affected leg, resulting in an inability to bear weight.[13]

*Tonic Labyrinthine Reflex (TLR)*

The patient exhibiting a poorly integrated TLR has severely limited movement. Examples of functional limitations are inability to lift the head in the supine position, inability to move from supine to sitting position using flexion of trunk and hips, inability to roll supine to prone (and vice versa), and inability to sit in a wheelchair for long periods.[6,13] In attempting to move from supine to sitting position, extensor tone initially is dominant until halfway up, when flexor tone begins to take over. Flexor tone continues until full sitting is reached, when the head falls forward, the spine flexes, and then the patient falls forward.[5] Sitting in a wheelchair for extended periods can result in increased extensor tone as the patient hyperextends the neck to view the environment. With the increased extensor tone the patient slips into a semisupine position with feet off footplates[13] (Figure 10-2).

*Positive Supporting Reflex (PSR)*

The patient who exhibits a PSR has difficulty placing the heel on the ground for standing and walking. A persistent PSR interferes with foot-flat lower extremity weight bearing and weight shifting.[6,13] The patient has difficulty arising from a chair and descending steps because the leg remains stiffly in extension. The rigid leg can carry the patient's body weight but cannot adjust in any balance reactions. Therefore all balance reactions are compensated with other body parts[5] (Figure 10-3).

*Crossed Extension Reflex (CER)*

The patient who has had a stroke and is influenced by the CER has difficulty with developing a normal gait pattern because strong extension occurs in the affected leg as the unaffected leg is flexed. The patient has difficulty bridging (lifting buttocks while supine with both legs flexed) in bed.[5,13]

*Palmar Grasp Reflex*

The patient with a poorly integrated grasp reflex cannot release objects placed in the hand, even if active finger extension is present.[13]

*Plantar Grasp Reflex*

The patient with a poorly integrated plantar grasp reflex has difficulty keeping toes from curling in the shoes. Normal equilibrium responses in the foot do not develop if the plantar grasp reflex is present.

*Functional Significance*

The occupational therapy practitioner must observe for the influence of the primitive reflexes as a part of the motor control evaluation. Observation of a patient engaging in occupational performance tasks will enhance the practitioner's understanding of the functional significance of the persistence of these reflexes in patients with CNS damage.

As the primitive reflexes become integrated in normal development, higher level protective extension, righting, and equilibrium reactions emerge. The following automatic reactions, which are normally part of the postural mechanism, are important for the occupational therapist to evaluate in patients with CNS dysfunction.

**Automatic Reactions**

*Protective Extension Reactions*

**Protective extension reactions** (extending the arms) are used to protect the head and face when a person is off balance or falling.[16,18] Without these reactions, the

Table 10-1

## Functional Implications with Persistence of Primitive Reflexes*

| *Reflex* | *Stimulus* | *Response* | *Examples of potential impact*[†] |
|---|---|---|---|
| Suck/swallow reflex | Light touch to lips or gums | Suckling (immature protrusion and retraction of tongue as observed in neonate) | • Difficulty performing oral hygiene activities<br>Excessive tongue protrusion during eating and drinking<br>Difficulty creating negative pressure to suck from a straw |
| Asymmetrical tonic neck reflex (ATNR) | Head turned to one side with chin over shoulder | Extension of arm and leg on face side; flexion on arm and leg on skull side | • Difficulty performing self-maintenance activities if head turned to one side |
| Symmetrical tonic neck reflex | Flexion of neck<br>Extension (hyperextension of neck) | Flexion of arms and extension of legs<br>Extension of arms and flexion of legs | • Difficulty bridging (lifting buttocks off supporting surface with hips and neck flexed)<br>Difficulty crawling reciprocally<br>Difficulty using arms to reach over head |
| Tonic labyrinthine reflex (TLR) | Supine position<br>Prone position | Extension of trunk and extremities or increased extensor postural tone<br>Flexion of trunk and extremities or increased flexor postural tone | • Difficulty performing all transitional movements that require dissociation between upper and lower body (flexion of upper body with extension of legs, e.g., moving from supine to long sitting in bed) |
| Positive supporting reflex (PSR) | Pressure to ball of foot | Extension in leg stimulated (hip and knee extension with plantar flexion of ankle, i.e., toe pointing downward) | • Difficulty bridging<br>Difficulty donning shoes or keeping them on<br>Difficulty with swing through phase of walking as it precedes toe off phase<br>Difficulty climbing stairs |
| Crossed extension reflex (CER) | Flexion of one leg | Extension of opposite leg | • Difficulty bridging with both legs flexed simultaneously<br>Difficulty walking with a reciprocal arm/leg gait pattern |
| Palmar grasp reflex | Pressure in palm of hand | Flexion of digits into palmar grasp | • Difficulty releasing objects from a palmar grasp, (e.g., drinking glass, hairbrush, mop) |
| Plantar grasp reflex | Pressure to ball of foot | Flexion of toes | • Curling of toes in shoes<br>Difficulty walking with foot flat<br>Absence of equilibrium responses in foot |

*In adults who have sustained an insult to the central nervous system (CNS), the emergence of primitive reflexes may interfere with motor control recovery. Typically, these reflexes are assessed while the patient is sitting or supine with the head initially in midline, with the exception of the tonic labyrinthine reflexes.

[†]In adults with CNS dysfunction while engaged in occupational performance tasks.

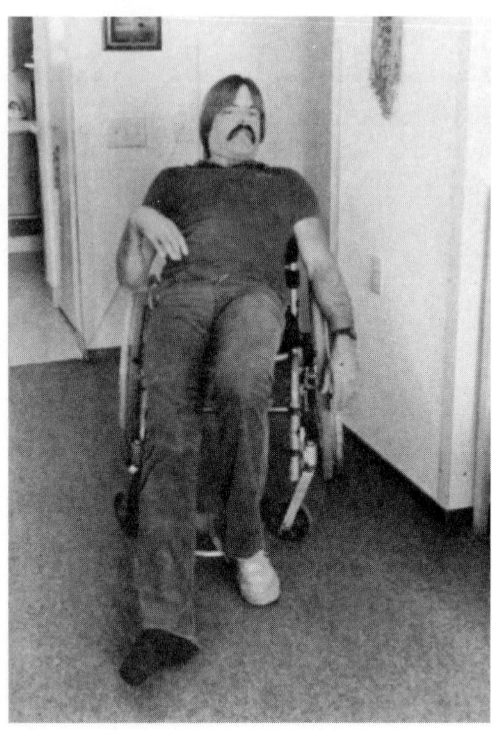

*Figure 10-2* Functional influence of tonic labyrinthine reflex (TLR) on sitting up in a wheelchair.

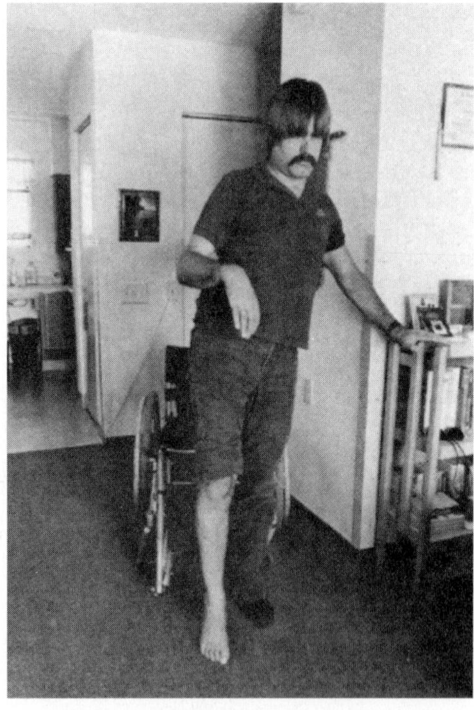

*Figure 10-3* Positive supporting reflex.

patient may be fearful of moving or reluctant to bear weight on the affected side during bilateral or two-handed activities such as using a rolling pin, cutting meat with a knife and fork, or playing a game of pool. The patient cannot break a fall without protective extension responses.

### *Righting Reactions*

The automatic **righting reactions** maintain or restore the normal position of the head in space (eyes parallel to the horizon) and its normal relationship with the trunk and limbs. Without effective righting responses, the patient has difficulty moving from one position to another, such as going from the supine position to sit or stand in order to arise from bed.[6]

### *Equilibrium Reactions*

**Equilibrium reactions** maintain and restore a person's balance in all activities.[6,23] They ensure sufficient postural alignment when the body's supporting surface is changed, altering a person's center of gravity. In mature equilibrium responses the patient's trunk elongates on the weight-bearing side. Without equilibrium responses, the patient has difficulty maintaining and recovering balance in all positions and activities. The patient with inadequate equilibrium reactions has difficulty sitting unsupported while performing dressing activities or standing at a sink while performing oral hygiene activities.

*Testing* Formal testing of the protective extension, righting, and equilibrium reactions may be difficult because of the patient's cognitive and physical limitations or the time constraints on the occupational therapy practitioner. The COTA develops observational skills so that the absence or presence of righting reactions may be noted during transfers and self-maintenance activities. Equilibrium and protective extension reactions can be observed when the patient shifts farther out of midline than necessary during functional activities. The COTA observes whether the patient is able to regain balance efficiently and effectively to complete the functional activity. Alternately, if the patient is unable to regain balance, the COTA should observe if protective responses are used to break a fall. The OT practitioner should be positioned to protect the patient if these responses fail.

Normal muscles allow for smooth and well-controlled mobility against the forces of gravity. If reflexes or stereotypical patterns are not integrated, however, and if protective extension, righting, and equilibrium reactions are impaired, the patient will have difficulty using the limbs for functional self-maintenance activities.

## EVALUATING UPPER EXTREMITY MOTOR RECOVERY

In addition to evaluating a patient's postural mechanism, the occupational therapist performs an evaluation of upper extremity movement and control. The therapist identifies where and to what extent the patient's motor control is dominated by stereotypical patterns of movement and where and under what conditions isolated movement is present. The therapist notes the degree to which the patient's abnormal postural mechanism interferes with selective volitional movement and determines in which direction of movement hypertonicity occurs and how it affects function.

Although upper extremity movement is the primary focus, the occupational therapy practitioner must examine the patient's general posture and movement. An understanding of how people move enhances the practitioner's skills in recognizing abnormal movements or postures that affect upper extremity function.

The upper extremity motor recovery evaluation begins by observing the patient's overall posture. Is the patient's posture symmetrical with equal weight on both hips (if sitting) or on both feet (if standing)? How does the patient move in general? Is the head in midline or tilted to one side? Is one shoulder higher than the other (elevated)? Is the trunk twisted or long on one side and short on the other? Asymmetries such as these impede the patient's ability to move the limbs normally and efficiently. Current therapy focuses on achieving normal functional movement to the extent possible to achieve maximal independence while engaged in occupational performance tasks.

Evaluation and treatment often occur together. For example, if asymmetry is noted, the OT practitioner attempts to correct the asymmetry before continuing with the assessment. This process provides valuable information about the patient's ability to respond to therapeutic touch and how the patient's posture affects muscle tone and movement.

After general observations of the patient's motor control and posture, the practitioner assesses more specifically the amount and type of motor recovery present in the upper extremities.

Testing is usually done while the patient is sitting. Observing upper extremity control in standing may provide the OT practitioner with a more realistic indication of the degree of impairment, especially if the patient will eventually be ambulatory. Functionally, many occupational performance tasks (e.g., donning slacks, sweeping the floor) are performed while standing.

### Brunnstrom's Stages of Motor Recovery

In the 1950s and 1960s Brunnstrom observed progressive changes in motor function and behavior during the motor recovery process after a CVA (Box 10-1).[8] Figure 10-4 provides a framework for assessing motor recovery as described by Brunnstrom. The various stages of motor function, as adapted from Brunnstrom, are described next.

#### *No Motion*

No motion can be elicited from the involved upper extremity(ies).

#### *Reflex Responses*

These movements are limited to generalized or localized motor responses to specific sensory stimuli.[21] For example, a patient with a positive palmar grasp reflex involuntarily holds an object placed in the palm of the hand. Table 10-1 provides additional examples.

*Box 10-1*

**Brunnstrom's Stages of Recovery After Cerebrovascular Accident (CVA, Stroke)**

1. No motion
2. Reflex responses
3. Associated reactions
4. Mass responses (synergistic)
5. Deviation from pattern
6. Wrist stability
7. Individual finger movement
8. Selected pattern with overlay
9. Selective movement

#### *Associated Reactions*

These abnormal increases in muscle tone in the involved extremity(ies) occur when activity requires intensive effort of the unaffected limbs. The involved extremity(ies) often move in a synergistic, mass pattern. Associated reactions can be elicited by resisting motion at a joint in an uninvolved limb or by having the patient squeeze an object with the unaffected hand. These reactions can also be observed during the patient's performance of transfers and other self-maintenance activities that require effort (Figure 10-5).[8]

#### *Mass Responses (Synergistic)*

Voluntary motion is limited to total limb movements in flexion or extension. The patient is unable to isolate individual joint motion or deviate from the stereotypical movement pattern.[8,21] This can be evaluated by asking the patient to move at only one joint and observing where the motion actually occurs. Patients who exhibit synergistic movement responses are unable to move one joint in isolation. The stereotypical patterns of movement may be seen partially or in full complement. The *flexion pattern response* consists of scapular adduction and elevation, humeral abduction and external rotation, elbow flexion, forearm supination, wrist flexion, and digit flexion (Figure 10-6). The *extension pattern response* consists of scapular abduction and depression, humeral adduction and internal rotation, elbow extension, forearm pronation, and wrist and finger flexion or extension (Figure 10-7).

#### *Deviation from Pattern*

Voluntary motor control deviates from the synergy through movement and is patterned predominantly when functional tasks are attempted. For example, a patient may be able actively to extend the wrist when asked but unable to use wrist extension while the shoulder is flexed (e.g., reaching for an item above the head). Testing involves asking the patient to perform movements that deviate from the synergies and observing the patient's ability to accomplish such movements successfully, as follows[21]:

**III. SENSORY MOTOR ASSESSMENT (continued)**

**OCCUPATIONAL THERAPY EVALUATION**

**F. Mass Pattern Responses:** key: 0 = zero, W = weak, M = moderate, S = strong.
Observer active R.O.M. and effect of heat and trunk position on motion.

| | ADMISSION | | DISCHARGE | |
|---|---|---|---|---|
| 1. FLEXION PATTERN | Right | Left | Right | Left |
| Shoulder abduction/elevation | | | | |
| Elbow flexions | | | | |

Comments: Note any motion occuring at forearm, wrist and band.

| | ADMISSION | | DISCHARGE | |
|---|---|---|---|---|
| 2. EXTENSION PATTERN | Right | Left | Right | Left |
| Shoulder Adduction/Internal Rotation | | | | |
| Elbow Extension | | | | |

Comments: Note any motions occuring at forearm, wrist and hand.

Key: N = normal, WE = with ease, WD = with difficulty, U = unable, NT = not tested

**G. Deviation From Patterns**

| | ADMISSION | | DISCHARGE | |
|---|---|---|---|---|
| | Right | Left | Right | Left |
| Shoulder add./Int. rot. with Elbow flexion | | | | |
| Shoulder abduction with Elbow extension | | | | |
| Forearm pronation with Elbow flexion | | | | |
| Forearm supination with Elbow extension | | | | |

Comments:

**H. Wrist and Hand Recovery: record grasp and pinch measurements**

| | ADMISSION | | DISCHARGE | |
|---|---|---|---|---|
| | Right | Left | Right | Left |
| Stable Wrist During Grasp | | | | |
| Mass Grasp: Notch # | | | | |
| Mass Release (3 inch cube) | | | | |
| Lateral Pinch | | | | |
| Palmar Pinch | | | | |
| Individual Finger Motions | | | | |

Comments:

**I. Selective With Pattern Overlay**

| | ADMISSION | | DISCHARGE | |
|---|---|---|---|---|
| | Right | Left | Right | Left |
| Integrate prox. to distal control (stack cones) | | | | |
| Reciprocal total U.E. motion (tether ball) | | | | |
| Rapid elbow flexion–extension | | | | |
| Rapid wrist flexion–extension | | | | |

Comments:

**HAND FUNCTION: (Functional Use Test)**

Class #

Involved Side:

Describe highest function:

*Figure 10-4* Upper extremity motor control assessment, part of the Occupational Therapy Stroke Evaluation. (Courtesy Occupational Therapy Department, Ranchos Los Amigos, Downey, Calif.)

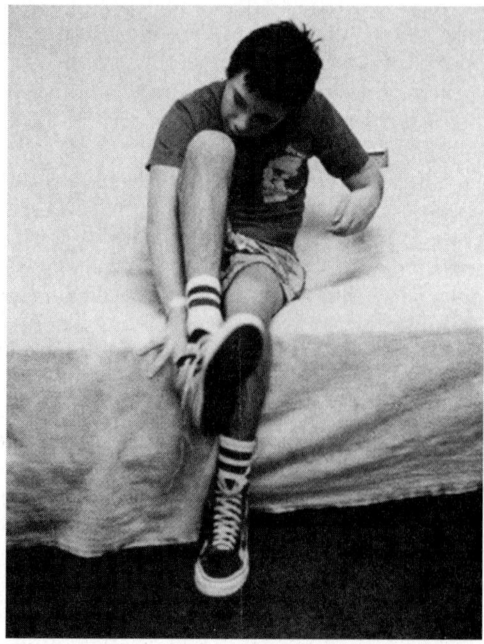

*Figure 10-5* Associated reaction elicited during lower extremity dressing.

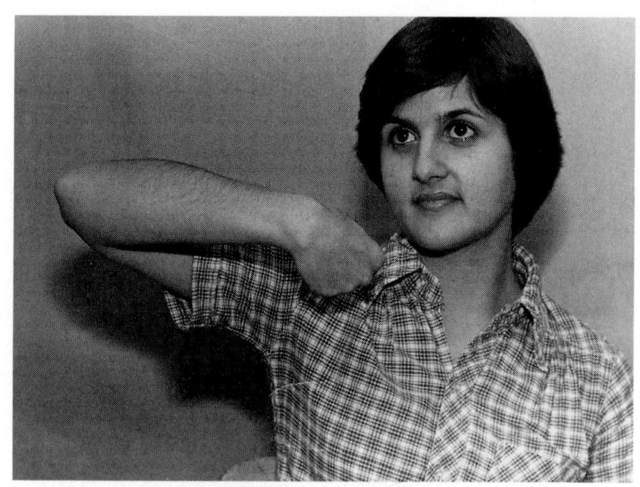

*Figure 10-6* Flexion synergy in upper extremity.

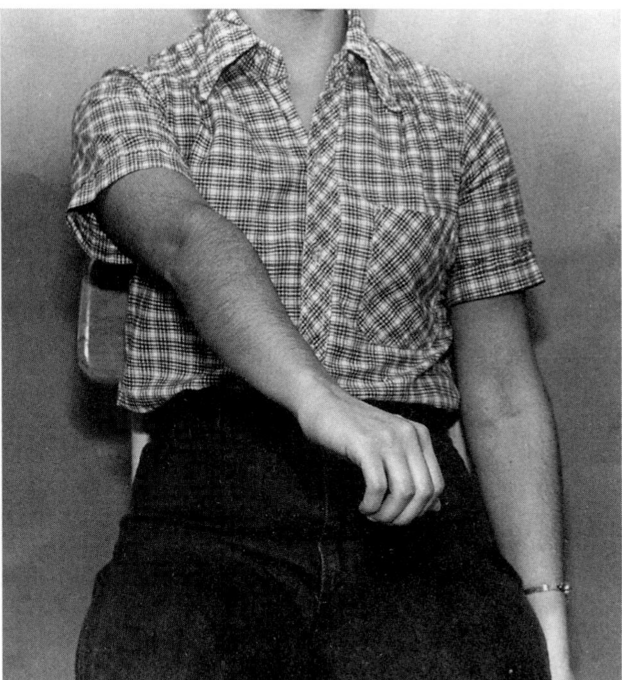

*Figure 10-7* Extension synergy in upper extremity.

1. Ask the patient to touch the back of the uninvolved shoulder with the involved hand (requires scapular abduction and humeral horizontal adduction or scapular abduction with elbow flexion).
2. Ask the patient to touch, using the involved hand, the therapist's finger, which is held out to the patient's involved side (requires shoulder or humeral abduction with elbow extension).
3. Ask the patient to use the involved hand to pick up an object from the therapist's hand, positioned approximately 4 inches (10 cm) above the patient's involved knee (requires elbow flexion with forearm pronation).
4. Ask the patient to reach out in front of the body using the involved hand to receive an object in the palm (requires elbow extension with forearm supination).

The occupational therapy practitioner can detect whether or not the patient is beginning to deviate from mass patterns by observing the patient performing these movements. Also, observations of the patient engaged in occupational performance tasks indicate when a patient is beginning to deviate from these patterns.

#### *Wrist Stability*

The OT practitioner asks the patient to make a fist and observes for stability of the wrist joint in extension. The patient must also be observed during the performance of tasks such as holding a toothbrush or holding a spoon during self-feeding.

#### *Individual Finger Movements*

The OT practitioner asks the patient to touch the tip of each finger with the tip of the thumb or to perform a tapping motion with the fingers against the table or the patient's leg. The practitioner observes for isolated selective movements. If muscle tone is normal, grasp and pinch strength can be measured by using a dynamometer, bulbometer, or pinch gauge.

#### *Selective Pattern with Overlay*

Joint movement in the affected limb may be isolated with voluntary control, and motion may occur in a variety of planes and directions. However, when the limb is functionally stressed (e.g., patient attempting to button small buttons on a shirt sleeve), synergistic patterns may be seen. The OT practitioner observes for compensatory movements being used during functional activities if the patient is in this stage of motor recovery. The patient may lean to the uninvolved side to raise the involved hand over the head. Shoulder elevation may be used to increase shoulder joint ROM on the involved side. The patient in this stage has difficulty performing rapid reciprocal motions, such as alternating wrist flexion and extension. During evaluation of rapid reciprocal movements, the patient's uninvolved limb should be compared to the involved limb.[21]

#### *Selective Movement*

**Selective movement** is the ability to control movements at each individual joint. The OT practitioner observes for selective movement and control while the patient is engaged in functional activities.

In summary, Brunnstrom provided a framework for the anticipated motor recovery in stroke patients. The last stage of motor recovery is selective movement. However, not all patients will reach this level of recovery.

### Evaluating Functional Use of the Limbs

The occupational therapy practitioner faces the challenge of maximizing patients' ability to return to purposeful and meaningful activities within their physical and social environments. The focus of functional outcomes must be maintained throughout the process of evaluating upper extremity motor control. Evaluating the functional status of the involved limb will guide the practitioner in selecting functional, realistic goals.

On the establishment of service competency, the COTA may be responsible for assessing a patient's functional abilities using simple, structured tests. The Functional Test for the Hemiplegic/Paretic Upper Extremity assesses the patient's ability to use the involved arm for occupational performance tasks. It contains items ranging from basic stabilization to more difficult tasks requiring distal fine manipulation with proximal stability. Examples of specific tasks include holding a pouch, stabilizing a jar, wringing a wet washcloth, interlocking and zipping a zipper, folding a sheet, and installing an overhead light bulb. This test provides objective data of the patient's functional abilities and is administered in 30 minutes or less.[43]

The OT practitioner also observes the patient during self-maintenance evaluation and training to determine functional use and potential for functional use of the involved extremity(ies). Whether the practitioner uses a simple structured test or observations during a checklist for activities of daily living (ADLs), the level of functional assist of the involved limb must be established to set realistic goals. The following descriptors are suggested[1]:

- *Minimal stabilizing assist.* The patient is able to use the involved upper extremity to stabilize objects being manipulated by the uninvolved extremity. The involved extremity is placed and stabilization accomplished by the limb's weight. For example, the involved upper extremity is placed on a piece of paper to stabilize it while the patient writes.
- *Minimal active assist.* The patient is able to use the involved upper extremity to assist actively in accomplishing a single part of an activity, for example, actively placing the hand on a piece of paper for writing or actively holding the involved arm away from the body for dressing or hygiene activities.
- *Maximal active assist.* The patient is able to use the involved arm and hand in all activities that require motor control for pushing or pulling, stabilizing, and gross grasp and release. For example, while writing a letter, the patient can push the paper upward using the involved arm and hand.
- *Incorporation of involved upper extremity in all bilateral tasks.* The patient is able to use the involved upper extremity to assist the uninvolved extremity in most occupational performance tasks, although speed and coordination may be impaired. For example, the patient is able to move both arms above the head to put on a pullover shirt, but movements are slow and cautious on the involved side.

### Occupational Therapy Considerations Based on Results of Motor Control Evaluation

Although the OT practitioner bases treatment on the patient's overall evaluation results, including cognition, vision, sensation, psychological aspects, and occupational needs,[33] the motor control evaluation results help to guide the program plan. Chapter 23 describes several approaches to motor control treatment in detail. The following are some general guidelines for treatment.

For hypotonia and limited to no motion in the upper extremity(ies), the OT practitioner needs to facilitate the increased tone necessary for stability. Weight-bearing and tactile and proprioceptive input may be used to increase muscle tone. The practitioner provides input in such a way as to avoid overstimulating specific muscles or encouraging abnormal patterns of movement. Therapeutic activities for improving strength may be used if motion is selective (i.e., not patterned) in the involved upper extremity. A primary goal of treatment should be to establish a balance of strength and tone between the agonist and antagonist muscles.[9] The involved arm can be positioned as normally as possible to provide appropriate sensory feedback while the patient is performing occupational tasks. Patient and family education in proper positioning and joint protection is important to prevent trauma to joint structures.

For hypertonia the OT practitioner uses inhibitive techniques to decrease the abnormal muscle tone and patterns of movement. The sensorimotor approaches described in Chapter 23 may be appropriate, depending on the disability, severity, and distribution of the hypertonia and the associated problems. The goal of treatment is to balance the tone for more normal movement. Therefore inhibition of the hypertonic muscles and facilitation of the antagonist muscles are necessary, using one of the sensorimotor approaches.

In some patients, hypertonicity is severe enough to require progressive inhibitory casting or splinting.[3,29,33,39] Casting provides the circumferential pressure necessary to prevent soft tissue contractures and maintain the muscle's normal length for functional ROM.[25,31]

Serial casting is most successful when a soft tissue contracture has been present for less than 6 months. A series of casts is applied to obtain the maximal end range of a contracted muscle. The final cast may be bivalved (cut into two halves) and used as a night positioner. However, many clinicians prefer bivalving *all* casts in the series because this prevents skin breakdown.[3] A bivalved cast also allows the practitioner to remove the cast for therapy on a regular basis. Various types of casts can be used to decrease hypertonicity in the adult with CNS damage.

A combination of peripheral nerve blocks and casting or splinting is often used.[3,25,28] Lidocaine blocks, which are short acting, can be administered by the physician before applying an inhibitory cast to make limb positioning easier. Phenol nerve blocks, also given by a physician, can last up to 3 months. Nerve blocks allow the therapist to increase antagonist control and strength to achieve a balance of muscle control between the agonist and antagonist muscles.[25,41]

Physical agent modalities, such as cold, heat, and neuromuscular electrical stimulation, can be used in preparation for or along with purposeful activity. These modalities must be provided by a practitioner with established service competency and can help temporarily to reduce hypertonicity to allow for the development of antagonistic control.

Patients with severe hypertonicity accompanied by severe pain may require evaluation of the cause of pain. Drug therapy (as prescribed by the physician) and other pain management techniques may be a part of the program plan. If a patient has a drug therapy regimen, the OT practitioner must be aware of the potential side effects of such drugs. It is crucial that the practitioner communicate to the medical staff any observed side effects that interfere with the patient's overall function.

Although motor control may be adequate for the performance of occupational tasks, sensory and perceptual deficits may limit the patient's success in performing functional activities. Perceptual deficits may alter the patient's abilities, requiring the occupational therapist to lower expected goals.[2] (See Chapters 11 and 24 for further discussions on perception.)

## COORDINATION

**Coordination** is the harmonious interaction of muscles throughout the limb that allows for the production of accurate controlled movement. Such movement is characterized by smoothness, rhythm, and appropriate speed. Voluntary control of muscle tone, postural tone, and balance among muscle groups is necessary for coordinated movement.

To effect coordinated movement, all the elements of the neuromuscular performance components must be intact. Coordinated movement depends on the contraction of specific agonist muscles with the simultaneous relaxation of the corresponding antagonist muscles, anchored by co-contraction of the joint-stabilizing muscles. In addition, proprioception, kinesthesia, and body schema must be intact. The patient must have the ability to judge space accurately and to direct body parts through space to the desired target with correct timing.[4]

### Occurrence of Incoordination

Coordination of muscle action is under the control of the cerebellum and is influenced by the extrapyramidal tracts. However, knowledge of body schema and body-to-space relationships is also essential to the production of coordinated movement. Therefore many types of lesions can cause disturbances of coordination.[4] These include diseases and injuries of muscles and peripheral nerves, lesions of the posterior columns of the spinal cord, and lesions of the cerebral cortex. Paralysis of the limbs caused by a PNS lesion prevents administering tests for coordination even though CNS mechanisms are intact.[28]

Common signs of incoordination seen by the occupational therapy practitioner include the following:

- **Ataxia** is impaired gross coordination and gait. The patient with ataxia may have visible tremor-like movements. Ataxia is seen in the delayed initiation of motor responses, in errors in range and force of movement, and in errors in rate and regularity of movement. For example, an ataxic patient cannot grade the force of grasp and might crush a styrofoam cup. In gait the patient demonstrates a wide base of support (legs far apart) with a reduced or absent arm swing. Step length may be uneven, and the patient may tend to fall toward one side. Ataxia results in a lack of postural stability, with patients tending to fixate or tighten specific muscle groups to compensate for the instability.[11,19,27]
- **Adiadochokinesia** ("not moving together") is an inability to perform rapidly alternating movements, such as forearm supination and pronation or elbow flexion and extension.[14] For example, a patient has difficulty dusting or washing windows.
- **Dysmetria** ("faulty distance between two points") is an inability to estimate the ROM necessary to reach the target of movement. It is evident when touching the finger to the nose or placing an object onto a table.[14] A patient has difficulty judging distances and may knock a cup while reaching for it.
- **Dyssynergia** ("faulty working together") is a "decomposition of movement" in which voluntary movements are broken into their component parts and appear jerky. Problems in articulation (see Dysarthria entry that follows) and phonation may be present.[14]
- **Tremor** is an involuntary shaking or trembling motion. Tremors are classified according to their type. An *intention tremor* occurs during voluntary movement, is often intensified at the termination of movement, and is often seen in patients with multiple sclerosis. The patient with an intention tremor may have difficulty performing tasks that require accuracy and precision of limb placement (e.g., drinking from a cup, inserting a key in a door). A *resting tremor* is present in the absence of voluntary movement (occurs while the patient is not moving). A *pill-rolling tremor,* in which the individual appears to be rolling a pill between the thumb and index and middle fingers, is a type of resting tremor often seen in patients with Parkinson's disease.
- **Rebound phenomenon of Holmes** ("to bounce or spring again") is a lack of the *check reflex,* or the inability to stop a motion quickly to avoid striking something. For example, if the patient's arm is bent against the resistance of the therapist and the resistance is suddenly and unexpectedly removed, the patient's hand will hit the face or body.[11,14]
- **Nystagmus** is an involuntary movement of the eyeballs in an up-and-down, back-and-forth, or rotating direction. After rotation or spinning of the body and head in space, nystagmus is the normal response that helps a person regain balance and orientation. Nystagmus can interfere with head control and fine adjustments required for balance.[14]
- **Dysarthria,** or faulty speech production, is explosive or slurred speech caused by the incoordination of the speech mechanism. The patient's speech may also vary in pitch, may appear nasal and tremulous, or both.[11,14]
- **Choreiform movements** are uncontrolled, irregular, purposeless, quick, jerky, and dysrhythmical movements of variable distribution that may also occur during sleep.[14]

- **Athetoid movements,** or movements without stability, are slow, wormlike, arrhythmical movements that primarily affect the distal portions of the extremities. *Athetosis* occurs in predictable patterns in the same subject and is not present during sleep.[14]
- **Spasms** are sudden, involuntary contractions of a muscle or large groups of muscles.[11] In a patient with a spinal cord injury, spasms often cause violent and involuntary straightening of the legs.
- **Dystonia** is faulty muscle tension or tone. Dystonic movements tend to involve large portions of the body and produce grotesque posturing with bizarre writhing movements.[4,11]
- **Ballism,** or projectile movement, is a rare symptom produced by continuous, gross, abrupt contractions of the axial and proximal musculature of the extremity. It causes the limb to fly out suddenly and occurs on one side of the body.[11,14]

### Clinical Evaluation of Coordination

**Incoordination** consists of errors in rate, rhythm, range, direction, and force of movement.[19] Observation is an important element of the evaluation. The neurological examination for incoordination may include the nose-finger-nose test, the finger-nose test, the knee pat (pronation-supination) test, and the finger wiggling test.[4,28] Such tests can reveal dysmetria, dyssynergia, adiadochokinesia, tremors, and ataxia. The neurologist usually performs these examinations.

### Occupational Therapy Evaluation of Coordination

Occupation is the hallmark of occupational therapy, and therefore the occupational therapist should seek to translate the clinical evaluation to a functional one. Selected activities and specific performance tests can reveal the effect of incoordination on function, which is the primary concern of the OT practitioner. The practitioner can observe for coordination difficulties during self-maintenance evaluation and training. The practitioner should observe for irregularity in the rate or force of the movement and sudden corrective movements in an attempt to compensate for incoordination. Thus movement during the performance of functional activities may appear irregular, jerky, and may overreach the target.[28]

The following general guidelines and questions can be used when evaluating incoordination:

1. The OTR evaluates the patient's muscle tone and joint mobility.
2. The OTR and the COTA provide manual stability to joints proximally to distally during functional tasks and note any differences in performance with and without stabilization.
3. The OTR and the COTA observe for resting or intention tremor during functional activities.
4. The OTR and COTA observe for any noticeable signs of incoordination during therapy sessions.
5. The OTR and the COTA observe whether the patient becomes more uncoordinated in distracting environments.

Several standardized tests of motor function and manual dexterity are available, as outlined by Smith.[38] These include the Purdue Pegboard,[35] The Minnesota Rate of Manipulation Test,[30] Lincoln-Oscretsky Motor Development Scale,[26] the Pennsylvania Bi-Manual Work Sample,[34] the Crawford Small Parts Dexterity Test,[12] and the Jebsen-Taylor Hand Function Test.[22] The OTR and the COTA with established service competency may administer one or more of these tests during the evaluation of coordination.

## SUMMARY

Motor control is the ability to make continuous postural adjustments and to regulate body and limb movements in response to functional situations. It is the result of the interaction of complex neurological systems. Evaluation of motor control includes assessment of the postural mechanism, selective movement, and coordination.

The presence of abnormal elements of motor control affects the quality of movements and the ability to perform functional tasks. The OTR evaluates muscle tone and upper extremity motor recovery. The COTA may assess aspects of the postural reflex mechanism and coordination using simple structured tests and observes for abnormal motor control while the patient is engaged in functional activities. The results of the motor control evaluation guide the practitioner in selecting the appropriate treatment approach(es), including sensorimotor approaches or rehabilitative and compensatory methods.

---

## *Selected Reading Guide Questions*

1. What are the roles of the OTR and the COTA in the evaluation and treatment of an adult with central nervous system (CNS) dysfunction who has a motor control deficit? How do these roles change with the establishment of service competency and with experience in a particular setting?
2. What are the components of the normal postural reflex mechanism?
3. Define *normal* muscle tone.
4. Describe the characteristics of normal muscle tone. Give an example of how normal muscle tone varies depending on the type of occupational performance task.
5. Describe the characteristics of hypotonicity.
6. Describe the characteristics of hypertonicity.
7. Diagrammatically depict the spectrum of normal and abnormal muscle tone.
8. Define *specific primitive reflexes,* and describe how the occupational therapy practitioner would assess for their presence.

9. Describe the functional difficulties encountered when the following primitive reflexes persist during the performance of functional activities in the adult who has sustained a CNS insult: (a) asymmetrical tonic neck reflex, (b) symmetrical tonic neck reflex, (c) tonic labyrinthine reflex, (d) crossed extension reflex, and (e) grasp reflex.
10. Define the expected stages of motor recovery in an adult after CNS dysfunction caused by a cerebrovascular accident (CVA).
11. Describe the upper extremity flexion and extension pattern responses typically observed in the patient who has sustained a CVA.
12. Define *fine coordination.* Analyze the stability and mobility necessary to perform specific occupational performance tasks, such as feeding and dressing.
13. List five types of incoordination, and describe the functional impact on an adult's performance of activities of daily living. For example, "Ataxia would interfere with self-feeding because. . . "

## REFERENCES


1. Andric M: Projecting the upper extremity functional level. In Professional Staff Association of Rancho Los Amigos Medical Center: *Stroke rehabilitation: state of the art, 1984,* Downey, Calif, 1984, Los Amigos Research and Education Institute.
2. Bernspang B, Viitanen M, Erickson S: Impairments of perceptual and motor functions: their influence on self-care ability 4-6 years after a stroke, *Occup Ther J Res* 9:27-37, 1989.
3. Berrol S: The treatment of physical disorders following brain injury. In Wood R, Eames P, editors: *Models of brain injury rehabilitation,* Baltimore, 1989, Johns Hopkins University Press.
4. Bickerstaff ER: *Neurological examination in clinical practice,* ed 3, London, 1973, Blackwell.
5. Bobath B: *Abnormal postural reflex activity caused by brain lesions,* ed 2, London, 1975, Heinemann.
6. Bobath B: *Adult hemiplegia: evaluation and treatment,* ed 2, London, 1978, Heinemann.
7. Bohannon RW, Smith MB: Interrater reliability of a modified Ashworth scale of muscle spasticity, *Phys Ther* 67:206-207, 1987.
8. Brunnstrom S: *Movement therapy in hemiplegia,* New York, 1970, Harper & Row.
9. Carr JH, Shepherd RB: *A motor relearning program for stroke,* ed 2, Rockville, Md, 1987, Aspen.
10. Charness A: *Stroke/head injury: a guide to functional outcomes in physical therapy management,* Rockville, Md, 1986, Aspen.
11. Chusid JG: *Correlative neuroanatomy and functional neurology,* ed 18, Los Altos, Calif, 1982, Lange.
12. Crawford Small Parts Dexterity Test, New York, Psychological Corporation.
13. Davies PM: *Steps to follow: a guide to treatment of adult hemiplegia,* New York, 1985, Springer Verlag.
14. deGroot J: *Correlative neuroanatomy,* ed 21, East Norwalk, Conn, 1991, Appleton & Lange.
15. DeMyer W: *Technique of the neurologic examination: a programmed text,* ed 2, New York, 1974, McGraw-Hill.
16. Farber S: *Neurorehabilitation: a multisensory approach,* Philadelphia, 1982, Saunders.
17. Felten DL, Felten SY: A regional and systemic overview of functional neuroanatomy. In Farber S: *Neurorehabilitation: a multisensory approach,* Philadelphia, 1982, Saunders.
18. Fiorentino M: *Normal and abnormal development: the influence of primitive reflexes on motor development,* Springfield, Ill, 1972, Thomas.
19. Ghez C: The cerebellum. In Kandel ER, Schwartz JH, Jessel TM: *Principles of neural science,* ed 3, New York, 1991, Elsevier.
20. Griffith ER: Spasticity. In Rosenthal M et al, editors: *Rehabilitation of the head injured adult,* Philadelphia, 1983, Davis.
21. Hazboun V: *Occupational therapy evaluation guide for adult hemiplegia,* Downey, Calif, 1991, Los Amigos Research and Education Institute.
22. Jebsen RH et al: An objective and standardized test of hand function, *Arch Phys Med Rehabil* 50:311-319, 1969.
23. Jewell MJ: Overview of the structure and function of the central nervous system. In Umphred DA, editor: *Neurological rehabilitation,* ed 2, St Louis, 1990, Mosby.
24. Johnstone M: *Restoration of motor function in the stroke patient,* ed 2, New York, 1983, Churchill Livingstone.
25. Keenan MA: The orthopedic management of spasticity, *J Head Trauma Rehabil* 2:62, 1987.
26. Lincoln-Oseretsky Motor Development Scale, Chicago, Stoelting Co.
27. Marsden CD: *The physiological basis of ataxia, Physiotherapy* 61:326, 1975.
28. Mayo Clinic and Mayo Clinic Foundation: *Clinical examinations in neurology,* ed 5, Philadelphia, 1981, Saunders.
29. McPherson JJ et al: A comparison of dorsal and volar resting hand splints in the reduction of hypertonus, *Am J Occup Ther* 36:664, 1982.
30. Minnesota Rate of Manipulation Test, Circle Pines, Minn, American Guidance Service.
31. Newton RA: Motor control. In Umphred DA, editor: *Neurological rehabilitation,* ed 2, St Louis, 1990, Mosby.
32. Okamoto GA: *Physical medicine and rehabilitation,* Philadelphia, 1984, Saunders.
33. Pelland MJ: Occupational therapy and stroke rehabilitation. In Kaplan PE, Cerrillo LJ: *Stroke rehabilitation,* Boston, 1986, Butterworth.
34. Pennsylvania Bi-Manual Work Sample, Circle Pines, Minn, Educational Test Bureau, American Guidance Service.
35. Purdue Pegboard, Chicago, Science Research Associates.
36. Ryerson S: Hemiplegia resulting from vascular insult or disease. In Umphred DA, editor: *Neurological rehabilitation,* ed 2, St Louis, 1990, Mosby.
37. Schneider F: Traumatic spinal cord injury. In Umphred DA, editor: *Neurological rehabilitation,* ed 2, St Louis, 1990, Mosby.
38. Smith HD: Occupational therapy assessment and treatment. In Hopkins HL, Smith HD: *Willard and Spackman's occupational therapy,* ed 8, Philadelphia, 1993, Lippincott.
39. Snook JH: Spasticity reduction splint, *Am J Occup Ther* 33:648, 1979.
40. Thilmann AF, Fellows SJ, Garms E: The mechanism of spastic muscle hypertonus, *BRN* 114:233-244, 1991.
41. Tomas ES et al: Nonsurgical management of upper extremity deformities after traumatic brain injury, *Phys Med Rehabil State Art Rev* 7, 1993.
42. Urbscheit NL: Cerebellar dysfunction. In Umphred DA, editor: *Neurological rehabilitation,* St Louis, 1990, Mosby.
43. Wilson DJ, Baker LL, Craddock JA: Functional Test for the Hemiplegic/Paretic Upper Extremity, Downey, Calif, 1984, Los Amigos Research and Education Institute.


## RECOMMENDED READING


Boehmer: *Improving upper body control,* Tucson, Ariz, 1988, Therapy Skills Builders.

Cech D, Martin ST: *Functional movement development across the life span,* Philadelphia, 1995, Saunders.

Pedretti LW: *Occupational therapy practice skills for physical dysfunction,* ed 4, St Louis, 1996, Mosby.

Shumway-Cook A, Woollacott MH: *Motor control: theory and practical applications,* Baltimore, 1995, Williams & Wilkins.

# Chapter 11

# Evaluation of Sensation, Perception, and Cognition

*Lorraine Williams Pedretti*
*Barbara Zoltan*
*Carol J. Wheatley*

## Chapter Objectives

*After studying this chapter, the student or practitioner will be able to:*

1. Differentiate the roles of the OTR and the COTA in the evaluation of sensation, perception, and cognition.
2. Define and describe various functions and deficits in the sensory, perceptual, and cognitive systems.
3. Explain the general principles for conducting tests of sensory, perceptual, and cognitive dysfunction.
4. Practice conducting specific sensory tests under supervision.
5. Describe the interrelationships among sensory, perceptual, and cognitive functions in the performance of everyday activities.

## Key Terms

sensation
feedback
feed-forward
light touch
pressure
thermal
pain
olfactory
gustatory
proprioception
perception
stereognosis
astereognosis
graphesthesia
agraphesthesia
body scheme
asomatognosia
praxis
apraxia
ideomotor apraxia
ideational apraxia
constructional apraxia
dressing apraxia
cognition
orientation
attention
memory
executive functioning
abstract thinking
concrete thinking
problem solving
reasoning
insight
dyscalculia

Occupational therapy practitioners help patients succeed in their daily life activities. When faced with a patient with physical dysfunction who is having difficulty performing a task such as donning a shirt, the certified occupational therapy assistant (COTA) may want to know the cause. Possible reasons include lack of sensation in the arm, neglect of body parts because of perceptual impairment, or an inability to understand the nature of the task. Each reason suggests dysfunction in a different performance component (sensory, perceptual, cognitive). Identification and correction of problems in performance components are often necessary for patients to achieve success in occupational performance areas such as daily living skills. Evaluation of dysfunction in sensory, perceptual, and cognitive performance components is the focus of this chapter.

As stated elsewhere in this text, evaluation is the responsibility of the registered occupational therapist (OTR). The COTA may assist, especially when the evaluation procedure is structured and the instructions and limitations are well understood. The performance components are generally viewed as complex, requiring additional advanced study for comprehension, and are therefore evaluated only by the OTR. Most clinicians agree that even entry-level OTRs require supervision and ample experience to gain service competency with some of the tests used to measure performance component dysfunction. However, some procedures for sensory evaluation are simple and straightforward and can easily be mastered by the entry-level practitioner. Therefore this chapter includes directions for procedures that can be administered by an entry-level COTA who has received the necessary training and supervision. The results would then be reported to the OTR for interpretation. More involved procedures that should be administered by an OTR are described so that the occupational therapy assistant can appreciate the value of these evaluations in the management of individual patients.

# *Section* I Evaluation of Sensation

LORRAINE WILLIAMS PEDRETTI

This section is concerned with somatosensory systems of touch, deep pressure, pain, proprioception, and thermal sensation (see Box 11-1 for definitions) and the special senses of taste and smell.

Humans and other animals receive sensory information from the environment; this information is critical to survival, and much of the nervous system is dedicated to registering, cataloging, processing, interpreting, and responding to sensation. Peripheral receptors in the skin (and other sense organs) transmit impulses to the central nervous system (CNS) by way of the peripheral and spinal nerves. Some sensation may produce a motor response before it is even registered by the brain. For example, the withdrawal of the hand from a hot object is driven by an automatic motor response before the object is perceived as being hot.[12]

*Box 11-1*

**Sensory Terms**

**Tactile** Referring to sensation received through the skin or hair receptors.

**Deep pressure** Tactile sensation of force applied to the skin, as in the feeling of the ischial tuberosities pressing into a chair seat.

**Pain** Unpleasant or noxious tactile sensation.

**Thermal sensation** Tactile sensation of heat or cold.

**Proprioception** Information about joint position and motion conveyed at an unconscious level from receptors in the muscles, joints, ligaments, and bone.

## SENSATION AND MOTOR PERFORMANCE

**Sensation** is the primary means of learning about the external world. People build an internal representation of the world based on their sensory experiences and use this model to guide their movements.[9] Motor performance in purposeful activity depends greatly on the continuous inflow of sensory information.[9,14] Sensory information helps people to manage effective movement and to correct errors in movement through feedback and feed-forward mechanisms.[9,13]

### Feedback

When performing a motor act, a person receives sensory feedback about the effectiveness of the motion through the various sensory systems. Sensations derived from the ongoing movement are sent back to the CNS, where a comparison is made between intended action and what is actually happening. Consider, for example, the act of writing; if a wrong word is used or misspelling occurs, visual and proprioceptive feedback signals that a motor error has occurred. The CNS processes this sensory feedback and revises the motor response, which is then carried out.

**Feedback** can be intrinsic or extrinsic. *Intrinsic feedback* arises from bodily sensations during movement. *Extrinsic feedback* comes from external sources, such as information about effectiveness of motor performance from a therapist or teacher. Feedback processes operate relatively slowly, and therefore feedback control is used primarily to maintain posture and to regulate slow movements.[9,13]

### Feed-Forward

**Feed-forward** control operates more quickly than feedback and is used to plan rapid movements before performing them. It uses sensory information (1) to predict what might happen to disturb movement and (2) to develop the motor plan.[9] For example, skiing is an activity that begins with feed-forward control. The skier must anticipate the sensory experience to plan the motor act of descending the ski run. The slope of the hill, the condition of the snow, the rate of speed, potential obstacles, and the path to be taken must be considered before the descent is begun. The skier anticipates the conditions and assumes a specific posture, sets muscles, initiates the motion, makes the appropriate balance responses, and directs movement along a given path toward the destination. As the motor act is being executed, the feedback system operates continuously to correct errors in the intended movement. The feed-forward system operates intermittently to anticipate or reevaluate the required action and to plan movement responses.[9,13]

### Effects of Sensory Loss on Movement

Proprioception and tactile sensation are essential for feedback and feed-forward control systems. Patients with impaired sensation have deficits in both feed-forward and feedback control. Those with proprioceptive dysfunction cannot sense position and motion of joints; those with tactile dysfunction cannot sense contact with objects. Consequently, motor performance is deficient. Vision can compensate somewhat for the loss of tactile and proprioceptive sensation. However, defects in feedback and feed-forward control still limit the patient's ability to use vision effectively. Because the patient cannot sense the tension in muscles and tendons or the resistance of the surface on which the hand is moving, and because visual feedback is processed slowly, any movement appears jerky and awkward. Errors in direction of movement cannot be corrected in time.[9]

When sensation is absent, the affected part(s) may be virtually paralyzed, even with adequate recovery of muscle function.[4] For example, patients with hemiplegia resulting from a cerebrovascular accident (CVA, stroke) tend not to use the affected hand unless proprioception is intact and two-point discrimination at the fingertip is less than inch (1 cm) apart, indicative of good discriminative sensation. Even slight sensory deficits result in persistent problems that limit the functional use of the affected hand in performing fine motor activities. The highly motivated patient may use visual compensation to engage the affected upper extremity in bilateral activities.[17] It is necessary to understand the patient's sensory status to appreciate fully the causes of apparent motor dysfunction and to plan appropriate treatment goals and methods.

## PRINCIPLES OF SENSORY EVALUATION

For the purposes of this chapter, the term *sensation* refers to the ability to identify the sensory modality (e.g., pain, thermal), its intensity, and its location.

Occupational therapists frequently evaluate sensation. Of utmost concern is whether sensation is adequate for the performance of activities of daily living (ADLs).[2] Any patient with CNS or peripheral nervous system (PNS) dysfunction should be routinely evaluated for sensory loss. Patients with CNS dysfunction tend to show loss of many sensory modalities over generalized areas, whereas those with PNS disorders tend to have loss of specific sensory modalities in circumscribed areas. Sensory testing may also be indicated in patients with burns (in which sensory receptors in the skin are destroyed), arthritis (in which joint swelling may cause compression of a peripheral nerve), and traumatic hand injuries (in which skin, muscles, tendons, ligaments, and nerves may be involved).

Other diagnoses that require sensory testing include peripheral nerve injuries and diseases, spinal cord injuries and diseases, brain injuries and diseases, and fractures. In patients with fractures, sensory testing may help to determine if there is peripheral nerve involvement.

### Sensory Supply to Specific Areas

Figure 11-1 illustrates the sensory distribution of the major peripheral nerves of the body and limbs. The peripheral nerves (e.g., ulnar nerve) lie outside the CNS. When performing sensory tests for peripheral nerve dysfunction, the therapist focuses on the area(s) supplied by the nerve(s) affected.

Figure 11-1 also shows the segmental or radicular distribution of nerve roots from the spinal cord. Each nerve root that exits from the spinal cord shows a specific area of sensory distribution known as a *dermatome.* When testing patients with spinal cord injury or disease, the therapist follows this dermatomal distribution. This can be helpful in determining the level(s) of spinal cord lesion and in detecting any sparing of spinal cord function.

### Purposes of Testing

A sensory test, done correctly, outlines areas of intact, impaired, or absent sensation. This information may help with the diagnosis and prognosis and serves as a baseline for the patient's progress. Results of the sensory evaluation indicate whether the patient should be taught to protect against injury and how to use compensatory techniques such as visual guidance for movement during activities. Results may also indicate

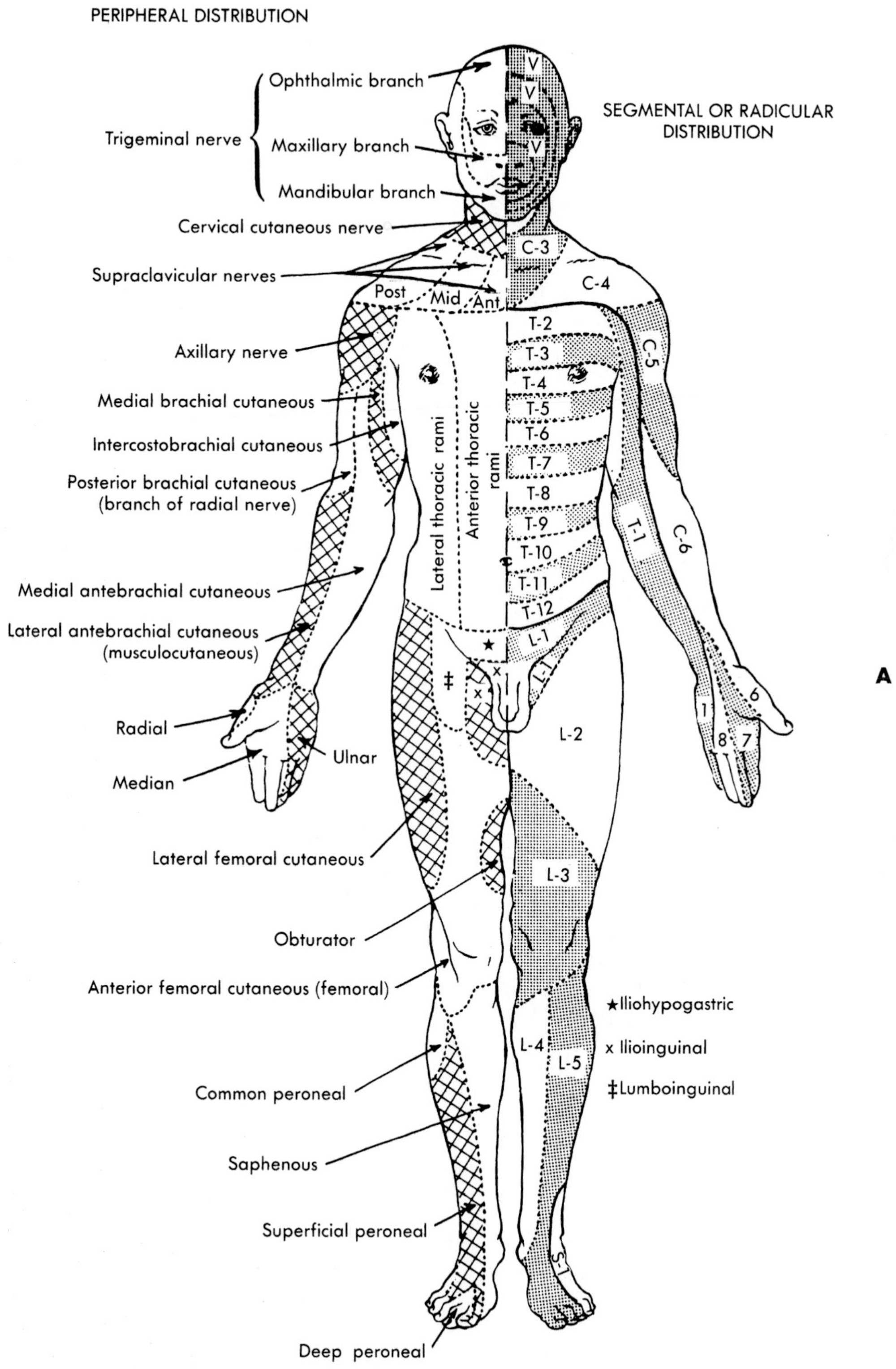


*Figure 11-1* **A,** Sensory distribution of major peripheral nerves and dermatomes corresponding to spinal cord segments, anterior view.

*Continued.*

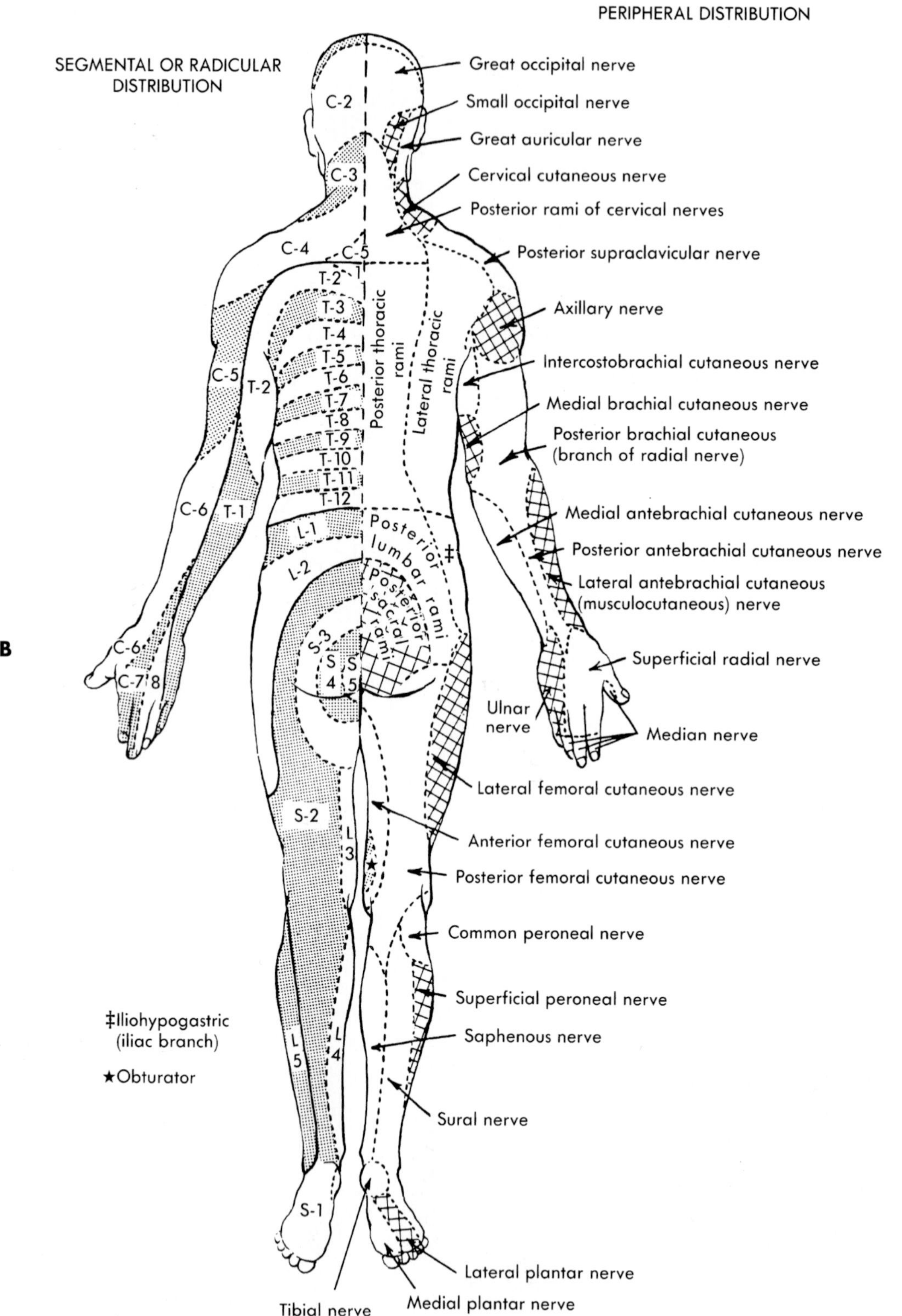


*Figure 11-1, cont'd.* **B,** Sensory distribution, posterior view. (From Chusid JG: *Correlative neuroanatomy and functional neurology,* ed 19, 1985, Lange Medical Publications).

whether a sensory retraining program is feasible.

Sensory loss may affect the use of splints and braces because the patient may be unaware of pressure points during use. Sensory loss may also affect controlled use of a dynamic splint, which requires good sensory feedback for effective operation.

Tests of sensory function do not always accurately predict functional use of the hand. One study of hand function in patients with median nerve problems showed that tests of touch, pain, temperature, and vibration did not correlate with hand function in simple manipulation activities. Some correlation was found between two-point discrimination and hand function.[4] This study underscores the importance of evaluating *function* as well as the sensory modalities. Therapists might use one of the several hand function tests to observe hand use under simulated conditions. For even more reliable evaluation, occupational therapy practitioners should observe the patient for spontaneous use of the affected part(s) in bilateral ADLs.

### Occluding Vision During Testing

Almost all the sensory tests described next require that the patient's vision be occluded so that the test stimuli cannot be seen. The *least* desirable methods of occluding vision are use of a blindfold or keeping the eyes shut. Many individuals with CNS dysfunction have difficulty keeping the eyes closed, and a blindfold can be a source of sensory distraction, producing anxiety in patients with sensory, perceptual, and balance disturbances.[7]

Several alternative methods are available for occluding vision. A small screen made by suspending a curtain between two posts is convenient and effective (see Fig. 11-3). If such a device cannot be constructed, something similar can be made by folding in the sides of a corrugated box and draping a cloth over one side (Figure 11-2, *A*), or a file folder can be held over the area being tested (Figure 11-2, *B*).

## TESTS FOR SENSATION

The following tests are based on evaluation tools of clinical neurology and are designed to test gross sensation of adults with CNS or PNS dysfunction.[1,11] The certified occupational therapy assistant can learn these tests. Service competency must be assured by good supervision and training before the COTA attempts these tests independently on patients. Additional sensory tests and tests of discrete sensation are found in the references, but generally these are performed by the OTR.[2,4,19]

### General Procedure

Testing should take place in a quiet, nondistracting environment. Extraneous noises from the examiner or testing instruments should be minimized. Tests should always be administered to *both sides* when unilateral dysfunction exists. This establishes a standard of accuracy for the individual patient and ensures that the patient has understood the directions for test administration. Parts to be tested should be positioned comfortably. In some cases the examiner will need to support the part manually or with putty, sandbags, or other cushioning material.[2] The subject's vision can be occluded by shielding the parts being tested from view.

It is important for the examiner (E) to orient the subject (S) to the test procedures and to the rationale for administering the tests. The examiner should be sure that the subject understands how to respond. Subjects who have receptive aphasia, known communication problems, or suspected cognitive difficulties should be tested by the OTR because of the compounding influence of these factors.

### Light Touch and Pressure Sensation

Tactile sensitivity is critical to the performance of all ADLs. For example, to know that there is an object in the hand depends on intact touch sensitivity, as does the ability to feel clothes on the body and know whether or not they are correctly adjusted. Pressure

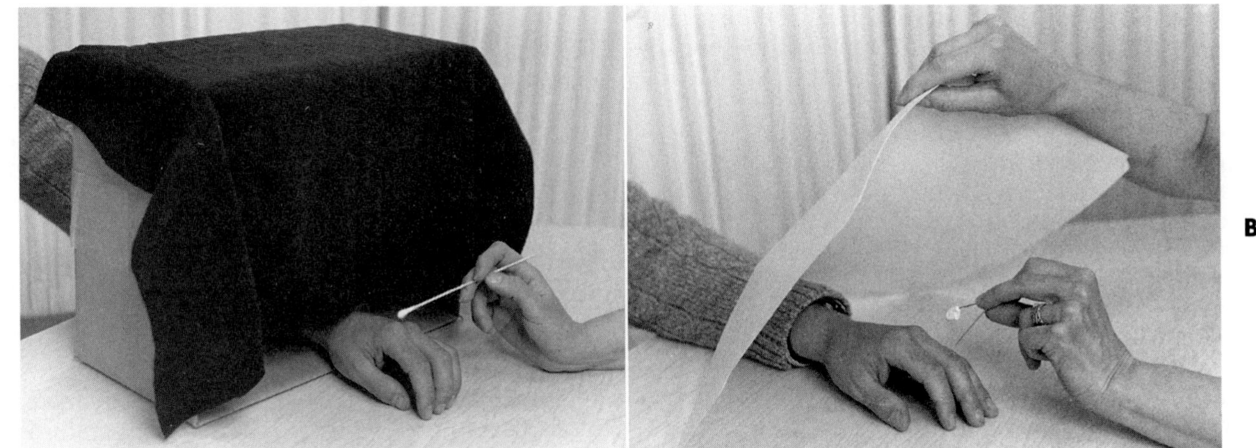

*Figure 11-2* Devices for occluding vision during sensory testing. **A,** Box with cloth drape. **B,** File folder.

sensation is also important in ADLs because it occurs continuously in activities such as sitting, pushing drawers and doors, crossing the knees, wearing belts and collars, and many other activities that stimulate pressure receptors. A patient may have intact pressure sensation when touch is impaired or absent because touch receptors are in the superficial layers of the skin and pressure receptors are in subcutaneous and deeper tissue. Touch sensation is necessary for fine discriminative activities. Pressure is a protective sensation because it warns of deep pressure or repetitive pressure that can lead to injury.[2] If touch sensation is impaired, pressure sensation can assist in the performance of ADLs and can substitute for touch feedback in some activities.

Examiners have employed various tools to apply stimuli for the **light touch** and **pressure** tests. These include a cotton ball, cotton swab, the fingertip, or a pencil eraser. All these objects can provide a gross or cursory evaluation of light touch or pressure sensation. Semmes-Weinstein monofilaments* may be used for more discrete and accurate testing of cutaneous pressure thresholds of light touch to deep pressure.[4,18]

### *Test for Light Touch Sensation[1,2,10,11]*

*Purpose* To determine S's ability to recognize and localize light touch stimuli.

*Limitations* Patients with receptive aphasia cannot be validly tested.

*Materials* Screen or manila folder to occlude vision; cotton swab.

*Conditions* Nondistracting environment where S is seated at a narrow table. Test may also be conducted at bedside or with S in wheelchair. Affected hand and forearm must be supported comfortably on table. E sits opposite S.

*Method* S's hand and forearm are hidden from S's view by placing them under screen or by E holding manila folder over them. E touches hand and forearm lightly with a cotton swab at random locations, covering area supplied by each peripheral nerve and each dermatome. A few trial stimuli should be administered with S watching to ensure S understands procedure and how to respond. Test should be administered on an uninvolved area first to establish a standard. If spasticity is a problem, E may support hand on dorsal surface and hold thumb in radial abduction and extension to secure relaxation of fingers for palmar testing (Figure 11-3).

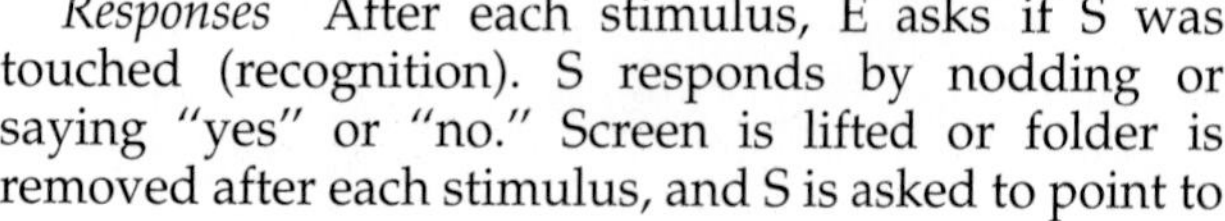

*Responses* After each stimulus, E asks if S was touched (recognition). S responds by nodding or saying "yes" or "no." Screen is lifted or folder is removed after each stimulus, and S is asked to point to

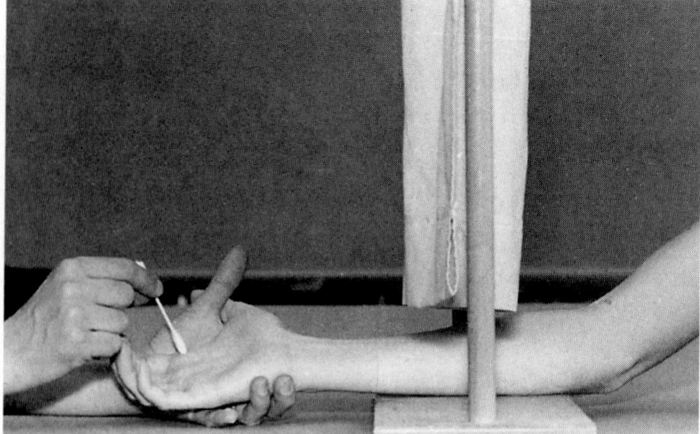

*Figure 11-3* Test for light touch sensation. Suspended curtain is used to occlude vision.

place where S was touched, using unaffected hand if possible. If S is unable to point, S is asked to describe location, and E should select locations that are easy to name (e.g., "knuckle of middle finger").

*Scoring* On scoring chart, E marks a plus (+) for ability to recognize and localize touch stimuli, a minus (−) for ability to recognize only, and a zero (0) for inability to recognize or localize a stimulus. Figure 11-4 shows a form that includes space for recording scores on a test for touch sensitivity.

*Interpretation of results* Results should be reported objectively to the OTR through scoring chart. Deviations of 3/5 to 1 1/5 inches (1.5 to 3 cm) from point of application of stimulus are normal for localization of stimuli, depending on area of hand or arm touched. Responses should be more accurate on hand than on forearm and more accurate on forearm than on upper arm. Ability to recognize and localize touch indicates intact sensation. Ability to recognize but not localize touch stimuli indicates sensory impairment. Inability to recognize or localize touch stimuli suggests that touch sensation is absent.

### *Test for Pressure Sensation*

Pressure sensitivity may be tested in exactly the same manner as described for light touch, except that E should press hard enough with the cotton swab to dent and blanch (whiten) the skin. Pressure sensitivity may be intact when light touch sensitivity is severely impaired or absent. Pressure sensation may provide important sensory feedback that can enhance function. Normally, pressure stimuli can be localized on the hand with 2.44 to 2.83 mg of pressure.[18]

## Thermal Sensation

**Thermal** sensation is another of the protective sensory modalities.[2] The ability to detect temperatures is essential for the prevention of injury in many ADLs, such as bathing, cooking, and ironing. The ability to detect temperature also contributes to the enjoyment of

*North Coast Medical, San Jose, Calif.

FORM FOR RECORDING SCORES ON
TESTS OF SENSATION

Department of Occupational Therapy

Name__________ Age_____ Sex_____

Diagnosis__________ Disability__________

Date__________

| TEST FOR LIGHT TOUCH SENSITIVITY | LEFT | RIGHT |
|---|---|---|
| Use a cotton swab and touch random locations on anterior and posterior surfaces.<br>Indicate on diagram:<br>Intact: +<br>Impaired: −<br>Absent: 0 | Anterior<br> 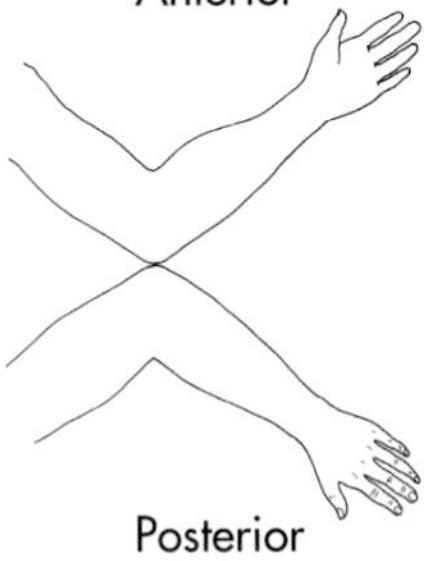<br>Posterior | Anterior<br> 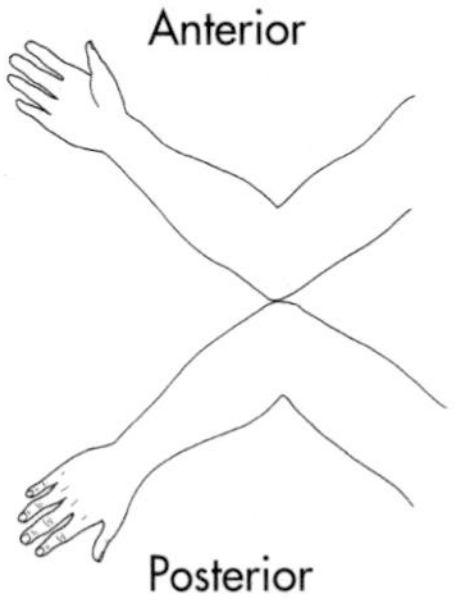<br>Posterior |

| TEST FOR PRESSURE SENSITIVITY | LEFT | RIGHT |
|---|---|---|
| Use a cotton swab and press random locations on anterior and posterior surfaces.<br>Indicate on diagram:<br>Intact: +<br>Impaired: −<br>Absent: 0 | Anterior<br> 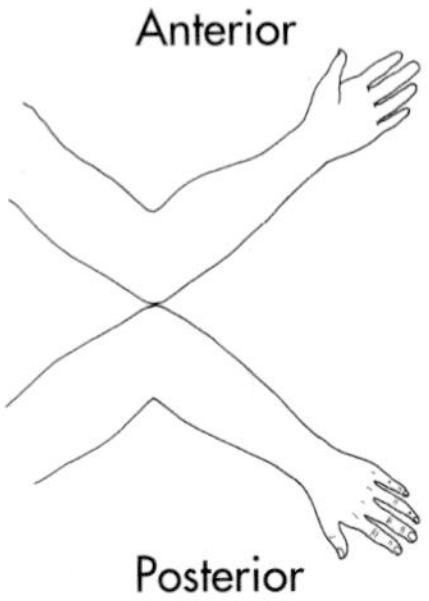<br>Posterior | Anterior<br> 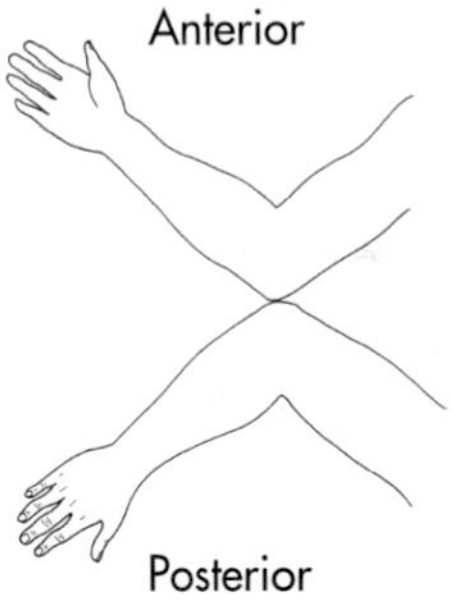<br>Posterior |

| TEST FOR SUPERFICIAL PAIN | LEFT | RIGHT |
|---|---|---|
| Use a large safety pin and touch random locations with sharp and dull ends on anterior and posterior surfaces.<br>Indicate on diagram:<br>Sharp:<br>Correct response +S<br>Sharp reported dull D<br>No response −S<br>Dull:<br>Correct response +D<br>Dull reported sharp S<br>No response −D | Anterior<br> 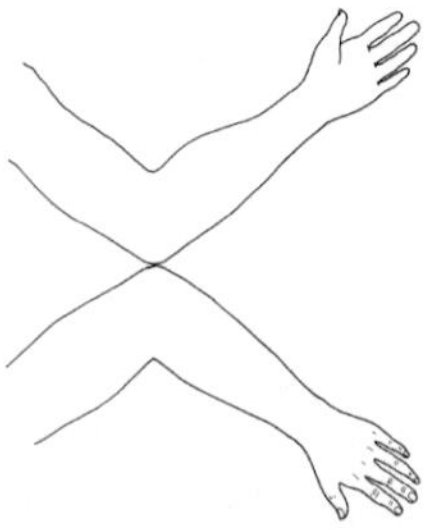<br>Posterior | Anterior<br> 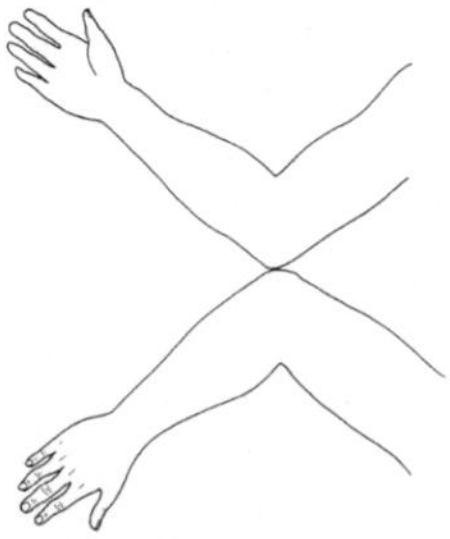<br>Posterior |

Remarks:__________

*Figure 11-4* Form for recording scores on tests for light touch and superficial pain sensation.

food and the detection of uncomfortable environmental temperatures. The patient who lacks accurate thermal discrimination must be taught burn prevention methods and precautions against injury in ADLs. As in the other sensory tests, the results can serve as a baseline for the patient's progress. Changes in sensory status may be used to measure recovery or degeneration, depending on the diagnosis.

Tests for thermal sensation have employed techniques such as touching the skin with test tubes filled with hot and cold water, immersing the fingers or hand into hot or cold water, and touching small hot or cold compresses to the area being tested. Another method is the Hot/Cold Discrimination Kit.* This kit includes two metal temperature probes with a thermometer at the head of each, two thermal cups, and a single stem thermometer. One thermal cup is filled with ice and water and the other with hot tap water. The single thermometer is inserted in the thermal cup. When the desired temperature is reached, the probe is inserted into the thermal cup and allowed to reach the desired testing temperature. The metal probes, which resemble test tubes, then are put in contact with the skin surface to be tested. This kit makes it possible to control temperatures accurately and to maintain constant temperature stimuli for the duration of the test.

### *Test for Thermal Sensation*[1,3,5,10]

*Purpose* To determine S's ability to discriminate between extremes of hot and cold and to detect variations in temperature at four levels.

*Limitations* Persons with receptive aphasia cannot be validly tested. Water temperature may change during the administration of the test and cannot be controlled accurately without a thermometer. Because of subjective element, this test can detect only ability to discriminate gross differences in temperature.

*Materials* Four test tubes (¾-inch [2 cm] diameter) with stoppers; hot, warm, tepid, and cold water.

*Conditions* Nondistracting environment where S is seated comfortably at a table with both hand and forearm supported on table, or alternative positioning described for light touch test.

*Method—Subtest I* Two test tubes are used, one filled with cold water (45° F or 7° C) and one with hot water (110° F or 43° C). Extreme temperatures should *not* be used because they can stimulate pain receptors. Stoppers are placed in tubes. E touches sides of test tubes to skin surfaces to be tested in random order and at random locations, being sure to cover test area thoroughly (Figure 11-5).

*Method—Subtest II* Four test tubes are used, one filled with cold water, one with tepid water, one with warm water, and one with hot water. E should color-code stoppers as follows: yellow—hot, green—warm, orange—tepid, and red—cold. E places stoppers in tubes. E asks S to touch or hold test tubes with affected hand(s) in random order. If S is unable to hold tubes, E may touch each one to S's palm and fingertips.

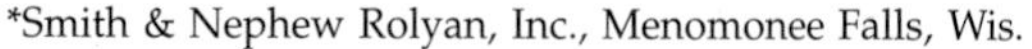

*Smith & Nephew Rolyan, Inc., Menomonee Falls, Wis.

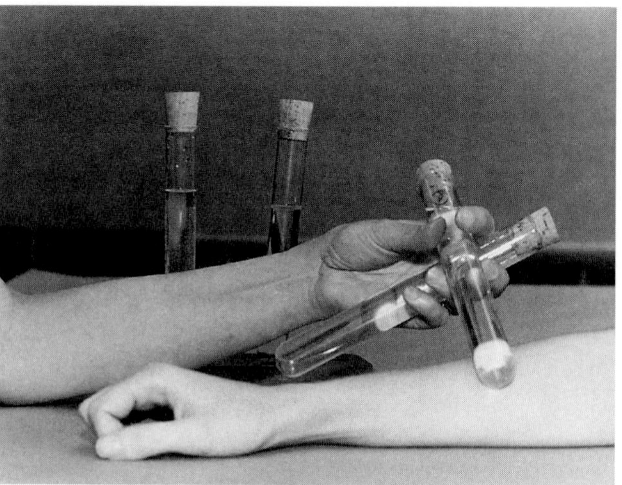

*Figure 11-5* Test for thermal sensation.

*Responses—Subtest I* S says "hot" or "cold" in response to each stimulus. If S is aphasic, E should work out alternate nonverbal response before beginning tests.

*Responses—Subtest II* S is asked to arrange test tubes on table from hottest to coldest in order from left to right. E checks correctness of order by checking color-coded stoppers or feeling tubes.

*Scoring (Figure 11-6) Subtest I:* E marks a plus (+) if temperature is correctly identified and marks a zero (0) if S cannot distinguish hot from cold. Subtest II is not administered if S cannot succeed at subtest I.

*Scoring—Subtest II:* E marks appropriate blanks on form with a check and the appropriate letter to indicate S's responses.

*Interpretation of results* Results should be reported objectively to OTR through scoring chart. Normal adults should be able to complete all items on this test successfully. Normal hand can distinguish temperatures 1° to 5° apart.[2]

### Superficial Pain Sensation

**Pain** is one of the protective sensations that allows the detection of stimuli potentially harmful to the skin and subcutaneous tissue.[2] The ability to detect painful stimuli is critical to the avoidance of injury during performance of ADLs and to the prevention of skin breakdown while wearing splints and braces and using wheelchairs, crutches, and other adaptive devices. In normal circumstances, pain sensation warns

FORM FOR RECORDING SCORES ON
TESTS OF THERMAL SENSITIVITY

Department of Occupational Therapy

Name____________________ Age________ Sex________

Diagnosis/Disability____________________

Date of Onset______________ Date of Test______________

TEST FOR THERMAL SENSITIVITY

SUBTEST I.

Touch sides of hot and cold test tubes to skin surfaces in random order and at random locations. Record scores on diagrams for tests of arms and hands or list site tested and record scores in columns.

| Test site (fill in location tested) | Score (+, 0) | | |
|---|---|---|---|
| Dates | | | |
| | | | |
| | | | |
| | | | |
| | | | |

Use diagram to record scores on test of arms and hands

| LEFT | RIGHT |
|---|---|
| Anterior | Anterior |
| Posterior | Posterior |

SUBTEST II.

| | Date | Date | Date |
|---|---|---|---|
| Arrange test tubes in correct order. | | | |
| Arrange test tubes in wrong order. | | | |

Indicate arrangement of test tubes by filling in spaces below with H for hot, W for warm, T for tepid, and C for cold.

Date: _____ _____ _____ _____ _____

_____ _____ _____ _____ _____

_____ _____ _____ _____ _____

*Figure 11-6* Form for recording scores on test for thermal sensation.

the individual, for example, to move quickly (as when withdrawing a finger from a hot surface), to adjust the position of clothing (as when an elastic leg band is binding), or to remove an offending article of apparel (e.g., shoe that is rubbing a blister on the foot). The patient who lacks the ability to detect such painful stimuli is more likely to be injured. If pain sensation is absent or impaired, it is important to teach sensory compensation and safety awareness in the treatment program.

The following test uses a safety pin to apply light pain stimuli. A new safety pin should be used for each patient and should be sterilized before testing and discarded after the test.

Special care must be taken if *skin atrophy* (wasting of the skin) exists, such as after peripheral nerve injury. The interruption of the nerve supply interferes with normal tissue nutrition and causes the atrophy.[2] The examiner should be aware that atrophic skin is particularly susceptible to injury and that a pinprick stimulus (which would not break normal skin) could produce a tiny break in atrophic skin. If this possibility is a concern, the end of a straightened paper clip may be used for the test.

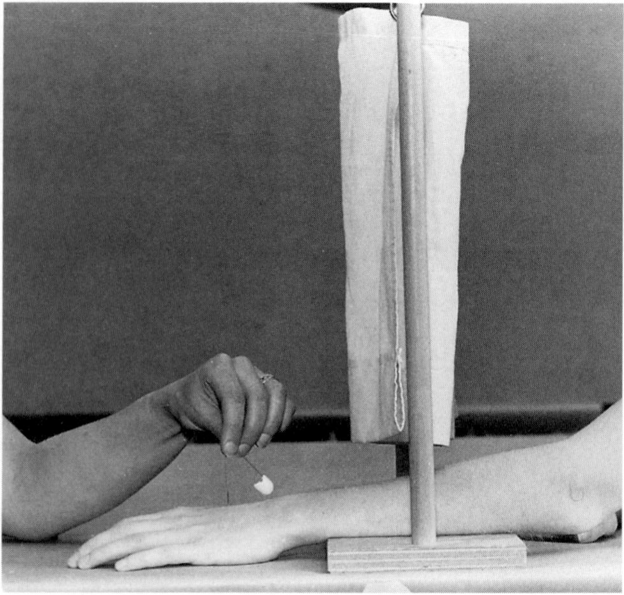

*Figure 11-7* Test for superficial pain sensation.

### *Test for Superficial Pain*[1,10,11,14]

*Purpose* To make a gross evaluation of superficial pain sensitivity.

*Limitations* Persons with receptive aphasia cannot be validly tested. The pulp of fingertips is relatively insensitive to a pinprick. Calloused or toughened areas (e.g., palms) normally are less sensitive to pinprick than other areas. If S is fearful of a safety pin, straightened paper clip may be used.

*Materials* Screen or manila folder to occlude S's vision; large safety pin or straightened paper clip.

*Conditions* Nondistracting environment where S is seated at a narrow table. Affected hand and forearm should be supported comfortably on table. E sits opposite S on other side of table. If S cannot be positioned in this manner, test may be administered while S is in bed or sitting in wheelchair with arms resting on a lapboard.

*Method* Hand and forearm to be tested are hidden from S's view by placing them under screen or by E holding a manila folder over them. Affected hand and forearm are touched lightly at random locations, using sharp and dull stimuli in random order and at random speed. Each stimulus should be applied with the same degree of pressure (Figure 11-7). It is important to apply stimuli to the area supplied by each peripheral nerve and each dermatome.[2] A few trial stimuli should be conducted with S watching to be sure that S understands test and knows how to respond. If spasticity is a problem, E may support hand on dorsal surface and hold thumb in radial abduction and extension to secure relaxation for palmar testing, as shown in Figure 11-3.

*Responses* S says "sharp" or "dull" in response to each stimulus. If S has trouble communicating verbally, E should ask S to indicate a response by pointing to appropriate side of an open safety pin in S's view.

*Scoring* Callahan[2] recommends the following coding system for responses: E marks a plus S (+S) at stimulus point on scoring chart for a correct response to a sharp stimulus, a minus S (–S) for no response to a sharp stimulus, a D when a sharp stimulus is reported as dull, a plus D (+D) for a correct response to a dull stimulus, a minus D (–D) for no response to a dull stimulus, and an S when a dull stimulus is reported as sharp.[2] Figure 11-4 shows a form for recording results of evaluation.

*Interpretation of results* Results should be reported objectively to OTR through scoring chart. Correct responses to both sharp and dull indicate that protective sensation is intact. Incorrect responses to both sharp and dull indicate absent protective sensation.

### Olfactory Sensation (Smell)

The sense of smell is conveyed by receptors that lie deep in the nasal cavity. Normal individuals can detect thousands of odors and at very low concentrations, making smell discrimination quite extraordinary. Olfactory acuity varies greatly among normal persons. **Olfactory** acuity normally declines with age.[6] The sense of smell is associated with the pleasure of taste and is important for detection of noxious and pleasant odors. Smell is also connected to neuronal circuits that influence emotional states and evoke memories.

*Hyposmia* is a diminished sense of smell. It may occur in patients with cystic fibrosis of the pancreas, Parkinson's disease, and untreated adrenal insufficiency. Loss of the sense of smell is known as *anosmia.* Anosmia may be specific (referring to lowered sensitivity to a specific odorant while perception of most others remains intact) or general.[6] Anosmia may result from local chronic or acute inflammatory nasal disease or from intracranial lesions that may be the result of a CVA, head injury, tumors, and infections. In some disturbances the sense of smell is distorted. The person may perceive odors that do not exist. Pleasant odors may be distorted or perceived as noxious, a condition known as *parosmia.*[1]

Anosmia interferes with detection of household gas, chemicals, smoke, car exhaust, and noxious environmental odors. Anosmia is a liability for the patient who has an occupation in which the sense of smell is critical to safety. The disturbance may interfere with the perception and enjoyment of food odors and taste because decreased sense of smell affects the ability to taste.

### *Test for Olfactory Sensation*

*Purpose* To determine if sense of smell is intact, impaired, or lost and whether loss is unilateral or bilateral.[1]

*Limitations* Persons with receptive aphasia cannot be validly tested. Persons with expressive aphasia who cannot communicate using symbols (e.g., pictures or words) to indicate responses cannot be validly tested. Test is subjective, and E must rely on S's self-report for results.

*Materials* Five small opaque or dark-colored bottles containing essences, powders, or crystalline material of familiar and natural odors. Coffee, almond, chocolate, lemon oil, and peppermint are suitable.[1] Vinegar, ammonia, or other irritating chemical odors should *not* be used in a test of olfaction because they stimulate all receptors of the mucous membranes and tend to be irritating.[5,8] If S cannot respond verbally, small cards with the word or a picture for each odor on them will be needed.

*Conditions* Nondistracting environment where no strong odors are present. S should be seated or semireclining.

*Method* S is asked to compress one nostril (or this may be done by E). S is then asked to take a breath to demonstrate that remaining nostril is open. If substances can be recognized from their appearance, vision is occluded. Cork of bottle or cotton swab moistened with essence is held under open nostril; with solid substances, container may be held under S's nostril. S is asked to take two moderate sniffs. Each substance is tried with a short delay between testing, and nostrils are tested alternately using the same and different substances.[1,3,11]

*Responses* E asks if S can (1) detect an odor, (2) identify odor, and (3) distinguish if odors are the same or different to both nostrils.[1,11]

*Scoring (Figure 11-8)* E marks a plus (+) on the form if odor is detected and correctly identified, a minus (–) if an odor is detected and incorrectly identified, and a zero (0) if no odor is detected. Whether or not the same odors are perceived as the same by both nostrils and whether S can differentiate between dissimilar odors presented to each nostril should be noted on the form.

*Interpretation of results* Results should be reported objectively to OTR through scoring chart. Ability to detect and identify odors quickly, ability to detect odor but not identify it, and ability to detect and differentiate odors without identification all may be regarded as normal responses. Distortion of odor (parosmia) and inability to detect odors are regarded as dysfunctional. If test responses are vague and variable, results are unreliable, and it is best to postpone test until a more favorable time.[1]

### Gustatory Sensation (Taste)

Taste receptor cells are located in the taste buds of the tongue, in the palate, and in the pharynx, epiglottis, and esophagus. Taste sensation is conveyed to the brain by way of the facial, glossopharyngeal, and vagus nerves (cranial nerves VII, IX, and X). Generally, four basic tastes can be detected: sweet, sour, salty, and bitter. Detection of more complex taste sensations is thought to result from activation of combinations of receptors for these four basic tastes.[6]

Taste is not only basic to the enjoyment of food but also is one of the sensory stimuli that triggers salivation and swallowing.[16] As with smell, taste is connected to neural circuits that control emotional states and trigger specific memories.[6] Taste sensation may be a consideration for the occupational therapist as part of a comprehensive evaluation of oral-motor mechanisms and for planning feeding training programs.[16] Disturbances of taste may be caused by PNS or CNS lesions.[11] Smokers may demonstrate a decreased sense of taste with aging.[8]

The test for **gustatory** sensation is usually performed by the OTR. Stimulation of the tongue may cause choking or other reactions that are potentially harmful to dysphagic patients. Pedretti[15] provides the directions for this test.

### Proprioception (Position and Motion Sense)

**Proprioception** refers to *unconscious* information about joint position and motion that arises from receptors in the muscles, joints, ligaments, and bone. (The *conscious* sense of motion may be referred to as *kinesthesia.*) A partial or complete loss of position and motion senses seriously impairs movement, even if muscle function is

RECORDING SCORES OF OLFACTORY AND GUSTATORY SENSATION

Name: ______________________________

Age: __________ Diagnosis: ______________________

Date: ______________

Key: + = Can detect and identify odor
− = Can detect odor, cannot identify odor
0 = Cannot detect or identify odor
S = Can detect same odors, both nostrils
D = Can detect different odors, both nostrils

OLFACTORY SENSATION

| | Left nostril | | Right nostril | | Comparisons | |
|---|---|---|---|---|---|---|
| Dates | | | | | | |
| Coffee | | | | | | |
| Almond | | | | | | |
| Chocolate | | | | | | |
| Lemon | | | | | | |
| Peppermint | | | | | | |

GUSTATORY SENSATION

Key: + = Identifies taste correctly
− = Cannot identify taste

| Dates | | | | Remarks |
|---|---|---|---|---|
| Sweet | | | | |
| Salt | | | | |
| Sour | | | | |
| Bitter | | | | |

*Figure 11-8* Form for recording scores on olfactory and gustatory sensation.

within normal limits. Therefore the occupational therapist must know if the patient has the sensory loss so that the motor dysfunction can be more fully understood. Results of the evaluation suggest whether treatment should employ compensatory methods or sensory retraining. Evaluation of position and motion sense requires specific training and the development of sensitivity in handling and positioning the patient. Pedretti[15] provides additional information on this component of evaluation.

## SUMMARY

Sensation provides the background information to perform essential daily activities. Without intact sensation, motor performance is inefficient, in addition to being fatiguing, and discouraging. Evaluation of sensation is important for patients with CNS disorders and peripheral nerve injuries. The occupational therapy assistant may be asked to assist the registered therapist in administering some portions of the sensory assessment.

# Section II Evaluation of Perceptual and Perceptual Motor Deficits

LORRAINE WILLIAMS PEDRETTI, BARBARA ZOLTAN, CAROL J. WHEATLEY

**Perception** is the mechanism by which the brain recognizes and interprets sensory information received from the environment. Perceived information is then further processed by the various cognitive functions. The end result may be a verbal expression or motor act. For example, a man searching for a pen to write something may feel in his pockets. His hand encounters a hard, smooth, cylindrical, oblong object (sensation). These sense data are translated into an image of a pen (perception). The man may then choose (cognitive) to remove it (motor) from his pocket or instead to use a pen provided by someone else.

This section describes the evaluation of perception, including higher level tactile discriminative sensations, body scheme, and praxis. Evaluation of these functions is most accurate when the examiner has a thorough understanding of higher cognitive functions, their anatomical representations, and their interrelationships. For this reason, evaluation of perception is the responsibility of the OTR. Selected tests may be delegated to the experienced COTA with established service competency in administering the test to the particular population being served.

## GENERAL PRINCIPLES OF EVALUATION

The registered occupational therapist may evaluate perception separately or in combination with evaluation of ADL performance.[2,28] The therapist uses a battery of perceptual tests that have varied response modes: verbal response, motor response, or flexible response (either mode). These variations in response mode allow the therapist to determine whether the patient has a deficit in the reception of information or in the verbal or motor output. This information will influence the treatment goals and approach. Occupational therapy practitioners obtain further data on the patient's perceptual abilities by observing performance in ADLs. Analyzing the perceptual motor demands of the patient's functional activities may provide yet more information.

Before administering the perceptual evaluation, the therapist has evaluated the patient's sensory and motor functions. The therapist should also be aware of language deficits and the patient's general level of alertness and responsiveness.

The patient's age and premorbid status are considered in the interpretation of performance in perceptual testing. For example, the majority of patients who have sustained a cerebrovascular accident (CVA) also are elderly. Numerous changes in visual, auditory, perceptual, and cognitive functions are associated with the natural aging process.[11] Similarly, a young, traumatically injured patient may have a history of learning disabilities before the head injury. To interpret test results accurately and to establish realistic treatment goals, the therapist requires a clear picture of the patient's premorbid status. If the patient is unable to supply the necessary information, the practitioner consults the family, friends, and educators.

## PERCEPTUAL FUNCTIONS AND METHODS OF EVALUATION

Stereognosis and graphesthesia are tactile discriminative skills. That is, they involve discrimination of different touch sensations at a higher level of CNS synthesis than the basic tactile sensory functions of light touch and pressure described in Section I.

### Stereognosis

**Stereognosis** is the perceptual skill that enables an individual to identify common objects and geometric shapes through touch (without the aid of vision). Stereognosis requires the integration of the sense of touch, pressure, position, motion, texture, weight, and temperature. The parietal cortex of the brain contains some of the operational centers for stereognosis.[13]

Stereognosis is essential to daily living because the ability to "see with the hands" is critical to many activities. This skill makes it possible to reach into a pocket or purse and find keys and to reach into a dark room and find the light switch. Stereognosis, along with proprioception, enables the use of hand tools and the performance of hand activities without the need to concentrate visually on the implements being used. Examples are knitting while watching television, sawing wood while focusing on the wood rather than the saw, and using a fork while conversing. A deficit in this perceptual function is called **astereognosis.** Patients who have astereognosis but who retain much of their motor function must visually monitor their hands' activities. Thus they become very slow and deliberative in their movements and generally tend to be less active.

The test for stereognosis (and the one after it for graphesthesia) can be learned by the COTA. Once service competency is assured, the occupational therapy assistant can administer these tests (in uncomplicated cases) when directed to do so by the OTR.

#### *Test for Stereognosis*[5,10,15,17]

*Purpose* To evaluate a subject's (S's) ability to identify common objects and perceive their tactile properties.

**FORM FOR RECORDING TEST OF STEREOGNOSIS**

Department of Occupational Therapy

Name ______________________ Age ________ Sex ________ Onset ______

Diagnosis/disability ______________________

Date ______________________

TEST OF STEREOGNOSIS

| COMMON OBJECTS | + − 0 | DESCRIPTION |
|---|---|---|
| Pencil | | |
| Fountain pen | | |
| Sunglasses | | |
| Key | | |
| Nail | | |
| Safety pin | | |
| Teaspoon | | |
| Quarter | | |
| Leather coin purse | | |

Remarks:

*Figure 11-9* Form for recording scores on tests for stereognosis.

*Materials* Means to occlude S's vision, such as a curtain or folder as described in Section I. Typical objects that could be used for identification include a pencil, fountain pen, sunglasses, key, nail, large safety pin, metal teaspoon, quarter, and small leather coin purse. Any common objects may be used, but the examiner (E) must consider S's social and ethnic background to ensure that S has had previous experience with the objects. Three-dimensional geometric shapes (square, sphere, pyramid, etc.) can also be used to test shape and form perception.

*Conditions* Test should be conducted in privacy in an environment with minimal distractions. S should be seated at a table in a position that accommodates affected hand and forearm comfortably. E should sit opposite S. If S is unable to manipulate test objects because of motor weakness, E should assist S to manipulate them in as near normal a manner as possible.

*Method* S's vision is occluded. Dorsal surface of S's hand is resting on table. Objects are presented in random order. Manipulation of objects is allowed and encouraged. E assists with manipulation of items if S's hand function is impaired.

*Responses* S is asked to name object, or if unable, to describe its properties. Aphasic patients may view a duplicate set of test objects after each trial and point to a choice.

*Scoring* A form similar to the one in Figure 11-9 may be used to score the patient's responses. E marks plus (+) if object is identified quickly and correctly and minus (−) if there is a long delay before identification

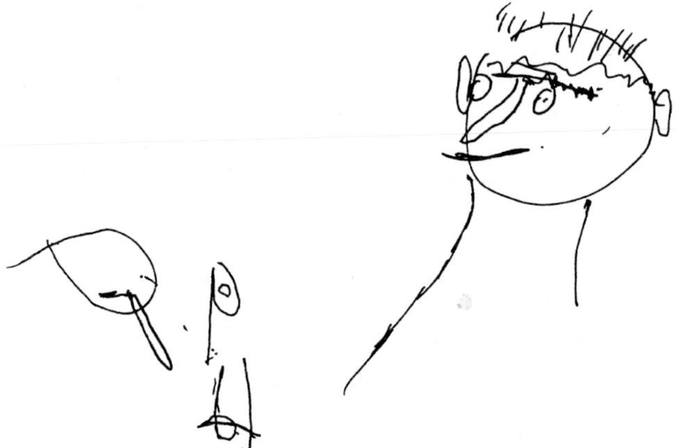

*Figure 11-10* Example of impaired body scheme. Drawing on the left is patient's first attempt to draw a face. Therapist asked patient to try again. Patient's second effort is drawing on the right.

of object or if S can only describe its properties (e.g., size, texture, material, shape). E marks zero (0) if S cannot identify object or describe its properties.

### *Test for Graphesthesia*

An additional test of discriminative sensation that measures parietal lobe function is the test for **graphesthesia.** This is the ability to recognize numbers, letters, or forms written on the skin.[8,13,22] The loss of this ability is called **agraphesthesia.** To test graphesthesia, vision is occluded, and letters, numbers, or geometric forms are traced on the fingertips or palm with a dull, pointed pencil or similar instrument. The subject tells the examiner which symbol was written.[22] If the patient is aphasic, pictures of the symbols may be used for the patient to indicate a response after each test stimulus.

## Body Scheme

An individual's **body scheme** is a postural model related to how the person perceives the position of the body and the relationship of the body parts.[16] It includes knowledge of body construction, the anatomical elements, and their spatial relationships; ability to visualize the body in movement and its parts in different positional relationships; ability to differentiate between right and left; and ability to recognize body health and disease.[3,28] The individual's body scheme is considered the foundation for development of future skills in the perception of environmental space.[29]

### *Tests for Body Scheme Disorders*

Body scheme evaluation is best performed by an experienced OTR. The therapist often must rule out constructional apraxia or other intervening factors as the cause of poor test performance. During the evaluation the therapist will be able to identify various

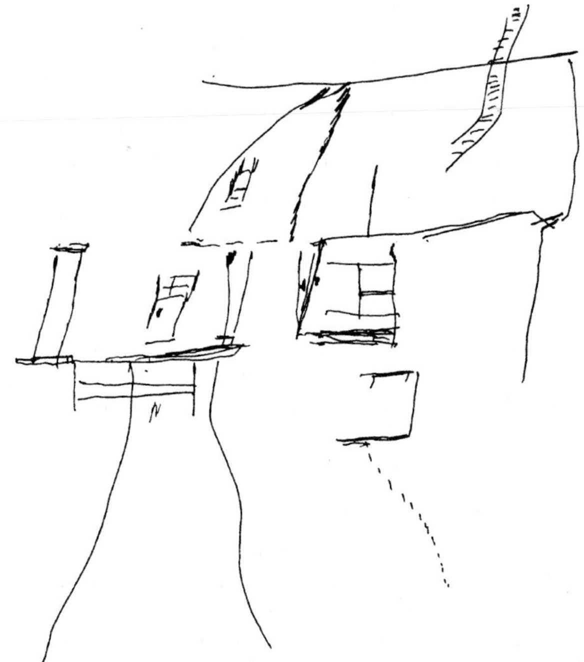

*Figure 11-11* Example of two-dimensional constructional apraxia and inattention to the left side in a patient's drawing of a house. Patient was a retired architect.

body scheme disorders, including asomatognosia, right/left discrimination deficits, unilateral inattention or neglect, and finger agnosia.

**Asomatognosia** refers to a loss of body scheme[16] and is usually evaluated by having the patient point to body parts on command or by imitation.[19,24,28,29] In addition, many examiners use the draw-a-person test and body and face puzzles.[19,28,29] Figure 11-10 illustrates an impairment in body scheme.

*Right/left discrimination deficits* can occur in extrapersonal space, intrapersonal space, or both. The most basic testing of right/left discrimination abilities is intrapersonal; the patient is asked to point to a body part, specifying the right or left side, on self. On a more advanced (extrapersonal) level, the patient is asked to identify right and left body parts on the examiner.[6]

*Unilateral inattention* or *unilateral neglect* is a failure to integrate perceptions from one side of the body or one side of body space. Left-sided neglect is more prevalent than neglect or inattention to the right side.[26] Figure 11-11 illustrates evidence of left-sided neglect. *Tactile inattention* refers to a decreased sensitivity to sensory input to one side of the body.[23] The patient may exhibit an attention deficit with or without associated visual and sensory impairments (e.g., homonymous hemianopia).

The evaluation of unilateral neglect is often done through table-top tasks such as body or face puzzles, scanning worksheets, or the draw-a-person test.[29] The most effective evaluation of unilateral neglect as it relates to a body scheme disorder is direct observation

Box 11-2

## Screening Evaluation for Praxis (Motor Planning)

**Procedure**

Examiner (E) sits directly in front of the subject (S). E asks S to demonstrate or copy actions in the following sequence. First, E asks S to demonstrate each verbal command listed below. If S is unable to perform the action, E demonstrates the action and asks S to imitate it. After all items are completed to command and imitation, items 1 to 5 are repeated, with E asking S to use real object.

**Time**

10 seconds for each item (E times S from start of gesture to end of gesture)

**Directions**

"I am going to ask you to try some different actions. In some of them, I will ask you to demonstrate or copy my movements, and in some I will ask you to use objects."

*To command*

1. "Show me how you blow out a match."
2. "Show me how you drink a glass of water."
3. "Show me how you brush your teeth with a toothbrush."
4. "Show me how you cut paper with scissors."
5. "Show me how you throw a ball."
6. "Show me how you salute."
7. "Show me how you wash your hands."
8. "Show me how you act like a boxer."

*To demonstrate*

E carries out the actions for each test item, stating, for example, "I am blowing out a match. Now you show me how you . . . ."

*With the object*

E presents real object for items 1 to 5 and states, "Show me how you . . . ."

NOTE: During this portion of test, E should ensure S's safe handling of objects. For bilateral tasks (command 4), E may assist by holding paper.

*Observe for*

1. Type of apraxia indicated:
   a. Blowing out match (buccal-facial)
   b. Drinking from glass (buccal-facial, unilateral limb kinetic)
   c. Brushing teeth (buccal-facial, unilateral limb kinetic)
   d. Cutting with scissors (unilateral limb kinetic)
   e. Throwing a ball (unilateral or bilateral limb kinetic)
   f. Saluting (cultural, unilateral limb kinetic)
   g. Washing hands (bilateral limb kinetic)
   h. Boxing (bilateral limb kinetic)
2. Use of body part as object
3. Performance in correct plane of movement
4. Which body parts the patient uses to carry out verbal/imitation commands
5. Which movements are easier toward or away from body
6. Differences in performance: unilateral vs. bilateral, objects vs. no object, verbal vs. imitation

*Scale*

Rate each item separately:

3 = Unable to perform; unable to attempt response
2 = Severely impaired; poor approximation of accurate response, uses trial and error, response greater than allotted time
1 = Impaired; able to approximate accurate response for majority of task, quality or response compromised or response greater than allotted time
0 = Intact; response accurate and within allotted time

Modified from Zoltan B et al: *Perceptual motor evaluation for head injured and other neurologically impaired adults,* rev ed, San Jose, Calif, 1987, Santa Clara Valley Medical Center.

during dressing and other ADLs. The astute occupational therapy assistant will easily identify such patients by simply watching their ADL performance.

The patient with *finger agnosia* has difficulty naming fingers on command or identifying which finger has been touched.[21] The evaluation of finger agnosia is accomplished through finger localization, or naming on command, or having the patient imitate finger movements made by the therapist.[19,24]

### Praxis

**Praxis** is the ability to plan and perform purposeful movement. An impairment in the ability to perform purposeful movement, with no loss of motor power, sensation, or coordination and with normal comprehension, is called **apraxia.**[16] Types of apraxias include ideational, ideomotor, constructional, oral, and dressing apraxia.

Any one or a combination of the apraxias can be seen in a patient. Because all aspects of ADLs require the effective planning and performance of skilled purposeful movement, the apraxic patient is faced with a frustrating and devastating residual deficit of brain injury. Evaluation of praxis disorders is reserved for the OTR. Parts of these tests may be delegated to the experienced COTA who has demonstrated service competency with the particular instrument and population.

### *Tests for Ideomotor and Ideational Apraxia*

**Ideomotor apraxia** is an inability to perform a motor act on command, although the patient is able to perform the act automatically. The patient may be able to describe the intended motion in words but is unable to execute the motor act at will. Observation of the patient in activity performance is critical to the identification of this deficit.

**Ideational apraxia** is an inability to form the concept of the movement or to execute the act in response to a command or automatically.[16] The distinction between ideational and ideomotor apraxia is often difficult. Thus some authors recommend simply using the term *apraxia*[18] or applying more descriptive terms, such as *apraxia of symbolic actions* or *apraxia of utilization of objects*.[9]

Full test batteries for ideational and ideomotor apraxia have been developed.[7,14] Each of these evaluations differentiates praxis abilities with certain body parts (e.g., unilateral limb, bilateral limb, or total body movements) and by level of concreteness (e.g., on command, by imitation). Box 11-2 shows a sample praxis evaluation developed at Santa Clara Valley Medical Center.[29] This screening evaluation is used to indicate the need for a more complete praxis evaluation.

### *Tests for Constructional Apraxia*

**Constructional apraxia** is a deficit in the ability to copy, draw, or construct a design, whether on command or spontaneously.[16] It is the inability to organize or assemble parts into a whole, as in putting together block designs (three dimensional) or drawings (two dimensional). This perceptual motor impairment is often seen in persons with severe head injury or CVA and is related to a dysfunction of the parietal lobes. Constructional apraxia causes significant dysfunction in ADLs that require constructional ability. Examples of such tasks include dressing, following instructions for assembling a toy, and stacking a dishwasher.[11] Figure 11-11, which shows evidence of left-sided neglect, demonstrates constructional apraxia as well.

Traditional tests of constructional praxis are the Test of Visual Motor Skills (TVMS),[12] the copy administration section of the Benton Visual Retention Test,[25] and the Rey Complex Figure.[18] The Three-Dimensional Block Construction[4] evaluates three-dimensional constructional praxis. Nonstandardized tests that may be used are drawing, constructing matchstick designs, assembling block designs, or building a structure to match a model. In daily living, tasks such as dressing or table setting require constructional skills.

### *Dressing Apraxia*

**Dressing apraxia,** or the inability to plan and perform the motor acts necessary to dress oneself, has been linked with problems of body scheme, spatial orientation, and constructional apraxia.[20,27] Clinically the patient may have difficulty initiating dressing or may make errors in orientation by putting the clothes on the wrong side of the body, upside down, or inside out.[1]

## SUMMARY

Perceptual motor deficits affect the patient's overall function. Problems vary in intensity and diversity, depending on the patient's diagnosis and area of brain damage. A systematic, comprehensive evaluation of perceptual motor functions by the OTR is crucial to facilitating achievement of the patient's highest functional potential. The COTA contributes to the evaluation of perception by administering structured tests as directed and by carefully observing the patient in the performance of activities.

# Section III Evaluation of Cognitive Dysfunction

CAROL J. WHEATLEY

Cognitive deficits may be the most devastating residual problems after brain damage from a cerebrovascular accident (CVA), traumatic brain injury (TBI), or acquired disease. **Cognition** involves the skills of understanding and knowing, the ability to judge and make decisions, and an overall awareness of the individual's surroundings.[8] Cognition may use information from external sources or can be internally generated. Cognition allows individuals to use and process sensed and perceived information.

The identification and clinical evaluation of individual cognitive deficits are challenging and complex. Deficit areas are rarely seen in isolation, and the interpretation of a patient's behavior is difficult. Typic ally, evaluation of cognition is conducted by the OTR along with other allied health professionals. Areas assessed by occupational therapy include attention, memory, initiation, planning and organization, mental flexibility, abstraction, insight, problem solving, and calculation abilities.

## UNDERLYING PRINCIPLES OF COGNITIVE EVALUATION

The occupational therapist evaluating cognition must consider several important principles. Because the

COTA may contribute by administering structured evaluation instruments, these principles are included here.

1. Cognition should always be seen in relation to other potential deficit areas. The quality of cognitive processes and skills depends on the integrity of the patient's sensory, language, visual, and perceptual systems. For example, the patient may be unable to attend to and concentrate on a particular task because of an underlying deficit in visual scanning. Because of this interrelationship, the occupational therapist administers the sensory, visual, and perceptual evaluations before beginning cognitive testing.

2. Discussions of the occupational therapy evaluation results with health professionals from other disciplines will enhance the OT practitioner's understanding of the patient's capacity. The occupational therapy approach to cognitive skills tends to emphasize the processing of visual, tactile, and spatial information, functions that are mediated primarily by the right hemisphere of the brain. Consultation with the speech pathologist concerning the patient's auditory, language, and linguistic/cognitive abilities is essential because these skills are processed mostly by the left brain hemisphere. Physical therapists can provide observations of the patient's visual perceptual functioning during gross motor and ambulation tasks. The psychologist or neuropsychologist can provide information regarding the individual's intellectual range, with an overview of the relative strengths and weakness of the various skills. In addition, the family can provide the team with a description of the patient's functioning before the onset of the disability. Without prior knowledge of all these areas, interpretation of the occupational therapy cognitive evaluation risks being inaccurate and invalid.[19,27]

3. The testing environment also influences the results of the cognitive evaluation. The concept of environment includes not only the physical features but also the time of day and amount of structure and feedback provided by the examiner. Patients' behavior in the foreign environment of the hospital or rehabilitation facility may be different from their performance in a familiar home setting.

4. The optimal test battery involves a selection of tests, standardized and normed for the population, and a variety of functional activities (e.g., homemaking). Therapists need standardized tests to provide objective, quantifiable data to measure the extent of the deficit compared with an established norm, to document progress, and to determine discharge planning. In addition, use of standardized tests facilitates communication between practitioners, with common terminology, concepts, and testing conditions. The use of functional activities provides opportunities to observe the practical implications of the deficits revealed by the standardized tests, known as *ecological validity*,[13,17] and allows the therapist to predict better the person's functioning in a home environment. It is in this area—observation of functional performance in ADLs—that the COTA can best contribute to the evaluation of cognitive skills.

5. When introducing a cognitive test to a patient, the therapist or assistant should avoid a condescending attitude or a too cheerful, false-positive approach. Regardless of the level of functioning, the patient still deserves to be approached on an age-appropriate level. The examiner should not offer choices when the patient has no choice ("Would you like to do some tests today?"). Instead, choices should be offered between tests ("Would you prefer to perform coordination tests or cognitive tests?") while acknowledging that all the tests must be completed eventually. The practitioner should not ask for cooperation as a personal favor ("I would like you to . . . ") or imply that the test is a joint effort ("Let's do some testing today"). Instead, the examiner must recognize each person's responsibility (e.g., "Here are some geometric shapes, and your job is . . . "). Also, the examiner must not provide cues as to the patient's right or wrong responses. Instead, the examiner should randomly reward the patient's effort throughout the test (e.g., "Good job" or "You put a lot of effort into that test").[15]

It is essential that the OT practitioner adhere to the instructions that accompany standardized tests so that the results will be valid.

## COMPOSITE BATTERIES OF COGNITIVE FUNCTIONS

Several test batteries are available to the OTR to screen a range of cognitive skills: the Middlesex Elderly Assessment of Mental State,[11] the Cognitive Assessment of Minnesota,[22] and the Neurobehavioral Cognitive Status Screening Examination.[14] The Arnadottir OT-ADL Neurobehavioral Evaluation (A-ONE) provides an analysis of functional activities to determine cognitive skill deficit areas.[2] The Cognitive Skills Workbook provides a pretest and posttest as well as treatment exercises for community living skills such as constructing a schedule, and reading a map.[9]

## EVALUATION OF SPECIFIC DEFICIT AREAS

Cognitive functions are evaluated in a particular order because certain cognitive skills depend on others. For example, individuals will be unable to display effective problem-solving skills when they cannot attend to or remember a particular task. The following functions are discussed in the order of the recommended progression of testing.

### Orientation and Attention

**Orientation** refers to an individual's ongoing awareness of the current situation, the environment, and the passage of time. Immediately after any traumatic injury, a person must develop an awareness of the events that preceded the accident and those occurring since then. After a CVA, for example, the individual is frequently disoriented initially but becomes more aware as healing occurs.

An unimpaired person is typically oriented to person (Who am I?), to place (Where am I?), and to time (What year, month, day, and time of day is it?). Orientation is related to an individual's memory capacity, because a person must be able to remember past occurrences to place current events in their proper perspective. After a severe TBI or CVA, a person initially may be confused regarding personal identity, which indicates a *disorientation to person.* This is a more global deficit than an inability to speak one's name, which may occur in the case of aphasia, when a person has difficulty with the verbal expression of any message. The patient may also confuse the identities of other individuals, for example, thinking that the therapist or assistant is a family member. *Orientation to place* refers to an individual's awareness of being in a hospital (if appropriate) or knowing the name of the immediate town, city, and state. Difficulty in monitoring the passage of time can result in *time disorientation.* Patients may confuse the sequence of events in time. For example, a patient may report that a family member visited the previous day when that person actually came to the hospital to see the patient a week earlier.

*Topographical orientation* describes an individual's awareness of the position of self in relationship to the environment, for example, the room, building, and city. Functional examples of this disorder are noted when a patient becomes confused when attempting to leave a room and locate another therapy department or travel to the cafeteria. These patients may perform better in the familiar environment of home and community, but deficits may still be apparent.

**Attention** is an active process that allows the individual to focus on the environmental information and sensations that are relevant at a particular time. Attention involves the simultaneous engagement of alertness, selectivity, sustained effort, flexibility, and mental tracking.[28] A patient must be alert and awake and be able to select a relevant focus of interest. The patient must be able to maintain this focus for as long as needed but be able to shift the focus if another event of interest or importance occurs. In addition, the patient must ignore information if it is not relevant and be able to track several types of information simultaneously. Because these skills underlie all aspects of cognitive functioning, they are frequently affected by TBI or CVA, and deficits may undermine performance in many areas. For example, a patient who is unable to attend to a task for more than a few seconds will not be able to take in all the necessary information to perform a higher level reasoning task.

The two types of information processing relevant to attention are automatic and controlled processing.[34] *Automatic processing* is used by the individual at a subcortical (not deliberately conscious) level. *Controlled processing* is used when new information is being considered. Two disorders, focused attentional deficit and divided attentional deficit, are related to these two types of information processing. A *focused attentional deficit* occurs when an automatic response is replaced by a controlled response. For example, walking (an automatic response) may require focused attention and deliberate control in a patient with a CVA concentrating on trying to walk.

A *divided attentional deficit,* however, occurs when the individual is unable to process all the information required for task completion. This deficit results in the patient becoming "overloaded." The patient typically responds by reverting to focused attention. For example, if a patient with a CVA is asked a question while ambulating, the patient will frequently stop movement to engage in conversation.

*Concentration* requires that an individual sustain focused attention for a period of time. Patients with difficulties in this area may be highly distractible or very sensitive to events occurring in the immediate environment that pull the focus away from the task at hand. It is important to note which types of stimuli (e.g., visual, auditory, tactile, gustatory) appear to distract the patient easily. A low-stimulus environment or "quiet room" is frequently available in the hospital or rehabilitation center.

Other patients have the opposite problem: they can become deeply focused on a given stimulus or activity and have difficulty maintaining general awareness of events occurring around them. Neither extreme is desirable. Effective functioning in daily life demands the ability to focus, to remain aware of (but not distracted by) peripheral events, and to disengage and reengage concentration as needed.

### *Tests for Orientation and Attention*

Assessment of orientation to person, time, and place can be conducted informally by asking the patient basic questions about personal identity, the date, time of day, season of the year, and the name of the hospital, city, and state. Because levels of orientation can vary with time of day and other conditions, these questions must be asked several times to determine the consistency of the patient's awareness. Topographical orientation is assessed by observing a patient's travel from one site to another or by asking the patient to draw a floor plan of the room, the therapy area, or the patient's home, verifying the latter with the family.

Examples of standardized tests of attention include Knox's Cube Test[25] and the Trail Making Test.[1] The OT practitioner's evaluation of attention should include structured clinical observation and activity analysis during functional tasks.

## Memory

**Memory** is the cognitive function that allows a person to retain and recall information. Figure 11-12 summarizes the memory process. A breakdown in the memory process can occur at any level. If a patient is unable to attend to information, it may never enter the system. Some patients are able to process information in

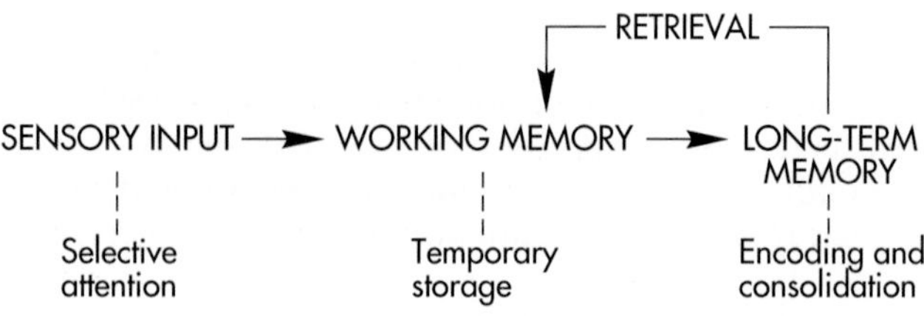


*Figure 11-12* The memory process.

short-term, or working, memory but never encode the material into long-term storage. Still others can store the information but have trouble retrieving it. Patients with memory deficits, who need to expend additional effort to learn new material, may also have difficulty forgetting information when it is no longer needed. Therefore the practitioner should avoid forcing such patients to unlearn and then relearn new information or procedures.

A person's ability to recite or reproduce information is generally taken as an indication of recall and is referred to as *declarative memory.* Tests of declarative memory may require a patient to repeat a word list or draw a set of geometric designs. Less formally, the practitioner may ask a patient about events occurring earlier in the day. Declarative memory is subdivided into two categories. *Episodic memory* refers to an individual's personal history and lifetime of experiences. *Semantic memory* describes the general fund of knowledge shared by groups of people, such as language and rules of social behavior. This type of memory is generally less affected after an injury.[12]

Some patients may have a significant deficit in declarative memory, but *procedural memory,* or memory for a skill or series of actions,[12] may be less impaired. For example, a patient who is unable to tell a therapist the steps to make a sandwich and cup of coffee may be able to perform the activity adequately. Procedural memory may enable a patient to learn new self-care techniques despite severe declarative memory deficits on standardized tests.

*Everyday memory* refers to a person's ability to remember information pertinent to daily life.[32] In the hospital or rehabilitation facility, this refers to learning the names and faces of the physicians, nurses, and therapy staff who are working regularly with the patient. Learning a schedule of appointments or the locations of various departments may be difficult and further complicated by frequent changes; therefore the hospital escort staff often assumes this responsibility for the patient. Everyday memory also includes the ability to keep track of daily events in their proper sequence. *Prospective memory* refers to the ability to remember events that are set to occur at some future time, such as an appointment scheduled for later in the day.[32]

Patients with memory deficits may tend to *confabulate,* or to fill in memory gaps with imaginary material.[30] They are unaware that they are adding erroneous information to the factual data and thus can become very confused regarding past events. Some patients with memory-deficits may deliberately try to "fake it," to cover embarrassment at the extent of the memory loss, but usually this is not considered confabulation.

Activities or topics of interest or of personal relevance to the patient are generally performed better than other, less interesting activities. This leads to a tendency for the family to minimize the deficit, for example, "He can remember if he *wants* to." Staff members need to explain this inconsistent performance and educate family members to the reality of the underlying deficit.

### *Tests for Memory Functions*

The OTR may employ any of several standardized tests for the evaluation of visual memory: the Benton Visual Retention Test,[23] the Rey Complex Figure,[15] and selected subtests of the Test of Visual Perceptual Skills (TVPS).[10] The Learning Efficiency Test provides comparison of auditory versus visual recall.[31] The Rivermead Behavioural Memory Test[33] is an evaluation of everyday memory skills. The Contextual Memory Test provides information on awareness of the deficits and use of strategies.[29]

Questionnaires such as the Subjective Memory Questionnaire can also be valuable and can be filled out by both the patient and a family member to determine the patient's level of awareness of memory deficits.[4]

Tests can be used to determine where the breakdown in the process occurs. For example, a patient may be unable to remember information in a free recall trial (with no or minimal cues) but may score high on a recognition task of the same information. This would suggest that the information was adequately stored, but that the patient has a deficit in retrieval. Treatment would then focus on the development of retrieval strategies.

## Executive Functioning

Specific components of **executive functioning** include goal formation, planning, implementing the plan, and effective performance.[15] An example of deficits in goal formation is seen in the patient who cannot think of anything to do but who responds well to an established routine. Occasionally the structured schedule of a hospital or rehabilitation facility may mask deficits in this area, which then become very apparent once the patient is discharged home, where there is less of a routine. Some patients may be able to verbalize an intended goal and plan a course of action but are unable to implement it. These patients often seem much more capable than their behavior actually demonstrates.

When attempting to implement the plan, a patient may demonstrate poor mental flexibility, resulting in perseverative or stimulus-bound behavior. *Perseveration* refers to the continuation or repetition of an action

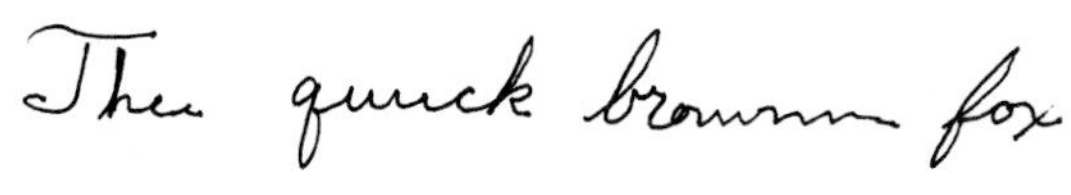

*Figure 11-13* Example of writing perseveration.

beyond its purpose. Perseveration can be seen in motor acts, verbalizations, or thought processes. A person might say that the patient is having difficulty "changing mental set." Figure 11-13 provides an illustration of writing perseveration. An example of *stimulus-bound behavior* can be seen in the patient who impulsively begins the task before receiving instruction or who is unable to draw attention away from a task when necessary.

Effective performance requires that the patient continually monitor and adjust performance activities throughout the execution of the task. Some patients demonstrate an inability to perceive their errors, and others may recognize the error but make no effort to correct the mistake.

#### *Tests for Executive Functioning*

Family members are frequently the best source of information about the patient's executive functioning. Formal evaluation may include a standardized test such as the Profile of Executive Control System (PRO-EX).[24] Skills are also evaluated through close clinical observation. For example, a homemaking evaluation that involves planning and simultaneously preparing a variety of dishes for a meal may be useful. Perseverative or stimulus-bound behavior would be noted as it relates to both a specific environment and particular tasks.

Perseveration may be related to other clinical deficits, such as poor comprehension or apraxia, or may be a sign of depression. Ongoing close observation, evaluation, and consultation with other team members is essential.

### Reasoning and Problem-Solving Skills

**Abstract thinking** enables a person to see relationships between objects, events, or ideas; to discriminate relevant from irrelevant detail; or to recognize absurdities.[15] Patients with frontal lobe damage often lose this ability and think only in the most concrete, literal manner. This literal thinking is often paired with mental inflexibility. These cognitive deficits and resultant behaviors create difficulty in problem solving and transfer of knowledge to new situations.[36]

The following example illustrates **concrete thinking.** A patient is asked the interview question, "What brought you to this hospital?" The patient responds, "My parents' car." The patient is interpreting the question literally rather than in reference to the accident that resulted in the brain injury.

**Problem solving** is a complex process involving many cognitive skills. It requires attention, memory, planning and organization, and the ability to reason and make judgments. Various types of **reasoning** can be used in the problem-solving process. *Convergent reasoning* enables a person to arrive at the central idea, such as when a patient notices a tendency to drop items grasped in the affected right hand and thus concludes that the hand is not reliable for such activities. *Divergent reasoning* is aimed at generating alternatives, as when the patient decides to begin using the left hand more often to avoid dropping objects.[5] *Deductive reasoning* refers to the ability to arrive at conclusions, and *inductive reasoning* enables a person to draw generalizations from experiences.[35] The patient must be able to process complex information in order to plan strategies and to evaluate established strategies.[6]

#### *Tests for Reasoning and Problem Solving*

Abstract conceptual thinking can be evaluated in a number of ways. The Test of Nonverbal Intelligence (TONI),[7] the Space Visualization subtest of the Employee Aptitude Series,[21] and the Minnesota Paper Formboard Test[16] all assess complex spatial reasoning skills. Object sorting tasks[26] are used as well, particularly with patients whose linguistic skills are limited.

### Insight and Awareness

Consider the paralyzed patient with brain damage who falls out of bed trying to walk to the bathroom. This behavior results from a lack of awareness or blatant denial of the paralysis. Limited **insight** results in impulsive and unsafe behavior. The patient with this deficit is unable to monitor, correct, and regulate the quality of the behavior.[36] A patient's insight frequently increases as body scheme is modified in response to the changes imposed by the disability. This is a long and complex process.

Memory deficits may also complicate the patient's awareness of the problem or the frequency with which it occurs. For example, the patient may remember having difficulty recalling a nurse's name only two or three times in a given day and thus make the judgment that the memory problem is minimal. However, the incidence actually may be closer to 12 to 15 times a day. Sometimes the use of a frequency checksheet, recorded by the patient under the supervision of the therapist or assistant, may help the patient more fully understand the severity of the problem.

A patient may have a total inability to recognize deficits; this is termed *anosognosia.*[20] A team approach is needed to distinguish between neurological and psychological (e.g., denial) types of awareness deficits.[3] An example of this is a patient (with intact basic perceptual and language abilities) who cannot recognize her own handwriting on a task performed earlier in the day and accuses the clinician of falsifying the work. This patient may not be responsive to the most carefully designed awareness training program and may be unable to live independently without supervision.

Other patients are able to recognize and discuss their inappropriate behavior but may not be unable to control it. This trait is referred to as *disinhibited behavior;* the person is unable to exert the usual level of inhibition that prevents people from acting on impulses. The person may laugh or cry or express other emotions that have no relationship to the actual emotional context of the situation. Other patients may respond with the correct category of emotion, such as to laugh at a humorous situation, but the extent and forcefulness of their laughter may be an exaggeration beyond what is appropriate.

#### *Evaluation of Awareness*

Assessment of these awareness disorders is made by behavioral observation and interviews with the family. Subjective questionnaires[4] can be completed by both the patient and a family member and the results compared and discussed with both parties.

### Dyscalculia

A deficit in the ability to perform simple calculations, or **dyscalculia,** can have strong implications for an individual's independent functioning in the community. Various types of calculation disorders have been identified.[18] A patient may have difficulty reading *(alexia)* or writing *(agraphia)* the numbers. The speech/language pathologist may evaluate these functions further. *Spatial dyscalculia* refers to a deficit in the spatial arrangement of the numbers.

Assessment may include number recognition and simple to complex mathematical problems, as well as functionally oriented items such as calculating change, recognition of coins, and budgeting. The *Cognitive Rehabilitation Workbook*[9] includes everyday calculation tasks, providing both pretest and posttest measures along with training exercises.

## SUMMARY

Cognition is a complex, hierarchical, interwoven process. Many different cognitive functions are involved in performing daily life activities. Assessment of specific cognitive deficits is the responsibility of the OTR and other members of the rehabilitation team, such as the psychologist and the speech/language pathologist. By observing the patient performing ADLs and other tasks in the rehabilitation treatment plan, the COTA will be able to identify behaviors that may indicate cognitive deficits.

## *Selected Reading Guide Questions*

1. Why is sensory and perceptual evaluation necessary and important to occupational therapy?
2. Discuss the relationship between sensation and motor performance.
3. In what types of disabilities are sensory evaluations routinely given?
4. What are some methods for occluding the patient's vision? What are the alternatives to blindfolding or asking the patient to keep eyes closed?
5. What is the functional significance of olfactory sensation?
6. Define *perception* and describe its role in everyday activities.
7. Define *body scheme.*
8. Describe how unilateral neglect can be observed.
9. List four types of apraxia, and discuss how each can affect the ability to perform daily living skills.
10. What are the implications of a deficit in attention and concentration on an individual's functioning in everyday activities?
11. Differentiate between procedural and declarative memory.
12. Define *confabulation* and explain why patients with memory problems may confabulate.
13. What behaviors will the patient with poor mental flexibility and abstraction display?

## *Exercises*

1. With a partner, learn the distribution of the dermatomes and the sensory distribution of the peripheral nerves. Washable body tattoo markers may be used, if involved parties are willing.
2. Practice performing each of the evaluations described in this chapter. Have a third person observe to check performance.

### *REFERENCES*


**Section I**

1. Bickerstaff ER, Spillane JA: *Neurological examination in clinical practice,* ed 5, London, 1989, Blackwell.
2. Callahan AD: Sensibility testing: clinical methods. In Hunter JM et al, editors: *Rehabilitation of the hand,* ed 3, St Louis, 1990, Mosby.
3. deGroot, J: *Correlative neuroanatomy,* East Norwalk, Conn, 1991, Appleton & Lange.
4. Dellon AL: *Evaluation of sensibility and re-education of sensation in the hand,* Baltimore, 1981, Williams & Wilkins.
5. De Myer W: *Technique of the neurologic examination: a programmed text,* ed 2, New York, 1974, McGraw-Hill.
6. Dodd J, Castellucci VF: Smell and taste: the chemical senses. In Kandel ER, Schwartz JH, Jessel TM: *Principles of neural science,* New York, 1991, Elsevier.
7. Eggers O: *Occupational therapy in the treatment of adult hemiplegia,* Rockville, Md, 1984, Aspen.
8. Farber SD: *Neurorehabilitation: a multisensory approach,* Philadelphia, 1982, Saunders.
9. Ghez C: The control of movement. In Kandel ER, Schwartz JH, Jessel TM: *Principles of neural science,* New York, 1991, Elsevier.
10. Gilroy J, Meyer JS: *Medical neurology,* London, 1969, Macmillan.
11. Mayo Clinic and Mayo Foundation: *Clinical examinations in neurology,* Philadelphia, 1981, Saunders.
12. Martin JH: Coding and processing sensory information. In Kandel ER, Schwartz JH, Jessel TM: *Principles of neural science,* New York, 1991, Elsevier.
13. Montgomery PC: Perceptual issues in motor control. In *Contemporary management of motor control problems.* Proceedings of the II Step Conference, Alexandria, Va, 1991, Foundation for Physical Therapy.

14. Occupational Therapy Department, Rancho Los Amigos Hospital: *Upper extremity sensory evaluation: a manual for occupational therapists,* Downey, Calif, 1985, The Department.
15. Pedretti LW: *Occupational therapy: practice skills for physical dysfunction,* ed 4, St Louis, 1995, Mosby.
16. Silverman EH, Elfant IL: Dysphagia: an evaluation and treatment program for the adult, *Am J Occup Ther* 33:382, 1979.
17. Waters RL, Wilson DJ, Gowland C: Rehabilitation of the upper extremity after stroke. In Hunter JM et al, editors: *Rehabilitation of the hand,* ed 3, St Louis, 1990, CV Mosby.
18. Werner JL, Omer GE: Evaluating cutaneous pressure sensation of the hand, *Am J Occup Ther* 24:347, 1970.
19. Wynn-Parry CB: *Rehabilitation of the hand,* London, 1981, Butterworth.

**Section II**

1. Archibald YM, Wepman JM: Language disturbance and nonverbal cognitive performance in eight patients following injury to the right hemisphere, *Brain* 91:117, 1968.
2. Arnadottir G: *The brain and behavior: assessing cortical dysfunction through activities of daily living,* St Louis, 1990, Mosby.
3. Ayres AJ: *Sensory integration and learning disorders,* Los Angeles, 1972, Western Psychological Services.
4. Benton AL, Fogel ML: Three-dimensional constructional praxis: a clinical test, *Arch Neurol* 7:347, 1962.
5. Benton AL, Schultz LM: Observations of tactile form perception (stereognosis) in pre-school children, *J Clin Psychol* 5:359, 1949.
6. Boone P, Landes B: Right-left discrimination in hemiplegic patients, *Arch Phys Med Rehabil* 49:533, 1968.
7. Brown J: *Aphasia, apraxia, agnosia,* Springfield, Ill, 1972, Thomas.
8. Chusid JG: *Correlative neuroanatomy and functional neurology,* ed 19, Los Altos, Calif, 1985, Lange.
9. Dee HL: Visuoconstructive and visuoreceptive deficit in patients with unilateral cerebral lesions, *Neuropsychologia* 8:305, 1970.
10. DeJong R: *The neurologic examination,* New York, 1958, Hoeber.
11. Fall CC: Comparing ways of measuring constructional praxis in the well elderly, *Am J Occup Ther* 41:500, 1987.
12. Gardner MF: The Test of Visual Motor Skills (TVMS), Burlingame, Calif, 1992, Psychological and Educational Publications.
13. Gilroy J, Meyer JS: *Medical neurology,* London, 1969, Macmillan.
14. Goodglass H, Kaplan E: *Assessment of aphasia and related disorders,* ed 2, Philadelphia, 1972, Thomas.
15. Head H et al: *Studies in neurology,* London, 1920, Oxford University Press.
16. Hécaen H, Albert ML: *Human neuropsychology,* New York, 1978, Wiley.
17. Kent BE: Sensory-motor testing: the upper limb of adult patients with hemiplegia, *Phys Ther J Am Phys Ther Assoc* 45:550, 1965.
18. Lezak MD: *Neuropsychological assessment,* ed 2, New York, 1983, Oxford University Press.
19. MacDonald J: An investigation of body scheme in adults with cerebral vascular accident, *Am J Occup Ther* 14:72, 1960.
20. Miller N: *Dyspraxia and its management,* Rockville, Md, 1986, Aspen.
21. Neistadt ME: Occupational therapy for adults with perceptual deficits, *Am J Occup Ther* 42:434, 1988.
22. Occupational Therapy Department, Rancho Los Amigos Hospital: *Upper extremity sensory evaluation: a manual for occupational therapists,* Downey, Calif, 1985, The Department.
23. Okkema K: *Cognition and perception in the stroke patient: a guide to functional outcomes in occupational therapy,* Gaithersburg, Md, 1993, Aspen.
24. Sauget J, Benton AL, Hécaen H: Disturbances of the body scheme in relation to language impairment and hemispheric locus of lesion, *J Neurol Neurosurg Psychiatry* 34:496, 1971.
25. Sivan AB: The Benton Visual Retention Test, San Antonio, Tex, 1992, Psychological Corporation.
26. Walsh K: *Neuropsychology: a clinical approach,* Edinburgh, Scotland, 1987, Churchill Livingstone.
27. Warren M: Relationship of constructional apraxia and body scheme disorders to dressing performance in adult CVA, *Am J Occup Ther* 35:431, 1981.
28. Zoltan B, Siev E, Freishtat B: *Perceptual and cognitive dysfunction in the adult stroke patient,* ed 2, Thorofare, NJ, 1986, Slack.
29. Zoltan B et al: *Perceptual motor evaluation for head injured and other neurologically impaired adults,* rev ed, San Jose, Calif, 1987, Santa Clara Valley Medical Center.

**Section III**

1. *Army individual test battery: manual of directions and scoring,* Washington, DC, 1944, Adjutant General's Office, US War Department.
2. Arnadottir G: *The brain and behavior: assessing cortical dysfunction through activities of daily living,* St Louis, 1990, Mosby.
3. Barco PP et al: Training awareness and compensation in postacute head injury rehabilitation. In Kreutzer JS, Wehman PH: *Cognitive rehabilitation for persons with traumatic brain injury,* Baltimore, 1991, Brookes.
4. Bennett-Levy J, Powell G: The Subjective Memory Questionnaire (SMQ): an investigation into the self-reporting of "real life" memory skills, *Br J Soc Clin Psychol* 19:177, 1980.
5. Beyer BK: *Practical strategies for the teaching of thinking,* Boston, 1987, Allyn & Bacon.
6. Bolger J: Cognitive retraining: a developmental approach, *Clin Neuropsychol* 4:66, 1982.
7. Brown L, Sherbenou RJ, Johnsen SK: The Test of Nonverbal Intelligence (TONI), Austin, Tex, 1982, Pro-Ed.
8. Craine JF: Principles of cognitive rehabilitation. In Trexler LE: *Cognitive rehabilitation: conceptualization and intervention,* New York, 1982, Plenum.
9. Doughtery PM, Radomski MV: *The cognitive rehabilitation workbook,* Rockville, Md, 1987, Aspen.
10. Gardner MF: The Test of Visual Perceptual Skills (TVPS), Burlingame, Calif, 1992, Psychological and Educational Publications.
11. Golding E: The Middlesex Elderly Assessment of Mental State, Thames, England, 1989, Thames Valley Testing.
12. Harrell M et al: *Cognitive rehabilitation of memory: a practical guide,* Gaithersburg, Md, 1992, Aspen.
13. Hart T, Hayden ME: The ecological validity of neuropsychological assessment and remediation. In Uzzell BP, Gross Y: *Clinical neuropsychology of intervention,* Boston, 1986, Martinus Nijihoff.
14. Kiernan RJ et al: The Neurobehavioral Cognitive Status Examination: a brief but differentiated approach to cognitive assessment, *Ann Intern Med* pp. 481-485, 1987.
15. Lezak MD: *Neuropsychological assessment,* New York, 1983, Oxford University Press.
16. Likert R, Quasha WH: *The revised Minnesota paper formboard test,* New York, 1970, Psychological Corporation.
17. Lynch WJ: Ecological validity of cognitive rehabilitation software, *J Head Trauma Rehabil* 7:36, 1992.
18. McCarthy RA, Warrington EK: *Cognitive neuropsychology: a clinical introduction,* San Diego, 1990, Academic.
19. Morse PA, Morse AR: Functional living skills: promoting the interaction between neuropsychology and occupational therapy, *J Head Trauma Rehabil* 3:33, 1988.
20. Prigatano GP: *Neuropsychological rehabilitation after brain injury,* Baltimore, 1986, Johns Hopkins University Press.
21. Ruch FL, Ruch M: Employee Aptitude Survey, San Diego, 1963, Educational and Industrial Testing Service.
22. Rustad RA et al: The Cognitive Assessment of Minnesota, Tucson, Ariz, 1993, Therapy Skill Builders.
23. Sivan AB: The Benton Visual Retention Test, San Antonio, Tex, 1992, Psychological Corporation.
24. Sohlberg MM: The Profile of Executive Control System (PRO-EX), Puyallup, Wash, 1992, Association for Neurological Research and Development.
25. Stone MH, Wright BD: Knox's Cube Test, Wood Dale, Ill, 1980, Stoelting.
26. Strauss AA, Werner H: Disorders of conceptual thinking in the brain injured child, *J Nerv Ment Dis* 96:153, 1942.
27. Tankle RS: Application of neuropsychological test results to interdisciplinary cognitive rehabilitation with head injured adults, *J Head Trauma Rehabil* 3:24, 1988.

28. Toglia JP: Attention and memory. In Royeen CB, editor: *AOTA self study series: Cognitive rehabilitation,* Rockville, Md, 1993, American Occupational Therapy Association.
29. Toglia JP: *The contextual memory test manual,* Tucson, 1993, Therapy Skill Builders.
30. Walsh K: *Neuropsychology: a clinical approach,* Edinburgh, Scotland, 1987, Churchill Livingstone.
31. Webster RE: The Learning Efficiency Test, ed 2, Novato, Calif, 1992, Academic Therapy.
32. Wilson BA, Moffat N, editors: *Clinical management of memory problems,* Rockville, Md, 1984, Aspen.
33. Wilson B, Cockburn J, Baddeley A: The Rivermead Behavioural Memory Test, Suffolk, United Kingdom, 1985, Thames Valley Testing.
34. Wood RL: Management of attention disorders following brain injury. In Wilson BA, Moffat N, editors: *Clinical management of memory problems,* Rockville, Md, 1984, Aspen.
35. Ylvisaker M et al: Topics in cognitive rehabilitation therapy. In Ylvisaker M, Gobble EM: *Community re-entry for head injured adults,* Boston, 1987, Little, Brown.
36. Zoltan B, Siev E, Frieshtat B: *The adult stroke patient: a manual for evaluation and treatment of perceptual and cognitive dysfunction,* rev ed 2, Thorofare, NJ, 1986, Slack.

## RECOMMENDED READING

Brand P, Yancy P: *The gift nobody wants,* New York, 1993, Harper Collins.

Royeen CB, editor: *AOTA self study series: cognitive rehabilitation,* Rockville, Md, 1993, American Occupational Therapy Association.

*Part* **IV**

# *Broad Aspects of Treatment*

*Chapter* 12

# Infection Control and Safety Issues in the Clinic

*Wendy S. Buckner*

## *Chapter Objectives*

*After studying this chapter, the student or practitioner will be able to:*

1. Recognize the role of occupational therapy personnel in preventing accidents.
2. Identify recommendations for safety in the clinic.
3. Describe preventive positioning for patients with lower extremity amputations, rheumatoid arthritis, burns, and hemiplegia.
4. Describe the purpose of special equipment.
5. Identify precautions when treating patients who require special equipment.
6. Identify universal precautions and recognize the importance of following them with all patients.
7. Describe proper techniques of handwashing.
8. Recognize the importance of having all health care workers understand and follow isolation procedures used in patient care.
9. Identify procedures for handling patient injuries.
10. Describe guidelines for handling various emergency situations.

## *Key Terms*

Fowler's position
turning frame
ventilator
endotracheal tube
electrocardiogram
pulmonary artery catheter
intracranial pressure monitor
arterial monitoring line
nasogastric tube
gastric tube
intravenous feeding
total parenteral nutrition (TPN)
hyperalimentation
infusion pump (IMED, IVAC)
intravenous (IV) line
urinary catheter
universal precautions
human immunodeficiency virus (HIV)

## Key Terms—cont'd

acquired immunodeficiency syndrome (AIDS)
hepatitis B virus
sterilization
autoclave
disinfectant
isolation
shock
seizure
insulin reaction
acidosis
cardiopulmonary resuscitation

The certified occupational therapy assistant (COTA) must ensure that patients remain safe within the health care setting. Medical technology and cost control methods have forced seriously ill patients into the OT clinic early in their illness and for shorter lengths of treatment. This increases the potential for injury to the patient.

Occupational therapy personnel are legally liable for negligence if a patient is injured because the staff failed to follow proper procedures.[4] This chapter reviews safety precautions associated with selected diagnoses. It also identifies precautions to consider when using equipment typically found in treatment settings. Guidelines for handling various emergency situations are reviewed. This chapter is only an overview and cannot substitute for training in procedures specific to a particular facility. In addition to following these procedures, the COTA should teach patients and their families applicable techniques to follow at home.

## SAFETY RECOMMENDATIONS FOR THE CLINIC

The prevention of accidents and subsequent injuries begins with consistent use of the following safety recommendations for the clinic:

1. Wash your hands for at least 30 seconds[3] before and after treating each patient to reduce cross-contamination.
2. Make sure adequate space is available to maneuver equipment. Avoid placing patients where they may be bumped by equipment or passing personnel. Keep the area free from clutter.
3. Do not attempt to transfer patients in congested areas or areas where your view is blocked.
4. Routinely check equipment to be sure it is working properly.
5. Ensure that furniture and equipment in the clinic are stable. When not in use, store items out of the way of the treatment area.
6. Keep the floor free of cords, scatter rugs, litter, and spills. Avoid highly polished floors, which may be very slippery.
7. Do not leave patients unattended. Use restraint belts properly to protect the patients when they are not closely observed.
8. Have the treatment area and supplies ready before the patient arrives.
9. Allow only properly trained personnel to provide patient care.
10. Follow the manufacturer's and facility's procedures for handling and storage of potentially hazardous material. Be sure such materials are marked and stored in a place in clear view. Do not store items above shoulder height.
11. Ensure that emergency exits and evacuation routes are clearly indicated.
12. Have emergency equipment, such as fire extinguishers and first-aid kits, readily available.

## PREVENTIVE POSITIONING FOR SPECIFIC DIAGNOSES

Many patients require proper positioning to prevent complications and maintain function. Staying in one position for a long time can lead to the development of contractures and bedsores (decubitus ulcers).

Specific patient conditions, such as impaired sensation, paralysis, poor skin integrity, poor nutrition, impaired circulation, and spasticity, require special attention. The patient's skin, especially bony prominences over the sacrum, ischium, trochanters, elbows, and heels, should be inspected. Reddened areas may develop from pressure within 30 minutes. Other indicators of excessive pressure are complaints of numbness or tingling and localized swelling.

Pillows, towel rolls, or similar devices may be used to provide comfort and stability but should be used cautiously to prevent secondary complications. The following examples of patient conditions demonstrate the need for specific positioning techniques. It is important to review these with both the patient and caregiver.

Patients with *above-knee* lower extremity amputations should avoid hip flexion and hip abduction. The time the patient may sit is limited to 30 minutes per hour. When the patient is supine, the stump is elevated on a pillow only for a few minutes. Prone lying is recommended to help avoid contracture of the hip flexor muscles.

Patients with *below-knee* lower extremity amputations should avoid prolonged hip and knee flexion to prevent contractures. Again, the patient may sit only 30 minutes per hour, and when supine, the patient should not keep the stump elevated for more than a few minutes. When elevated, the knee is maintained in extension. The patient is instructed to keep the knee extended throughout the day. Prone lying is recommended.

To avoid contractures resulting from muscle spasticity, patients with hemiplegia should avoid the following positions for prolonged periods: shoulder adduction and internal rotation, elbow flexion, forearm supination or pronation, wrist flexion, finger and thumb flexion and adduction, hip and knee flexion, hip external rotation, and ankle plantar flexion and inversion. Both the arm and the leg should be moved through the available range of motion (ROM) several times per day.

Patients with rheumatoid arthritis should avoid prolonged immobilization of the affected extremity joints. Gentle active range of motion (AROM) or passive range of motion (PROM) of the joints should be performed several times per day if the joints are not acutely inflamed.

As burns heal, scars and contractures are likely to form. Therefore it is important to avoid prolonged positioning of the joints affected by the burn or skin graft, especially positions of comfort. The positions comfortable to the patient do not produce the stress or tension needed to maintain mobility of the wound area. When the burn is located on the flexor or adductor surface of a joint, positions of flexion and adduction should be avoided. Passive or active exercise should be done frequently to both the involved and the uninvolved joints. The patient will probably have to endure great pain to restore normal joint function.

## PRECAUTIONS WITH SPECIAL EQUIPMENT

When seeing patients at the bedside, the COTA first should contact the nurses' station to determine if any specific instructions exist regarding positioning. For example, a patient may need to follow a turning schedule and may be limited in time allowed to remain in one position. If the patient's current position in bed is not suitable for treatment, the treatment might be rescheduled. Other options would be to change the patient's position temporarily or to treat the patient as much as possible in the current position. If the patient's position is changed, the COTA makes sure the patient is returned to the preferred position at the end of treatment.

### Hospital Beds

Two of the more frequently used beds in hospitals are the standard manually operated bed and the electrically operated bed. Both beds are designed to make it easier to support the patient and to change a patient's position. Other more specialized beds are needed for patients with more traumatic conditions. Whatever type is used, the bed should be positioned so that the patient is easily accessed and the OT practitioner can use good body mechanics (see Chapter 18).

Most standard adjustable beds are adjusted by using electrical controls attached to the head or the foot of the bed or to a special cord that allows the patient to operate them. The controls are marked according to their function and can be operated by using the hand or foot. The entire bed can be raised and lowered, or the upper portion of it can be raised while the lower portion remains unchanged. When the upper portion is raised slightly, the patient's position is referred to as **Fowler's position.** Most beds allow the lower portion to be adjusted to provide knee flexion, which in turn causes hip flexion.

Side rails are on most beds as a protective measure. Some rails are lifted upward to engage the locking mechanism, whereas others are moved toward the upper portion of the bed until the locking mechanism is engaged. If a side rail is used for patient security, the practitioner ensures (before leaving the patient) the rail is locked securely and has not compressed or stretched any intravenous (IV) lines or other tubing.

A **turning frame** (e.g., Stryker wedge frame) has a front and back frame covered with canvas. The support base allows the head or foot ends of the frames or the entire bed to be elevated. One person can easily turn the patient horizontally from prone to supine or from supine to prone positions. This bed is used most frequently with patients who have a spinal cord injury and require immobilization. The turning frame allows access to patients and permits moving them from one place to another without removing them from the frame. The skin of patients using this type of bed must be monitored frequently because the bed allows only two basic positions.

The *circular turning frame* (Circ-O-Lectric bed) has a front and back frame attached to two circular supports. The frames on which the patient is positioned move the patient vertically from supine to prone or from prone to supine. The circular support frames are moved by an electric motor and can be stopped at any point within their half-circle range. The patient or other persons can operate a control switch to adjust the position. This bed has similar uses to the Stryker frame and also provides the benefit of frequent position changes to relieve skin pressure. However, a patient is still at risk of developing skin problems because of the pressure forces that may occur when the bed is turned or rotated vertically. Patients may also experience symptoms of motion sickness such as vertigo, nausea, or hypotension when being turned.

The *air-fluidized support bed* (Clinitron) is an expensive bed that contains 1600 pounds of silicone-coated glass beads called *microspheres.* Heated, pressurized air flows around the beads to suspend a polyester cover that supports the patient. When set in motion, the microspheres develop the properties associated with fluids. Patients feel like they are floating on a warm waterbed. The risk of developing skin problems is reduced because of the minimal contact pressure of the patient's body against the polyester sheet. This bed is used with patients who have several infected lesions or who require skin protection and whose position cannot be altered easily. Caution should be used to prevent puncturing the polyester cover, thus causing the microspheres to be expelled.

### Ventilators

A **ventilator** (respirator) moves gas or air into the patient's lungs and is used to maintain adequate air exchange when normal respiration is decreased. Two frequently used types are *volume-cycled ventilators* and *pressure-cycled ventilators.* Both ventilators deliver a predetermined volume of gas ("air") during inspiration and allow for passive expiration. Usually the gas from the ventilator is delivered to the patient through an **endotracheal tube** (ETT). When the tube is in place, the patient is considered to be *intubated.* Insertion of the ETT prevents the patient from talking. When the ETT is removed, the patient may complain of a sore throat and have a distorted voice for a short time. It is important to avoid disturbing, bending, kinking, or occluding the tubing or accidentally disconnecting the tube of the ventilator from the ETT. The patient who uses a ventilator may participate in various bedside activities, including sitting and ambulation. The tubing should be of sufficient length to allow the activity to be performed. Because the patient has difficulty talking, the OTR or COTA should use questions that can be answered with head nods or other nonverbal means. A patient using a ventilator may have reduced tolerance for activities and should be monitored for signs of respiratory distress, such as a change in the respiration pattern, fainting, or lips turning blue.

### Monitors

Various monitors are used to observe the physiological state of patients requiring special care. Therapeutic activities can be performed by patients who are being monitored, provided care is taken to avoid disruption of the equipment. Many of the units have an auditory and/or visual signal that is activated by a change in the patient's condition or position or by a change in the equipment's function. A nurse may need to evaluate and correct the cause of the alarm unless the COTA has received special instruction.

The **electrocardiogram** (ECG, EKG) monitors the patient's heart rate, blood pressure, and respiration rate. Acceptable or safe ranges for the three physiologic indicators can be set in the unit. An alarm is activated when the upper or lower limits of the ranges are exceeded or if the unit malfunctions. A monitoring screen provides a graphic and digital display of the values for observation of the patient's responses to treatment.

The **pulmonary artery catheter** (PAC) (e.g., Swan-Ganz catheter) is a long, plastic IV tube inserted into the internal jugular or the femoral vein and passed through to the pulmonary artery. It then provides accurate and continuous measurements of pulmonary artery pressures and detects even very subtle changes in the patient's cardiovascular system, including responses to medications, stress, and activity. Activities can be performed with the PAC in place, as long as they do not interfere with the location of the catheter's insertion. For example, if the catheter is inserted into the subclavian vein, elbow flexion should be avoided and shoulder motions restricted.

The **intracranial pressure** (ICP) **monitor** measures the pressure exerted against the skull by brain tissue, blood, or cerebrospinal fluid (CSF). It is used for patients who have experienced a closed head injury, cerebral hemorrhage, brain tumor, or an overproduction of CSF in order to monitor ICP. Some of the complications associated with this device are infection, hemorrhage, and seizures. Two of the more frequently used ICP monitoring devices are the *ventricular catheter* and the *subarachnoid screw.* Both are inserted in a hole drilled in the skull. Physical activities should be limited when these devices are in place. The patient avoids activities that would cause a rapid increase in ICP, such as isometric exercises. Positions to avoid include neck flexion, hip flexion greater than 90°, and the prone position. The patient's head should not be lowered more than 15° below the horizontal plane. Care must be taken to avoid disturbing the plastic tube.

The **arterial monitoring line** (A line) is a catheter inserted into an artery to measure blood pressure continuously or to obtain blood samples without repeated needle punctures. Treatment can be provided with an A line in place, but care should be taken to avoid disturbing the catheter and inserted needle.

### Feeding Devices

Special feeding devices may be necessary to provide nutrition for patients who are unable to chew, swallow, or ingest food. Some of the more common devices are the nasogastric tube, gastric tube, and IV feedings.

The **nasogastric** (NG) **tube** is a plastic tube inserted through a nostril and terminating in the patient's stomach. The tube may cause the patient to have a sore throat and an increased gag reflex. The patient cannot eat food or drink fluids through the mouth while the NG tube is in place. Movement of the patient's head and neck, especially forward flexion, should be avoided.

The **gastric tube** (G tube) is a plastic tube inserted through an incision in the patient's abdomen directly into the stomach. During treatment the OT practitioner must avoid disturbing or removing the tube.

**Intravenous feeding, total parenteral nutrition (TPN),** and **hyperalimentation** devices are used to infuse the total calories (TPN) or nutrients (hyperalimentation) needed to promote tissue growth. A catheter is inserted directly into the subclavian or another vein and then passed through the subclavian vein. The catheter may be connected to a semipermanently fixed cannula or sutured at the point of insertion. The COTA should carefully observe the various connections to be certain they are secure before and after treatment. A disrupted or loose connection may result in the development of an air embolus, which could be life threatening to the patient.

The system usually includes an **infusion pump (IMED, IVAC)**, which administers fluids and nutrients at a preselected, constant flow rate. An audible alarm is activated if the system becomes imbalanced or when the fluid source is empty. Treatment activities can be performed as long as the tubing is not disrupted, disconnected, or occluded and undue stress on the infusion site is avoided. Motions of the shoulder on the side of the infusion site may be restricted, especially abduction and flexion.

Most **intravenous (IV) lines** are inserted into superficial veins. Various sizes and types of needles or catheters are used, depending on the purpose of the IV therapy, the infusion site, the need for prolonged therapy, and site availability. During treatment the COTA must be careful to avoid disrupting, disconnecting, or occluding the tubing. The infusion site should remain dry, the needle should remain secure and immobile in the vein, and no restraint should be placed above the infusion site (e.g., no blood pressure cuff applied above the site). The total system should be observed to ensure it is functioning properly when treatment begins and ends. If the infusion site is in the antecubital area, the elbow should not be flexed. The patient who ambulates with an IV line in place should be instructed to grasp the IV support pole so the infusion site will be at heart level. If the infusion site is allowed to hang lower, blood flow may be affected. Similar procedures to maintain the infusion site in proper position should be followed when the patient is treated while in bed or at a treatment table. The patient should avoid activities requiring the infusion site to be elevated above the level of the heart for a prolonged period. Problems related to the IV system should be reported to nursing personnel. Simple procedures such as straightening the tubing may be performed by the properly trained COTA.

### Urinary Catheters

A **urinary catheter** is used to remove urine from the bladder when the patient is unable to control its retention or release. The urine is then drained through plastic tubing into a collection bag, bottle, or urinal. Any form of trauma, disease, condition, or disorder affecting the neuromuscular control of the bladder sphincter may require the use of a urinary catheter. The catheter may be used temporarily or for the remainder of the patient's life.

A urinary catheter can be applied internally *(indwelling catheter)* or externally. Female patients require an indwelling catheter inserted through the urethra and into the bladder. Males may use an *external catheter.* A condom is applied over the shaft of the penis and is held in place by an adhesive applied to the skin or by a padded strap or tape encircling the proximal shaft of the penis. It is connected to a drainage tube and bag.

When treating patients with urinary catheters, the COTA must remember the following precautions:

1. Avoid disrupting or stretching the drainage tube, and do not put tension on the tubing or the catheter.
2. Do not allow the bag to be placed above the level of the bladder for more than a few minutes.
3. Do not place the bag in the patient's lap when being transported.
4. Observe the production, color, and odor of the urine.
5. Report the following observations to a physician or nurse: foul-smelling, cloudy, dark, or bloody urine or a reduction in the flow or production of urine.
6. Be sure to empty the collection bag when it is full.

Infection is a major complication for persons using catheters, especially indwelling catheters. Everyone involved with the patient should maintain cleanliness during treatment. The COTA should not attempt to replace or reconnect the tubing unless properly trained. Health care settings that routinely treat patients with catheters have specific protocols for catheter care.

Two types of internal catheters frequently used are the Foley and suprapubic catheters. The *Foley catheter* is a type of indwelling catheter held in place in the bladder by a small balloon that is inflated with air, water, or sterile saline solution. To remove the catheter, the balloon is deflated and the catheter withdrawn. The *suprapubic catheter* is inserted directly into the bladder through incisions in the lower abdomen and bladder. The catheter may be held in place by adhesive tape, but care should be taken to avoid its removal, especially during self-care activities.

## INFECTION CONTROL

Infection control procedures are used to prevent the spread of diseases and infection among patients, health care workers, and others. They are designed to interrupt or establish barriers to the infection cycle. **Universal precautions** (Box 12-1 and Figure 12-1) were first established by the Centers for Disease Control and Prevention (CDC) to protect the health care worker from infectious diseases such as **human immunodeficiency virus (HIV), acquired immunodeficiency syndrome (AIDS),** and **hepatitis B virus (HBV).** However, these precautions are effective only when used with *all* patients, not only those identified as infected.

The U.S. Occupational Safety and Health Administration (OSHA) has issued regulations to protect the employees of health care facilities. All treatment settings must comply with the following federal regulations:

1. Educate employees on the methods of transmission and the prevention of HBV and HIV.
2. Provide safe and adequate protective equipment, and teach the employees where it is located and how to use it.

*Box 12-1*

## Summary of Universal Precautions

1. Use extreme care to prevent injuries caused by sharp instruments.
2. Cover minor, nondraining, noninfected skin lesions with a bandaid.
3. Report infected or draining lesions and weeping dermatitis to the supervisor.
4. Avoid personal habits (e.g., nail biting) that increase the potential for oral mucous membranes coming in contact with body substances.
5. Perform procedures involving body substances carefully to minimize splatters and aerosols.
6. Cover environmental surfaces with moisture-proof barriers if possible splattering with body substances may occur.
7. Wash hands regularly, especially after gloves are worn.
8. Avoid unnecessary use of protective clothing. Use alternate barriers whenever possible.
9. Wear gloves to touch the mucous membranes or nonintact skin of any patient and when direct contact with visible body substances is anticipated.
10. Wear protective clothing (gown, mask, goggles) when splashing of body substances is anticipated.
11. Remove protective clothing after each use and before leaving the area where the contact occurred. Discard disposable items and routinely process nondisposable items.

3. Teach the employees about work practices used to prevent occupational transmission of disease, including (but not limited to) universal precautions, proper handling of patient specimens and linens, proper cleaning of body fluid spills (Figure 12-2), and proper waste disposal.
4. Provide proper containers for the disposal of waste and sharp items, and teach the employees the color-coding system used to distinguish infectious waste.
5. Post warning labels and biohazard signs (Figure 12-3).
6. Offer the hepatitis B vaccine to employees at substantial risk of occupational exposure to HBV.
7. Provide education and follow-up care to employees who are exposed to communicable disease.

OSHA has also outlined the responsibilities of health care employees, including the following:

1. Use protective equipment and clothing provided by the facility whenever the employee comes in contact, or anticipates coming in contact, with body fluids.
2. Dispose of waste in proper containers, using knowledge and understanding of the handling of infectious waste and color-coded bags or containers.
3. Dispose of sharp instruments and needles into proper containers without attempting to recap, bend, break, or otherwise manipulate them before disposal.

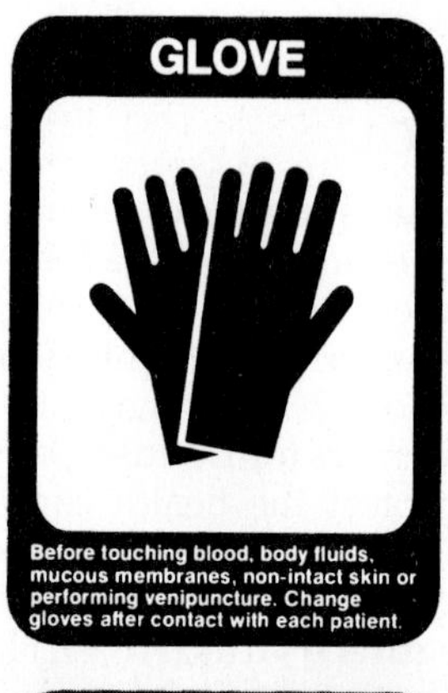

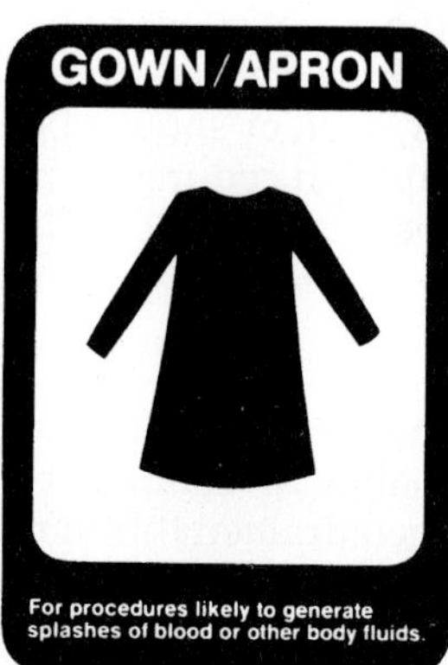

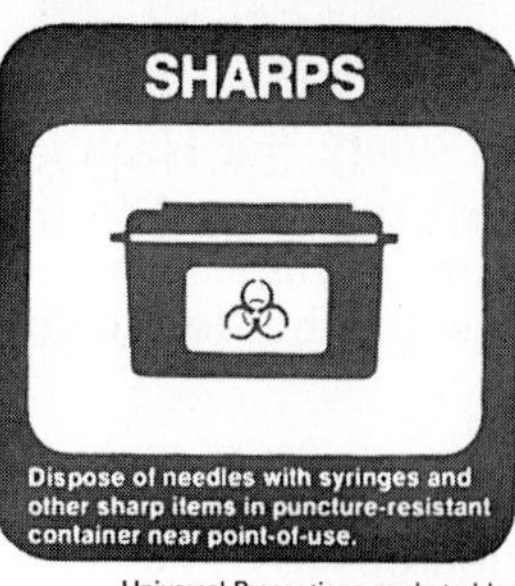


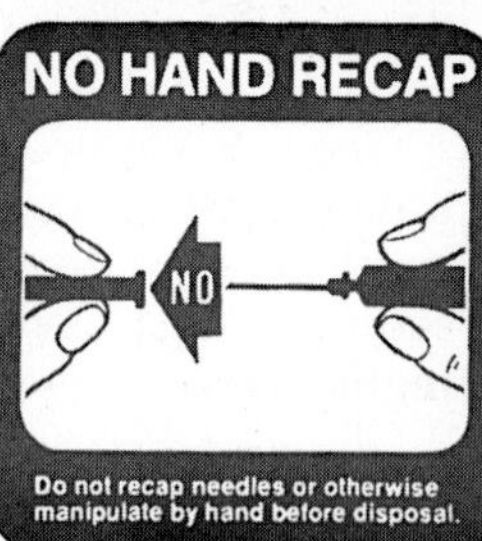


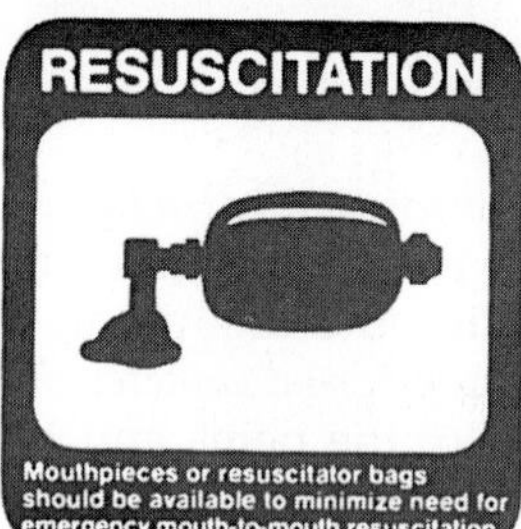


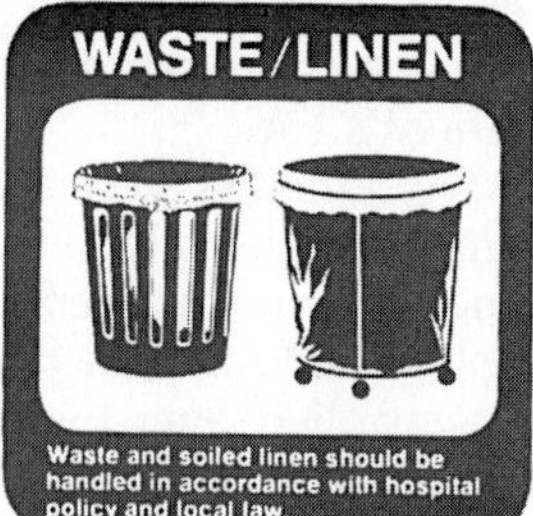


Universal Precautions apply to blood, visibly bloody fluid, semen, vaginal secretions, tissues and to cerebrospinal, synovial, pleural, peritoneal, pericardial and amniotic fluids.

*Figure 12-1* Universal blood and body fluid precautions. (Courtesy Brevis Corp, Salt Lake City, Utah.)

4. Keep the work and patient care area clean.
5. Wash hands immediately after removing gloves and at all other times required by hospital or agency policy.
6. Immediately report any exposures (e.g., needle sticks, blood splashes) or any personal illnesses to the supervisor and receive instruction about any further follow-up action.

Although it is impossible to eliminate all pathogens from an area or object, the likelihood of an infection occurring can be greatly reduced. The largest source of preventable patient infection is contamination from the hands of health care workers. Handwashing (Box 12-2) and the use of gloves are the most effective barriers to the infection cycle. Additional measures include wearing caps, masks, and gowns and properly disposing of sharp instruments, contaminated dressings, and bed linens.

In the clinic, general cleanliness and proper control of heat, light, and air are also important for infection control. Spills should be cleaned up promptly. Work

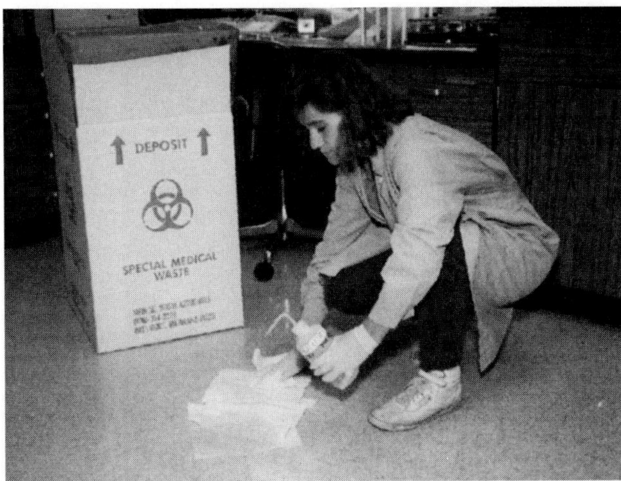


*Figure 12-2* Spills of body fluids must be cleaned up by a gloved employee, using paper towels, which should then be placed in an infectious waste container. Then 5.25% sodium hypochlorite (household bleach) diluted 1:10 should be used to disinfect the area. (From Zakus SM: *Clinical procedures for medical assistants,* ed 3, St Louis, 1995, Mosby.)

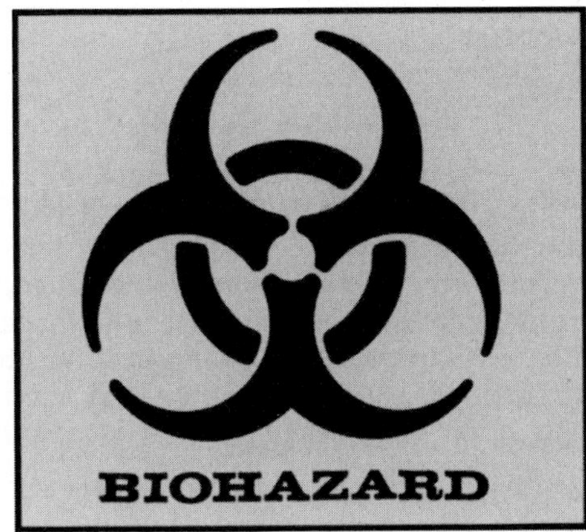


*Figure 12-3* Biohazard label. (From Zakus SM: *Clinical procedures for medical assistants,* ed 3, St Louis, 1995, Mosby.)

*Box 12-2*

### Technique for Effective Handwashing

1. Remove all jewelry, except plain band-type rings. Remove watch or move it up the arm. Provide complete access to area to be washed.
2. Approach the sink, and avoid touching the sink or nearby objects.
3. Turn on the water, and adjust it to a lukewarm temperature and a moderate flow to avoid splashing.
4. Wet wrists and hands with fingers directed downward, and apply approximately 1 teaspoon of liquid soap or granules.
5. Begin to wash all areas of hands (palms, sides, backs), fingers, knuckles, and between each finger using a vigorous rubbing and circular motions (Figure 12-4). If wearing a band, slide it up or down the finger and scrub skin underneath it. Interlace fingers and scrub between each finger.
6. Wash for at least 30 seconds, keeping the hands and forearms at elbow level or below and hands pointed down. Wash longer if a patient known to have an infection was treated.
7. Rinse hands well under running water.
8. Wash as high up wrists and forearms as contamination is likely.
9. Rinse hands, wrists, and forearms under running water (Figure 12-5).
10. Use an orangewood stick or nail brush to clean under each fingernail at least once a day when starting work and each time hands are highly contaminated. Rinse nails well under running water (Figure 12-6).
11. Dry hands, wrists, and forearms thoroughly with paper towels. Use a dry towel for each hand. Water should continue to flow from tap as hands are dried.
12. Use another dry paper towel to turn water faucet off (Figure 12-7). Discard all towels in an appropriate container.
13. Use hand lotion as necessary.

Modified from Zakus SM: *Clinical procedures for medical assistants,* ed 3, St Louis, 1995, Mosby.

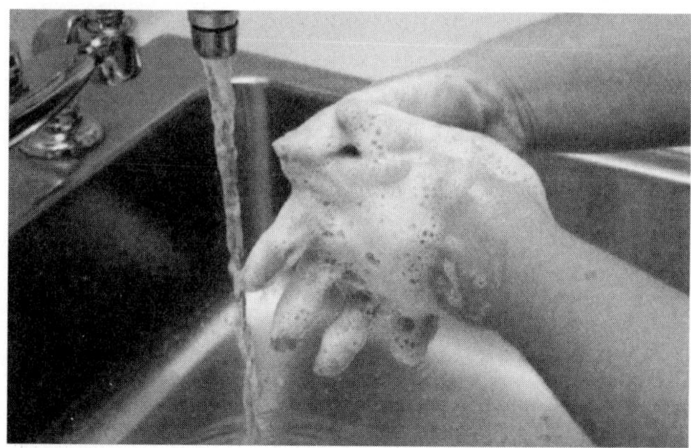

*Figure 12-4* Handwashing technique. Interlace fingers to wash between them. Create a lather with soap. Keep hands pointed down. (From Zakus SM: *Clinical procedures for medical assistants,* ed 3, St Louis, 1995, Mosby.)

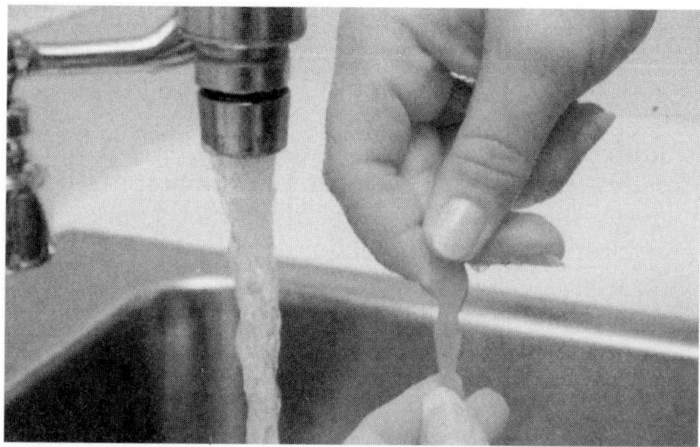

*Figure 12-6* Use blunt edge of an orangewood stick to clean under fingernails. (From Zakus SM: *Clinical procedures for medical assistants,* ed 3, St Louis, 1995, Mosby.)

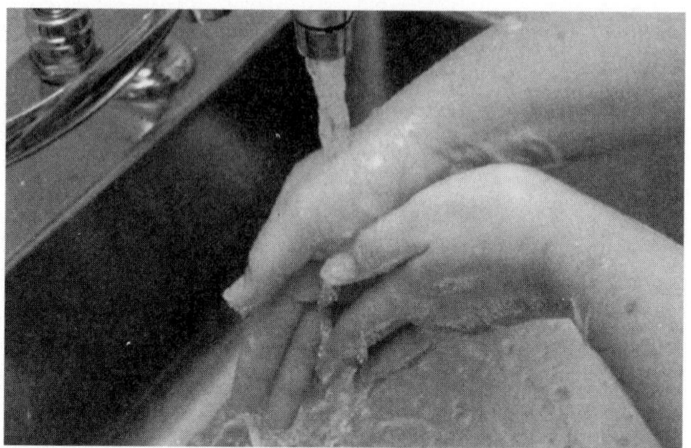

*Figure 12-5* Rinse hands well, keeping fingers pointed down. (From Zakus SM: *Clinical procedures for medical assistants,* ed 3, St Louis, 1995, Mosby.)

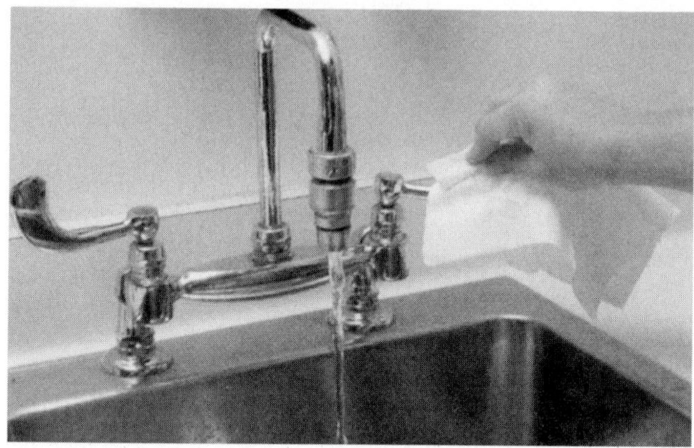

*Figure 12-7* After drying hands, turn water faucet off, using a dry paper towel. (From Zakus SM: *Clinical procedures for medical assistants,* ed 3, St Louis, 1995, Mosby.)

areas and equipment should be kept free from contamination.

*Decontamination* means "to remove, inactivate, or destroy blood-borne pathogens on a surface or item to the point where they are no longer capable of transmitting infectious particles and the surface or item is rendered safe for handling, use, or disposal."[2] Items to be sterilized or decontaminated should first be thoroughly cleaned to remove any residual matter. **Sterilization** is used to destroy all forms of microbial life, including highly resistant bacterial spores. An **autoclave** is used to sterilize items by steam under pressure. Ethylene oxide, dry heat, and immersion in chemical sterilants are other methods of sterilization.

A variety of **disinfectants** may be used to clean environmental surfaces and reusable instruments. When using liquid disinfectants and cleaning agents, gloves are worn to protect the skin from repeated or prolonged contact. The CDC, local health department, or hospital infection control department can provide information regarding the best product and method to use.

Instruments and equipment used to treat a patient should be cleaned or disposed of according to institutional or agency policies and procedures. Contaminated reusable equipment should be placed carefully in a container, labeled, and returned to the appropriate department for sterilization. Contaminated disposable items should be placed carefully in a container, labeled, and disposed of properly.

Contaminated or soiled linen should be disposed of with minimal handling, sorting, and movement. It can be placed in an appropriate bag and labeled before transport to the laundry, or the bag can be color-coded to indicate the type or condition of linen it contains. Other contaminated items, such as toys, magazines, personal hygiene articles, dishes, and eating utensils, should be disposed of or disinfected. They should not be used by others until they have been disinfected.

### Isolation Systems

Isolation systems are designed to protect a person or object from becoming contaminated or infected by transmissible pathogens. Various isolation procedures are used in different institutions. All health care workers must understand and follow the isolation approach used in their facilities to ensure protection.

Generally, patients are isolated from other patients and the hospital environment because they have a transmissible disease. **Isolation** involves placing the patient in a room alone or with one or more patients with the same disease to reduce the possibility of transmitting the disease to others. Specific infection control techniques must be followed by all who enter the patient's room. These requirements are listed on a color-coded card and placed on or next to the door of the patient's room. Boxes 12-3 and 12-4 list strict isolation and respiratory isolation procedures. Protective clothing, including gown, mask, cap, and gloves, may be required. When leaving the patient, it is important to remove the garments in the proper sequence.

Occasionally, patients' conditions (e.g., burns, systemic infections) make them more susceptible to infection. They may be placed in *protective isolation.* With this approach, persons entering the patient's room may have to wear protective clothing to prevent the transmission of pathogens to the patient. In this case, the sequence and method of donning the protective garments are more important than the sequence used to remove them.

Box 12-3

### Strict Isolation*

**Visitors: Report to nurses' station before entering room.**

1. Masks are indicated for all persons entering room.
2. Gowns are indicated for all persons entering room.
3. Gloves are indicated for all persons entering room.
4. Hands *must* be washed after touching the patient or potentially contaminated articles and *before* taking care of another patient.
5. Articles contaminated with infective material should be disregarded or bagged and labeled before being sent for decontamination and reprocessing.

*Card will be color-coded yellow.

Box 12-4

### Respiratory Isolation*

**Visitors: Report to nurses' station before entering room.**

1. Masks are indicated for those who come close to patient.
2. Gowns are not indicated.
3. Gloves are not indicated.
4. Hands *must* be washed after touching patient or potentially contaminated articles and *before* taking care of another patient.
5. Articles contaminated with infective material should be discarded or bagged and labeled before being sent for decontamination and reprocessing.

*Card will be color-coded blue.

## INCIDENTS AND EMERGENCIES

Occupational therapy assistants should be able to respond to a variety of medical emergencies and to recognize when it is better to receive assistance from the most qualified individual available, such as a physician, emergency medical technician, or nurse. This should be relatively easy in a hospital but may require an extended time if the treatment is conducted in a patient's home or outpatient clinic. The assistant should keep emergency telephone numbers close at hand. The COTA needs to determine at the time of the incident whether it is best to ask for assistance before or after beginning emergency care. In most cases it is advisable to call for assistance before initiating emergency care, unless the delay is life threatening to the patient.

Many accidents can be prevented by consistently following safety measures. However, occupational therapy practitioners should always be alert to the possibility of an injury and should "expect the unexpected" to happen. Most institutions have specific policies and procedures to follow. In general, when a patient is injured, the COTA should do the following:

1. Ask for help. Do not leave the patient alone. Prevent further injury to the patient and provide emergency care.
2. When the "emergency" is over, document the incident according to the institution's policy. Do not discuss the incident with the patient or significant others. Do not admit to negligence or provide information suggestive of negligence to anyone.[3]
3. Notify the supervisor of the incident, and file the incident report with the appropriate person within the organization.

### Falls

Injury from falls can be prevented by staying alert and reacting quickly when patients lose their balance. Proper guarding techniques must be practiced. In many instances it is unwise to try to keep the patient upright. Instead, the practitioner should carefully assist the patient to the floor or onto a firm support.

If a patient begins to fall forward, the COTA should do the following:

1. Restrain the patient by firmly holding the gait belt.
2. Push forward against the pelvis, and pull back on the shoulder or anterior chest.
3. Help the patient to stand erect once you determine the patient is not injured. The patient may briefly lean against you for support.

4. If the patient is falling too far forward to be kept upright, guide the patient to reach slowly for the floor.
5. Slow the momentum by gently pulling back on the gait belt and the patient's shoulder.
6. Step forward as the patient moves toward the floor.
7. Tell the patient to bend the elbows when the hands contact the floor to help cushion the fall.
8. Ensure the patient's head is turned to the side to avoid injury to the face.

If the patient begins to fall backward, the procedure is as follows:

1. Rotate your body so that one side is turned toward the patient's back, and widen your stance.
2. Push forward on the patient's pelvis, and allow the patient to lean against your body.
3. Assist the patient to stand erect.
4. If the patient falls too far backward, continue to rotate your body to stay upright until it is turned toward the patient's back, and widen your stance.
5. Instruct the patient to lean briefly against your body or to sit on your thigh.
6. Consider lowering the patient into a sitting position on the floor, using the gait belt and good body mechanics.

### Burns

Generally, only minor first-degree burns are likely to occur in occupational therapy practice. These can be treated with basic first-aid procedures. The COTA should contact skilled personnel for immediate care if the burn has any charred or missing skin or shows blistering. For first-degree burns, where the skin is only reddened, the following steps are taken:

1. Rinse or soak the burned area in cold (not iced) water.
2. Cover with a clean or sterile dressing or bandaid. A moist dressing may be more comfortable for some patients.
3. Do not apply any cream, ointment, or butter to the burn because this will mask the appearance and may lead to infection or a delay in healing.

### Bleeding

A laceration may result in minor or serious bleeding. The objectives of treatment are to prevent contamination of the wound and to control the bleeding. To stop the bleeding, the COTA should do the following:

1. Wash hands and apply protective gloves. Continue to wear protective gloves during treatment of the wound.
2. Place a clean towel or sterile dressing over the wound, and apply direct pressure to the wound. If no dressing is available, use the gloved hand.
3. Elevate the wound above the level of the heart to reduce blood flow to the area.
4. In some cases, consider cleansing the wound with an antiseptic or by rinsing it with water.
5. Encourage the patient to remain quiet and to avoid using the extremity.
6. If arterial bleeding occurs, as evidenced by spurting blood, apply intermittent, direct pressure to the artery above the level of the wound as necessary. The pressure point for the brachial artery is on the inside of the upper arm, midway between the elbow and armpit. The pressure point for the femoral artery is in the crease of the hip joint, just to the side of the pubic bone.
7. Do not apply a tourniquet unless you have been trained to do so.

### Shock

Patients may experience **shock** as a result of excessive bleeding, as a reaction to changing from a supine to an upright position, or as a response to excessive heat. Signs and symptoms of shock include pale, moist, and cool skin; shallow, irregular breathing; dilated pupils; a weak or rapid pulse; and dizziness or nausea. Shock should not be confused with fainting, which would result in a slower pulse, paleness, and perspiration. Patients who faint generally recover promptly if allowed to lie flat. The OT practitioner who notices a patient experiencing symptoms of shock should intervene with the following actions:

1. Determine the cause of shock, and correct it if possible. Monitor the patient's blood pressure and pulse rate.
2. Place the patient in a supine position, with head slightly lower than the legs. If head and chest injuries are present or respiration is impaired, consider keeping the head and chest slightly elevated.
3. Do not add heat, but prevent loss of body heat, if necessary, by applying a cool compress to the patient's forehead and covering the patient with a light blanket.
4. Keep the patient quiet, and ensure the patient avoids exertion.
5. After the symptoms are relieved, gradually return the patient to an upright position, and monitor the patient's condition.

### Seizures

Seizures may result from a specific disorder, brain injury, or medication. The COTA should be able to recognize a seizure and take appropriate action to keep the patient from being injured. A patient experiencing a **seizure** usually becomes rigid and statuelike for a few seconds, then begins to convulse with an whole-body jerking motion. The person will most likely turn blue and may stop breathing for up to 50 or even 70 seconds. Some patients' sphincter control may be lost during or at the end of the seizure, and they may involuntarily void urine or feces. The COTA who suspects a patient is about to have a seizure should initiate the following interventions:

1. Place the person in a safe location, away from anything that might cause injury. *Do not* attempt to restrain or restrict the convulsions.
2. Assist in keeping the patient's airway open, but do not attempt to open the mouth by placing any object between the teeth. Never place your finger or a wooden or metal object in the patient's mouth, and do not attempt to grasp or position the tongue.
3. If the patient's mouth is open, place a soft object between the teeth to prevent the patient from accidentally biting the tongue. A sturdy cloth object or a tongue depressor wrapped with several layers of gauze and fastened with adhesive tape may be used.
4. When the convulsions subside, turn the patient's head to one side in case of vomiting.
5. After the convulsions cease, have the patient rest. It may be helpful to cover the patient with a blanket or screen to provide privacy.
6. Obtain medical assistance.

### Insulin-Related Illnesses

Many patients seen in occupational therapy practice may experience insulin-related episodes. The COTA must be able to differentiate between the conditions of hypoglycemia (insulin reaction) and hyperglycemia (acidosis), as shown in Table 12-1.

An **insulin reaction** can be caused by too much systemic insulin, the intake of too much food or sugar, or too little physical activity. If the patient is conscious, some form of sugar is provided (e.g., candy, orange juice). If the patient is unconscious, glucose may have to be provided intravenously. The patient should rest, and all physical activity should be stopped. This condition is not as serious as acidosis, but the patient should be given the opportunity to return to a normal state as soon as possible.

**Acidosis** can lead to a diabetic coma and eventual death if not treated. It should be considered a medical emergency requiring prompt action, including assistance from qualified personnel. The patient should not be given any form of sugar. Usually an injection of insulin is needed, and a nurse or physician should provide care as quickly as possible.

### Choking and Cardiac Arrest

All health care practitioners should be trained to treat patients who are choking or having a cardiac arrest. Specific training courses are offered by both the American Heart Association and the American Red Cross. The following information is presented as a *reminder* of the basic techniques and is *not* meant to substitute for training.

The urgency of choking cannot be overemphasized. Immediate recognition and proper action are essential. When assisting a conscious adult or child older than 1 year, the COTA should do the following:

*Table 12-1*

**Warning Signs and Symptoms of Insulin-Related Illnesses**

| | *Insulin reaction* | *Acidosis* |
|---|---|---|
| Onset | Sudden | Gradual |
| Skin | Moist, pale | Dry, flushed |
| Behavior | Excited, agitated | Drowsy |
| Breath odor | Normal | Fruity |
| Breathing | Normal to shallow | Deep, labored |
| Tongue | Moist | Dry |
| Vomiting | Absent | Present |
| Hunger | Present | Absent |
| Thirst | Absent | Present |

Modified from Pierson FM: *Principles and techniques of patient care*, Philadelphia, 1994, Saunders.

1. Ask the patient, "Are you choking?" If the patient can speak, or cough effectively, *do not* interfere with the patient's own attempts to expel the object.
2. If the patient is unable to speak, cough, or breathe, check the mouth and remove any visible foreign object.
3. If the patient is unable to speak or cough, position yourself behind the person. Clasp your hands over the patient's abdomen, slightly above the umbilicus but below the diaphragm.
4. Use the closed fist of one hand, covered by your other hand, to give three or four abrupt thrusts against the person's abdomen by compressing the abdomen in and up forcefully *(Heimlich maneuver).* Continue to apply the thrusts until the obstruction becomes dislodged or is relieved or the person becomes unconscious.
5. Obtain medical assistance.

When assisting an unconscious adult or child older than 1 year, the COTA should take the following steps:

1. Place the patient in a supine position, and call for medical help.
2. Open the patient's mouth, and use your finger to attempt to locate and remove the foreign object (finger sweep).
3. Open the airway by tilting the head back and lifting the chin forward. Attempt to ventilate using the mouth-to-mouth technique.
4. If step 3 is unsuccessful, deliver up to five abdominal thrusts (Heimlich maneuver), repeat the finger sweep, and attempt to ventilate. It may be necessary to repeat these steps.
5. Be persistent and continue these procedures until the object is removed or medical assistance arrives.
6. Consider initiating cardiopulmonary resuscitation (CPR) techniques to stabilize the patient's cardiopulmonary functions after the object has been removed.

The following procedures are recommended for **cardiopulmonary resuscitation**[1]:

1. Determine the patient's condition by gently shaking the person and asking, "Are you all right?" or "How do you feel?"
2. If there is no response, place the patient in a supine position on a firm surface. Open the patient's airway by lifting up on the chin and pushing down on the forehead to tilt the head back.
3. Check for respiration by observing the chest or abdomen for movement, listening for sounds of breathing, and feeling for breath by placing your cheek close to the patient's mouth. If none of these signs is present, the patient is not breathing; proceed to initiating breathing techniques.
4. Pinch the patient's nose closed, and maintain the head tilt to open the airway. Place your mouth over the patient's mouth and form a seal with your lips; perform two full breaths, then proceed to evaluate the circulation. Some persons prefer to place a clean cloth over the patient's lips before initiating mouth-to-mouth respirations. If available, a plastic intubation device can be used to decrease the contact between the caregiver's mouth and the patient's mouth and any saliva or vomitus.
5. Palpate the carotid artery for a pulse. If there is no pulse, begin external chest compressions.
6. To initiate chest compressions, kneel next to the patient, place the heel of one hand on the inferior portion of the sternum just proximal to the xiphoid process, and place your other hand on top of the first hand. Position your shoulders directly over the patient's sternum, keep your elbows extended, and press down firmly, depressing the sternum approximately 1½ to 2 inches (4 to 5 cm) with each compression. Relax after each compression, but do not remove your hands from the sternum. The relaxation and compression phases should be equal in duration. This can be accomplished by mentally counting "1001," "1002," "1003," and so on, for each phase.
7. If doing all CPR procedures without assistance, perform 15 chest compressions and then two breaths. Compress at the rate of 80 to 100 times per minute. Continue these procedures until qualified assistance arrives or the patient is able to sustain independent respiration and circulation. If alone, attempt to gain assistance from other persons by calling loudly for help. If a second person is present, the person should contact an advanced medical assistance unit before beginning to assist with CPR. The patient usually requires hospitalization and evaluation by a physician. (NOTE: Extreme care must be used to open an airway in a patient who may have a cervical spine injury. For such patients, use the chin lift, but avoid the head tilt. If the technique does not open the airway, tilt the head slowly and gently until the airway is open.)

These procedures are appropriate for adults and children 8 years of age and older to use. A pamphlet or booklet containing diagrams and instructions for CPR techniques can be obtained from most local offices of the American Heart Association. Courses of instruction in first aid and CPR are offered through the American Heart Association, the American National Red Cross, and other organizations.

## SUMMARY

All occupational therapy personnel have a legal and professional obligation to promote safety for self, the patient, visitors, and others. The COTA should be prepared to react to emergency situations quickly, decisively, and calmly. The consistent use of safe practices helps reduce accidents to patients and workers and decreases the time and cost of treatment.

## *Selected Reading Guide Questions*

1. Why is it important to teach the patient and significant others guidelines for handling various emergency situations?
2. Describe at least four behaviors the COTA can adopt to improve patient safety.
3. Describe the consequences of improper positioning of patients.
4. Define the following: IV line, A line, NG tube, TPN, hyperalimentation, and ventilator.
5. Describe *universal precautions.*
6. Why is it important to follow universal precautions with all patients?
7. Describe the proper technique for handwashing.
8. How should the COTA respond to a patient emergency?
9. How would you help a patient falling forward? A patient falling backward?
10. What emergency situations might require obtaining advanced medical assistance, and what situations could a COTA handle alone?

### *REFERENCES*

1. Adult basic life support, *JAMA* 268:2184-2198, 1992.
2. Occupational Safety and Health Administration, US Department of Labor: Occupational exposure to bloodborne pathogens: final rule, *Fed Register* 56:64175, 1991.
3. Pierson FM: *Principles and techniques of patient care,* Philadelphia, 1994, Saunders.
4. Steich TJ: Malpractice and occupational therapy personnel, *Occup Ther News* 39:8, 1985.
5. Zakus SM: *Clinical procedures for medical assistants,* ed 3, St Louis, 1995, Mosby.

### *RESOURCES*

Centers for Disease Control and Prevention (CDC), Occupational Safety and Health Administration (OSHA), Environmental Protection Agency (EPA): Contact for information on infection control.

American Heart Association local offices, American National Red Cross: Contact for information on first aid, choking, and CPR.

Chapter 13

# Psychosocial Aspects of Physical Disability

*Lorraine Williams Pedretti*
*Mary Beth Early*

## Chapter Objectives

*After studying this chapter, the student or practitioner will be able to:*

1. Relate the psychosocial experience of physical disability to the model of human occupation and to human development.
2. Discuss expected personal reactions to the experience of physical dysfunction.
3. Describe common societal reactions to physically disabled persons, and discuss the origins of these reactions.
4. Describe the process of adjustment to the experience of physical disability, and list the expected stages of the adjustment process.
5. Name and describe specific interventions used in occupational therapy to help patients cope with and adjust to psychosocial effects of physical dysfunction.
6. Discuss substance abuse in relation to physical disability.
7. Describe the most effective methods for changing negative societal attitudes toward physically disabled persons.

## Key Terms

personal causation
locus of control
social support
identity versus role confusion
generativity versus stagnation
intimacy versus isolation
apparent acceptance
spread factor
depression
denial
displacement
dependency
regression
passing
compromise body image
milieu therapy
self-help group
substance abuse

The effects of physical disability extend beyond the physical body, impacting the spirit and the soul. To be truly effective, occupational therapy must consider the psychological, social, and spiritual person as well as the presenting physical problem. OT practitioners must accustom themselves to approaching the situation from the patient's point of view, to helping patients process and integrate what has happened to them, and to involving patients as much as possible in setting goals.

Physical dysfunction is initially an experience of loss: loss of function of a physical part, loss of body image dependent on the "normal" functioning of that part, and loss of social roles and personal identity.

Independence, self-sufficiency, and autonomy may be lost, partially or totally and permanently or temporarily.[43]

The content and quality of daily life change dramatically; the new environment and lifestyle of the health care facility enforce passivity and dependence. The schedule, people, and activities are new and are not self-chosen. Privacy must be surrendered and virtual strangers allowed to probe the body. Familial, social, and vocational roles are interrupted and may be seriously altered by the disability experience.

Not only is the disabled individual affected, but also the others with whom the person has contact. The responses of the disabled person and significant others significantly affect the outcome of rehabilitation.[43] The disabled adult must first learn to survive, then to regain essential physical skills, and finally to resume meaningful life roles. These are monumental tasks that require significant adjustment.[38]

Psychological consequences of physical disability depend on many factors. The range of personal reactions varies from one individual to another. Some factors that may influence the patient's response to the dysfunction are (1) time of life and developmental stage in which the disability was acquired, (2) the extent and location of the defect, (3) whether or not it is obvious, (4) the social definition of the defect, (5) the attitudes of significant others toward the individual and the defect, (6) the extent to which the disability interferes with functioning, and (7) the disruption of valued goals.

This chapter considers the relationship between the psychosocial and the physical self in the context of physical disease and disability. It begins with a review of concepts from the model of human occupation and from human developmental theory. These concepts frame the rest of the chapter. The personal and social reactions to disability and the nature of adjustment to disability are examined. The chapter concludes with some interventions and techniques to facilitate psychosocial adjustment and optimal functioning in the community.

The model of human occupation is described in detail in Chapter 3, which the reader is encouraged to review. The following is only a summary, with particular emphasis on physical disability and its effects.

## A CONTEXT: THE MODEL OF HUMAN OCCUPATION

Physical disability disrupts the occupational life of the individual in many ways and on many levels.[33] Initially (and most obviously) the disability impairs the performance subsystem—the skills and components of skills used in activities of daily living (ADLs). However, this disruption reverberates into the habituation subsystem; the loss of skills prevents the performance of habits (e.g., bathing, dressing) and occupational roles (e.g., homemaker, worker, student). Because of physical disability, the person may be able to handle only a few roles, and these may be different from those previously held.[14] Interestingly, occupational therapy assessment of role changes is relatively rare in physical dysfunction settings, where therapists focus predominantly on physical restoration.[63]

Effects on the volition subsystem, that is **personal causation**, values, and interests, may be profound. Physical disability occurs most often as a result of some external agent (e.g., accident, infection, disease) rather than any personal action (e.g., suicide attempt, recklessness, substance abuse). The power of an outside agency to alter a person's life so dramatically may challenge the individual's sense of self-direction (locus of control). Being unable to perform in customary roles may engender uncertainty about long-held values (e.g., economic self-sufficiency, social productivity) and may prevent realization of valued goals (e.g., to hike the length of the Appalachian Trail during retirement). Previously held interests may be incompatible with physical restrictions. All these consequences are potentially negative and damaging but can be ameliorated by intrapersonal, social, and environmental factors.

### Intrapersonal Factors

Evidence strongly indicates that the individual's premorbid personality, particularly a strong sense of locus of control and social efficacy, may promote positive adjustment to physical disability.[17,23,28] In other words, people who have an internal orientation of **locus of control** (a strong sense that they, rather than fate, are in control of their lives) are more likely to overcome their limitations and to achieve the maximal possible quality of life. In some individuals, physical disability becomes a challenge to meet, and the effort involved reinforces and may increase the personal sense of competence and efficacy.

### Social Factors

The family and other close **social supports** are critical in adjustment to physical dysfunction. To rebuild a meaningful occupational life, the physically disabled individual must be able to count on the support of others to compensate for lost skills and roles. Previously able to provide for personal needs in areas such as bathing and dressing, the severely disabled individual may need assistance (permanently or temporarily) from others. The availability and willingness of significant others to perform these functions are crucial. The psychological messages (e.g., acceptance, resentment, revulsion) sent consciously or unconsciously by the caregiver will affect the patient's psychosocial adjustment.

### Environmental Factors

The human-made environment is designed for able-bodied people. Although legislative and social pressures have introduced accessible features into banks, sidewalks, restaurant toilets, and other public environments, disabled individuals must still determine how to move and communicate in a world that perhaps only minimally meets their needs. Altering physical features (e.g., installing ramps and handrails) and providing appropriate communication devices (e.g., computers) and adaptive equipment often make adjustment easier.[48] Despite their functional assets, new devices can be stressful to learn and may cause the person to feel somewhat "odd," especially compared with the premorbid self.[33]

Human occupation is a useful model for considering the effects of disability on a patient. The OT practitioner who frames the approach to the patient around this model ask questions such as the following:

- What skills, habits, and roles has this patient lost as a result of this disability?
- What is the patient's sense of personal causation?
- What values and interests does the patient have?
- What is the patient's social and object environment?
- Most importantly, which interventions will assist in increasing the patient's sense of personal causation and in putting the environment more within this person's control?

## ANOTHER CONTEXT: DEVELOPMENTAL STAGES

Physical disability may be congenital (from birth) or may occur at any time of life, with its effects varying with the developmental stage. Table 13-1 summarizes the stages of psychosocial development according to Erikson.[16] Without reviewing all of human development, this section briefly examines just two stages, adolescence and middle adulthood, and the possible effects of disability occurring at these stages.

Adolescence is the stage of **identity versus role confusion.** The adolescent is learning, comparing, and "trying on" various adult roles. Vocational choice, gender identification, and identification with peers rather than the family are key issues. Many of the occupational therapy studies of psychosocial adjustment to

*Table 13-1*

**Erikson's Eight Stages of Psychosocial Development**

| *Approximate age* | *Psychosocial stage* | *Explanation* |
|---|---|---|
| Birth-18 months | Basic trust versus mistrust | Infant needs nurturance from mother. If infant perceives mother as reliable, infant will develop the capacity to trust others. If not, infant will tend to mistrust others, will feel anxious about their willingness to meet infant's needs, etc. |
| 2-4 years | Autonomy versus shame and doubt | During this period, child learns to control bowel and bladder and becomes more independent in exploring the environment. Child's sense of motivation and will are shaped by parents' attitudes toward bodily functions and their willingness to allow child to practice self-control. |
| 3-5 years | Initiative versus guilt | Preschool and kindergarten child begins to combine skills and plan activities to accomplish goals. Child begins to imitate adult roles and to try out new ways of doing things. Child develops a sense of self-direction. |
| 6-12 years | Industry versus inferiority | During elementary school, child acquires skills and work habits and compares self to peers. Attitudes to parents, teachers, and other children contribute to child's sense of personal competence. |
| Adolescence | Identity versus role confusion | Adolescent experiments with a variety of adult roles. Key issues include vocational choice and gender identification. Rebellion against parents is common as teenagers try to assert a separate identity. |
| Young adulthood | Intimacy vesus isolation | Central concern of this period is to find a suitable partner with whom to share the person's life. |
| Middle adulthood | Generativity versus stagnation | Adult looks toward future and tries to make a contribution to it through work, community leadership, childrearing, etc. |
| Old age | Ego integrity versus despair | Faced with prospect of death, older adult reviews and evaluates life's choices to determine if what the person meant to do has been accomplished. |

Modified from Early MB: *Mental health concepts and techniques for the occupational therapy assistant,* ed 2, New York, 1993, Raven.

disability have focused on adolescence,[11,28,34,48] perhaps because of the dramatic effects of disability on personal identity. Reactions of peers and authorities, perceived lack of romantic appeal, worries over scholastic competence, and continued dependence on parents are some of the concerns of disabled individuals at this developmental stage.[34,48]

Each developmental stage carries its own tasks and will be affected differently by disability. A spinal cord injury occurring in later life is devastating but usually does not affect the *development* of personal identity, because this task normally has been achieved during adolescence. Rather, the current developmental task is challenged while previously achieved tasks are revisited and reevaluated. For example, a married 56-year-old male school teacher typically is in Erikson's stage of **generativity versus stagnation,** with an emphasis on making a contribution to the future through work, community activity, and raising children (who may be college age or older). A spinal cord injury to this individual requires an adjustment in the way generativity is addressed, perhaps with retirement from employment and a shift in ADLs, often to a more sedentary, intellectual, computer-based lifestyle. However, each preceding developmental task is also reevaluated. For example, the adolescent task of developing an identity may reemerge as individuals consider their new role of "patient" and ponder who they will "be" now that they cannot perform the activities they once identified as part of their "being." They also question their sexual identity and performance and their ability to be an intimate partner. Thus the task of **intimacy versus isolation** resurfaces as well.

The OT practitioner approaching the patient with physical disability must keep in mind the following questions:

- What is this person's developmental stage?
- What developmental task(s) might this person be grappling with?
- Based on this, what concerns or responses might I expect from this patient?
- How can I assist this individual to recognize and state personal goals and achieve them?

With the context of human occupation and human development in mind, we now turn to the personal and social consequences of physical dysfunction.

## PSYCHOSOCIAL CONSEQUENCES OF PHYSICAL DYSFUNCTION

### Personal Reactions

Individual reactions to physical dysfunction depend on the psychological meaning of the specific dysfunction in relation to the individual's personality and life history.[20] For example, paraplegia is likely to have a different meaning to an athlete (who defines self-worth in terms of physical performance and physique) than to an office worker (whose sense of self may be defined more in terms of using mental and hand activities).[35]

Paradoxically, some persons may evaluate the physical disability as positive. A dysfunction viewed as a well-deserved punishment may lead to a greater sense of well-being. A dysfunction viewed as an opportunity to depend on a caring person may gratify dependency wishes or allow the patient to avoid responsibility.[30,60]

Productivity and physical attractiveness are highly valued in American culture. Deficiencies in these areas may lead to feelings of low self-worth. Feelings of low worth tend to be "all-or-none" in quality. The individual may focus on only one characteristic and generalize from this to a belief that the entire self is worthless. The feelings of low self-worth also extend into the past and into the future so that the person can neither conceive of self as ever having been productive or attractive nor contemplate the possibility of future change.

The conclusions of worthlessness are in a sense true, because they fit society's definition of the self in terms of productivity and attractiveness. This is a distortion because it bases self-worth on deficits and overlooks remaining assets and intrinsic worth. Although the concept of intrinsic worth (i.e., the person valued for self alone without external comparisons) is desired and ideal, it is probably difficult or impossible to achieve for most people. In general, people in American society value themselves according to external standards of attractiveness, productivity, and achievements.

Disabled persons may conclude that they are worthless and of negative value and therefore believe that they are "awful" as well. They may expect and think that they deserve the rejection of others based on that notion. If they are not of any value to themselves, others will not see them as valuable and therefore will reject them. This type of thinking can persist and may lead to withdrawal or an intense search for approval and love. Some persons will draw from this thinking process what seems to be a logical conclusion: they are worth nothing to self or to others, therefore life is meaningless and empty, and they should not exist. This feeling may be especially strong in those who have intense guilt feelings.[21]

The meaning of the disability to the patient is the crucial factor in planning a sound approach in treatment and in aiding with the adjustment process. Therefore treatment directed to aid psychosocial adjustment must be based on individual reactions to the circumstances rather than on reactions and characteristics assumed to be similar among patients with the same physical disability or the same degree of severity of disability.[56]

### Societal Reactions

Historically, American culture's predominant reaction to disabled persons has been negative. Political action, including the passage of the Americans with Disabilities Act of 1990, has somewhat altered public perceptions of acceptable behavior toward these individuals.[1,6] However, prejudices persist, even among health care providers, and may significantly affect the disabled individual.

### Avoidance and Rejection

Attitudes of others toward physical disability affect attitudes of disabled persons toward themselves. In newly disabled individuals, devaluing attitudes toward the disabled population, once an out-group, may now be directed to the self, with very serious consequences.[56] Few people are really comfortable with disabled or deformed individuals. Their presence confronts nondisabled persons with their own vulnerability. To avoid feeling threatened, nondisabled individuals reject or avoid disabled or deformed persons.[60]

The appearance of the injury or disability also engenders nonacceptance. If the disability is unsightly, this tends to be overestimated by nondisabled persons and is a factor that prompts rejection or avoidance. They may display unwarranted pity or excessive curiosity. The disabled person feels set apart from most "normal" people and is constantly striving to fight the negative implications of the physical dysfunction and to gain genuine social acceptance.[39]

### Nonacceptance

Nonacceptance by nondisabled persons stems from negative attitudes. The disabled person feels ostracized when others are resistant or reluctant to interact socially.

**Apparent acceptance** by nondisabled persons is equally disturbing. In this case the person conveys the socially correct forms of acceptance and inclusion, but this is not genuine social acceptance. Apparent acceptance may be perceived as motivated by pity or duty and may seem devoid of meaning or real pleasure in the interchange. In both nonacceptance and apparent acceptance, disabled persons sense the underlying inability or unwillingness of nondisabled persons to know them as they really are.

Disabled individuals perceive a lack of patience on the part of nondisabled persons toward slowness and difficulties in performance. Whether this attitude is maintained by the nondisabled population or is projected by the disabled population, it engenders the same feeling of nonacceptance in the disabled person.[39]

### Spread Factor

Nondisabled persons also tend to judge disabled individuals not only in terms of the apparent physical limitation but also in terms of psychological factors assumed to be associated with the disability.[39] Nondisabled people may treat physically disabled individuals as if they are limited mentally and emotionally as well.[15] The evaluation of the visible disability is "spread" to other characteristics that are not necessarily affected. The frequent assumption that a person who has cerebral palsy is also mentally retarded and the practice of speaking loudly to blind persons as if they are also deaf are examples of this phenomenon. This **spread factor** is generally a devaluing process, and the disabled person is thereby stigmatized and considered of lower social status and unworthy of acceptance.[39]

Nondisabled persons also tend to view limitations as more severe and restrictive than they actually are. They may judge that a given physical dysfunction prevents the disabled person's participation in a given activity or social situation; however, the nondisabled person cannot know the disabled person's capabilities. It is better for nondisabled persons to invite disabled individuals to participate and to allow them to determine whether or not participation is feasible. Even when the situation appears totally impossible, an invitation still signals acceptance and allows for the disabled person to participate in restructuring the situation. The changes required may be simple or complex but should be left to the discretion of the disabled person and not structured by the preconceived notions of nondisabled persons.[39]

### Labeling

Words exist in the language of American culture that have a stigmatizing effect on the disabled person. Expressions such as "retard," "crip," and "psycho" are examples. Within the language of the medical and allied health professions, these terms become formalized to "mentally retarded," "physically disabled," and "mentally ill." These terms have value for the classification of persons into diagnostic categories, but they stigmatize as well.[15] It follows that when rehabilitation workers refer to their patients as a diagnosis or disability (e.g., "quad" or "hemi"), they are contributing to the stigmatization of those who they set out to help.

### Minority Group Status

Stigma may be considered as negative perceptions or behaviors of normal people toward physically disabled individuals or toward all persons different from themselves. Physically disabled persons are regarded in much the same way as other minority groups in the population. They are subject to both overt and covert stereotyping and a reduced social status. Stigmatization is a basic fact of life for almost all disabled persons. Interpersonal relationships between nondisabled and disabled people tend to follow a superior-inferior pattern or not to exist at all. Nondisabled persons tend to demonstrate stereotyped, inhibited, and overcontrolled behavior in interactions with disabled persons. They tend to show less variable behavior, terminate interactions sooner, and express opinions less representative of their actual beliefs.[15,48]

### Segregation

There is still substantial segregation of the physically disabled population, despite the passage in 1990 of the Americans with Disabilities Act. Although some of this segregation is necessary (e.g., institutionalization, special schools) and designed to assist disabled persons, it nevertheless sets them apart psychologically and evokes feelings of inferiority in relation to nondisabled peers.

### *Unfounded Positive Images*

In some instances, disabled persons are also subjected to unfounded positive images. The belief that the other senses of blind people are sharpened to compensate for the loss of vision is such an example. This is the myth of "automatic compensation." The fact is that blind and deaf individuals learn to use their other senses more efficiently.[24]

### Attitudes in the Health Care Facility

The health care facility can be considered a microcosm of society. Health care workers tend to believe that societal prejudices toward disabled patients do not exist in the facility. The assumption is that rehabilitation personnel are immune from discriminatory attitudes and that patients are accepted as persons when they are accepted as patients.[22]

The attitudes of the professionals involved with the rehabilitation of disabled patients are of great importance and may be highly influential in the disabled person's response to rehabilitation. Negative reactions will result in a negative response in the patient. Such reactions increase the patient's suffering and decrease motivation, leading to uncooperative behavior.[30]

Although the staff may hold the view that prejudice does not exist in the facility, in reality the staff's view is that the patient is a person to be helped, a malleable individual who can be shaped and educated into a specific health status and behavior. Convictions of superiority are reinforced by the emergence of a teacher-student relationship, a superior-inferior pattern.[22] Practitioners seeking to protect themselves from the pain experienced by those in their care may engage in "distancing behaviors."[54] This pattern is further reinforced by the segregated dining areas, the staff's uniforms, and the institution's organizational hierarchy.

The patients view themselves as disabled and unable to perform. They perceive themselves as applicants asking the knowledgeable, powerful, and authoritative others if they can regain the characteristics and skills of nondisabled persons. The patients confront a closed, self-sufficient subculture with an unfamiliar value system and are actually outsiders in the facility seeking acceptance from omnipotent persons in authority. The patients occupy the lowest level in the status hierarchy of the institution and are manipulated by many forces over which they have no control. Individual life goals may be partly or completely determined by others and choices and decisions imposed under a facade of personal involvement and self-determination.

To change this, the occupational therapy practitioner must shed the role of teacher and authority to engage authentically with the patient as an equal and to assume the role of facilitator and guide. Segregation in the facility needs to be abandoned to the extent possible, for example, in the dining and recreation areas. Recognition and respect for different needs, goals, and value systems can change the attitudes of health care workers toward patients. Involvement of the patient in the decision-making process for treatment and in patient government can also be helpful in reducing prejudice and equalizing the status of residents of the health care facility.[49,50]

## ORIGINS OF ATTITUDES TOWARD PHYSICALLY DISABLED PERSONS

Aversion to disabled persons is not natural or instinctive as has been thought. Studies by animal psychologists and cultural anthropologists suggest that the existence of instinctive hostile attitudes toward disabled individuals is a myth.[12]

### History

All societies probably have discriminated positively or negatively against disabled persons. Examples of extreme forms of prejudice are the attribution of supernatural powers to physically different individuals on the positive end and the elimination of physically deformed infants on the negative end. More modern societies have expressed their prejudice in more subtle ways, such as excluding disabled persons from employment opportunities and social interactions.[57]

The popularity of "freak" shows in circuses was testimony to paradoxical repulsion-attraction of nondisabled people toward disabled and deformed persons. Negative attitudes toward disabled people are rooted in ancestral superstitions and mythologies and have evolved into the sophisticated bigotry of the present age.[24]

Because of the primacy of group survival, "primitive" societies did not tolerate those who were physically impaired. The physically weak individuals were expendable, and the law of survival of the fittest prevailed.[24]

Superstitions and folklore guided primitive peoples before the advent of organized religions. Evil spirits were thought to reside in the bodies of those who were sick or deformed. Therefore such individuals were to be avoided. Mental illnesses and physical afflictions were thought to be the work of evil spirits. If the spirits did not exit the afflicted body after considerable effort, it was believed that the individual was being punished, and thus such individuals were avoided or killed.[24]

In discussing the history and psychology of amputation, Friedmann[20] noted that in ancient civilizations, self-mutilation was practiced to appease the gods and thus was a form of "religious rehabilitation." Few civilizations encouraged the survival of deformed infants. In some societies, transgressions of rules or crimes were punished by the amputation of a limb or part. Thus the concepts that disability is a deserved punishment for misdeeds, that disabled persons are not acceptable in society, and that disability is reparation for sin have ancient roots.

As societies became more civilized, methods of dealing with disabled people began to change. In a few societies, they were accepted and treated well. During the Middle Ages, blind persons occupied a privileged position in France. In both Asia and the Mediterranean regions, progressive physicians called for humane treatment of the disabled population. In most countries, however, inhumane treatment of the disabled individual persisted. Infants with disabilities were abandoned, drowned, or killed. Infanticide was practiced by nobility to maintain the purity of the bloodline. Children who escaped the fate of death roamed the country as beggars; some were subjected to slavery or forced into prostitution.[24]

During the Renaissance, more tolerant attitudes toward and improved treatment of physically different persons developed. The Elizabethan English Poor Laws (1597-1601) were the legal foundation for the protection of poor and disabled people from degrading treatment and provided financial support for unemployed persons, including those with disabilities. Gradually the perception of the disabled individual began to shift from one of total worthlessness to one of marginal productivity in society.[24]

Despite this progress, early American historical records indicate little knowledge of and few resources available to disabled persons. Medical care was limited in the colonies but began to improve in the nineteenth century. Medical personnel began to demand better facilities to treat disabled patients. However, this attitude was not widespread, and many physicians continued to demonstrate negative attitudes toward and inhumane treatment of physically disabled patients. The myth that such afflictions were the result of evil spirits continued, as did treatment with "bleeding," potions, and ostracism.[24]

A few hospitals in New York and Philadelphia provided treatment to physically disabled persons before the Civil War; the first sheltered workshop for disabled patients was established in 1837. At the end of the nineteenth century, the Cleveland Rehabilitation Center was established and was the forerunner of present-day rehabilitation centers. Among private organizations to help disabled persons that began during this period were The Salvation Army (1880) and Goodwill Industries (1902).[24]

Ancient myths and stereotypes persist. Many people still associate disabilities with sin and the Devil or with evil.[19] Disability becomes associated with *bad* and able-bodied with *good.* Metaphorical use of these associations appear in the Bible, as well as in both ancient and contemporary literature. This concept is communicated to children through books, television, and religious training.[24]

### Literature and Media

Media images of disabled persons are molded from early childhood through fairy tales and classical literature. Physical deformity, illness, and unattractiveness often symbolize inner defects, evil natures, and villainous behavior.[61] Some of the oldest and best known children's stories convey prejudices. These stories subtly teach children scorn for disabled persons. Characters such as Cinderella's stepsisters (who were obese and unattractive), Captain Hook of *Peter Pan* (who wore a prosthesis), the wicked witch of *Hansel and Gretel* (who was aged, arthritic, and had a kyphosis), and the evil character in *Jack and the Beanstalk* (afflicted by gigantism) set up an association between physical difference and evil.[8]

An examination of these and other well-known stories reveals that physical attractiveness, health, and intactness of the body are usually features of the heroes and heroines, the noble, and the good person. Conversely, villains are often portrayed with some infirmity or unattractive feature, such as large noses, wrinkles, and warts. Moral character and personality are thus associated with external appearance.

Some stories show physical disability as a consequence of a misdeed. Pinocchio's nose grew as a result of his failure to tell the truth, whereas pirates lost eyes and limbs as a result of their violent behavior.[61]

There have been almost no average, ordinary physically abnormal individuals in children's stories in the past. More recently, several children's books that portray disabled persons in a more favorable and matter-of-fact manner have been published.*

Although classical children's literature cannot be eliminated, parents and others reading this literature to children need to be aware of the biases that may be conveyed and to discuss and reflect on them with the children to minimize the unquestioned acceptance of these portrayals.[61] Fortunately, children today are much more matter-of-fact about disability, because they are likely to have disabled classmates, and disability is openly discussed in the classroom.[8]

This same type of stereotyping occurs in television programs, movies, cartoons, comic strips, and adult fiction.

Currently, disabled persons are being portrayed in more positive ways, performing ordinary life roles in movies, television programs, and television advertising.

### Religion

The image of the physically disabled individual varies from society to society, and the dominant religion in a society may translate the disability into spiritual terms. The disability may be assigned a spiritual cause, such as possession, the consequences of sin, a special sign of God's grace, or a blessing.[12] Thurer[61] believes that the stereotyping in literature reflects the subtle prejudice of the Judeo-Christian ethic that fosters the notion that God has smiled on those who are whole and successful, whereas those who are wrongdoers are punished with suffering and physical defects.

Many people have grown up with the notion that God is all-wise, all-loving, and all-powerful. He is seen

*References 5, 7, 10, 40, 46, 52, 53, 55, 56, 61.

as a parent figure who rewards obedience and disciplines disobedience. He protects those in His favor from harm and arranges for each person to receive what that individual deserves in life. If this premise is accepted, the question must be considered: "Why do bad things happen to good people?"[37] This question is raised when personal tragedy is experienced and when daily media confrontations occur with seemingly senseless tragedies that occur everywhere and to all types of people. It is troubling to know that suffering is distributed unfairly in the world. For many, this awareness raises questions about the goodness and even the existence of God. Kushner[37] outlines various popular explanations of suffering based on this notion of God and discusses the faulty reasoning in each.

Some of the most common notions of the causes of suffering that are based on scripture are that (1) suffering is punishment for sin (Isaiah 3:10-11, Proverbs 3:7-8), (2) suffering is for personal growth or testing of spiritual strengths (Genesis 22), and (3) suffering is a cure for personality flaws (Proverbs 3:11-12).[9,37]

The New Testament introduces the concept of suffering as a share in the glory of Jesus Christ (Romans 8:17). Illness and disability are also sometimes shown as associated with the presence of demons (Matthew 8:16, 8:28; Luke 9:37-43, 11:14, 13:10-14). However, there are also many accounts of healings in which no association exists with sin or evil spirits (Matthew 8:8-13, Mark 8:22-26, Luke 17:11-18[9]).

Someone who believes that suffering is punishment for sin will believe that the sufferers have received what they deserve. The difficulty arises when the individual cannot find a misdeed that deserves the punishment and may become angry at God or repress that anger to protect the perceived reputation of God as the fair and just parent.[37]

If a person accepts the notion that suffering is for the enoblement of people to repair faulty aspects of the personality, it follows that suffering is for the individual's own good. Associated ideas are that God teaches a lesson with suffering and that everything happens for a purpose, although that purpose may be obscure and known only to God. Another explanation of suffering is that God tests only those whom he knows are strong of spirit.[37] This generates the idea that those with afflictions are privileged or chosen by God for a special role and are therefore elevated in God's sight. This idea does not explain all those who break under the strain of their suffering or those who do not appear strong enough to deal with it.[37]

If the presence of demons as a cause of illness and disability is accepted, it may follow that some spiritual illness or defect exists, and if the demons are driven out with prayers of healing, the sufferer will surely get well. Although there are documented accounts of sudden and unexplained healings, it cannot be said that a "formula" exists that works in every instance.

All these responses or attempts at explaining tragedy assume that God is the cause of suffering. They attempt to explain why God would mete out suffering. Is it for the individual's own growth, is it divine punishment, or is it that God does not care what happens to humans? Some approaches lead the believer to self-blame and foster the denial of reality and repression of true feelings. Kushner[37] asks his readers to consider the possibility that God does not cause suffering and that maybe it occurs for reasons other than the result of the will of God. Perhaps God does not cause bad things to happen, and the question is not "Why me?" but rather, "God, see what is happening to me, can you help?" (Psalms 121:1-2).[9,37] God may not control some events. Some misfortunes that befall people may be the result of "bad luck," bad people, human weakness, random events, and the inflexible laws of nature.[37] Any health care worker or patient who is wrestling with this question is advised to read Kushner's book, *When Bad Things Happen to Good People.*[37]

Spiritual counseling is a necessary aspect of the treatment program for many patients. Occupational therapy practitioners should recognize this need and make the appropriate referrals.

## ADJUSTMENT TO PHYSICAL DYSFUNCTION

Physical illness or injury resulting in disability is a significant life stressor to which the individual brings a unique repertoire of coping mechanisms and response patterns.[59] Minimal or no prolonged effect on personality usually results from physical dysfunction. Behavior and emotions may be temporarily disordered by the crisis of physical change, but the personality appears to be capable of drawing on its resources and integrating the crisis experience.[58]

The individual with physical dysfunction is faced with the problem of coping with fears and anxieties and maintaining a balance between conflicting needs and tendencies at a time when defenses are weakened and it is most difficult to cope. Anxieties are typically managed through a variety of coping mechanisms.[30]

### Reactions and Coping Mechanisms

#### *Depression*

Mourning the loss of function or loss of a part invariably occurs after the onset of physical dysfunction. **Depression** is a feeling of sadness often accompanied by changes in behavior, such as sleeplessness or excessive sleeping and disinterest in previously enjoyed activities.[2] Depression often occurs with the realization of the limitations imposed by the disability and may last a year or longer.[60] The individual realizes that recovery will not be complete and that returning to "normal" is not possible. This confrontation with reality is likely to evoke a depression, which may occur early or late in the course of the illness or injury. It may have occurred before the patient entered the rehabilitation phase of the treatment regimen.

While the patient is depressed, progress in rehabilitation will be limited. During this time, occupational therapy personnel must maintain good communication with the patient. Areas for discussion are the patient's emotional pain, self-concept and self-esteem, goals and potential capabilities, and plans for the occupational therapy program. Such discussions need to be reinforced often and should focus on both the present and the future.[24] Patients with depression may respond to treatment with antidepressant drugs, psychotherapy, and stress management.[41]

### Denial

The person with an acquired disability may unconsciously deny its reality as a means of reducing its impact. Initially, the individual may believe that the situation will turn out to be just a bad dream. As the disability persists and is recognized as reality, the person may deny the permanence of the disability.[12] **Denial** may be manifested by cheerfulness and an unrealistic lack of concern about the disabling condition.[30]

The failure to accept the reality of the circumstances results in unproductive behavior, such as shopping for miracle cures or the "right" experts. Patients in this stage may be difficult to work with in occupational therapy.[12,24] They do not accept the role of the disabled person and see little relevance in working toward restorative and compensatory activities that would lead them to a productive life.[24]

Denial can also be helpful. It may assist the patient to restore some emotional equilibrium and is usually followed by a more realistic attitude toward the disability.[24]

### Repression

Repression is the mechanism that removes painful memories from awareness. This mechanism may be necessary to the readjustment of some disabled persons. Selective forgetting of one's former attitudes toward the disabled may be necessary to self-acceptance.[12] On the other hand, discussion of painful thoughts and memories may be necessary to achieving progress in restoring psychic equilibrium and in occupational therapy. Such discussion should be carried out only by well-trained persons.[24]

### Projection

The unconscious mechanism of projection allows what is unacceptable to the self to be shifted onto others. The patient with an acquired disability may project previously held negative attitudes about disabled persons onto OT personnel and family. An important goal in rehabilitation is helping patients to acknowledge their feelings and to accept responsibility for them so that they can gain control of their rehabilitation.[12,24]

### Displacement

In **displacement,** energy associated with one object or person is directed to a secondary target. For example, anger about the cause of the disability may be directed to the occupational therapy practitioners, who had nothing to do with its onset. The disabled person does not know who to blame and is asking the question, "Why did this happen to me?" Negative energy associated with such inner conflict is often released on family, friends, and OT personnel. Sometimes the anger is internalized and leads to depression. Vacillation between anger and depression may occur.

Patients displaying displacement should be confronted about their behavior and made aware of its negative effect on significant others and those engaged in their therapy efforts. A disability does not give the patient the right to be rude or uncivil to others.[24]

### Sublimation

Sublimation is the process of channeling energy from prohibited goals to more socially acceptable ones. In occupational therapy, anger and aggression should be channeled into constructive activities. However, it is important to leave time and opportunity for interaction with others as well. Resolution of interpersonal conflict is an important part of the OT process.[24]

### Aggression

Bravado and aggressiveness may be used to cover helplessness and dependency and to hide deep fears and anxieties.[30] Aggression can be directed inward to self or outward to others. As a coping style, it may take one of two forms: hostile aggression or aggressive behavior. Hostile aggression is not constructive in the therapeutic process and is disruptive. Aggressive behavior, on the other hand, can be productive, as in aggressively pursuing rehabilitation goals. Aggressive behavior can be a way of asserting the self. For some disabled persons, assertive behavior should be encouraged.[24]

### Dependency

**Dependency** may be manifested by keeping family and personnel close by and having more attendant care than is realistically needed.[30]

The individual who uses dependency relies on others to perform ADLs. This is the behavioral symbol of a helpless attitude. All people are dependent to some extent; no person is capable of meeting all needs without some outside assistance. Dependent persons may be thought of as lazy or lacking in initiative, but dependency really is surrendering independent problem-solving and looking to others to find solutions to problems.[24]

Some patients react against independence after some rehabilitation gains have been made. This is most likely to occur in late adolescents and young adults and those with longstanding, latent conflicts of dependency-versus-independence in the developmental phase of separation and individuation. The OT staff must understand the patient's developmental issues to plan appropriate intervention strategies.[35]

Patients whose premorbid personalities tended to be passive and dependent may have difficulty in therapy and may resist efforts to end the sick role and associated dependency. For these patients, limits must be placed on regression, and the staff must consistently express clear expectations for cooperation and participation in the occupational therapy program.[35]

Some disabled persons present themselves as unable to do anything about their problems. OT practitioners must guard against allowing patients to become overly dependent on them. A balance between control and assistance must be maintained, because the ultimate goal of occupational therapy is to facilitate self-help.[24]

#### *Regression*

Reverting to feelings, thoughts, and behaviors that worked well for coping in the past is sometimes used to relieve anxiety. **Regression** is a way of denying reality. Helpers may be seen as parents, lovers, or friends who met the patient's needs earlier in life. If the patient does not accept helpers for who they really are, the disability is not accepted, and the occupational therapy process is delayed. OT practitioners must be careful not to think that they can replace others in the patient's life.[24] When some of the more significant problems are solved, the disabled person may regain enough confidence to resume more mature behavior.[12]

#### *Rationalization*

Unconscious justification of thoughts or behavior with reasons that are more acceptable to the ego than the actual reasons are is rationalization. Rationalization may take four forms: (1) blaming incidental causes for problems, (2) devaluing unobtainable goals, (3) finding some advantage in an undesirable situation, and (4) mentally balancing negative and positive traits. An example of the first form occurs when disabled persons believe others do not like them because they are disabled. In the second form, an example is persons who convince themselves that it was all right to lose a job because the salary was too low. An example of the third form can be found in the fable of the blind man who stated that being blind made him a better person because he no longer judged others by external factors such as clothing or skin color. Beliefs such as "pretty women are dumb" or "disabled persons have more human understanding" are examples of the fourth form.[12]

#### *Compensation*

Compensation is a way of making up for a deficit in one area by capitalizing on strengths in another. For example, a disabled person may excel in academics to compensate for the inability to excel in sports. Compensation is often an unconscious decision. Deliberately bringing it to consciousness can help the patient make a self-assessment of strengths and weaknesses. Compensation may be helpful and wholesome if adjustment is personally and socially satisfying.[12,24]

#### *Fantasy*

Fantasy is the substitution of imaginary activities for actual activities.[24] It is a way to gain satisfactions not available in real life.[12] Continuous fantasy can be a sign of serious problems, and patients should not be allowed to abandon the actual world for fantasy.[12,24] However, the disabled person can use fantasy to cope until better solutions are found.[24] The use of fantasy can be channeled constructively in role-playing situations. The disabled person who is afraid to be seen in public or of participating in social situations can imagine doing so in role playing and become desensitized. Fantasy can be used to help the individual develop a repertoire of functional behaviors.

#### *Passing*

The denial of difference and attempts to conceal it is known as **passing.** This is a conscious behavior and not a true defense mechanism. Passing indicates shame and is a source of interaction strain. It requires constant vigilance, and denying the disability becomes a central focus of life. Acceptance, rather than denial, of the disability frees the person to use internal and external resources toward maximal functioning.[24] Those whose disabilities are not apparent to others, such as persons with epilepsy or cardiac dysfunction, can use passing to some advantage. It allows the person to manage the initial stages of social interaction so that essential personal traits make the first impression in relationships.

When a disability is visible, passing is impossible. The person must manage tension in social encounters. The person who uses passing must manage tension as well as information about the disability. If the hidden disability is ultimately revealed, the person must deal with the discomfort when others learn the truth.[12]

Whether passing is a negative or positive behavior depends on the reasons for adopting this coping strategy. If it serves a practical purpose and is not caused by a negative self-concept, it can be a sign of adjustment and of concern for the discomfort of others. If it is used because the person is ashamed of the disability, it can be a sign of low self-esteem.[12]

### The Compromise Body Image

The ultimate adjustment to physical dysfunction requires developing a new **compromise body image.**[60] This new body image comes to substitute for the premorbid body image, which is no longer compatible with the present body.

During development the body image is formed from multiple perceptions of the body based on past experience, current sensations, and the attitudes and values of the culture. Parental attitudes contribute significantly, as do the comments and fantasies of peers and others. Particular body parts may be overvalued and the body perceived as good or bad, attractive or repugnant, and lovable or unlovable. A person needs only to glance at the magazine covers on a newsstand to absorb the prevailing ideal body image of American culture.

For newly disabled persons, comparisons of their bodies to those of others may lead to self-denigration. Shame, anxiety, and disgust may provoke defenses such as denial and repression. Depression and mourning for the lost body part or function may ensue. With time, attachment to the former body image is gradually surrendered, often through the use of positive coping mechanisms such as compensation and sublimation. A new compromise body image evolves, incorporating the features once considered unacceptable. Anger vanishes, and psychic energy is freed for new activity, including occupational therapy efforts.[60]

### Stages in Adjustment to Physical Dysfunction

Adjustment to physical dysfunction was described by Kerr[32] and others[26,34,35] as progressing through five stages. The adjustment process is analogous to the grief process described by Kübler-Ross.[36]

Occupational therapy practitioners must remember that the stages are points on a continuum and that all stages are not inevitable for all disabled persons. They also must understand the adjustment process, because a relationship seems to exist between the person's attitude toward the physical disability and the success of rehabilitation.

The stages as described by Kerr[32] are as follows:

1. Shock: "This isn't me."
2. Expectancy of recovery: "I'm sick but I'll get well."
3. Mourning: "All is lost."
4. Defensive A—healthy: "I'll go on in spite of it."
   Defensive B—pathological: Marked use of defenses to deny the effects of the disability.
5. Adjustment: "It's different but not bad."

#### *Shock*

Shock is an immediate reaction to trauma and occurs during the early diagnostic and treatment period. It includes a sense of numbness and the inability to integrate or comprehend the magnitude of the event.[35]

The person lacks understanding that the body is ill or of the extent of the seriousness of the illness or injury. Because of these factors, the person may show an apparent lack of anxiety that appears to be unrealistic. As the reality of the situation becomes more apparent to the person, the reaction is "This can't be me. It's a bad dream. I'll wake up, and this will all be gone." The disabled person is likely to blame the hospital and medical personnel for the lost ability to function. The feeling is "If I could only get out of here, I'd be all right." Psychologically, the person is still a normal, able-bodied person, pursuing the same goals and doing the same things as before the onset of the disabling condition.

An incompatibility exists between the person's real physical situation and the mental image. This incompatibility may account for the person's apparently inappropriate references to the disability, situation, recovery, and future performance. At this stage, perceptions incompatible with the self-image are rejected.

Inevitably the person also tests reality. This occurs after the onset of disability, and when the fact of changed function comes into focus, the psychological situation changes. A pathological "denial of illness" may occur, and some persons previously considered psychologically healthy remain in this stage.[32]

#### *Expectancy of Recovery or Denial*[26,32]

This stage lasts from a few days to 2 or 3 months. The patient may maintain that recovery will be quick and complete. This is a defense mechanism against the sudden, drastic change in functioning and the realization that the condition is generally permanent. Denial of the severity and irreversibility of the situation is maintained, and the person hopes that the situation will be reversed in the future.[35] The patient may make frequent references to getting well or being whole again and may discuss future plans in which full recovery or a normally functioning body is essential.

The individual's only goal is to get well. This may lead to the search for a cure and "shopping" from one physician or health care agency to another. The person is preoccupied with the physical condition. Small improvements may be overestimated or misinterpreted. The person will do anything perceived as aiding recovery because this is the primary goal. The person believes that recovery will take place, so motivation toward learning to function with a disability is minimal.[32]

The person believes realistically that the disability is a barrier to everything in life that is important and worthwhile. A whole body is needed to attain important personal goals. Therefore full recovery must be achieved before anything else can be undertaken.[32]

Family, friends, and medical personnel may encourage denial by urging the individual not to think of the losses and may make false promises of recovery. The persistence of denial delays the healing process of grief.[26]

A change in this belief system or progress toward the next stage occurs when the person is moved toward a condition more similar to normal living. Being transferred from an acute care setting to the occupational therapy unit, being discharged in a wheelchair, having therapy terminated, having therapy redirected to learning to live with the disability, or being told that full recovery will not occur are some of the events that may precipitate mourning.[32]

#### *Mourning or Depression*

Mourning occurs when expectancy of recovery shifts to the realization that the disability is permanent. This realization may be overwhelming and may require the intervention of specialists in psychiatry or psychology.[32]

Depression is a response to a sense of helplessness and a loss of self-esteem. Anxiety, sadness, and grief are natural and appropriate and are to be expected in the adjustment process. Self-esteem may be low, and the individual may have a sense of helplessness and of being a burden to others. The initial depression involves difficulty in integrating the residual disability into a new self-concept.[35] All seems lost, and all former goals seem unattainable. Motivation to cope with the disability is gone. The person wants to give up and may contemplate suicide.[32,35]

Sadness is not easily expressed, and any overt expression may be associated with childishness. Occupational therapy practitioners must assure the patient that such sadness is normal and natural and should be expressed if the patient is to move beyond this stage. The mourning patient needs the opportunity to work out such feelings.[26] If the individual is not allowed to express grief for the lost function or part because of the reprimands and attitudes of OT practitioners and others, discussion of these feelings may be avoided. Hostility toward those who forbid the expression of feelings may result in a "problem patient" who will not work and who spends much time complaining about the health care agency procedures and personnel.[32]

The patient may subsequently externalize hostility and blame for the loss to family, friends, physicians, and other clinicians. Hostility and anger must be channeled to productive activity to make functional gains.[35]

Patients may become resigned to this fate, believing they are worthless and inadequate, and may remain at this stage in the process. They may adopt the role of the invalid and become permanent residents of a health care institution.[38] Such patients simply live and remain dependent and possibly hostile.

The disability is now seen as an impenetrable barrier to important life goals, and unlike the hope for recovery that characterized the previous stage, the goal of recovery is now seen as unrealistic.

To effect progress to the next stage, the barrier imposed by the disability must be reduced. To the degree that this is possible, progress in adjustment and therapy can be made. It may be possible to create situations in which previously held goals can be attained. However, because self-care activities were probably taken for granted, adults may not view their accomplishment as a positive goal.[32]

The person in this stage may also begin to mourn the loss of some psychological characteristics. Patients may believe they have lost their "fight," "pride," or "faith," which can be more distressing than the physical loss. When this occurs, it may be important to expose the person to situations in which disabled persons can be observed demonstrating these qualities. The person can then begin to realize that the disability is irrelevant for the attainment of more basic goals.[32]

### *Defensive A—Healthy*

The defensive stage may be considered healthy if the person begins to deal with the disability. Motivation to learn to function with the disability increases significantly. The person is pleased with accomplishments and takes an active interest in being as normal as possible.

The disability barrier is being reduced and becomes less impenetrable. The person attains some goals that were held as a nondisabled person. Some treasured experiences, although minor, are still possible. The barrier is still present, however, but ways are discovered to circumvent it. The person learns to achieve previously held goals by other routes. Other goals may remain unattainable, and the person may remain distressed by the areas perceived to be unachievable.[32]

The movement toward adjustment comes through a changed need system. The need for a whole or normal body may be relinquished when important goals can be attained despite the disability. The goals are attainable, so the disability becomes less relevant. When physical impairment does interfere with goal attainment, the person must relinquish the goals and discover equally satisfying ways of meeting important needs.[32]

### *Defensive B—Pathological*

The defensive stage may be considered pathological if the person uses defense mechanisms to deny the continued existence of a partial barrier imposed by the disability. Diverse behavior may be displayed, depending on the defense mechanisms used. Patients may attempt to conceal the disability; may rationalize and say they do not want the things that are now unattainable to them; may project negative feelings to others, claiming that they cannot accept the disability although the patients have; and may try to convince others that they are well adjusted. The existence of barriers imposed by the disability is denied.[32] A new compromise body image that can be accepted both consciously and unconsciously fails to develop. Psychotic reactions may result. Passive, dependent reactions may be manifested by a complete loss of motivation and a surrendering of all ambition. Psychological regression may become apparent, and pathological denial may be manifested by an inability to express negative feelings and by a repression of anger.[60]

Under some additional stress, the person may regress to an earlier stage and remain there permanently, or the person may progress to adequate adjustment after a temporary regression.

### *Adaptation or Adjustment*

After grief, mourning, and hope of return are relinquished, new roles based on new functions can be achieved. An understanding of the patient's defense mechanisms and coping strategies will help facilitate the process of adaptation to functioning with a physical difference. The therapist or assistant can assess coping strategies by finding out how the patient customarily managed stresses. Coping strategies tend to be consistent, and stresses are handled by intensified use of previous strategies. Once identified, those strategies that can be used to enhance occupational therapy efforts can be maximized, whereas those that deter such efforts can be rechanneled.[35] If an adequate adjustment is attained, the person considers the disability as merely one of many personal characteristics.

The disability is no longer considered a major barrier to be overcome, because satisfying ways to meet personal needs and goals have been found.

Practitioners cannot assume that teaching the disabled patient to perform activities will automatically lead to an adequate adjustment. Two other goals, held by many people, need to be attained before adjustment is possible. The first goal lies in religion or personal philosophy. The person with religious beliefs must feel "right with God." All the beliefs about the role of suffering in relation to God's influence on life must be resolved. The disability will be a barrier between the person and God if the person regards it as a punishment or believes that God will heal those who love Him. The second goal involves achieving a feeling of personal adequacy. Because of the tendency in society to relegate the disabled person to an inferior status, this person must be helped to discriminate between adequate and inferior on the basis of intrinsic worth rather than physique and productivity.[32,62]

### Sexual Adjustment

After pain, fear of death, and major discomforts of the disability have subsided, newly disabled persons begin to reassess life and relationships. Social concerns become more intense. Questions about attractiveness and the possibility of sexual relationships arise.[12] The sex-related limitations imposed by the disability and sexual taboos and prohibitions generate anxiety in the disabled person. Anxiety can be intensified by misunderstanding and misinformation. Anxiety increases if the patient's questions are not answered or concerns are not discussed. If such silence prevails, patients receive the message that they are asexual beings and that sex should not be a concern.[25] Uncertainties about sexual matters are influenced by the attitudes of health care professionals and the premorbid beliefs of the disabled individual about the sexuality of disabled persons.[12]

Practitioners who are reluctant to address the patient's sexual concerns send the message that the patient's fears are well founded and that interest or efforts that do not focus directly on the disabling condition are of minor concern.[12,13] The predisability attitudes of disabled persons make them aware that others may regard them as asexual or incapable of any satisfying sexual activity.[12] Because sexual matters are regarded as very personal and private, patients are reluctant to discuss them. The patient may consider sexual concerns as separate from the disability and think that they are to be borne in silence and handled without assistance.[13]

Chapter 14 discusses sexuality and sexuality counseling of physically disabled patients.

## PSYCHOSOCIAL CONSIDERATIONS IN TREATMENT OF PHYSICAL DYSFUNCTION

### Assessment and Evaluation

Psychosocial aspects of the person should be assessed as part of the evaluation of the patient with physical disabilities. Interest inventories, activity configurations, role assessments, occupational histories, and similar tools may be used.[4,18,44,45,51] These instruments may be administered by the service-competent certified occupational therapy assistant (COTA). On a less formal level, the COTA may obtain much useful information about the patient's premorbid lifestyle, goals, and interests through casual conversation with the patient during the course of treatment activities.

### Interpersonal Approaches in Treatment

#### *Attitudes Toward the Patient*

The patient must be regarded as a whole person. The individual's capabilities, problems, interests, experiences, needs, fears, prejudices, beliefs, cultural influences, and reactions to the physical dysfunction are as important as the physical considerations in planning interaction strategies and the treatment program.[66]

To facilitate self-acceptance, the occupational therapy practitioner can demonstrate to patients that they are accepted as total persons and that feelings of shame or guilt need not be associated with the disability. The clinician reacts to the patient as a person who happens to have a disability. Such an approach reduces the fear and anxiety associated with being different. The COTA should demonstrate genuineness, empathy, and concern for the patient as a unique human being.[62]

Becoming disabled alters a person's social interactions with others. The newly disabled person knows that selfhood has not changed because of the disability but may find that responses from others are very different. This may cause questioning of personal identity, appropriate roles, and expectations in performance ability. The early answers to such questions come from the OT practitioners in everyday treatment situations. By their words and actions, clinicians may communicate answers to critical and perhaps unspoken questions from the disabled person.[31]

Behavior of practitioners that reflects respect for the rights, capabilities, and abilities of the disabled person to make judgments and be involved in the occupational therapy process communicates faith in the disabled individual as a human and a fully functioning adult. The COTA should accord patients equal status and avoid treating them as dependent children. The communication of a belief in the patient's capacities is essential. An attitude of helping the disabled person to explore and discover possibilities in performance skills and social interchange is much more helpful than preconceived notions and conclusions about the patient's capacities. Involvement of the patient on the occupational therapy team to the extent possible communicates the belief that the disabled person can be a self-determining agent in the OT process.[31]

The focus of therapy and rehabilitation should be on helping the person to reformulate an approving self who wants to continue with life despite important discontinuity with past identity. This requires the development of a new self-image based on a sense of worth rather than on deficiency and self-contempt.[59]

Adverse or negative reactions of OT workers toward patients may stem from a number of causes. Personality incompatibility or prejudicial reactions to a particular age, gender, ethnic group, or physical dysfunction are some of the factors that can evoke a negative reaction. Awareness and admission of adverse reactions are the first steps in coping with them constructively. Some signs of adverse reactions to patients are (1) failure to keep appointments; (2) offering less treatment time; (3) frequently arranging for the patient to be treated by an aide, student, or other therapist; (4) unnatural and excessive politeness and service to the patient; (5) a feeling of boredom when the patient is present; (6) a tendency to ignore the patient when others are present; (7) unrealistic optimism or pessimism about the patient's prognosis or potential achievements; and (8) giving the patient inadequate answers and instructions.[30]

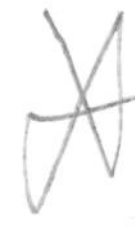

To deal with adverse reactions to patients, OT practitioners who become aware of these reactions may undertake a self-analysis or analysis with the aid of peers or a counselor to identify the underlying cause of the negative reaction, if it is not readily apparent. Discussion of such reactions with the patient who evokes them is sometimes appropriate. If the reaction is caused by an asocial or inappropriate behavior that is within the patient's capacity to change and if changed would aid in acceptance by others, discussion of the feeling with the patient may be helpful. Clinicians may be able to change their reactions and reconstruct interaction with the patient more positively through ongoing counseling with peers or a professional counselor. If these measures fail and the negative reactions cannot be resolved, transferring the patient to the care of another is essential to the patient's progress.[30,60]

### *Self-Definition*

Geis[21] stresses self-definition and a sense of personal worth as critical factors in successful rehabilitation and suggests some methods for helping patients to value themselves positively. The disabled person cannot adjust and adapt while maintaining an unrealistic self-image.

The individual's definition of self is the crucial factor, determining the degree of sense of worth and self-satisfaction that can be achieved. The goal of occupational therapy is to help the patient to change a self-defeating definition to one that is self-enhancing. Fixed beliefs about attractiveness, productivity, or achievement will cause the patient to define the self and measure individual value in terms of these standards. Therapy involves helping the patient to challenge fixed beliefs and to feel worthwhile in other ways. The patient needs to be directed to satisfactions that are attainable and helped to value goals and self preferentially rather than by some absolute standard.

In treatment the traditional focus has been on assisting the patient to develop better modes of "doing." An emphasis on doing only or becoming efficient at reaching performance goals may focus self-valuation on an extrinsic standard of productivity. Techniques for helping the patient simply to "be" and to value aspects of themselves need to be added to treatment modalities. Geis[21] describes "being" as a spontaneous expressive activity that may be purposeless and nonstriving. It exists during such pursuits as fiestas, ballet, dancing, and leisure activities and enjoying theatrical performances, comic events, and sports events, in which gratification is intrinsic and linked with the process rather than with the goal or result of the activity. In contrast, "doing" activity has its satisfaction linked with the effect or ultimate achievement of the goal of the activity process. Before the onset of physical disability the patient's self-definition and sense of personal worth usually have been based largely on "doing" behavior. With the onset of physical dysfunction, a major loss occurs in the self-satisfaction derived from "doing." This may evoke feelings of reduced self-worth, which can be ameliorated by helping the patient derive gratification from "being" experiences. Treatment methods that emphasize the patient's exploration, manipulation, personal interests and choices, enjoyment, delight, and play can facilitate self-satisfaction from "being."[21]

### *Preventing Maladjustment*

Pathological reactions in adjustment may be prevented if OT practitioners can recognize the stage of adjustment that the patient is experiencing and structure approaches and activities to accommodate the patient's particular emotional needs at that point in the adjustment process. Patients should be encouraged to express their fears, anxieties, worries, and sense of loss. This must be done with tact and understanding. Therapists and assistants must expect that the patient has strong emotions and must be prepared to invite the expression of these emotions and to cope with them. Practitioners should not minimize the problems or enter into the patient's denial. Attitudes of acceptance of individuals with physical dysfunction will facilitate their self-acceptance. A cheerful and optimistic attitude from the staff is useful, but appropriately expressing irritation and anger may help the patient realize that such expressions are allowed and will be accepted.[30,60]

Early recognition of pathological reactions is important.[30,42] OT practitioners should observe for deep depression, suicidal tendencies, undue guilt or preoccupation with symptoms, bizarre behavior, confusion, paranoid symptoms, or other evidence of psychosis.[30]

Therapists and COTAs should share their observations for reality testing and for referral of problems to the appropriate specialists with other members of the rehabilitation team. All should make a concerted effort to deal with the normal adjustment process and minor problems. Assistance and special treatment by psychiatry or psychology specialists may be required to manage pathological reactions. Counseling of personnel by these specialists may be helpful in dealing effectively with the patient, coping with feelings toward the patient, and helping the patient progress toward a healthy adjustment.[29]

### *Enhancing Adjustment*

The goal of occupational therapy is to promote ego integrity and feelings of self-worth. Early OT efforts should be directed toward shaping basic life goals, and later efforts should shift to the emotional, physical, and technical resources necessary for their accomplishment.[59]

A focus of OT practitioners is to help disabled persons believe that their "inner self" still exists. Functional aid should be seen in the larger context of enhancing self-respect. Functional and physical progress can be ego builders and aid in the adjustment process. Functional efforts in the early stages of therapy should be designed to help the patient see that performance is possible and that the future holds some promise. Emphasis on functional achievements as ends in themselves for specific skill development, however, can divert energy and attention from feelings about physical dysfunction that must be manifested and resolved.

Therefore the OT practitioner's proper role is that of assistant to the patient. Unfortunately, most treatment settings are founded on the medical model. The professionals assume the expert and authoritarian role, whereas the patients assume a passive, dependent, and compliant role. Passivity and authoritarian direction are inappropriate for patients with chronic, permanent conditions. Their role should be primary and the roles of clinicians secondary.[59]

The patient's self-enhancement is supported when practitioners abandon their sense of omnipotence and see themselves as assistants to patients as they work toward restoring their lives. The clinician's role must shift from that of active authoritarian to a more passive mode of professional behavior. The patient's role must shift from passive recipient of services to active doer. The occupational therapy approach is more suitable than the medical model approach when treating physically disabled persons, whose issues are social, emotional, functional, and vocational performance problems to be solved.[59]

The occupational therapy practitioner plays an important role in facilitating psychosocial adjustment to physical dysfunction. A primary and concrete role is that of teaching the patient to cope with ADLs. The frustrations of dealing with minor ADLs can make the OT process unbearable. The COTA teaches the patient to master ADLs and to deal with the problems of everyday life. Through the process of the ADL program, the patient learns to solve problems and gains confidence that frustrations associated with the disability can be overcome.[62] The COTA is in a unique position to observe the patient's psychological functioning when working closely with the patient and observing the performance of a variety of tasks. Psychological factors such as motivation, initiative, creativity, originality, and persistence can be assessed by performance observation.[42]

Watson[65] described a psychiatric consultation-liaison program in an acute physical disabilities setting. This is a method of delivering psychiatric services to physically ill or disabled patients and addresses problems that interfere with the patient's treatment. The program's goal was to facilitate adjustment to a lifestyle compatible with the patient's value system, disability, and prognosis. Depression was the most common reason for referral to the program. A team approach was used, and the members were the psychiatrist, psychiatric nurse, and occupational therapist.

The registered occupational therapist (OTR) used functional activities to help the patient explore the meaning of the disability or illness. Participation in activity and the accompanying discussion ultimately had a positive outcome, although the patient sometimes directed negative behavior or attitudes toward the therapist as limitations were confronted. The therapist used informal discussion to address fears, anxieties, feelings of helplessness, and vulnerability. The treatment program helped the patient redefine problems and assets.[63]

The goals of occupational therapy were to provide opportunities for mastery and control, reduce emotional distress, promote psychological competence, and help to maintain or establish an active support network. The OT evaluation assessed premorbid competencies and level of functioning; previously used coping methods; roles, responsibilities, values, and goals; past history and interests; available support network; and discharge plans. This information was attained through interviews and observation during participation in activities. The OTR encouraged the discussion and helped the patient to evaluate the situation.

The therapist's primary concern was to build rapport. This was accomplished by meeting the patient on the patient's level, showing an understanding of the patient's emotional distress, and structuring the environment to promote psychological competence. Activities related to the patient's roles, interests, values, and responsibilities were important to promote psychological competence. Activities such as homemaking, cooking, crafts, games, and work simulations proved to be gratifying and motivating.

The focus in treatment was on ability rather than disability. The OTR structured treatment to ensure success. Making objects for others helped the patient resume the role of contributor. The treatment program focused on doing and giving rather than on symptoms and complaints and helped to reestablish significant relationships and restore engagement in meaningful activities. The therapist gradually transferred responsibility for choice and control to the patient in the treatment situation. The OTR had to be continuously aware of the patient's emotional status and changing psychosocial needs. Easily accomplished, pleasant, and familiar activities were initially used to motivate and engage the patient. As emotional stresses decreased, more demanding physical rehabilitation activities were introduced.[63]

## Group Approaches

Besides interpersonal interaction strategies to facilitate adjustment to physical dysfunction, several group approaches have been proposed and can be applied in occupational therapy. Therapeutic communities, self-help groups, milieu therapy, group counseling, and sensitivity training may be helpful to facilitate the patient's adjustment and the development of a positive self-image.[59] Coping skills, problem-solving exercises, and role playing can be used effectively in groups.

Kutner[38] states that "in the diagnostic work-up and medical treatment plan of the recently disabled patient, it is rather rare to include a listing of 'role disorders' accompanying the illness or injury.... They require not the cursory attention typically accorded them but specific and purposeful therapy." This statement has important implications for occupational therapy. The OT practitioner, concerned with the patient's occupational performance in self-maintenance, work, play, and leisure roles, is the expert in role definition, role analysis, and role change. Indeed a list of "role disorders" should appear in the medical record contained in the OT reports.

### *Milieu Therapy*

Kutner[38] suggests that milieu therapy may offer a solution for acquiring new roles, readapting old ones, and gaining the social and physical skills necessary to reach goals.

**Milieu therapy** is particularly appropriate as an occupational therapy method because it uses environmental or residential settings as a training ground for patients to practice social, interpersonal, and functional skills and to test their ability to deal with problems frequently encountered in the community. This approach to treatment has always been fundamental to OT practice.

The milieu therapy program engages the patient in a variety of social encounters, both group and individual, and exposes the patient to increasingly challenging problems. This same gradation can be applied simultaneously to performance skills. The experiences are structured to test social competence, judgment, problem-solving ability, and social responsibility.

The major therapeutic objective of milieu therapy is the maintenance of the achievements acquired in the OT program. It attempts to provide the patient with the necessary social, psychological, and performance skills to overcome frustration, to deal effectively with new or risky social situations, to cope with rebuff or rejection, and to remain independent.

Most therapeutic efforts have been concentrated on physical restoration, with the assumption that personal and social readjustment follow automatically when physical integrity is restored. When adjustment difficulties occur, it has been customary to call on social, psychological, and psychiatric services to manage these special problems. In contrast, milieu therapy deals with the problems of adjustment to new or changed roles by structuring situations and environments to allow the patient to adopt and test roles as part of the treatment process.[38]

### *Self-Help Group*

The self-help group model is another approach to managing psychosocial adjustment to physical dysfunction. Jaques and Patterson[29] reviewed the growth and development of self-help groups in the United States and described their effectiveness in the aid and rehabilitation of their members. The **self-help group** is one that provides aid for each group member around specific problems or goals. Positive benefits to members of self-help groups include (1) gaining information and knowledge about the dysfunction or the problem, (2) learning coping skills from group members who are living successfully with the condition, (3) gaining motivation and support through communication with others who have similar experiences, (4) modeling the successful problem-solving behaviors of group members, (5) evaluating personal progress, (6) belonging to and identifying with a group, and (7) finding self-help in a situation of mutual concern.

The mutual aid or self-help group is an excellent means of maintaining therapeutic gains and preventing deterioration of function. It provides modeling by members who are coping with stigma and problems of functioning and reintegrating life roles.

Certain operational assumptions are characteristic of the self-help approach. Individuals with shared problems come together. All group members maintain peer status. Peers come together expecting to help themselves or one another. Behavior change is expected in each patient at that person's own pace. Group members identify with the program, are committed to it, and practice its principles in daily life. There are regularly scheduled group meetings, but peers are available to one another as needed outside of group meetings. This allows for both individual and group modes of contact. The group process includes acknowledging, revealing, and relating problems; receiving and giving feedback; and sharing hopes, experiences, encouragement, and criticism. Members are responsible for themselves and their behavior. Leadership develops and changes within the group on the basis of giving and receiving help. Status comes from giving and receiving help effectively.

Many persons who were not helped in professional relationships and experiences turned to and received aid in self-help groups, which arose to meet needs that professionals could not meet. The professional process and self-help group models can share experiences with one another under certain conditions. The professional must meet the conditions of common problems, peer relationship, and mutual aid, and those professionals who cannot meet these conditions can act only as visitors or observers. A professional can act as a consultant or speaker to self-help groups if invited to do so by the group; however, professional therapeutic skills cannot be used as such within the self-help group.[29]

The self-help group model, or some modification of it, has application in occupational therapy. It may have most potential for use in long-term rehabilitation programs, extended care facilities, or community day-care programs. Self-help groups could be initiated from the common needs of patients in the program. The focus on solving problems in functional performance can provide a safe area for sharing. Ultimately, as group relationships are cemented and mutual support is achieved, group members may move freely to emotional and social concerns and to problems of community reintegration. The COTA and other concerned professionals could act as consultants, invited speakers, or group members, if the necessary conditions outlined previously are met.

### *Group Counseling*

A group counseling approach to psychological rehabilitation for patients with spinal cord injuries has been described by Mann, Godfrey, and Dowd.[42] The group was based on the proposition that self-concept is one of the factors determining psychological adjustment to physical disability. The goals of the group were (1) to assist each patient in increasing self-concept to facilitate total rehabilitation, (2) to overcome depression, (3) to provide a setting where problems with interpersonal relationships could be discussed and plans for their resolution could be made, and (4) to modify perceptual distortions that patients may have about staff or other patients.

In the group, established patients assisted new patients in coming to terms with their disability and planning a new life. Former patients assumed leadership roles. Patients were given feedback about their strengths and assets by leaders and other patients. This was done to correct negative self-evaluation. Group interaction focused on how each patient could make maximum use of remaining function rather than on concentrating on lost abilities. Patients were encouraged to share feelings with the group and reaped the benefit of knowing that others had similar feelings and experiences.

The group operated on an open basis, with members coming and going at will. Initially, patients were selected by the therapists, based on perceived need for psychological assistance, verbal ability, and ideas and resources that potential members could offer the group. Subsequently, members began to bring other patients with them, and they were allowed to join.

The sessions were informally structured and presented to the patients as an opportunity to discuss feelings and concerns. The sessions progressed from general discussion to the discussion of people, interpersonal relationships, and self-exploration. The general focus of the sessions remained on the situational aspects of the disabilities rather than on psychodynamics. The leaders of the group were two occupational therapists and a psychologist.[42]

## SUBSTANCE ABUSE

A major national report states that more disabilities result from substance abuse than from any other preventable health condition.[27] The COTA should therefore expect to find both active and former (inactive) substance abusers among patients treated in rehabilitation settings. **Substance abuse** is a recognized psychiatric disorder.[2] Active substance abuse is often associated with other maladaptive behaviors such as denial, projection, and rationalization, which form the *preferred defensive structure* (PDS) of the alcoholic patient.[47] In addition, persons with physical disabilities may use alcohol or other substances to cope with anxiety and depression.[41] The physically disabled person who abuses alcohol or other substances requires treatment for both the physical disability *and* the substance abuse disorder. This is not usually a focus of occupational therapy intervention in physical medicine and rehabilitation settings, but the COTA should be alert to the possibility of substance abuse and should report any suspicions to the OTR supervisor and attending physician.

## CHANGING NEGATIVE SOCIETAL ATTITUDES

Studies have suggested that society's attitudes and expectations toward disabled persons may critically influence their mental health. If this is so, health professionals should seek ways to influence attitudes positively.

Anthony[3] cited several studies that involved contact, information, and contact plus information to effect change in attitudes toward disabled individuals. Attitudes of nondisabled toward disabled persons can be positively influenced by providing them with an experience that involves both contact with disabled persons and information about the disability. Contact without information has only a limited positive effect and may actually reinforce negative attitudes. Information alone increases knowledge but has little effect on attitudes. Anthony recommended that health care professionals design contact plus information programs to facilitate attitude change in employers, school personnel, and students of various age groups.[3]

## SUMMARY

The occupational therapy program for patients with physical dysfunction must include assessments, objectives, and methods designed to facilitate psychosocial adjustment. The treatment approaches include using therapeutic relationships, structuring a therapeutic environment, and using group and dyadic interpersonal experiences. Activities should assist the patient in adjusting to the physical dysfunction and in restructuring lifestyle to achieve the maximal independence possible.

Occupational therapy uses methods that demand the action and involvement of the patient in the rehabilitation process. In the initial stages, when depression and denial are present and ego strength is poor, formal teaching or discussion groups fail because the patient cannot integrate verbal material that addresses psychological exploration. Therefore social, recreational, special interest, and activity groups can be used to facilitate participation in therapeutic tasks.

The group process may include discussion of needs and feelings, mutual support, and learning skills for working with the health care agency, its personnel, and the community. The OTR and COTA should plan and structure group experiences that enhance the development of social skills, allow opportunities to test interaction strategies, discover assets and new or modified roles, and practice problem-solving behavior.

The COTA can facilitate a collaborative treatment program through the use of individual and group processes. The patient's involvement in treatment planning is critical because the patient who uses individual skills in planning, sharing, playing, socializing, and making judgments is more likely to want to pursue ADL skills and other modalities for physical and functional improvements.

If the patient is involved in this type of programming, no need exists to point out that all skills have not been lost and that assets and capabilities still can be used. The patient usually undergoes a concomitant and gradual increase in self-esteem and progress toward healthy adjustment and accommodation to the physical dysfunction.[64]

Professional health care workers must facilitate the achievement of self-acceptance and the development of coping strategies in their disabled patients. Negative public attitudes toward disabled persons are a deterrent to successful psychosocial rehabilitation. These attitudes will be slow to change, but the COTA can help a person apply physical and psychological resources to cope in a difficult world.[62]

## *Selected Reading Guide Questions*

1. Why should occupational therapy practitioners evaluate and consider the patient's environment, including physical, social, and cultural elements?
2. Define the following terms as they apply to societal reactions to disabled persons: avoidance and rejection, nonacceptance, spread factor, labeling, minority group status, segregation, and unfounded positive images.
3. Give an example of a *distancing behavior* by a health care provider.
4. Describe the behaviors that might be seen in a depressed person.
5. Give an example of each of the following, as they may be expressed or exhibited by a patient with a physical dysfunction: denial, repression, projection, displacement, sublimation, aggression, dependency, regression, rationalization, and compensation.
6. Describe *passing* as a strategy used by disabled persons. Is this an effective strategy or not? Explain.
7. What is the *compromise body image,* and how does it develop?
8. Name and describe the expected stages in adjustment to physical dysfunction.
9. Why is it important for OT practitioners to be aware of their own reactions to patients and disabilities?
10. Explain what the COTA should do when a patient becomes emotional and upset about the disabling condition.
11. Why is this the correct response?
12. Give three reasons why group approaches are useful in treating patients with physical disabilities.

## *Exercises*

1. Using a case example from your own clinical experience or one provided by the instructor, identify the patient's chronological age and expected psychosocial stage (according to Erikson). Discuss the effects of the disability on the achievement of the developmental task of this stage.
2. Imagine that you had a severe and disfiguring impairment such as an extensive facial burn. Discuss with a peer partner how you would feel about your self (self-image), your relationships with others, and your expectations for the rest of your life (e.g., relationships, work, social roles).

### *REFERENCES*


1. American Occupational Therapy Association. White paper: occupational therapy and the Americans with Disabilities Act, *Am J Occup Ther* 45:470-471, 1992.
2. American Psychiatric Association: *Diagnostic and statistical manual of mental disorders,* ed 4, Washington, DC, 1994, American Psychiatric Press.
3. Anthony WA: Societal rehabilitation: changing society's attitudes toward the physically and mentally disabled. In Marinelli RP, Dell Orto AE, editors: *The psychological and social impact of physical disability,* ed 2, New York, 1984, Springer.
4. Barris R, Oakley F, Kielhofner G: The role checklist. In Hemphill BJ, editor: *Mental health assessment in occupational therapy: an integrative approach to the evaluation process,* Thorofare, NJ, 1988, Slack.
5. Blume J: *Deenie,* Scarsdale, NY, 1973, Bradbury.
6. Bowman O: Americans have a shared vision: occupational therapists can help create the future reality, *Am J Occup Ther* 46:391-396, 1992.
7. Bunnett R: *Friends in the park,* New York, 1992, Checkerboard.
8. Burtoff B: Fairy tale stereotypes can harm, *San Jose Mercury News,* Jan 26, 1980, p 1C.

9. Catholic Biblical Association of America, Bishops' Committee of the Confraternity of Christian Doctrine: *The New American Bible,* Nashville, Tenn, 1971, Nelson.
10. Corcoran B: *A dance to still music,* New York, 1974, Atheneum.
11. Curtin C: Psychosocial intervention with an adolescent with diabetes using the model of human occupation, *Occup Ther Mental Health* 11:23-36, 1991.
12. De Loach C, Greer BJ: *Adjustment to severe disability,* New York, 1981, McGraw-Hill.
13. Diamond M: Sexuality and the handicapped. In Marinelli RP, Dell Orto AE, editors: *The psychological and social impact of physical disability,* ed 2, New York, 1984, Springer.
14. Dickerson AE, Oakley F: Comparing the roles of community living persons and patient populations, *Am J Occup Ther* 49:221-228, 1995.
15. English RW: Correlates of stigma toward physically disabled persons. In Marinelli RP, Dell Orto AE, editors: *The psychological and social impact of physical disability,* New York, 1977, Springer.
16. Erikson E: *Childhood and society,* New York, 1963, Norton.
17. Fine SB: Resilience and human adaptability: who rises above adversity?—1990 Eleanor Clarke Slagle Lecture, *Am J Occup Ther* 45:493-503, 1991.
18. Florey L, Michelman SM: Occupational role history: a screening tool for psychiatric occupational therapy, *Am J Occup Ther* 36:301-308, 1982.
19. Frank G: Life histories in occupational therapy clinical practice, *Am J Occup Ther* 50:251-264, 1996.
20. Friedmann LW: *The psychological rehabilitation of the amputee,* Springfield, Ill, 1978, Thomas.
21. Geis HJ: The problem of personal worth in the physically disabled patient: In Marinelli RP, Dell Orto AE, editors: *The psychological and social impact of physical disability,* New York, 1977, Springer.
22. Gellman W: Roots of prejudice against the handicapped, excerpted from *J Rehabil* 25:4, 1959. In Stubbins J, editor: *Social and psychological aspects of disability,* Baltimore, 1977, University Park.
23. Goleman D: *Emotional intelligence,* New York, 1995, Bantam.
24. Henderson G, Bryan WV: *Psychological aspects of disability,* Springfield, Ill, 1984, Thomas.
25. Hohman GW: Reactions of the individual with a disability complicated by a sexual problem. In Marinelli RP, Dell Orto AE, editors: *The psychological and social impact of physical disability,* ed 2, New York, 1984, Springer.
26. Hughes F: Reaction to loss: coping with disability and death. In Marinelli RP, Dell Orto AE, editors: *The psychological and social impact of physical disability,* ed 2, New York, 1984, Springer.
27. Institute for Health Policy, Brandeis University: *Substance abuse: the nation's number one health problem—key indicators for policy,* Princeton, NJ, 1993, Robert Wood Johnson Foundation.
28. Janelle S: Locus of control in nondisabled versus congenitally physically disabled adolescents, *Am J Occup Ther* 46:334-342, 1992.
29. Jaques ME, Patterson K: The self help group model: a review. In Marinelli RP, Dell Orto AE, editors: *The psychological and social impact of physical disability,* New York, 1977, Springer.
30. Jeffress EJ: *Psychological implications of physical disability,* San Jose, Calif, Instructional Resources Center, San Jose State University (videotape).
31. Kerr N: Staff expectations for disabled persons: helpful or harmful. In Marinelli RP, Dell Orto AE, editors: *The psychological and social impact of physical disability,* New York, 1977, Springer.
32. Kerr N: Understanding the process of adjustment to disability. In Stubbins J, editor: *Social and psychological aspects of disability,* Baltimore, 1977, University Park.
33. Kielhofner G, editor: *A model of human occupation: theory and application,* Baltimore, 1985, Williams & Wilkins.
34. King GA et al: Self-evaluation and self-concept of adolescents with physical disabilities, *Am J Occup Ther* 47:132-140, 1993.
35. Krueger DW: Emotional rehabilitation: an overview. In Krueger DW, editor: *Emotional rehabilitation of physical trauma and disability,* New York, 1984, Medical and Scientific Books.
36. Kübler-Ross E: *On death and dying,* New York, 1969, Macmillan.
37. Kushner HS: *When bad things happen to good people,* New York, 1981, Avon.
38. Kutner B: Milieu therapy. In Marinelli RP, Dell Orto AE, editors: *The psychological and social impact of physical disability,* ed 2, New York, 1984, Springer.
39. Ladieu-Leviton G, Adler DL, Dembo T: Studies in adjustment to visible injuries: social acceptance of the injured. In Marinelli RP, Dell Orto AE, editors: *The psychological and social impact of physical disability,* New York, 1977, Springer.
40. Lasker J: *He's my brother,* Morton Grove, Ill, 1974., Whitman.
41. Leary WE: As fellow traveler of other illnesses, depression often goes in disguise, *New York Times,* Jan 17, 1996.
42. Mann W, Godfrey ME, Dowd ET: The use of group counseling procedures in the rehabilitation of spinal cord injured patients, *Am J Occup Ther* 27:73, 1973.
43. Marinelli RP, Dell Orto AE, editors: *The psychological and social impact of physical disability,* ed 2, New York, 1984, Springer.
44. Matsutsuyu JS: The interest checklist, *Am J Occup Ther* 23:323-328, 1969.
45. Moorhead L: The occupational history, *Am J Occup Ther* 23:329-334, 1969.
46. Moran G: *Imagine me on a sit ski,* Morton Grove, Ill, 1995, Whitman.
47. Moyers PA: An organizational framework for occupational therapy in the treatment of alcoholism, *Occup Ther Ment Health* 8:27-46, 1988.
48. Mulcahey MJ: Returning to school after a spinal cord injury: perspectives from four adolescents, *Am J Occup Ther* 46:305-312, 1992.
49. Nelson CE, Payton OD: The issue is . . . a system for involving patients in program planning, *Am J Occup Ther* 45:753-755, 1991.
50. Northen JG et al: Involvement of adult rehabilitation patients in setting occupational therapy goals, *Am J Occup Ther* 49:214-220, 1995.
51. Oakley F: Role checklist, parts 1 and 2. In Hemphill BJ, editor: *Mental health assessment in occupational therapy: an integrative approach to the evaluation process,* Thorofare, NJ, 1988, Slack.
52. O'Dell S: *Sing down the moon,* Boston, 1970, Houghton Mifflin.
53. Osofsky A: *My buddy,* New York, 1992, Holt.
54. Peloquin SM: The depersonalization of patients: a profile gleaned from narratives, *Am J Occup Ther* 47:830-837, 1993.
55. Powers ME: *Our teacher's in a wheelchair,* Morton Grove, Ill, 1986, Whitman.
56. Robinson V: *David in silence,* Philadelphia, 1956, Lippincott.
57. Safilios-Rothschild C: Prejudice against the disabled and some means to combat it. In Stubbins J, editor: *Social and psychological aspects of disability,* Baltimore, 1977, University Park.
58. Shontz F: Six principles relating disability and psychological adjustment. In Marinelli RP, Dell Orto AE, editors: *The psychological and social impact of physical disability,* ed 2, New York, 1984, Springer.
59. Siller J: Psychological situation of the disabled with spinal cord injuries. In Stubbins J, editor: *Social and psychological aspects of disability,* Baltimore, 1977, University Park.
60. Simon JI: Emotional aspects of physical disability, *Am J Occup Ther* 15:408, 1971.
61. Thurer S cited by Burtoff B: Fairy tale stereotypes can harm, *San Jose Mercury News,* Jan 26, 1980.
62. Vargo JW: Some psychological effects of physical disability, *Am J Occup Ther* 32:31, 1978.
63. Vause-Earland T: Perceptions of role assessment tools in the physical disability setting, *Am J Occup Ther* 45:26-31, 1991.
64. Versluys H: Psychological adjustment to physical disability. In Trombly CA, Scott AD: *Occupational therapy for physical dysfunction,* Baltimore, 1977, Williams & Wilkins.
65. Watson LJ: Psychiatric consultation-liaison in the acute physical disabilities setting, *Am J Occup Ther* 40:338, 1986.
66. Willard HS, Spackman CS, editors: *Occupational therapy,* ed 4, Philadelphia, 1971, Lippincott.

## RECOMMENDED READING

Brand P, Yancey P: *The gift no one wants,* New York, 1993, Harper Collins.

Carr SH: Adaptation to loss: occupational therapy as a way of life, *Am J Occup Ther* 45:167-170, 1991.

Early MB: *Mental health concepts and techniques for the occupational therapy assistant,* New York, 1993, Raven.

Frankl VE: *Man's search for meaning,* New York, 1984, Washington Square.

Hockenberry J: *Moving violations,* New York, 1995, Hyperion.

Mairs N: *Plaintext: deciphering a woman's life,* New York, 1986, Perennial.

Price R: *A whole new life,* New York, 1994, Macmillan.

Resman M: Unspoken needs, *OT Week* 10:14, 1996.

Sharrott GW, Cooper-Fraps C: Theories of motivation in occupational therapy: an overview, *Am J Occup Ther* 40:249-257, 1986.

Chapter 14

# Sexuality: An Activity of Daily Living

*Gordon Umphred Burton*

## Chapter Objectives

*After studying this chapter, the student or practitioner will be able to:*

1. Discuss how issues of sensuality and sexuality are relevant to occupational therapy services and activities of daily living.
2. Discuss the potential impact of a physical disability on the concept of self as a sexual being.
3. Describe the relevance of sexuality to occupational therapy practice in terms of at least one frame of reference or model of practice.
4. Discuss the relationship of sexuality to self-esteem, self-image, and interpersonal relationships.
5. Explain how occupational therapy practitioners can assist patients in clarifying their values about sexuality.
6. Identify the effects of sexual abuse in childhood on the normal development of sexuality.
7. Discuss how occupational therapy clinicians can facilitate the patient's ownership of the body and establishment of personal boundaries.
8. List signs that may indicate sexual abuse of adults.
9. List the effects of aging on sexual function.
10. Describe strategies for dealing with emotional factors and sexuality education of patients.

## Key Terms

sexual history
sensuality
sexual abuse
lubrication
erection
reflexogenic erection
adaptive aids
sexual harassment

Why should the certified occupational therapy assistant (COTA) be concerned with issues of sensuality or sexuality when dealing with a patient? The answer is that sensuality and sexuality are aspects of everyone's activities of daily living (ADLs) and directly relate to the quality of each person's life. This places sexuality within occupational performance, the domain of occupational therapy. Occupational therapy clinicians work with patients in many areas related to sensuality and sexuality (Box 14-1).

Any physical limitations may make patients question whether they will physically be able to make love

*Box 14-1*

**Aspects of Occupational Performance Related to Sexuality**

- Quality of life
- Role delineation
- Positioning
- Cultural aspects
- Impulse control
- Energy conservation
- Muscle weakness
- Hypertonicity/hypotonicity
- Appreciation of body
- Psychosocial issues
- Range of motion
- Joint protection
- Motor control
- Cognition
- Increased or decreased sensation

or have sex. In becoming disabled, patients become detached from the typical roles and practices of the able-bodied population.[4,35] The disabled individual is often incorrectly seen as asexual, an object of pity, and unattractive.[25] The image alone would be disabling even in the absence of physical disability. Being perceived as unattractive and possibly unlovable is devastating and may lead to the conclusion that the disabled individual will never be intimate emotionally or physically with anyone. Total despair for the patient and all significant others may result.

Two studies of females who had acquired spinal cord injuries reported that they felt less than half as attractive after they became disabled.[5,24] This is surprising because spinal cord injury is usually not associated with an observable physical change in the body. However, the person's *perceived* attractiveness does greatly decrease. Males have reported that they feel emasculated by a disability and that their male "macho" role is threatened.[34] This is just a sample of the feelings and perceptions that may affect the patient's sensuality and sexuality, which must be assessed and treated by the occupational therapy practitioner. Sexuality is an essential aspect of rehabilitation of the person with an acquired disability and the habilitation of a person with a congenital disability.

This chapter examines these and other issues related to sexuality and sensuality.

## FRAMES OF REFERENCE

Occupational therapy attempts to integrate patients' physical being with their emotional and psychological being to attain a higher quality of life through the use of purposeful activities.[31] Two frames of reference can be explored in relation to sexuality.

### Developmental Frame of Reference

The developmental frame of reference states that development is horizontal, that is, simultaneously occurring in psychosocial, physical, neurophysiological, and cognitive growth and in sociocultural skills. The individual also develops chronologically, with further maturation of earlier development and skills. Integration of the senses starts before birth and develops into an organization of body schema and body awareness that helps in acquiring not only skills but also the feeling of sensualness and sexuality. Disability can damage this feeling of sensualness during its development or may distort already formed perceptions of sensuality.[28] When physical expression of affection, sensuality, and sexuality is impaired, the individual may feel incompetent in self-expression and consequently isolated and inadequate.

### Model of Human Occupation

The model of human occupation takes into consideration volition, habituation, performance, and environment (see Chapter 3).[25] Volition has three components: personal causation, values, and interests. Disabled persons who have learned to believe that disabled individuals are not sensual or sexual or physically and emotionally lovable tend not to develop interests of a sexual and sensual nature easily. If the person has been taught that the role of disabled people is asexual and not sensual, this will influence the way the person performs ADL. This asexual role may interfere with normal dating, marital life, or procreation. The performance subsystem in the model of human occupation performance includes skills and the rules for using skills. Disabled patients may have some impaired skills, but sex is often not thought of as a skill. However, it is most definitely a purposeful activity both in intimate relationships and in the role of procreation. Human occupation is carried out within the environment. Braces, wheelchairs, splints, and mobility deficits negatively affect the everyday environment of the disabled person.

## REACTIONS TO SEXUAL ASPECTS OF DISABILITY

Sexuality or sensuality can be an expression of confidence, a validation of the self, and an expression of a person's perceived lovability. The person who becomes disabled or is born with a disability may feel less positive about self and less lovable.[34] Sexuality alone is not what is important, but sexuality is often used as a barometer of how patients feel about themselves. The OT practitioner who helps the patient feel as positive as possible about the physical and other qualities of the self will note an increase in motivation for all aspects of therapy.

The patient's perceived self seldom matches the views of others. All persons think they have imperfections that everyone else sees, such as a large nose, big thighs, too hairy or not hairy enough, or too tall or too short. The clinician must attempt to help the patient adjust these negative perceptions to enable functioning within the normal parameters of life. The goal is to enable the patient to feel lovable, which is what most people want to be. If people feel lovable they usually feel a sense of self-worth, attractiveness, sensuality,

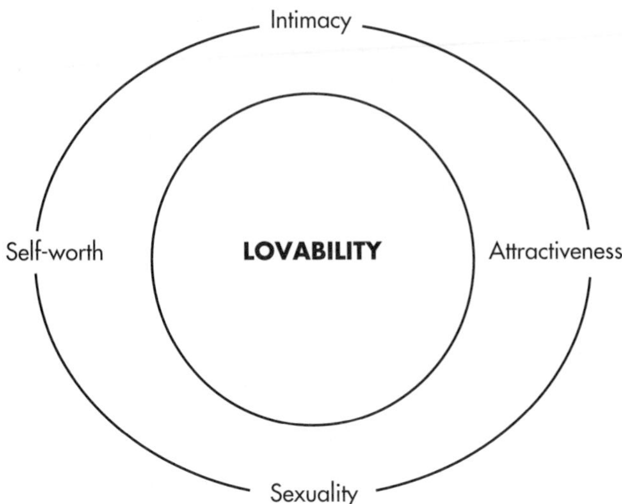


*Figure 14-1* Sexuality in context.

and capacity for intimacy. All these aspects must work together to accomplish a realistic balance in a person's life (Figure 14-1).

Sexuality affects marital satisfaction, adjustment to physical disability, and success of vocational training. People often judge others by their physical attractiveness. In Western civilization, physical intimacy is closely associated with love; someone who perceives the self as incapable of expressing sensuality or sexuality may feel incapable of loving and being loved. Without the capacity of loving and being loved, the individual may feel isolated and valueless. The occupational therapy practitioner should work with the patient to prevent feelings of worthlessness and hopelessness and to encourage self-worth and productivity.[35]

One of the first questions that arises when a person has a major injury or disability is whether or not sex is still possible. This question quickly is buried in the hospital and adjustment activities that make up the daily routine, but the patient does not forget it. A common complaint of people with disabilities is that the medical staff never dealt with or allowed the disabled person to deal with the topic of sexuality. People with disabilities believe that if their sensuality and sexuality are negated, a significant percentage of their person is being negated. This lack of acceptance results in their feeling that they are not treated as a whole person.

Males who are newly disabled report that they feel emasculated.[34] They may not be as capable of lifting weights or of performing other physical activities as they previously were. Sports may not be easily accessible. Looking up at others from a wheelchair and needing others to have needs met may increase dependent feelings. In both males and females, increased dependence often results in a decrease in their sex life.[12,26,40] The COTA needs to be sensitive and help the patient deal appropriately with these feelings.

Conversations regarding sexuality may create situations where these feelings may arise. Another possible reaction to the feelings of dependency and emasculation[34] may be trying to "flirt" to prove masculinity. Flirting may be attempted with a female or a male clinician depending on the patient's sexual orientation. The COTA should be alert to the issues the patient is working on to help preserve the patient's sense of self. At the same time, the COTA should not allow harassment, discussed later, or exploitation of either a clinician or a patient.

Females may interpret and react to these feelings differently. Women report feeling unattractive and fear that they may not be desirable to anyone again. This may lead to despair if a woman feels that unattractiveness will stop her from achieving some of her major goals in life. Thus she may flirt to see if she is perceived as still attractive. Discussion of the topic of sexuality is a way to explore feelings of dependency, attractiveness, and unattractiveness as they affect ability to function. If the patient's perceived sexual roles are threatened, the effects may be profound and should be dealt with as early in treatment as possible.

Patients often ask occupational therapy practitioners about sexual issues relating to their disability because the OTR and COTA often deal with other intimate issues such as self-care and personal hygiene. The trust built up in the relationship allows for this communication. Because the COTA deals with activities such as bathing, dressing, or toileting, the patient may feel safe asking questions regarding sex. The COTA should be prepared for this with information and resources, but it is not necessary that the COTA know everything or that the COTA be a sex counselor. The COTA has an obligation to help the patient obtain the information needed.

## VALUES CLARIFICATION

Sexual values of the significant other, the patient, and the COTA[11] must be examined in order for the COTA to interact with the patient in the most effective and positive manner regarding sexual matters.[35] Unless the COTA is aware of the thoughts and feelings of all the individuals involved, the COTA may make assumptions that are inaccurate and that could be devastating.[7] One of the most direct ways of gaining information is through a sexual history interview.[7,34] The goals of a **sexual history** are for the clinician to understand how the individual thinks and feels about sex and bodily functions and to discover the needs of all parties affected.[8,27] According to some researchers, many disabled individuals may have had a sexual dysfunction before they became physically disabled, and this may be determined during the sexual history interview.[28] Box 14-2 provides some questions that could be asked. All questions should not be asked at the same time, and every patient is not asked all questions.

After taking the sexual history, the interviewer may be able to ascertain whether the patient associates guilt

*Box 14-2*

### Sexual History Interview

The interviewer should create an environment that will allow for confidentiality, comfort, and self-expression. In early intervention the interviewer should ask about the patient's concerns regarding contraception, "safe sex," homosexuality, masturbation, sexual health, aging, menopause, or physical changes. For a more in-depth sexual history, the interviewer can ask the following:

- How did you first find out about sexuality?
- In what situation did you first learn about heterosexuality and homosexuality?
- Who furnished you with information about sexuality when you were young?
- Were you ready for the information when you first heard about sexuality?
- Is sexuality important to you at this point in your life?
- How would you describe your sexual activities at this point in your life?
- How do you think sexuality expresses your feelings and meets your and others' needs?
- If you could change aspects of your current sexual situation, what would you change and how would you change them?
- What concerns do you have about birth control, disease control, and your sexual safety?
- What physical, medical, or drug-related concerns do you have relating to your sexuality?
- Have you ever been pressured, threatened, or forced into a sexual situation?
- What sexual practices have you performed in the past (oral, anal, genital, etc.)?
- What sexual activities have you engaged in that you would consider "kinky"?
- How important do you think sexuality will be in your future?
- Are there questions or concerns that you have regarding this interview?

with the sex act, body parts, or sexual alternatives (e.g., masturbation techniques, oral sex, sexual positions, or equipment unfamiliar to the patient). The interviewer may learn, for example, that some patients report feelings of guilt or fear regarding sex after a heart attack or a stroke (fear that sex may "cause" a stroke or guilt at "causing" the first episode).

Another fear is that because the disabled person may have catheters, adaptive equipment, or scars, the partner will not accept the alterations and will reject the person. Performance is often an issue. "Can the disabled person do it?" is the question asked by able-bodied and disabled persons alike.

The COTA can furnish the necessary information regarding sexuality, directing the patient to other professionals, providing magazines and books, showing movies, or providing role models. In all these cases the COTA must remember that the patient's values and preconceived notions are probably being assaulted, and the COTA must be tactful in approaching these issues. Personal care such as toileting, hygiene (care during menstruation, bathing, etc.), and birth control are issues that reflect values regarding sexuality and body image. These self-care issues are often not emphasized enough during acute illness and rehabilitation. Discussing such issues once or twice is insufficient. The situation (environment) in which these issues are discussed is critical. A personal (intimate) conversation cannot take place in a crowded treatment room, during a rushed and impersonal treatment session, or with a clinician with whom the patient has no ongoing relationship (e.g., in facilities where clinicians are constantly rotated). The clinician must create the environment that will allow for or facilitate intimate discussion. Discussions will help the patient explore feelings about having a new body and adapting to ongoing degeneration of the body (if the patient has a progressive disability). Conversations can take place during other therapeutic activities, so billing for time should not be a concern.

Before considering interventions that the COTA might use to work with disabled persons in the area of sexuality, this discussion first describes how sensuality and sexuality develop.

## DEVELOPMENT OF SENSUALITY AND SEXUALITY

The sense of **sensuality** and sexuality begins to develop before birth. The fetus responds to stimuli within the first 8 weeks after conception. As the child develops after birth, a major focus becomes the craving and demand for sensation, as well as the relief of anxiety that accompanies sensory input.[37] The sensation of touch is interpreted as pleasurable or not pleasurable. Pleasurable sensations are comforting, and the child attempts to prolong them. This can be observed in a baby who cries when nursing ceases. If pleasure in interaction with others is developed, the ability to maintain the warmth of being close and being nourished is translated into trust, lovability, and bonding with the caregiver.[23,37] A sense of intimacy is initiated at this point in life. Thus trust, intimacy, sensuality, lovability, and later sexuality appear to have a basis in sensory organization.

As a toddler or preschooler (1½ to 4 years), the child will put anything in the mouth and actively seeks oral and tactile sensory input. The child develops the ability to stimulate and satisfy the self and the ego, and sensuality starts to be refined. The ability to explore surroundings using the hands, mouth, and other parts of the body allows the child to develop communication, self-gratification, and a feeling of competence. This feeling of competence is derived from the effective use of the body to feel good and accomplish tasks. The child learns the names of body parts and body processes and perceives the body as good. Simultaneously, intimacy between the self and another person is refined, as are sex roles.[13]

Between this early phase in development and adulthood, these roles are tested and retested. To some degree the child develops improved motor skills to obtain positive sensory input. Children normally start exploring their own and others' bodies at this stage. They explore their genitals when their diapers are being changed and in the bathtub.[13,37] They may be interested in looking at nude people. They explore the differences between males and females. They may ask about genitals, breasts, and "how babies are made." They often like the sensation of being nude and may display their genitals. Ownership of the body and what is done to it is starting to develop at this point. Toileting activities for self and others are usually seen as very interesting. Often the child uses "dirty" words for body parts and body functions at this stage.[23] In general the child is in an exploratory stage, and minimal or no shame and anxiety is attached to these activities.

Young school-age children (about 5 to 9 years) engage in most of the previous activities with greater sophistication but also develop other interests in this area. They often think of relations, especially sexual relations between opposite-gender partners, as being negative and unacceptable. They talk with friends about sex and sexual matters. They want privacy when toileting, often "play doctor" with others, and may compare genitals with peer-age friends. Body changes and sexual tension are heightened, and the child may have fantasies of marrying one of the parents.[23] Their sense of ownership of their bodies should be well developed, and they start to feel more control over their bodies and lives. These feelings of adequacy and self-acceptance are based on how well the person perceives that the previous tasks were accomplished.

This early development of sensuality and sexuality sets the foundation for later perceptions of the body and sense of self. COTAs must remember aspects of normal development when working with children who have a disability so that they may encourage age-appropriate activities. When working with adults of all ages, COTAs must remember these aspects of development and note that some of the therapy activities may stimulate remembrances of these past events. Some activities may be perceived as infantile or may bring up unresolved issues for the patient or clinician. This is especially true of ADL activities such as dressing, toileting, hygiene, and general self-care.

### Sexual Abuse of Children

The life of a child is shaped by an evolving barrage of experiences. Many experiences, both positive or negative, can lead to growth and learning. This in turn helps the child mature into a well-adjusted, caring adult member of society. One type of experience that does not lead to potential growth and adjustment of a child toward adulthood is **sexual abuse.** Although most adults hesitate to discuss it because it is so emotional, the problem still exists. The helplessness of a normal child toward advances from a larger, stronger, more authoritative, and often caregiving adult is well documented.[1]

Although abuse does not occur in all disabled individuals, the development of normal sensuality and sexuality may be hindered and even halted because of the attitude the disabled child may develop toward the disabled body.[1,14] To evolve from a giggling child toward a mature sensual adult, the child needs normal relationships, normal experiences, and (when mature and ready) normal sensual and sexual interactions with a significant other.

Clinicians must increase their awareness of what constitutes sexual abuse. Children with disabilities have long been forced to undress and be examined or treated as part of their care. This is sometimes necessary, but the wishes and dignity of the person should be respected at all times. An occupational therapy student with an upper extremity amputation related a horrifying story. When she was 16 years old and well developed, she was told to undress down to the waist and walk in front of a room full of men (physicians and medical students) to be examined in a pediatric prosthetic clinic. She described how humiliated and ashamed she was and how this only happened because of the disability. This served to increase her hatred of her disability and her body that had started when she was younger and made her even more self-conscious about her body.

The many obstacles encountered by disabled patients should not stop them from expressing the same sensuous and sexual needs expressed by all people. As an informed professional, the COTA can help to eliminate unnecessary obstacles and teach patients to remove those for which they are responsible.

Another example comes from an interview with an adult who had cerebral palsy as a child; the person stated that therapy was either so painful or so clinical that she disassociated herself from sensations in her body during and after therapy. Later in life this became a problem when she was married. She stated that it took 7 years of marriage before she could enjoy the sensations of being touched by her husband. She also stated that it was a revolutionary concept for her to realize that a vibrator could be used to give sexual pleasure rather than to activate muscles in therapy.

The therapy session should help the patient develop a sense of personal ownership of the body.* This is often neglected in working with adults but is especially neglected by health professionals when working with children. The clinician often does not ask permission to touch a patient, thus connoting that the patient lacks the right to control being touched by others. What is being communicated, however, uintentionally, is that any person has the right to handle and touch the

*References 1, 2, 7, 14, 27, 32, 37.

patient. It is difficult to think of more likely victims than persons who have learned that they do not have the right to say "no!" to being touched, especially when they cannot physically resist unwanted advances and in some cases cannot even communicate that abuse has occurred.[1] The effects of this can be seen in adults. When one patient was asked why tone increased in her lower extremities when she was touched, she responded, "I was sexually abused by my father in the name of therapy, and therapy and sexual abuse are synonymous at this point." Understandably, she had been resistant to reentering therapy.

One way of helping patients "own" their bodies (besides asking permission to touch) is through naming body parts and body processes. Once the body parts and processes are named using correct terminology as opposed to slang, it is possible for the patient to communicate and to relate in an appropriate manner.[7,10,37] The use of dignified language also presents the body in a more positive way (because people tend to use slang only to identify "negative" things—toes are toes, but a penis is a "prick").[7,10,37]

Children often think that bad things happen only to bad people and that being disabled is punishment for bad behavior. The adult client who has lost cognitive abilities may be thinking at the same level. This may have a cultural component but should be dealt with early to ensure that this notion does not become fixed in the patient's self-perception and erode self-image. To develop the concept that the body (with congenital disabilities) or the "new" body (with acquired disabilities) is acceptable and good may be one of the goals of therapy.[1,7,32,37,41] This attitude can be encouraged by pointing out a particularly positive aspect of the patient's body and mentioning this regularly. The feature could be the hair or eyes or a smile but should be an aspect of the patient that can be seen and commented on by others as well.[9] Commenting on how well the body feels when it is relaxed or how good the sun feels on the body helps the patient recognize that the body can be a positive source of pleasure.

Another message that can affect the young disabled patient in later life is the notion that disabled persons are asexual and will never have sexual needs or partners.[7,26,27,32,37] Although it may be difficult to discuss this question directly, the COTA can mention that other people with similar disabilities are married and have children. In this way the COTA is communicating that the possibility exists of fulfilling or continuing "normal" sex roles in the future. Without this possibility being presented, the patient may think that all the movies, books, and television programs that deal with normal adult interactions *do not* apply to disabled persons. Such attitudes may discourage socialization and alienate the disabled population from the able-bodied population.

### Adult Sexuality

Adaptive devices (e.g., leg braces, wheelchairs, communication devices) can be an impediment to sexuality. It can be difficult to perceive the self as sexy with an indwelling catheter or leg braces. Through discussion, the patient can develop some ideas regarding how to handle the situation when it arises.[26,27,29,32,41] Discussing positioning to reduce pain and spasticity or to enable the patient to engage in sexual relations more comfortably will help the patient anticipate and deal with problems before they arise.[17,27,32,33] Sexual hygiene may be considered as an ADL and thus may be considered in the domain of therapy.

The patient may believe that femininity or masculinity is threatened by the newly acquired disability[9,34,35] and try to assert sexuality through jokes, flirting, or even "passes" at the COTA. In these cases the COTA must realize that what is being sought is often just the confirmation that the patient is still a sexual and sensual person; thus the COTA's response is very important. If the COTA rejects or ridicules the patient, it may be a long time before the patient will again consider seeking confirmation of personal attractiveness. The patient may believe that rejection by the clinician (who is familiar with disabled persons) means that no one else could accept the patient as lovable. The COTA should not be surprised by such advances and should deal with the situation in a professional manner. The COTA should also realize that approximately 10% of the population is homosexual and should be prepared for advances from patients of the same gender. The clinician should be aware that this is not the time to attempt to change the patient's sexual orientation and that it is not respectful to be offended. Instead, the COTA should be equally professional in dealing with this patient as with any other patient. All the COTA's interactions should be directed toward creating an environment that will promote a stronger and better adjusted patient.

A technique for helping the female patient to discuss rather intimate matters would be to ask her how she will perform a breast self-examination with her disability. With a male the COTA might ask how he will perform a testicular self-examination. If the facility does not have information about these examinations, the local Planned Parenthood office should. Each of these activities falls into the domain of important hygiene and may not have been discussed by others. This interaction will set the stage for other intimate interactions, will impress on patients that they still need to be concerned about such daily personal matters, and will reaffirm patients' sexual identity.

### Sexual Abuse of Adults

Sexual abuse of adults is not often thought of as an area that relates to patients or disabled persons, but sufficient evidence indicates that this problem is more pervasive than believed.[1,2,3] Some persons with disabilities have reported being approached by "pimps" representing prostitution rings that specialize in providing disabled people for their customers. Some people appear to be attracted by the idea of having sex with disabled persons and are willing to pay for this. Patients should be warned about this form of exploitation. Some patients have also mentioned that medical staff have taken inappropriate liberties with them and that aides on whom the patients depended have demanded sexual favors as part of the "fringe benefits." Patients must be aware that they can and should report such assaults to Adult Protective Services. The COTA must do the same if reason exists to suspect abuse. If this is reported, patients may be concerned that they may be without another aide or that during the time an aide is being hired, they will be without essential assistance. These are major concerns for patients dependent on others for care and should be respected.

As a general rule, health care practitioners are often not suspicious of other caregivers, medical staff, aides, transportation assistants, or volunteers, but the COTA should be alert to signs of possible abuse.[3,14,27] It is an unfortunate fact that some individuals prey on and victimize disabled patients, both adults and children, and are drawn to the health care fields for this reason.[1] The clinician should watch for signs of patients being upset after interacting with a specific person; caregivers consistently taking patients off alone for no apparent reason; caregivers excessively touching patients, especially in a sensuous manner; patients being particularly agitated when around a specific individual; or patients being overly compliant with a certain caregiver. All these may be signs of trouble.

## DEALING WITH PHYSICAL SYMPTOMS OF DYSFUNCTION

This section discusses specific symptoms that may create problems with sexual functioning for disabled persons and their partners (Table 14-1).

### Hypertonia

Hypertonia can increase tightness when muscles are stretched. To avoid quick stretching of muscles involved in a movement pattern, motion should be performed slowly. The OTR may advise specific inhibition techniques to reduce muscle tone further. Patients with hypertonia may need to discuss options for different positions in which to have sexual intercourse. Alternate ways of dealing with personal hygiene (e.g., toileting, inserting tampons, gynecological examinations, birth control) may need to be explored in relation to hypertonicity.

### Flaccidity (Hypotonia)

With low tone the patient may lack endurance and may need physical support using pillows or towels or even bolsters to prop up body parts. This helps to protect the body from overstretching and fatigue. Sexual positions that allow support of involved joints need to be explored, as well as the patient's and partner's attitudes about the positions.

### Low Endurance

Low endurance can create problems during sex because the individual may not be able to tolerate

*Table 14-1*

**Conditions and Possible Effects on Sexual Functioning**

| *Diagnoses* | *Anxiety/fear* | *Contractures* | *Cultural barriers* | *Decreased libido* | *Depression* | *Impotence* | *Incontinence* | *Limited ROM* | *Loss of mobility* | *Loss of sensation* | *Low endurance* | *Medication* | *Paralysis/spasticity* | *Poor body image* | *Tremor* | *Catheter/ostomy* |
|---|---|---|---|---|---|---|---|---|---|---|---|---|---|---|---|---|
| Amputations | x | x | x | | x | | | | x | x | | | | x | | |
| Arthritis | x | x | x | x | x | | | x | x | | x | x | | x | | |
| Burns | x | x | x | | x | | | x | x | x | x | | x | x | | |
| Cardiac condition | x | | x | x | x | x* | | | x | | x | x | | x | | |
| Cerebral palsy | x | x | x | | x | | x | x | x | x | x | | x | x | x | x |
| CVA | x | x | x | x | x | x | x | x | x | x | x | x | x | x | x | x |
| Diabetes | x | | x | x | x | x | | | x | x | x | | | x | x | |
| Hand injury | x | x | x | | x | | | x | x | x | | | x | x | | |
| Head injury | x | x | x | x+ | x | x | x | x | x | x | x | x | x | x | x | x |
| Musculoskeletal injury | x | x | x | | x | | x | x | x | x | x | x | x | x | x | |
| Spinal cord injury | x | x | x | | x | x | x | x | x | x | x | x | x | x | x | x |

*x*, Possible involvement; *ROM*, range of motion; *CVA*, cerebrovascular accident; *, fear or medication as possible causes; +, increased or decreased.

prolonged activity. Some techniques for dealing with these problems are work simplification, timing of sex during points of the day when energy is highest, and positions that take less energy to perform.

### Loss of Mobility and Contractures

Many movement patterns are restricted, and sex positions will be limited by reduced range of motion (ROM). Activity analysis can reveal positions that will allow for sexual activity without focusing on the limitations. Creative problem solving is important, and a sense of humor is helpful.

### Joint Degeneration

Conditions such as arthritis can cause pain, damage to the joints, and contractures. Joint damage can be lessened by avoiding situations that put stress and repetitive weight bearing on the joints. This can be accomplished by finding a position (e.g., missionary) that can take weight and stress off the knees or hips (Figure 14-2). The position must not put undue stress on the back. This position may not be acceptable for the patient who has limited hip abduction, in which case a side-lying position may be more acceptable. This patient should try to avoid positions such as those portrayed in Figures 14-2, 14-5, and 14-9.

### Pain

Pain limits the enjoyment of sexual activities.[20,32] These sexual activities may be scheduled for a time of day when pain is diminished and energy is at its highest. Most people find that pain is diminished soon after taking medication, and sexual activity can be pursued at that time. Communication between partners is especially important when pain is involved. Often the unaffected partner feels that her or his needs are not being considered or met. This may be because the partner does not understand the strong negative effect that pain has and cannot see a physical problem. The partner may start to believe that the person in pain is just not interested. A referral for counseling may help resolve the emotional aspects (if the counselor understands the effects of pain), but the OTR or COTA may help the patient think of acceptable ways of meeting the partner's physical (sexual) needs so that this does not cause pain for the patient. A possible example of this may be masturbating the partner. If this activity stimulates pain, the patient may consider verbally describing or reading a sexually stimulating fantasy while the partner masturbates. In this way the partners are interacting, and neither person is feeling so isolated.

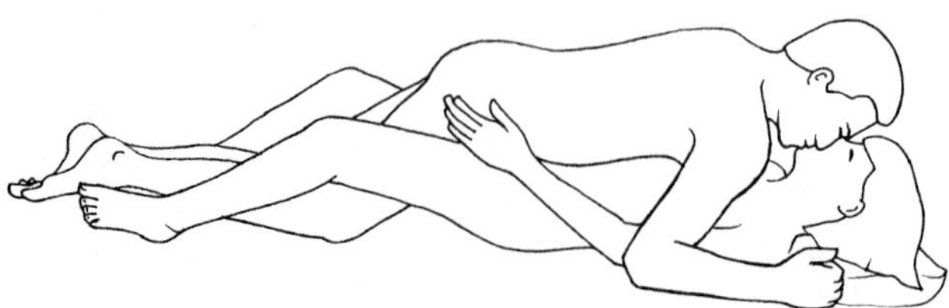

*Figure 14-2* This position places pressure on female's bladder and requires hip abduction but little energy expenditure for her.

### Loss of Sensation

Loss of sensation can affect the sexual relationship through the lack of erogenous stimulation in the affected area. The loss can block proper warning that an area is being damaged either through abrasion (e.g., vagina not being sufficiently lubricated) or breakage (e.g., bladder or even bones if the partner is on top and being too forceful for the situation). Lack of sensation may signify a break in the reflex loop, which may hamper reflexogenic erections (in the male) or lubrication (in the female); either of these issues can be dealt with but first must be recognized. Information on skin care, erections, and lubrication is discussed later in this chapter.

### Aging and Sexuality

Aging results in changes that can affect sexuality (Box 14-3). Menopause and the resulting hormonal changes may cause vaginal atrophy and slowed reactions to sexual stimulation. In the male, greater stimulation may be needed to develop and maintain an erection, and reaction time between erections may be greater. Partners often need to be informed of ways to increase stimulation and to realize that quality, not quantity, of sexual activity is important in the relationship. The patient should be made aware of the aging process and its normal effect on sexuality to prevent the patient

*Box 14-3*

**Effects of Aging on Sexuality**

**Female**

Vaginal lubrication decreases and is delayed.
Size and elasticity of vagina decreases.
Size of uterus decreases.
Thickness of vaginal wall decreases.
Reaction of muscle tone decreases.
Vaginal itching increases.
Chance of infection increases.
Orgasm decreases in length.

**Male**

Strength of orgasm decreases.
Spontaneous erection decreases (needs extra stimulation).
Length of time needed before ejaculation increases.
Length of time needed before second act increases.
Size and firmness of testes decrease.
Sperm count and quantity of seminal fluid decreases.
Hardness of erection decreases.
Decreased steroids may result in decreased muscle strength and drive.

from blaming all the problems on the disability. This is important because the disability is damaging enough to the patient without attributing more, unrelated problems to it.

## DEALING WITH OTHER BARRIERS TO SEXUALITY

### Isolation

The environment is composed of objects, persons, and events that have an impact on the individual and on which the individual has an impact. Some of the objects with which disabled persons interact are wheelchairs, braces, canes, crutches, and splints. These objects are all hard, cold, and angular and generally communicate a "hard exterior" and a fragile interior, which is viewed as not "huggable" and soft or safe to hug because a person in a wheelchair, in braces, or on crutches may be "hurt" or knocked down. Thus the disabled person may grow up feeling isolated because of appliances or, as one patient expressed it, "in a plastic bubble." People may relate to the objects around the patient in a nonsensual manner, and thus everyday events may reinforce isolation and lack of sensuousness in the patient. The feeling of isolation is seen to a greater degree in patients who have been discharged from the health care facility for a time. Even in the relatively acute phase of the disability, the clinician and patient may role-play how to deal with a new partner and how to explain the equipment used by the patient (e.g., catheters). This may help ease the patient's anxieties and promote comfort with such issues. At the same time the clinician is communicating the message to the patient that sex is a possibility in the future. The patient should be reminded that disabled people have existed throughout human history. Thus disability is normal, and it is not abnormal to be disabled (from a societal point of view). If people live long enough, they will all become disabled. Mr. Ed Roberts, founder of the Center for Independent Living, is noted for calling able-bodied persons "TABs," or *t*emporarily *a*ble *b*odied.

### Medications

The side effects of medications may cause impotence or delayed sexual response and other problems. Side effects of medication should be discussed with the physician or pharmacist to determine if medications can be changed. If they cannot, simply acknowledging that the problem is organic may be helpful to the patient. Diuretics, antihypertensives, and blood pressure medication may cause impotence, decreased libido, and loss of orgasm. Tranquilizers and antidepressants may contribute to decreased libido and impotence.

### Performance Anxiety

At times of great emotional stress the male may find that the reflexogenic erection may be inhibited. This may lead to increased anxiety in relation to sexuality and create a cycle of dysfunctional inhibition. Taking the focus off of erection and genital intercourse and focusing on sensuality and making each other feel good (e.g., with a massage) often induce more normal physiological reactions. If this does not work, a trained counselor may be needed to help deal with this problem (assuming it is not organic in nature).

### Skin Care

The person with a disability should be informed that position may need to be modified to protect the skin better and prevent skin breakdown, as well as to increase pleasure. Repeated rubbing on the skin may cause abrasions or burns and result in damage. The COTA should attempt problem solving with the patient to find ways either to prevent the friction or to find a position that will not allow this to happen. Pressure on bony prominences or a partner exerting pressure in a specific spot may also cause problems with skin irritation and must be avoided.

### Lubrication

Stimulation of natural **lubrication** in females is important, but this may not be considered in a woman with paralysis because she may not be able to feel the stimulation. Reflexive stimulation to cause lubrication should occur even though the woman may not feel it. Without proper lubrication, damage may occur without the parties being aware of the problem. If needed, artificial water-based lubricants (e.g., K-Y jelly) should be introduced. The individual should be warned that only water-based lubricants should be used because petroleum-based lubricants may cause irritation and attack latex in condoms, causing condom failure. In heterosexual sex the female is many times more likely to be infected with the human immunodeficiency virus (HIV) than the male in any given encounter; thus condom failure should be a major concern.

### Erection

To the male the ability to achieve an **erection** may be one of the most significant signs of his masculinity.[35] If awareness of sensory stimulation to the penis is blocked by paralysis, the male may think he is impotent. This may not be the case, and the patient may go through much anguish for no reason. The patient should be encouraged to explore his body in an effort to stimulate a **reflexogenic erection.** Rubbing the penis, thighs, or anus may be effective. Even rubbing the big toe has been reported by some men with quadriplegia to stimulate an erection. If the reflex loop is broken, it may not be possible to achieve an erection, and alternative methods may need to be explored. The first alternative may be forms of sex that do not require an erect penis, such as using a vibrator or engaging in oral or digital sex. If the patient believes that penile intercourse is the only acceptable alternative, several interventions are available. Injections of hormones that stimulate erections may be used, but this may lead to problems if the patient does not have good judgment and good hand dexterity or has adverse reactions. Use of a vacuum tube is sometimes effective and is one of the less invasive techniques.[37] Surgical implants can be used but may have drawbacks, such as infection and skin breakdown. An excellent discussion of these alternatives can be found in the journal *Sexuality and Disability* (see Recommended Reading).

## OTHER ASPECTS OF SEXUALITY

### Birth Control

Disabled persons must be aware of many issues regarding birth control.[6,18,27,32] The patient and partner first should realize that most disabling conditions do not impair fertility; this is especially true for females. Therefore the patient must consider birth control issues and complications. Condoms require hand use, although an applicator can be adapted in some cases (someone with good hand dexterity must assemble the device at an earlier time). Diaphragms are not feasible for people who have poor hand function unless the partner does have hand dexterity and both parties feel comfortable with the partner placing the diaphragm as an aspect of foreplay. The contraceptive sponge requires good use of hands. Using oral contraceptives (the "pill") may increase the risk of clotting, especially when the woman has impaired mobility or paralysis. If the patient has decreased sensation, the intrauterine device (IUD) may result in increased complications from bleeding, cramping, puncturing of the uterus, or infection. Spermicides require good hand control or the assistance of a partner with good dexterity. At all times the patient must think of decreasing the chance of infection and using safe sex.

### Adaptive Aids

Disabled patients may need to use **adaptive aids,** especially if they lack hand function. One aid may be a vibrator for foreplay or masturbation.[27,32] Special vibrators have been adapted for males and females.[27,32] Pillows can be used for positioning, and other devices can be used for patients with special needs. The counselor must prepare the patient for the concept of using sexual aids before asking the person to use such devices. For example, the COTA might ask the patient to explore the sensation that the vibrator produces in the lower extremities (in private). In this way the patient may discover the possible use of the vibrator or at least will be more open to the idea of using a vibrator as a sexual aid when told about potential functional benefits.

### Safe Sex

The issue of "safe sex" has been prominent since the advent of acquired immunodeficiency syndrome (AIDS). Safe sex is important to protect against all forms of sexually transmitted diseases (STDs).[27] Patients need to be informed that this is an important issue for several reasons. If a sensory impairment exists in and around the genital area, the patient may not be aware of the infection, which can lead to massive damage. Having a genital infection provides an easy entrance for diseases such as HIV, herpes virus, or any other STD. Disabled patients must recognize this possible increased risk for HIV and STD infections so that they will be extra cautious and thus empowered.

### Hygiene Concerns

Catheter care should be addressed, especially when hand function is impaired. Questions may arise regarding if (or how) a person with an indwelling catheter can have sex. The answer for both males and females is yes, but they should use some precautions. If at any time the catheter becomes kinked or closed off (this will definitely happen in a catheterized male having vaginal intercourse), pressure should not be placed on the bladder. The length of time that flow of urine is restricted should be kept as short as possible (about 30 minutes), and the bladder should be fully voided before sexual activity. Damage to the bladder and kidneys could result if these precautions are not followed. As a preventive measure, the patient should not drink fluids at least 2 hours before sex to avoid the bladder filling during this time. Sexual positions that avoid pressure on the bladder should be used (Figures 14-3 to 14-10). Many of the same positions may be used if the patient has a stoma appliance.

It is not unusual for a person with impaired bowel or bladder function to have an "accident" during sexual activities. If the patient and clinician discuss this possibility and how it could be handled, some of the patient's awkwardness at the time may be averted. This form of role playing can also be used to review other scenarios (e.g., "You are heading to the bedroom

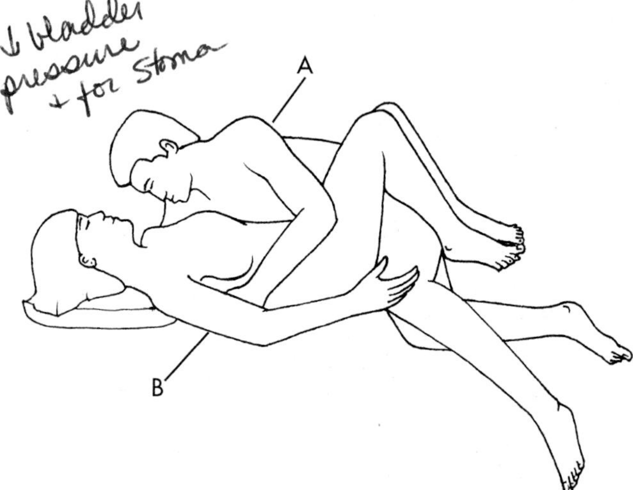


*Figure 14-3* Vaginal entry of partner *B* requires no hip abduction, and hip flexion tightness would not impede performance. Energy requirements for both parties are minimal. Bladder pressure and safety of catheter and stoma appliance should not be concerns with this position for partner *B*. This position may be recommended if partner *B* has back pain or is paralyzed. A roll can be used to support lumbar spine.

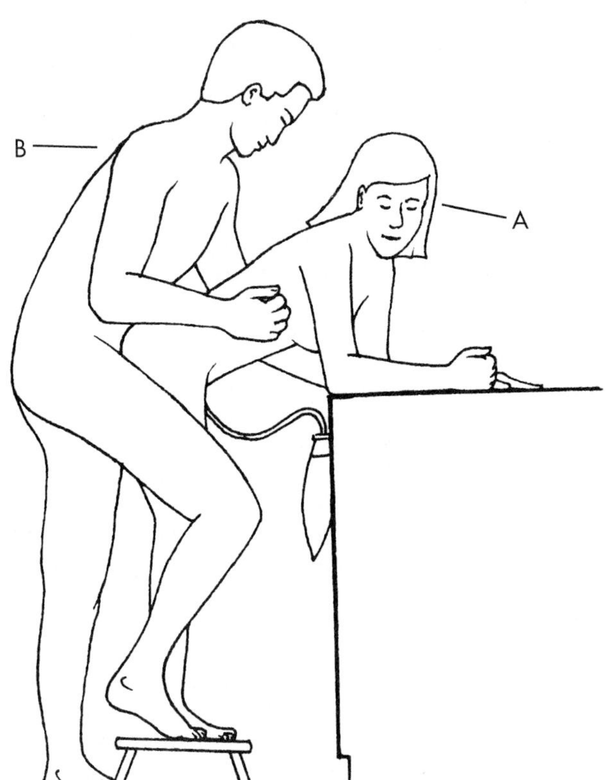


*Figure 14-4* Partner *A* needs little hip abduction but good strength. Partner *B* may find decreased strain on his back. Position cannot be used if either partner has hip, knee, or ankle joint dysfunction.

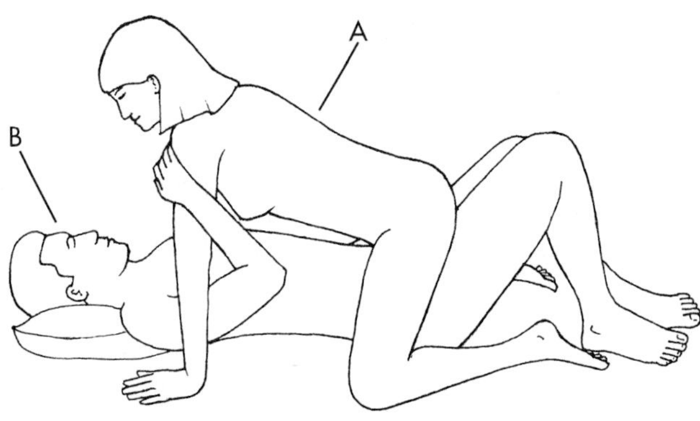


*Figure 14-5* Partner *A* must have hip abduction, balance, and endurance, but there is no pressure on bladder or stoma. If catheter is used, it would be unrestricted. Back pain may be avoided by keeping trunk vertical. Partner *B's* hip flexors could be contracted. If low back pain is a problem, legs should be flexed and a roll placed under lower back. If stoma appliance is used, this position would avoid interference. This position is effective if low endurance is a problem for partner *B*.

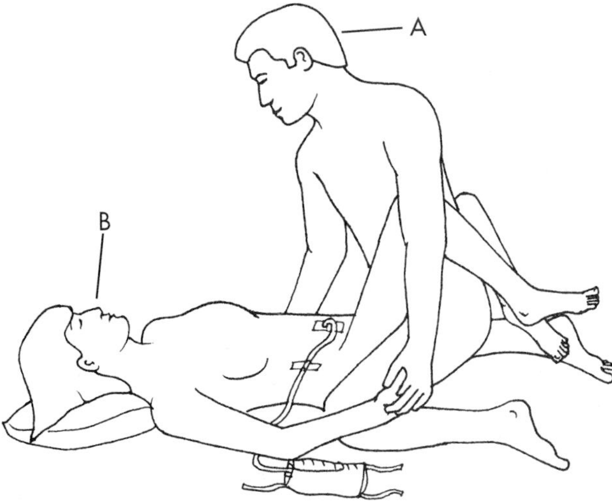


*Figure 14-6* This position keeps pressure off bladder, lessens the risk of tubing becoming bent, reduces pressure on back (especially if a small roll is used under low back), and does not require partner *B* to use much energy. Legs do not need to be as high as shown. This may be a comfortable position if hip flexors are contracted.

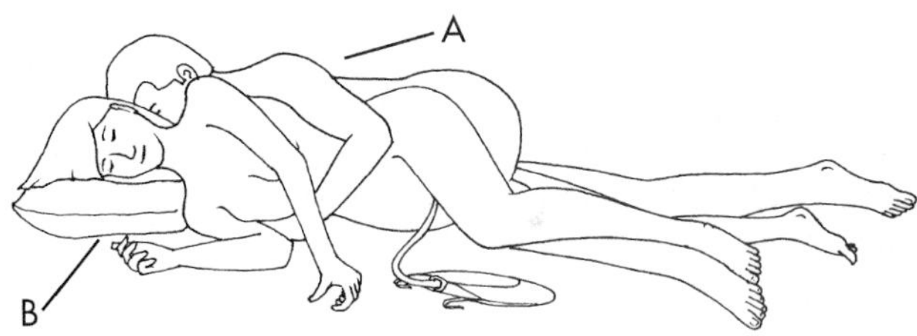


*Figure 14-7* Partner *B* does not need to expend much energy in this position, and both partners may avoid swayback. Either person may have hemiparesis. Partner *B* does not need hip abduction, and pressure on stoma bag may be avoided.

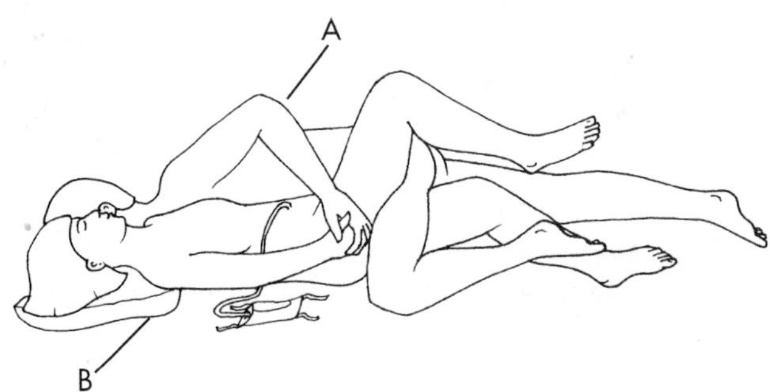


*Figure 14-8* This position can be used if either partner has hemiparesis or if low endurance is a problem. Partner *A* may avoid swayback in this position.

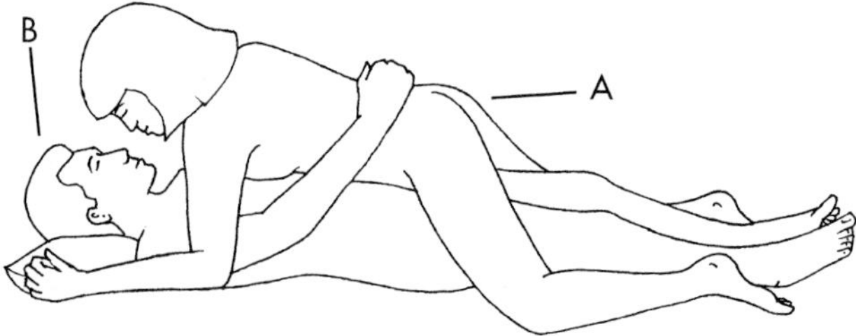


*Figure 14-9* This position can be used if partner *B* is paralyzed or has limited range of motion. Partner *B's* back may need a roll for support, and *B* must be concerned about pressure on his bladder.

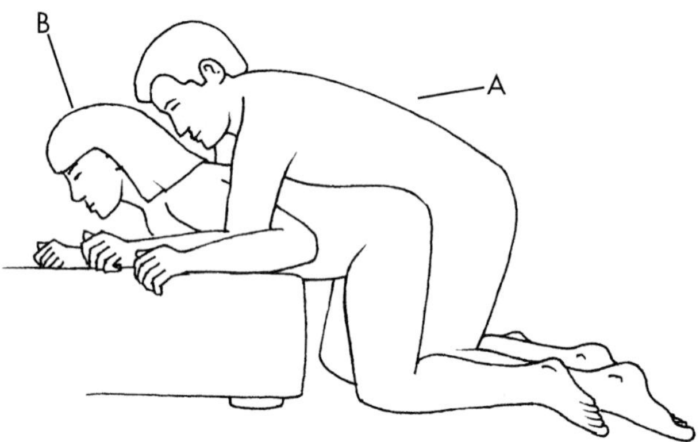


*Figure 14-10* Partner *B* does not need much energy and little or no abduction of hips for this rear vaginal entry position. This would not be a good position for persons with back, hip, or knee joint degeneration because of weight on knees and inevitable movement at hips.

with a new partner. How will you explain your catheter and appliances to this person?"). These may be awkward conversations for the clinician and patient, but it is usually easier to deal with the situation before it occurs than to wait for the inevitable accident.

### Pregnancy, Birth, and Child Care

Pregnancy may result in complications that may affect the patient's function and mobility. Increased weight impedes transfers and increases the possibility of *dysreflexia* (autonomic hyperreflexia) or increased bladder and bowel care.[6,7] The birth may present unique situations. For example, induction of labor may be contraindicated, and the medical staff may not be trained in this area. After the birth, the disabled parent may need to have the wheelchair modified. Consultations may be needed for the disabled patient to achieve an optimal level of functioning in the parenting role.[18]

## TECHNIQUES FOR RESPONDING TO EMOTIONAL ASPECTS OF DYSFUNCTION

The following techniques or approaches have been effectively used to deal with selected sexuality problems of the disabled patient.

### Repetition of Information

Mentioning sexuality issues once is not sufficient to change the patient's functional performance. Most people, whether disabled or not, need to have information repeated. This is especially true for persons in crisis or in the process of adjustment. The COTA should approach the patient using the following guidelines:

- Do not try to give too much information at one time, or more than is asked for, because the patient may become overwhelmed.
- Do not assume the patient understands what is being said.
- Have the patient ask questions and paraphrase what you have said, or you can ask questions to see if the information is being processed.

### Discovery of the "New" Body

With any disability, the patient develops an altered perception of the body. That is, the patient has a "new" body and must find altered ways of moving, interpreting sensations, and performing even mundane ADLs. A major focus of the therapeutic experience is to help the patient discover how to use this new body as effectively as possible and to process sensory information optimally. The COTA can facilitate this exploration of the new body by creating situations that will encourage body awareness through the input of sensation and function.[27] This can be accomplished through exercises that encourage exploration of the body by the patient or both patient and partner. Exercises such as gentle tapping or rubbing of a specific area can be attempted to see if sensation exists or if the stimulation causes a change in tone (through reflex activity if no sensation present). Many people with a disability (e.g., paralysis) report that they have experienced nongenital orgasms[24,27] by stimulating other, new erogenous areas, often in the region just above where sensation starts to appear. If sensation or a change in tone occurs, the occupational therapy practitioner may give suggestions on how to use this change in ADLs. The clinician may ask the patient to think of ways this change in tone could be used. One example is triggering reflex leg extension to assist with putting on pants. This stimulates problem solving in the patient and leads to empowerment.

### PLISSIT

This acronym stands for *p*ermission, *l*imited *i*nformation, *s*pecific *s*uggestions, and *i*ntensive *t*herapy. It is a progressive approach to guide the clinician to help the patient deal with sexual information. *Permission* refers to allowing the patient to feel new sensations and experiment with new thoughts or ideas regarding sexual functioning. *Limited information* refers to explaining, on a superficial level, what effect the disability may have on sexual functioning. At this point an explanation with great detail is not usually necessary and may complicate the process. The next level of information is providing *specific suggestions*. Depending on the clinical situation, it may be the COTA's domain to give specific suggestions on how to deal with specific problems that relate to the disability, such as positioning. This is the highest level the COTA should attempt without continued education and training because an extensive counseling background is needed to help the patient undergo *intensive therapy.* Intensive therapy should be reserved for the rare patient who has an abnormal coping pattern in dealing with sexuality.

### Communication

During rehabilitation the patient will need to learn how to communicate changed needs, including sexual needs. This can be facilitated by the COTA simply giving the patient permission to discuss these issues. The patient may need to learn how to communicate sexual needs and desires and position options to a partner accurately, either verbally or nonverbally, in order to have a mutually satisfactory sexual relationship.[24,32] Each patient will have unique problems or issues in this area that may be related to the nature of the disability. In Parkinson's disease, for example, the lack of facial expression impedes the nonverbal communication of intimacy. The patient may need to be taught to communicate verbally to a partner the feelings that were previously communicated through facial expression.

### Activity Analysis

To assess the patient's positioning needs, the occupational therapy practitioner must analyze the components of the activity. This entails examining the physical, psychological, social, cultural, and even the cognitive components of the patient and partner. The clinician must examine the activity from an objective and professional perspective because the patient usually lacks such a viewpoint. The clinician must realize that the sex act itself is only a small part of the act of making love. At the same time the clinician must treat this as just one more ADL that may need professional assistance and must be analyzed accordingly. The clinician must also remember that frequency of sex may have been daily or very infrequent before the disability occurred. The clinician's biases should not be imposed on the patient. This is especially true if the partners are of the same sex or multiple partners are involved, if masturbation was or is the preferred method of release of sexual tension, or if the patient never had a need to release sexual tension.

### Sexuality Education

Some patients may need sex (sexuality) education because they may never have received the information even before the disability occurred. Some patients may not have been informed because of the disability or were misinformed about sexual practices.[1] Research has shown that even people with hearing impairments have significantly less information regarding sexuality than those without hearing losses.[39] The COTA may not be the practitioner who educates the patient or partner, but the COTA is in a position to anticipate this need and may have knowledge of the resources available for the patient to acquire this information (see resource list at the end of this chapter). The COTA should provide a range of resources and not only books about sexuality and disabled persons. Such books are very useful but, because of their nature, focus on the disability. Disabled patients should also refer to books written for able-bodied persons.[19,21,22] These not only give patients an understanding of sex, but also allow them to see how normal they are. Excellent books are available for the disabled patient.*

### Staff Training

Many schools do not allocate the time to train the health care professional on the subject of sexuality.[16] In-service programs can be arranged to help staff recognize disabled patients' needs.[16,23] Many books, articles, videotapes, and training packets are available.[3,10,11] The staff must be educated about the significance of this issue so that they are able to present positive feelings about dealing with sexuality.[2]

### Harassment of Staff

As mentioned earlier, patients may have difficulty confronting their feelings regarding attractiveness, and the staff should not overreact or reject the patient. At the same time, COTAs should *never* permit patients to harass them sexually.[30,38] **Sexual harassment** occurs when the clinician feels threatened, intimidated, or treated as a sexual object. This is damaging not only to staff morale, but also to the patient if it is allowed.[21,38] Direct feedback should emphasize that the clinician feels offended and that the patient's behavior is inappropriate and must cease. All staff members should be informed and agree on a plan to stop the patient's behavior if it persists.

## SUMMARY

For most people, sexuality is entwined with personal identity. The ability to give and receive love is interwoven with the person's self-concept. Sexuality is classified as an activity of daily living in the uniform terminology of the American Occupational Therapy Association, and thus the COTA should anticipate that disabled patients will require evaluation, assistance, information, and intervention in this area. Communicating with patients about sexuality requires professional dignity and the greatest possible flexibility from the practitioner. Among the specific qualities the practitioner should possess are knowledge of sexual theory and practices; tolerance; appreciation for the needs, views, and practices of others; excellent verbal and nonverbal communication skills; utmost discretion; and an understanding of the limitations of the COTA's role. The COTA is encouraged to seek additional training in this area and to obtain appropriate supervision when providing services to disabled patients related to issues of sexuality.

*References 10, 17, 18, 20, 27, 32, 33.

## Selected Reading Guide Questions

1. Discuss the factors that contribute to the asexual image of the disabled person.
2. Explain why the newly disabled patient might flirt with a staff member. Describe appropriate and helpful ways to respond.
3. Why might a patient ask the COTA, rather than the physician, about sexual aspects of a disability?
4. What is the purpose of a sexual history interview?
5. Describe the conditions (environment) in which an sexual history interview or other discussion of sexual matters is best conducted.
6. Describe how the sense of sensuality and sexuality develops in the growing child.
7. Discuss how a clinician's insensitivity to personal ownership of the body may affect disabled children as they mature.
8. List and discuss methods that the COTA can use to help disabled individuals develop a positive attitude toward their bodies.
9. List signs that may indicate sexual abuse.
10. Give specific suggestions for dealing with the following physical symptoms in sexual activities: hypertonia, hypotonia, low endurance, loss of mobility or contractures, joint degeneration, pain, and loss of sensation.
11. List and discuss the effects of aging on sexuality for both males and females.
12. Discuss isolating aspects of the disabled patient's environment, and suggest methods to reduce isolation.
13. Describe effects of medications on sexuality.
14. Discuss ways to prevent skin breakdown during sexual activity.
15. Differentiate between safe and unsafe artificial lubricants that can substitute for natural lubrication during sexual activities.
16. Describe how an erection may be achieved by reflexogenic means in a male who has no direct sensation in the penis.
17. Discuss some of the problems the disabled person might encounter with common birth control methods.
18. Identify what PLISSIT stands for, and explain each component. Identify which components can be performed by the COTA and which require more education.

### REFERENCES


1. Andrews AB, Veronen LJ: Sexual assault and people with disabilities, *J Soc Work Hum Sex* 8:137-159, 1993.
2. Annon JS: *The behavioral treatment of sexual problems*, vols 1 and 2, Honolulu, 1974, Enabling Systems.
3. Boyle PS: Training in sexuality and disability: preparing social workers to provide services to individuals with disabilities, *J Soc Work Hum Sex* 8:45-62, 1993.
4. Braithwaite DO: From majority to minority: an analysis of cultural change from ablebodied to disabled, *Int J Intercult Relat* 14:465-483, 1990.
5. Charlifue SW et al: Sexual issues of women with spinal cord injuries, *Paraplegia* 30:192-199, 1992.
6. Cole SS, Cole TM: Sexuality, disability, and reproductive issues for persons with disabilities. In Haseltine FP, Cole SS, Gray DB, editors: *Reproductive issues for persons with physical disabilities*, Baltimore, 1993, Brookes.
7. Cole SS, Cole TM: Sexuality, disability, and reproductive issues through the life span, *Sex Disabil* 11:189-205, 1993.
8. Cole TM: Gathering a sex history from a physically disabled adult, *Sex Disabil* 9:29-37, 1991.
9. Corbett K, Klein S, Bregante JL: The role of sexuality and sex equity in the education of disabled women, *Peabody J Educ* 64:198-211, 1987.
10. Cornelius DA et al: *Who cares? A handbook on sex education and counseling services for disabled people*, Baltimore, 1982, University Park.
11. Ducharme S, Gill KM: Sexual values, training, and professional roles, *J Head Trauma Rehabil* 5:38-45, 1991.
12. Edwards DF, Baum CM: Caregivers burden across stages of dementia, *Occup Ther Pract* 2:17-31, 1990.
13. Fitz-Gerald M, Fitz-Gerald DR: Involvement in sex education, *Volta Rev* 89:96-110, 1987.
14. Froehlich J: Occupational therapy interventions with survivors of sexual abuse, *Occup Ther Psychosoc Dysfunct* pp. 1-25, 1992.
15. Gender AR: An overview of the nurse's role in dealing with sexuality, *Sexual Disabil* 10:70-71, 1992.
16. Goldstein H, Runyon C: An occupational therapy education module to increase sensitivity about geriatric sexuality, *Phys Occup Ther Geriatr* 11:57, 1993.
17. Griffith ER, Lemberg S: *Sexuality and the person with traumatic brain injury: a guide for families*, Philadelphia, 1993, Davis.
18. Haseltine FP, Cole SS, Gray DB: *Reproductive issues for persons with physical disabilities*, Baltimore, 1993, Brookes.
19. Hayden N: *How to satisfy a woman every time . . .*, New York, 1982, Bibli O'Phile.
20. Hebert L: *Sex and back pain*, Bloomington, Minn, 1987, Educational Opportunities.
21. Hite S: *The Hite report*, New York, 1976, Macmillan.
22. Hite S: *The Hite report on male sexuality*, New York, 1981, Knopf.
23. Johnson TC: Understanding the sexual behaviors of young children, *Sexuality Information and Education Council of the United States Report*, 1991.
24. Kettl P et al: Female sexuality after spinal cord injury, *Sex Disabil* 9:287-295, 1991.
25. Kielhofner G: *A model of human occupation*, Baltimore, 1985, Williams & Wilkins.
26. Krause JS, Crewe NM: Chronological age, time since injury, and time of measurement: effect on adjustment after spinal cord injury, *Arch Phys Med Rehabil* 72:91-100, 1991.
27. Kroll K, Klein EL: *Enabling romance*, New York, 1992, Harmony.
28. Lefebvre KA: Sexual assessment planning, *J Head Trauma Rehabil* 5:25-30, 1990.
29. Lemon MA: Sexual counseling and spinal cord injury, *Sex Disabil* 11:73-97, 1993.
30. McComas J et al: Experiences of students and practicing physical therapists with inappropriate patient sexual behavior, *Phys Ther* 73:762-769, 1993.
31. Miller BR et al: *Six perspectives on theory for the practice of occupational therapy*, Rockville, Md, 1988, Aspen.
32. Neistadt ME, Freda M: *Choices: a guide to sex counseling with physically disabled adults*, Malabar, Fla, 1987, Krieger.
33. Rabin BJ: *The sensuous wheeler*, Long Beach, Calif, Rabin.
34. Romeo AJ, Wanlass R, Arenas S: A profile of psychosexual functioning in males following spinal cord injury, *Sex Disabil* 11:269-276, 1993.
35. Sandowski C: Responding to the sexual concerns of persons with disabilities, *J Soc Work Hum Sex* 8:29-43, 1993.
36. Scott R: Sexual misconduct, *PT Mag Phys Ther* 1:78, 1993.
37. Smith M: Pediatric sexuality: promoting normal sexual development in children, *Nurse Pract* 18:37-44, 1993.

38. Stockard S: Caring for the sexually aggressive patient: you don't have to blush and bear it, *Nursing '91* 21:72-73, 1991.
39. Swartz DB: A comparative study of sex knowledge among hearing and deaf college freshmen, *Sex Disabil* 11:129-136, 1993.
40. Verduyn WH: Spinal cord injured women, pregnancy, and delivery, *Sex Disabil* 11:29-43, 1993.
41. Zani B: Male and female patterns in the discovery of sexuality during adolescence, *J Adolesc* 14:163-178, 1991.

## RECOMMENDED READING

Gregory MF: *Sexual adjustment: a guide for the spinal cord injured,* Bloomington, Ind, 1992, Accent on Living.

Kempton W, Caparulo F: *Sex education for persons with disabilities that hinder learning: a teacher's guide,* Santa Barbara, Calif, 1989, Stanfield.

Leyson JF: *Sexual rehabilitation of the spinal-cord-injured patient,* Clifton, NJ, 1991, Humana.

*Resources for people with disabilities and chronic conditions,* ed 2, Lexington, Ky, 1993, Resources for Rehabilitation.

Sandowski C: *Sexual concern when illness or disability strikes,* Springfield, Ill, 1989, Thomas.

*Sexuality and Disability,* vol 1, no 1, 1994.

Shortridge J, Steele-Clapp L, Lamin J: Sexuality and disability: a SIECUS annotated bibliography of available print materials, *Sex Disabil* 11(2):159-179, 1993.

Sobsey D et al: *Disability, sexuality, and abuse,* Baltimore, 1991, Brookes.

## AGENCIES AND SUPPORT CENTERS

American Association of Sex Education Counselors and Therapists
435 N. Michigan Avenue, Suite 1717, Chicago, IL 60611
(312) 644-0828

Association for Sexual Adjustment in Disability
P.O. Box 3579, Downey, CA 90292

Coalition on Sexuality and Disability
122 East Twenty-third Street, New York, NY 10010
(212) 242-3900

Sex Information and Education Council of the United States (SIECUS)
130 West Forty-second Street, Suite 2500, New York, NY 10036
(212) 819-9770

Sexuality and Disability Training Center
University of Michigan Medical Center
Department of Physical Medicine and Rehabilitation
1500 E. Medical Center Drive, Ann Arbor, MI 48109
(313) 936-7067

The Task Force on Sexuality and Disability of the American Congress of Rehabilitation Medicine
5700 Old Orchard Road, Skokie, IL 60077
(708) 966-0095

# Chapter 15

# Purposeful Activities, Therapeutic Exercise, and Therapeutic Modalities

*Lorraine Williams Pedretti*
*Ingrid Wade*

## *Chapter Objectives*

*After studying this chapter, the student or practitioner will be able to:*

1. Differentiate purposeful activity from other modalities used in occupational therapy.
2. Identify the eight characteristics that should be present in any activity used for therapeutic purposes.
3. Contrast the focus of activity analysis under the biomechanical and sensorimotor approaches.
4. Grade an activity to accommodate changes in a variety of factors, such as strength, range of motion, endurance, coordination, and perceptual and cognitive skills.
5. Identify the necessary characteristics of activities used for physical restoration.
6. Discuss the appropriate use of enabling activities and adjunctive modalities.
7. Describe the uses of therapeutic exercise for a variety of occupational therapy goals.
8. Understand the indications, contraindications, procedures, and precautions for a variety of exercise protocols.
9. Discuss the appropriate uses of various physical agent modalities in occupational therapy.
10. Identify appropriate modalities in the continuum of care.

## *Key Terms*

modality
purposeful activity
activity configuration
activity analysis
adaptation of activity
gradation of activity
therapeutic exercise
engram
isometric (static) contraction
isotonic (concentric) contraction
eccentric contraction
isotonic resistive exercise
isotonic active exercise
active-assisted exercise
passive exercise
passive stretch
active stretch
isometric exercise
neuromuscular control
physical agent modalities
conduction
convection
conversion
ultrasound
cryotherapy
transcutaneous electrical nerve stimulation (TENS)
functional electrical stimulation (FES)

Historically, arts and crafts have been identified as the primary therapeutic modalities of occupational therapy. In the 1954 second edition of *Principles of Occupational Therapy*[37] by Helen Willard and Clare Spackman, Spackman wrote: "In occupational therapy, exercise of the muscles or motion of the joints is obtained by having the patient himself use the disabled part in the course of some constructive procedure, such as woodworking. Occupational therapy may not be indicated for some patients until they are capable of sustained active motion for brief periods." She stated that the physical therapist uses physical agent modalities and exercise, and the occupational therapist uses complementary purposeful activity. She urged that treatment be coordinated between the two disciplines and suggested that it was usually beneficial for occupational therapy to follow physical therapy.[37]

Arts and crafts are still in use as treatment methods and remain an effective and significant element of some occupational therapy programs.[13] However, the scope of OT treatment methods has broadened considerably over the years. Today, registered occupational therapists (OTRs) are qualified in a variety of therapeutic modalities.[1] Their competence is gained through entry level and graduate education, specialty certification, continuing education, and work experience. Certified occupational therapy assistants (COTAs) may be exposed to a variety of modalities through their academic education and clinical fieldwork. Depending on the area in which they practice and the availability of health care services and specialized health care practitioners, COTAs may need to achieve service competency in a number of different modalities.

The term **modality** was defined for purposes of the American Occupational Therapy Association (AOTA) policy statement "according to *Webster's New World Dictionary,* second College Edition, [as] the employment of, or method of employment of, a therapeutic agent."[1] In the context of this chapter, modality includes both media and methods, as defined by Reed.[32] A *medium* is "the means by which a therapeutic effect is transmitted." For example, a vestibular ball is a medium. *Methods* are "the steps, sequence or approach used to activate the therapeutic effect of a medium," such as the handling and movements used with the vestibular ball to effect the desired motor responses.[32]

Modalities chosen for professional practice are influenced by eight factors, according to Reed.[32] These are cultural practices, social acceptance or nonacceptance, economics of health care, available technology, influences of a given theoretical model, historical influences, and research. Chapter 1 reviews the evolution of treatment modalities in physical disabilities practice.

In addition to arts, crafts, and other purposeful activities, therapists and assistants have become increasingly skillful in applications of therapeutic exercise, physical agent modalities, and the facilitation and inhibition techniques associated with the sensorimotor approaches to treatment, all of which traditionally belonged to the field of physical therapy. Many occupational therapy practitioners use these modalities because they promote the development of the individual's abilities to engage in occupational performance, a primary aim of occupational therapy. Principles of therapeutic exercise and sensorimotor approaches are also applied to purposeful activities, with adaptations and gradations to achieve desired treatment goals.

This chapter presents the theory and principles of purposeful activity, enabling activities, and the adjunctive modalities: therapeutic exercise and physical agents.

## PURPOSEFUL ACTIVITY

One of the first principles of occupational therapy, stated by Dunton in 1918, is that occupation must have some useful end for it to be effective in the treatment of mental and physical disability.[39] This principle implies that the activity or occupation has a purpose and that purposeful activity has an intrinsic or inherent goal beyond the motor function required to perform the task.[7] An individual engaged in purposeful activity focuses attention on the goal rather than the processes required to reach the goal.[2,5] Conversely, *nonpurposeful activity* has been defined as activity in which no inherent goal exists other than the motor function used to perform the activity.[39] The performer's attention is likely to be focused on the movements. By this definition, adjunctive methods (e.g., therapeutic exercise) and enabling activities (e.g., moving cones and stacking blocks) cannot be considered purposeful activity. Nonetheless, these media have a place in the treatment continuum.

Purposeful activity is the "cornerstone of occupational therapy" and its primary treatment modality.[39,41] AOTA has defined **purposeful activity** as "... goal-directed behaviors or tasks that comprise occupations. An activity is purposeful if the individual is an active, voluntary participant and if the activity is directed toward a goal that the individual considers meaningful."[5] The uniqueness of occupational therapy lies in its emphasis on the extensive use of purposeful activity. This emphasis gives occupational therapy the theoretical foundation for its broad application to psychosocial, physical, and developmental dysfunction as well as to health maintenance.[2]

Purposeful activity has both inherent and therapeutic goals. For example, sawing wood may have the inherent goal of securing parts for construction of a bookshelf, whereas the therapeutic objectives may be to strengthen shoulder and elbow musculature. Sawing wood employs the neuromuscular system to accomplish the inherent or intrinsic goal of the activity being performed. The conscious effort of the patient performing the activity is focused on the ultimate outcome and not on the movement itself.[7] The patient directs and is in control of the movement. As the patient becomes absorbed in the performance of the activity, it is assumed that the affected parts are used more naturally and with less fatigue.[38] It has been shown that concentration on motion has a detrimental effect on that motion and that muscles controlled by conscious attention and focused effort fatigue rapidly. Therefore it is more effective to focus attention on the activity and its inherent goal rather than on the muscles or motions being used to accomplish the activity.[7]

Studies have shown the efficacy of purposeful activity. The results of a study by Steinbeck[39] supported the assumption that patients performing purposeful activity are motivated to perform for a longer period than when they are performing nonpurposeful activity. A study of motivation for product-oriented versus non–product-oriented activity by Thibodeaux and Ludwig[41] indicated the need to determine the patient's level of interest in the process and in the activity end product and the patient's enjoyment of the activity in treatment planning. Rocker and Nelson[34] studied the importance of keeping or not keeping the activity product. They found that not being allowed to keep an activity product can elicit hostile feelings in normal subjects. Yoder, Nelson, and Smith[44] studied the effects of added-purpose versus rote exercise in female nursing home residents. The added-purpose exercise resulted in significantly more movement repetitions than rote exercise. These studies suggest that goal-directed, purposeful activity increases motivation for participation in sustained activity. Therefore the patient's level of interest in the activity and the meaning of the activity and activity product to the patient are important considerations in selecting media and methods for treatment.

Purposeful activities are used or adapted for use to meet one or more of the following therapeutic objectives: (1) to develop or maintain strength, endurance, work tolerance, range of motion (ROM), and coordination; (2) to practice and use voluntary, automatic movement in goal-directed tasks; (3) to provide for purposeful use of and general exercise to affected parts; (4) to explore vocational potential or train in work skills; (5) to improve sensation, perception, and cognition; (6) to improve socialization skills and enhance emotional growth and development; and (7) to increase independence in occupational role performance. Arts, crafts, games, sports, leisure, self-care, home management, mobility, and work-related activities are considered purposeful activities. This section focuses on theory and general principles for selecting and applying purposeful activities as therapy.

### Theory of Activity

Occupational therapy was founded on the concept that humans have an *occupational nature;* that is, it is natural for humans to engage in activity, and the process of being occupied contributes to their health and well-being.[7,11,17] Activity is valuable for the maintenance of health in the healthy person and for the restoration of health after illness and disability. By engaging in relevant, meaningful, and purposeful activity, change is possible and dysfunction is reversible.[11] The OT practitioner acts as facilitator of the change process.[10] Therefore physical dysfunction can be reversed, corrected, or eased when the patient participates in goal-directed (purposeful) activity.[7]

The value of purposeful activity lies in the patient's mental and physical involvement in a task that exercises the affected parts in a functional context while simultaneously meeting emotional, social, and personal gratification needs.[7,38] Cynkin and Robinson[11] pointed out that for the attainment of optimal function and health, the person must be consciously involved in problem solving and creative activity, which are processes linked with the use of the hands. Virtually all occupational performance tasks involve the use of the hands.

The activities that form the pattern of one's life, that are performed routinely and automatically, are taken for granted until some dysfunction occurs to disrupt their performance. Occupational therapy is founded on the concept that dysfunction can be modified, altered, or reversed toward function through engagement in activities of real life.[11]

Cynkin and Robinson[11] make several assumptions about activities, human nature, and change. These are summarized as follows:

1. People require a variety of activities to fulfill their needs and wants, to develop physically and psychosocially, and to achieve mastery and competence.
2. Activities are socioculturally regulated by the values and beliefs of the culture. A culture may be rigid or flexible in its interpretation of acceptable behaviors for various groups. Whether rigid or flexible, however, every culture sets a point beyond which deviations in behavior or activities patterns are deemed unacceptable.
3. Changes in activities-related behavior can move from dysfunctional toward more functional. People desire change and are able to change.
4. Change in activities-related behavior takes place through motor, cognitive, and social learning.

### Activity Configuration

Selecting appropriate and meaningful activities for the patient requires knowledge of the patient, as gained through evaluation. This should begin with obtaining and analyzing the individual's **activity configuration.**[41] This model (Figure 15-1), adapted from Cynkin,[10] includes information about the patient's values, educational history, work history, leisure interests and activities, and vocational interests and plans. It concludes with a daily schedule, a list of life roles, an analysis of the activity balance, and an assessment of developmental tasks. If the person is an outpatient and is in an advanced rehabilitation program, a daily schedule for the present and a schedule reflecting activity before the injury or illness can be constructed and compared. If the patient is acutely ill or in the early stages of rehabilitation, a daily schedule reflecting activity before the injury or illness should be made. This information may be obtained from interviews with the patient and significant friends and family members.

Requirements of funding sources and budget restrictions may not permit the OTR or COTA to spend time with a patient for the sole purposes of this lengthy interview. Much of this information can be obtained gradually during regular treatment sessions. It is not necessary to gather the information all at once or through a formal interview.

### Activity Analysis

A careful activity analysis is essential to the selection of appropriate activities for use in treatment. An **activity analysis** should yield information about the usefulness and application of purposeful activities as intervention strategies for physical dysfunction and health maintenance. Activities can be analyzed from three perspectives: the field of action, the actor, and the activity.

The *field of action* involves the objects and environment relevant to the performance of the activity and the explicit and implicit rules for performance of the activity in the environment. The *actor* is the person performing the activity. The performance components required of that person, the relevance of the activity to the person, the influencing sociocultural norms, and the importance of the activity in the person's everyday life require analysis. When doing an analysis from the *activity* perspective, the intrinsic properties and characteristics of the activity and its relationship to the real world need to be examined.[11]

#### *Principles of Activity Analysis*

If activities are to be used as the core of occupational therapy, their usefulness as therapeutic modalities must be defined, analyzed, and classified.[10] Activities selected for therapeutic purposes should (1) be goal directed; (2) have some significance and meaning to the patient to meet individual needs in relation to social roles; (3) require the patient's mental or physical participation; (4) be designed to prevent or reverse dysfunction; (5) develop skills to enhance performance in life roles; (6) relate to the patient's interests; (7) be adaptable, gradable, and age appropriate; and (8) be selected through knowledge and professional judgment of the OT practitioner with the patient's input.[15]

*Analysis for biomechanical approach* The biomechanical approach to treatment is likely to be used in lower motor neuron and orthopedic dysfunctions. Improvement of strength, ROM, and muscle endurance are the goals of occupational therapy for patients with such dysfunctions. Thus activity analysis focuses on muscles, joints, and motor patterns required to perform the activity. An activity should be analyzed in the context in which it is to be performed. Steps of the activity must be identified and broken down into the motions required to perform each step. ROM, degree of muscle strength, and type of muscle contraction to perform each step should be identified. The activity analysis model at the end of this chapter is based on the biomechanical approach.

*Analysis for sensorimotor approaches* Sensorimotor approaches to treatment are likely to be used for upper motor neuron disorders such as cerebral palsy, cerebrovascular accident (stroke), and head injury. Activity analysis for these dysfunctions should focus on the movement patterns required in the particular treatment approach. The therapist must also consider the effect of the activity on balance, posture, muscle tone, and the facilitation or inhibition of abnormal reflexes and movements. For example, if using the *proprioceptive neuromuscular facilitation* (PNF) approach, the occupational therapy practitioner must incorporate PNF patterns in the activity or select activities that naturally use these patterns. For the *neurodevelopmental (Bobath) approach,* postures and movements that inhibit abnormal reflexes and tone are important. Chapter 23

Patient's Name____________________ Age__________ Sex________

Life Stage__________________________________________________

*Educational History*

1. Highest educational level achieved
2. Location and type of schools (public, private, parochial)
3. Subjects of greatest interest
4. Subjects of least interest
5. Average grades achieved
6. Likes/dislikes about school
7. Leisure interests during school years
8. Social groups to which subject belonged
9. Educational level of parents, siblings
10. Future educational plans
11. Career aspirations

*Work History*

1. Most recent work/job performed
2. Previous jobs
3. Special job training (past, present)
4. Likes and dislikes about jobs, past and present
5. Most preferred jobs (real or imagined)
6. Preferences for working alone or with others
7. Works alone or with others
8. Socializes with co-workers (on the job, off the job)
9. Job supervisor
10. Type of supervision received (close, distant)
11. Most effective/desirable type of supervision
12. Plans for future work or job changes

*Leisure Interests and Activities*

1. Interest in sports, games, hobbies (specify)
2. Participation in sports, games, hobbies (when, how long)
3. Other leisure interests that would be pursued given adequate time
4. Are leisure skills considered important to life? Why or why not?

*Values and Cultural Influences*

1. Cultural group with which the patient identifies
2. Describe cultural customs which are important (e.g., celebrations, holiday festivals, foods, religious practices, garments, family traditions).
3. Health practices unique to this culture. Special beliefs about health and illness. Respective roles of ill and well members of family. If raised in another country, attitudes toward health care system in United States. Experiences with U.S. health care system.
4. Describe things (concrete and abstract) that are most valued (e.g., cars, jewels, toys, pictures, family traditions, honesty, integrity, fairness). Why are they valuable?

*Daily Schedule*

Construct a daily schedule for a typical weekday and typical weekend day in the patient's life. Give details for hour-by-hour activities.

*Life Roles*

List all occupational roles of the patient (e.g., worker, father, brother, sportsman, gardener).

*Life Balance*

Approximate percent of time spent by the patient in each of the performance areas of self-maintenance, home and child management, work, and play/leisure.

*Life Tasks*

Review the patient's life stage and adaptive tasks in progress during this stage. Consider how these tasks influence the use of time and choice of activities.

*Figure 15-1* Activity configuration/daily schedule. Outline for interview. (Modified from Cynkin S: *Occupational therapy: toward health through activities,* Boston, 1979, Little, Brown.)

discusses these and other sensorimotor approaches and their applications to activity.

Analysis of the perceptual and cognitive requirements of the activity is particularly important for patients with upper motor neuron disorders, in whom these functions are often disturbed. The OT practitioner must select activities that meet the requirements for motor performance *and* can be performed with some success by these patients.

### *Adapting and Grading Activity*

*Adapting activity* It may be necessary to adapt activities to suit the special needs of the patient or the environment. An activity may need to be performed in a special way to accommodate the patient's residual abilities. Eating with one hand using a special splint with a utensil holder is such an adaptation. An activity may need to be adapted to the patient's positioning or to the environment. An example is setting up a special reading stand and the use of prism glasses to enable a patient to read while in a supine position in bed. **Adaptations of activity** require the OT practitioner to analyze the patient's needs and abilities, the environment, and positioning in relation to the goals of the activity and the treatment program. Problem-solving ability, creativity, and ingenuity in making adaptations are some of the occupational therapy profession's unique skills in rehabilitation.

Adaptation of activity can be a challenge. The OT practitioner should remember that for the adaptations to be used effectively, the patient must be able to use them in a good, comfortable position. The patient must understand the need for and purpose of the activity and the adaptations and be willing to perform the activity with the simple modifications. Peculiar and complicated adaptations that require frequent adjustment and modification should be avoided.[38]

*Grading activity* Activities or the manner in which they are performed may be modified for purposes of grading. **Gradation of activity** allows for gradual improvement by increasing demands for higher and higher levels of performance as the patient's capacity increases. This requires that the activity be appropriately paced and modified to demand the maximal performance from the patient at any point in the treatment process.

At first the demands of the activity often must be reduced to enable performance by the patient with limited capacity. For example, if the required movement patterns or degree of resistance cannot be obtained when the activity is performed in the usual manner, the OT practitioner may make simple modifications. These are usually accepted by the patient provided they are not complex and do not require motions that feel strained and unnatural. The patient's motivation for the activity may fade if artificial movements or excessive resistance are involved. These factors discourage participation and interfere with the development of coordination.[20,38] They also require that the patient focus on movements rather than on the activity's goal. This reduces satisfaction and undermines one of the primary purposes and benefits of purposeful activity described earlier.

Activities may be graded in many ways to accommodate the patient's needs and the treatment objectives. Activities can be graded for increasing strength, ROM, endurance and tolerance, coordination, and perceptual, cognitive, and social skills.

STRENGTH. Strength may be graded by increasing resistance. This is accomplished by changing the plane of movement from gravity decreased to against gravity and by adding weights to the equipment or to the patient, using tools of increasing weight, grading the texture of the materials from soft to hard or fine to rough, or changing to another, more or less resistive activity. For example, a wrap sandbag attached to the wrist could be used to increase resistance to arm movements during macramé. A pulley-and-weight system can be attached to an inclined-plane sanding board to increase resistance to the bi-ceps when the sanding block is pulled downward. Springs may be used to increase resistance on a block printing press. When grasp strength is inadequate, grasp mitts may be used to fasten the hand to a tool or equipment handle to assist grip strength and allow arm motion.

RANGE OF MOTION. Activities for increasing or maintaining joint ROM may be graded by (1) positioning materials and equipment to demand greater reach or excursion of joints or (2) adapting equipment with lengthened handles to facilitate active stretching.

An example of a simple adaptation is positioning a large checkerboard in a vertical orientation to achieve the desired range of shoulder flexion while playing the game (Figure 15-2). Positioning an object, such as a mosaic tile project, at increasing or decreasing distances from the patient on the table top can affect the shoulder and elbow ROM needed to reach the materials. Tool handles may be increased in size by using a larger dowel or by padding the handle with foam rubber to accommodate limited ROM or to facilitate grasp.

ENDURANCE AND TOLERANCE. Endurance may be graded by moving from light to heavy work and increasing the length of the work period. Standing and walking tolerance may be graded by increasing the time spent standing to work, perhaps initially at a stand-up table (Figure 15-3), and increasing the time and distance spent in activities requiring walking. These may include home management and workshop activities.

COORDINATION. Coordination and muscle control may be graded by decreasing gross resistive movements and increasing fine, controlled movements required in a purposeful activity. An example is progressing from sawing wood with a crosscut saw, to using a coping saw, then a jewelers' saw. Dexterity and speed of movement may be graded by practice at increasing speeds once movement patterns have been mastered

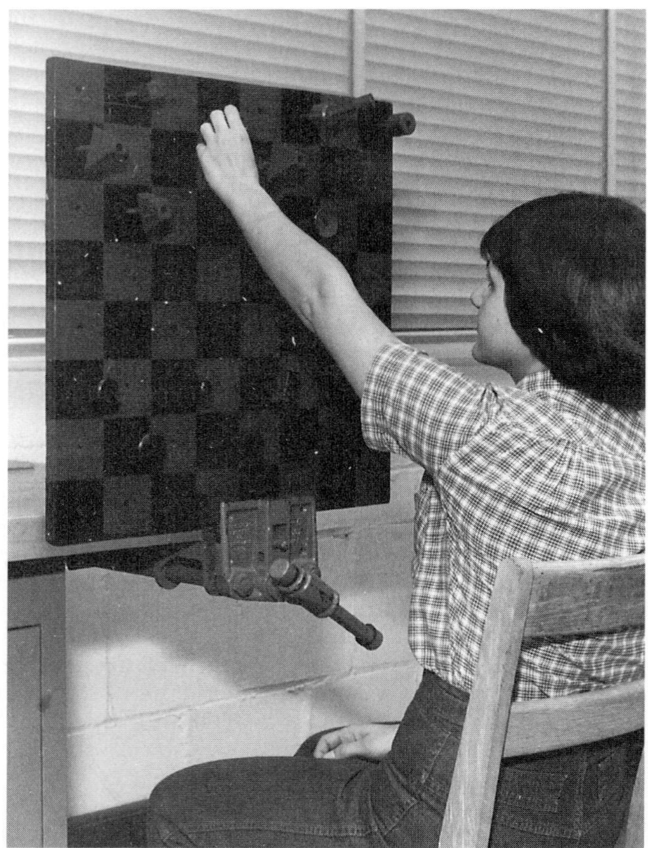

*Figure 15-2* Checkerboard is positioned vertically to increase range of motion (ROM) of shoulder flexion while playing game.

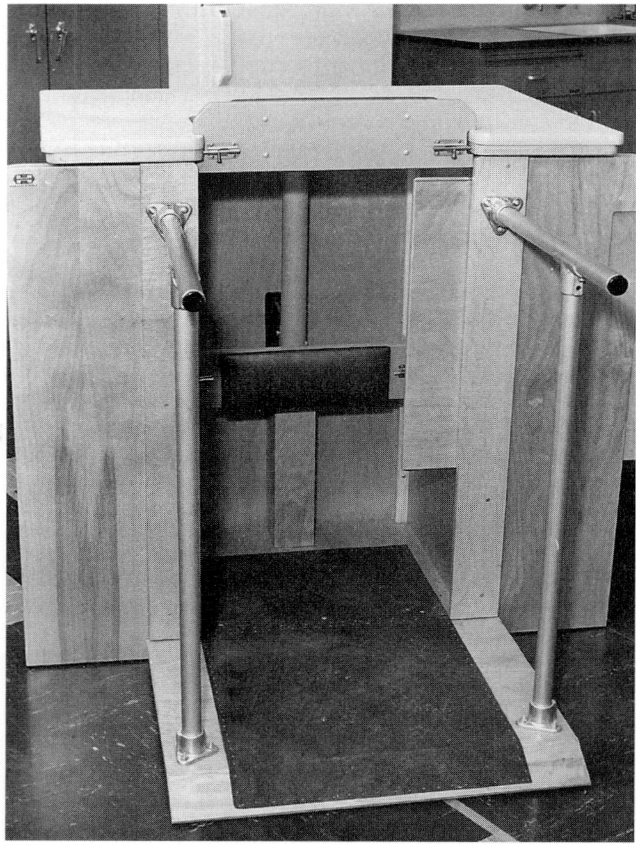

*Figure 15-3* Stand-up table with sliding door, padded knee support, and backrest.

through coordination training and neuromuscular education.

PERCEPTUAL, COGNITIVE, AND SOCIAL SKILLS. Grading activity for increasing cognitive demands requires an analysis of those demands in the given activity. For example, in grading cognitive skills, the treatment program can begin with simple one-step or two-step activities that require minimal judgment, decision making, or problem solving and progress to activities with several steps that require some judgment or problem-solving processes. For example, a patient in a lunch preparation group may be assigned the task of buttering bread that has already been lined up on the work surface. This could be graded to lining up the bread, then buttering it and placing a slice of lunch meat on it, and ultimately to making sandwiches.

Similarly, for grading social interaction, the treatment program may begin with an activity that demands interaction only with the therapist or assistant. The patient can progress to activities requiring dyadic interaction with another patient and eventually to small-group activities. The practitioner can facilitate the patient's progression from the role of observer to that of participant and then to leader. At the same time the OT practitioner would decrease supervision, guidance, and assistance to promote more independent functioning in the patient.

### Selection of Activity

In the treatment of physical dysfunction, activities are usually selected for their potential to improve sensorimotor, neuromusculoskeletal, and psychosocial components. Activities selected for improvement of physical performance should provide targeted exercise or purposeful use of affected parts. They should enable the patient to transfer the motion, strength, and coordination gained in adjunctive and enabling modalities to useful, normal daily activities. If activities are to be used for physical restoration, they must have certain characteristics, as follows[15,38]:

1. Activities should provide action rather than position of involved joints and muscles; that is, they should allow alternate contraction and relaxation of the muscles being exercised and allow the joints to move through their available ROM.
2. Activities should provide repetition of motion. This means that activities should allow for an indefinite but controllable number of repeti-

tions of the desired movement patterns sufficient to be of benefit to the patient.
3. Activities should allow for one or more types of grading, such as for resistance, range, coordination, endurance, or complexity.

The type of exercise needed must be considered. Active and resistive exercises are most often used in the performance of purposeful activity.[38] Requirements for passive and assistive exercise are less easily applied to purposeful activities.

Other important considerations in the selection of activity are (1) the objects and environment required to perform the activity; (2) safety factors; (3) preparation and completion time; (4) complexity; (5) type of instruction and supervision required; (6) structure and controls in the activity; (7) learning requirements; (8) independence, decision making, and problem solving required; (9) social interaction potential; (10) communication skills required; and (11) potential gratification to the patient.

It is assumed that if the OT practitioner selects an activity in which the patient has an interest, the patient will experience enough satisfaction to continue performing the activity. Purposeful activity is thought to provide intrinsic motivation to sustain performance.[39]

Therapy must be individualized for each patient, using evaluative tools such as the interest checklist, activity configuration, occupational history, interview, and activity analysis.[41]

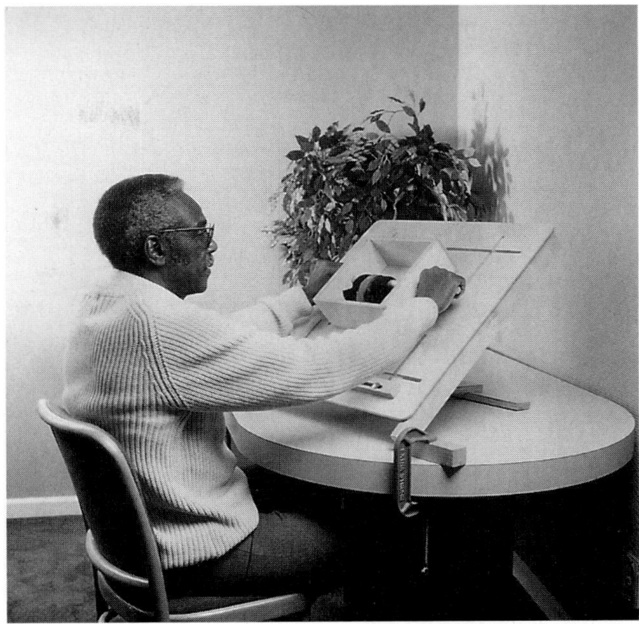

*Figure 15-4* Inclined plane sanding board simulates sanding wood on an inclined plane and is used to exercise elbow and shoulder musculature. (From S & S Worldwide, adapt-Ability, 1995.)

## ENABLING ACTIVITIES

The term *enabling activities* designates a variety of simulations created by occupational therapy practitioners for patients not yet able to engage in purposeful activity. Enabling activities are considered nonpurposeful by the definition given earlier because they generally do not have an inherent goal. Even so, these activities may engage the patient's mental and physical participation, depending on their nature and the patient's motivation.

The purposes of enabling activities are to practice specific motor patterns, train in perceptual and cognitive skills, and practice sensorimotor skills that will be encountered in purposeful activities necessary for functioning in the home and community.

Among the more common enabling activities in occupational therapy is using the inclined sanding board as an exercise (Figure 15-4), probably derived from the activity of woodworking. The activity has no end product and simulates sanding wood on an inclined plane, exercising elbow and shoulder muscles. Moving a series of cones from one side of a table top to the other or stacking cones are other such activities. Cones may be used to train the patient in gross coordination and a combined (out of synergy) movement pattern in the Brunnstrom approach (Figure 15-5). Puzzles and other table-top perceptual and cognitive training media are used to practice visual perceptual functions, motor planning skills, memory, sequencing, and problem solving (Figure 15-6). Use of clothing fastener boards and household hardware boards provides experience in manipulation of everyday objects before the patient is confronted with the

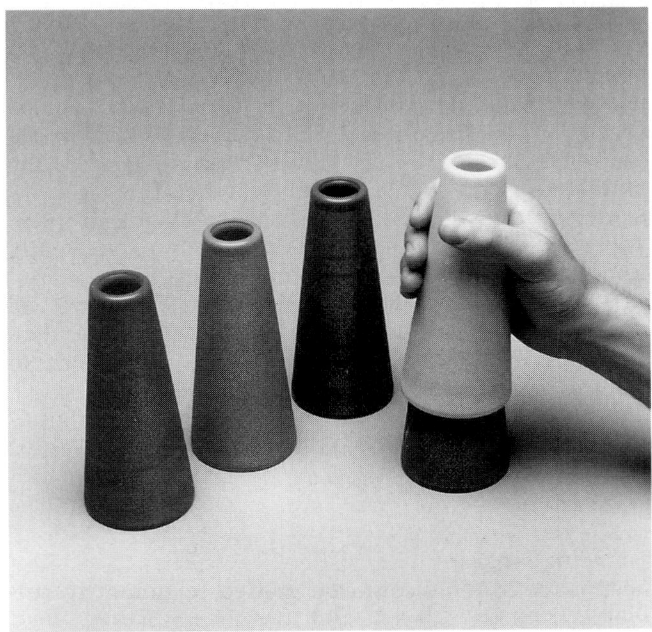

*Figure 15-5* Stacking cones are used to train coordination or specific movement patterns such as reaching and grasping. (Courtesy North Coast Medical, Inc., San Jose, Calif.)

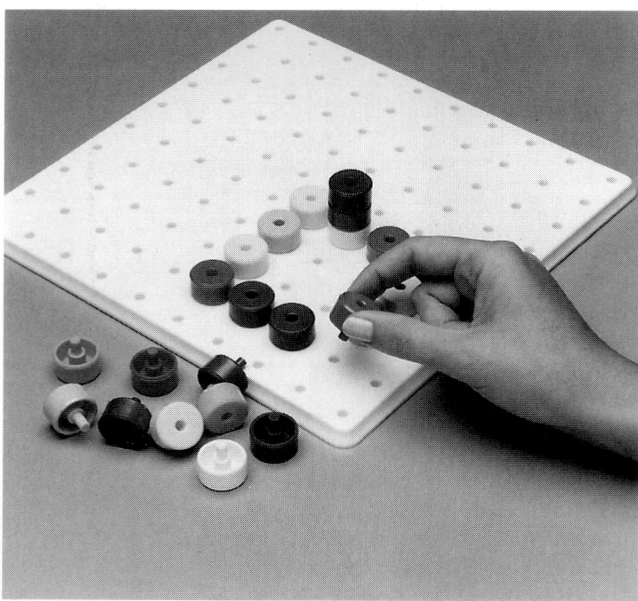

*Figure 15-6* Form, color, pattern, and sequencing skills can be practiced with pegboards and puzzles. (Courtesy North Coast Medical, San Jose, Calif.)

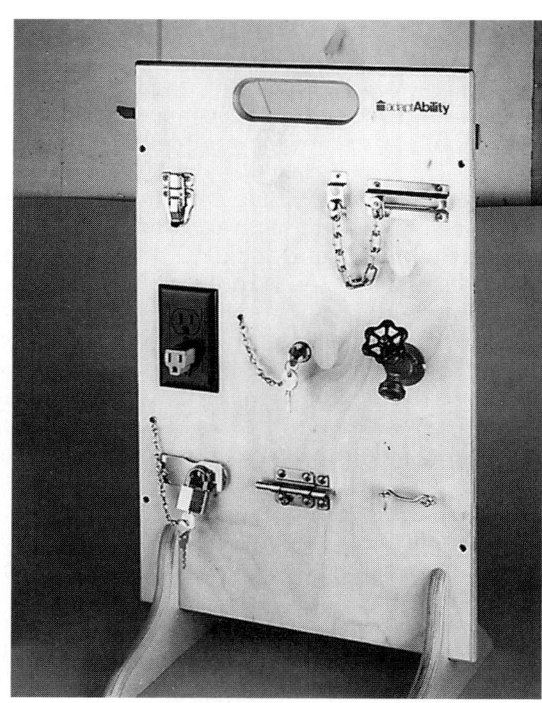


*Figure 15-7* Boards built with household fasteners can be used to practice management of common hardware in the home. (From S & S Worldwide, adaptAbility, 1995.)

real task (Figure 15-7). At a higher level of technological sophistication, commercially available work simulators and computer programs to train patients in using cognitive skills are examples of enabling modalities.

Many enabling modalities in OT practice have been created to facilitate perceptual, cognitive, and motor learning. Such activities may be appropriate for the skill acquisition stage of learning, when the patient is understanding the movement and practicing problem solving. Practice should occur daily or more frequently and feedback given often so that errors are decreased and skills refined to prepare for performance of real-life purposeful activity. These activities should be used judiciously, and their place in the sequence of treatment and motor learning should be well planned. They are often used along with adjunctive modalities and purposeful activities as part of a comprehensive treatment program.

## ADJUNCTIVE MODALITIES

Adjunctive modalities are used before purposeful activity is given. They are meant to prepare the patient for occupational performance. Examples are exercise, orthotics, sensory stimulation, and physical agent modalities.[29] This section presents therapeutic exercise and physical agent modalities in the context of occupational therapy practice. Orthotics is presented separately in Chapters 20 and 22.

### Therapeutic Exercise

Early in the history of occupational therapy, the psychological effects of performing purposeful activity were considered a primary focus in the treatment of persons with physical dysfunction.[17] It was later recognized that physical benefits accrued from the performance of activity. Therapists began to apply kinesiological concepts in selecting appropriate therapeutic activities. To do this, they needed to understand the principles of therapeutic exercise.

As treatment methods evolved, occupational therapists began to use therapeutic exercise alone to prepare patients for purposeful activity and to expedite treatment in a health care system constrained by budget and time. The use of therapeutic exercise as a modality raised considerable controversy.[14] The treatment of patients in acute stages of illness and disability imposed new demands and role responsibilities on OT practitioners. Brief treatment sessions in acute care, the extent of the patient's physical incapacities, and shortened length of stay in hospitals and rehabilitation facilities resulted in occupational therapists expanding the range of modalities used in treatment. It was feared that if OT practitioners used exercise or other preparatory modalities, purposeful activity would be forgotten. Although the principles of exercise had been applied to purposeful activity from early in the history of occupational therapy, exercise now was seen as antithetical (directly opposite) to purposeful activity. Exercise (preparation) and activity (application) are *complementary* to one another in the treatment continuum, and both may be used in a single treatment plan. If only pure exercise is used, the patient has not received occupational therapy.[14] When used by OT practitioners, the purposes of therapeutic exercise should be to remediate sensorimotor dysfunction, augment purposeful activity, and prepare the patient for doing tasks in performance areas.

### *Definition*

**Therapeutic exercise** is any body movement or muscle contraction to prevent or correct a physical impairment, improve musculoskeletal function, and maintain a state of well-being.[9,19] Specific exercise protocols are used to achieve specific goals. Many exercise options are available, and each should be tailored to meet the goals of treatment and the specific capacities and precautions relative to the patient's physical condition. Exercise can be used to increase ROM and flexibility, strength, coordination, endurance, and cardiovascular fitness.[19]

### *Purposes*

The general purposes of therapeutic exercise are to accomplish the following[31]:

1. Develop awareness of normal movement patterns and improve voluntary, automatic movement responses.
2. Develop strength and endurance in patterns of movement that are acceptable and necessary and do not produce deformity.
3. Improve coordination, regardless of strength.
4. Increase specific power of desired isolated muscles or muscle groups.
5. Assist in overcoming ROM deficits.
6. Increase strength of muscles needed to use hand splints, mobile arm supports, and other devices.
7. Increase work tolerance and physical endurance through increased strength.
8. Prevent or eliminate contractures developing as a result of imbalanced muscle power by strengthening the antagonistic muscles.

### *Prerequisites for Use*

For therapeutic exercise to be effective, the patient must meet certain criteria. Therapeutic exercise is most effective in the treatment of orthopedic disorders (e.g., fractures, arthritis) and lower motor neuron disorders that produce weakness and flaccidity (e.g., peripheral nerve injuries and diseases, poliomyelitis, Guillain-Barré syndrome, infectious neuronitis, spinal cord injuries and diseases).

Therapeutic exercise is contraindicated for patients who have poor general health or inflamed joints or who have had recent surgery.[30] It may not be useful in patients with severely limited joint ROM caused by well-established, permanent contractures. As defined and described here, therapeutic exercise cannot be used effectively with those who have spasticity and lack voluntary control of isolated motion or those who cannot control dyskinetic movement (involuntary movements such as tics). Dyskinetic movement is likely to occur with upper motor neuron disorders; these are more amenable to exercise regimens of the sensorimotor approaches to treatment (see Chapter 23).

The candidate for therapeutic exercise must be medically able to participate in the exercise regimen, be able to understand the directions for the exercise and its purposes, and be interested and motivated to perform the exercise. The patient must have available motor pathways and the potential for recovery or improvement of strength, ROM, coordination, or movement patterns, as applicable. It is important that some sensory feedback is available to the patient. This means that sensation must be at least partially intact so that the patient can perceive motion and position of the exercised part and have some sense of superficial and deep pain. Muscles and tendons must be intact, stable, and free to move. Joints must be able to move through an effective ROM for those types of exercise that use joint motion as part of the procedure. The patient should be relatively free of pain during motion and should be able to perform isolated, coordinated movement. If any dyskinetic movement occurs, the patient should be able to control it so that the exercise procedure can be performed as prescribed.[30]

### *Types of Exercise*

*Exercise to increase muscle strength* Active-assisted, active, and resistive isotonic and isometric exercises are used to increase strength. After partial or complete denervation of muscle and during inactivity or disuse, muscle strength decreases. When strength is inadequate, substitution patterns are likely to develop.[43] A *substitution* is the use of muscle groups and patterns of motion not ordinarily used because of loss or weakness of the muscles normally used to perform a movement. An example is using shoulder abduction to achieve a hand-to-mouth movement if elbow flexors cannot perform against gravity (Figure 15-8). When muscle loss is permanent, some substitution patterns may be beneficial as a compensatory measure to improve performance of functional activities. Many are not beneficial, however, and the aim of therapeutic exercise often is to prevent or correct substitution patterns.[43]

To increase strength, a muscle must contract at or near its maximal capacity and for enough repetitions and length of time. Strengthening programs generally are based on having the muscle contract against a large resistance for a few repetitions. Strengthening exercises are *not* effective if the contraction is insufficient.[9,21]

Excess strengthening, however, may result in muscle fatigue, pain, and temporary reduction of strength. If a muscle is overworked, it becomes fatigued and is not able to contract. Selection of the type of exercise must suit the muscle grade and the patient's fatigue tolerance level. Fatigue level varies from individual to individual, and the threshold for muscle fatigue decreases in pathological states.[21] Many patients may not be sensitive to fatigue or may push themselves beyond tolerance in the belief that this

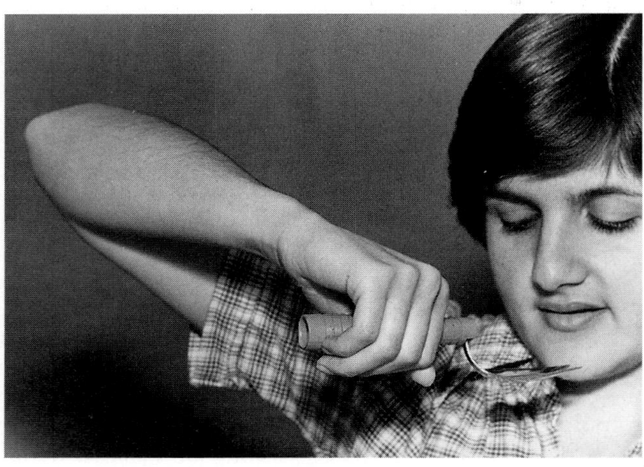

*Figure 15-8* Shoulder abductors may substitute for weak elbow flexors in hand-to-mouth movements.

hastens recovery. This means that the OTR must make a careful evaluation of the patient's muscle power and capacity for exercise. The OTR or COTA providing treatment must also supervise the patient closely and observe for signs of fatigue. These signs may be slowed performance, distraction, perspiration, increase in rate of respiration, performance of exercise pattern through a decreased ROM, and inability to complete the prescribed number of repetitions.

*Exercise to increase muscle endurance* *Endurance* is the ability of the muscle to work for prolonged periods and resist fatigue. Whereas a high-load, low-repetition regimen is effective for muscle strengthening, a low-load, high-repetition exercise program is more effective for building endurance.[9,12] Having determined the patient's maximal capacity for a strengthening program, the practitioner can reduce the maximum resistance load and increase the number of repetitions to adapt the strengthening program to build endurance. This approach is used to build endurance in specific muscles or muscle groups. The strength-versus-endurance training may be seen on a continuum. Resistance and number of repetitions can be modulated to achieve gains in both strength and endurance.[9]

*Exercise for physical conditioning and cardiovascular fitness* Exercise to improve general physical endurance and cardiovascular fitness uses large muscle groups in sustained, rhythmical aerobic exercise or activity. Examples are swimming, walking, bicycling, jogging, and some games and sports. This type of exercise is often used in cardiac rehabilitation programs, in which the parameters of the patient's physical capacities and tolerance for exercise should be well defined and medically supervised. To improve cardiovascular fitness, exercise should be done 3 to 5 days per week, at 60% to 90% of maximum heart rate or 50% to 85% of maximum oxygen uptake. From 15 to 60 minutes of exercise with rhythmical activities using large muscle groups is recommended.[9]

*Exercise for range of motion and joint flexibility* Active and passive ROM exercises are used to maintain joint motion and flexibility. Active exercise is done by the performer and passive exercise by an outside force, such as the therapist or assistant or a device such as the continuous passive motion machine. This is a mechanical device that can be preset to provide continuous passive motion throughout the joint ROM. The device must be used cautiously and must be carefully monitored to prevent mishaps and possible harm to the patient.[9]

Stretching or forced exercise is necessary to increase ROM. Some type of force is applied to the part when soft tissue (muscles, tendons, ligaments) is at or near its available length. The use of a low-resistance stretch of sustained duration is more effective than high-resistance, repetitive, quick bouncing movements. Low-resistance, sustained stretch is less likely to produce tissue tearing, trauma, or activation of stretch reflexes in hypertonic muscles. The use of thermal agents (see later discussion) or neuromuscular facilitation techniques (see Chapter 23) may enhance static stretching.[9]

*Exercise to improve coordination* *Coordination* is the combined activity of many muscles into smooth patterns and sequences of motion. Coordination is an automatic response monitored primarily through proprioceptive sensory feedback. Kottke[20] differentiated neuromuscular control from coordination. He defined *control* as "the conscious activation of an individual muscle or the conscious initiation of a preprogrammed engram." Control involves conscious attention to and guidance of an activity.

An **engram** is a preprogrammed pattern of muscular activity as it is represented in the central nervous system (CNS). An engram is formed only after many repetitions of a specific motion or activity. With repetition, conscious effort decreases, and the motion becomes more and more automatic. Ultimately the motion can be performed with little conscious attention. When an engram is excited, the same pattern of movement is produced automatically. Brushing one's teeth is an example of an engram.

Procedures for the development of neuromuscular control and neuromuscular coordination are briefly outlined in the section on exercise classification. The reader is referred to the original sources for a full discussion of the neurophysiological mechanisms underlying these exercises. Neuromuscular education or control training involves teaching the patient to control individual muscles or motions through conscious attention. Coordination training is used to develop preprogrammed multimuscular patterns (engrams).[20]

### *Types of Muscle Contraction Used in Therapeutic Exercise*[16,21]

*Isometric or static contraction* During an **isometric (static) contraction,** no joint motion occurs, and the muscle length remains the same. The muscle is set (contracted), or a muscle and its antagonist are contracted at a point in the ROM to stabilize a joint. This may occur without resistance or against some outside resistance, such as the practitioner's hand or a fixed object. An example of isometric exercise of the triceps against resistance is pressing against a table top with the ulnar border of the forearm while the elbow remains at 90° flexion.

*Isotonic or concentric contraction* During an **isotonic (concentric) contraction,** joint motion occurs and the muscle shortens. This may be done with or without resistance. Isotonic contractions may be performed in positions with gravity decreased or against gravity, according to the patient's muscle grade and the goal of the exercise. An isotonic contraction of the biceps is used when lifting a fork to the mouth for eating.

*Eccentric contraction* When muscles contract eccentrically, the tension in the muscle increases or remains constant while the muscle lengthens. This may be done with or without resistance. An example of an **eccentric contraction** performed without resistance is the slow lowering of the arm to the table. The biceps is contracting eccentrically in this instance. An example of eccentric contraction against resistance is the controlled return of a pail of sand lifted from the ground. In this case the biceps is contracting eccentrically to control the rate and coordination of the elbow extension in setting the pail on the ground.

### *Exercise Classification*

The occupational therapist selects from the following types of exercise, considering the patient's muscle grade, muscle endurance, joint mobility, diagnosis and physical condition, treatment goals, position, and the desired plane of movement.

*Isotonic resistive exercise* Resistive exercise uses isotonic muscle contraction against a specific amount of weight to move the load through a given range of motion.[9,16,21] Eccentric contraction may also be used against resistance. **Isotonic resistive exercise** is used primarily for increasing strength of fair plus (F+) to normal (N) muscles but may also be helpful for producing relaxation of the antagonists to the contracting muscles. This latter purpose can be useful if increased ROM is desired for stretching or relaxing hypertonic antagonists.

The patient performs muscle contraction against resistance and moves the part through the available ROM. The resistance applied should be the maximum against which the muscle is capable of contracting. Resistance may be applied manually or by weights, springs, elastic bands, sandbags, or special exercise devices. It is graded by progressively increasing the amount of resistance (Figure 15-9).[9,16,21] The number of repetitions that are possible will depend on the patient's general physical endurance and the endurance of the specific muscle. A variety of strength training programs exist, based on the principle that to increase strength, the muscle must contract against its maximal resistance. The number of repetitions, rest intervals, frequency of training, and speed of movement vary with the particular approach and the patient's ability to accommodate to the exercise regime.[9]

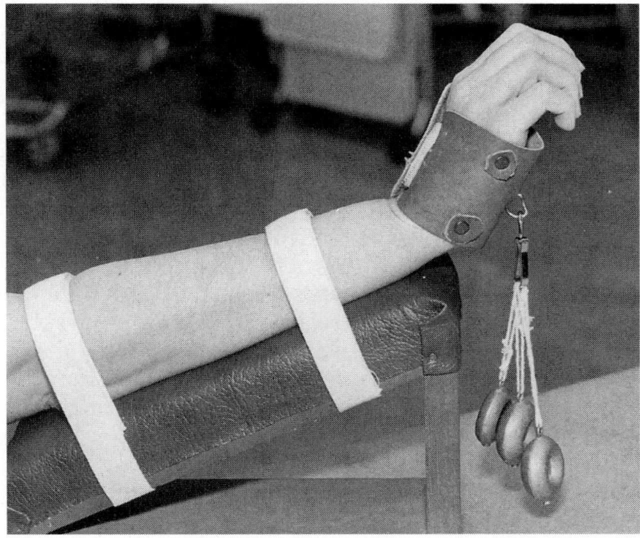

*Figure 15-9* Resistive exercise for wrist extensors. Forearm is stabilized, and a handcuff compensates for weak grasp.

One specialized type of resistive exercise is the DeLorme method of *progressive resistive exercise* (PRE).[12,36] PRE is based on the overload principle: muscles perform more efficiently if given a "warm-up" period and must be taxed beyond usual daily activity to improve in performance and strength.[12]

During the exercise procedure, small loads are used initially. These are increased gradually after each set of 10 repetitions of the desired movement. The muscle is thus warmed up to prepare to exert its maximal power for the final 10 repetitions. The exercise procedure consists of three sets of 10 repetitions each, with resistance applied as follows: (1) first set, 10 repetitions at 50% of maximal resistance; (2) second set, 10 repetitions at 75% of maximal resistance; and (3) third set, 10 repetitions at maximal resistance.[9,12,36] The load must be chosen carefully so that the patient can perform all 10 repetitions. As strength improves, resistance is increased so that 10 repetitions can always be performed.[9] The patient is instructed to inhale during the shortening contraction and exhale during the relaxation or eccentric contraction.[12,36]

An example of a PRE is a triceps, capable of 12 pounds maximal resistance, extending the elbow, first against 6 pounds, then against 9 pounds, and the final 10 repetitions against 12 pounds. *Maximal resistance,* the amount of resistance the muscle can lift through the ROM 10 times, is determined by the following procedure. The patient is instructed to contract the muscle and move the part through the full ROM against progressively increasing loads for sets of 10 repetitions until the maximal load that can be lifted 10 times is reached.

At the start of the treatment program, the OT practitioner often has difficulty determining the maximal resistance the patient can handle. This may be because the patient (1) may not know how to exert maximal effort, (2) may be reluctant to exercise strenuously for fear of pain or reinjury, (3) may be unwilling or unable to endure discomfort, and (4) may have difficulty with timing of exercises.

The practitioner's experience and trial and error help in determining maximal resistance. The practitioner should estimate the amount of resistance the patient can take based on the muscle test results and then add or subtract resistance (weight or tension) until the patient can perform the sets of repetitions adequately.

The exercises should be performed once daily four or five times weekly. Rest periods of 2 to 4 minutes should be allowed between each set of 10 repetitions. Modifications of the exercise procedure may be made to suit individual needs. Some possibilities are 10 repetitions at 25% of maximal resistance, 10 repetitions at 50%, 10 repetitions at 75%, and 10 repetitions at maximal resistance. Another possibility is five repetitions at 50% and 10 repetitions at maximal resistance. Still another possibility is to omit the second set of exercises. Adjustments in the first two sets of exercises may be made to suit the individual's capacity.[12]

Another approach is the *Oxford technique,* essentially a reverse of the DeLorme method. The exercise sequence begins with 100% resistance, decreases to 75%, then to 50% on subsequent sets of 10 repetitions each.[12,36] The greatest gains may be made in the early weeks of the treatment program, with smaller increases occurring at a slower pace in the subsequent weeks or months. During the performance of any strengthening exercise, the OT practitioner should ensure joint alignment of the exercise device, proper fit and adjustment of the device; no substitute movements, and clear instructions on the patient's speed, ROM, and proper breathing.[12,31]

APPLICATION TO ACTIVITY. Many purposeful activities are performed using resistive exercise. For instance, leather lacing, if the lace is pulled in an upward direction, can offer slight resistance to the anterior deltoid. Sanding with a weighted sand block can provide significant resistance to the anterior deltoid and triceps if done on an inclined-plane sanding board. Activities such as sawing and hammering offer resistance to upper extremity musculature. Kneading dough and forming clay objects present varying degrees of resistance to hand muscles. Rolling pie crust, cookie dough, or clay with a rolling pin can provide resistive exercise to shoulder and elbow motions.

*Isotonic active exercise* Isotonic muscle contraction is used in active exercise. Eccentric contraction may also be used. **Isotonic active exercise** is done when the patient moves the joint through its available ROM against no outside resistance.

Poor (P) to fair (F) muscles can gain strength and maintain ROM through active motion exercise of the complete ROM with gravity decreased or against gravity. Active motion may be used with higher muscle grades to maintain strength and ROM when resistance is contraindicated. Active exercise is *not* used to *increase* ROM because this requires added force not present in active exercise.

In active exercise the patient moves the part through the complete ROM independently. If the exercise is performed in a gravity-decreased plane, the resistance produced by friction may be reduced by using a powdered surface, skateboard, deltoid aid, or free-moving suspension sling. Exercise is graded by changing to a more resistive form as strength improves.[16,21]

APPLICATION TO ACTIVITY. Activities that offer little or no resistance can be used as active exercise. A needlework activity performed in the gravity-decreased plane can provide active exercise to the wrist extensors or elbow extensors. When a grade of F or 3 is reached, the wrist can be moved against gravity in an activity such as picking up and placing tiles for a mosaic tile project.

*Active-assisted exercise* Isotonic muscle contraction is used in active-assisted exercise. The patient moves the joint through partial ROM, and the range is completed by the occupational therapy practitioner (Figure 15-10) or a mechanical device. Mechanical assistance may be supplied by slings, pulleys, weights, springs, or elastic bands (Figure 15-11).[36] The goal of **active-assisted exercise** is to increase strength of trace (T), poor minus (P–), and fair minus (F–) muscles while maintaining ROM. With T muscles the patient may contract the muscle, and the therapist or assistant completes the entire ROM. This exercise is graded by decreasing the amount of assistance until the patient can perform active exercises.[16,21]

APPLICATION TO ACTIVITY. If assistance is required to complete the movement, an activity must be structured so that assistance can be offered by the OT practitioner, the patient's other arm or leg, or a mechanical device. Various bilateral activities are performed using active-assisted exercise, such as bilateral sanding, bilateral sponge wiping, using a sweeper, and sawing. In bilateral activities the unaffected arm or leg can perform the major portion of the work, and the affected arm or leg can assist to the extent possible.

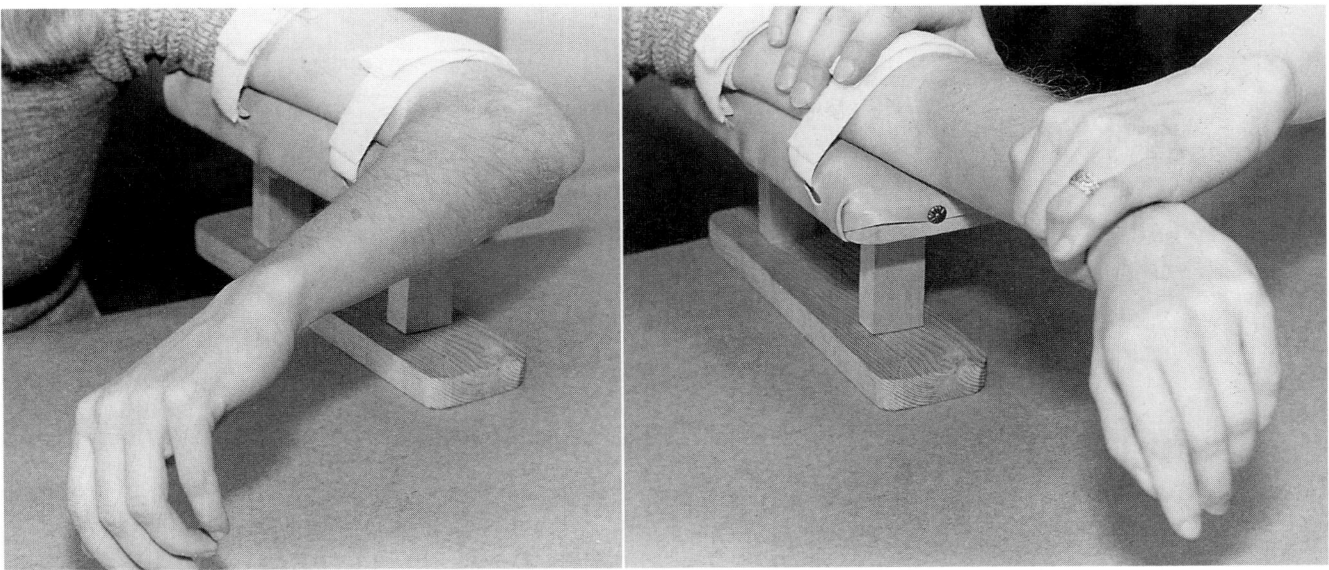


*Figure 15-10* Active-assisted exercise. **A,** Patient actively extends elbow toward extension from position of full flexion. Gravity-decreased position maximizes active movement. **B,** OT practitioner assists patient to complete range of motion.

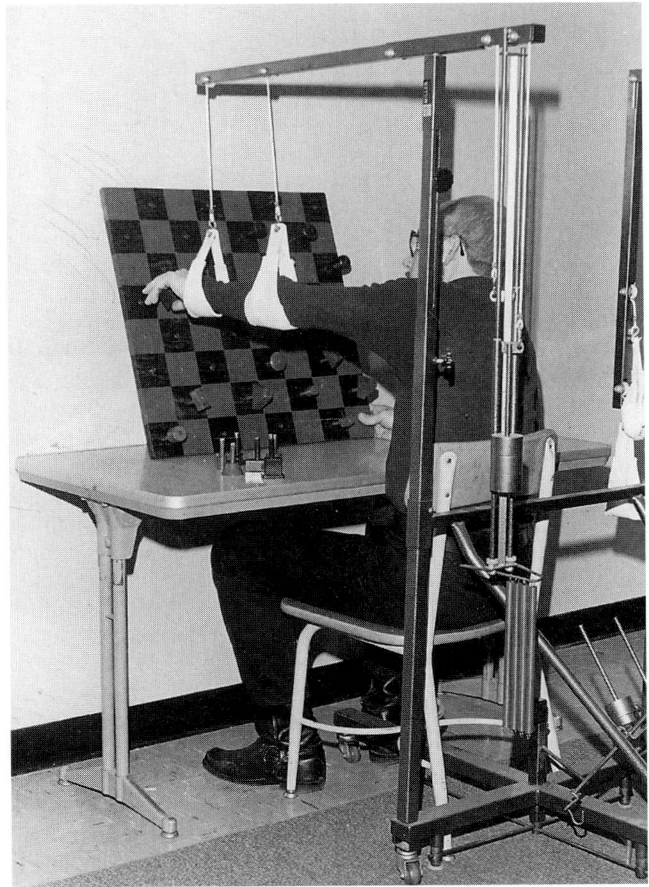

*Figure 15-11* Active-assisted exercise. Deltoid aid reduces effects of gravity, thus permitting greater range of active reaching in shoulder movements.

*Passive exercise* In passive exercise, *no* muscle contraction occurs. Muscle strength cannot be increased by passive exercise. Passive exercise is not useful to increase ROM because no force is applied to the joint. The purpose of **passive exercise** is to maintain ROM, thereby preventing contractures and adhesions and deformity.

To achieve this goal, passive exercise should be performed for at least three repetitions, twice daily.[19] It is used when absent or minimal muscle strength (grades 0 to T) precludes active motion or when active exercise is contraindicated because of the patient's physical condition. During the exercise procedure the joint or joints to be exercised are moved through their normal ROMs manually by the therapist/assistant or patient or mechanically by an external device, such as a pulley or counterbalance sling. The joint proximal to the joint being exercised should be stabilized during the exercise procedure[16] (Figure 15-12).

APPLICATION TO ACTIVITY. A passive limb often can be included in a bilateral activity if the contralateral limb is unaffected. Several of the activities described earlier for active-assisted exercise can be used for passive exercise as well.

*Passive stretch* When doing passive stretching, the OT practitioner moves the joint through the available ROM and holds momentarily at the end of the ROM, applying a gentle but firm force or stretch. The patient should have no residual pain when the stretching is discontinued. **Passive stretch,** or forced exercise, increases ROM. It is used when a loss of joint ROM occurs, and when stretching is not contraindicated.

If the patient's muscle grades are adequate, the patient can move the part actively through the avail-

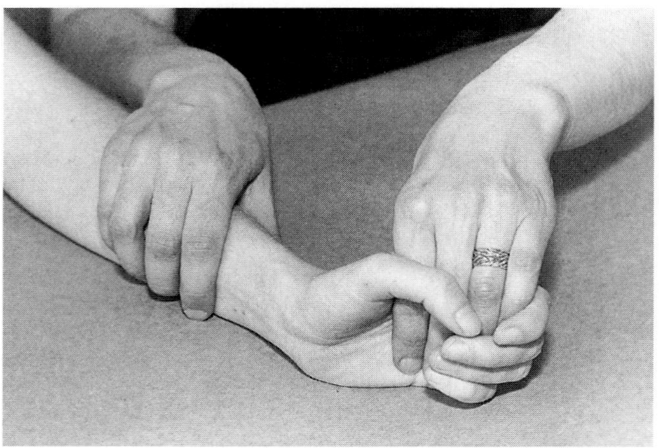

*Figure 15-12* Passive exercise. OT practitioner manually moves patient's wrist through range of motion. Proximal bone (forearm) is stabilized by clinician's other hand.

able ROM, and the OTR or COTA can take it slightly farther, thus forcing or stretching the soft tissue structures around the joint.

Passive stretching requires a good understanding of joint anatomy and muscle function (Box 15-1). It should be performed cautiously under proper medical supervision and with medical approval. Muscles to be stretched should be in a relaxed state.[21] The OT practitioner should never force muscles when pain is present unless the physician prescribes that the patient work through pain. Gentle, firm stretching held for several seconds is more effective and less hazardous than quick, short stretching. The parts around the area being stretched should be stabilized and compensatory movements prevented. Incorrect stretching procedures can produce muscle tearing, joint fracture, and inflammatory edema.[19]

APPLICATION TO ACTIVITY. Passive stretching may be incorporated into an activity if an unaffected part guides the movement of the affected part and forces it slightly beyond the available ROM. One example is the passive stretch of wrist flexors during a block-printing activity if the block is pressed down with the open hand while the patient is standing.

*Active stretch* The purpose of **active stretch** is the same as for passive stretch, that is, to increase joint ROM, especially in a contracted muscle. In active stretching the patient uses the force of antagonist muscles to increase the length of the contracted agonist muscle (Box 15-2). Active stretching requires good to normal strength of the antagonist, good coordination, and motivation of the patient. For example, forceful contraction of the triceps will stretch the biceps muscle. Because the exercise may produce discomfort, the patient tends to avoid the stretching component of the movement. Therefore supervision and frequent evaluation of its effectiveness are necessary.

*Box 15-1*

## Passive Stretching

**Guidelines**

1. Work under medical supervision and with medical approval.
2. Understand joint anatomy and muscle function.

**Procedure**

1. Stabilize parts around area to be stretched.
2. Prevent compensatory movements.
3. Make sure muscle is relaxed before stretching.
4. Apply gentle, firm, prolonged stretch, holding for several seconds up to 45 seconds.

*Box 15-2*

## Active Stretching

**Guidelines and procedure**

1. Make sure that antagonist muscles have good to normal muscle strength.
2. Educate patient as to proper position so as to prevent compensatory movements.
3. Observe patient carefully, and correct as needed.
4. Evaluate effectiveness frequently.

APPLICATION TO ACTIVITY. Many activities can be used to incorporate active stretching. Slowly sawing wood, for example, requires a forceful contraction of the triceps with a concomitant stretch of the biceps.

*Isometric exercise without resistance* Isometric exercise uses isometric contractions of a specific muscle or muscle group. In **isometric exercise** a muscle or group of muscles is actively contracted and relaxed without producing motion of the joint that it usually mobilizes.

The purpose of isometric exercise without resistance is to maintain muscle strength when active motion is not possible or is contraindicated. It may be used with any muscle grade above trace. It is especially useful for patients in casts, after surgery, and with arthritis or burns.[9]

The patient is taught to "set" or contract the muscles voluntarily and to hold the contraction for 5 or 6 seconds (Box 15-3). The OT practitioner's fingers may be placed distal to the joint on which the muscles act. Without offering resistance, the fingers provide a kinesthetic image of resistance and help the patient learn to set the muscle. If passive motion is allowed, the practitioner may move the joint to the desired point in the ROM and ask the patient to hold the position.

Isometric exercise affects the cardiovascular system, which may be a contraindication for some patients. It

Box 15-3

### Isometric Exercise Without Resistance

**Guidelines and procedure**

1. Observe precautions because this exercise may increase blood pressure suddenly. *Do not use* in patients with hypertension or cardiovascular problems.
2. Teach patient to set or hold muscles voluntarily.
3. To increase patient awareness of muscle contraction, apply light fingertip input distal to joint on which muscles act.
4. Instruct patient to hold contraction for specified time and to perform specified number of repetitions.

Box 15-4

### Isometric Exercise Against Resistance

**Guidelines and procedure**

1. Observe precautions because this exercise may increase blood pressure suddenly. *Do not use* in patients with hypertension or cardiovascular problems.
2. Use with muscles graded fair plus (F+) and above.
3. Apply resistance manually, or use weights or other graded resistive devices.
4. Teach patient to set or hold muscles voluntarily at a fixed position (generally neutral).
5. Instruct patient to hold contraction for 5 or 6 seconds and to perform specified number of repetitions.
6. Instruct or supervise patient to perform exercises once a day, 5 days a week.

may cause a rapid, sudden increase in blood pressure, depending on the patient's age, intensity of contraction, and muscle mass being contracted. Therefore this exercise should be performed with caution.[9]

*Isometric exercise with resistance* Isometric exercise with applied resistance uses isometric muscle contraction performed against some outside resistance. Its purpose is to increase muscle strength of muscles graded fair plus or 3+ to normal or 5. The patient sets the muscle or muscle group while resistance is applied and holds the contraction for 5 or 6 seconds. Isometric exercises should be performed for one exercise session per day, 5 days a week. Besides manual resistance, the patient may hold a weight or resist against a solid surface, depending on the muscle group being exercised. A small weight held in the hand while the wrist is stabilized in a neutral position requires isometric contractions of the wrist flexors and extensors (Box 15-4).

Muscle strength is graded by increasing the amount of outside resistance or the degree of force against which the patient resists. A tension gauge should be used to monitor accurately the amount of resistance applied. Isometric exercises are effective for increasing strength and endurance, but isotonic exercise usually is the method of choice for these purposes. Isometric exercise has several specific applications, as in arthritis, when joint motion may be contraindicated but muscle strength must be increased or maintained.[16,31] The cardiovascular precautions previously stated are particularly important with isometric resistive exercise.

APPLICATION TO ACTIVITY. Any activity that requires holding or static posture incorporates isometric exercise. Holding tool handles or holding the arm in elevation while painting are examples. This type of exercise, if contraction is sustained, can be very fatiguing.

*Exercise for neuromuscular control* In this form of exercise the patient is taught to control individual prime movers that are too weak to be used normally. The purpose of exercise for **neuromuscular control** is to improve muscle strength and muscle coordination toward normal motor patterns. To achieve these ends, the patient must learn precise control of the muscle.

To participate successfully, the patient must be able to learn and follow instructions, cooperate, and concentrate on the muscular retraining. Before beginning, the patient should be comfortable and securely supported. The exercises should be performed in a nondistracting environment, and the patient must be alert, calm, and rested. There should be an adequate pain-free arc of motion of the joint on which the muscle acts, as well as good proprioception. Visual and tactile sensory feedback may be used to compensate or substitute for limited proprioception, but the coordination achieved will never be as great as when proprioception is intact (Box 15-5).

PROCEDURE. Passive motion is used to stimulate the proprioceptive stretch reflex and to develop the patient's awareness of the desired motion and the muscles involved. This passive movement may be repeated several times. The patient's awareness may be enhanced if the OT practitioner also demonstrates the desired movement and if the movement is performed by the analogous unaffected part. The skin over the muscle belly and tendon insertion may be stimulated to enhance the effect of the stretch reflex. Stroking and tapping over the muscle belly may also be used by practitioners trained in this technique to facilitate muscle action.[20]

The OTR or COTA should explain the location and function of the muscle, its origin and insertion, line of pull, and action on the joint. The practitioner should then demonstrate the motion and instruct the patient to think of the pull of the muscle from insertion to origin. The skin over the muscle insertion can be stroked in the

Box 15-5

## Exercise for Neuromuscular Control of Individual Muscles

**Guidelines**

1. Ascertain that patient is capable of learning and following directions, is cooperative, and is able to concentrate on muscle retraining.
2. Eliminate distractions in environment.
3. Make sure that patient is calm, alert, and rested.
4. Make sure that sufficient pain-free range of motion (ROM) exists in joint on which targeted muscle acts.
5. Ascertain whether patient has adequate proprioception. If not, compensate through visual and tactile feedback.

**Procedure**

1. Explain to patient the muscle's location and function, origin and insertion, line of pull, and action on joint.
2. Instruct patient to think about motion while therapist or assistant performs it passively and strokes skin over muscle's insertion, stroking in direction of motion.
3. Instruct patient to assist by contracting muscle while OT practitioner performs passive motion and stimulates skin as before.
4. Instruct patient to move part through ROM with assistance and cutaneous stimulation while therapist or assistant emphasizes contraction of prime mover only.
5. Instruct patient to perform movement independently, using prime mover.

direction of the pull while the patient concentrates on the sensation of the motion during the passive movement performed by the therapist or assistant.

The exercise sequence begins with instructing the patient to think about the motion while the practitioner performs it passively and strokes the skin over the muscle's insertion in the direction of the motion. The patient is then instructed to assist by contracting the muscle while the clinician performs passive motion and stimulates the skin as before. Next, the patient moves the part through the ROM with assistance and cutaneous stimulation while the clinician emphasizes contraction of the prime mover only. Finally, the patient carries out the movement independently, using the prime mover.

Coordination exercises must begin with minimal or no resistance if activity is to be isolated to prime movers. If the muscle is very weak (trace to poor), the procedure may be carried out entirely in an active-assisted manner so that the muscle contracts against no resistance and can function alone.

Progression from one step to the next depends on successful performance of each step without substitutions. Each step is performed three to five times per training session for each muscle to be exercised, depending on the patient's exercise tolerance.

*Exercise for training coordination* The goal of coordination training is to develop the ability to perform multimuscular motor patterns that are faster, more precise, and stronger than those performed when only control of individual muscles is used. The development of coordination depends on repetition. Initially the movement must be simple and slow so that the patient can be consciously aware of the activity and its components. Good coordination does not develop until repeated practice results in a well-developed activity pattern that no longer requires the patient's conscious effort and attention.

PROCEDURE. Training should take place in an environment in which the patient can concentrate and perform the given exercise accurately. The exercise is divided into components that the patient can perform correctly. It is important to keep the effort low by reducing speed and resistance to prevent the spread of excitation to muscles that are not part of the desired movement pattern (Box 15-6).

When the motor pattern is divided into units that the patient can perform successfully, each unit is trained by practicing it under voluntary control. The OTR or COTA instructs the patient in the desired movement and uses sensory stimulation and passive movement. The patient must observe and voluntarily modify the motion. Slow practice is imperative to make this monitoring possible. The OT practitioner must offer enough assistance to ensure precise movement and patient concentration on the sensations produced by the movements. With concentration on movement, fatigue occurs rapidly, and the patient should be allowed frequent, short rests. As the patient masters the components of the pattern and performs them precisely and independently, the exercise sequence is graded to subtasks or several components that are practiced repetitively. As the engrams for the subtasks are perfected, they are progressively linked together until the movement pattern can be performed.

The exercise can be graded for speed, force, or complexity, but the OT practitioner must remember that this increases the patient's effort and may result in incoordinated movement. Therefore the grading must remain within the patient's capacity to perform the precise movement pattern.

The motor pattern must be performed correctly, or faulty engrams will develop. Constant repetition of an incoordinated pattern reinforces it, resulting in persistent incoordination. Factors that increase incoordination are fear, poor balance, too much resistance, pain, fatigue, strong emotions, and prolonged inactivity.[20]

APPLICATION TO ACTIVITY. Occupational therapy can be used to develop coordination, strength, and endurance. OT activities have the advantage of engaging the patient's attention and interest. Activities should be structured to enable the patient to use the precise

Box 15-6

**Exercise for Training Coordination of Multiple Muscles**

**Guidelines**

1. Ascertain that patient is capable of learning and following directions, is cooperative, and is able to concentrate.
2. Eliminate distractions in environment.
3. Make sure that patient is calm, alert, and rested.
4. Divide exercise into component segments that patient can perform correctly. Practice *one* component at a time.
5. Reduce speed and resistance to keep effort low so that other muscles (outside targeted pattern) are not excited. Keep speed *slow.*
6. Mental fatigue occurs rapidly because patient is required to concentrate intensely. Provide *frequent* short rests.
7. Do *not* permit patient to repeat incorrect or incoordinated patterns. Instead, have patient rest, determine source of error, and reinstruct.

**Procedure**

1. Instruct the patient in the movements of the first component segment.
2. Use sensory stimulation and passive movement (see steps 2 through 5 of boxed material on exercise for neuromuscular control of individual muscles).
3. Assist patient as needed to make sure movement is precise.
4. Add new components as patient masters previous ones. Link components into subtasks or sequences of components by chaining.

movement pattern and to work at speeds sufficiently slow to maintain precision.

OTRs, often consulting with physical therapists, may initiate coordination training with neuromuscular education and progress to repetitive activities requiring desired coordinated movement patterns. The COTA can acquire service competency in this area, given sufficient information on muscle actions and synergies and sufficient time to integrate and apply this information. Examples of enabling activities that demand repetitive patterns of nonresistive movement are placing small blocks, marbles, cones, paper cups, or pegs. These can later be translated to more purposeful activities, such as leather lacing, mosaic tile work, needlecrafts, and repetitive tasks (e.g., sanding, polishing, wiping, sweeping, dusting).

## Physical Agent Modalities

The introduction of **physical agent modalities** (PAMs) into occupational therapy practice generated considerable discussion and controversy.[40,42] Occupational therapists specializing in hand rehabilitation first began including physical agents in a comprehensive treatment program because this seemed necessary and expedient.[33,35] After much study and discussion, AOTA issued an official statement on the use of PAMs by OT practitioners. This document stated that OTRs may use PAMs as adjuncts to or preparation for performance of purposeful activity. Further, it stipulated that the OT practitioner must have documented evidence of the theoretical background and technical skills to apply the modality and integrate it into an OT intervention plan.[3]

Subsequently, AOTA published a position paper on PAMs.[4] The official statement was reiterated, physical agents were defined, and their use as adjuncts to or in preparation for purposeful activity was elaborated. AOTA stated, "The exclusive use of physical agent modalities as a treatment method during a treatment session without application to a functional outcome is not considered occupational therapy." Further, AOTA stated that use of PAMs is not considered an entry-level practice; rather, their use requires appropriate postprofessional education to ensure competence of the OT practitioner.[4]

PAMs are used by OTRs (and some COTAs), who have received specialized training in the physiology and the implementation of modalities. The OT practitioner must be able to demonstrate competency in the use of modalities incorporated into the treatment plan.

PAMs are used in the context of occupational therapy intervention programs by OT practitioners before or during functional activities to enhance the effects of treatment. The purpose of this section is to introduce the basic techniques and when and why they might be applied. Examples of the treatment of upper extremity injuries are presented because PAMs are most often used in occupational therapy for treatment of hand injuries and diseases. However, the use of the techniques described are not limited to the treatment of hands.

### *Thermal Modalities*

*Heat* is used to increase motion, decrease joint stiffness, relieve muscle spasms, increase blood flow, decrease pain, and assist in the reabsorption of exudates and edema in a patient with a chronic condition.[22] Applying heat before a prolonged stretch, as in dynamic splinting, allows the permanent elongation of collagen fibers. In the absence of heat, these fibers return to their original length when stretched.

The blood flow maintains a person's core temperature at 98.6° F (37° C). To attain maximum benefits from heat, tissue temperature must be raised to 105° to 113° F (40.5° to 45° C). Precautions must be taken with temperatures above this range to prevent tissue destruction.

Contraindications to the use of heat include acute conditions, sensory losses, impaired vascular structures, malignancies, and application to very young or old persons. The use of heat may significantly enhance

CA

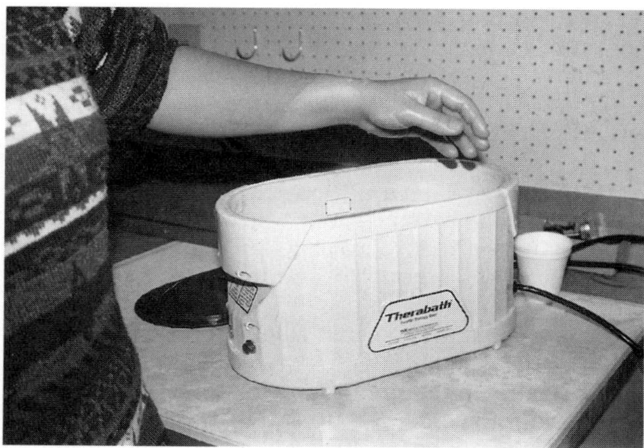


*Figure 15-13* Patient's hand is dipped in warm paraffin to prepare hand for performance of therapeutic activities.

*Box 15-7*

## Physical Agent Modality: Paraffin

**Guidelines**

1. Before using, obtain training to ensure service competency.
2. Protect areas of sensory impairment to avoid burns.
3. Do not use on areas with open wounds or moderate to severe edema.

**Procedure**

1. Verify temperature of paraffin.
2. Instruct patient to dip affected part slowly and repeatedly until desired thickness is obtained.
3. Wrap affected part in plastic bag and towel for 15 to 20 minutes.
4. Peel off paraffin casting, and prepare paraffin for reuse as directed.

the effects of splinting and therapeutic activities that attempt to increase ROM and functional abilities.

*Three modes of heat generation* **Conduction** occurs when heat is transferred from one object to another through direct contact. The use of paraffin and hot packs are examples of conduction.

*Paraffin* is stored in a tub that maintains a temperature of 125° to 130° F (51.5° to 54.5° C). An insulating layer of paraffin is applied to the extremity by having the patient repeatedly dip the hand into the tub until a thick layer of paraffin is applied (Figure 15-13). The hand is then wrapped in a plastic bag and towel for 10 to 20 minutes (Box 15-7).[22] Paraffin conforms well to surfaces, so it is ideal for use on the hands and digits. Partial hand coverage is possible. The paraffin transfers its heat to the hand and then acts as an insulator against dissipation of heat to the air. Care must be taken to protect insensate parts to avoid burns. To avoid excessive vasodilation, paraffin should not be applied when moderate to severe edema is present. It cannot be used if open wounds are present. Paraffin can be used in the clinic or incorporated into a home program. The tubs are small, and the technique is safe and easy to use in a home environment. It is an excellent adjunct to a home program of dynamic splinting, exercises, or general activities of daily living (ADLs). It may be used in the clinic before therapeutic exercises and functional activities.

*Hot packs* contain either a silicate gel or a clay bentonite wrapped in a cotton bag that is submerged in a hydrocollator. The hydrocollator is a water tank that maintains the temperature of the packs at 160° to 175° F (71° to 79.5° C).[22] Since tissue damage may occur at this temperature, the packs are separated from the skin by layers of towels. As with paraffin, precautions should be taken when applying to insensate skin or tissue that has sustained vascular damage.

Hot packs are typically used for myofascial pain, before soft tissue mobilization, and before any activities performed to elongate contracted tissue.[8] With a patient who has sustained a hand injury, the packs may be applied to the extrinsic musculature (muscles whose bellies lie outside the hand but that act on the hand). Heat to the extrinsic muscles can decrease muscle tone caused by guarding without heating the hand. Unlike paraffin, hot packs can be used when open wounds are present.

**Convection** is another source of heat generation in which heat is supplied to the tissues by way of fluid motion around the tissues. Examples of this are whirlpool and fluidotherapy. The *whirlpool* is used more often for wound management than heat application. In *fluidotherapy,* warm air is blown through finely ground corn husk, agitating the corn particles. This is similar to the whirlpool, but the corn particles are used instead of water. The temperature is thermostatically maintained, with the therapeutic range up to 125° F (51.5° C).

Studies have shown fluidotherapy to be an excellent technique for raising tissue temperature in the hands and feet.[8] Fluidotherapy is also effective for desensitization. The agitator can be adjusted to decrease or increase the flow of the corn particles, thus controlling the amount of stimulation to the skin. An extremity can be heated, and therefore this technique is effective as a warm-up method before exercises, dexterity tasks, functional activities, and work simulation tasks.

**Conversion** occurs when heat is generated internally by friction. This occurs with the use of **ultrasound.** The sound waves penetrate the tissues and create vibration of the molecules. Because of the friction generated, heat occurs. Sound is therefore converted to heat.

The sound waves are applied with a transducer that glides across the skin in slow, continuous motions. Gel is used to improve the transmission of the sound to the tissues. Ultrasound is considered a deep-heating agent.[26] Ultrasound at intensities higher than the recommended standards can destroy tissue. In addition, precautions must be taken to avoid heating growth plates in the bones of children, an unprotected spinal cord, and freshly repaired structures such as tendons and nerves. Practitioners must not use this modality until service competency has been obtained through appropriate training and supervision by a registered and service-competent therapist.

### *Cooling Modalities*

**Cryotherapy** is the use of cold and is often applied in the treatment of edema, pain, and inflammation. Cold produces vasoconstriction, which decreases the amount of blood flow into the injured tissue. Cold is used to decrease muscle spasms by cooling the muscle and decreasing the amount of firing from the afferent muscle spindles. Cryotherapy is contraindicated for patients with cold intolerance or vascular repairs. The use of cryotherapy may be incorporated into clinical treatment, but it is especially useful in a home program.

*Cold packs* can be applied in several ways. Many packs are available commercially, ranging in size and cost. An alternative to purchasing a cold pack is to use a bag of frozen vegetables. A reusable "slush bag" can be made by combining crushed ice and alcohol in a plastic bag. Ice packs should be covered with a moist towel to prevent tissue injury. The advantage of commercial packs is that they are easy to use, especially if the patient must use them frequently during the day. When patients are working, it is recommended that they keep cold packs at home and at their work for convenience. The optimum temperature to store a cold pack is 45° F(7.2° C).

Other forms of cryotherapy include ice massage and the use of cooling machines. *Ice massage* is used when the area to be cooled is small and very specific. An example would be inflammation of a tendon specifically at its insertion or origin. The procedure entails using a large piece of ice (e.g., water frozen in a paper cup) and massaging the area with circular motions until numbness of the skin occurs, usually within 4 to 5 minutes.

*Cooling devices* that circulate cold water through tubes in a pack are available through vendors. These devices maintain their cold temperatures for a prolonged time, but they are expensive to rent or purchase. They are very effective at reducing edema immediately after surgery or injury during the inflammatory phase of wound healing.

### *Contrast Baths*

Contrast baths combine the use of heat and cold. The physical response is alternating vasoconstriction and vasodilation of the blood vessels. The patient is asked to submerge the arm, alternating between two tubs of water. One contains cold water (59° to 68° F, or 14.5° to 20° C), and the other contains warm water (96° to 105° F, or 35.5° to 40.5° C). The purpose is to increase collateral circulation, which effectively reduces pain and edema. As with cold packs, contrast baths are a beneficial addition to a home therapy program. This technique is contraindicated for patients with vascular disorders or injuries.

### *Electrical Modalities*

Electrical modalities are used by an OTR to decrease pain, decrease edema, increase motion, and "reeducate" muscles to increase a patient's functional abilities. Many techniques are available; this discussion focuses on those used most often. Electrical modalities should *not* be used on patients with pacemakers or cardiac conditions.

Electrical modalities are beyond the range of service competency of entry-level COTAs. If directed to use these modalities, the COTA must immediately seek advice and direction from a supervising OTR and should not proceed alone with the modality until achieving service competency.

**Transcutaneous electrical nerve stimulation (TENS)** employs constant electrical stimulation with a modulated current to decrease pain. Pain is classified in three categories: physical, physiological, and psychological. When trauma occurs, an individual responds to the initial pain by guarding the painful body part. This guarding may result in muscle spasms and fatigue of the muscle fibers, especially after prolonged guarding. The supply of blood and oxygen to the affected area is decreased, and soft tissue and joint dysfunction results.[25] These reactions magnify and compound the problems associated with the initial pain response. The therapist's goal after an acute injury is to prevent this cycle from occurring. In the case of chronic pain, the goal is to stop the cycle that has been established. TENS is an effective technique for controlling pain without the side effects of medications. Pain medications are frequently used with TENS, which often reduces the duration of their administration. TENS is safe to use, and patients can be educated in independent home use.

TENS can be used for acute or chronic pain and is frequently used after surgery when motion must be initiated within 72 hours. TENS can be especially helpful to patients who have a low threshold to pain, making exercising easier. TENS is also beneficial in treating patients with reflex sympathetic dystrophy because continued active motion is crucial. TENS is also used for treating trigger points for pain, with direct electrode application to the trigger point to decrease its irritability.[27]

TENS can be employed to decrease pain from an inflammatory condition, such as tendonitis or a nerve impingement. For safe use, the patient must be educated in tendon/nerve protection and rest, with a proper home program of symptom management, positioning, and ADL/work modification. Without the sensation of pain, the patient may "overdo" and stress the inflamed tissues.

**Functional electrical stimulation (FES)** provides a continuous interrupted current. It is applied through an electrode to the motor point of innervated muscles to provide a muscle contraction. The current is interrupted to enable the muscle to relax between contractions, and the OTR can adjust the durations of the on and off times.

FES is used to increase ROM, facilitate muscle contractions, and strengthen muscles.[28] It may be used after surgery to provide a stronger contraction for increased tendon gliding, to strengthen a muscle that has become weakened because of disuse, or during the reinnervation phase after a nerve injury.

Other techniques that use an electrical current include *high-voltage galvanic stimulation (HVGS)* and *interferential electrical stimulation.* These techniques are applied to treat pain and edema.[28]

## SELECTING APPROPRIATE MODALITIES IN THE CONTINUUM OF CARE

Many years ago, roles and responsibilities for occupational therapy were more circumscribed and limited. Occupational therapists treated patients only after they were capable, at least to some degree, of performing purposeful activity.[14]

However, evolution of treatment methods, trends in health care, and the rapid development of medical technology have significantly altered the roles of the various rehabilitative therapies and expanded the repertoire of treatment modalities that OTRs are competent to practice.

Patients are now referred to occupational therapy long before they are capable of performing purposeful activity. Therapists and assistants are treating patients in the very acute stages of illness and disability. Treatment is directed toward preparing the patient for the time when purposeful activity is possible. For example, the OTR applies a positioning splint to a patient immediately after hand surgery in anticipation of how the hand will be used later in treatment and in real life; the COTA uses sensory stimulation on the comatose patient to elicit arousal and a return to interacting with persons and objects in the environment; and the OT practitioner applies paraffin to decrease joint stiffness and increase mobility of finger joints before performance of a macramé project.

The unique perspective of occupational therapy envisions the potential for performance and uses modalities that lead incrementally to performance. Implementing procedures that enhance readiness for performance of purposeful activity is also the concern of the OT practitioner.[6]

Dutton[14] outlined guidelines for use of both activity and exercise in the same treatment program. She proposed that exercise is a preparation phase, and purposeful activity is the application stage in treatment. Within the biomechanical frame of reference, she stated that movements more easily achieved through exercise are isolated, rhythmical, linear, and reciprocal movements. Exercise is appropriate for increasing ROM and for applying extreme resistance for the purpose of strengthening. However, purposeful activity is more appropriate for maintaining ROM, increasing endurance, and performing coordinated, arrhythmical, diagonal, and asymmetrical movements.[14]

Purposeful activity is not appropriate for every phase of treatment. Occupational therapists have developed expertise in handling techniques, facilitation/inhibition, splinting, positioning, massage, exercise, sensory stimulation, physical agent modalities, and other nonpurposeful modalities that meet the needs of the acutely ill or seriously impaired patient. If used by competent practitioners, these skills can be integrated into a comprehensive treatment program that includes purposeful activity[14] (Figure 15-14).

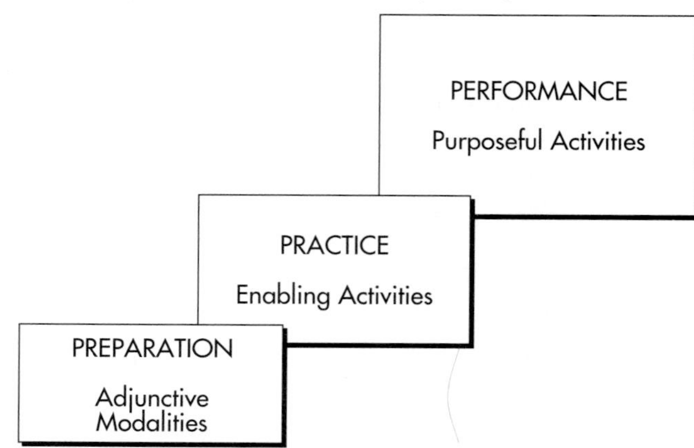


*Figure 15-14* Building blocks of occupational performance: preparation, practice, and performance.

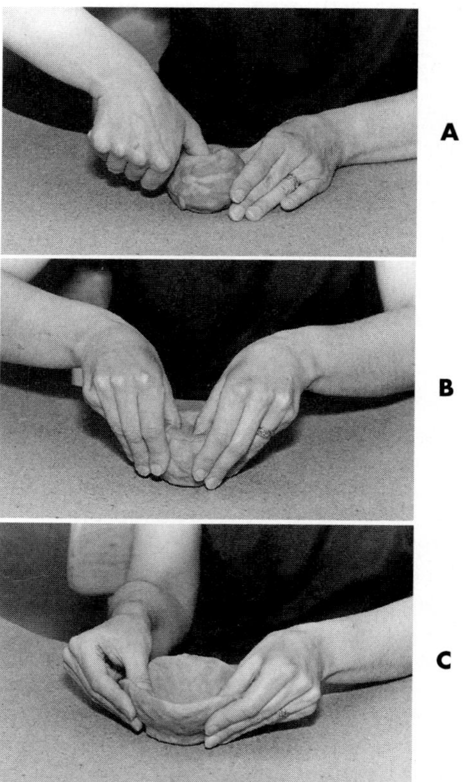


*Figure 15-15* **A,** Opening pinch pot with thumb. **B,** Walls of pot are gradually spread with pinching motion of fingers. **C,** Pinching continues in circular direction until desired size of pot is reached.

# Activity Analysis Model

The activity analysis offers one systematic approach for examining the therapeutic potential of activities. This model includes factors that must be considered regarding the performer, the field of action, and the activity in the selection of purposeful, therapeutic activity. In this example, only two steps (pinch, release) of a multistep activity are analyzed. The reader is encouraged to complete the motor analysis by considering movements of the shoulder, forearm, and wrist that accompany the pinch and release pattern analyzed.

I. **Preliminary information**
   - A. Name of activity: pinch pottery
   - B. Components of task
     1. Roll some clay into a ball 3 to 4 inches (7.5 to 10 cm) in diameter.
     2. Place ball centered on work table in front of performer.
     3. Make a hole in center of ball with right or left thumb (Figure 15-15, *A*).
     4. With thumb and first two fingers of both hands, pinch around and around hole from base to top of ball.
        - a. Pinch by pressing thumb against index and middle fingers.
        - b. Release pinch by extending thumb and index and middle fingers slightly.
     5. Continue pinching in this way, gradually spreading walls of clay until a small bowl of the desired size is formed.
   - C. Steps of activity being analyzed
     1. Pinch
     2. Release
   - D. Equipment and supplies needed
     1. Ball of soft ceramic clay
     2. Wood table 30 to 32 inches (75 to 80 cm) high or wood work surface fastened to table with C clamps
     3. Chair at work table
     4. Sponge and bowl of water
     5. Ceramic smoothing tool
   - E. Environment field of action[10]: Occupational therapy workshop or craft activity room. Sink and damp storage area should be available in work area. Ample room should be available around work table so that performer is not crowded and can move freely between table and sink and damp storage-closet. Lighting should be adequate for clear visualization of clay object and work area.
   - F. Position of performer in relation to work surface/equipment: Performer is seated in chair at table, at a comfortable distance for reaching and manipulating clay and tools. Clay is centered in front of performer, and tool, sponge, and water bowl are to right and near top of work area.
   - G. Starting position of performer: Sitting erect with feet flat on floor; shoulders are slightly abducted and in slight internal rotation, bringing both hands to center work surface; elbows are flexed to about 90°; forearms are pronated about 45°; wrists are slightly extended and in ulnar deviation; and thumbs are opposed to index and middle fingers, ready to pinch posterior surface of opened clay ball (Figure 15-15, *B*).
   - H. Movement pattern used to perform steps under analysis: Flexion of metacarpophalangeal (MP) and interphalangeal (IP) joints of index and middle fingers; opposition and flexion of thumb (pinch), followed by extension of MP and IP joints of index and middle fingers; and extension and palmar abduction of thumb (release). Repeat pattern around ball of clay until a small bowl of desired size and thickness is formed (Figure 15-15, *C*).

II. **Motor analysis[18]**
   - A. Joint and muscle activity: List joint motions for all movements used during performance of activity. For each, indicated amount of range of motion (ROM) used (minimal, moderate, full), muscle group used to perform motion, strength required (minimal [poor plus to fair], moderate [fair plus to good], full [good plus to normal]), and type of muscle contraction (isotonic, isometric, eccentric). Joints and muscles: (*MP,* metacarpophalangeal; *PIP,* proximal interphalangeal; *DIP,* distal interphalangeal; *FDP,* flexor digitorum profundus; *FDS,* flexor digitorum superficialis; *FPL,* flexor pollicis longus; *FPB,* flexor pollicis brevis; *ED,* extensor digitorum; *EI,* extensor indicis; *APL,* abductor pollicis longus; *APB,* abductor pollicis brevis; *EPL,* extensor pollicis longus; *EPB,* extensor pollicis brevis):

| *Joint motion* | *ROM* | *Muscle group* | *Muscle strength* | *Type of muscle contraction* |
|---|---|---|---|---|
| **Motions for pinch** | | | | |
| *Index and middle fingers* | | | | |
| MP flexion | Minimal | FDP, FDS, lumbricales | Moderate | Isotonic |
| PIP flexion | Minimal | FDP, FDS | Moderate | Isotonic |
| DIP flexion | Minimal | FDP | Moderate | Isotonic |
| Finger adduction | Maximal | Interossei palmares | Moderate | Isometric |
| *Thumb* | | | | |
| Opposition | Full | Opponens pollicis, FPL, FPB | Moderate | Isotonic |
| **Motions for release** | | | | |
| *Index and middle fingers* | | | | |
| MP extension | Minimal | ED, EI | Minimal | Isotonic |
| PIP and DIP extension | Minimal | ED, EI | Minimal | Isotonic |
| Finger adduction | Maximal | Interossei palmares | Moderate | Isometric |
| *Thumb* | | | | |
| Radial abduction | Moderate | APL, APB | Minimal | Isotonic |
| MP and IP extension | Full | EPL, EPB | Minimal | Isotonic |

Adapted from Killingsworth A: 0T120 Activity Module, San Jose State University, San Jose, Calif.

*Continued.*

B. Grading: Grade this activity for one or more of the following factors:
   1. ROM: Cannot be graded for ROM.
   2. Strength: Grade for strength by stiffening consistency of clay.
   3. Endurance: Grade for sitting tolerance by increasing length of activity sessions; grade for sitting balance by decreasing sitting support.
   4. Coordination: Requires fine coordination as performed. Grade coordination by adding scored or painted designs to surface; grade to sculpture of small clay figures.

C. Criteria for activity as exercise
   1. Action of joints: Movement localized to flexion and extension of MP and IP joints of index and middle fingers and carpometacarpal (CMC), MP, and IP joints of thumb.
   2. Repetition of motion: Pinch and release sequence is repeated until bowl has reached desired height and thickness.
   3. Gradable: Activity is gradable for strength and endurance.

**III. Sensory analysis**[23,24]: Check sensory stimuli received by performer. These are any sensory experiences obtained from position, motion, materials, or equipment. Describe how sensation is received, as follows:

| *Sensory modality* | *How received during activity* |
|---|---|
| 1. Tactile | x Touching clay and tools |
| 2. Proprioception (joint motion, position sense) | x Awareness of joint position and motion during pinch/release |
| 3. Vestibular (balance, sense of body, head motion) | x Maintenance of posture in chair while performing activity |
| 4. Visual | x See clay object and environment |
| 5. Olfactory (smell) | x May be slight odor of damp clay |
| 6. Pain | x 0 |
| 7. Thermal (temperature) | x Coldness of clay felt by hands |
| 8. Pressure | x Fingertips pressing against walls of clay bowl |
| 9. Auditory (hearing) | x 0 |
| 10. Other | |

**IV. Cognitive analysis**[24]: Check all that apply and justify your answer, as follows:

| *Cognitive skill* | *Justification* |
|---|---|
| Memory | x Memory for instructions |
| Sequencing (steps in order) | x Perform steps in order |
| Problem-solving | x What to do if clay is too wet or too dry and walls of bowl are too thin or too thick |
| Following instructions: | |
| Verbal | x Ability to comprehend and follow verbal instructions |
| Demonstrated | x Ability to follow demonstrated instructions |
| Written | 0 |
| Concentration/attention required | x Moderate: Focusing on bowl and knowing when its walls are thin enough and high enough |

**V. Safety factors:** What are the potential hazards of this activity? Describe the safety precautions that would be necessary when using this activity, as follows:

There are few hazards in this activity. Ingesting clay and using smoothing tool inappropriately are possible. Sitting balance must be adequate to maintain upright posture to perform the activity. Precautions to be taken are adequate supervision to ensure appropriate use of clay and tool and having performer accomplish task from a wheelchair with supports if sitting balance is impaired.

**VI. Interpersonal aspects of activity**[2]

A. Solitary activity: May be done alone.

B. Potential for dyadic interaction: May be done in parallel with one other person, but does not require interaction.

C. Potential for group interaction: May be done in a parallel group, but does not require interaction.

**VII. Psychological/psychosocial factors**

A. Symbolism in performer's culture[10]: Activity may be seen as more feminine than masculine in mainstream American culture. It may be associated with artistic, liberal, naturalist groups of people in American society.

B. Symbolic meaning of activity to performer: Activity may be seen as a leisure skill rather than work. Some persons may regard it as "child's play."

C. List feelings/reactions evoked in performer during performance of activity[24]: Soft, moist, pliable, and plastic properties of the clay may evoke soothing feelings in many persons. Others may regard it as messy or dirty. Potential for personal gratification is good because an attractive end product is easy to achieve, creative, individualistic, and useful.

**VIII. Therapeutic use of activity**

A. List intrinsic goal of activity: To make a small clay bowl.

B. List possible therapeutic objectives for the activity.
   1. To increase pinch strength.
   2. To improve coordination of opposition.
   3. To increase sitting tolerance.

## SUMMARY

Occupational therapy practitioners use purposeful activity, therapeutic exercise, enabling activities, and adjunctive modalities in the continuum of treatment and may use them simultaneously. In many treatment facilities the physical therapy practitioner is responsible for application of physical agent modalities and the formal therapeutic exercise regimen. The OT practitioner provides more general exercise and helps the patient apply newly gained strength, ROM, and coordination during performance of purposeful activities. In other settings the roles of the respective disciplines are less sharply defined, with each discipline (and practitioners within each discipline) sharing in exercise and activity aspects of the treatment program according to their expertise, interests, and the roles and responsibilities assigned by the treatment facility.

Purposeful activity is the core of occupational therapy practice. Its value lies in its health-giving and remedial nature. The selection of appropriate therapeutic activities is based on the patient's activity configuration and on careful activity analysis. Appropriate therapeutic activity is individualized and designed to be meaningful and interesting to the patient while meeting therapeutic objectives.

Therapeutic activity may be adapted to meet special needs of the patient or the environment. It may be graded for physical, perceptual, cognitive, and social purposes to keep the patient functioning at maximal potential at any point in the treatment program. The uniqueness of occupational therapy lies in its extensive use of goal-directed purposeful activities as treatment modalities.

## *Selected Reading Guide Questions*

1. What is meant by *substitution patterns?* Why do they occur?
2. What demand must be made on a muscle for its strength to increase?
3. List four signs of fatigue from excess exercise.
4. List at least four purposes of therapeutic exercise.
5. List four precautions or contraindications to therapeutic exercise, and explain why each can preclude the use of therapeutic exercise.
6. What type of exercise should be used if muscle grades are fair plus to good? Why?
7. If a patient has joint pain and inflammation with good muscle strength, what type of exercise should be used? Why?
8. How is passive stretching different from passive exercise?
9. Describe the procedure and precautions for passive stretching.
10. When beginning progressive resistive exercise, how is the patient's maximal resistance determined?
11. Describe the steps in coordination exercises.
12. List at least five requirements that activities must meet to be used for therapeutic purposes.
13. How can activities be adapted to meet specific therapeutic objectives and to allow for grading the therapeutic program?
14. List four ways in which activities may be graded.
15. What are the three criteria an activity must meet to be useful for exercise purposes?
16. How can the application of physical agent modalities enhance the patient's performance of activities?
17. Name and discuss at least five factors that should be considered in the selection of activities.
18. What is the physiological effect of the application of heat to soft tissue? When might heat be used in occupational therapy?
19. List and describe three physical agent modalities, and discuss their use as preparatory modalities for functional activity.

### *REFERENCES*


1. American Occupational Therapy Association: Association policy: occupational therapists and modalities, *Am J Occup Ther* 37:816, 1983.
2. American Occupational Therapy Association: Position paper on purposeful activities, *Am J Occup Ther* 37:805, 1983.
3. American Occupational Therapy Association: Official AOTA statement on physical agent modalities, *Am J Occup Ther* 45:1075, 1991.
4. American Occupational Therapy Association: Position paper: physical agent modalities, *Am J Occup Ther* 46:1090, 1992.
5. American Occupational Therapy Association: Position paper: purposeful activity, *Am J Occup Ther* 47:1081-1082, 1993.
6. Ayres AJ: Basic concepts of clinical practice in physical disabilities, *Am J Occup Ther* XII:300-302, 1958.
7. Ayres AJ: Occupational therapy for motor disorders resulting from impairment of the central nervous system, *Rehabil Lit* 21:302, 1960.
8. Cannon NM, Mullins PT: *Manual on management of specific hand problems,* Pittsburgh, 1984, American Rehabilitation Educational Network.
9. Ciccone CD, Alexander J: Physiology and therapeutics of exercise. In Goodgold J, editor: *Rehabilitation medicine,* St Louis, 1988, Mosby.
10. Cynkin S: *Occupational therapy: toward health through activities,* Boston, 1979, Little, Brown.
11. Cynkin S, Robinson AM: *Occupational therapy and activities health: toward health through activities,* Boston, 1990, Little, Brown.
12. De Lateur BJ, Lehmann J: Therapeutic exercise to develop strength and endurance. In Kottke FJ, Stillwell GK, Lehmann JF, editors: *Krusen's handbook of physical medicine and rehabilitation,* ed 4, Philadelphia, 1990, Saunders.
13. Drake M: *Crafts in therapy and rehabilitation,* Thorofare, NJ, 1992, Slack.
14. Dutton R: Guidelines for using both activity and exercise, *Am J Occup Ther* 43:573-580, 1989.
15. Hopkins HL, Smith HD, Tiffany EG: The activity process. In Hopkins HL, Smith HD, editors: *Willard and Spackman's occupational therapy,* ed 7, Philadelphia, 1988, Lippincott.
16. Huddleston OL: *Therapeutic exercises,* Philadelphia, 1961, Davis.
17. Kielhofner G: A heritage of activity: development of theory, *Am J Occup Ther* 36:723, 1982.

18. Killingsworth A: Activity module for OCTH 120, Functional kinesiology, San Jose, Calif, 1989, San Jose State University (unpublished).
19. Kottke FJ: Therapeutic exercise to maintain mobility. In Kottke FJ, Stillwell GK, Lehmann JF, editors: *Krusen's handbook of physical medicine and rehabilitation,* ed 4, Philadelphia, 1990, Saunders.
20. Kottke FJ: Therapeutic exercises to develop neuromuscular coordination. In Kottke FJ, Stillwell GK, Lehmann JF, editors: *Krusen's handbook of physical medicine and rehabilitation,* ed 4, Philadelphia, 1990, Saunders.
21. Kraus H: *Therapeutic exercise,* Springfield, Ill, 1963, Thomas.
22. Lehmann JF: *Therapeutic heat and cold,* ed 3, Baltimore, 1982, Williams & Wilkins.
23. Llorens L: *Activity analysis for sensory integration (CPM) dysfunction,* 1978, (unpublished).
24. Llorens LA: Activity analysis: agreement among factors in a sensory processing model, *Am J Occup Ther* 40:103, 1986.
25. Mannheimer JS, Lampe GN: *Clinical transcutaneous electrical nerve stimulation,* Philadelphia, 1984, Davis.
26. Michlovitz SL: *Thermal agents in rehabilitation,* ed 2, Philadelphia, 1990, Davis.
27. Moran CA, Saunders SR, Tribuzi SM: Myofascial pain in the upper extremity. In Hunter JM et al, editors: *Rehabilitation of the hand: surgery and therapy,* ed 3, St Louis, 1990, Mosby.
28. Mullins PT: Use of therapeutic modalities in upper extremity rehabilitation. In Hunter JM et al, editors: *Rehabilitation of the hand: surgery and therapy,* ed 3, St Louis, 1990, Mosby.
29. Pedretti LW et al: Use of adjunctive modalities in occupational therapy, *Am J Occup Ther* 46:1075-1081, 1992.
30. Rancho Los Amigos Hospital: *Muscle reeducation,* Downey, Calif, 1963, Rancho Los Amigos Hospital (unpublished).
31. Rancho Los Amigos Hospital: *Progressive resistive and static exercise: principles and techniques,* Downey, Calif, Rancho Los Amigos Hospital (unpublished).
32. Reed KL: Tools of practice: heritage or baggage? *Am J Occup Ther* 40:597, 1986.
33. Reynolds C: OTs and PAMs: a physical therapist's perspective, *OT Week* 8:17, 1994.
34. Rocker JD, Nelson DL: Affective responses to keeping and not keeping an activity product, *Am J Occup Ther* 41:152, 1987.
35. Rose H: Physical agent modalities: OT's contribution, *OT Week* 8:16-17, 1994.
36. Schram DA: Resistance exercise. In Basmajian JV, editor: *Therapeutic exercise,* ed 4, Baltimore, 1984, Williams & Wilkins.
37. Spackman CS: Occupational therapy for patients with physical disabilities. In Willard HS, Spackman CS: *Principles of occupational therapy,* Philadelphia, 1954, Lippincott.
38. Spackman CS: Occupational therapy for the restoration of physical function. In Willard HS, Spackman CS, editors: *Occupational therapy,* ed 4, Philadelphia, 1971, Lippincott.
39. Steinbeck TM: Purposeful activity and performance, *Am J Occup Ther* 40:529, 1986.
40. Taylor E, Humphrey R: Survey of physical agent modality use, *Am J Occup Ther* 45:924-931, 1991.
41. Thibodeaux CS, Ludwig FM: Intrinsic motivation in product-oriented and non-product-oriented activities, *Am J Occup Ther* 42:169, 1988.
42. West WL, Weimer RB: The issue is: should the representative assembly have voted as it did, when it did, on occupational therapist's use of physical agent modalities? *Am J Occup Ther* 45:1143-1147, 1991.
43. Wynn-Parry CB: Vicarious motions. In Basmajian JV, editor: *Therapeutic exercise,* ed 3, Baltimore, 1982, Williams & Wilkins.
44. Yoder RM, Nelson DL, Smith DA: Added-purpose versus rote exercise in female nursing home residents, *Am J Occup Ther* 43:581-586, 1989.

## *RECOMMENDED READING*

Neistadt ME et al: An analysis of a board game as a treatment activity, *Am J Occup Ther* 47:154-160, 1993.

Sten DB: Issues affecting PAMs in hand therapy, *OT Week* 6:16-17, 1992.

Zimmerer-Branum S, Nelson DL: Occupationally embedded exercise versus rote exercise: a choice between occupational forms by elderly nursing home residents, *Am J Occup Ther* 49:397-402, 1995.

Part V

# Treatment Interventions

Chapter 16

# Teaching and Learning in Occupational Therapy

*Lorraine Williams Pedretti*
*Darcy Ann Umphred*

## Chapter Objectives

*After studying this chapter, the student or practitioner will be able to:*

1. Identify some of the main concepts of motor learning.
2. Consider the effects of various practice schedules and practice methods on motor learning.
3. Contrast various types of feedback and their effects on learning.
4. Identify the characteristics of an effective teacher.
5. Identify the stages of the teaching/learning process.
6. Name and discuss the four basic steps in good instruction.
7. Contrast various methods of teaching, and match these to characteristics of individual learners.

## Key Terms

learning
motor learning
procedural learning
declarative learning
whole learning
progressive-part learning
pure-part learning
whole-to-part-to-whole learning
skill acquisition stage
skill refinement stage
skill retention stage
mass practice schedule
distributed practice schedule
random practice schedule
random sequence practice method
blocked practice method
transfer
intrinsic feedback
extrinsic feedback
summary feedback
reinforcement

Teaching and learning are the core of the therapeutic process. **Learning** can be defined as the acquisition of skills or information that results in a change in a person's behavior, attitudes, insights, or perceptions.[4] Learning takes place within the learner.

The occupational therapy practitioner, as teacher, provides the environment and designs and guides the experiences that facilitate learning.[14] The practitioner instructs the patient or learner in the skills that facilitate independence and personal development. The practitioner may be a registered occupational therapist (OTR) or a certified occupational therapy assistant (COTA).

Teaching of motor skills is a large part of the work of OT practitioners working in physical dysfunction settings. This chapter explores the concepts of motor learning, especially as these might apply to skills taught to patients. It considers the effects of various practice regimens and feedback models and reviews the basic steps in good instruction that apply to all occupational therapy teaching. Finally, some methods used to instruct patients who cannot learn easily through visual or auditory channels are discussed.

## CONCEPTS OF MOTOR LEARNING

**Motor learning** is the acquisition of motor skills. It is "a set of processes associated with practice or experience leading to relatively permanent changes in the capability for responding."[17] The desired outcome of motor learning is a permanent change in motor behavior or skill as a result of practice and experience. This change in behavior leads to the formatting of motor programs (a brain blueprint of a motor sequence) that are at first highly specific to the immediate activity learned, but that in time generalize to similar tasks in different environments.

The ability to retain what is initially learned is essential in motor learning.[7] Once a motor pattern is learned, encoding for long-term retention and retrieval depends on the context of the activity, the amount and type of practice performed, the motivation and attention of the learner, and the feedback given the learner from both the therapist and the learner's inherent feedback mechanisms.[15]

Learning of motor skills can be relatively straightforward and does not always involve intense thinking or complex cognitive processes. Learning necessary for motor execution is referred to as **procedural learning.** Procedural learning becomes automatic or habitual. An example is transferring from a wheelchair to a bed. This is contrasted with **declarative learning,** which depends more on memory and other analytical skills.[10] Declarative learning can be recalled by the learner and told as a story ("First, I do this . . . next, I do that . . . ," etc.). Learning to use a computer is an example of this type of learning. The areas of the brain involved in the storage and retrieval of procedural learning and declarative learning are different. For this reason, the environments and teaching procedures that enhance optimal learning vary according to the type of learning desired.[2,17] Often a task that will become procedural must first be learned in a declarative way. Tying shoelaces or typing at a keyboard are examples of these tasks, which first require intense concentration on the sequence of the steps and on *how* and *where* and *when* to move each body part. Once learned, however, speed and efficiency of movement are possible only when the doer operates on a *procedural* level, without too much conscious control or attention.

Because the profession of occupational therapy and the fields of motor learning and motor control are so intricately interwoven, the OT practitioner will benefit from understanding the various stages of motor learning and the effects of different reinforcement schedules and practice environments. In addition, the practitioner must anticipate how the characteristics and limitations of each patient will influence the content and speed of learning.

Occupational therapy is concerned with the acquisition of relevant life skills, including both procedural and declarative tasks. The measurement tools used to evaluate these skills require motor output from the patient. During assessment or evaluation, the patient demonstrates motor programs used to perform independent functional activities of daily living (ADLs). The focus in occupational therapy is on learning specific functional tasks or skills so that the patient can achieve personal goals for occupational performance. Motor learning, on the other hand, focuses more on *how* motor skills are learned, controlled, and retained, with the primary focus on the learner. Motor learning and occupational therapy are both concerned with learning motor skills; however, occupational therapy emphasizes functional outcomes, whereas motor learning emphasizes the learner and the process.

Two core concepts of occupational therapy theory are the use of purposeful activities as treatment modalities and the patient's active participation in the treatment process.[7] Gliner[3] proposed that purposeful activity could be the common ground between the fields of motor learning and occupational therapy. He proposed an "ecological" or event approach to motor learning in which the environment (object and task) and the performer must be considered as a unit, with the "environment providing meaning and support to the performer's actions." In this approach the skill is considered in relation to the immediate object or environment, and the focus is on adaptation to the environment. The learner can attempt different skills using different strategies for adaptation. The learner discovers appropriate muscular organizations for the motor skill to be performed. Many different possibilities exist for performing the same task. The performer discovers these possibilities and, with many trials and much practice, refines the muscular organization of the task until the motor skill can be performed in the most efficient way.[3]

In occupational therapy the patient interacts with the task and the environment. The OT practitioner structures the patient-environment interaction and learning experiences to maximize achievement of occupational performance goals. The context within which the patient learns and practices the task dramatically affects the outcome. For example, assume a patient needs to learn to sit in a chair while eating dinner. The cognitive tasks of selecting which food to eat first, how small to cut the meat, and whether to interact with someone else while eating require declarative memory. The tasks of cutting the meat and maintaining postural balance while sitting are procedural. These procedural tasks need to become very automatic without much cognitive energy expenditure. Thus, to make maintaining balance while sitting automatic, the practitioner needs to incorporate the context of the environment (sitting on a hard surface while eating) and distract the patient's attention from the motor strategies needed to sit. To facilitate carryover into real-life experiences, the practitioner also needs to include the cultural and psychological dimensions appropriate to the specific patient.

### Acquisition of Motor Skills

In the treatment process, patients engage in instruction and practice to perform motor behaviors that are beyond their present skill level. Many general factors affect motor learning: arousal of the central nervous system (CNS), attention to the task, motivation of the patient, the type of memory needed (declarative versus procedural; verbal, visual, or kinesthetic), type of movement required (simple to complex), practice schedule used, type of practice chosen, type and timing of reinforcement used by the clinician, and the specific environmental context within which the task must be accomplished. The motor skills being learned and practiced may have been learned before but because of the disability must be relearned or learned differently. The OT practitioner acts as teacher and facilitator by providing instruction, giving physical and verbal guidance, providing feedback about faulty performance, suggesting modifications, and providing reinforcement. The practitioner must decide which activities are to be mastered, how to structure the therapy session, the order of presentation of treatment tasks, and how to provide practice that will result in the greatest retention of learning.[17] For the patient to receive optimal learning, all these decisions should be made by the patient whenever possible or with the patient's consent and cooperation. By empowering the patient, the OT practitioner incorporates arousal, attention, and motivational components into the motor learning environment.

The type of movement required to succeed at the task plays a significant role in the type of practice or practice context selected. Simple and discrete tasks usually are learned best by introduction of **whole learning,** in which the patient practices the entire task at one time. A transfer from bed to chair would be considered a simple task and often can be learned as one procedure. Contrast this with learning the task in components such as (1) lock the chair, (2) move weight forward to edge of chair, (3) shift weight over feet, (4) stand up, (5) pivot, and (6) sit down. By teaching six different components or procedural programs as part of the transfer, the clinician may increase the difficulty level unnecessarily.

However, intermediate skills and serial tasks often are learned easier if taught in a **progressive-part learning** context. For example, teaching a dance might be considered an intermediate skill. It may require walking or stepping to a beat, along with various movements between and within limbs, while moving on a diagonal and with a partner. If the dance has a specific sequence, learning the first few movements and then adding more steps, always starting from the beginning, would be considered a progressive-part practice schedule.

Some skills can be learned in a **pure-part learning** context. If the skill is cutting food on a plate, whether the individual cuts the meat or the vegetables first does not matter. All types of cutting are required, and thus pure-part learning can be used. **Whole-to-part-to-whole learning** generally leads to the best retention when the patient must learn a complex skill. Putting on a necktie using one hand is an example of this type of skill. Knowing the whole while working on component parts helps with long-term retention.

The patient always is a critical variable when determining the complexity of the task. The demands on memory, information processing, task organization, and number of separate components interacting with the state of the patient's CNS after injury are the ultimate determinants of the type of practice selected.[17,20,21]

### Stages of Motor Learning

The stages of motor learning are skill acquisition, skill refinement, and skill retention. The practice schedule (practice versus rest periods or time between practice) selected for therapy should match the stage of motor learning. During the **skill acquisition stage** the patient is understanding the idea of the movement to begin to acquire the skill. Errors are frequent and performance inefficient and inconsistent. Thus frequent repetition and feedback are necessary. Generally at this stage of motor learning, a **mass practice schedule** is used. Mass practice is performed frequently, on a daily schedule; this is similar to the type of scheduling done in a rehabilitation department. As the patient moves to a **skill refinement stage,** both the patient and the clinician should recognize an improvement in performance, a reduction in the number and size of errors, and an increase in consistency and efficiency of the movement. The practice requires some delay between sessions, and often a **distributed practice schedule** is advised. This distributed practice might be three times per week, to two times or one time. This is similar to a fixed home program or fixed outpatient program.

When the stage of motor learning progresses to the **skill retention stage,** with patients developing the ability to perform movement and achieve functional goals, a **random practice schedule** is most effective. This empowers patients to practice at their own pace. The objective is to retain the skill and to transfer that skill to different settings. In these varied contexts, patients must modify the timing, force, sequencing, balance, postural integrity, and ongoing excitation of all the neurons in the brain stem and the spinal motor neurons (the motor pool) to succeed at the task. This could be considered motor problem solving and is a hallmark of true motor learning.

The more novel the task, the more intensive is the mass practice necessary. For some activities, mass practice leads to higher performance and better retention, whereas for others, distributed or random practice may lead to the best retention. Factors such as memory loss, low levels of cognition, and severe emotional distress can influence motor learning and behavior. These need to be considered when selecting the specific practice schedule appropriate for each patient.

### Measures of Learning

In traditional learning models, when a motor skill (e.g., putting on shoes) was being practiced, performance was observed or measured during the practice session. If performance was successful during practice, it was assumed that the task was learned. However, this method of evaluation does not ensure that skills are retained or that they can be generalized to other situational contexts. For example, if the patient learns to don trousers, can he also put on undershorts? If he can put on trousers in the hospital room, can he also don them at home? If the instruction takes place on Monday, will he be able to perform the same skill on Thursday if no opportunity exists to practice during the intervening days?[7,17] To obtain a true measure of learning and skill retention, performance must be assessed again later, outside of the practice sessions and in as realistic a setting as possible.[9,16]

Although the process of skill acquisition by normal humans is not yet fully understood, specific factors that could facilitate learning and enhance long-term retention and generalization of motor tasks can be inferred from studies.[17] These factors are type of practice, practice context, stages of motor learning, and the type and frequency of feedback. These factors apply to the motor learning that occurs in therapy sessions.[7,8,13]

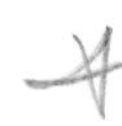

### Practice Methods

#### *Random Sequence Practice*

If several tasks are planned for the treatment session, it is most effective to present them in random order. For example, the patient may be asked to pick up cones, cubes, buttons, and spheres in random order. The prehension (grasping) pattern for each is different. This requires that the patient reformulate the solution to the motor problem each time a different object is approached. The **random sequence practice method** involves not only repetition of the same motor patterns, but also the formulation of plans to solve motor problems.[16] If motor skill acquisition is measured by performance during a random practice session, learning may not appear to be occurring as rapidly as when the repetitive or blocked practice model is used. However, the repeated regeneration of the solution to motor problems has been shown to be more beneficial to retention than repetitive practice of the same motor skills.[17]

#### *Blocked Practice*

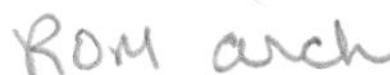

The **blocked practice method** involves repeated performance of the same motor skill. For example, the patient is asked to pick up a cup from the left side and place it on a saucer on the right side of a table. The patient only needs to solve the motor problem once or twice and then repeat the same motor skill over and over again. If measured during the practice session, performance improves faster with blocked practice. In blocked practice, however, the patient does not need to attend to the task, once learned, because it no longer requires novel solutions. No opportunity exists for alternative activities to cause some forgetting and the reformulation of the solution to the motor problem, a process that enhances long-term learning and retention.[16,17]

In early learning or with confused patients, blocked practice may be necessary to promote learning. The patient needs to practice the same movements over and over to establish the motor pattern. For example, it may be helpful at the outset to practice with the same open-front shirt repeatedly before introducing a jacket or housecoat that requires similar movement patterns.[16]

### Practice Contexts

Generalization or transfer of learning occurs more reliably with practice in different contexts. **Transfer** enables an individual to perform similar tasks in a new context by drawing on past experience. This indicates that the skill not only was performed in a single situation, but also has been acquired and retained; this would be considered the motor retention stage of motor learning.[16] For example, the patient who learns to sponge-bathe the upper body in the hospital lavatory and can perform the task in the bathroom in her own home has transferred the learning to a new context. Although the motor skills and the practice environment are not identical in the new context, the memory of performing similar motor skills in a similar environment enables the patient to perform the task.

Practice under variable conditions can increase generalization of learning to new situations. Dressing training, for example, can occur in the patient's room some of the time and in the occupational therapy clinic's area for activities of daily living (ADLs) at other times. Various types of clothing requiring similar motor patterns should be used. Undershorts could be varied with trousers and shirts with cardigan sweaters in dressing practice. Training should be done in the environment most appropriate and most realistic for the task being performed. For example, eating should occur at a table with the appropriate utensils and real food.[16]

## Feedback

Information about whether a movement has been successful in achieving the goal of acting on the environment is a critical ingredient in motor learning.[16,17] If learners do not obtain the intrinsic feedback necessary to estimate the success of their own motor performance, learning may be poor or not occur at all. In such instances an alternative means of providing feedback must be found. Feedback must be provided by some extrinsic source, such as the therapist or teacher or even some mechanical device (e.g., biofeedback machine).[17]

### *Intrinsic Feedback*

**Intrinsic feedback** is information received by the learner as a result of performing the task itself.[17] Intrinsic feedback arises from sensory stimulation to tactile receptors, proprioceptors, and visual and vestibular systems while performing the task. Intrinsic feedback occurs during performance of the task (i.e., information about the movements) and after the task is completed (i.e., results of the action).[16] This feedback may not be brought to conscious awareness and may be processed at a preconscious level within the CNS to determine whether the motor patterns selected for task accomplishment were accurate or needed refinement. For example, a male patient putting on a shirt receives knowledge of performance when he can feel the movements of joints and muscles and the sensation of the shirt on the skin as the task progresses. He can sense whether arms and hands are in the correct position to grasp the edge of a shirt front or push an arm through a sleeve. He can feel the fabric on the arms and trunk and thus knows whether a sleeve is pulled up over the shoulder. When the task is completed, he can see the results by looking in the mirror and seeing that the shirt is properly adjusted, the buttons are buttoned, and the collar is lying flatly.

The patient actually does not attend to all these variables but does recognize whether the task is accomplished. If the goal of the task has been attained, the patient will decide whether the quality of the accomplishment met the criteria for acceptable behavior. If the CNS determines that corrections are appropriate, those modifications in the plan will be made and practiced the next time the task arises. The capacity for intrinsic feedback may be mildly to severely limited in patients with sensory, perceptual, or cognitive impairments. If intrinsic feedback is not possible or is distorted by sensory or motor dysfunction, more extrinsic feedback is needed for motor learning.[16,17]

### *Extrinsic Feedback*

Feedback about performance from an outside source such as an OT practitioner or a mechanical device is called **extrinsic feedback.** It is used to augment intrinsic feedback.[16,17] Two types of extrinsic feedback are (1) knowledge of performance and (2) knowledge of results.

*Knowledge of performance* Verbal feedback about the process or performance provides the patient with information about the movements progressing toward the goal of a motor skill.[9,16,17] The therapist or assistant might say, "You need to raise your arm a little higher" or "You are not holding on to the edge of the shirt tightly enough." Such feedback informs the performer about the quality of movement and its effectiveness in achieving the goal.

*Knowledge of results* The OT practitioner provides feedback about the outcome, product, or results of the motor actions.[9,16,17] The practitioner might say, "The shirt is put on correctly; it looks neat, and each button is lined up with its buttonhole." Such feedback can also be used to point out faulty performance and facilitate the revision of movement patterns. The practitioner could point out that the buttons are not lined up with the correct buttonhole or that the body of the shirt is twisted to one side. The patient then can revise the movement plan to correct the faulty performance.[16]

Feedback is essential to learning and enhances the learning process. Knowledge of performance should be given more frequently than knowledge of results during treatment sessions. This is because knowledge of performance is directed toward correcting faulty movement patterns. More feedback should be given frequently in early stages of learning so that the patient can correct performance errors.[16] Studies have demonstrated that when enough feedback has been provided for the patient to correct significant errors in movement, it should be gradually decreased.

**Summary feedback,** which is given after a series of trials with no feedback, has a more positive effect on retention than more frequent feedback given after each trial. This might be explained by the absence of extrinsic feedback early in learning requiring the patient to use intrinsic feedback to correct errors in the movement activity. A declining schedule of feedback actually enhances long-term retention of activities learned in the rehabilitation program because the patient will use intrinsic feedback to self-correct.[17]

## Components of Motor Control

The motor control system involves the interaction of many components, such as range of motion (ROM), muscle strength, synergy patterns, balance, postural integrity, rate, direction, speed, and context of the environment. Each component affects the performance of the entire system. With a problem, deficit, or imbalance in one component, the other aspects of the system compensate and modify their function to allow the patient to succeed at the desired task.

If musculoskeletal aspects such as ROM, muscle strength, and joint integrity are deficient, the CNS components may need to adjust so that a task may be completed. For example, if lack of joint stabilization at the shoulder causes unsteadiness in use of the hand, the CNS may increase the firing rate of motor neurons going to muscles that normally would provide this stabilization. That is, the CNS would make the neurons that control the muscles stabilizing the shoulder (e.g., pectoralis minor, trapezius) more sensitive to stimulation so that they would contract with only a small stimulus. In that scenario, a hypertonic muscle or synergy may develop and limit motor function but correct the instability. During treatment, the clinician needs to decide whether to allow the patient to use dysfunctional motor components to compensate for instability. This scenario may lead to the patient being able to succeed at the task in a limited environmental context. Alternatively, the clinician can give extrinsic feedback and provide a contrived environment so that the patient can experience success at the task. However, this approach may lead to dependency on the clinician for task success unless the clinician at some time relinquishes the control of the motor patterns and the patient begins to use intrinsic feedback to self-correct. Neither method will automatically lead to better performance or retention of motor learning.

## PRINCIPLES AND METHODS OF TEACHING

### Characteristics of an Effective Teacher

The effective teacher is enthusiastic about the learning content and enjoys teaching. The teacher is positive, realistic, accepting, empathetic, and nonjudgmental toward the learners. This person is consistent in approach and expectations, flexible, adaptable, attentive, and able to motivate learners. The effective teacher gives positive and honest reinforcement to learners and observes and analyzes their behaviors to evaluate the outcome of learning. Such characteristics enhance the possibility of moving the learner toward independence and thus to successful treatment outcomes.[4]

The effective teacher remains in the teaching role and does not become friend, mother, brother, or confidant to the learner.[14] Thorough knowledge of the skill to be taught and the ability to present it in an understandable way are essential.[4] Poor preparation or uncertainty about the skill causes the patient to lose confidence in the clinician. For the effective teacher to also be a *master clinician,* additional personality characteristics are required. A master clinician dealing with motor learning problems acts as a guide to the patient, directing the patient's learning through an interaction that is compassionate, bonding, and accepting of the individual as a unique and worthwhile person. The master clinician is constantly empowering patients to take control over their cognitive, psychosocial, and motor systems. Personal control leads to occupational independence and a better quality of life.[21]

### Individual and Group Treatment

The OTR is responsible for planning individual and group instruction, although aspects of this may be delegated to the COTA. Treatment plans and group protocols, analogous to lesson plans, are designed to include problems, goals, teaching methods, and ways to evaluate treatment outcomes. The OTR assumes responsibility for seeing that treatment goals are achieved.

In physical disabilities practice, most treatment is carried out on an individual basis. However, some treatment is done in groups. Group treatment may be used in physical disabilities practice when treatment goals are best reached through group interaction, when the OT practitioner is treating two or more patients with similar problems, and as a way to cut costs and to allow the patient to practice without the need for extensive extrinsic feedback. A therapeutic group may come together to share and resolve problems, explore interests, perform tasks, or participate in common activities.[4,14] In group treatment the OT practitioner must understand group structure, process, and function; act as a group leader; and facilitate group roles.

Several types of groups may be used in a treatment program, including conversational, decision-making, discovery, and instructional groups. In an *instructional group* situation the leader teaches or demonstrates a skill, and the members share a common need to learn it.[4] If the skill, task, or activity is practiced within a limited context, this may be the time to practice skill acquisition and refinement. Instructional groups may be divided into project and parallel types.[4,14] In physical disabilities practice, group treatment is likely to be based on the parallel or project group model, with task performance rather than group process as the primary focus. With the group activity having multiple goals and varied contexts, the skill retention phase of motor learning might be the focus.

In a *parallel group,* members work in the presence of one another with minimal sharing of tasks. Examples are the reality orientation group and hemiplegia exercise group. In a *project group,* members are involved in a common short-term or long-term task that requires some sharing or interaction with one another. The task may be competitive or cooperative. Little interaction is involved, other than that necessary for completion of the task.[14] Examples are a cooking group or a ball toss game.[18] Patient members might be at various stages of motor learning. To perform an altered task in a group context, the patient must develop and rely on intrinsic feedback to modify the existing motor plans. This elicits adaptation and should lead to better retention and retrieval of motor plans in the future.

Generally the group size should be no less than 4 or more than 20, with some compatibility among members' problems and characteristics. The environment where the group treatment occurs should be appropriate for the activities to be performed. Space should be adequate and comfort of each group member assured. The style of leadership, group format, group roles, and communications should reflect the stated group treatment goals and patients' learning needs.[4]

## The Teaching/Learning Process

The teaching/learning process is a systematic problem-solving process designed to facilitate learning. The teaching/learning sequence involves four basic steps: assessment, design of the plan, instruction, and feedback/evaluation (Figure 16-1).[9]

### *Assessment*

The teacher (assistant or therapist) must assess characteristics of self, learner characteristics, learning needs, learning skills and style, and the situation.[4,9] This assessment is made by the OTR and COTA during the evaluation phase of patient treatment. During the evaluation the OTR can assess the patient's cognitive status, perceptual deficits, and physical limitations. Psychosocial readiness also should be considered. The patient's attitudes, feelings, and emotional state in relation to the task, the practitioner who will do the teaching, and the teaching process need to be assessed.[4] Such information is essential to estimating the patient's readiness for learning, planning appropriate treatment activities, and selecting methods of teaching.

Readiness for learning implies that the learner is prepared for the learning process. The person possesses the necessary cognitive, perceptual, and physical skills to perform and master the learning task. Of primary importance is the condition of the brain and CNS to accommodate learning. This means that the OTR must assess CNS functions to select appropriate learning tasks and teaching methods.[4] OT practitioners sometimes begin with tasks at too high a level for the patient to perform because the patient's cognitive, perceptual, motivational, or physical capacities have been overestimated.[14]

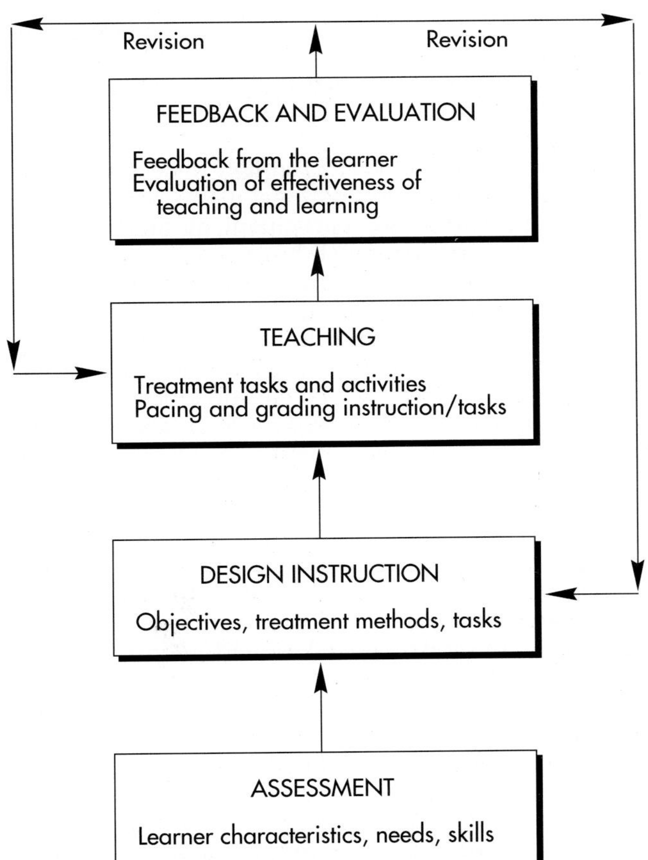


*Figure 16-1* Systems model of teaching-learning process. (Modified from Kemp JE: *The instructional design process,* New York, 1985, Harper & Row.)

### *Design of Teaching Plan*

The OTR is responsible for planning treatment or instruction. This can be done only after some assessment of the learner has been completed. Specific learning or treatment objectives must be written. Instructional tasks are planned, and methods of instruction to suit the learner are designed. The most appropriate learning environment is selected and prepared,[4] with a focus on accommodating the various components of motor learning and the patient's stage of learning.[17]

In selecting treatment tasks, the patient's motivation to perform them significantly affects participation in the learning process. The learner's perception of the relevance, value, and meaning of the learning task at hand influences involvement in performance. Motivation may be intrinsic or extrinsic. *Intrinsic motivation* derives from an internal drive, is self-initiated, and occurs when the learner has a need to know something and is ready to learn. *Extrinsic motivation,* on the other hand, derives from an external stimulus to act, such as the therapist deciding what the learner needs to learn and presenting this information. Extrinsic motivation engages the learner in a learning process that requires more effort, concentration, and time than learning that is motivated intrinsically. Much learning is probably driven by a combination of intrinsic and extrinsic motivation.[4] Again, the OT practitioner must differentiate whether the task to be learned requires declarative or procedural memory. If it is a cognitive task, attention and focus on the task may be very appropriate. If it is a motor task, however, cognitive attention may be detrimental to motor learning and must be drawn away from the motor activity.

The patient's age, gender, interests, and cultural group must be considered in selecting relevant treatment activities. If the patient is part of this decision-making process, the task selected will closely match the patient's goals. Choosing age-appropriate tasks and considering possible gender-role identification of activities and the value of specific activities in the patient's culture are helpful in engaging the patient's motivation to perform treatment tasks.[14] The importance of cultural considerations cannot be overemphasized and plays a major role in the attainment of functional carry-over into real-life situations.[12] Selecting activities that are relevant to life roles and meaningful in the patient's family or social group ensures a higher level of motivation and participation than activities that seem irrelevant. This relevance needs to be determined by patients and their support systems and not by the practitioner's inherent beliefs. The learner needs to understand why the activity is to be done and how it is relevant to recovery and resumption of important life activities.[4]

### *Instruction*

The therapist or assistant teaches the task or activity to the individual or group in an understandable and meaningful way. Repetition of instruction may be important to the learning process, especially with patients who have cognitive or perceptual limitations. Patients should be given opportunities for questions and clarification.[4]

Patients must be challenged in task performance and still experience some success. Tasks that are too difficult for success may be at a learning level incompatible with the patient's learning abilities and are detrimental to motivation. Tasks that are too easy will fail to help the patient move forward to higher levels of accomplishment. The OT practitioner must find activities that provide some challenge to the patient but are not so difficult as to cause discouragement. Activities may be graded according to the complexity of their physical and cognitive demands and the levels of supervision and assistance provided by the therapist.[4] Tasks are most appropriately taught in a relevant environment and activities context. For example, practice in brushing hair is most appropriately done as part of the normal morning hygiene activities in the patient's bathroom rather than in the middle of the afternoon in the occupational therapy clinic.[14]

*Pacing and grading instruction* *Pacing* refers to structuring the instruction and the practice so that learners can progress at their own speed. Tasks should be taught in a manner and at a pace that learners can handle. Once the patient is beyond the skill acquisition phase, practice that is distributed over time and spaced with intervening rests or alternative activities tends to be more effective for retention than long periods of concentrated practice on the same task.[4,17]

Learning should also be graded in complexity because learning is enhanced if it progresses from simple to complex. Simple tasks requiring simple motor plans should be taught as a whole-movement activity. In designing the learning experience, the therapist or assistant should analyze the activity and break it down into its component steps when appropriate. When the type of practice selected is pure-part learning, steps can be taught singly, and as each step is mastered, another step in the sequence is added to the learning process until the patient masters the whole task.[13,14,17]

One way to grade the patient's independent performance of an activity is to use backward or forward chaining as a method of instruction. In *backward chaining* the OT practitioner provides assistance through all the steps of the activity, then allows the patient to perform the last step independently. This is then graded to the last two steps, three steps, and so forth, until the patient can perform the whole activity independently. The process would be consistent with a whole-to-part-to-whole type of practice environment. In *forward chaining* a similar process is used, except the practitioner allows the patient to perform the first step independently and then assists the patient to perform the rest of the steps. Then the patient performs the first two steps, then three steps, and so on, until the activity can be performed independently. A sequential-step approach to structuring the motor learning environment would match this forward chaining.[6,11,19] Chaining may be helpful for patients with memory deficits and difficulty with sequencing or remembering the steps of the activity. Again, the OT practitioner needs to analyze the task considering not only motor plans needed to perform it but also patients' motivation and cognitive abilities. If the task requires constant cognitive judgment, the clinician would not want to have patients practice unless they were capable of making these judgments.

*Active participation and repetition* One of the primary principles of occupational therapy is for the patient to be an active participant in the treatment process. The patient must be actively engaged in learning. This means that the patient may help to set treatment goals, plan activities, and participate in the performance processes of learning. It is not enough to be told or shown an activity. The patient must perform it and learn the activity at a tactile and kinesthetic level to ensure retention.[10,14] Active participation enhances learning and enables the patient to be in control of the process, the director of action.

*Feedback and evaluation* Feedback and reinforcement are closely connected. Confirmation of successful responses encourages the person to continue learning.[9] The person also needs feedback during the learning process to recognize mistakes and modify performance. It is best to correct the learner as soon as an error is noted so that erroneous patterns do not develop.[4]

**Reinforcement** may be derived intrinsically from the personal satisfaction of observing the results of successful performance or may be provided extrinsically by the OT practitioner. Verbal reinforcement in a cognitive task may be direct and very meaningful. In the cognitive arena, behavior that is reinforced tends to be repeated. In a motor task, however, external reinforcement may override the intrinsic mechanism and not allow for innate self-correction. When extrinsic feedback is used to assist in motor learning, feedback should be realistic, honest, and appropriate to the task. That is, the practitioner does not need to exclaim loudly in superlatives when a shoe has been tied effectively. A more appropriate reinforcer would be a low-key, positive statement that the lace is correctly tied and will effectively keep the shoe on the foot. Similarly, if the motor performance is not going to reach the identified goal, the practitioner might suggest an alternative plan of action and repeat the instruction, possibly in a different sensory mode.[14]

Constructive criticism must be given thoughtfully and tactfully and should be delivered in a nonthreatening but honest manner. False praise can be just as confusing and insulting as criticism. Constructive suggestions for alternative action that may be more successful should be included with any correction.[4] Considerable reinforcement may be needed in the early stages of learning regardless of whether the task is based on cognitive or motor components. As tasks are mastered, less reinforcement is necessary.[14,17]

In evaluating the effectiveness of the teaching/learning process, the OT practitioner must ask, How did it go? Were treatment objectives achieved? What was the extent or quality of achievement of specific objectives? This is an opportunity for the OTR or COTA to receive feedback from the learner(s). Feedback can be *verbal,* reflecting the learners' affective reactions to a group activity, or *behavioral,* reflecting the ability to perform tasks or behaviors that were not possible before the instruction.[4] Progress can be evaluated by repeating tests that were administered on the initial evaluation. The results can provide objective evidence of the effectiveness of treatment. A muscle test may show a change in grade of strength, and a self-care reevaluation can demonstrate a change in the level of independent dressing. The OT practitioner needs to ensure that all measurements submitted for billing and as a part of the medical record are objective and quantifiable. A separate record of descriptive or subjective impressions often helps the practitioner remember behaviors that cannot be measured objectively but that reflect change in the cognitive, psychosocial, or motor systems.

### Instruction: The Teaching Process

The instruction phase of the teaching/learning process just discussed can be subdivided into four specific steps (Figure 16-2). This process would need to be modified or dramatically altered if the patient was at a low cognitive level and unable to interact with the external world. The following teaching process relates *only* to patients who have the ability to comprehend and interact with the environment. Given this premise, the OT practitioner can prepare for treatment systematically, using this process as a guide. A standard procedure, such as the following, for planning treatment is helpful for consistency and evaluation of treatment outcomes.

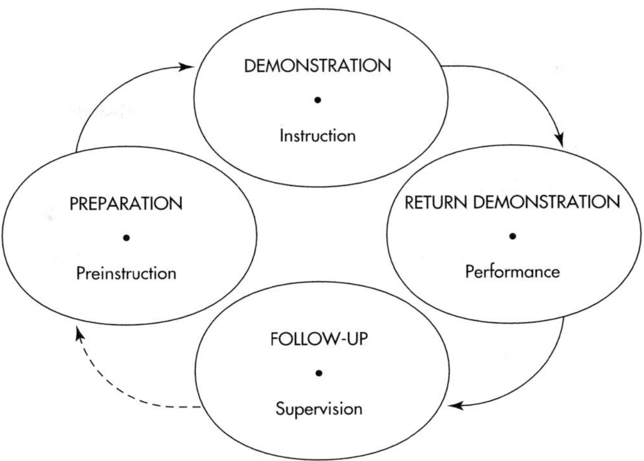


*Figure 16-2* Four basic steps in good instruction. Dotted line shows that cycle must begin again for each new activity introduced.

### *Preparation: Preinstruction Phase*

Preparation should occur before instruction. Assuming that the patient has been evaluated and problems identified, the therapist or assistant planning instruction selects the purposes and objectives of the treatment or activity with the patient's input. What is the patient to learn or be able to do? How much skill and competence is the learner expected to achieve? How long will it take to achieve each learning objective? The clinician may also analyze potential treatment activities at this stage, considering the activity's physical and cognitive demands and breaking the activity down into its component steps. This helps in estimating the patient's potential for learning the activity. Methods of teaching (discussed in more detail later) are then selected.

The final stage of the preinstruction process is to prepare the environment for the therapy session before the patient arrives. Treatment time should not be wasted while the OT practitioner prepares for treatment. Furniture should be arranged, areas cleared, and equipment and materials gathered. On arrival, the patient should be positioned comfortably and correctly for the activity.[5]

### *Demonstration: Motivation and Instruction Phase*

Once the preparations are complete, instruction begins. The practitioner should put the patient at ease and arouse the patient's interest in the activity. Explanation of the activity's purposes and potential benefits can help to motivate participation. The therapist or assistant then demonstrates the activity to the patient. The demonstration can take many forms (discussed next), but in general the practitioner should tell and show the patient how to do the activity, illustrating one step at a time. Key points are stressed,and instruction is given clearly, completely, and patiently. Repetition and review are often necessary. The clinician should not present any more than the patient can successfully master at one time. Words should be kept few and simple. Some patients require tactile and kinesthetic cues or gentle manual guidance along with verbal and demonstrated instruction.[5]

### *Return Demonstration: Performance Phase*

Once the therapist or assistant has taught the activity, the patient should perform the skill, demonstrating whether or not the instruction has been grasped. Asking "Do you understand?" after the demonstration is not enough. The practitioner should observe the performance and correct errors as they occur. If the patient can verbally list the key points as the activity is performed, this can reinforce understanding of the activity process. The OTR or COTA should observe until the patient clearly is performing the activity correctly.[5]

### *Follow Up: Guided Independence Phase*

When the OT practitioner is certain the patient is performing the activity in the prescribed manner, it may be possible to move on to attend to other patients or duties. However, some continuous supervision is necessary. The OTR or COTA may periodically observe the patient's performance from a distance or may attend to the patient from time to time to offer assistance and recheck performance. The practitioner gives the patient opportunities to ask questions, corrects faulty performance, and provides realistic, positive, and appropriate feedback. The degree of independent performance may be graded by tapering off coaching and close supervision as the patient masters the skills.[5]

## METHODS OF TEACHING

The methods of instruction chosen by the occupational therapy practitioner depend on the patient's cognitive level, perceptual functions, physical status, and motivation. The teaching methods discussed here require different levels of perceptual and cognitive function and access one or more sensory systems in transmitting data to the cerebral cortex for information processing and execution of the motor plan. In therapy, the methods may be combined. The practitioner must find the method that best suits the patient's learning style and level of comprehension.

### Teaching Through the Auditory System: Verbal Instruction

When using verbal instruction, the clinician speaks an instruction and expects the patient to carry it out. For example, the COTA says, "Brush your hair." Such a command assumes that the patient understands the words spoken, has previous experience with the activity, can retain the memory of the command, can retrieve it from memory, has retained the motor patterns associated with the hairbrush and the act of brushing hair, can plan and execute the motor task associated with the command, and is motivated to brush the hair. Patients with, for example, deficits in receptive language, auditory perception, auditory or visual memory, and motor planning (praxis), will have considerable difficulty following verbal instructions only. Generally, this is the least effective method of teaching.

### Teaching Through the Visual and Auditory Systems: Verbal Instruction and Demonstration

Demonstrating an activity while giving verbal instruction can enhance learning significantly. Two sensory systems are engaged, the auditory and the visual. The clinician not only describes or instructs in the steps of the activity, but demonstrates them as well. Practitioners may brush their own hair and ask patients to imitate what was shown or may ask them to perform in parallel, one step at a time. With this method of instruction, receptive language skills and auditory memory are not as critical, but the ability to imitate motor acts of another person must be intact. Patients with motor-planning deficits (apraxia) will have difficulty because they will not be able to plan movements to imitate the clinician's demonstration. Poor visual or auditory memory may also hamper the learning process when using this method.

### Teaching Through the Somatosensory and Vestibular Systems: Touch, Proprioception, and Motion

For patients who have deficits in the ability to follow auditory and demonstrated instructions, the COTA may need to augment instruction with input to the somatosensory system. If using tactile, proprioceptive, or movement stimuli to cue the patient, the COTA may choose to use no words or just short simple commands. Some demonstration may also be appropriate. The COTA may say, "Brush your hair," then may touch the patient's hand and move the hand to the hairbrush. This alone may be enough to cue the patient to perform the task. If it is not, the COTA may lift the patient's hand holding the hairbrush and simulate the movement pattern of hair brushing on the patient's head. Often the feeling of the correct movements and the tactile cue to pick up the brush facilitate the auditory and visual input of the demonstration and enhance learning.

*Guiding* is a special form of tactile, proprioceptive, and vestibular input.[1] The patient is guided through the activity with the close physical contact of the practitioner throughout the movement process. Little or no verbal instruction is given. The patient maintains contact with a reference point of solid support (e.g., table, counter surface) while performing the activity rather than moving through space unsupported. The purpose of guiding is to give the patient familiar sensory input.

During the guiding process the patient may take over some of the movement as the brain recognizes it from past experience.[1] As learning occurs, the clinician may decrease the amount of guiding and use less intense sensory input. When guiding, the clinician stands behind the patient and places the arms along the surfaces of the patient's arms. The clinician places the hand over the patient's hand and guides it along the surface of the table or vanity to reach the brush. The brush is grasped by the patient's hand, with the clinician's hand over top. The hand is guided back along the vanity surface and to the patient's body. The body may be used as a solid surface of support as the arm is guided toward the head. The clinician then guides the patient's arm through the brushing movements with the head now as the solid support.

The sensorimotor approaches described in Chapter 23 all use somatosensory input in the methods of teaching motor skills. The use of tactile and proprioceptive cues is helpful for patients who are apraxic and cannot imitate movements or have "forgotten" motor patterns associated with common implements such as a hairbrush. The effectiveness of this approach may be limited with patients who have severe tactile and proprioceptive sensory losses or who resist being touched.

## SUMMARY

The fields of motor learning and occupational therapy are concerned with the acquisition and retention of motor skills. It is important to focus on both how the skills are acquired and the end results of performance. Occupational therapy goals often involve learning motor skills for independent living. Although it is assumed that the OT practitioner is the instructor and the patient is the learner, the therapist or assistant must be open to learning from the patient.

Learning and retention are influenced by the structure and quality of practice and feedback. Random practice and summary feedback during motor learning have a positive effect on long-term retention. Blocked practice is useful in the early stages of learning to establish motor patterns and increase performance. Long-term skill retention is best measured at a later time after practice sessions to eliminate practice effects and the influence of short-term learning.

Instruction and practice should be appropriately paced for the learner and graded in complexity. Backward and forward chaining in instruction are two ways of grading toward independent performance. Practice is best done in the context most appropriate to the activity. Practice under variable conditions facilitates the patient's ability to transfer and generalize learning.

Feedback is necessary to correct faulty motor performance. Two types of feedback that enhance learning are intrinsic and extrinsic feedback. The learner receives intrinsic feedback through the sensory information from task performance and the outcome and receives extrinsic feedback from an outside source (e.g., therapist, mechanical device). Extrinsic feedback should be realistic, honest, and appropriate and provided in ways that allow the patient to revise erroneous motor acts. The frequency of extrinsic feedback should be decreased as performance is mastered. Summary feedback, given after several trials at a task, is more helpful for long-term retention than immediate or frequent feedback. Feedback about how the task is performed can help the patient develop the capacity for intrinsic feedback.

In occupational therapy for physical dysfunction, most treatment is done in individual sessions. However, group treatment may be used. Groups are usually project or parallel types, with the primary focus on task performance rather than group process. Successful learning in a group situation depends on the patient's level of cognitive and psychosocial function. The OTR is responsible for planning individual and group treatment, with contributions by the COTA to this process. The COTA may be given significant responsibility for carrying out the treatment.

The treatment plan is analogous to an instructional lesson plan and should be developed using the four steps in the teaching/learning process: (1) assessment, (2) design of a plan, (3) instruction, and (4) evaluation. The instruction phase can be further subdivided into four phases: preinstruction/preparation, instruction/demonstration, performance/return demonstration, and supervision/follow-up.

Methods of instruction selected by the OT practitioner depend on the patient's physical and cognitive status and motivation. Instruction may be given using the auditory, visual, and somatosensory systems. The use of multisystem input is often helpful to facilitate learning. Teaching methods can be graded to accommodate characteristics of the learner's cognitive and perceptual abilities.

To achieve the desired goals of accomplishing performance of essential motor skills, the patient must have a readiness for learning and must be prepared and have enough physical and cognitive resources and motivation to perform the task. Relevance of the task to the patient's life is essential to motivation.

The clinician also actively participates in the learning process. This involves evaluating the patient, setting goals and selecting appropriate activities with the patient, providing instruction and feedback, and evaluating treatment outcomes.

## *Selected Reading Guide Questions*

1. What is the result of learning?
2. Define *motor learning.*
3. What is the difference between procedural and declarative learning?
4. What is meant by the *ecological* approach to motor learning?
5. What is the difference between *whole learning* and *progressive-part learning?* Give examples illustrating when it is appropriate to use each.

6. List and define the stages of motor learning.
7. Identify the different practice schedules, and explain the conditions under which each is most effective.
8. How is learning measured?
9. What is meant by *transfer* of learning? How is it measured?
10. Describe two methods of practice. What are the advantages and disadvantages of each?
11. What is meant by *practice context?*
12. Why is feedback/reinforcement important to learning?
13. Identify and contrast two types of feedback.
14. List the components of motor control.
15. List at least eight characteristics of an effective teacher.
16. What are some reasons to use group treatment?
17. List and define the steps in the teaching/learning process.
18. What are some of the important factors a practitioner must consider about the patient when designing the instructional (treatment) plan?
19. What is meant by *pacing* and *grading instruction?*
20. List three major methods of teaching, accessing the sensory systems used as the mode of instruction. Give examples of how you would teach a patient to use a spoon to eat mashed potatoes using each method.

## REFERENCES

1. Bonfils K: The Affolter approach. In Pedretti LW: *Occupational therapy: practice skills for physical dysfunction,* ed 4, St Louis, 1995, Mosby.
2. Cai Z: The neural mechanism of declarative memory consolidation and retrieval: a hypothesis, *Neurosci Biobehav Rev* 14:295-304, 1990.
3. Gliner JA: Purposeful activity in motor learning theory: an event approach to motor skill acquisition, *Am J Occup Ther* 39:28, 1985.
4. Hames CC, Joseph DH: *Basic concepts of helping,* ed 2, East Norwalk, Conn, 1986, Appleton-Century-Crofts.
5. Hopkins HL, Tiffany EG: *Occupational therapy: base in activity.* In Hopkins HL, Smith HD: *Willard and Spackman's occupational therapy,* ed 7, Philadelphia, 1988, Lippincott.
6. Humphrey R, Jewell K: Developmental disabilities. Section 1. Mental retardation. In Hopkins HL, Smith HD: *Willard and Spackman's occupational therapy,* ed 8, Philadelphia, 1993, Lippincott.
7. Jarus T: Motor learning and occupational therapy: the organization of practice, *Am J Occup Ther* 48:810, 1994.
8. Kaplan M: Motor learning: implications for occupational therapy and neurodevelopmental treatment, *Dev Disabil Special Interest Sect Newslett* 17:1, 1994.
9. Kemp JE: *The instructional design process,* New York, 1985, Harper & Row.
10. Kupfermann I: Learning and memory. In Kandel ER, Schwartz JH, Jessell TM: *Principles of neural science,* ed 3, New York, 1991, Elsevier.
11. Levy LL: Behavioral frame of reference. In Hopkins HL, Smith HD: *Willard and Spackman's occupational therapy,* ed 8, Philadelphia, 1993, Lippincott.
12. Llorens L et al: Ethnogeriatrics: implication for occupational therapy and physical therapy, *Phys Occup Ther Geriatr,* vol 11, 1993.
13. Mathiowetz V, Haugen JB: Motor behavior research: implications for therapeutic approaches to central nervous system dysfunction, *Am J Occup Ther* 48:734-745, 1994.
14. Mosey AC: *Activities therapy,* New York, 1973, Raven.
15. Newton R: Contemporary issues and theories of motor control: assessment of movement and balance. In Umphred DA: *Neurological rehabilitation,* ed 3, St Louis, 1995, Mosby.
16. Poole J: Application of motor learning principles in occupational therapy, *Am J Occup Ther* 45:530, 1991.
17. Schmidt RA: Motor learning principles for physical therapy. In *Contemporary management of motor control problems.* Proceedings of the II Step Conference, Alexandria, Va, 1991, Foundation for Physical Therapy.
18. Schwartzberg S: Tools of practice. Section 2. Group process. In Hopkins HL, Smith HD: *Willard and Spackman's occupational therapy,* ed 8, Philadelphia, 1993, Lippincott.
19. Umphred DA: Classification of treatment techniques based on primary input systems: inherent and contrived feedback/loop systems included. In Umphred DA, editor: *Neurological rehabilitation,* ed 3, St Louis, 1995, Mosby.
20. Umphred DA: Introduction and overview: multiple interactive conceptual models: frameworks for clinical problem solving. In Umphred DA, editor: *Neurological rehabilitation,* ed 3, St Louis, 1995, Mosby.
21. Umphred DA: Limbic complex: influence over motor control and learning. In Umphred DA, editor: *Neurological rehabilitation,* ed 3, St Louis, 1995, Mosby.

Chapter 17

# Activities of Daily Living

Diane Foti
Lorraine Williams Pedretti

## Chapter Objectives

*After studying this chapter, the student or practitioner will be able to:*

1. Describe the role of the occupational therapy practitioner in providing activities of daily living (ADLs) services.
2. Discuss the factors that affect the role of the certified occupational therapy assistant in the practice area of ADLs.
3. Name, objectively describe, and contrast differing levels of independence in ADLs.
4. Describe the procedures for performing an ADL evaluation, including instruments to be used, techniques, timing, strategies, and reporting procedures.
5. Identify recommended adaptive devices to facilitate ADLs for individuals with specific functional losses.
6. Sequence and carry out training programs to enable individuals with specific functional losses to perform their own ADLs to the maximal possible level of independence.
7. Relate ADLs to other performance areas, and discuss the role of play and leisure in the life of the physically disabled individual.

## Key Terms

activities of daily living (ADLs)
instrumental activities of daily living (I-ADLs)
mobility
self-care
environmental hardware
communication
home management
community living skills
performance evaluation
safety management
bedside commode
transfer tub bench
health management
dressing stick
stocking aid
buttonhook
reacher
swivel spoon
universal cuff
plate guard
scoop dish
suction brush
nonskid mat
bridging
rocker knife
wand mouthstick

Activities of daily living (ADLs—sometimes called *basic ADLs*) and instrumental activities of daily living (I-ADLs) are the skills that support personal independence.[10,14] Self-maintenance, mobility, communication, home management, and community living skills are taken for granted by the average person. In persons with physical dysfunction, loss of the ability to care for personal needs and manage the environment can damage self-esteem and provoke feelings of dependence and even infantilism. Family roles may be disrupted, requiring partners to assume the role of caregiver when a person loses the ability to perform ADLs or I-ADLs independently.[20]

Occupational therapy programs provide evaluation and training in ADL and I-ADL task performance in virtually every type of healthcare service. The role of occupational therapy is to assess ADL and I-ADL performance skills, determine problems that interfere with independence, determine treatment objectives, and provide training or equipment to enhance the achievement of a higher level of independence. The occupational therapy practitioner may also be involved in removing or reducing physical, cognitive, social, and emotional barriers that interfere with performance. A given patient's need to learn new methods or to use assistive devices to perform daily tasks may be temporary or permanent, depending on the particular dysfunction and the prognosis for recovery. Both registered occupational therapists (OTRs) and certified occupational therapy assistants (COTAs) may be involved in providing ADL services; this is an area in which the COTA with proven service competency may function autonomously.

## DEFINITIONS

Daily activities can be separated into ADLs (or basic ADLs) and I-ADLs. ADLs require basic skills, whereas I-ADLs require more advanced problem-solving skills, social skills, and complex environmental interactions. ADL tasks are categorized according to the following areas: mobility, self-care, management of environmental hardware and devices, communication, and sexual expression. **Mobility** includes movement in bed, transfers, wheelchair mobility, and ambulation with or without walking aids. **Self-care** consists of dressing, self-feeding, toileting, bathing, and grooming activities. Management of **environmental hardware** and devices may include the ability to use telephones, keys, faucets, light switches, windows, doors, and scissors. **Communication** skills include the ability to write, operate a personal computer, read, type, or use a telephone, tape recorder, or special communications device. Sexual expression consists of engaging in desired sexual and intimate activities.

I-ADLs are divided into categories of home management, community living skills, health management, and safety preparedness. **Home management** activities include shopping, meal planning and preparation, cleaning, laundry, child care, recycling, and operating household appliances. **Community living skills** include money and financial management, management of public or private transportation, shopping, and access to recreation and leisure activities. Table 17-1 provides more detail on the subskills for these and other categories of I-ADLs.

## EVALUATION OF PERFORMANCE AREAS

ADLs represent one of the major performance areas in the occupational performance domain of concern (see Chapter 2). To review, the three occupational perfor-

*Table 17-1*

### Activities of Daily Living (ADLs) and Instrumental ADLs (I-ADLs)

| *ADLs* | *I-ADLs* |
|---|---|
| **Mobility** | **Home management** |
| Bed mobility | Shopping |
| Wheelchair mobility | Meal planning |
| Transfers | Meal preparation |
| Ambulation | Cleaning |
| | Laundry |
| | Child care |
| | Recycling |
| **Self-care** | **Community living skills** |
| Dressing | Money/financial management |
| Self-feeding | Use of public transportation |
| Toileting | Driving |
| Bathing | Shopping |
| Grooming | Access to recreation activities |
| **Communication** | **Health management** |
| Writing | Handling medication |
| Typing/computer use | Knowing health risks |
| Telephoning | Making medical appointments |
| Using special communication devices | |
| | **Safety management** |
| | Fire safety awareness |
| | Ability to call 911 |
| | Response to smoke detector |
| | Identification of dangerous situations |
| **Environmental hardware** | **Environmental hardware** |
| Keys | Vacuum cleaner |
| Faucets | Can opener |
| Light switches | Stove/oven |
| Windows/doors | Refrigerator |
| | Microwave oven |

mance areas are (1) work and productive activities, (2) play and leisure, and (3) ADLs, or self-maintenance. A primary purpose of occupational therapy is to facilitate skill in performing these essential tasks of living. The OT practitioner must help the individual with a disability to balance chosen activities in these three performance areas, taking into account personality, skills, limitations, needs, cultural values, and lifestyle.

The OT practitioner can begin evaluating the client's performance profile by charting a daily or weekly schedule (see Chapter 5), an activities configuration, an interest checklist, or an occupational role history.[6,9,21,23,28] The activities configuration protocol can be used to gather data about the client's values, educational history, and work history, including current or recent work experience, past work experience, and vocational interests and plans. The interest checklist indicates degree of interest in five categories of activities: (1) manual skills, (2) physical sports, (3) social recreation, (4) ADLs, and (5) cultural and educational activities.[21] The history of occupational roles gathers data about past and current occupational roles and the balance between work and leisure roles.[9] Although the interest checklist and the occupational role history were developed for a psychiatric population, they can be adapted for application to clients with a physical dysfunction.

An interview and performance evaluation can yield a well-rounded picture of the client's occupational performance. Deficits and imbalances in occupational performance will be apparent. The **performance evaluation** is fundamental to the development of a comprehensive treatment plan, which deals with performance components that underlie those skills. The performance evaluations addressed in this chapter are ADLs and I-ADLs. Resources to improve access or ability to participate in play and leisure activities are also presented. Chapter 19 discusses the evaluation of motor vehicle driving skills.

The patient's performance in ADLs and other occupational performance areas is critical. Practitioners who focus on remedying specific performance components may lose sight of this. For example, increasing fine motor control cannot be an end in itself. It must be applied to the individual's occupational role performance, including independence with handling clothing fasteners, using computer keyboard skills, and performing mechanical repairs. The outcome of improving a performance component should be linked to a functional task.

## FACTORS TO CONSIDER IN ADL/I-ADL EVALUATION AND TRAINING

Before ADL/I-ADL performance evaluation and training can begin, the OTR must assess performance components and consider several factors about the client and the environment. Physical resources, such as strength, range of motion (ROM), coordination, sensation, and balance, should be evaluated to determine potential skills and deficits in ADL performance and the possible need for special equipment. Perceptual and cognitive functions should be evaluated to determine potential for learning ADL skills. General mobility in a bed or wheelchair or ambulation should be assessed.

In addition to these relatively concrete and objective evaluations, the OT practitioner should be familiar with the client's culture and its values and mores in relation to self-care, the sick role, family assistance, and independence. The client's values and the client's peer group and culture should be considered in selecting objectives and initial activities in the ADL program. The balance of activities that demand time and energy in the client's day may influence how many ADLs may be performed independently.

The environment to which the client will return is an important consideration. Will the client live alone or with the family or a roommate? Will the client be going to a skilled nursing facility (SNF) or to a boarding and care home permanently or temporarily? Will the client return to work and community activities? The type and amount of assistance available in the home environment must be considered if the caregiver is to receive orientation and training in the appropriate supervision and assistance required.

The finances available for assisted care, special equipment, and home modifications are important considerations. For example, a wheelchair-bound client who is wealthy may be willing and able to make major modifications in the home, such as installing an elevator, lowering kitchen counters, widening doorways, and replacing deep pile carpeting to accommodate a wheelchair lifestyle. A client with fewer financial resources may need the assistance of an OT practitioner in making less costly modifications, such as removing scatter rugs and door sills, installing a plywood ramp at the entrance, and attaching a hand-held shower head to the bathtub faucet.

The ultimate goal of any ADL and I-ADL training program is for the client to achieve the maximal level of independence. The *maximal level of independence* is defined differently for each client. For the client with mild muscle weakness in one arm caused by a peripheral neuropathy, complete independence in ADLs may be the maximal level. For the client with high-level quadriplegia, however, self-feeding, oral hygiene, and communication activities with devices and assistance may be the maximal level of independence that can be expected. Therefore the potential for independence should be based on each client's unique personal needs, values, capabilities, limitations, and environmental resources.

American culture strongly values independence. Rehabilitation personnel and the patient's family or friends may unwittingly push for independence inappropriately. Achieving independence must be important to the client and within the realm of possibility. The physical prognosis and long-term prospects must be considered.

## ADL/I-ADL EVALUATION

### General Procedure

When data have been gathered about the client's physical, psychosocial, and environmental resources, the feasibility of ADL evaluation or training should be determined by the OT practitioner together with the client, supervising physician, and other rehabilitation team members. In some cases, ADLs should be delayed because of client limitations or in favor of more immediate treatment objectives that require the client's energy and participation.

Evaluation of ADL and I-ADL performance may be accomplished by the OTR or service-competent COTA. Evaluation often begins with an interview, using a checklist as a guide for questioning the client about individual capabilities and limitations. Several types of ADL I-ADL checklists and evaluations are available, covering similar categories and performance tasks.[5]

The interview may be used for screening to determine whether further evaluation is needed. The OTR usually makes this determination. The interview alone can lead to inaccurate assumptions about performance, because the client may recall performance before the onset of the dysfunction, may have some confusion or memory loss, and may overestimate or underestimate individual abilities because the client has had little opportunity to perform routine ADLs after the onset of the physical dysfunction. To assess ADL performance accurately, observation of performance is necessary. The phrase "one look is worth a thousand words" applies well here.

Ideally the OT practitioner should evaluate ADL performance when and where the client usually performs the activities. For example, a dressing evaluation could be arranged early in the morning in the treatment facility, where the client may be dressed by nursing personnel, or in the client's home. Self-feeding evaluation should occur at regular meal hours. If normal scheduling is not possible because of personnel and environmental constraints, the evaluation may be conducted during regular treatment sessions in the occupational therapy clinic under simulated conditions. However, simulation requires the client to perform routine self-maintenance tasks at noncustomary times in an artificial environment. Clients who have difficulty generalizing learning concepts may have problems transferring learning from simulations to actual daily activities.

The OT practitioner should begin by selecting relatively simple and safe tasks from the ADL/I-ADL checklist and should progress to more difficult and complex items. The evaluation should be completed over several sessions to avoid fatigue and reduce confusion resulting from an artificial situation. Those tasks that would be unsafe or obviously cannot be performed should be omitted and the appropriate notation made on the evaluation form.

During the performance evaluation the OT practitioner should observe the methods the client is using or attempting to use to accomplish the task and attempt to determine causes of performance problems. Common causes include weakness, spasticity, involuntary motion, perceptual deficits, and low endurance. If problems and their causes can be identified, the clinician has a good foundation for establishing training objectives, priorities, and methods and for determining the need for assistive devices.

Other important aspects of this evaluation that should not be overlooked are the client's need for respect and privacy and the ongoing interaction between the client and practitioner. The client's feelings about having the body viewed and touched should be respected. Privacy should be maintained for toileting, grooming, and dressing tasks. The clinician with whom the client is most familiar and comfortable may be the appropriate person to conduct the ADL evaluation and training. As the clinician interacts with the client during performance of ADLs, it may be possible to elicit the client's attitudes and feelings about the particular tasks, individual priorities in training, dependence and independence, and cultural, family, and personal values and customs about ADL performance.

### Recording Results

During the interview and performance evaluation the clinician makes the appropriate notations on the checklists. Separate checklists may be used for self-care, home management, mobility, and home environment evaluations. When describing levels of independence, OT practitioners often use such terms as moderate independence, maximal assistance, and minimal skill. Such terms must be defined or illustrated by supporting statements if they are to be meaningful and useful descriptors of performance. The practitioner must specify whether the level of independence refers to a single activity, a category of activities such as dressing, or all ADLs. In designating levels of independence, an agreed-on performance scale, such as that shown in Table 17-1, should be used to mark the ADL checklist. Definitions usually are broad and general. They can be modified to suit the program plan and approach of the particular treatment facility.

The information is then summarized succinctly for inclusion in the client's permanent records so that co-workers can refer to it. Figures 17-1 and 17-2 provide a sample case study, ADL and home management checklists, and summaries of an initial evaluation and progress report. The reader should keep in mind that the evaluation and progress summaries relate to the ADL portion of the treatment program only.

### Home Management

Home management tasks are I-ADLs and are evaluated similarly to self-care ADL tasks. The client should first be interviewed to elicit a description of the home and former and present home management responsibilities. Those tasks the client will need to perform when returning home, as well as those the client would like to perform, should be ascertained during the interview. If the client has a communication disorder or a cognitive deficit, assistance from friends or family members may be enlisted to obtain the information needed. The client may also be questioned about the ability to perform each task on the activities list. However, the evaluation is much more meaningful and accurate if the interview is followed by a performance evaluation in the treatment facility's ADL kitchen or apartment or in the client's home if possible.

It is assumed at this point that motor, sensory, perceptual, and cognitive skills have already been evaluated. Therefore the OT practitioner should select tasks and exercise safety precautions consistent with the client's capabilities and limitations. The initial tasks should be simple one-step or two-step procedures that are not hazardous, such as wiping a dish, sponging off a table, and turning the water on and off. As the evaluation progresses, tasks graded in complexity and involving safety precautions should be performed, such as making a sandwich and a cup of coffee and vacuuming the carpet.

Home management skills apply to women, men, and sometimes adolescents and children. Individuals may live independently or share home management responsibilities with their partners. In some homes, roles may have to be reversed after the onset of a physical disability, with the partner who usually stays at home seeking outside employment and the disabled individual remaining at home.

If a client is going to be home alone, several basic ADL and I-ADL skills are needed for safety and independence. ADL skills include independence with toileting, transfers or alternative plans to allow for rest periods, and use of the telephone or special call system in case of emergency. Minimal I-ADL skills required to stay at home alone include abilities to (1) prepare or retrieve a simple meal, (2) employ safety precautions and exhibit good judgment, (3) take medication, and (4) obtain emergency aid if needed. The practitioner can evaluate potential for remaining at home alone through the activities of home management evaluation. **Safety management** is also part of the home management evaluation (see Table 17-1).

A child with a permanent disability also needs to be considered for evaluation of and training for I-ADL skills as the need for independence increases with development and maturation.

## HOME EVALUATION

When discharge from the treatment facility is anticipated, a home evaluation should be performed to facilitate the client's maximal independence in the living environment. Ideally, physical and occupational therapy practitioners should perform it together on a visit to the client's home. The client and family members or roommates should be present. However, time and budget limitations may not allow two clinicians to go to the client's home. Therefore one rehabilitation professional may perform the evaluation, or the evaluation may be referred to the home

### Sample case study

J.V. is a 48-year-old married woman who suffered a cerebral thrombosis resulting in a CVA 6 months ago. She lives in a modest home with her husband and teenage daughter and was a full-time homemaker before the onset of her stroke. She was a cheerful and active woman who enjoyed cooking, baking, gardening, and visiting her neighbors and friends. The stroke resulted in the disturbance of cerebellar and brain stem functions. J.V. has a severe motor apraxia for speech, cannot close her mouth, drools, and walks with a broad-based ataxic gait. Since the onset of her disability J.V. has been very depressed, weeps frequently, is dependent for much of her self-care, and sits idly for long periods of time. She was referred to occupational therapy for evaluation and training in ADL, adjustment to disability, and development of drooling and swallowing control to facilitate feeding.

**SAMPLE ADL PROGRESS REPORT**

J.V. has attended occupational therapy 3 times weekly for 3 weeks since the initial evaluation. Further evaluation of self-care skills revealed that J.V. is capable of some hygiene skills, except a tub bath, nail care, hair care, and makeup application. However, at home she remains almost entirely dependent on Mr. V. for self-care, while crying and complaining of feeling weak.

Home management evaluation revealed considerable difficulty with most tasks except table setting, dusting, dishwashing, and sweeping, which she can perform if given cues and supervision. Performance of more complex tasks is limited by psychomotor retardation, incoordination, distractibility, inability to sequence a process, and apraxia for fine hand activities. It was necessary to supervise J.V. closely and give step-by-step instructions while she performed household tasks. A few simple homemaking tasks were performed for several training sessions, but performance did not improve.

J.V. appears to be very depressed and lacks intrinsic motivation. It was suggested to her family that they offer less assistance for self-care, and involve her with them in household tasks that she can perform, under their supervision, if possible.

The occupational therapy program will continue with greater emphasis on achieving control of mouth musculature, a primary goal of J.V. ADL training will be delayed until J.V. is moving toward the achievement of this primary goal.

*Figure 17-1* Activities of daily living (ADLs) evaluation. (Modified from Activities of Daily Living Evaluation Form 461-1, Hartford, Conn, 1963, The Hartford Easter Seal Rehabilitation Center.)

*Continued.*

OCCUPATIONAL THERAPY DEPARTMENT

ACTIVITIES OF DAILY LIVING EVALUATION

Name J. V. Age 48 Diagnosis CVA Dom. Right

Disability Bilateral incoordination, ataxia, apraxia of mouth musculature

Mode of ambulation Independent

Grading key:
- I = Independent
- MiA = Minimal assistance
- MoA = Moderate assistance
- MaA = Maximal assistance
- D = Dependent
- NA = Not applicable
- 0 = Not evaluated

TRANSFERS AND AMBULATION

| | Date | Independent | Assisted | Dependent |
|---|---|---|---|---|
| Tub or shower | 8/1 | | | D |
| Toilet | 8/1 | | MiA | |
| Wheelchair | NA | | | |
| Bed and chair | | I | | |
| Ambulation | | | MiA | |
| Wheelchair management | NA | | | |
| Car | | | MiA | |

BALANCE FOR FUNCTION

| | Adequate | Inadequate |
|---|---|---|
| Sitting | I | |
| Standing | I | |
| Walking | | MiA |

ADL SKILLS

| EATING | Date 8/1 (Grade) | 8/25 | | | REMARKS |
|---|---|---|---|---|---|
| Butter bread | I | | | | |
| Cut meat | I | | | | |
| Eat with spoon | I | | | | |
| Eat with fork | I | | | | |
| Drink with straw | D | | | | Mouth apraxia |
| Drink with glass | D | | | | prevents performance |
| Drink with cup | D | | | | of these activities |
| Pour from pitcher | D | | | | |

| UNDRESS | Date 8/1 | 8/25 | | | REMARKS |
|---|---|---|---|---|---|
| Pants or shorts | I | | | | Is physically |
| Girdle or garter belt | MaA | | | | capable of |
| Brassiere | MiA | | | | performing the |
| Slip or undershirt | I | | | | activities as |
| Dress | I | | | | indicated but |
| Skirt | I | | | | Mr. V. reports |
| Blouse or shirt | I | | | | that J.V. is |
| Slacks or trousers | I | | | | dependent on him |
| Bandana or necktie | NA | | | | for much assistance, |
| Stockings | MoA | | | | pleading fatigue, |
| Nightclothes | I | | | | whining, and |
| Hair net | NA | | | | crying for help |
| Housecoat/bathrobe | I | | | | |
| Jacket | I | | | | |
| Belt and/or suspenders | I | | | | |
| Hat | I | | | | |
| Coat | I | | | | |
| Sweater | I | | | | |
| Mittens or gloves | I | | | | |
| Glasses | NA | | | | |
| Brace | NA | | | | |
| Shoes | MoA | | | | |
| Socks | MoA | | | | |
| Overshoes | MoA | | | | |

| DRESS | Date 8/1 | 8/25 | | | REMARKS |
|---|---|---|---|---|---|
| Pants or shorts | MiA | | | | |
| Girdle or garter belt | MoA | | | | |
| Brassiere | MoA | | | | |
| Slip or undershirt | I | | | | |
| Dress | I | | | | |
| Skirt | I | | | | |
| Blouse or shirt | I | | | | |
| Slacks or trousers | I | | | | |
| Bandana or necktie | NA | | | | |
| Stockings | MoA | | | | |
| Nightclothes | I | | | | |
| Hair net | NA | | | | |
| Housecoat/bathrobe | I | | | | |
| Jacket | I | | | | |
| Belt and/or suspenders | I | | | | |
| Hat | I | | | | |
| Coat | I | | | | |
| Sweater | I | | | | |
| Mittens or gloves | I | | | | |
| Glasses | NA | | | | |
| Brace | NA | | | | |
| Shoes | MoA | | | | |
| Socks | MoA | | | | |
| Overshoes | MoA | | | | |

| FASTENINGS | Date 8/1 (Grade) | 8/25 | | | REMARKS |
|---|---|---|---|---|---|
| Button | I | | | | |
| Snap | MoA | | | | |
| Zipper | MiA | | | | |
| Hook and eye | MaA | | | | |
| Garters | D | | | | |
| Lace | D | | | | |
| Untie shoes | D | | | | |
| Velcro | MiA | | | | |

| HYGIENE | Date 8/1 | 8/25 | | | REMARKS |
|---|---|---|---|---|---|
| Blow nose | 0 | I | | | |
| Wash face, hands | 0 | I | | | |
| Wash extremities, back | 0 | MaA | | | |
| Brush teeth or dentures | 0 | I | | | |
| Brush or comb hair | 0 | I | | | |
| Set hair | 0 | D | | | |
| Shave or put on makeup | 0 | MiA | | | |
| Clean fingernails | 0 | I, D | | | |
| Trim fingernails, toenails | 0 | D | | | |
| Apply deodorant | 0 | I | | | |
| Shampoo hair | 0 | D | | | |
| Use toilet paper | 0 | I | | | |
| Use tampon or sanitary napkin | 0 | NA | | | |

| COMMUNICATION | Date 8/1 | 8/25 | | | REMARKS |
|---|---|---|---|---|---|
| Verbal | D | | | | |
| Read | I | | | | |
| Hold book | I | | | | |
| Turn page | I | | | | |
| Write | I | | | | Writes name and few words |
| Use telephone | D | | | | |
| Type | D | | | | |

| HAND ACTIVITIES | Date 8/1 | 8/25 | | | REMARKS |
|---|---|---|---|---|---|
| Handle money | 0 | | | | |
| Handle mail | 0 | | | | |
| Use of scissors | 0 | | | | |
| Open cans, bottles, jars | 0 | | | | |
| Tie package | 0 | | | | |
| Sew (baste) | 0 | | | | |
| Sew button, hook and eye | 0 | | | | |
| Polish shoes | 0 | | | | |
| Sharpen pencil | 0 | | | | |
| Seal and open letter | 0 | | | | |
| Open box | 0 | | | | |

| COMBINED PERFORMANCE ACTIVITIES | Date 8/1 | 8/25 | | | REMARKS |
|---|---|---|---|---|---|
| Open-close refrigerator | 0 | I | | | |
| Open-close door | 0 | I | | | |
| Remove and replace objects | 0 | I | | | |
| Carry objects during locomotion | 0 | D | | | |
| | 0 | | | | |
| Pick up object from floor | 0 | D | | | |
| Remove, replace light bulb | 0 | D | | | |
| Plug in cord | 0 | 0 | | | |

| OPERATE | Date 8/1 (Grade) | 8/25 | | | REMARKS |
|---|---|---|---|---|---|
| Light switches | 0 | I | | | |
| Doorbell | 0 | I | | | |
| Door locks and handles | 0 | D | | | |
| Faucets | 0 | I | | | |
| Raise-lower window shades | 0 | D | | | |
| Raise-lower venetian blinds | 0 | D | | | |
| Raise-lower window | 0 | D | | | |
| Open-close drawer | 0 | I | | | |
| Hang up garment | 0 | I | | | |

SUMMARY OF EVALUATION RESULTS

Date 8/1

| Intact | Impaired | | REMARKS |
|---|---|---|---|
| | | SENSORY STATUS | |
| X | | Touch | |
| X | | Pain | |
| X | | Temperature | |
| | X | Position sense | More marked on left |
| | X | Olfaction | |
| | X | Stereognosis | More marked on left |
| | X | Visual fields (hemianopsia) | |
| | | PERCEPTUAL/CONCEPTUAL TESTS | |
| X | | Follow directions | Verbal |
| X | | Visual spatial (form) | |
| | X | Visual spatial (block design) | Minimal impairment |
| X | | Make change | |
| | X | Geometric figures (copy) square, circle, triangle, diamond | Some difficulty with triangle & diamond |
| | X | Praxis | Mild apraxia evident on fine hand activities |
| | | FUNCTIONAL RANGE OF MOTION | |
| X | | Comb hair—two hands | |
| X | | Feed self | |
| X | | Button collar button | |
| X | | Tie apron behind back | |
| X | | Button back buttons | |
| X | | Button cuffs | |
| X | | Zip side zipper | |
| | X | Tie shoes | Poor balance limits |
| | X | Stoop | Reach and bending for these activities |
| | X | Reach shelf | |

*Figure 17-1, cont'd.* For legend see p. 241.

OCCUPATIONAL THERAPY DEPARTMENT

ACTIVITIES OF HOME MANAGEMENT

Name *J. V.* Date *8/25*

Address *Anytown, U.S.A.*

Age *48* Weight *135* Height *5'5"* Role in family *Wife, mother*

Diagnosis *CVA* Disability *Bilateral ataxia, apraxia of mouth musculature*

Mode of ambulation *Independent, no aids, mild ataxic gait*

Limitations or contraindications for activity ______

DESCRIPTION OF HOME

1. Private house *✓*
   - No. of rooms *6 - kitchen, dining room, living room, 3 bedrooms*
   - No. of floors *2*
   - Stairs *14 - bedrooms on second floor*
   - Elevators *0*
2. Apartment house ___
   - No. of rooms ___
   - No. of floors ___
   - Stairs ___
   - Elevators ___
3. Diagram of home layout (attach to completed form)

Will patient be required to perform the following activities? If not, who will perform?

| | | |
|---|---|---|
| Meal preparation | *No* | *Daughter* |
| Baking | *No* | *Daughter (J.V. used to bake a lot)* |
| Serving | *Yes* | |
| Wash dishes | *Yes* | |
| Marketing | *No* | *Husband* |
| Child care (under 4 years) | *No* | |
| Washing | *Yes* | |
| Hanging clothes | *NA* | *Has dryer* |
| Ironing | *No* | *Daughter* |
| Cleaning | *Yes* | *Light cleaning* |
| Sewing | *No* | *Does not sew* |
| Hobbies or special interest | *Yes* | *Baking and gardening would be desirable activities* |

Does patient really like housework? *No*

Sitting position: Chair *X* Stool *X* Wheelchair *NA*

Standing position: Braces *NA* Crutches *NA* Canes *NA*

Handedness: Dominant hand *Right* Two hands *X* One hand only ___ Assistive ___

Grading key:
- I = Independent
- MiA = Minimal assistance
- MoA = Moderate assistance
- MaA = Maximal assistance
- D = Dependent
- 0 = Not evaluated

| CLEANING ACTIVITIES | Date *8/25* Grade | | | | REMARKS |
|---|---|---|---|---|---|
| Pick up object from floor | *D* | | | | |
| Wipe up spills | *D* | | | | |
| Make bed (daily) | *D* | | | | |
| Use dust mop | *I* | | | | |
| Shake dust mop | *D* | | | | |
| Dust low surfaces | *I* | | | | |
| Dust high surfaces | *D* | | | | |
| Mop kitchen floor | *D* | | | | |
| Sweep with broom | *I* | | | | |
| Use dust pan and broom | *MiA* | | | | |
| Use vacuum cleaner | *D* | | | | |
| Use vacuum cleaner attachments | *D* | | | | |
| Carry light cleaning tools | *I* | | | | |
| Use carpet sweeper | *I* | | | | |
| Clean bathtub | *D* | | | | |
| Change sheets on bed | *D* | | | | |
| Carry pail of water | *D* | | | | |

| MEAL PREPARATION | Date *8/25* | | | | REMARKS |
|---|---|---|---|---|---|
| Turn off water | *I* | | | | |
| Turn off gas or electric range | *I* | | | | |
| Light gas with match | *D* | | | | |
| Pour hot water from pan to cup | *D* | | | | |
| Open packaged goods | *I* | | | | |
| Carry pan from sink to range | *D* | | | | |
| Use can opener | *D* | | | | |
| Handle milk bottle | *I* | | | | |
| Dispose of garbage | *D* | | | | |
| Remove things from refrigerator | *D* | | | | |
| Bend to low cupboards | *D* | | | | |
| Reach to high cupboards | *D* | | | | |
| Peel vegetables | *D* | | | | |
| Cut up vegetables | *D* | | | | |
| Handle sharp tools safely | *D* | | | | |
| Break eggs | *D* | | | | |
| Stir against resistance | *D* | | | | |
| Measure flour | *D* | | | | |
| Use eggbeater | *D* | | | | |
| Use electric mixer | *D* | | | | |
| Remove batter to pan | *D* | | | | |
| Open oven door | *I* | | | | |
| Carry pan to oven and put in | *D* | | | | |
| Remove hot pan from oven to table | *D* | | | | |
| Roll cookie dough or piecrust | *D* | | | | |

*Figure 17-2* Activities of home management. (Modified from Activities of Home Management Form, Occupational Therapy Department, University Hospital, Ohio State University, Columbus, Ohio.)

| MEAL SERVICE | Date *8/25* | | | | REMARKS |
|---|---|---|---|---|---|
| Set table for four | *I* | | | | |
| Carry four glasses of water to table | *D* | | | | |
| Carry hot casserole to table | *D* | | | | |
| Clear table | *I* | | | | |
| Scrape and stack dishes | *I* | | | | |
| Wash dishes (light soil) | *I* | | | | |
| Wipe silver | *I* | | | | |
| Wash pots and pans | *MiA* | | | | |
| Wipe up range and work areas | *MoA* | | | | |
| Wring out dishcloth | *I* | | | | |

| LAUNDRY | Date *8/25* | | | | REMARKS |
|---|---|---|---|---|---|
| Wash lingerie (by hand) | *D* | | | | |
| Wring out, squeeze dry | *D* | | | | |
| Hang on rack to dry | *I* | | | | |
| Sprinkle clothes | *I* | | | | |
| Iron blouse or slip | *D* | | | | |
| Fold blouse or slip | | | | | |
| Use washing machine | | | | | |

| SEWING | Date *8/25* | | | | REMARKS |
|---|---|---|---|---|---|
| Thread needle and make knot | | | | | |
| Sew on buttons | | | | | |
| Mend rip | | | | | |
| Darn socks | | | | | |
| Use sewing machine | | | | | |
| Crochet | | | | | |
| Knit | | | | | |
| Embroider | | | | | |
| Cut with shears | | | | | |

HEAVY HOUSEHOLD ACTIVITIES. WHO WILL DO THESE?

| | Date *8/25* | | | | REMARKS |
|---|---|---|---|---|---|
| Wash household laundry | | | | | |
| Hang clothes | | | | | |
| Clean range | | | | | |
| Clean refrigerator | | | | | |
| Wax floors | | | | | |
| Marketing | | | | | |
| Turn mattresses | | | | | |
| Wash windows | | | | | |
| Put up curtains | | | | | |

WORK HEIGHTS

SITTING/STANDING
Wheelchair ___ Chair *X* Stool *X*

| | |
|---|---|
| Best height for | |
| Ironing | *17½" seated* |
| Mixing | *26" on high stool at counter* |
| Dish washing | *26" on high stool at counter* |
| General work | |
| Maximal depth of counter area (normal reach) | *25"* |
| Maximal useful height above work surface | *33" if standing* |
| Maximal useful height without counter surface | *68" if standing* |
| Maximal reach below counter area | *20" if standing* |
| Best height for chair | *17½"-can be used at adjustable ironing board* |
| Best height for stool with back support | *24"-can be used at sink or food preparation counter* |

SUGGESTIONS FOR HOME MODIFICATION

*Remove scatter rugs in bedroom*
*Install guard rail on both sides of toilet*
*Install grab bars on wall next to bathtub*
*Place nonskid strips on bottom of bathtub*

*Figure 17-2, cont'd*

health agency that will be providing home care services to the client. The client and a family member should be interviewed to determine the client's and family's expectations and the roles the client will assume in the home and community. The cultural or family values regarding a disabled member may influence role expectations and whether or not independence will be encouraged. Willingness and financial ability to make modifications in the home can also be determined.[27]

Sufficient time should be scheduled for the home visit so that the client can demonstrate the required transfer and mobility skills. The clinician may also ask the client to demonstrate selected self-care and home management tasks in the home environment. During

## HOME EVALUATION CHECKLIST

Name________________________________________ Date______________
Address__________________________________________________________
Diagnosis_______________________________

**Mobility Status** ❑ ambulatory, no device ❑ cane ❑ walker ❑ wheelchair

*Exterior*

**Home located on** ❑ level surface ❑ hill

**Type of House** ❑ owns house ❑ apartment ❑ mobile home ❑ board and care

**Number of floors** ❑ one story ❑ two story ❑ split level

**Driveway surface** ❑ inclined ❑ level ❑smooth ❑ rough

Is the DRIVEWAY negotiable? ❑ yes ❑ no
Is the GARAGE accessible? ❑ yes ❑ no

*Entrance*

**Accessible entrances** ❑ front ❑ back ❑ side

**Steps** number ______ height of each ______ width ______ depth ______

Are there HANDRAILS? ❑ yes ❑ no

If yes, where are they located? ❑ left ❑ right

HANDRAIL height from step surface? ______

If no, how much room is available for HANDRAILS? ______

**Are landings negotiable?** ❑ yes ❑ no

Briefly describe any problems with LANDINGS:______________________________

**Ramps** ❑ yes ❑ no
❑ front ❑ back
height ______
width ______
length ______

Are there HANDRAILS? ❑ yes ❑ no

If yes, where are they located? ❑ left ❑ right height_______

If no ramp, how much room is available for one? ______________________

**Porch**
width ______
length ______
Level at threshold? ❑ yes ❑ no

**Door**
width ______
threshold height ______ Negotiable? ❑ yes ❑ no
❑ swing in
❑ swing out
❑ sliding

*Interior*

**Living Room**

Is furniture arranged for easy maneuverability? ❑ yes ❑ no

Is frequently used furniture accessible ❑ yes ❑ no

Type of floor covering: ______________________

Comments ______________________________________

**Hallways**

Can wheelchair or walking aide be maneuvered in hallway? ❑ yes ❑ no

hall width ______
door width ______

Sharp turns ❑ yes ❑ no

Steps? ❑ yes ❑ no
number ______

Are there HANDRAILS? ❑ yes ❑ no

If yes, where are they located? ❑ left ❑ right height_______

**Bedroom**
❑ single
❑ shared

Is there room for a W/C? ❑ yes ❑ no

Door:
width ______
threshold height ______ Negotiable? ❑ yes ❑ no
❑ swing in
❑ swing out

Bed:
❑ twin
❑ double
❑ queen
❑ king
❑ hospital bed

Overall height ______ Accessible? ❑ yes ❑ no

Would hospital bed fit into room if needed? ❑ yes ❑ no

Clothing:

Are drawers accessible? ❑ yes ❑ no ❑ on right ❑ on left

Is closet accessible? ❑ yes ❑ no ❑ on right ❑ on left

Comments: ______________________________________

**Bathroom**

Door:
width ______
threshold height ______ Negotiable? ❑ yes ❑ no

Tub:
height, floor-rim ______
height, tub bottom rim ______
tub width inside ______

glass doors? ❑ yes ❑ no
width of tub doors ______

overhead shower? ❑ yes ❑ no

Is tub accessible? ❑ yes ❑ no

Stall Shower: ❑ yes ❑ no
door width ______
height of bottom rim ______
accessible? ❑ yes ❑ no

Sink:
height ______
faucet type ______
❑ open
❑ closed
accessible? ❑ yes ❑ no

Toilet:
height from floor ______
location of toilet paper ______
distance from toilet to side wall L ______ R ______

Grab bars: ❑ yes ❑ no
Location ______________________

Comments: ______________________________________

**Kitchen**

Door:
width ______
threshold height ______ Negotiable? ❑ yes ❑ no

Stove:
height ______
Location of controls ❑ front ❑ back
Is stove accessible for use? ❑ yes ❑ no

Oven:
Height from floor to door hinge & door handle ______
Location of oven ______________________

Sink:
Will w/c fit underneath? ❑ yes ❑ no
Type of faucets ___________

Cupboards:
accessible from w/c? ❑ yes ❑ no

Refrigerator:
hinges on ❑ left ❑ right
accessible from w/c? ❑ yes ❑ no

Switches / Outlets:
accessible? ❑ yes ❑ no

Kitchen Table:
height from floor ______
accessible? ❑ yes ❑ no

Comments: ______________________________________

**Laundry**

Door: width ______
threshold height ______ Negotiable? ❑ yes ❑ no

Steps: ❑ yes ❑ no
number ______
height ______
width ______

Are there HANDRAILS? ❑ yes ❑ no

If yes, where are they located? ❑ left ❑ right height_______

*Figure 17-3* Home visit checklist. (Modified from *Occupational/Physical Therapy Home Evaluation Form,* San Francisco, Ralph K. Davies Medical Center; and *Occupational Therapy Home Evaluation Form,* Albany, Calif, 1993, Alta Bates Hospital.)

*Continued.*

Washer:
- ❑ Topload
- ❑ Front load
- accessible? ❑ yes ❑ no

Dryer:
- ❑ Topload
- ❑ Front load
- accessible? ❑ yes ❑ no

*Safety*

Throw rugs
❑ yes ❑ no
Location ______

Phone
accessible? ❑ yes ❑ no
Location ______

Emergency phone numbers
❑ yes ❑ no
Location ______

Mailbox
accessible? ❑ yes ❑ no
Location ______

Thermostat
accessible? ❑ yes ❑ no
Location ______

Electric Outlets / switches
accessible? ❑ yes ❑ no

Imperfect floor?
❑ yes ❑ no
Location ______

Sharp Edged furniture?
❑ yes ❑ no
Location ______

Insulated hot water pipes: ❑ yes ❑ no
Location ______

Cluttered areas?
❑ yes ❑ no
Location ______

Fire extinguisher?
❑ yes ❑ no
Location ______

**Equipment present:** ______

**Problem list:** ______

**Recommendations for modifications:** ______

**Equipment Recommendations:** ______

*Figure 17-3, cont'd.* For legend see opposite page.

the evaluation the client should demonstrate the use of any ambulation aids and assistive devices. The clinician should bring a tape measure to measure width of doorways, height of stairs, height of bed, and other dimensions.

The evaluator can begin by explaining the purposes and procedures of the home evaluation to the client and others present, if this was not done before the visit. The evaluator can proceed to take the required measurements while surveying the general arrangement of rooms, furniture, and appliances. It may be helpful to sketch the size and arrangement of rooms for later reference and to attach the sketch to the home visit checklist (Figure 17-3). (For more information on a variety of checklists, see Letts et al.[18])

Once the record of the home arrangement and dimensions is completed, the client is asked to demonstrate mobility and transfer, essential self-care, and home management skills. If relevant, the client's ability to use the entrance to the home and transfer to and from an automobile should be included in the home evaluation.

During the performance evaluation the clinician should be observing safety factors, ease of mobility and performance, and limitations imposed by the environment. If the patient requires assistance for transfers and other activities, the caregiver should be instructed in appropriate methods. The patient may also be instructed in methods to improve maneuverability and simplify performance of tasks in a small space.

At the end of the evaluation the clinician can make a list of problems, modifications recommended, and additional safety equipment and assistive devices. The most frequently needed changes are installation of a ramp or railings at the entrance to the home; removal of scatter rugs, extra furniture, and bric-a-brac; removal of door sills; addition of safety grab bars around the toilet and bathtub; rearrangement of furniture to accommodate a wheelchair; rearrangement of kitchen storage; and lowering of the clothes rod in the closet.[27]

Access into the bathroom and maneuvering with a wheelchair or walker frequently cause problems. The clinician may recommend a **bedside commode** until a bathroom can be made accessible or modified to allow for independence with toileting (Figure 17-4). Shower seats can be used in the tub (if the client is able to transfer safely over the edge of the tub) and may also be used in a shower. A **transfer tub bench** (Figure 17-5) is recommended for individuals who cannot step over the edge of the tub safely or independently. Installation of a hand-held shower increases access to the water and also eliminates the need for standing or risky turns while bathing.

When the home evaluation is completed, the evaluator should write a report summarizing the information on the form and describing the client's performance in the home. The report should conclude with a summary of the environmental barriers and the client's functional limitations. Recommendations should include equipment or alterations, with specifics in terms of size, building specifications, costs, sources, and specialized training required for use. Recommendations may also include further functional goals to improve independence in the home environment.

Home evaluation recommendations must be carefully reviewed with the client and family. The OT practitioner must use tact and diplomacy to present options and must grant the client freedom to refuse or consider alternative possibilities. Cultural values, aesthetic preferences, and family finances may be limiting factors in implementing needed changes. The social worker may be involved in handling funding for equipment and alterations, and the client should be made aware of this service when cost is discussed.[27]

The evaluator should include recommendations regarding the feasibility of the client remaining in or

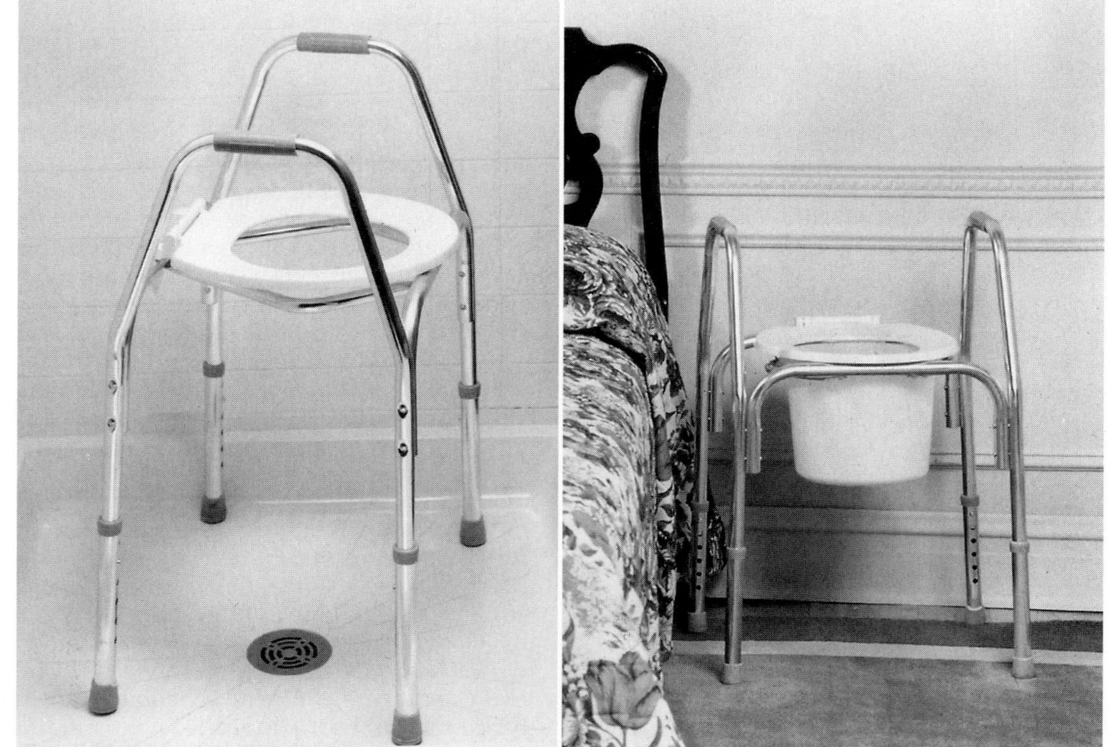


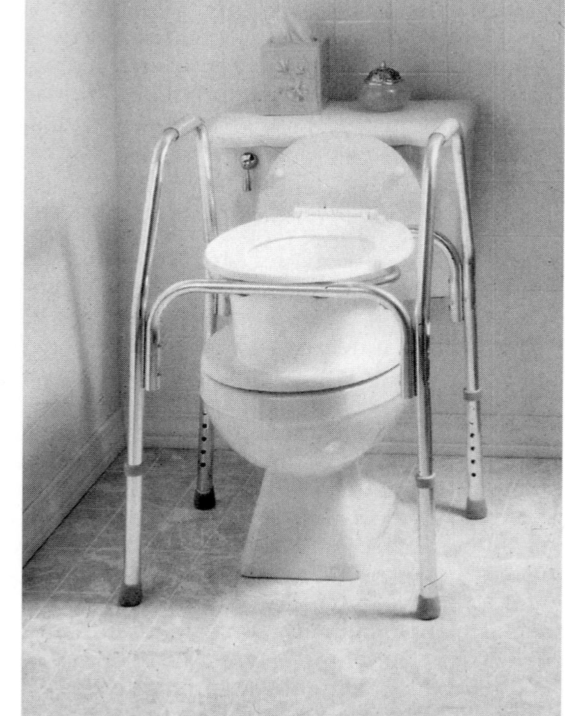


*Figure 17-4* All-purpose commode. **A,** In shower; **B,** bedside; **C,** over toilet. (Courtesy Sammons, a BISSELL Co.)

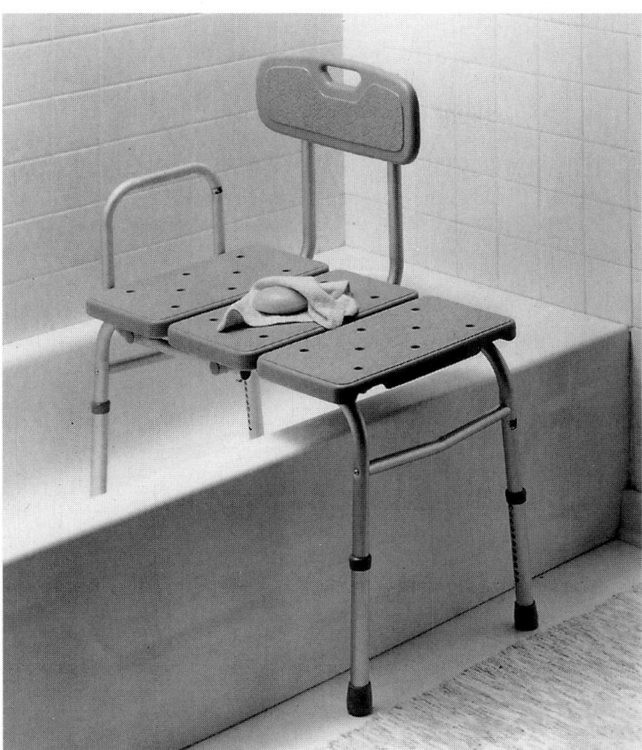

*Figure 17-5* Transfer tub bench. (Courtesy Sammons, a Bissell Co.)

managing the home alone or being discharged to the home environment, as applicable. If any question exists regarding the client's ability to return home safely and independently, the home evaluation summary should include the functional skills the client needs to return home.

If a home visit is not possible, some information can be obtained by interviewing the client and family member after a trial home visit. The family member or caregiver may be instructed to complete the home visit checklist and to provide photographs or sketches of the rooms and their arrangements. Problems encountered by the client during the home visit should be discussed and the necessary recommendations for their solution made, as described earlier.[27]

## COMMUNITY LIVING SKILLS

### Money and Financial Management

If the client is to resume management of money and financial matters independently, the skills required for these tasks must be assessed. The evaluator must consider the effects of any cognitive, perceptual, or judgment problems on performance. The client may be capable of handling only small amounts of money or may need retraining with activities that require money management, such as shopping, balancing a checkbook, or making a budget. Adaptive writing devices can allow the client with a physical limitation to handle the paperwork aspects of money management. Caregivers who are new to the role of financial manager may require training and support in acquiring an unfamiliar role.

### Community Mobility

Some clients are capable of driving and can afford to have their own vehicle adapted or purchase an adapted van (see Chapter 19). The client who cannot drive or who cannot afford an adapted vehicle must learn to use public transportation or travel on foot or in a wheelchair. The occupational therapy practitioner must then consider the client's physical, perceptual, cognitive, and social capabilities to be independent and safe with community mobility.

Physical capabilities to be considered are (1) whether the client has the endurance to be mobile in the community without fatigue and (2) whether the client is adequately independent with walker, cane, crutch, or wheelchair skills and transfers to go beyond the home environment. Skills needed include managing uneven pavement, curbs, steps, ramps, and inclines and crossing streets. Using accessible transportation such as buses with lifts may also be included. Other skills to be evaluated before considering community mobility are how to (1) handle money, (2) carry objects in a wheelchair or with a walker, and (3) manage toileting in a public restroom.

Cognitive skills needed for community mobility include having basic geographical orientation, knowing where and how to receive directions, and solving problems should they occur. If taking a bus, the client must know how to read a schedule and map. If the disability is new, the client may be developing new social skills, which initially will be stretched to the limit by community situations. Social skills include being assertive enough to obtain an accessible table at a restaurant, obtaining assistance with items that cannot be reached in the grocery store, and becoming comfortable with a new body image within the able-bodied community.

The client's community environment also needs to be assessed. Considerations include (1) how safe is the neighborhood for an individual who might be vulnerable because of physical limitations? (2) what is the terrain like? (3) are there curb cut-outs? (4) are the sidewalks smooth and even? and (5) how far away is the closest store and bus stop?

Accessibility of community transportation should also be considered. Some communities have door-to-door cab and van service provided the client meets certain requirements, which may include arranging transportation 1 week in advance; being able to go out the front door and to the curb independently; and being able to transfer independently into the vehicle. The client using a public bus must learn how to manage the electric lifts and how to lock a wheelchair into place. Neighboring bus stops must be evaluated because not all are wheelchair accessible.

Community mobility requires preplanning by the OT practitioner and client, accurate assessment of the client's abilities, and awareness of potential physical, cognitive, and social barriers. A valuable resource by Armstrong and Lauzen, *Community Integration Program*,[2] provides practical treatment protocols for a community living skills program. Efforts toward independence in community mobility are worth the investment because the client can expand life tasks beyond the home and interact with the community.

## HEALTH MANAGEMENT

**Health management** includes the client's ability to understand the medical condition and to make reasonable decisions to maintain good health. Some practical aspects of health management include the client's abilities to handle medications, know when to call a physician, and how to make medical appointments. The evaluation of the client's ability to perform these activities will probably include other team members (e.g., nurse, physician).

The OTR or COTA must assess each health management task separately, considering the performance components required. The occupational therapy assessment can be helpful in determining which specific aspects of the task need to be modified for the client to be independent. For example, the OT practitioner may work jointly with a nurse to ensure that a client with hemiplegia and diabetes is able to manage insulin shots. The OT evaluation considers the client's cognitive and perceptual abilities to make judgments on drawing the insulin out of the bottle, measuring the insulin, and injecting the insulin. The COTA may address physical concerns, such as how to stabilize the insulin bottle and handle the syringe with one hand. Different strategies for opening the medication and measuring liquids may be needed.

The OT practitioner may also evaluate and train the client in subskills needed to make a medical appointment, such as using the phone, finding the appropriate phone numbers, and providing the needed information.

## ADL/I-ADL TRAINING

When ADL/I-ADL training is indicated, appropriate short-term and long-term objectives must be established, based on the evaluation and the client's priorities and potential for independence. The following sequence of training for self-care (ADL) activities is suggested: feeding, grooming, continence, transfer skills, toileting, undressing, dressing, and bathing. This sequence is based on the normal development of self-care independence in children.[27] This sequence may need to be modified to accommodate the specific dysfunction and the client's capabilities, limitations, and personal priorities.

The OT practitioner should estimate which ADL/I-ADL tasks are possible and which are impossible for the client to achieve. The clinician should explore with the client the possibility of alternate methods of performing the activities and using assistive devices. The level of assistance needed for each task should be determined. It may not be possible to estimate these factors until training is underway.

The ADL/I-ADL training program may be graded by beginning with a few simple tasks, which are gradually increased in number and complexity. Training should progress from dependent, to assisted, to supervised, to independent, with or without assistive devices.[27] The rate at which grading can occur depends on the client's potential for recovery, endurance, skills, and motivation.

### Methods of Teaching ADLs

The methods of teaching the client to perform ADLs must be tailored to suit each client's learning style and ability. Clients who are alert and grasp instructions quickly may be able to perform an entire process after a brief demonstration and verbal instruction. Clients who have perceptual problems, poor memory, or difficulty following instructions require a more concrete, step-by-step approach in which the amount of assistance is reduced gradually as success is achieved. For these persons it is important to break down the activity into small steps and to progress through them slowly, one at a time. Slow demonstration by the clinician of the task or step in the same plane and in the same manner in which the client is expected to perform is very helpful. Verbal instructions to accompany the demonstration may or may not be helpful, depending on the client's receptive language skills and ability to process and integrate two modes of sensory information simultaneously.

Helpful tactile and kinesthetic modes of instruction include (1) touching body parts to be moved, dressed, bathed, or positioned; (2) passively moving the part through the desired pattern to achieve a step or task; and (3) gently guiding the part manually through the task (see Chapters 16 and 23). Such techniques can augment or replace demonstration and verbal instruction, depending on the client's best avenues of learning. Skill, speed, and retention of learning require repeated task performance. Tasks may be repeated several times during the same training session, if time and the client's physical and emotional tolerance allow, or they may be repeated daily until desired retention or level of skill is achieved.

The process of *backward chaining* can be used in teaching ADL skills (see Chapter 16). This method is particularly useful in training clients with brain damage.[27]

Before beginning training in any ADL, the clinician must prepare by providing adequate space and arranging equipment, materials, and furniture for maximal convenience and safety. The clinician should be thoroughly familiar with the task to be performed and any special methods or assistive devices that will be used. The OT practitioner should be able to perform the task as the client is expected to perform it—skillfully. This may include, for example, performance with the practitioner's nondominant hand.

Next the activity is presented to the client, usually in one or more modes of guidance, demonstration, and verbal instruction described earlier. The client then performs the activity either along with the clinician or immediately after being shown, with supervision and assistance as required. Performance is modified and corrected as needed, and the process is repeated to ensure learning. Because other staff or family members frequently will be the individuals reinforcing the newly learned skills, family training is critical to reinforce learning and to ensure that the client carries over the skills from previous treatment sessions.

In the final phase of instruction, after mastering the task or several tasks, the client attempts to perform them independently. The OT practitioner should follow up by checking on performance in progress. Finally, the practitioner must check on adequacy of performance and carry-over of learning with nursing personnel, the caregiver, or the supervising family members.[12]

### Recording Progress in ADL Performance

The ADL checklists used to record performance on the initial evaluation usually have one or more spaces for recording changes in abilities and results of reevaluation during the training process. The sample checklist described earlier is designed and completed in this way (see Figure 17-1). Progress is usually summarized for inclusion in the medical record. The progress record should summarize changes in the client's abilities and current level of independence and estimate the client's potential for further independence, attitude, motivation for ADL training, and future goals for the ADL program. The progress record should also reflect how the client's current level of independence or assistance may affect discharge plans. For example, the client who continues to need moderate assistance with self-care may need to hire an attendant. Alternately, the OT practitioner may justify a need for ongoing treatment when the client has potential for further independence.

## SPECIFIC ADL TECHNIQUES

Standard techniques to solve specific ADL problems are not practical in every situation. The occupational therapy practitioner may have to explore a variety of methods or assistive devices to reach a solution. The OT practitioner sometimes needs to design a special device, method, splint, or piece of equipment to allow the client to perform a particular activity. Many assistive devices available today through rehabilitation equipment companies were originally created by OT practitioners and clients. Many special methods used to perform specific activities also evolved through trial-and-error approaches of clinicians and their clients. Clients often have good suggestions because they live with the limitation and are confronted regularly with the need to adapt the performance of daily tasks.

The purpose of the following summary of techniques is to provide some general ideas about how to solve ADL problems for specific classifications of dysfunctions. (See References for more detailed instuction in ADL methods.)

### Limited Range of Motion and Strength

The major problem for clients with limited joint ROM is the lack of reach and joint excursion. Environmental adaptation and assistive devices are used to compensate. Individuals who lack muscle strength may require some of the same devices or techniques to conserve energy and to compensate for weakness. Some adaptations and devices are outlined here.[19,22,24,27]

#### *Dressing Activities*

General suggestions for facilitating dressing include the following:

1. Use front-opening garments, one size larger than needed and made of fabrics with some stretch.
2. Use **dressing sticks** with a garter on one end and a neoprene-covered coat hook on the other for pushing and pulling garments off and on feet and legs (Figure 17-6) and to push a shirt or blouse over the head. Use a pair of dowels with a cup hook on the end of each to pull on socks to which a loop tape has been sewn at the top.
3. Use larger buttons or zippers with a loop on the pull tab.
4. Replace buttons, snaps, hooks, and eyes with Velcro or zippers (for those patients who cannot manage traditional fastenings).
5. Eliminate the need to bend and tie shoelaces or to use finger joints in this fine motor activity by using elastic shoelaces or other adapted shoe fasteners.
6. Facilitate donning stockings without bending to the feet by using **stocking aids** made of garters attached to long webbing straps or by buying those commercially available (Figure 17-7).
7. Use one of several types of commercially available **buttonhooks** if finger ROM is limited (Figure 17-8).
8. Use **reachers** for picking up socks and shoes, arranging clothes, removing clothes from hangers, picking up objects on the floor (Figure 17-9), and donning pants.

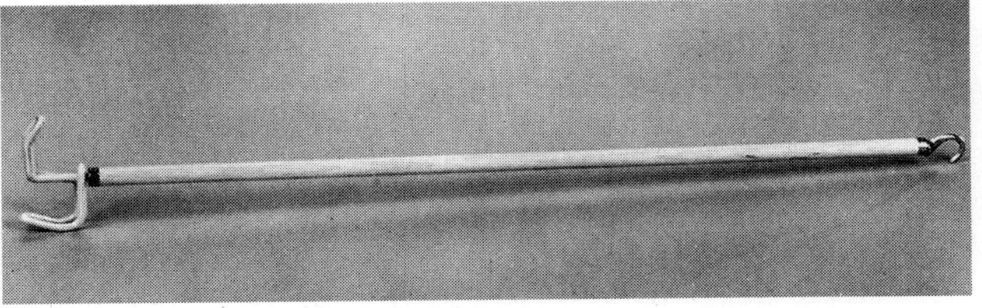

*Figure 17-6* Dressing stick or reacher. (Courtesy Sammons, a BISSELL Co.)

### *Eating Activities*

Assistive devices that can facilitate feeding include the following:

1. Built-up handles on eating utensils can accommodate limited grasp or prehension (Figure 17-10).
2. Elongated or specially curved handles on spoons and forks may be needed to reach the mouth. A **swivel spoon** or spoon-fork combination can compensate for limited supination (Figure 17-11).
3. Long plastic straws and straw clips on glasses or cups can be used if neck, elbow, or shoulder ROM limits hand-to-mouth motion or if grasp is inadequate to hold the cup or glass.
4. **Universal cuffs** or utensil holders can be used if grasp is very limited and built-up handles do not work (Figure 17-12).
5. Plate guards or scoop dishes may be useful to prevent food from slipping off the plate.

### *Hygiene and Grooming*

Environmental adaptations that can facilitate bathing and grooming include the following:

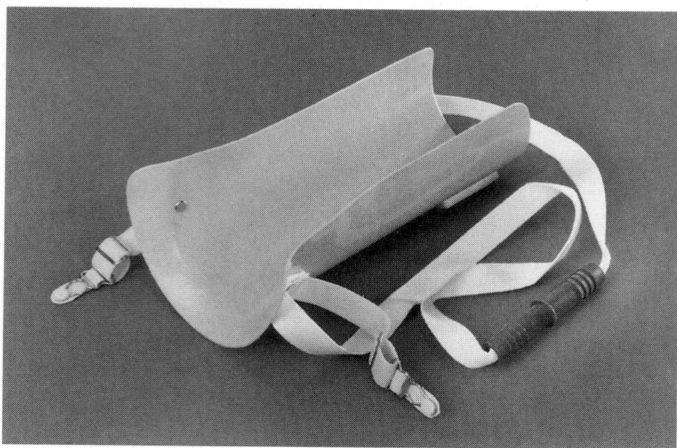

*Figure 17-7* Sock aid. (Courtesy Sammons, a BISSELL Co.)

1. A hand-held shower head on a flexible hose for bathing and shampooing hair can eliminate the need to stand in the shower and offers the user control of the direction of spray. The handle can be built up or adapted for limited grasp.
2. A long-handled bath brush or sponge with a soap holder (Figure 17-13) or long cloth scrubber can allow the user to reach legs, feet, and back. A wash mitt and soap on a rope can aid limited grasp.
3. A position-adjustable hair dryer may be helpful for those who prefer a hairstyle more elaborate than one that can be air-dried.[8] This device is useful for clients with limited ROM, upper extremity weakness, incoordination, and use of only one upper extremity. The dryer is adapted from a desk lamp with spring-balanced arms and a tension control knob at each joint. The lamp is removed and the hair dryer is fastened to the spring-balanced arms. The device is mounted on a table or counter top and can be adjusted for various heights and direction of airflow. This frees the client's hands to manage brushes or combs used to style the hair. Specifications are available for constructing this device.[8]
4. Long handles on a comb, brush, toothbrush, lipstick, mascara brush, and safety or electric razor may be useful for limited hand-to-head or hand-to-face movements. Extensions may be constructed from inexpensive wooden dowels or pieces of PVC pipe found in local hardware stores.
5. Spray deodorant, hair spray, and spray powder or perfume can extend the reach by the distance the material sprays. Some persons may require special adaptations to operate the spray mechanism (Figure 17-14).
6. Electric toothbrushes and a Water-Pik may be easier to manage than a standard toothbrush.

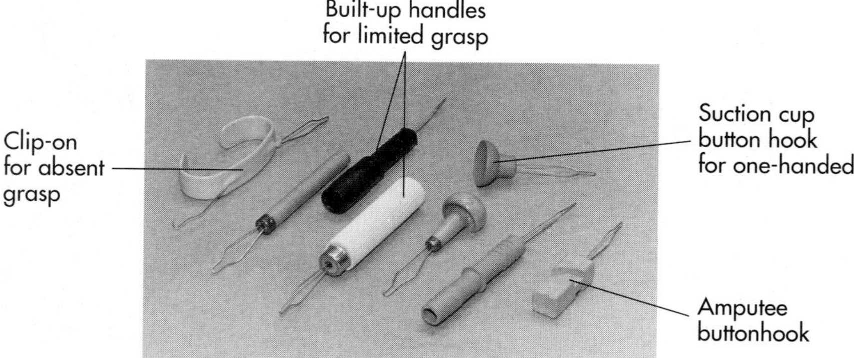


*Figure 17-8* Buttonhooks to accommodate limited grasp, special types of grasp, or amputation.

7. A short reacher can extend reach for using toilet paper. Several types of toilet aids are available in catalogs of assistive devices.
8. Dressing sticks can be used to pull garments up after using the toilet. An alternative is the use of a long piece of elastic or webbing with garters on each end that can be hung around the neck and fastened to pants or panties, preventing them from slipping to the floor during use of the toilet.

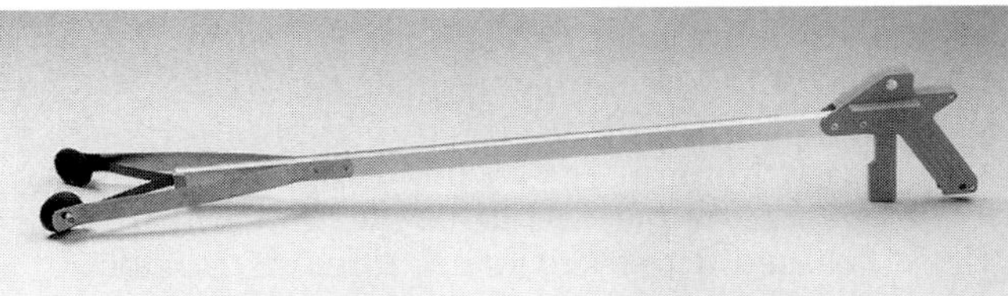

*Figure 17-9* Extended-handle reacher.

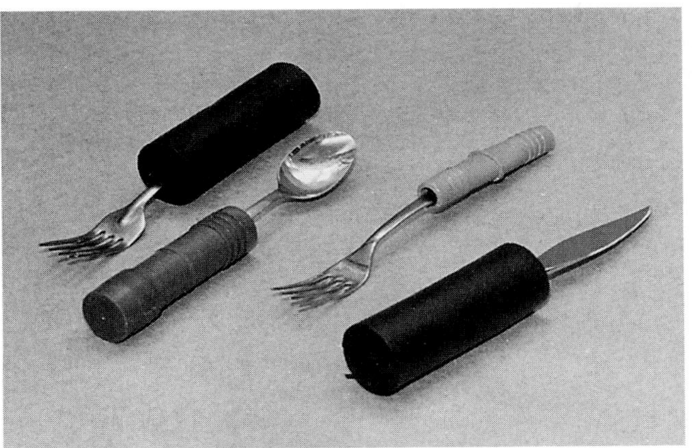

*Figure 17-10* Eating utensils with built-up handles.

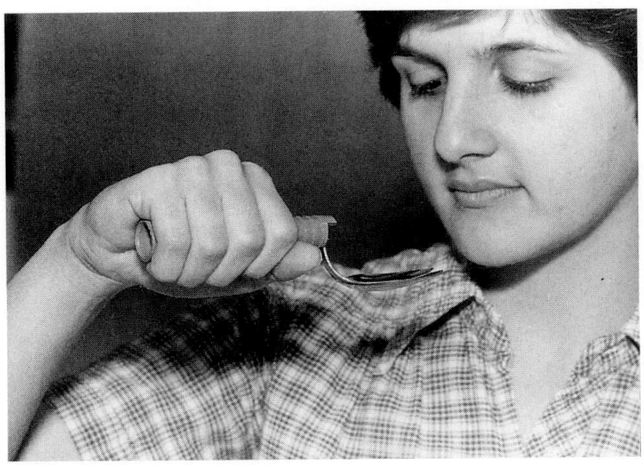

*Figure 17-11* Swivel spoon compensates for limited supination or incoordination.

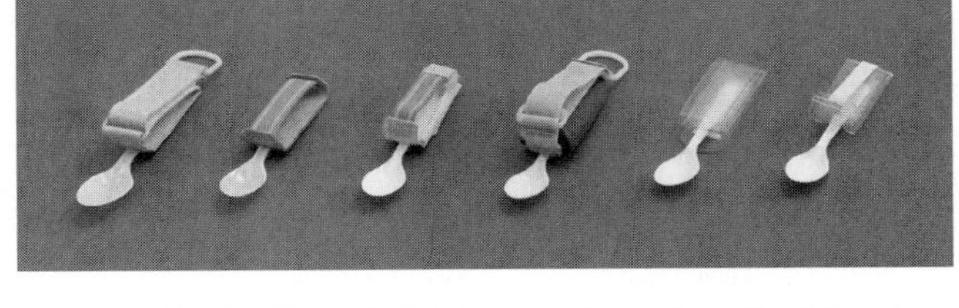

*Figure 17-12* Utensil holders/universal cuffs. (Courtesy Sammons, a BISSELL Co.)

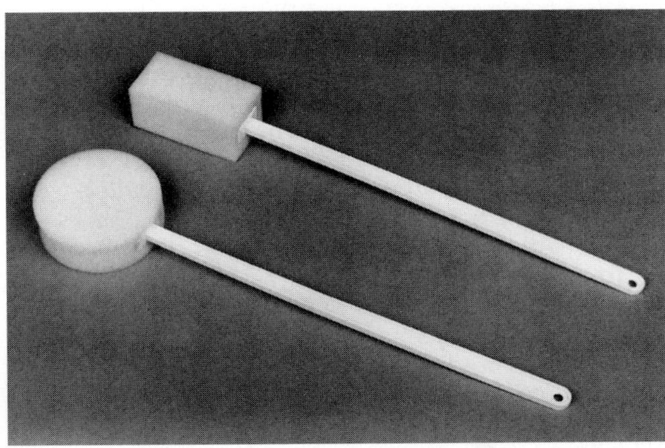

*Figure 17-13* Long-handled bath sponges. (Courtesy Sammons, a BISSELL Co.)

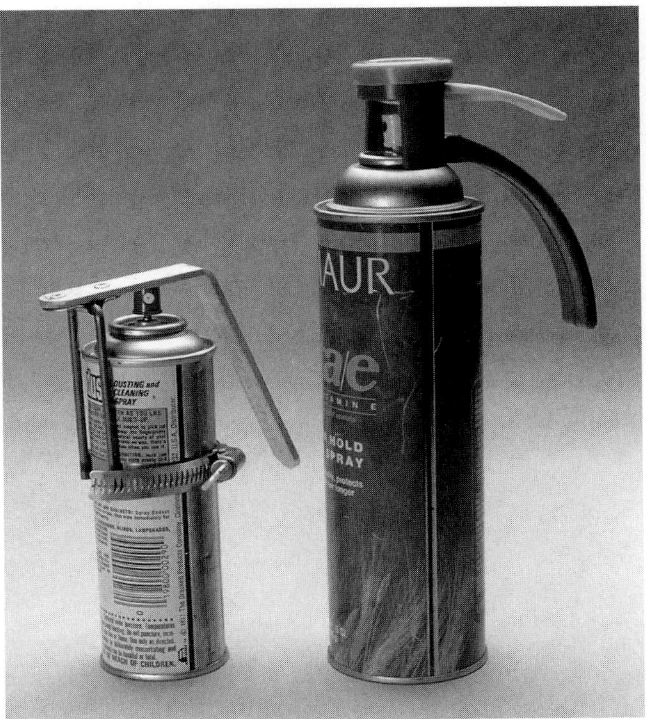

*Figure 17-14* Spray can adapters. (Courtesy Sammons, a BISSELL Co.)

9. Safety rails (Figure 17-15) can be used for bathtub transfers, and safety mats or strips can be placed in the bathtub bottom to prevent slipping.
10. A transfer tub bench (see Figure 17-5), shower stool, or regular chair set in the bathtub or shower stall can eliminate the need to sit on the bathtub bottom or stand to shower, thus increasing safety.
11. Grab bars can be installed to prevent falls and to ease transfers.

### *Communication and General Environment*

Adaptations that can facilitate communication and use of common household fixtures include the following:

1. Telephones should be placed within easy reach. A clip-type receiver holder (Figure 17-16), extended receiver holder, large-button phone, speakerphone, or voice-activated phone may be necessary. A dialing stick or push-button phone are other adaptations.
2. Built-up pens and pencils to accommodate limited grasp and prehension can be used. A Wanchik writer and several other commercially available or custom-fabricated writing aids are helpful (Figure 17-17).
3. Electric typewriters or personal computers and book holders can facilitate communication for those with limited or painful joints.
4. Lever-type doorknob extensions (Figure 17-18), car door openers, and adapted key holders can compensate for hand limitations.
5. Extended or built-up handles on faucets can accommodate limited grasp.

### *Mobility and Transfers*

The individual who has limited ROM *without* significant muscle weakness may benefit from the following assistive devices:

1. A glider chair operated by the feet can facilitate transportation if hip, hand, and arm motions are limited.
2. Platform crutches can prevent stress on hand or finger joints and can accommodate limited grasp.
3. Enlarged grips on crutches, canes, and walkers can accommodate limited grasp.
4. A raised toilet seat can be used if hip and knee motion is limited.
5. A walker with padded grips and forearm troughs can be used if marked hand, forearm, or elbow joint limitations are present.
6. A walker or crutch bag and basket can facilitate carrying objects.

### *Home Management Skills*

Home management activities can be facilitated by a variety of environmental adaptations, assistive devices, energy conservation methods, and work simpli-

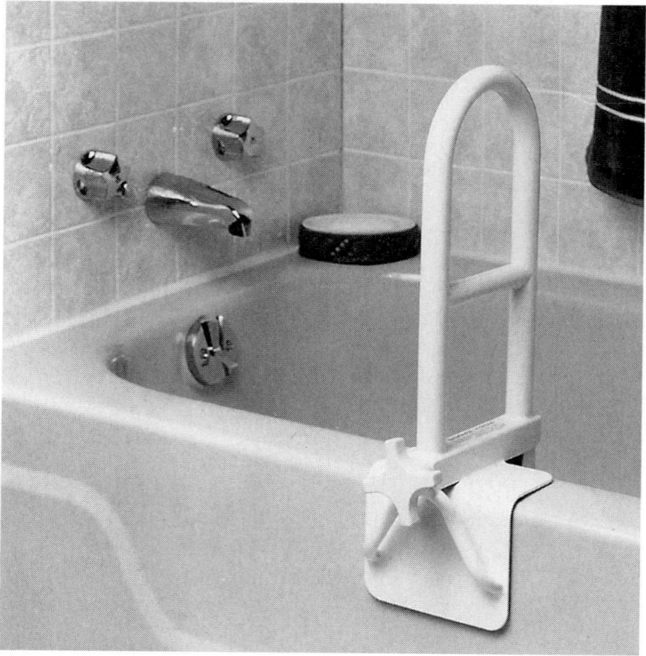

*Figure 17-15* Bathtub safety rail. (Courtesy Sammons, a BISSELL Co.)

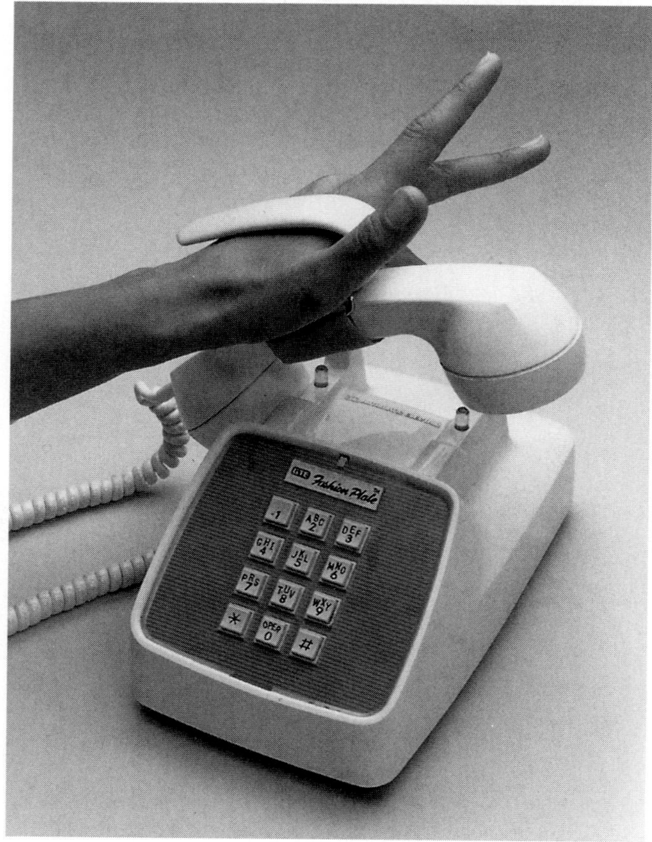

*Figure 17-16* Telephone clip holder. (Courtesy Sammons, a BISSELL Co.)

fication techniques.[16,24] Persons with rheumatoid arthritis should use the principles of joint protection (see Chapter 26). Home management for persons with limited ROM may be eased and improved by the following:

1. Store frequently used items on counters where possible or on the first shelves of cabinets (just above and below counters).
2. Use a high stool to work comfortably at counter height. Alternately, if a wheelchair is used, attach a drop-leaf table to the wall for planning and meal preparation.
3. Use a utility cart of comfortable height to transport several items at once.
4. Use reachers to pull down lightweight items (e.g., cereal box) from high shelves.
5. Stabilize mixing bowls and dishes with nonslip mats.
6. Use lightweight utensils, such as plastic or aluminum bowls and aluminum pots.
7. Use electric can openers and electric mixers.
8. Use electric scissors or adapted loop scissors to open packages (Figure 17-19).
9. Eliminate bending by using extended, flexible plastic handles on dust mops, brooms, and dustpans.
10. Use adapted knives for cutting (Figure 17-20).
11. Use pull-out shelves to organize cupboards and eliminate bending.
12. Eliminate bending by using wall ovens, countertop broilers, and microwave ovens.
13. Eliminate leaning and bending by using a top-loading automatic washer and elevated dryer. Front-loading appliances are more easily operated by wheelchair users.
14. Use an adjustable ironing board to make it possible to sit while ironing.
15. For child care by the ambulatory parent or caregiver, elevate the playpen and diaper table and use a bathinette or a plastic tub on the kitchen counter for bathing. These adaptations reduce the amount of bending and reaching. The crib mattress can be in a raised position until the child is 3 or 4 months old.

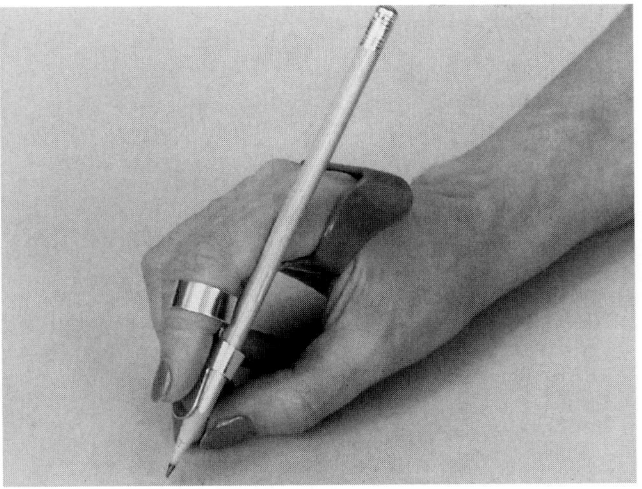

*Figure 17-17* Wanchik writing aid. (Courtesy Sammons, a BISSELL Co.)

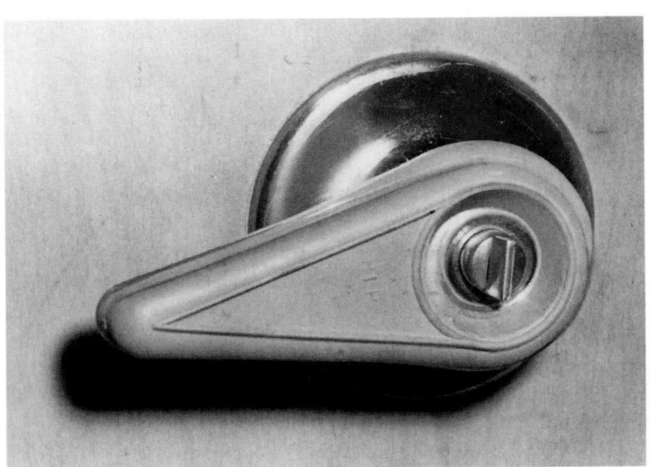

*Figure 17-18* Rubber doorknob extension. (Courtesy Sammons, a BISSELL Co.)

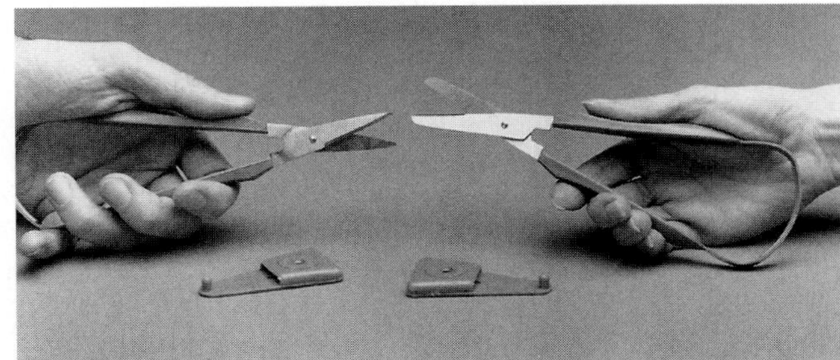

*Figure 17-19* Loop scissors. (Courtesy Sammons, a BISSELL Co.)

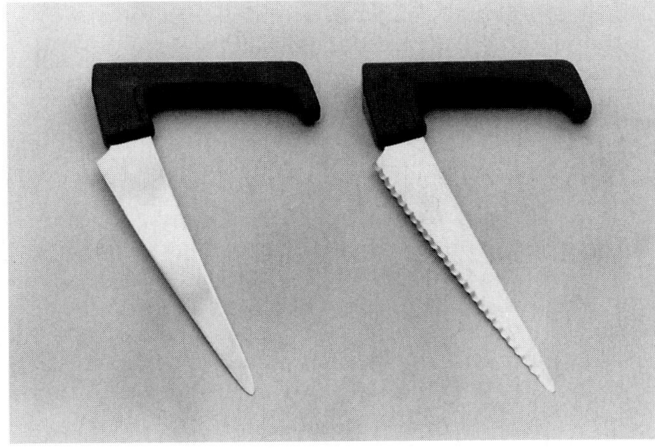

*Figure 17-20* Right-angle knife. (Courtesy Sammons, a BISSELL Co.)

16. Use larger, looser-fitting garments with Velcro fastenings on children.
17. Use a reacher to pick up clothing and children's toys.

### Problems of Incoordination

Incoordination can result from a variety of central nervous system (CNS) disorders, such as Parkinson's disease, multiple sclerosis, cerebral palsy, and traumatic brain injuries (TBIs). Incoordination may take the form of tremors or ataxia or athetoid or choreiform movements. Persons with incoordination may have difficulty maintaining safety and achieving adequate stability of gait, body parts, and objects to complete ADLs.

Fatigue, emotional factors, and fears may increase the severity of incoordinated movement. The client must be taught appropriate energy conservation and work simplification techniques, along with appropriate work pacing and safety methods. The client who learns to avoid and reduce fatigue and fear will perform tasks better and with increased coordination.

The incoordinated individual with reasonable muscle strength can use weighted devices to help stabilize objects. A Velcro-fastened weight can be attached to the client's arm to decrease ataxia. Objects such as eating utensils, pens, and cups can be weighted.

Another technique that can be used throughout all ADL tasks is stabilizing the upper part of the involved upper extremity. This is accomplished by propping the elbow on a counter or table top, pivoting from the elbow and moving only the forearm, wrist, and hand in the activity. Stabilizing the arm reduces some of the incoordination and may allow the individual to accomplish gross and fine motor movements without assistive devices.[1,19,27]

#### *Dressing Activities*

Dressing difficulties typically encountered with incoordination can be reduced by using the following adaptations:

1. Front-opening garments that fit loosely can facilitate donning and removing garments.
2. Large buttons, Velcro, or zippers with loops on the tab can facilitate opening and closing fasteners. A buttonhook with a large, weighted handle may be helpful.
3. Elastic shoelaces, Velcro closures, other adapted shoe closures, and slip-on shoes eliminate the need for bow tying.
4. Trousers with elastic tops for women or Velcro closures for men are easier to manage than those with hooks, buttons, and zippers.
5. Brassieres with front openings or Velcro replacements for the usual hook and eye may be used with more ease. A slipover elastic-type brassiere or bra-slip combination also may eliminate the need to manage brassiere fastenings. Regular (back-fastening) brassieres may be fastened in front at waist level, then slipped around to the back. Next the arms are put into the straps, which are worked up over the shoulders.
6. Clip-on ties can be used by men.
7. To compensate for balance problems, dressing should be performed while sitting on or in the bed or in a wheelchair or chair with arms.

#### *Eating Activities*

For clients with problems of incoordination, eating can be a challenge. Lack of control during eating is not only frustrating but can cause embarrassment and social rejection. Therefore it is important to make eating safe, pleasurable, and as neat as possible. Some suggestions for achieving this goal include the following:

1. Use plate stabilizers, such as nonskid mats, suction bases, or damp dish towels.
2. Use a **plate guard** or **scoop dish** to prevent food being pushed off the plate. The plate guard can be taken from home and clipped to any ordinary dinner plate (Figure 17-21).
3. Prevent spills during the plate-to-mouth movement by using weighted or swivel utensils to offer stability. Weighted cuffs may be placed on the forearm to decrease involuntary movement (Figure 17-22).
4. To eliminate the need to carry the glass or cup to the mouth (which may cause spills), use long plastic straws with a straw clip on a glass or cup with a weighted bottom. Plastic cups with covers and spouts can also reduce spillage.
5. Use a resistance or friction-type arm brace similar to a mobile arm support to help control patterns of involuntary movement during feeding activities of adults with cerebral palsy and athetosis.[11] Such a brace may help many clients with severe incoordination to achieve some degree of independence in feeding.

#### *Hygiene and Grooming*

The client may be helped to stabilize and handle toilet articles by using the following techniques:

1. If frequent dropping is a problem, articles such as a razor, lipstick, and toothbrush can be attached to a cord. An electric toothbrush may be more easily managed than a regular one.
2. Weighted wrist cuffs may be helpful during the finer hygiene activities, such as applying makeup, shaving, and hair care.
3. The position-adjustable hair dryer described earlier for clients with limited ROM can be useful for those with incoordination as well.[8]
4. An electric razor rather than a blade razor offers stability and safety. A strap around the razor and hand can prevent dropping.
5. A **suction brush** attached to the sink or counter can be used for nail or denture care (Figure 17-23).

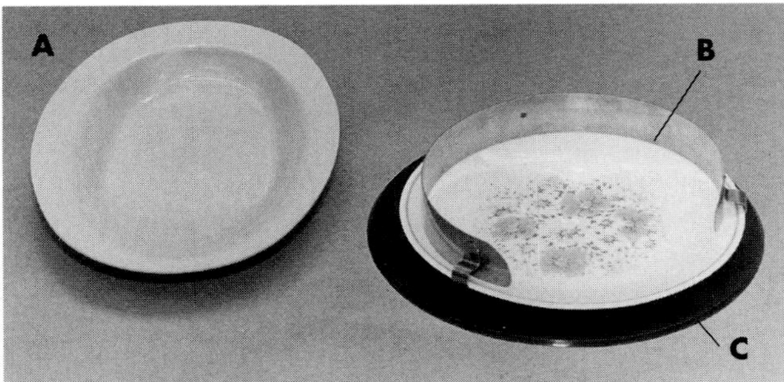


*Figure 17-21* **A,** Scoop dish. **B,** Plate with plate guard. **C,** Nonskid mat.

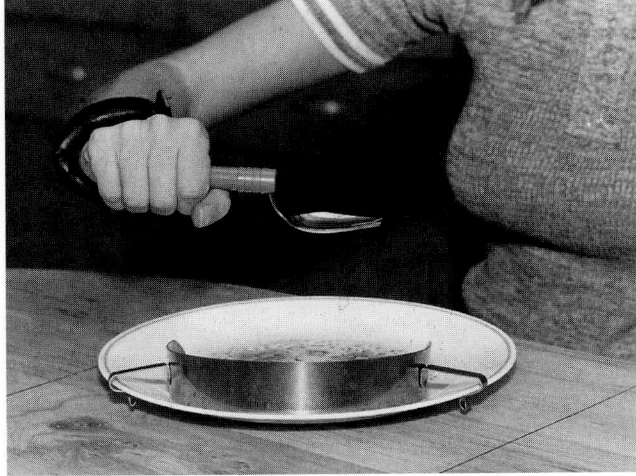

*Figure 17-22* Weighted wrist cuff and swivel utensil can sometimes compensate for incoordination or involuntary motion.

6. Soap should be on a rope and can be worn around the neck or hung over a bathtub or shower fixture during the bath or shower to keep it within easy reach. A leg from a pair of pantyhose tied over a faucet, with a bar of soap in the toe, will stretch for use and keep soap within reach.
7. An emery board or small piece of wood with fine sandpaper glued to it can be fastened to the table top for filing nails. A nail clipper can also be stabilized in the same manner.
8. Large-size roll-on deodorants are used more easily than sprays or creams.
9. Sanitary pads that stick to undergarments may be easier to manage than tampons.
10. A bath mitt with a pocket to hold the soap can be used for washing and eliminates the need for frequent soaping and rinsing and wringing a washcloth.
11. **Nonskid mats** should be used inside and outside the bathtub during bathing. Their suction bases should be fastened securely to the floor and bathtub before use. Safety grab bars should be installed on the wall next to the bathtub or fastened to the edge of the bathtub. Sitting on a bathtub seat or shower chair is safer than standing while showering or transferring to a bathtub bottom. Many uncoordinated clients require supervisory assistance during bathing. Sponge bathing while seated at a bathroom sink may substitute for bathing or showering several times a week.

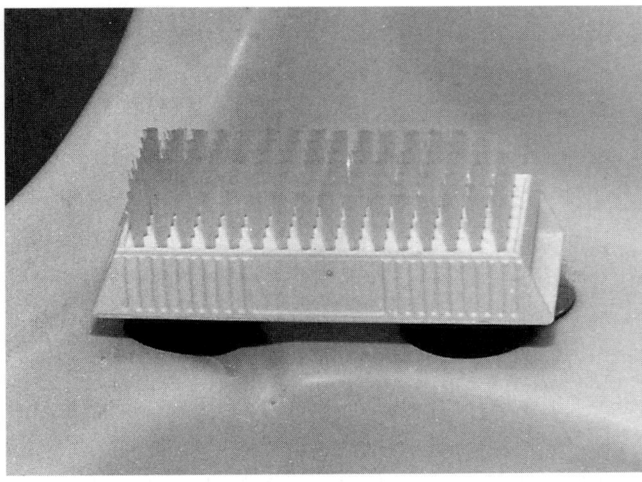

*Figure 17-23* Suction brush attached to bathroom sink for dentures or fingernails. Brush can also be used in kitchen to wash vegetables and fruit.

### *Communication and General Environment*

Adaptations that can facilitate communication and the use of common household fixtures by clients with incoordination include the following:

1. Doorknobs may be managed more easily if adapted with lever-type handles or covered with rubber or friction tape (see Figure 17-18).
2. A holder for a telephone receiver, large-button phones, or speakerphones may be helpful.
3. Writing may be managed by using a weighted, enlarged pencil or pen. An electric typewriter or computer with a keyboard guard is helpful for communication. A computer mouse (or trackball or joystick) may be substituted for the keyboard.
4. Keys may be managed by placing them on an adapted key holder that is rigid and extends leverage for turning the key. However, inserting the key in the keyhole may be very difficult unless the incoordination is relatively mild.
5. Extended lever-type faucets are easier to manage than are push-pull spigots and knobs that turn. To prevent burns during bathing and kitchen activities, cold water should be turned on first and hot water added gradually.
6. Lamps can be wired with switches that respond to light touch or to a remote signal. Wall switches

can also eliminate the need to turn a small switch manually.

### Mobility and Transfers

Clients with problems of incoordination may use a variety of ambulation aids, depending on the type and severity of incoordination. Sometimes the OT practitioner must help the client with degenerative diseases recognize the need for ambulation aids and accept their use. This may mean switching from a cane to crutches to a walker and finally to a wheelchair for some persons. Clients with incoordination can improve stability and mobility by using the following techniques:

1. Instead of lifting objects, slide them on floors or counters.
2. Use ambulation aids as appropriate.
3. Use a utility cart, preferably a custom-made cart that is heavy and has some friction on the wheels.
4. Remove door sills, throw rugs, and thick carpeting.
5. Install banisters on indoor and outdoor staircases.
6. Substitute ramps for stairs wherever possible.

### Home Management Activities

The occupational therapy practitioner should make a careful assessment of homemaking activities performance to determine (1) which activities can be done safely, (2) which activities can be done safely if modified or adapted, and (3) which activities cannot be done adequately or safely and therefore should be assigned to someone else. The major problem areas are stabilization of foods and equipment to prevent spilling and accidents and the safe handling of appliances, pots, pans, and household tools to prevent cuts, burns, bruises, electric shock, and falls. Suggestions for improving safety and function in home management tasks include the following[16,19,27]:

1. Use a wheelchair and wheelchair lapboard (even if ambulation is possible with devices). This saves energy and increases stability when balance and gait are unsteady.
2. If possible, use convenience and prepared foods to eliminate processes such as peeling, chopping, slicing, and mixing.
3. Use easy-open containers or store foods in plastic containers once opened. A jar opener is also useful.
4. Use heavy utensils, mixing bowls, and pots and pans to increase stability.
5. Use nonskid mats on work surfaces.
6. Use electrical appliances such as crock pots, electric frypans, toaster ovens, and microwave or convection ovens because they are safer than using the range.
7. Use a blender and counter-top mixer because they are safer than hand-held mixers and easier than mixing with a spoon or whisk.
8. If possible, adjust work heights of counters, sink, and range to minimize leaning, bending, reaching, and lifting, whether the client is standing or using a wheelchair.
9. Use long oven mitts, which give greater protection than potholders.
10. Use pots, pans, casserole dishes, and appliances with bilateral handles because they may be easier to hold and manage than those with one handle.
11. Use a cutting board with stainless-steel nails (Figure 17-24) to stabilize meats, potatoes, and vegetables while cutting or peeling. When not in use, the nails should be covered with a large cork. To prevent slippage when in use, the bottom of the board should have suction cups, be covered with stair tread, or placed on a non-skid mat.
12. Use heavy dinnerware, which offers stability and control to the distal part of the upper extremity and may be easier to handle. If dropping and breakage are problems, unbreakable dinnerware may be more practical.
13. Cover the sink, utility cart, and counter tops with protective rubber mats or mesh matting to stabilize items.
14. Use a serrated knife for cutting and chopping because it is easier to control.
15. To eliminate the need to carry and drain pots of hot liquids, use a steamer basket or deep-fry basket for preparing boiled foods.
16. Use tongs to turn foods during cooking and to serve foods because they may offer more control and stability than a fork, spatula, or serving spoon.
17. Use blunt-ended loop scissors to open packages.
18. The ambulatory client may find it easier to vacuum with a heavy upright cleaner. The wheelchair user may be able to manage a light-

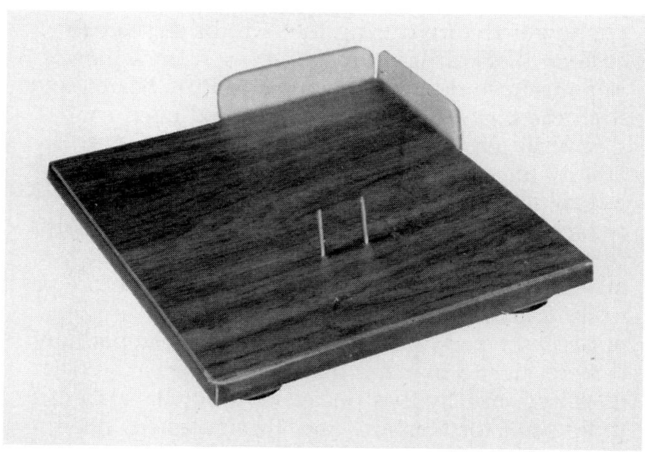

*Figure 17-24* Cutting board with stainless-steel nails, suction-cup feet, and corner for stabilizing bread is useful for patients with incoordination or lacking use of one hand. (Courtesy Sammons, a BISSELL Co.)

weight tank-type vacuum cleaner or electric broom.
19. Use dust mitts for dusting.
20. Eliminate objects that are easily broken or difficult to manage, such as fragile knickknacks, unstable lamps, and dainty doilies.
21. Eliminate ironing by using no-iron fabrics or a timed dryer or by assigning this task to other members of the household.
22. Use front-loading washers, a laundry cart on wheels, and premeasured detergents, bleaches, and fabric softeners.
23. Sit while working with an infant. Use foam-rubber bath aids, an infant bath seat, and a wide, padded dressing table with safety straps with Velcro fastening to offer enough stability for bathing, dressing, and diapering an infant. (Child care may not be possible unless the incoordination is mild.)
24. Use disposable diapers with tape fasteners because they are easier to manage than cloth diapers and pins.
25. Do not feed the infant with a spoon or fork unless the incoordination is very mild or does not affect the upper extremities. It may be safer for another household member to feed the infant.
26. Dress the child in clothing that is large, loose, stretchy, nonslippery, and fastened with Velcro.

### Hemiplegia or Use of Only One Upper Extremity

It is tempting but misleading to classify together all conditions that may result in the dysfunction of one upper extremity. Unilateral upper extremity amputations and temporary disorders such as fractures, burns, and peripheral neuropathy may lead to unilateral upper extremity (UE) dysfunction. Patients with unilateral UE dysfunction resulting from such disorders are likely to learn compensatory techniques quickly and easily, assuming normal functioning of sensory, perceptual, and cognitive systems. However, the most common diagnosis in which unilateral UE dysfunction is likely to be seen by the COTA is hemiplegia, and this is a different case.

Clients with hemiplegia require specialized methods of teaching; many have greater difficulty in learning and performing one-handed skills than do persons with orthopedic or lower motor neuron dysfunction. This is because the head, trunk, and leg are involved as well as the arm; consequently, ambulation and balance difficulties may be impaired. In addition, sensory, perceptual, cognitive, and speech disorders may affect the ability to learn and retain learning and performance. Finally, the presence of motor and ideational apraxia sometimes seen in this group of clients limits their potential for learning new motor skills and remembering previous ones. The client with hemiplegia needs to be evaluated for sensory, perceptual, and cognitive deficits to determine potential for ADL performance and to establish appropriate teaching methods to facilitate learning.

The major problems for the one-handed worker are reduced work speed and dexterity and poor stabilization, a task usually assumed by the nondominant arm. The major problems for the client with hemiplegia are unsteady balance and the risk of injury because of sensory and perceptual loss.[1,16,19,27]

#### *Dressing Activities*

If balance is a problem, the client should dress while seated in a locked wheelchair or sturdy armchair. Clothing should be within easy reach. Reaching tongs may be helpful for securing articles and assisting in some dressing activities. Dressing and other ADLs should be approached with a minimum of assistive devices.

*One-handed dressing techniques* Some dressing techniques for the client with hemiplegia employ neurodevelopmental (Bobath) treatment principles (see Chapter 23). The following one-handed dressing techniques can facilitate dressing for clients with use of one upper extremity. A general rule is to begin with the affected arm or leg first when donning clothing. When removing clothing, start with the unaffected extremity.[1]

SHIRTS. Front-opening shirts may be managed by any one of three methods. The first method can be used for jackets, robes, and front-opening dresses.

*METHOD 1: BASIC OVER HEAD—DONNING (FIGURE 17-25)*
1. Grasp shirt collar with unaffected hand and shake out twists *(a)*.
2. Position shirt on lap with inside facing up and collar toward chest *(b)*.
3. Position sleeve opening on affected side so it is as large as possible and close to affected hand, which is resting on lap *(c)*.
4. Using unaffected hand, place affected hand in sleeve opening and work sleeve over elbow by pulling on garment *($d_1$, $d_2$)*.
5. Put unaffected arm into its sleeve and raise up to slide or shake sleeve into position past elbow *(e)*.
6. With unaffected hand, gather shirt up middle of back from hem to collar and raise shirt over head *(f)*.
7. Lean forward, duck head, and pass shirt over it *(g)*.
8. With unaffected hand, adjust shirt by leaning forward and working it down past both shoulders. Reach in back and pull shirttail down *(h)*.
9. Line shirt fronts up for buttoning and begin with bottom button *(i)*. Button sleeve cuff of affected arm. Sleeve cuff of unaffected arm may be prebuttoned if cuff opening is large. Button may be sewn on with elastic thread or sewn onto a small tab of elastic and fastened inside shirt cuff. A small button attached to a crocheted loop of elastic thread is another alternative. Slip button on loop through buttonhole in garment so that

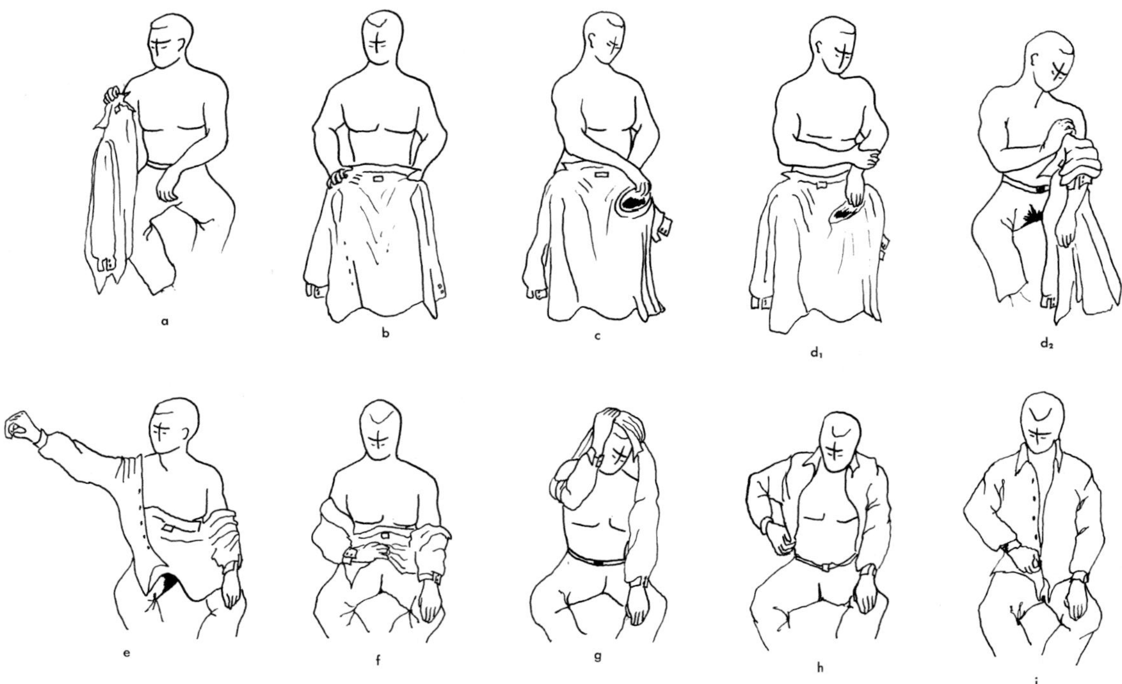

*Figure 17-25* Steps in donning shirt: method 1 (basic over head). (Courtesy Christine Shaw, Metro Health Center for Rehabilitation, Metro Health Medical Center, Cleveland, Ohio.)

elastic loop is inside. Stretch elastic loop to fit around original cuff button. This simple device can be transferred to each garment and positioned before the shirt is put on. The loop stretches to accommodate width of hand as it is pushed through end of sleeve.[26]

*METHOD 1: BASIC OVER HEAD—REMOVING*

1. Unbutton shirt.
2. Lean forward.
3. With unaffected hand, grasp collar or gather material up in back from collar to hem.
4. Lean forward, duck head, and pull shirt over head.
5. Remove sleeve from unaffected arm and then from affected arm.

*METHOD 2: OVER HEAD ON/SHRUG OFF—DONNING*

Method 2 may be used by clients who have shirt twisted or have trouble sliding the sleeve down onto unaffected arm.

1. Position shirt as described in method 1, steps 1 to 3.
2. With unaffected hand, place involved hand into shirt sleeve opening and work sleeve onto hand, but do *not* pull up over elbow.
3. Put unaffected arm into sleeve and bring arm out to 180° of abduction. Tension of fabric from unaffected arm to wrist of affected arm will bring sleeve into position.
4. Lower arm and work sleeve on affected arm up over elbow.
5. Continue as in steps 6 to 9 of method 1.

*METHOD 2: OVER HEAD/SHRUG OFF—REMOVING*

1. Unbutton shirt.
2. With unaffected hand, push shirt off shoulders, first on affected side, then on unaffected side.
3. Pull on cuff of unaffected side with unaffected hand.
4. Work sleeve off by alternately shrugging shoulder and pulling down on cuff.
5. Lean forward, bring shirt around back, and pull sleeve off affected arm.

*METHOD 3: OVER SHOULDER—DONNING (FIGURE 17-26)*

1. Position shirt and work onto arm as described in method 1, steps 1 to 4.
2. Pull sleeve on affected arm up to shoulder *(a)*.
3. With unaffected hand, grasp tip of collar that is on unaffected side, lean forward, and bring arm over and behind head to carry shirt around to unaffected side *(b)*.
4. Put unaffected arm into sleeve opening, directing it up and out *(c)*.
5. Adjust and button as described in method 1, steps 8 and 9.

*METHOD 3: OVER SHOULDER—REMOVING*

The shirt may be removed using the same procedure described for method 2.

*METHOD 4: DONNING PULLOVER SHIRT (OVER HEAD)*

1. Position shirt on lap, with bottom toward chest and label facing down.

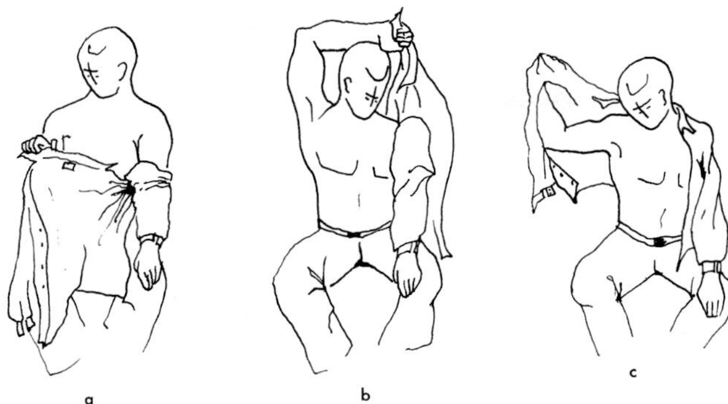

*Figure 17-26* Steps in donning shirt: method 3 (over shoulder). (Courtesy Christine Shaw, Metro Health Center for Rehabilitation, Metro Health Medical Center, Cleveland, Ohio.)

2. With unaffected hand, roll up bottom edge of shirt back up to sleeve on affected side.
3. Position sleeve opening so it is as large as possible, and use unaffected hand to place affected hand into sleeve opening. Pull shirt up onto arm past elbow.
4. Insert unaffected arm into sleeve.
5. Adjust shirt on affected side up and onto shoulder.
6. Gather shirt back with unaffected hand, lean forward, duck head, and pass shirt over head.
7. Adjust shirt.

*METHOD 4: REMOVING PULLOVER SHIRT (OVER HEAD)*

1. Gather shirt up with unaffected hand, starting at top back.
2. Lean forward, duck head, and pull gathered fabric in back over head.
3. Remove from unaffected arm and then affected arm.

TROUSERS. Trousers may be managed by one of the following methods. These may be adapted for shorts and women's panties as well. It is recommended that trousers have a well-constructed button-fly front opening; this may be easier to manage than a zipper. Velcro may be used to replace buttons and zippers. Trousers should be worn in a size slightly larger than worn previously and should have a wide opening at the ankles. They should be put on after the socks have been put on but before the shoes. The client who is dressing in a wheelchair should place feet flat on the floor, not on the footrests of the wheelchair.

*METHOD 1: PARTIAL STANDING—DONNING*

1. Sit in sturdy armchair or in locked wheelchair (Figure 17-27) *(a)*.
2. Position unaffected leg in front of midline of body with knee flexed to 90°. Using unaffected hand, reach forward and grasp ankle of affected leg or sock around ankle *($b_1$)*. Lift affected leg over unaffected leg to crossed position *($b_2$)*.
3. Slip trousers onto affected leg up to position where foot is completely inside of trouser leg *(c)*. Do *not* pull up above knee, or it will be difficult inserting unaffected leg.
4. Uncross affected leg by grasping ankle or portion of sock around ankle *(d)*.
5. Insert unaffected leg and work trousers up onto hips as far as possible *($e_1$, $e_2$)*.
6. To prevent trousers from dropping when pulling pants over hips, place affected hand in pocket or place one finger of affected hand into belt loop. If able to do so safely, stand and pull trousers over hips *($f_1$, $f_2$)*.
7. If standing balance is good, remain standing to pull up zipper or button *($f_3$)*. *Sit down to button front (g)*.

*METHOD 1: PARTIAL STANDING—REMOVING*

1. Unfasten trousers and work down on hips as far as possible while seated.
2. Stand, letting trousers drop past hips or work them down past hips.
3. Remove trousers from unaffected leg.
4. Sit and cross affected leg over unaffected leg, remove trousers, and uncross leg.

*METHOD 2: SEATED BRIDGING—DONNING*

Method 2 is used for clients who are in wheelchairs (brakes locked, footrests swung away) or in sturdy, straight armchairs (back against wall) and for patients who cannot stand independently.

1. Position trousers on legs as in method 1, steps 1 to 5.
2. Elevate hips by leaning back against chair and pushing down against floor with unaffected leg; this is called **bridging.** As hips are raised, work trousers over hips with unaffected hand.
3. Lower hips back into chair and fasten trousers.

*METHOD 2: SEATED BRIDGING—REMOVING*

1. Unfasten trousers and work down on hips as far as possible while sitting.
2. Lean back against chair, push down against floor with unaffected leg to elevate hips, and with unaffected arm, work trousers down past hips.
3. Proceed as in method 1, steps 3 and 4.

*METHOD 3: RECUMBENT BRIDGING—DONNING*

Method 3 is done in a recumbent position, that is, lying down or reclining. It is more difficult to perform than those methods done sitting. If possible, the bed should be raised to a semireclining position for partial sitting.

1. Using unaffected hand, place affected knee in flexed position and cross over unaffected leg, which may be partially flexed to prevent affected leg from slipping.
2. Position trousers and pull onto affected leg first, up to knee. Then uncross leg.
3. Insert unaffected leg and work trousers up onto hips as far as possible.
4. With unaffected leg flexed, press down with foot and shoulder to elevate hips from bed. While in

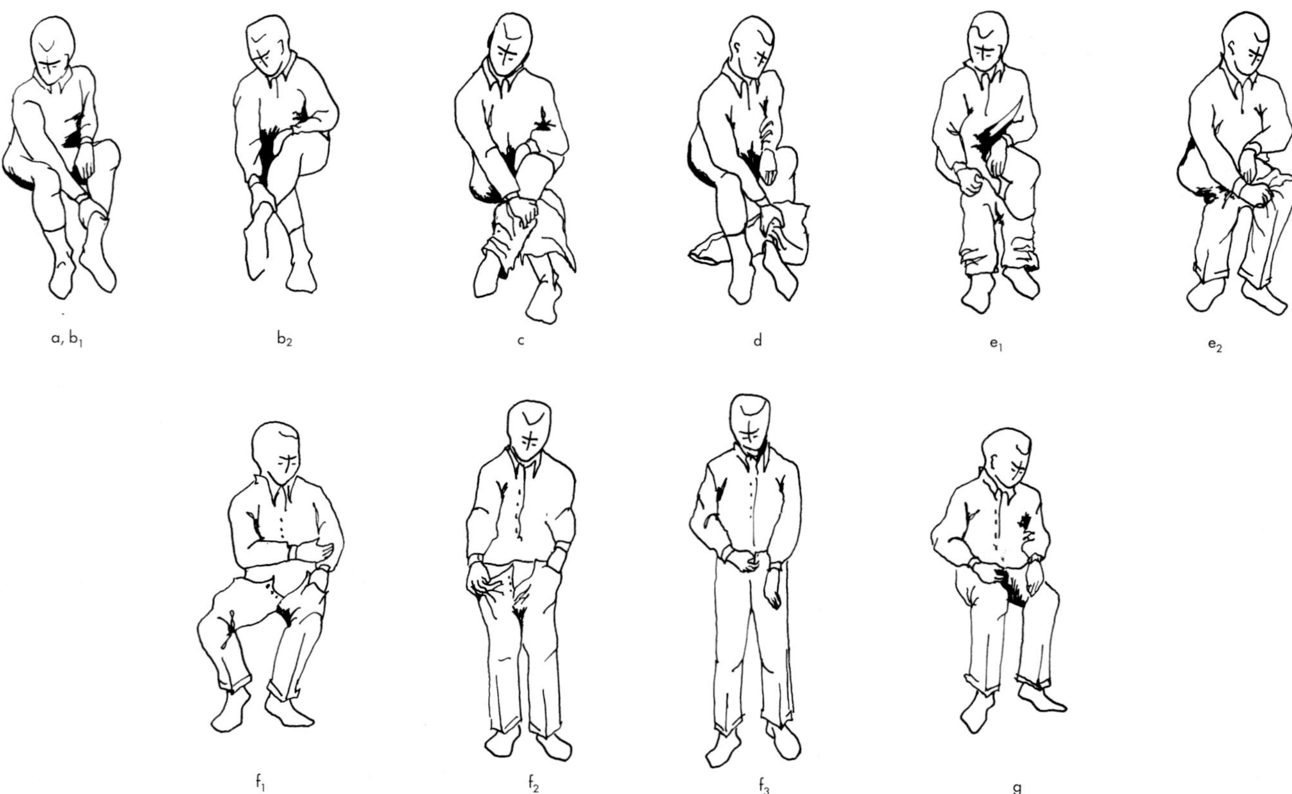


*Figure 17-27* Steps in donning trousers: method 1 (partial standing). (Courtesy Christine Shaw, Metro Health Medical Center, Cleveland, Ohio.)

this bridged position, with unaffected arm, pull trousers over hips or work trousers up over hips by rolling from side to side.

5. Fasten trousers.

*METHOD 3: RECUMBENT BRIDGING—REMOVING*

1. Bridge hips as in putting trousers on in method 3, step 4.
2. Work trousers down past hips, remove unaffected leg, and then remove affected leg.

**BRASSIERE (BACK OPENING)**

*DONNING*

Clothing items such as brassieres, neckties, socks, stockings, and braces may be difficult to manage with one hand. The following methods are recommended.

1. Position brassiere on lap so that shoulder strap side is toward knees and inside is facing up. Tuck one end of brassiere into pants, girdle, or skirt waistband and wrap other end around waist (wrapping toward affected side may be easiest). Hook brassiere in front at waist level and slip fastener around to back (at waistline level).
2. Place affected arm through shoulder strap, then place unaffected arm through other strap.
3. Work straps up over shoulders. Pull strap on affected side up over shoulder with unaffected arm. Put unaffected arm through its strap and work up over shoulder by directing arm up and out and pulling with hand.
4. Use unaffected hand to adjust breasts in brassiere cups.

If the client has some function in the affected hand, a fabric loop may be sewn to back of brassiere near fastener. Affected thumb may be slipped through this to stabilize brassiere while unaffected hand fastens it. Front-opening bras may also be adapted in this way.

In all cases, it is helpful if the brassiere has elastic straps and is made of stretch fabric. All-elastic brassieres, prefastened or without fasteners, may be put on using method 1 described previously for shirts.

*REMOVING*

1. Slip straps down off shoulders, unaffected side first.
2. Work straps down over arms and off hands.
3. Slip brassiere around to front with unaffected arm.
4. Unfasten and remove.

**NECKTIE**

*DONNING*

Clip-on neckties are attractive and convenient. If a conventional tie is used, the following method is recommended:

1. Place collar of shirt in up position, bring necktie around neck, and adjust it so that smaller end is at length desired when tying is completed.
2. Fasten small end to shirt front with tie clasp or spring-clip clothespin.
3. Loop long end around short end (one complete loop) and bring up between V at neck. Then bring tip down through loop at front and adjust tie, using ring and little fingers to hold tie end and thumb and forefingers to slide knot up tightly.

*REMOVING*

Pull knot at front of neck until small end slips up enough for tie to be slipped over head. Tie may be hung up in this state and replaced by slipping it over head, around upturned collar, with knot tightened as described in step 3 of donning.

SOCKS OR STOCKINGS

*DONNING*

1. Sit in straight armchair or in wheelchair with brakes locked, feet on floor, and footrest swung away.
2. With unaffected leg directly in front of midline of body, cross affected leg over it.
3. Open top of stocking by inserting thumb and first two fingers near cuff and spreading fingers apart.
4. Work stocking onto foot before pulling over heel. Care should be taken to eliminate wrinkles.
5. Work stocking up over leg. Shift weight from side to side to adjust stocking around thigh.
6. Thigh-high stockings with elastic band at top are often an acceptable substitute for pantyhose, especially for nonambulatory clients. Elastic should not be so tight as to impair circulation.
7. Pantyhose may be donned and doffed as a pair of slacks, except legs would be gathered up, one at a time, before placing feet into leg holes.

*REMOVING*

1. Work socks or stockings down as far as possible with unaffected arm.
2. With unaffected leg directly in front of midline of body, cross affected leg over it.
3. Remove sock or stocking from affected leg. Some clients may require dressing stick to push sock or stocking off heel and foot.
4. Lift unaffected leg to comfortable height or seat level and remove sock or stocking from foot.

SHOES. If possible, select slip-on shoes to eliminate lacing and tying. The client who uses an ankle-foot orthosis (AFO) or short leg brace usually needs shoes with fasteners.

1. Use elastic laces and leave shoes tied.
2. Use adapted shoe fasteners such as "kno-bows."
3. Use one-handed shoe-tying techniques (Figure 17-28).
4. Client can learn to tie a standard bow with one hand, but this requires excellent visual perceptual and motor planning skills along with much repetition.

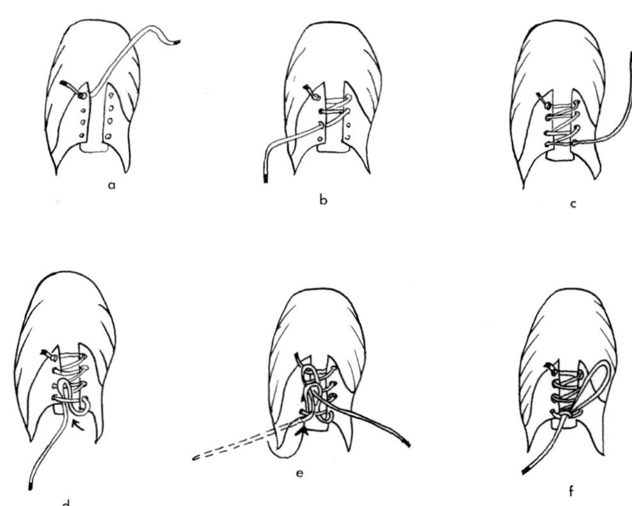


*Figure 17-28* One-handed shoe-tying method. (Courtesy Christine Shaw, Metro Health Center for Rehabilitation, Metro Health Medical Center, Cleveland, Ohio.)

ANKLE-FOOT ORTHOSIS. An AFO is frequently used by the client with hemiplegia who lacks adequate ankle dorsiflexion to walk safely and efficiently.

*DONNING (FIGURE 17-29)*

1. Sit in straight armchair or wheelchair with brakes locked and feet on floor *(a)*. Fasteners are loosened and tongue of shoe pulled back to allow AFO to fit into shoe *(b)*.
2. AFO and shoe are placed on floor between legs but closer to affected leg, facing up *(c)*.
3. With unaffected hand, lift affected leg behind knee and place toes into shoe *(d)*. It is important to keep or reposition affected leg, shoe, and AFO as much as possible directly under affected knee.
4. Reach down with unaffected hand and lift AFO by the upright. Simultaneously, use unaffected foot against affected heel to keep shoe and AFO together *(e)*.
5. Heel is not pushed into shoe at this point. With unaffected hand, apply pressure directly downward on affected knee to force heel into shoe, if leg strength is not sufficient *(f)*.
6. Fasten Velcro calf strap and fasten shoes *(g)*. Affected leg may be placed on footstool to assist with reaching shoe fasteners.
7. To fasten shoes, one-handed bow tying may be used. Elastic shoelaces, Velcro-fastened shoes, or other commercially available shoe fasteners may be required if client is unable to tie shoes.

*REMOVING: VARIATION 1*

1. While seated as for donning an AFO, cross affected leg over unaffected leg.

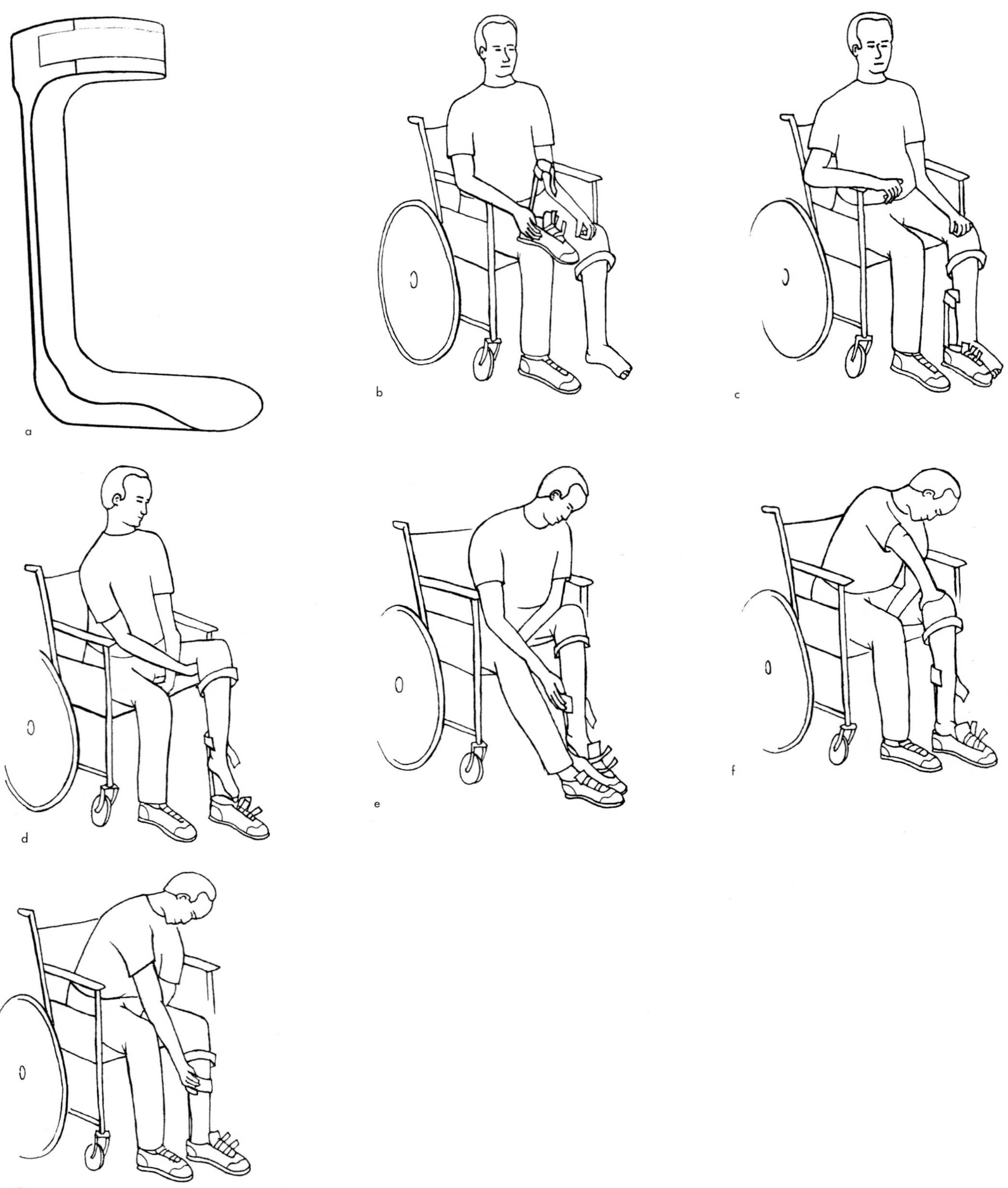


*Figure 17-29* Steps in donning ankle-foot orthosis (AFO).

2. Unfasten straps and laces with unaffected hand.
3. Using unaffected hand, push down on AFO upright until shoe is off foot.

REMOVING: VARIATION 2

1. Unfasten straps and laces.
2. Straighten affected leg by putting unaffected foot behind heel of shoe and pushing affected leg forward.
3. Push down on AFO upright with unaffected hand and at same time push forward on heel of AFO shoe with unaffected foot.

### *Eating Activities*

The only significant eating problem when using one-handed techniques is managing a knife and fork simultaneously for meat cutting. This problem can be solved by the use of a **rocker knife** for cutting meat and other foods (Figure 17-30). The knife cuts with a rocking motion rather than a back-and-forth slicing action. Use of a rocking motion with a standard table knife or a sharp paring knife may be adequate to accomplish cutting tender meats and foods. If such a knife is used, the patient is taught to hold the knife handle between the thumb and the third, fourth, and fifth fingers, and the index finger is extended along the top of the knife blade. The knife point is placed in the food in a vertical position, and then the blade is brought down to cut the food. The rocking motion, using wrist flexion and extension, is continued until the food is cut.

The OTR or COTA should keep in mind that one-handed meat cutting involves learning a new motor pattern and may be difficult for clients with hemiplegia and apraxia.

### *Hygiene and Grooming*

With the use of alternate methods and some assistive devices, hygiene and grooming activities can be accomplished by clients using one hand or one side of the body. Suggestions for achieving hygiene and grooming with one hand include the following:

1. Use an electric razor rather than a safety razor.
2. Use a bathtub seat or chair in the shower stall or bathtub. Use a suction-based bathmat, wash mitt, long-handled bath sponge, safety rails on the bathtub or wall, soap on a rope or suction soap holder, and suction brush for fingernail care.
3. Sponge-bathe while sitting at the lavatory (washbowl), using the wash mitt, suction brush, and suction soap holder. The uninvolved forearm and hand may be washed by placing a soaped washcloth on the thigh and rubbing the hand and forearm on the cloth.
4. Use the position-adjustable hair dryer previously described. Such a device frees the unaffected upper extremity to hold a brush or comb to style the hair during blow-drying.[8]
5. Care for fingernails as described previously for clients with incoordination.

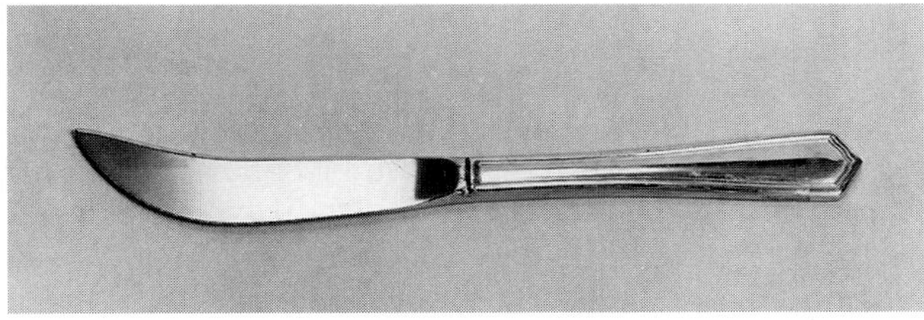

*Figure 17-30* One-handed rocker knife. (Courtesy Sammons, a BISSELL Co.)

6. Use spray deodorants rather than creams or roll-ons because they can be applied more easily to the uninvolved underarm.
7. Use a pump-action toothpaste dispenser rather than a tube.
8. Use a suction denture brush for care of dentures. The suction fingernail brush may also serve this purpose (see Figure 17-23).

### *Communication and General Environment*

Suggestions to facilitate writing, reading, and using the telephone include the following:

1. The primary problem in writing is stabilization of the paper or tablet. This can be overcome by using a clipboard or paperweight or by taping the paper to the writing surface. In some instances the affected arm may be positioned on the table top to stabilize the paper passively.
2. The patient who must shift dominance to the nondominant extremity may need to practice to improve speed and coordination in writing. One-handed writing and typing instruction manuals are available.
3. Book holders may be used to stabilize a book while reading or holding copy for typing and writing practice. For reading while seated in an easy chair, the client can position a soft pillow on the lap to stabilize a book.
4. The telephone is managed by lifting the receiver to listen for the dial tone, setting it down, dialing or pressing the buttons, then lifting the receiver to the ear. To write while using the telephone, a telephone receiver holder that is on a stand or that rests on the shoulder must be used. A speakerphone can also leave hands free to take messages. Alternative input-output devices such as wired or remote headsets can also be used.

### *Mobility and Transfers*

Chapter 18 describes principles of transfer techniques for patients with hemiplegia.

### *Home Management Activities*

A variety of assistive devices are available to make home management activities easier to perform.[16] The nature and severity of the disability are the determining factors in how many home management activities can realistically be performed, which methods can be used, and how many assistive devices can be managed. Whether the client is disabled solely by the loss of function of one arm and hand (as in amputation or peripheral neuropathy) or whether both arm and leg are affected along with possible visual, perceptual, and cognitive dysfunctions (as in hemiplegia) makes a significant difference in planning treatment. Suggestions regarding home management for the client with use of one hand include the following (see References for further details)[16]:

1. Stabilization of items is a major problem for the homemaker who can use only one hand. Stabilize foods for cutting and peeling by using a board with two stainless-steel or aluminum nails in it. A raised corner on the board stabilizes bread while making sandwiches or spreading butter. Suction cups or a rubber mat under the board will keep it from slipping. Rubber stair tread may be glued to the bottom of the board (see Figure 17-24).
2. Use sponge cloths, nonskid mats or pads, wet dishcloths, or suction devices to keep pots, bowls, and dishes from turning or sliding during food preparation.
3. To open a jar, stabilize it between the knees or in a partially opened drawer while leaning against it. Break the air seal by sliding a bottle opener under the lid until the air is released, then use a Zim jar opener (Figure 17-31).
4. Open boxes, sealed paper bags, and plastic bags by stabilizing between the knees or in a drawer, as just described, and cutting open with a household shears. Special box and bag openers are also available from ADL equipment vendors.
5. Open an egg by holding it firmly in the palm of the hand, hitting it in the center against the edge of the bowl, and then using the thumb and index finger to push the top half of the shell up and the ring and little fingers to push the lower half down. Separate whites from yolks by using an egg separator or a funnel.
6. Eliminate the need to stabilize the standard grater by using a grater with suction feet, or use an electric counter-top mincer.
7. Stabilize pots on the counter or range for mixing or stirring by using a pan holder with suction feet (Figure 17-32).
8. Eliminate the need to use hand-cranked or electric can openers requiring two hands by using a one-handed electric can opener.
9. Use a utility cart to carry items from one place to another. A cart that is weighted or constructed of wood may be used as a minimal support during ambulation for some clients.
10. Transfer clothes to and from the washer or dryer by using a clothes carrier on wheels.
11. Use electrical appliances that can be managed with one hand to save time and energy. Some of these are a lightweight electrical hand mixer, blender, and food processor. Safety factors and judgment need to be evaluated carefully when electrical appliances are considered.
12. Floor care becomes a problem if ambulation and balance are affected (in addition to the arm). For clients with involvement of one arm only, a standard dust mop, carpet sweeper, or upright vacuum cleaner should present no problem. A self-wringing mop may be used if the mop handle is stabilized under the arm and the wringing lever operated with the unaffected arm. Clients with balance and ambulation prob-

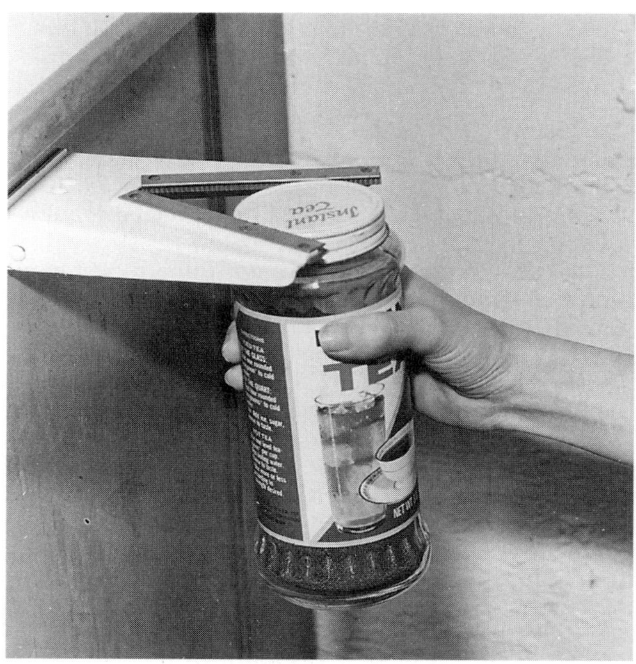


*Figure 17-31* Zim jar opener.

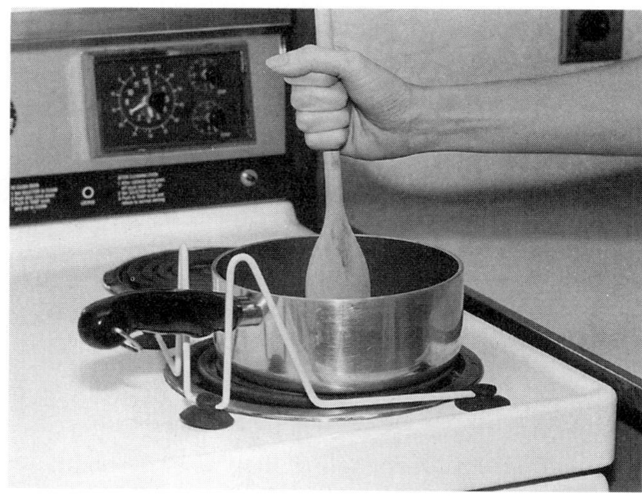

*Figure 17-32* Pan stabilizer.

lems may manage some floor care from a sitting position. Dust mopping or using a carpet sweeper may be possible if gait and balance are adequate without the aid of a cane.

These are just a few of the possibilities to solve home management problems for clients with use of one hand. The OT practitioner must evaluate each client to determine how the dysfunction affects performance of homemaking activities. One-handed techniques require more time and may be difficult for some clients to master. Activities should be paced to accommodate the client's physical endurance and tolerance for one-handed performance and use of special devices. Work simplification and energy conservation techniques should be employed.

New techniques and devices should be introduced on a graded basis as the client masters one technique and device and then another. Family members must be oriented to the client's skills, special methods used, and work schedule. The clinician may facilitate the planning of homemaking responsibilities with the family and client, focusing on which tasks are to be shared by other family members and the procedures for supervising the client, if needed.

If special equipment and assistive devices are needed for ADLs, it is advisable to acquire these through the health agency, if possible. The OT practitioner can then train the client in their use and demonstrate to a family member before the items are used at home. After training, the clinician should provide the client with sources to replace items independently, such as a consumer catalog of adaptive equipment.

### Wheelchair-Dependent Clients With Good to Normal Arm Function (Paraplegia)

Clients who are confined to a wheelchair need to find ways to perform ADLs from a seated position, to transport objects, and to adapt to an environment that is predesigned for standing and walking. Given normal upper extremity function, the wheelchair ambulator can probably perform independently. The client should have a stable spine, and mobility precautions should be clearly identified.

#### *Dressing Activities*

It is recommended that wheelchair-dependent clients put on clothing in this order: stockings, undergarments, braces (if worn), trousers or slacks, shoes, shirt, or dress.[1]

*Dressing techniques using both hands*

SOCKS OR STOCKINGS

*DONNING*

1. Put on socks or stockings while seated on bed.
2. Pull one leg into flexion with one hand and cross over other leg.
3. Use other hand to slip sock or stocking over foot and pull it on.

Soft stretch socks or stockings are recommended. Pantyhose that are slightly large may be useful. Elastic garters or stockings with elastic tops may lead to skin breakdown and should be avoided. Dressing sticks or a stocking device may be helpful to some clients.

*REMOVING*

Remove socks or stockings by flexing leg as described for donning, then pushing sock or stocking down over heel. Dressing sticks may be needed to push sock or stocking off heel and toe and to retrieve it.

TROUSERS. Trousers and slacks are easier to fasten if they button or zip in front. If braces are worn, zippers in the side seams may be helpful. Wide-bottom slacks of stretch fabric are recommended. The following procedure is for putting on trousers, shorts, slacks, and underwear.

*DONNING*

1. Use side rails or trapeze to help pull up to sitting position.
2. Sit on bed and reach forward toward feet, or sit on bed and pull knees into flexed position.
3. Holding top of trousers, flip pants down to feet.
4. Work pant legs over feet and pull up to hips. Crossing ankles may help work pants on over heels.
5. In semireclining position, roll from hip to hip and pull up garment.

Reaching tongs may be helpful to pull garment up or position garment on feet if the client has impaired balance or limited ROM in the lower extremities or trunk.

*REMOVING*

Remove pants or underwear by reversing procedure for putting on. Dressing sticks may be helpful to push pants off feet.

SLIPS AND SKIRTS

*DONNING*

1. Sit on bed, slip garment over head, and let it drop to waist.
2. In semireclining position, roll from hip to hip and pull garment down over hips and thighs.

Slips and skirts slightly larger than usually worn are recommended. A-line, wraparound, and full skirts are easier to manage and look better on a person seated in a wheelchair than do narrow skirts.

*REMOVING*

1. In sitting or semireclining position, unfasten garment.
2. Roll from hip to hip, pulling garment up to waist level.
3. Pull garment off over head.

SHOES. If the client has sensory loss and is at risk for bruising during transfers, shoes should be put on in bed. Shoes may be slipped on using one of the following variations.

*DONNING: VARIATION 1*

1. On bed, in full-leg sitting position, pull one knee at a time into flexed position with hands.
2. While supporting leg in flexed position with one hand, use free hand to put on shoe.

*DONNING: VARIATION 2*

1. Sit on edge of bed or in wheelchair (for back support).
2. Bend one knee up to flexed position, supporting leg with arm, and slip shoe on with free hand.

*DONNING: VARIATION 3*

1. Sit on edge of bed or in wheelchair.
2. Cross one leg over other and slip shoe on.
3. Put foot on footrest and push down on knee to push foot into shoe.

*REMOVING*

1. Flex or cross leg as described for appropriate variation.
2. For variations 1 and 2, remove shoe with one hand while supporting flexed leg with other hand.
3. For variation 3, remove shoe from crossed leg with one hand while maintaining balance with other hand, if necessary.

SHIRTS. Shirts, pajama jackets, robes, and dresses that open completely down the front may be put on while the client is seated in a wheelchair. If it is necessary to dress while in bed, the following procedure can be used.

*DONNING*

1. Balance body by putting palms of hands on mattress on either side of body. If balance is poor, assistance may be needed or bed backrest elevated. (If backrest cannot be elevated, one or two pillows may be used to support back.) With backrest elevated, both hands are available.
2. If difficulty is encountered in customary methods of applying garment, open garment on lap with collar toward chest. Put arms into sleeves and pull up over elbows. Then hold on to shirttail or back of dress, pull garment over head, adjust, and button.

Fabrics should be wrinkle-resistant, smooth, and durable. Roomy sleeves and backs and full skirts are more suitable styles than more closely fitted garments.

*REMOVING*

1. Sitting in wheelchair or bed, open fastener.
2. Remove garment in usual manner.
3. If step 2 is not feasible, grasp collar with one hand while balancing with other hand. Gather material up from collar to hem.
4. Lean forward, duck head, and pull shirt over head.
5. Remove sleeve from supporting arm and then from the working arm.

### *Eating Activities*

Eating activities can generally be performed easily by the wheelchair-dependent client with good to normal arm function. Wheelchairs with desk arms and swing-away footrests are recommended so that the client can sit close to the table.

### *Hygiene and Grooming*

Face and oral hygiene and arm and upper body care should present no problem. Researchers may be helpful to secure towels, washcloths, makeup, deodorant, and shaving supplies from storage areas, if necessary. Tub baths or showers require some special equipment. Chapter 18 discusses transfer techniques for the toilet and bathtub. Suggestions to make bathing activities easier for the wheelchair-dependent client include the following:

1. Use a hand-held shower head, and keep a finger over the spray to determine sudden temperature changes in water.
2. Use long-handled bath brushes with soap insert for ease in reaching all parts of the body.
3. Use soap bars attached to a cord around the neck.
4. For sponge bath in a wheelchair, cover the chair with a sheet of plastic.
5. Use shower chairs or bathtub seats.
6. Increase safety during transfers by installing grab bars on wall near the bathtub or shower and on the bathtub.
7. Fit bottom of the bathtub or shower with nonskid mat or adhesive material.
8. Remove doors on the bathtub and replace with a shower curtain to increase safety and ease of transfers.

### *Communication and General Environment*

With the exception of reaching difficulties in some situations, wheelchair-dependent patients should have no problem using the telephone. Short-handled reachers may be used to grasp the receiver from the cradle. Entering numbers can be accomplished with a short, rubber-tipped, ¼-inch dowel stick. A cordless telephone eliminates reaching except when the phone needs recharging. These clients should be able to use writing implements, typewriter, tape recorder, and personal computer with no difficulty.

Managing doors may present some problems. If the door opens toward the client, opening it can be managed by the following procedure:

1. If doorknob is on the right, approach door from right and turn doorknob with left hand.
2. Open the door as far as possible and move wheelchair close enough so that it helps keep door open.

3. Holding door open with left hand, turn wheelchair with right hand and wheel through door.
4. Start closing door when halfway through.

If the door is heavy and opens out or away from the client, the following procedure is recommended[4]:

1. Back up to door so knob can be turned with right hand.
2. Open door and back through so that large wheels keep it open.
3. Also use left elbow to keep door open.
4. Wheel backward with right hand.

### *Mobility and Transfers*

Chapter 18 discusses principles of transfer techniques.

### *Home Management Activities*

When performing homemaking activities from a wheelchair, the major problems are work heights, adequate space for maneuverability, access to storage areas, and transfer of supplies, equipment, and materials from place to place. If funds are available for kitchen remodeling, lowering counters and range to a comfortable height for wheelchair use is recommended. However, such extensive adaptation is often not feasible. Suggestions for home management are as follows[16]:

1. Remove cabinet doors to eliminate the need to maneuver around them for opening and closing. Frequently used items should be stored on counters or toward the front of easy-to-reach cabinets above and below the counter surfaces.
2. If entrance and inside doors are not wide enough, use a narrower wheelchair or make doors slightly wider by removing strips along the door jambs. Offset hinges can replace standard door hinges and increase the door jamb width by 2 inches (5 cm) (Figure 17-33).
3. Increase the client's height with a wheelchair cushion so that standard counters may be used.
4. Use detachable desk arms and swing-away detachable footrests to allow the client to roll as close as possible to counters and tables and also to stand at counters, if possible (Figure 17-34).
5. Transport items safely and easily by using a wheelchair lapboard. The lapboard may also serve as a work surface for preparing food and drying dishes. It also protects the lap from injury from hot pans and prevents utensils from falling into the lap (Figure 17-35).
6. Fasten a drop-leaf-type board to a bare wall or a slide-out board under a counter to give the wheelchair-bound homemaker one work surface that is at a comfortable height in an otherwise standard kitchen.
7. Fit cabinets with custom-made or ready-made lazy Susans or pull-out shelves to eliminate

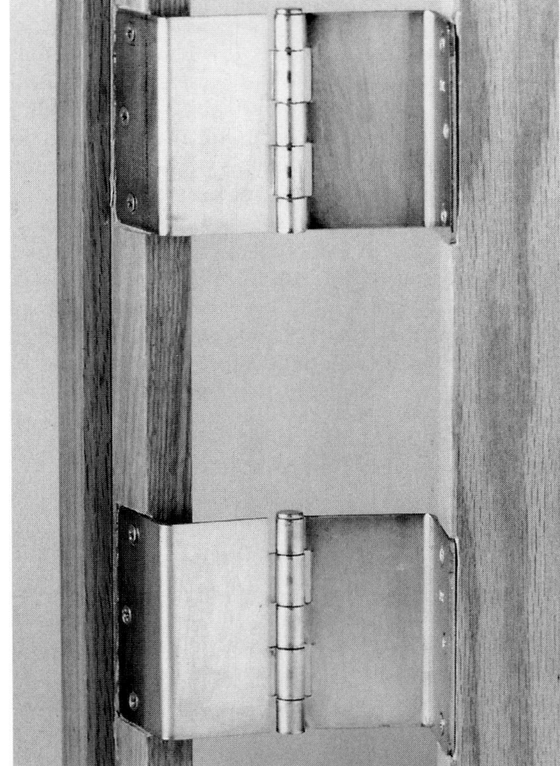


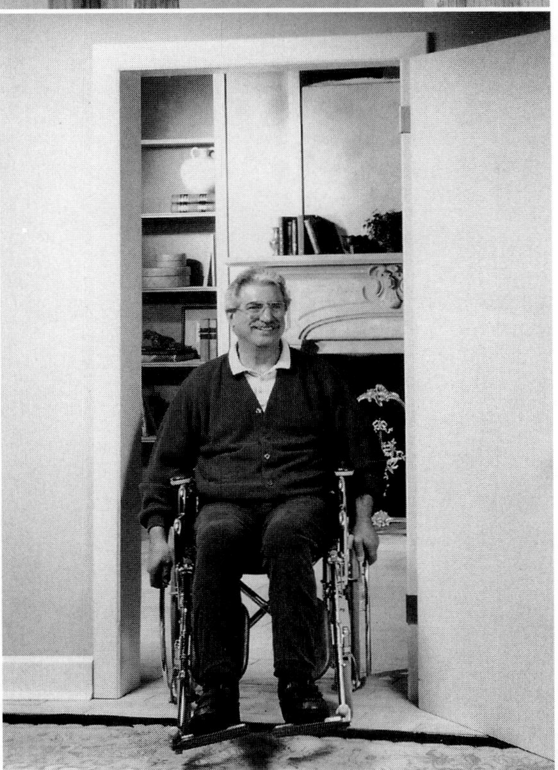


*Figure 17-33* **A,** Offset hinges. **B,** Offset hinges widen doorway for wheelchair-dependent patient. (Courtesy Sammons, a BISSELL Co.)

need to reach to the rear of the space (Figure 17-36).
8. Ranges ideally should be at a lower level than standard height. If this is not possible, place controls at the front of the range and hang a mirror over the range, angled at such a degree that the homemaker can see contents of pots.
9. Substitute small electric cooking units and microwave ovens for the range if it is not safely manageable.
10. Use front-loading washers and dryers.
11. Vacuum carpets with a carpet sweeper or tank-type cleaner that rolls easily and is lightweight or self-propelled. A retractable cord may be helpful to prevent tangling of cord in wheels.

### Wheelchair-Dependent Client with Upper Extremity Weakness (Quadriplegia)

In general, clients with muscle function from spinal cord levels C7 and C8 can follow the methods just described for paraplegia. Clients with muscle function from C6 can be relatively independent with adaptations and assistive devices. However, those with muscle function from C4 and C5 require considerable special equipment and assistance. Clients with muscle function from C6 may benefit from the use of a wrist-driven flexor hinge splint. Externally powered

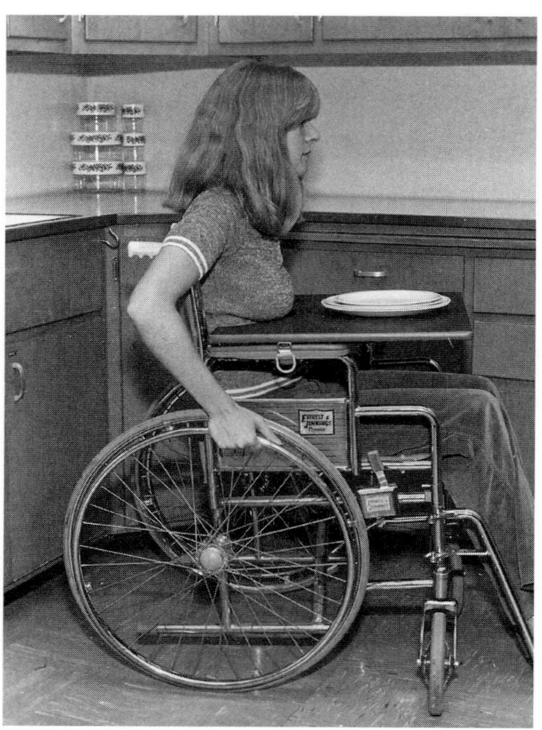

*Figure 17-35* Wheelchair lapboard is used to transport items.

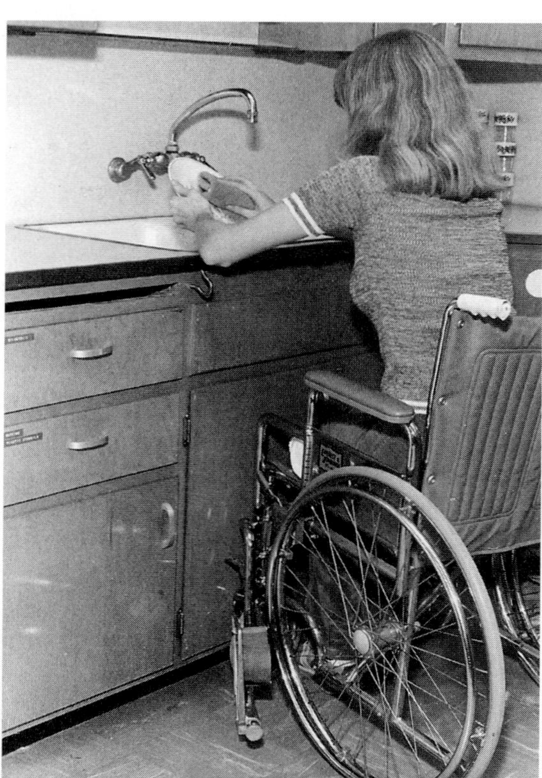

*Figure 17-34* Wheelchair footrests are swung away to allow close access to sink.

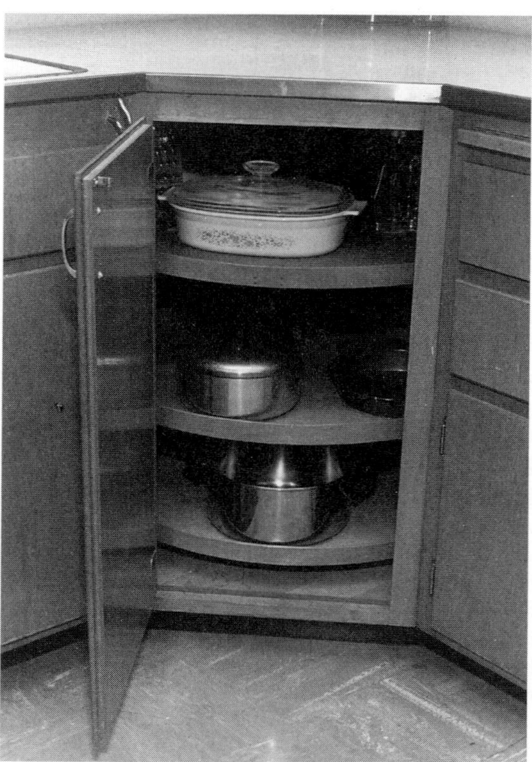

*Figure 17-36* Lazy Susan in kitchen storage cabinet.

splints and arm braces or mobile arm supports are recommended for C3, C4, and C5 levels of muscle function.[1]

### Dressing Activities

Determining whether or not a patient meets the criteria for beginning dressing activities is a professional-level responsibility. However, the COTA can assist in the determination and always should closely observe patient readiness for this or any other activity.

*Criteria* Training in dressing can begin once the spine is stable.[3,25] Minimal criteria for upper extremity dressing are (1) fair to good muscle strength in deltoids, upper and middle trapezii, shoulder rotators, rhomboids, biceps, supinators, and radial wrist extensors; (2) ROM of 0° to 90° in shoulder flexion and abduction, 0° to 80° in shoulder internal rotation, 0° to 30° in external rotation, and 15° to 140° in elbow flexion; (3) sitting balance in bed or wheelchair, which may be achieved with the assistance of bed rails, an electric hospital bed, or wheelchair safety belt; and (4) finger prehension, achieved with adequate tenodesis grasp or a wrist-hand orthosis.

Additional criteria for dressing the lower extremities are (1) fair to good muscle strength in pectoralis major and minor, serratus anterior, and rhomboideus major and minor; (2) ROM of 0° to 120° in knee flexion, 0° to 110° in hip flexion, and 0° to 80° in hip external rotation; (3) body control for transfer from bed to wheelchair with minimal assistance; (4) ability to roll from side to side, balance in side lying, or turning from supine to prone position and back; and (5) vital capacity of 50% or greater.[25]

*Contraindications* Dressing is contraindicated if any of the following factors are present: (1) unstable spine at site of injury; (2) pressure sores or tendency for skin breakdown during rolling, scooting, and transferring; (3) uncontrollable muscle spasms in legs; and (4) less than 50% vital capacity.[3,25]

*Sequence of dressing* The recommended sequence for training to dress is to put on underwear and trousers while still in bed, then transfer to a wheelchair to put on shirts, socks, and shoes.[25] Some patients may choose to put the socks on before the trousers, because socks may help the feet slip through the trouser legs more easily.

*Expected proficiency* Total dressing, which includes both upper and lower extremity dressing skills, can be achieved by clients with spinal cord lesions at C7 and below. Although total dressing can be achieved by those with lesions at C6, lower extremity dressing may be difficult or impracticable in terms of time and energy.

Upper extremity dressing can be achieved by clients with lesions at C5 to C6, with some exceptions. It is difficult or impossible for these clients to put on a brassiere, tuck a shirt or blouse into a waistband, or fasten buttons on shirt fronts and cuffs. Factors such as age, physical proportions, coordination, concomitant medical problems, and motivation affect the client's degree of proficiency in dressing skills.[3]

*Types of clothing* Clothing should be loose and have front openings. Trousers need to be a size larger than usually worn to accommodate the urine collection device or leg braces, if worn. Wraparound skirts and rubber pants are helpful for women. The fasteners that are easiest to manage are zippers and Velcro closures. Because the quadriplegic client often uses the thumb as a hook to manage clothing, loops attached to zipper pulls, undershorts, and even the back of the shoes can be helpful. Belt loops on trousers are used for pulling and should be reinforced. Brassieres should have stretch straps and no boning in them. Front-opening brassiere styles can be adapted by fastening loops and adding Velcro closures; back-opening styles can have loops added at each side of the fastening.

Shoes can be one-half to one size larger than normally worn to accommodate edema and spasticity and to avoid pressure sores. Shoe fasteners can be adapted with Velcro, elastic shoelaces, large buckles, or flip-back tongue closures. Loose woolen or cotton socks without elastic cuffs should be used initially. As skill is gained, nylon socks, which tend to stick to the skin, may be introduced. If neckties are used, the clip-on type or a regular tie that has been preknotted and can be slipped over the head may be manageable for some clients.[3,25]

The following techniques can make dressing easier for clients with upper extremity weakness.

**TROUSERS AND UNDERSHORTS**

*DONNING*

1. Sit on bed with bed rails up (full-leg sitting position). Trousers are positioned at foot of bed with trouser legs over end of bed and front side up.[25]
2. Sit up and lift one knee at a time by hooking right hand under right knee to pull leg into flexion, then put trousers over right foot. Return right leg to extended or semiextended position and repeat procedure with left hand and left knee.[3]
   It is important to maintain one leg at a time in flexion by holding it with one arm or by taking advantage of spasticity. If neither of these strategies works, a dressing band may be used. This is a piece of elasticized webbing sewn into a figure-eight pattern, with one small loop and one large loop. Small loop is hooked around foot and large hoop anchored over knee. Band is measured for each client so that its length is appropriate to maintain desired amount of knee flexion. Once trousers are in place, knee loop is pushed off knee and dressing band removed from foot with dressing stick.[7]

3. Work trousers up legs, using patting and sliding motions with palms of hands.
4. While still sitting with pants at midcalf height, insert dressing stick in front belt loop. Dressing stick is gripped by slipping its loop over wrist. Pull on dressing stick while extending trunk, returning to supine position. Return to sitting position and repeat this procedure, pulling on dressing sticks and maneuvering trousers up to thigh level.[25] If balance is adequate, an alternative is for client to remain sitting and lean on left elbow and pull trousers over right buttock, then reverse process for other side. Another alternative is for client to remain in supine position and roll to one side; throw opposite arm behind back; hook thumb in waistband, belt loop, or pocket; and pull trousers up over hips. These maneuvers can be repeated as needed to pull trousers over buttocks.[3]
5. Using palms of hands in pushing and smoothing motions, straighten trouser legs.
6. In supine position, fasten trouser placket by hooking thumb in loop on zipper pull, patting Velcro closed, or using hand splints and buttonhooks if buttons present.[3,25]

*DONNING: VARIATION*

For step 2, substitute the following:
Sit up and lift one knee at a time by hooking right hand under right knee to pull leg into flexion, then cross foot over opposite leg above knee. This position frees up foot to place trousers more easily and requires less trunk balance. Continue with all other steps.

*REMOVING*

1. Lying supine in bed with bed rails up, unfasten belt and placket fasteners.
2. Placing thumbs in belt loops, waistband, or pockets, work trousers past hips by stabilizing arms in shoulder extension and scooting body toward head of bed.
3. Use arms as described in step 2 and roll from side to side to slide trousers past buttocks.
4. Coming to sitting position and alternately pulling legs into flexion, push trousers down legs.[25]
5. Trousers can be pushed off over feet with dressing stick or by hooking thumbs in waistband.

**CARDIGANS OR PULLOVER GARMENTS.** Cardigan and pullover garments include blouses, vests, sweaters, skirts, and front-opening dresses.[3,25] Upper extremity dressing is frequently performed in the wheelchair for greater trunk stability.

*DONNING*

1. Position garment across thighs with back facing up and neck toward knees.
2. Place both arms under back of garment and in armholes.
3. Push sleeves up onto arms past elbows.
4. Using a wrist extension grip, hook thumbs under garment back and gather material up from neck to hem.
5. To pass garment over head, adduct and externally rotate shoulders and flex elbows while flexing head forward.
6. When garment is over head, relax shoulders and wrists, and remove hands from back of garment. Most of material will be gathered up at neck, across shoulders, and under arms.
7. To work garment down over body, shrug shoulders, lean forward, and use elbow flexion and wrist extension. Use wheelchair arms for balance if necessary. Additional maneuvers to accomplish task are to hook wrists into sleeves and pull material free from underarms or lean forward, reach back, and slide hand against material to aid in pulling garment down.
8. Garment can be buttoned from bottom to top with aid of buttonhook and wrist-hand orthosis if hand function is inadequate.

*REMOVING*

1. Sit in wheelchair and wear wrist-hand orthosis. Unfasten buttons (if any) while wearing splints and using buttonhook. Remove splints for remaining steps.
2. For pullover garments, hook thumb in back of neckline, extend wrist, and pull garment over head while turning head toward side of raised arm. Maintain balance by resting against opposite wheelchair armrest or pushing on thigh with extended arm.
3. For cardigan garments, hook thumb in opposite armhole and push sleeve down arm. Elevation and depression of shoulders with trunk rotation can be used to have garment slip down arms as far as possible.
4. Hold one cuff with opposite thumb while elbow is flexed to pull arm out of sleeve.

**BRASSIERE (BACK OPENING)**

*DONNING*

1. Place brassiere across lap with straps toward knees and inside facing up.
2. Using a right-to-left procedure, hold end of brassiere closest to right side with hand or reacher and pass brassiere around back from right to left. Lean against brassiere at back to hold it in place while hooking thumb of left hand in a loop that has been attached near brassiere fastener. Hook right thumb in a similar loop on right side and fasten brassiere in front at waist level.
3. Hook right thumb in edge of brassiere, and using wrist extension, elbow flexion, shoulder adduction, and internal rotation, rotate brassiere around body so that front of brassiere is in front of body.
4. While leaning on one forearm, hook opposite thumb in front end of strap and pull strap over shoulder, then repeat procedure on other side.[3,25]

*REMOVING*

1. Hook thumb under opposite brassiere strap and push down over shoulder while elevating shoulder.
2. Pull arm out of strap and repeat procedure for other arm.
3. Push brassiere down to waist level and turn around as described previously to bring fasteners to front.
4. Unfasten brassiere.

Alternatives to a back-opening bra are (1) a front-opening bra with loops to use a wrist extension grip or (2) a fully elastic bra that has no fasteners and can be donned like a pullover sweater.

**SOCKS**

*DONNING*

1. Sit in wheelchair (or on bed if balance is adequate) in cross-legged position with one ankle crossed over opposite knee.
2. Pull sock over foot with wrist extension grip and patting movements with palm of hand.[3,25]
3. If trunk balance is inadequate and cross-legged position cannot be maintained, prop foot on stool, chair, or open drawer, keeping opposite arm around upright of wheelchair for balance. Fastening wheelchair safety belt or leaning against wheelchair armrest on one side are alternatives to maintain balance.
4. Use stocking aid (see Figure 17-7) or sock cone to assist in putting on socks while in this position. Powder sock cone and apply sock to it by using thumbs and palms of hands to smooth sock out on cone. Powder inside of cone to reduce friction against cone.
5. Place cord loops of sock cone around wrist or thumb and throw cone beyond foot.
6. Maneuver cone over toes by pulling cords using elbow flexion. Insert foot as far as possible into cone.
7. To remove cone from sock after foot has been inserted, move heel forward off wheelchair footrest. Use wrist extension of one hand behind knee, and with other hand continue pulling cords of cone until it is removed and sock is in place on foot. Use palms to smooth sock with patting and stroking motion.[25]
8. Two loops can also be sewn on either side of top of sock so that thumbs can be hooked into loops and socks pulled on.

*REMOVING*

1. While sitting in wheelchair or lying in bed, use dressing stick or long-handled shoehorn to push sock down over heel. Cross legs if possible.
2. Use dressing stick with cuphook on end to pull sock off toes.[4]

**SHOES**

*DONNING*

1. For putting on shoes, use same position as for donning socks.
2. Use extended-handle dressing aid and insert it into tongue of shoe; then place shoe opening over toes. Remove dressing aid from shoe and dangle shoe on toes.
3. Using palm of hand on sole of shoe, pull shoe toward heel of foot. Use one hand to stabilize leg while pushing other against sole of shoe to work shoe onto foot. Use thenar eminence and sides of hand for pushing motion.
4. With feet flat on floor or on wheelchair footrest and knees flexed 90°, place long-handled shoehorn in heel of shoe and press down on flexed knee.
5. Fasten shoes.[25]

*REMOVING*

1. Sitting in wheelchair as described for donning socks, unfasten shoes.
2. Use shoehorn or dressing stick to push on heel counter of shoe, dislodging it from heel; then shoe will drop or can be pushed to floor with dressing stick.

### *Eating Activities*

Eating may be assisted by a variety of devices, depending on the quadriplegic client's level of muscle function.[1] Levels C5 and above require mobile arm supports or externally powered splints and braces. A wrist splint and universal cuff may be used together if a wrist-hand orthosis (flexor hinge splint) is not used. The universal cuff holds the eating utensil, and the splint stabilizes the wrist. A nonskid mat and a plate with plate guard may provide adequate stability of the plate for pushing and picking up food (Figure 17-37).

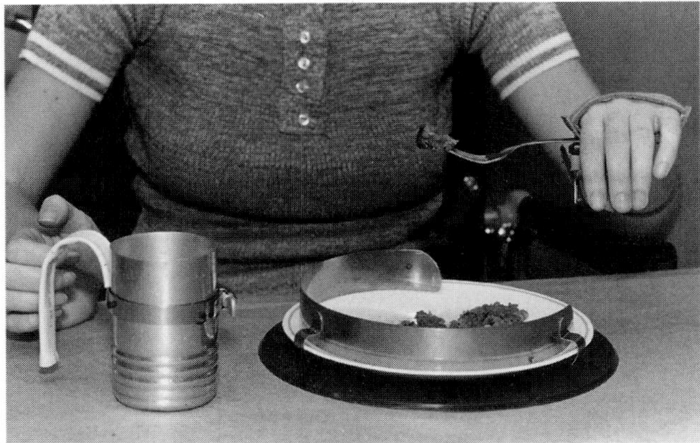

*Figure 17-37* Self-feeding with aid of universal cuff, plate guard, nonskid mat, and clip-type cup holder to compensate for absent grasp.

The *spoon-plate* is an option for independent feeding for clients with high spinal cord injuries.[29] It is a portable device that can be adjusted in height to the level of the client's mouth. The plate is made of a high-temperature thermoplastic and is formed over a mold that has a cupped rim shaped to the approximate depth and length of a spoon. The client rotates the device with mouth and neck control. Food is removed from the rim of the plate with the mouth. Successful use of the device depends on adequate oral control, head and trunk control, and motivation. (See Wykoff and Mitani[29] for information on making or obtaining this device.)

Also available for clients who have no use of their upper extremities is the electric self-feeder, which requires only slight head motion and is activated by a chin switch (Figure 17-38).

A regular or swivel spoon-fork combination can be used when the client has minimal muscle function (C4 to C5). A long plastic straw with a straw clip to stabilize it in the cup or glass eliminates the need for picking up these drinking vessels. A bilateral or unilateral clip-type holder on a glass or cup allows many clients with hand and arm weakness to manage liquids without a straw.

Built-up utensils may be useful for clients with some functional grasp or tenodesis grasp. Cutting food may be managed with a quad-quip knife if arm strength is adequate to manage the device (Figure 17-39).

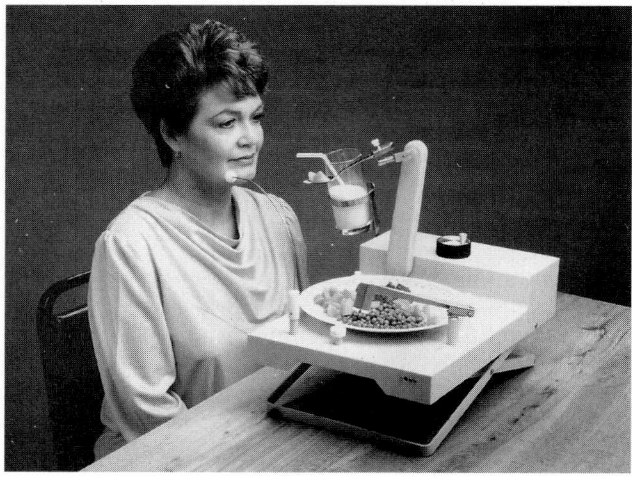

*Figure 17-38* Electric self-feeder. (Courtesy Sammons, a BISSELL Co.)

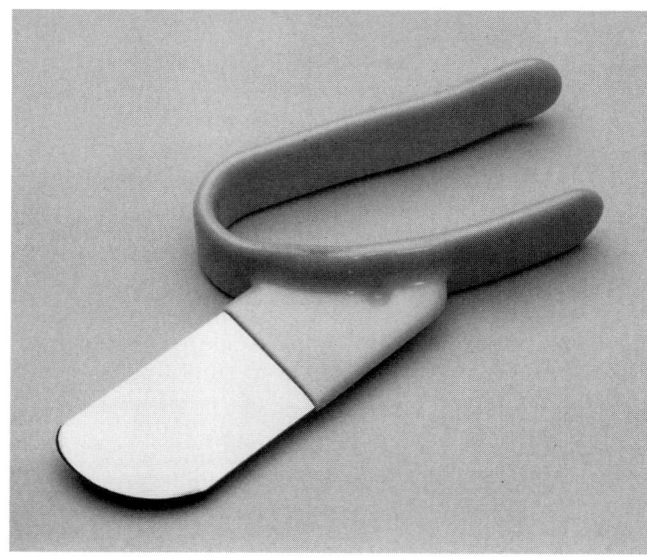

*Figure 17-39* Quad-quip knife.

### *Hygiene and Grooming*

General suggestions to facilitate hygiene and grooming are as follows[1]:

1. Use a shower or bathtub seat and transfer board for transfers.
2. Extend reach by using long-handled bath sponges with loop handle or built-up handle.
3. Eliminate need to grasp washcloth by using bath mitts.
4. Hold comb and toothbrush with a universal cuff.[1]
5. Use the position-adjustable hair dryer previously described.[8] Use a universal cuff to hold brush or comb for hair styling while using this mounted hair dryer.
6. Use a clip-type holder for electric razor.
7. Suppository inserters can be used by quadriplegic clients who can manage bowel care independently.
8. Use skin inspection mirror with long stem and looped handle for independent skin inspection (Figure 17-40). The degree of weakness for each client must be considered when selecting devices and selecting and adapting methods.
9. Adapted leg-bag clamps to empty catheter leg bags are also available for patients with limited hand function. Velcro straps may substitute for elastic leg-bag straps.

### *Communication and General Environment*

Suggestions for facilitating communication include the following:

1. Turn pages with an electric page turner, mouthstick, or head wand if hand and arm function are inadequate (Figure 17-41).
2. For typing, writing, operating a tape recorder, and painting, insert a pen, pencil, typing stick, or paintbrush in a universal cuff that has been positioned with the opening on the ulnar side of the palm (Figure 17-42).
3. Dial the telephone with the universal cuff and a pencil positioned with eraser down. The receiver may need to be stationed in a telephone arm and positioned for listening or adapted with a telephone clip holder (see Figure 17-16). Special adaptations are available to substitute for the need to replace the receiver in the cradle. For patients with no arm function, a speakerphone can

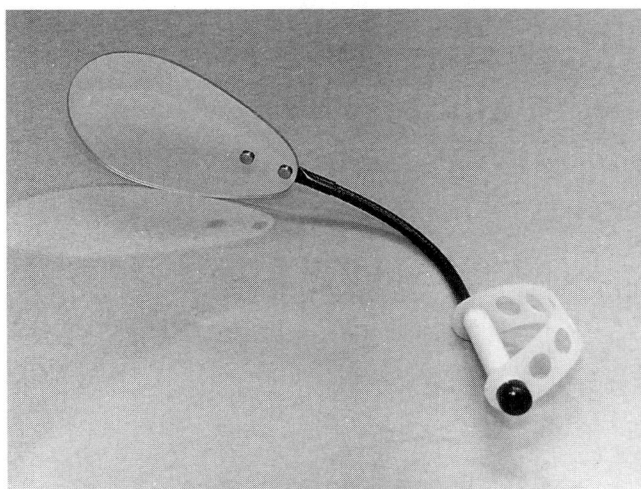

*Figure 17-40* Skin inspection mirror.

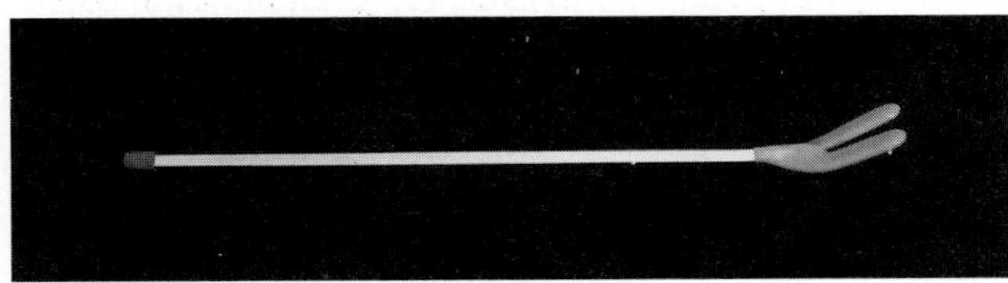

*Figure 17-41* Wand mouthstick. (Courtesy Sammons, a BISSELL Co.)

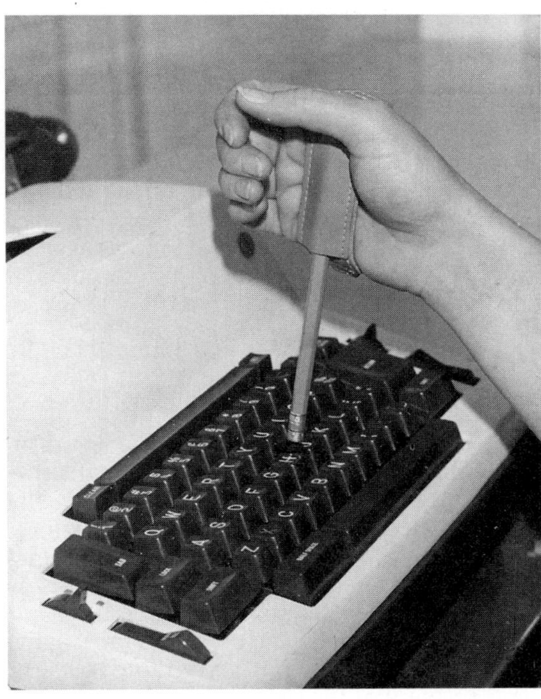

*Figure 17-42* Typing with aid of utensil holder and typing stick.

be used with a mouthstick to push the button to initiate a call; the operator assists with dialing. A voice-activated phone is also available for clients with little to no upper extremity function.
4. Use personal computers, word processors, or electric typewriters. A computer mouse may replace the keyboard.
5. Built-up pencils and pens or special pencil holders are needed for clients with hand weakness. The Wanchik writer is an effective adaptive writing device (see Figure 17-17).
6. Sophisticated electronic communication devices operated by mouth, pneumatic controls, and head control are available for clients with no upper extremity function.[27]
7. Kelly[13] described two mouthsticks and a cassette tape holder that allow persons with C3, C4, or C5 quadriplegia to operate a tape recorder or radio independently. The first mouthstick, a rod about 20 inches (50 cm) long with a friction tip, is used to depress the operating buttons and adjust the radio's volume and selector dials. The second mouthstick is a metal rod that separates into two prongs at its end. These prongs are 4 inches (10 cm) apart, and the mouthstick is used to insert cassettes from the cassette holder into the tape recorder and to remove cassettes from the recorder. The vertical cassette tape stand is made of metal, tilted backward at a 70° angle, and designed to hold eight tapes at its eight levels. (See Kelly[13] for specifications on construction of these devices.)
8. Environmental control units (ECUs) use a single panel to operate multiple devices such as televisions, radios, lights, telephones, intercoms, and hospital beds. ECUs are readily available at local electronic stores.

### *Mobility and Transfers*

Chapter 18 discusses principles of wheelchair transfer techniques for the quadriplegic client. Mobility depends on degree of weakness. Electric wheelchairs operated by hand, chin, or pneumatic controls have greatly increased the mobility of clients with severe upper and lower extremity weakness. Vans fitted with wheelchair lifts and stabilizing devices have provided such clients with transport to pursue community, vocational, educational, and avocational activities with an assistant. In addition, adaptations for hand controls have allowed many clients with at least C6-level function to drive independently.

### *Home Management Activities*

Many wheelchair-dependent clients with upper extremity weakness are dependent or partly dependent for homemaking activities. Clients with muscle function of C6 or better may be independent for light homemaking with appropriate devices, adaptations, and safety awareness. Many of the suggestions for wheelchair maneuverability and environmental adaptation outlined for the paraplegic client apply to these clients as well. In addition, the patient with upper extremity weakness needs to use lightweight equipment and special devices. The *Mealtime Manual for People with Disability and the Aging* contains many excellent and specific suggestions that apply to the homemaker with weak upper extremities.[16]

## ACCESS TO RECREATION AND LEISURE ACTIVITIES

A well-rounded occupational therapy treatment program must consider the client's recreation and leisure interests and needs. Participation in recreational activities frequently holds intrinsic value for the client, helps boost self-esteem, and may be important in the social life of the client, family, and friends.[5]

Assessment needs to include previous activities, new activities the client would be willing to learn, and the client's potential for participating in the activities. To determine the client's interests, the OT practitioner can use the interest checklist and activities configuration described earlier in the Evaluation of Performance Areas section.

The COTA's role in leisure and recreation will vary according to the type of program and the availability of other specialized personnel, such as a recreation therapist. The COTA may function as a resource person, referring the client to community agencies and support centers; may recommend the client be referred to a recreation therapist; or may teach the client some leisure tasks. The client's caregiver must be educated to help in purchasing items needed for the activity and to learn new methods to help the client become involved in leisure activities.

Resources available in the community vary but may include services to meet the physically limited individual's needs. Some examples of these services are sailing, skiing, white water rafting, camping, wheelchair basketball, and travel agencies that specialize in planning trips for the physically challenged person.

Adaptive equipment for leisure activities is also available, including adapted bicycle units to attach to wheelchairs, swimming aids, adapted bowling equipment, and fishing equipment to attach to a wheelchair or to use with one hand (Figure 17-43). For more sedentary activities, card holders, automatic card shufflers, pneumatic video game controls, camera holders to attach to a wheelchair, and needlework tools are available for one-handed use. Adaptive equipment for gardening can assist those who have difficulty bending, reaching, and grasping tools.[17]

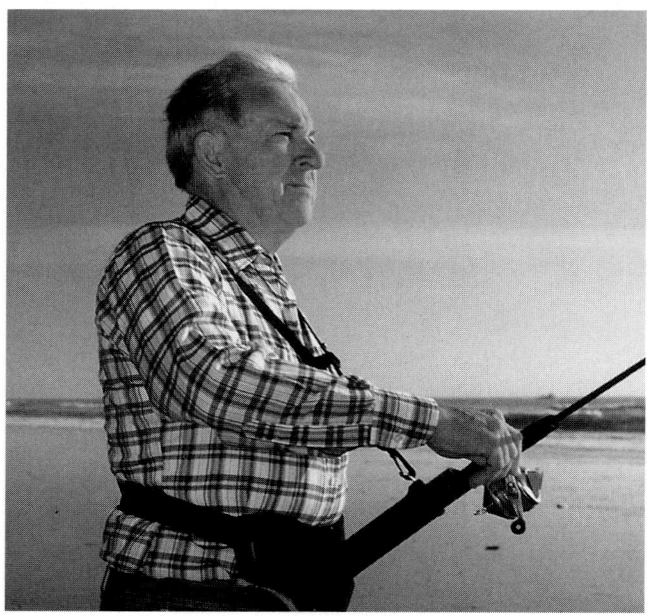

*Figure 17-43* Angler's rod holder. (Courtesy Don Krebs' Access to Recreation, Adaptive Recreation Equipment for the Physically Challenged, Thousand Oaks, Calif.)

Even during the initial treatment, with its focus on basic ADLs and I-ADLs, many clients will want to begin considering involvement in recreation and leisure activities. The COTA who is knowledgeable about resources and adaptive equipment for leisure activities may function as a resource person to help the client resume a balance of activities.

## SUMMARY

ADLs and I-ADLs are tasks of self-maintenance, mobility, communication, home management, and community living skills that allow a client to function independently and assume important occupational roles.

ADLs represent one of the performance areas in the occupational performance model. Occupational therapy practitioners routinely evaluate performance in ADLs to assess clients' level of functional independence. This is a practice area in which the COTA may establish service competency and special expertise. Evaluation is performed through the interview and observation of performance. Evaluation results and ongoing progress are recorded on one of many available ADL checklists, and the content is summarized for the permanent medical record.

Treatment is directed toward training in independent living skills using methods in such activity areas as eating, dressing, mobility, home management, communication, and community living. The COTA practicing in this area should be familiar with the special equipment and methods for performing ADLs needed by the client with specific functional problems.

## Selected Reading Guide Questions

1. Define and differentiate between activities of daily living (ADLs) and instrumental activities of daily living (I-ADLs). List three subcategories in both ADLs and I-ADLs.
2. Describe the role of occupational therapy in restoring ADL and I-ADL independence.
3. List at least three activities for each of the following subcategories of skills: self-care, mobility, communication, home management, and community living.
4. List three factors that the occupational therapy practitioner must consider before commencing ADL performance evaluation and training. Describe how each could limit or affect the client's ADL performance.
5. Discuss the concept of *maximal independence*, as defined in the text.
6. List the general steps in the procedure for ADL evaluation.
7. What is the purpose of the home evaluation?
8. List the steps in the home evaluation.
9. Who should be involved in a comprehensive home evaluation?
10. What other areas or factors are assessed in a home evaluation?
11. How does the OT practitioner record and report results of the home evaluation and make the necessary recommendations?
12. How does the OT practitioner, with the client, select ADL and I-ADL training objectives after an evaluation?
13. Describe three approaches to teaching ADL skills to a client with perception or memory deficits.
14. List the important factors to include in an ADL progress report.
15. Give an example of a health and safety management issue.
16. Explain how you, as a COTA, would establish service competency and maximal independence in providing ADL services within the legal guidelines of your state or other local jurisdiction.

## Exercises

1. Demonstrate the use of at least three assistive devices mentioned in the text.
2. Teach a person to don a shirt, using one hand.
3. Teach another person how to don and remove trousers, as if the person had hemiplegia.
4. Teach a different person how to don and remove trousers, as if the legs were paralyzed.

### REFERENCES


1. *Activities of daily living for patients with incoordination, limited range of motion, paraplegia, quadriplegia, and hemiplegia,* Cleveland, 1968, Division of Occupational Therapy, Highland View Hospital, Cuyahoga County Hospitals (unpublished).
2. Armstrong M, Lauzen S: *Community integration program,* ed 2, Washington, 1994, Idyll Arbor.
3. Bromley I: *Tetraplegia and paraplegia: a guide for physiotherapists,* ed 2, London, 1981, Churchill Livingstone.
4. Buchwald E: *Physical rehabilitation for daily living,* New York, 1952, McGraw-Hill.
5. Christiansen C: Occupational performance assessment. In Christiansen C, Baum C, editors: *Occupational therapy: overcoming human performance deficits,* Thorofare, NJ, 1991, Slack.
6. Cynkin S, Robinson AM: *Occupational therapy and activities health: toward health through activities,* Boston, 1990, Little, Brown.
7. Easton LW, Horan AL: Dressing band, *Am J Occup Ther* 33:656, 1979.
8. Feldmeier DM, Poole JL: The position-adjustable hair dryer, *Am J Occup Ther* 41:246, 1987.
9. Florey LL, Michelman SM: Occupational role history: a screening tool for psychiatric occupational therapy, *Am J Occup Ther* 36:301, 1982.
10. Guerette P, Moran W: ADL awareness, *Team Rehabil Rep,* June 1994.
11. Holser P, Jones M, Ilanit T: A study of the upper extremity control brace, *Am J Occup Ther* 16:170, 1962.
12. Hopkins HL, Smith HD, Tiffany EG: Therapeutic application of activity. In Hopkins HL, Smith HD, editors: *Willard and Spackman's occupational therapy,* ed 6, Philadelphia, 1983, Lippincott.
13. Kelly SN: Adaptations for independent use of cassette tape recorder/radio by high-level quadriplegic patients, *Am J Occup Ther* 37:766, 1983.
14. Kemp BJ, Mitchell JM: Functional assessment in geriatric mental health. In Birren JE et al, editors: *Handbook of mental health and aging,* ed 2, San Diego, 1992, Academic Press.
15. Kester DL: Prevocational and vocational assessment. In Hopkins HL, Smith HD, editors: *Willard and Spackman's occupational therapy,* ed 6, Philadelphia, 1983, Lippincott.
16. Klinger JL: *Mealtime manual for people with disabilities and the aging,* Camden, NJ, 1978, Campbell Soup.
17. Krebs D: *Adaptive recreation equipment for the physically challenged,* Thousand Oaks, Calif, 1995, Access to Recreation.
18. Letts L et al: Person-environment assessments in occupational therapy, *Am J Occup Ther* 48:608-618, 1994.
19. Malick MH, Almasy BS: Activities of daily living and homemaking. In Hopkins HL, Smith HD, editors: *Willard and Spackman's occupational therapy,* ed 7, Philadelphia, 1988, Lippincott.
20. Malick MH, Almasy BS: Assessment and evaluation: life work tasks. In Hopkins HL, Smith HD, editors: *Willard and Spackman's occupational therapy,* ed 6, Philadelphia, 1983, Lippincott.
21. Matsusuyu J: The interest checklist, *Am J Occup Ther* 23:323, 1969.
22. Melvin JL: *Rheumatic disease: occupational therapy and rehabilitation,* ed 2, Philadelphia, 1982, Davis.
23. Moorhead L: The occupational history, *Am J Occup Ther* 23:329, 1969.
24. Professional Manual Subcommittee of the Educational Committee, Allied Health Professional Section, Arthritis Foundation: *Arthritis manual for allied health professionals,* New York, 1973, The Foundation.
25. Runge M: Self-dressing techniques for clients with spinal cord injury, *Am J Occup Ther* 21:367, 1967.
26. Sokaler R: A buttoning aid, *Am J Occup Ther* 35:737, 1981.
27. Trombly CA: Activities of daily living. In Trombly CA, editor: *Occupational therapy for physical dysfunction,* ed 2, Baltimore, 1983, Williams & Wilkins.
28. Watanabe S: *Activities configuration,* Final report RSA-123-T-68, Regional Institute on the Evaluation Process, New York, 1968, American Occupational Therapy Association.
29. Wykoff E, Mitani M: The spoon plate: a self-feeding device, *Am J Occup Ther* 36:333, 1982.


### RECOMMENDED READING


Sine RD et al: *Basic rehabilitation techniques:* a self-instructional guide, ed 3, Gaithersberg, Md, 1988, Aspen.

Chapter 18

# Wheelchairs and Wheelchair Mobility, Functional Mobility and Transfer Training, and Ambulation Aids

*Carole Adler*
*Michelle Tipton-Burton*
*Regina M. Lehman*

## Chapter Objectives

*After studying this chapter, the student or practitioner will be able to:*

1. Describe the process of evaluation for wheelchair use.
2. List and discuss the factors that influence the selection of a wheelchair.
3. Describe the process by which a wheelchair is prescribed.
4. Appreciate the range of styles and types of wheelchairs available, and analyze for whom each would be most appropriate.
5. Describe the process of wheelchair measurement.
6. List the factors that influence wheelchair positioning.
7. Describe the elements of wheelchair safety for the wheelchair user and caregiver.
8. Apply the basic concepts of wheelchair mobility.
9. State and practice proper body mechanics used during transfers.
10. Describe the three most frequently used transfer techniques.
11. Describe the role of the occupational therapy practitioner with the patient who employs an ambulation aid.

## Key Terms

wheelchair
measurement
positioning
alignment
prescription
mobility
transfer
body mechanics
pelvic tilt
stand-pivot transfer
sliding-board transfer
bent-pivot transfer
dependent transfer
ambulation aid

## WHEELCHAIRS

**Wheelchairs** provide basic mobility for people with permanent or progressive disabilities of ambulation resulting from diagnoses such as cerebrovascular accident (CVA, stroke), cerebral palsy, brain injury, spinal cord injury, multiple sclerosis, and muscular dystrophy. Wheelchairs offer a temporary means of mobility for those with a short-term illness or orthopedic problem. The wheelchair is more than a method of transportation and significantly affects the user's body image, positioning, skin integrity, and overall functioning and general well-being. Regardless of the client's diagnosis, the occupational therapy practitioner must understand the complexity of wheelchair technology, the options and modifications available, the evaluation and measuring process, the procedures for use and care, and the process by which wheelchairs are funded.

Wheelchairs have evolved considerably in recent years, with significant advances in powered and manual wheelchair technology. Products are constantly changing. Many of the improvements have resulted from users' recommendations, but the therapists prescribing the equipment have had influence as well.

Registered occupational therapists (OTRs) and physical therapists, depending on their respective roles at the treatment facility, are usually responsible for evaluating, measuring, and selecting a wheelchair for the patient. They also teach wheelchair safety and mobility. In certain settings, such as long-term care facilities or nursing homes, one or more of these tasks may become the responsibility of the certified occupational therapy assistant (COTA).

Because of the increasingly sophisticated nature and variety of power and manual wheelchairs, it is advisable to include an experienced, knowledgeable rehabilitation technology supplier (RTS) and a durable medical equipment (DME) supplier on the ordering team. These specialists are proficient in ordering custom-made items and can offer an objective and broad mechanical perspective on the availability and appropriateness of the options being considered. The RTS is the client's resource for repairs and reordering when returning to the community.

Whether the client requires a non–custom-made rental wheelchair for temporary use or a custom-designed wheelchair for use over many years, an individualized prescription clearly outlining the specific features of the chair is needed to ensure optimal fit, performance, mobility, and enhancement of function.

A wheelchair that has been prescribed by an inexperienced or nonclinical person is potentially hazardous to the user. A poorly fitting wheelchair can contribute to unnecessary fatigue, skin breakdown, and trunk or extremity deformity and can inhibit function.[6] A wheelchair is an extension of the user's body[7] and therefore should support rather than inhibit good alignment, mobility, and function.

## WHEELCHAIR EVALUATION

The OT practitioner has considerable responsibility in recommending the wheelchair appropriate to meet not only the immediate needs of the patient, but the long-term needs as well. When evaluating for a wheelchair, the clinician must "know the patient" and have a broad perspective on the patient's clinical, functional, and environmental needs. Careful evaluation of physical status must include the specific diagnosis, prognosis, and current and future conditions that may affect wheelchair use (e.g., age, spasticity, loss of range of motion [ROM], muscle weakness, endurance). Functional use of the wheelchair in a variety of environments must be considered. Box 18-1 lists questions to ask before making specific recommendations.

All data must be considered before making recommendations. The information must be weighed for advantages and disadvantages of different models and options before preparing the final prescription.

The clinician must develop a good working relationship with the equipment supplier and the reimbursement sources to advocate successfully and secure payment for the mobility system most appropriate for the patient. The practitioner should focus on verbal and written skills to communicate clearly and effectively throughout the entire assessment and treatment process. In addition, the practitioner must cultivate an in-depth awareness of the specific requirements, reimbursement, and documentation. Thorough justification of medical necessity is imperative for authorization of payment. OT practitioners must substantiate clearly why particular features of a wheelchair are being recommended. They must be aware of standard versus "up charge" items, their cost, and how they will impact the end product.[1]

## WHEELCHAIR ORDERING CONSIDERATIONS

The following points should be carefully addressed when assessing a wheelchair and before determining a specific brand and specifications.[1,5,9]

### Patient Considerations

An in-depth evaluation of the patient's physical, cognitive/perceptual, and psychosocial status must precede any determination of the most appropriate wheelchair for the individual. This evaluation may be performed by the OTR with the assistance of the COTA. The final choice of wheelchair considers information from these evaluations, including the specific diagnosis and residual disability, prognosis, age, occupational roles, and areas of deficit that will affect the patient's performance in the chair.

### Environment

The environment within which the user will be expected to maneuver the wheelchair necessarily influences its selection. Patients who will be using their wheelchair in a hospital or nursing home will not require as many special features as those who will be at home or out in the community.

### Propelling a Wheelchair

Propelling a wheelchair may be accomplished in a variety of ways, depending on the patient's physical capacities. The client who is deemed capable of self-propulsion using the arms on the rear wheels of the wheelchair must possess sufficient bilateral grasp, arm strength, and physical endurance to maneuver the chair independently over varied terrain throughout the day.[9] Various push rims are available to facilitate self-propulsion, depending on the user's arm and grip strength. A hemiplegic patient may propel a wheelchair with the unaffected arm, using the ipsilateral leg to maneuver the wheelchair.

A power wheelchair should be considered to provide independent mobility for persons with minimal or no use of the upper extremities or with limited endurance. Power chairs are also recommended for uneven outdoor terrain.[9] Power chairs can be of belt-drive or direct-drive construction, have a variety of features and programmability, and be controlled by foot, arm, head, or neck switches or by pneumatic switches. Even individuals with the most severe disabilities can drive power wheelchairs using these sophisticated technologies.

If the chair is to be caregiver propelled, the OT practitioner must consider ease of maneuverability and handling by the caregiver as well as the patient's positioning and mobility needs.

Regardless of the method of propulsion, the chair should be chosen with a view to the user's current and future mobility and positioning needs. Lifestyle and environment, available resources such as ability to maintain the chair, transportation options, and available reimbursement sources are major determining factors.

*Box 18-1*

#### Questions to Ask Before Making Specific Wheelchair Recommendations

- What is the specific diagnosis/disability?
- What is the prognosis?
- Is range of motion (ROM) limited?
- Is abnormal muscle tone present?
- Is strength or endurance limited?
- What is the patient's respiratory status? Is oxygen or a ventilator required when the patient is in the wheelchair?
- Does the patient have any cognitive or perceptual deficits?
- How is the patient going to propel the chair?
- Will a caregiver be responsible for propelling the wheelchair?
- How old is the patient?
- How long will the patient be expected to use the wheelchair?
- What was the patient's lifestyle, and how has it changed?
- Is the patient active or sedentary?
- How will the dimensions of the chair affect the patient's ability to transfer to various surfaces?
- What is the maneuverability of the wheelchair in the patient's home: entrance, door width, turning radius in bathroom and hallways, floor surfaces?
- What is the ratio of indoor to outdoor activities?
- Where will the wheelchair primarily be used: in the home, at school, work, the community?
- Which mode of transportation will be used? Will the patient be driving from the wheelchair? How will it be loaded and unloaded from the car?
- Which special needs exist in the work or school environment (e.g., work heights, available assistance, accessibility of toilet facilities, parking facilities)?
- Does the patient participate in indoor or outdoor sports activities?
- How will the wheelchair affect the patient psychologically?
- Who will pay for the wheelchair?
- Can accessories and special modifications be justified, or are these luxury items?
- What are the patient's resources for equipment maintenance?

### Rental versus Purchase

The therapist or assistant should have an idea as to the length of time the user will require the chair and whether the chair should be rented or purchased. This will affect the type of chair being considered. This decision is based on several clinical and functional issues. A rental chair is appropriate for short-term or temporary use, such as when the user's clinical picture, functional status, or body size is changing. Rental chairs may be necessary when the permanent wheelchair is being repaired. A rental wheelchair also may be useful when the client cannot accept a wheelchair and needs to experience it initially as a temporary piece of equipment. Often the eventual functional outcome is not known. In this case a chair can be rented for several months until a reevaluation determines whether a permanent chair will be necessary.[1]

A permanent wheelchair is indicated for the full-time user and the client with a progressive need for a wheelchair over a long period. It may be indicated when custom features are required and also when body size is changing, as with the growing child.[1]

### Frame Style

Once method of propulsion and permanence of chair have been determined, the clinician must consider frame styles, focusing on the various features, advantages, and disadvantages of each and how these will affect the client in every aspect of life, both from a short-term and a long-term perspective.

## WHEELCHAIR SELECTION

The following points should be addressed before determining the specific type of chair.[1]

### Manual versus Power

*Manual* (Figure 18-1, *A*).

- Does user have sufficient strength and endurance to propel chair?
- Does manual mobility enhance functional independence and cardiovascular conditioning of user?
- Does user require manual mobility as an exercise modality?
- Does user demonstrate *insufficient* cognitive ability to propel an electric wheelchair safely?
- Will caregiver be propelling the chair at any time?

*Power* (Figure 18-1, *B*)

- Does user demonstrate *insufficient* endurance and functional ability to propel manual wheelchair independently?
- Does user demonstrate progressive functional loss, making powered mobility an energy-conserving option?
- Is powered mobility required to increase independence at school, at work, and in the community?
- Does user demonstrate cognitive and perceptual ability to operate a power-driven system safely?
- Do user and caregiver demonstrate responsibility for care and maintenance of equipment?
- Is a van available for transportation?

### Manual Recline versus Power Recline

*Manual Recline* (Figure 18-2, *A*)

- Is user unable to sit upright because of hip contractures, poor balance, and/or fatigue?
- Is caregiver available to assist with weight shifts and position changes?
- Is relative ease of maintenance a concern?
- Is cost a consideration?

*Power Recline (Power Only)* (Figure 18-2, *B*)

- Does client have the potential to operate independently?
- Are independent weight shifts and position changes indicated for skin care and increased sitting tolerance?
- Does client demonstrate safe, independent use of controls?
- Are resources available for care and maintenance of equipment?
- Will a power recline decrease or make more efficient use of caregiver's time?
- Will a power recline reduce the need for transfers to bed for catheterizations and rest periods throughout the day?

A

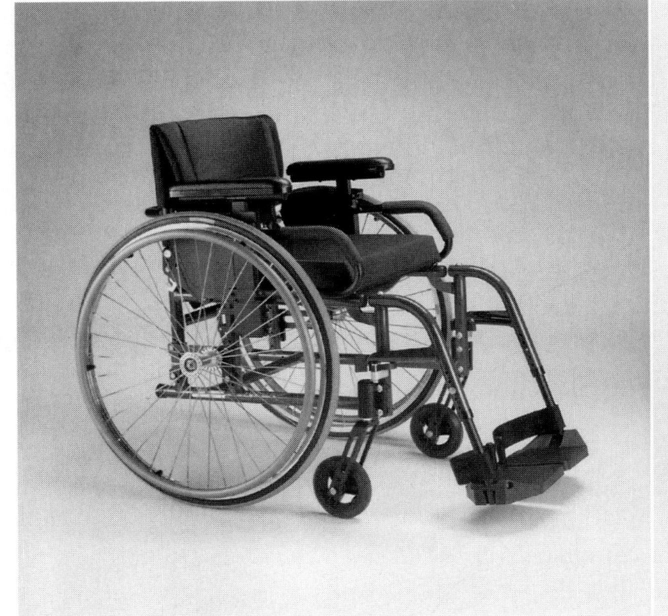

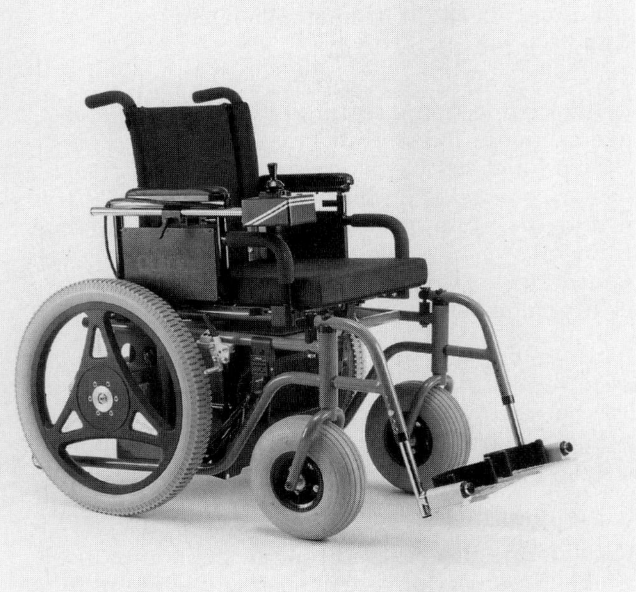

B

*Figure 18-1* Manual versus electric wheelchair. **A,** Rigid-frame chair with swing-away footrests. **B,** Power-driven wheelchair with hand control. (Courtesy Quickie Designs.)

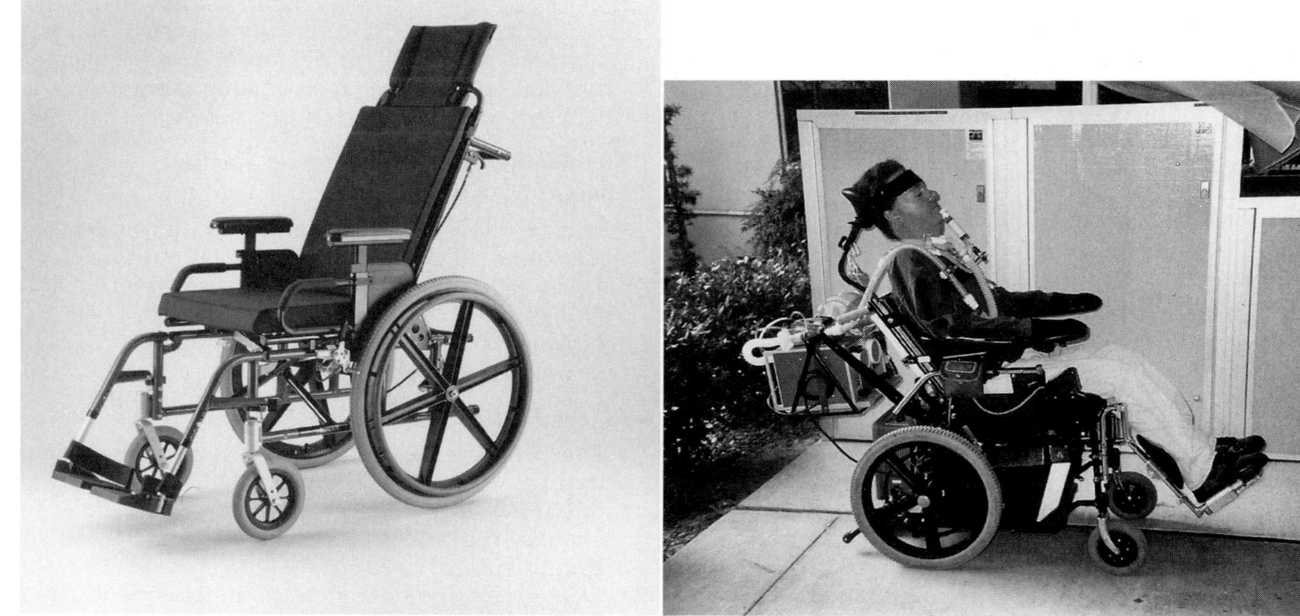


*Figure 18-2* Manual recline versus power recline wheelchair. **A,** Reclining back on folding frame. **B,** Power recliner with chin control on electric wheelchair. (**A,** courtesy Quickie Designs.)

- Will client require quick position changes in the event of hypotension and dysreflexia?
- Since a power recline is relatively "high tech" and expensive, has a reimbursement source been identified?

**Folding versus Rigid Manual Wheelchairs**

***Folding*** (Figure 18-3, *A*)

- Does client prefer a traditional-looking chair?
- Is the folding frame required for transport, storage, or home accessibility?
- Which footrest style is necessary for transfers, desk clearance, and other daily living skills? Elevating footrests may only be available on folding frames.
- Is client or caregiver able to load and fit into necessary vehicles?

Most equipment suppliers are knowledgeable and have a variety of brands available. Frame weight can range between 28 and 50 pounds (13 to 22 kg), depending on size and accessories. Frame adjustments and custom options depend on the model.

***Rigid*** (Figure 18-3, *B*)

- Considering the size and bulk of the nonfolding frame, does user or caregiver have the upper extremity function and balance to load and unload from a vehicle?
- Will user benefit from limited maintenance responsibilities because there are few moving parts?

Footrest options are limited, and the frame is more lightweight (20 to 35 pounds [10 to 16 kg]). Features include adjustable seat angle, rear axle, caster mount, and back height. Efficient frame design maximizes performance. Options in frame material composition, frame colors, and aesthetics are available. These chairs are usually custom-ordered; availability and expertise are usually limited to custom rehabilitation technology suppliers.

**Lightweight (Folding or Nonfolding) versus Standard Weight (Folding)**

***Lightweight (Less Than 35 lb [16 kg])*** (Figure 18-3, *A*)

- Does user have trunk balance and equilibrium necessary to avoid tipping lighter frame weight?
- Does lighter weight enhance mobility by reducing user's fatigue?
- Do lightweight parts such as armrests and footrests provide ease of management during activities of daily living (ADLs)?
- Are custom features necessary (e.g., adjustable height back, seat angle, axle mount)?

***Standard Weight (More Than 35 lb [16 kg])*** (Figure 18-4)

- Does user require the stability of a standard-weight chair?
- Does user have the ability to propel a standard-weight chair?

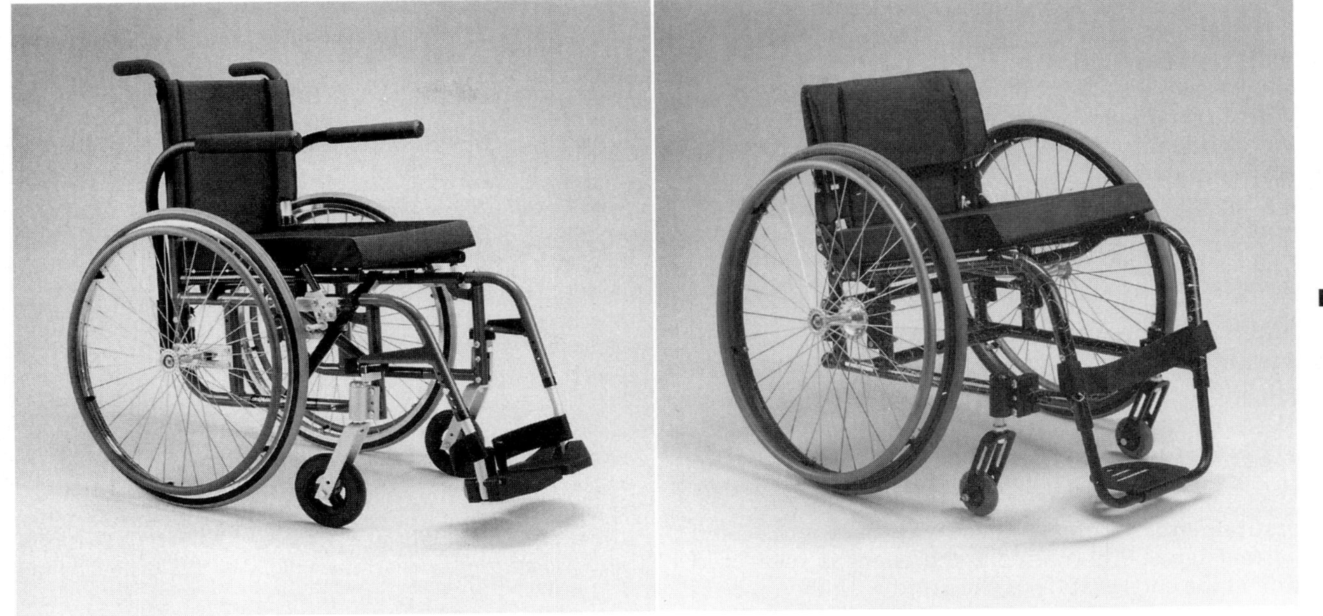


*Figure 18-3* Folding versus rigid wheelchair. **A,** Lightweight folding frame with swing-away footrests. **B,** Rigid (nonfolding) aluminum frame with tapered front end and solid foot cradle. (Courtesy Quickie Designs.)

- Can caregiver manage the increased weight when loading the wheelchair and fitting into a vehicle?
- Will the increased weight of parts *not* be a factor during performance of ADLs?

Custom options are limited, and these wheelchairs are usually less expensive (except heavy-duty models).

### "Bottom of the Line" versus "Top of the Line"

The price range, durability and warranty, and standard and custom features within a specific manufacturer's brand line must be considered.

#### *Bottom of the Line*

- Is chair required only for part-time use?
- Does user have a limited life expectancy?
- Is chair required as a second or transportation chair, used only 10% to 20% of the time?
- Will chair be primarily for indoor or sedentary use?
- Will the chair be propelled *only* by the caregiver?
- Are custom features or specifications *not* necessary?
- Is significant durability *not* an issue?

Bottom-of-the-line wheelchairs are limited in sizes, options, adjustability, and warranty available on the frame. Such chairs cost considerably less than top-of-the-line wheelchairs and may be chosen when reimbursement limitations exist.

#### *Top of the Line*

- Will client be a full-time user?

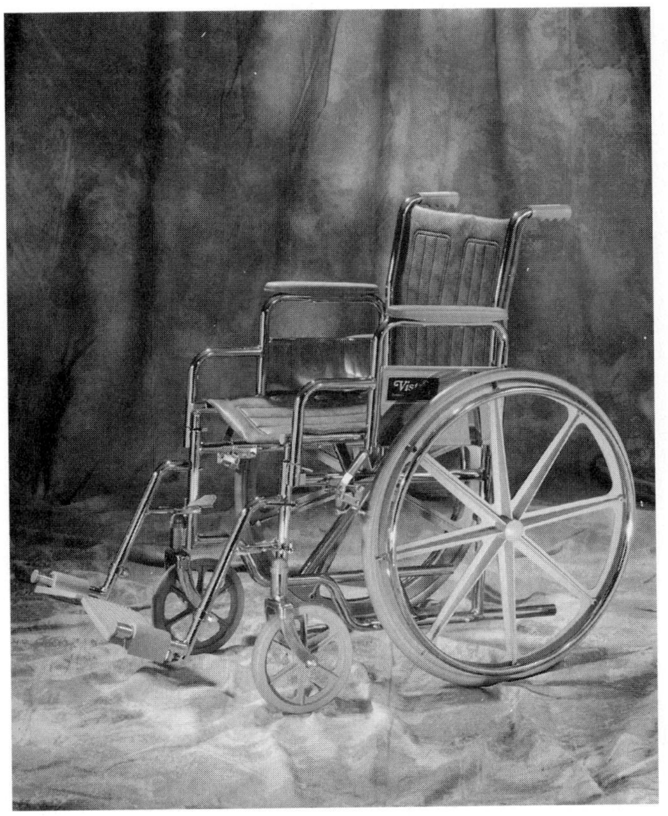

*Figure 18-4* Standard folding frame (more than 35 pounds [16 kg]) with swing-away footrests. (Courtesy Everest and Jennings.)

- Does a good chance exist for long-term use of the wheelchair?
- Will this be the primary wheelchair?
- Is user active both indoors and outdoors?
- Will this frame style improve the possibility for independent mobility?
- Is user a growing adolescent, or does patient have a progressive disorder requiring later modification?
- Are custom features, specifications, or positioning devices required?

Top-of-the-line wheelchairs generally have a long-term warranty on the frame and permit a high degree of custom specifications, options, and adjustability.

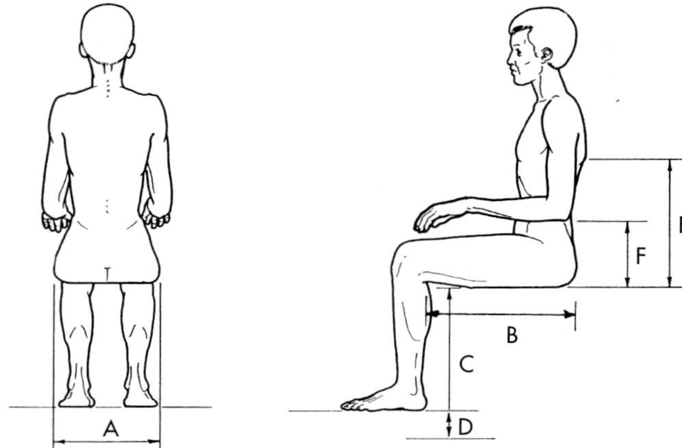


*Figure 18-5* Wheelchair measurement: what and where to measure. **A,** Seat width. **B,** Seat depth. **C,** Seat height from floor. **D,** Footrest clearance. **E,** Back height. **F,** Armrest height. (Modified from Wilson A, McFarland SR: *Wheelchairs: a prescription guide,* Charlottesville, Va, 1986, Rehabilitation Press.)

## WHEELCHAIR MEASUREMENT PROCEDURES

**Measurements** should be taken with the client seated on a mat table. Alternatively, the client is measured sitting in the chosen style of chair and with the cushion closest to those being ordered. If the client will be wearing a brace or body jacket or will require any additional devices in the chair, these should be in place during the measurement. Observation skills are very important during this process. *Do not* rely on measurements alone; "eyeball" entire body position *every step* of the procedure.[1,7]

**Seat Width** (Figure 18-5, *A*)

- *Objectives*
  1. To distribute user's weight over the widest possible surface.
  2. To keep overall width of chair as narrow as possible.
- *Measure:* Across widest part of either thighs or hips while client is sitting in a chair comparable to what is anticipated.
- *Wheelchair clearance:* Add ½ to 1 inch (1.3 to 2.5 cm) on each side of hip or thigh measurement taken. Consider how increasing overall width of chair will affect accessibility.
- *Check:* Palm between client's hip/thigh and skirt and armrest.
- *Consider:*
  1. Potential weight gain or loss.
  2. Accessibility of varied environments.
  3. Overall width of wheelchair.

**Seat Depth** (Figure 18-5, *B*)

- *Objective:* Distribute body weight along sitting surface by bearing weight along entire length of thigh to just behind knee. Distributed weight bearing assists in preventing pressure sores on buttocks and in normalizing optimal muscle tone throughout entire body.
- *Measure:* From rear of buttocks to inside of bent knee.
- *Wheelchair clearance:* 1 to 2 inches (2.5 to 5 cm) *less* than above measurement.
- *Check:* Clearance behind knees to prevent contact of front edge of seat upholstery with popliteal space.
- *Consider:*
  1. Braces or back inserts that may be pushing client forward.
  2. Postural changes throughout day from fatigue or spasticity.
  3. Thigh length discrepancy; depth of seat may be different for each leg.
  4. If considering a power recliner, assume client will slide forward slightly throughout day and make depth adjustments accordingly.
  5. Seat depth may need to be shortened to allow independent propulsion with the lower extremities.

**Seat Height from Floor and Foot Adjustment** (Figure 18-5, *C*)

- *Objectives:*
  1. To support user's body while maintaining thighs parallel to floor.
  2. To elevate footplates to provide ground clearance over varied surfaces and curb cuts (Figure 18-5, *D*).
- *Measure:* Top of seat post to floor and popliteal fossa to bottom of heel.
- *Wheelchair clearance:* Client's thighs are parallel to floor so that body weight is distributed evenly along entire depth of seat. Lowest point of footplates must clear floor by at least 2 inches (5 cm).
- *Check:* Slip fingers under client's thighs at front edge of seat upholstery. NOTE: A custom seat height

may be needed to obtain footrest clearance. One inch (2.5 cm) of increased seat height will raise the footplate 1 inch.
- *Consider:*
  1. If knees are too high, increased pressure at ischial tuberosities puts person at risk for skin breakdown and pelvic deformity.
  2. Sitting too high off ground can alter client's center of gravity, affect seat height for transfers, and impair visibility if client is driving a van from wheelchair.

**Back Height** (Figure 18-5, *E*)

- *Objective:* To provide back support consistent with physical and functional needs. Back should be low enough for maximal function and high enough for maximal support.
- *Measure:*
  1. For full trunk support, from top of seat post to top of shoulders.
  2. For minimal trunk support, top of back upholstery should be low enough to permit free arm movement without irritating skin or scapula but high enough to provide good total body alignment.
- *Check:* Client is not being pushed forward because back is too high or leaning backward over top of upholstery because back is too low.
- *Consider:*
  1. Adjustable height backs, usually 4-inch (10 cm) range.
  2. Adjustable upholstery.
  3. Lumbar support or other commercially available or custom back insert to prevent or reduce effects of kyphosis, scoliosis, or other long-term trunk deformity.

**Arm Height** (Figure 18-5, *F*)

- *Objectives:*
  1. To maintain posture and balance.
  2. To provide support and alignment for upper extremities.
  3. To allow change in position by pushing down on armrests.
- *Measure:* With client in comfortable position, from seat post to bottom of bent elbow.
- *Wheelchair clearance:* Height of top of armrest should be 1 inch (2.5 cm) higher than height from seat post to client's elbow.
- *Check:* Posture should look correct; shoulders should not slouch forward, be subluxed, or be forced into elevation when in normal sitting posture with flexed elbows slightly forward on armrests.
- *Consider:*
  1. Other uses of armrests, such as to increase functional reach or to hold a cushion in place.
  2. Certain styles of armrests can increase overall width of chair.
  3. Are armrests necessary at all?
  4. User's ability to remove and replace armrest from chair independently.

The OT practitioner reviews all measurements against standards for a particular model of chair. Manufacturers have listings of standard dimensions available and the costs for custom modifications.

### Pediatric Chairs

The goals in pediatric wheelchair ordering, as in all wheelchair ordering, should focus on obtaining a proper fit and facilitating optimal function. A standard wheelchair rarely meets a child's fitting requirements. Custom seating systems specific to the pediatric population are available.

Clinicians should consider a chair that will accommodate the child's growth. For children under 5 years of age, the clinician must decide whether to use a stroller base or a standard wheelchair base. Considerations are the child's ability to propel the chair relative to the developmental level and the parent's choice as to whether to have the child in a stroller or a wheelchair.

Many variables must be considered when customizing a wheelchair frame. The clinician should consult with an experienced RTS or the wheelchair manufacturer before assuming a custom request will be successful.

## ADDITIONAL SEATING AND POSITIONING CONSIDERATIONS

Regardless of the diagnosis, a wheelchair evaluation is not complete until selection and integration of seat cushion, back support, and other positioning devices are carefully analyzed.[1] The OT practitioner must appreciate the impact of body alignment on skin integrity, tone normalization, overall functional ability, and general well-being. The goals of a comprehensive seating and **positioning** assessment follow.[1]

### Prevention of Deformity

A symmetrical base of support preserves proper skeletal alignment and discourages spinal curvature and other body deformities.

### Tone Normalization

By providing proper body alignment and bilateral weight-bearing and adaptive devices as needed, tone normalization can be maximized.

### Pressure Management

Pressure sores can result from improper alignment and an inappropriate sitting surface. The proper seat cushion can provide comfort, assist in trunk and pelvic alignment, and create a surface that will minimize pressure, heat, and shearing (the primary causes of skin breakdown). Specialized seat cushions that use air (e.g., the Roho) or gels (e.g., the Jay) may be appropriate for clients with absent sensation or inability to shift weight in the wheelchair. These are available through the respective company vendors and can be prescribed at the same time as the wheelchair.

### Promotion of Function

Pelvic and trunk stability free the upper extremity for participation in all functional activities, including wheelchair mobility and ADLs.

### Maximal Sitting Tolerance

Wheelchair sitting tolerance will increase as support, comfort, and symmetrical weight bearing are provided.

### Optimal Respiratory Function

Support in an erect, well-aligned position can decrease compression of the diaphragm and thus contribute to an increase in vital capacity.

### Provision of Proper Body Alignment

Good body **alignment** is necessary for prevention of deformity, normalization of tone, and preparation for movement. Commercially available, custom-made, or in-house–fabricated positioning equipment is used for alignment. The client should be able not only to propel the wheelchair, but also to move around within the wheelchair.

Establishment of good body alignment should begin at the pelvis. Neutral pelvic alignment (pelvis square to the supporting surface) provides stability and facilitates orientation of the body toward midline (the optimal position for function). Once the pelvis is aligned, the lower extremities and the trunk are evaluated. Proper positioning of the legs provides a symmetrical, stable base of support on which trunk, head, and upper extremity control may be built. Alignment of the spine and trunk are required to maximize the functional capabilities of the head, neck, and upper extremities. The head and neck are generally positioned last.

### Contractures

Limitations in ROM because of soft tissue contracture need to be accommodated when considering both wheelchair and positioning needs. The use of appropriate positioning devices can compensate for alignment problems and increase comfort in the wheelchair.

### Positioning Devices

Positioning devices may be fabricated by the therapist or assistant if resources and work space are available. Cushions can be made from a variety of foams. The needs of the specific user will determine the density of foam chosen for the cushion. Most foams can be cut with an electric carving knife. Solid seat or back inserts, lateral supports, lapboards, and footplate modifications can be fabricated from wood or plastics. Power tools are required for cutting these materials, and appropriate safety precautions must be observed.

A variety of seating and positioning equipment is commercially available for all levels of disability. Custom modifications are continually being designed to meet user needs. In addition, technology in this area is constantly growing, and interest in wheelchair technology as a professional specialty is expanding as well. Skill of clinicians in this practice area ranges from negligible to extensive. Although an integral aspect of any wheelchair evaluation, the scope of seating and positioning equipment is much greater than can be addressed in this chapter. (See Recommended Readings list at the end of this chapter for additional resources.)

## WHEELCHAIR ACCESSORIES

Once the measurements and additional positioning devices have been determined, the clinician may select accessories to meet a user's individual needs. It is extremely important to understand the function of each accessory and how it interfaces with the rest of the wheelchair and seating and positioning equipment.

*Armrests* come in fixed, flip-up, detachable, desk, standard, reclining, and tubular styles. The fixed armrest is a continuous part of the frame and is not detachable. It limits proximity to table, counter, and desk surfaces and prohibits side transfers. Flip-up, detachable desk and standard-length arms allow for side-approach transfers. Reclining arms are attached to the back post and recline with the back of the chair. Tubular arms are found on lightweight frames.

*Footrests* may be standard, swinging detachable, solid cradle, and elevating. The standard footrests are fixed to the wheelchair frame and do not move. They prevent the person from moving close to counters and may make some types of transfers more difficult. The swinging detachable footrests can be moved to the side of the chair or removed entirely from the chair. They allow a closer approach to the bed, bathtub, and counters and, when removed, reduce the overall wheelchair length and weight for easy loading into a car. They lock into place with a locking device on the wheelchair.[9] A solid cradle footrest is found on rigid lightweight chairs and is not removable. Elevating legrests are available for those users with conditions such as edema, an arthrodesed knee, and orthopedic problems.

The *footplates* may have heel loops and toe straps to aid in securing the foot.[9] A calf strap can be used on a solid cradle or where additional support behind the calf is necessary. Additional accessories can include seat belts, various brake styles, brake extensions, antitip devices, caster locks, arm supports, and head supports.[1,9]

## PREPARATION OF PRESCRIPTION

Once specific measurements, modifications, and accessories have been determined, the wheelchair prescription must be completed. The **prescription** should be concise and very specific so that everything requested can be accurately interpreted by the equipment supplier who will be submitting a sales contract for payment authorization. "Before and after" pictures can be very helpful in illustrating medical necessity. The parameters for payment authorization from a particular reimbursement source must be known so that medical necessity can be demonstrated. The OT practitioner must be aware of the cost of everything being requested and be ready to explain why it is necessary. Payment can be denied if every item and modification requested is not clearly substantiated.

Before delivery of the wheelchair to the client, the OT practitioner should check the chair against the specific prescription and ensure that all specifications and accessories are correct. When ordering a custom chair, it is recommended that the user be fitted by the ordering therapist to ensure that the chair fits and that it provides all the elements that were anticipated when the prescription was generated.

## WHEELCHAIR SAFETY

Elements of safety for the wheelchair user and the caregiver are as follows:

1. Brakes should be locked during all transfers.
2. Footplates should never be stood on, and during most transfers should be in the up position.
3. In most transfers, footrests should be swung away if possible.
4. If pushing the chair, the caregiver should be sure that the patient's elbows are not protruding from the armrests and the hands are *not* on the hand rims. If approaching from behind to assist in moving the wheelchair, the caregiver should inform the patient of this intent and check the position of the feet and arms before proceeding.
5. If pushing the patient up a ramp, the caregiver should move in a normal, forward direction. If the ramp is negotiated independently, the client should lean slightly forward while propelling the wheelchair up the incline.[8]
6. If pushing the patient down a ramp, the caregiver should tilt the wheelchair backward by pushing the foot down on the tipping levers to its balance position, which is a tilt of approximately 30°. Then the caregiver should ease the wheelchair down the ramp in a forward direction while maintaining the chair in its balance position. The caregiver should move with knees slightly bent and the back straight.[8] The caregiver may also move down the ramp backward while the patient maintains some control of the large wheels to prevent rapid backward motion. This approach is useful if the grade is relatively steep. Ramps with only a slight grade can also be managed in a forward direction if the caregiver maintains grasp and pull on the handgrips, and the patient again maintains some control of the large wheels to prevent rapid forward motion. If the ramp is negotiated independently, the client should move down the ramp facing forward while leaning backward slightly and maintaining control of speed by grasping the hand rims. Gloves may be helpful to reduce the effect of friction.[8]
7. A caregiver can manage ascending curbs by approaching them forward, tipping the wheelchair back, and pushing the foot down on the tipping levers, thus lifting the front casters onto the curb and pushing forward. The large wheels then are in contact with the curb and roll on with ease as the chair is lifted slightly onto the curb.
8. To descend the curb using a forward approach, the wheelchair is tilted backward, and the large wheels are rolled off the curb in a controlled manner while the front casters are tilted up. When the large wheels are off the curb, the caregiver can slowly reduce the tilt of the wheelchair until the casters are once again on the street surface. The curb may be descended using a backward approach. When approaching the curb, the caregiver moves the chair and self around to a backward position and pulls the wheelchair to the edge of the curb. Standing below the curb, the caregiver can guide the large wheels off the curb by slowly pulling the wheelchair backward until it begins to descend. After the large wheels are safely on the street surface, the caregiver can tilt the chair back to clear the casters, move backward, lower the casters to the street surface, and then turn around.[8]

## WHEELCHAIR MOBILITY

The client's ability to mobilize the wheelchair is influenced by several factors. Physical capabilities, cognitive and perceptual skills, and the surface on which the wheelchair is propelled must be considered when teaching wheelchair **mobility** skills. If the wheelchair is to be used in the home, school, or work environment, the OT practitioner should evaluate the environment so appropriate skills can be taught before discharge. The following considerations should be taken into account.

### Indoor Mobility Considerations

- Will the client be required to maneuver the wheelchair in tight spaces, such as a kitchen or bathroom?
- Are there raised door saddles between rooms in the home?
- Will the client be required to mobilize the wheelchair over a variety of surfaces, such as carpet, tile, or wood flooring?

### Outdoor Mobility Considerations

- Will the client be using the wheelchair outdoors frequently and need to negotiate pavement, curbs, or grassy surfaces?
- Will the client need to use public transportation?

### Advanced Wheelchair Mobility Skills

If the client is highly active and will be using the wheelchair as the primary means of moving about, instruction in advanced wheelchair mobility skills is indicated. These skills include negotiation of rough terrain, such as grass, and the ability to go up and down ramps and curbs independently. The occupational therapist or assistant must include instruction in these areas before the client's reentry into the community.

With good strength and coordination, many clients can be trained to manage curbs independently. To mount and descend a curb, the client must have a good bilateral grip, arm strength, and balance. To mount the curb, the client tilts the chair onto the rear wheels and pushes forward until the front wheels hang over the curb, then lowers them gently. The client then leans forward and forcefully pushes forward on the hand rims to bring the rear wheels up on the pavement. To descend a curb, the client should turn the chair so that the back is toward the curb and then lean forward and push slowly backward until the rear and then the front wheels roll down the curb.[3]

The ability to lift the front casters off the ground and balance on the rear wheels ("pop a wheelie") expands the user's independence for curb management and movement over grassy, sandy, or rough terrain. Clients who have good grip, arm strength, and balance usually can master this skill and perform it safely. The technique involves being able to tilt the chair on the rear wheels, balance the chair on the rear wheels, and move and turn the chair on the rear wheels. The client should not attempt to perform these maneuvers without instruction and training in the proper techniques, which are beyond the scope of this chapter.[3] (See References for specific instructions on teaching these skills.)

## TRANSFER TECHNIQUES

During a **transfer** a patient is moved from one surface to another. Transferring includes the sequence of events that must occur both before and after the move, such as the pretransfer sequence of bed mobility and the posttransfer phase of wheelchair positioning. Assuming that a patient has some physical or cognitive limitations, the OT practitioner must assist in or supervise a transfer. Many therapists puzzle over which transfer type and technique to employ or feel perplexed when a particular one does not succeed with the patient. It is important to remember that each patient, therapist, and situation are different. The techniques outlined in this chapter are not all inclusive, but rather are basic ones with generalized principles. Each transfer must be adapted for the particular patient and the patient's needs. Directions for some transfer techniques that are most frequently employed in practice are outlined: the stand-pivot, bent-pivot, and two-person transfers.

### Preliminary Concepts

When selecting and performing transfer techniques to ensure safety for both patients and themselves, clinicians must be aware of the following concepts:

1. Clinicians should be aware of patients' assets and limitations, especially their physical, cognitive, perceptual, and behavioral abilities and deficits.
2. Clinicians should know their own physical abilities and limitations and whether they can communicate clear, sequential instructions to patients (and eventually to long-term caregivers).
3. Clinicians should be aware of and use correct moving and lifting techniques.

### Guidelines for Using Proper Mechanics

Clinicians should be aware of the following principles of basic **body mechanics**[2]:

1. Move close to patient or move patient closer to you.
2. Square off with patient (face head on).
3. Bend knees: use your legs, not your back.
4. Keep a neutral spine (not bent or arched back).
5. Keep a wide base of support.
6. Keep your heels down.
7. Ask for help when situation is more than you can handle.
8. Use simple movements in one axis. Avoid rotating at same time as bending forward or backward.

Before performing a transfer, the clinician should consider the following questions:

1. What are medical precautions that would affect patient's mobility or method of transfer?
2. Can transfer be performed safely by one person, or is assistance required?
3. Has enough time been allotted for safe execution of a transfer? Are you in a hurry?
4. Does patient understand what is going to happen? Does patient demonstrate fear or confusion? Have you adequately prepared patient?
5. Is equipment that patient is being transferred to and from in good working order and in a locked position?
6. What is height of bed (or surface) in relation to wheelchair? Can the heights be adjusted?
7. Is all equipment positioned correctly?
8. Is all bedding and equipment moved out of the way so you are working without obstructions?
9. Is patient dressed properly in case you need to use a waistband to assist? If not, do you need a transfer belt or other assistance?
10. What are other components of the transfer, such as leg management and bed mobility?

The clinician must be familiar with as many types of transfers as possible so that each situation can be resolved as it arises. Many classifications of transfers exist, based on the amount of participation by the clinician. Classifications can range from *dependent,* in which the patient is unable to participate and the clinician moves the patient, to *independent,* in which the patient moves independently while the clinician merely supervises, observes, or provides input for appropriate technique as related to the patient's disability.

Before attempting to move a patient, the clinician should understand the biomechanics of movement and the effect of the patient's center of positioning mass on transfers.

## Principles of Body Positioning

### *Pelvic Tilt*

Generally, after the acute onset of a disability and or prolonged time spent in bed, patients assume a posterior **pelvic tilt** (i.e., slouched position with lumbar flexion). This in turn moves the center of mass back toward their buttocks. The clinician may need to give verbal cues or physically facilitate the patient into a neutral or slightly anterior pelvic-tilt position to move the center of mass forward over the center of the patient's body (Figure 18-6).[5]

### *Trunk Alignment*

The clinician should note whether the patient's trunk alignment is shifted to the right or the left side. The patient may need verbal cues or physical assistance to come to and maintain a midline trunk position before and during the transfer. Otherwise the weight shift could throw both the patient and the clinician off balance.[5]

### *Weight Shifting*

To initiate the transfer, the patient's weight needs to be shifted forward, taking weight off the buttocks. This allows the patient to stand, partly stand, or be pivoted by the clinician. This step must be performed regardless of the type of transfer.[5]

### *Lower Extremity Positioning*

The patient's feet must be placed firmly on the floor with ankles stabilized and with knees aligned at 90° flexion over the feet. This allows the weight to be shifted easily onto and over the feet. Heels must be pointing toward the surface to which the patient is transferring. The patient should either be barefoot or

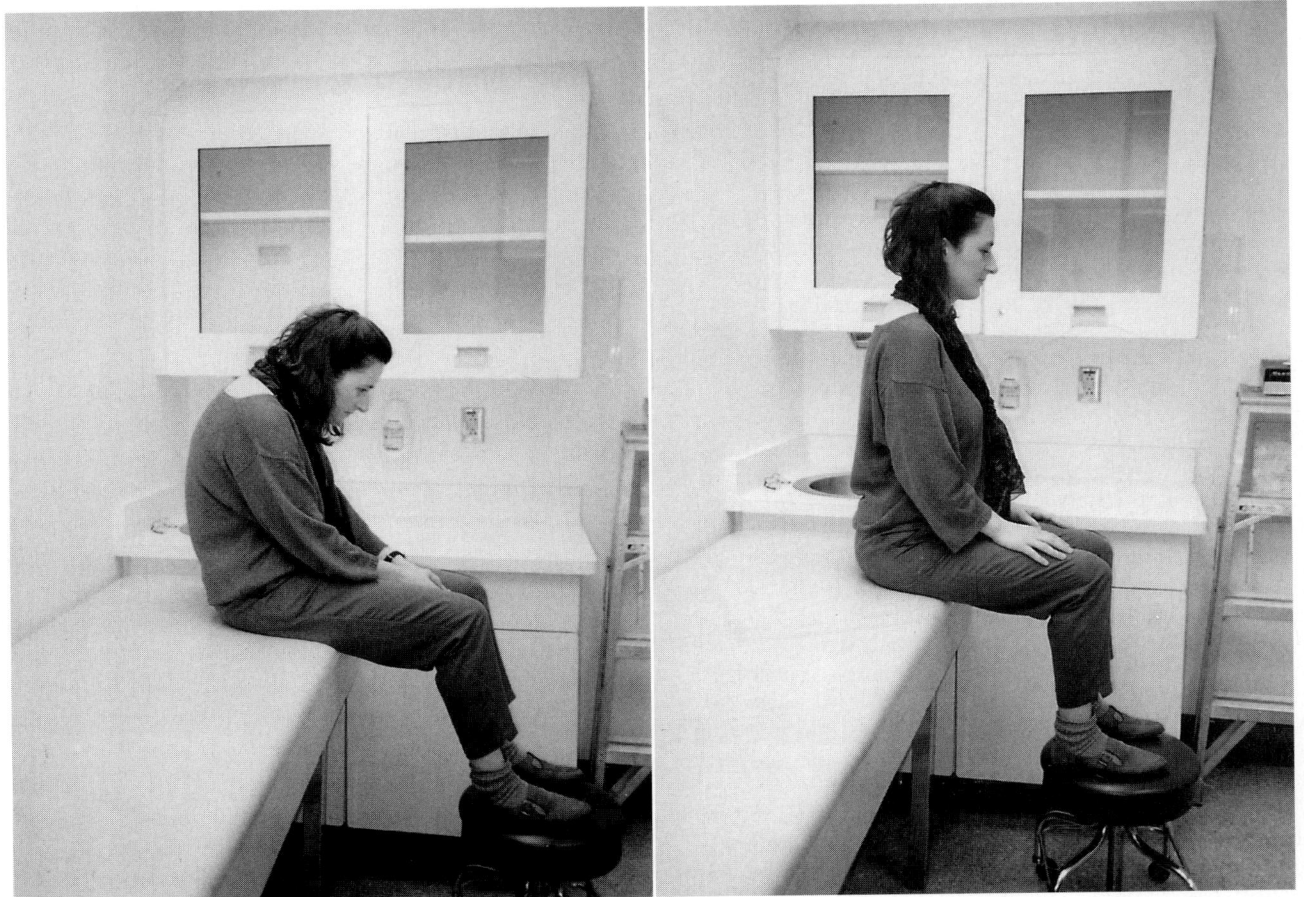


*Figure 18-6* **A,** Posterior pelvic tilt. **B,** Neutral pelvic position.

have shoes on to prevent slipping out of position. Feet can easily pivot in this position, and the risk of twisting or injuring an ankle or knee is minimized.[5]

### *Upper Extremity Positioning*

The patient's arms must be in a safe position or in a position where the patient can assist in the transfer. If one (or both) of the upper extremities is (are) nonfunctional, the arms should be placed in a position that is safe and will not be in the way during the transfer (i.e., in the patient's lap). If the patient has partial or full movement, motor control, and strength, the patient can assist in the transfer. The patient either reaches toward the transfer surface or pushes off from the starting surface.

## Preparing Equipment and Patient for Transfer

The OTR or COTA must realize that the transfer process includes setting up the environment, positioning the wheelchair, and assisting the patient into a pretransfer position. A general overview of these steps follows.

### *Positioning the Wheelchair*

1. Place wheelchair at an angle of approximately 45° to transfer surface.
2. Lock brakes.
3. Place both patient's feet firmly on floor, hip width apart and with knees over feet.
4. Remove armrest closest to bed.
5. Remove wheelchair seat belt.

### *Bed Mobility in Preparation for Transfer*

*Rolling*

1. Before rolling, clinician may need to put hand under patient's scapula on weak side and gently mobilize it forward to prevent patient from rolling onto shoulder, causing potential pain or injury.
2. Assist patient in clasping strong hand around wrist of weak arm, and lift upper extremities toward ceiling.
3. Flex knees.
4. Clinician may assist patient to roll onto side by moving arms, then legs, and by holding one hand at scapula area and other at hip, guiding the roll.

*Sitting up at edge of bed*

1. Bring patient's feet off edge of bed.
2. Assist patient to lift head and push up.
3. Shift patient's body to upright sitting position.
4. Place patient's hands on bed at sides of body to help maintain balance.

*Scooting to edge of bed*

When working with a patient who has had a CVA (stroke) or traumatic brain injury, the clinician walks the patient's hips toward the edge of the bed by shifting the patient's weight to the unaffected side, positioning the hand behind the opposite buttock, and guiding forward. The patient's weight is shifted to the affected side and the procedure repeated if necessary. The clinician moves the patient forward until the patient's feet are flat on the floor.

For a patient with spinal cord injury, the clinician grasps the patient's legs from behind the knees and pulls the patient forward, placing feet firmly on the floor and ensuring that ankles are in a neutral position.

## Stand-Pivot Transfers

The **stand-pivot transfer** requires that the patient be able to stand and pivot on one or both feet. It is most often used with patients who have hemiplegia, hemiparesis, or general loss of strength or balance.

### *Wheelchair-to-Bed/Mat Transfer*

1. Assist patient to scoot to edge of surface and put feet flat on floor (Figure 18-7). Ankles are pointed toward transfer surface.
2. Stand on patient's affected side with hands either on patient's scapulae or around waist or hips. Stabilize patient's foot and knee with own foot and knee. Assist by guiding patient forward as buttocks are lifted up and toward transfer surface (Figure 18-7, *A*).
3. Patient either reaches toward transfer surface or pushes off starting surface (Figure 18-7, *B*).
4. Guide patient toward transfer surface and gently assist patient down to a sitting position (Figure 18-7, *C*).

### *Variations: Stand-Ambulate Transfer*

This transfer is generally used when a patient can take small steps toward the surface goal rather than pivoting around. The clinician's interventions may range from physical assistance (to accommodate for potential loss of balance) to facilitation of near-normal movement, equal weight bearing, and maintenance of appropriate posture (for those with hemiplegia or hemiparesis). If a patient demonstrates impaired cognition or behavior deficits, including impulsiveness and poor safety judgment, the clinician may need to provide verbal cues or physical guiding.

## Sliding-Board Transfers

Individuals who cannot bear weight on the lower extremities and who have weakness or poor endurance in their upper extremities benefit from a **sliding-board transfer.** The transfer requires upper extremity strength and is most often used by patients with lower extremity amputations or those with spinal cord injuries who have adequate upper extremity strength.

### *Method*

1. Position and set up wheelchair as previously outlined (Figure 18-8).
2. Lift up patient's leg closest to transfer surface. Place the board at midthigh between buttocks and knee and angled toward the opposite hip.
3. Place board firmly under thigh and on transfer surface.

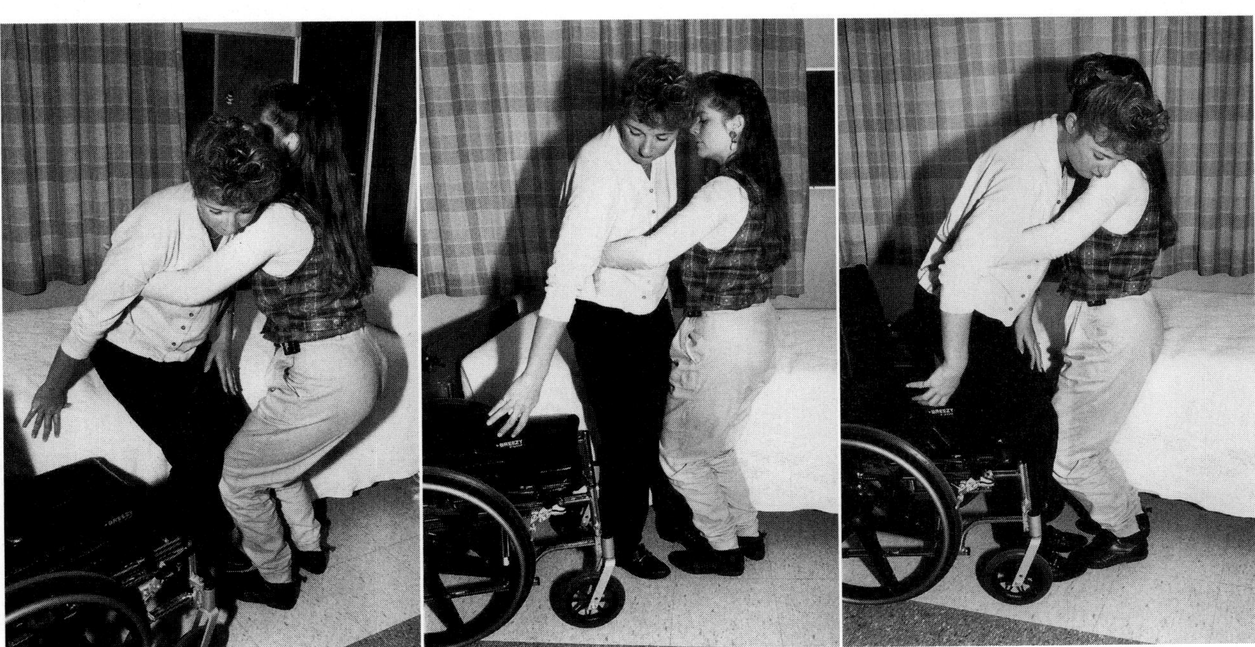


*Figure 18-7* Standing-pivot transfer: wheelchair to bed, assisted. **A,** Clinician stands on patient's affected side and stabilizes patient's foot and knee. Clinician assists by guiding patient forward and initiates lifting buttocks up. **B,** Patient reaches toward transfer surface. **C,** Clinician guides patient toward transfer surface. (Courtesy Luis Gonzalez, SCVMC.)

4. Block patient's knees with your knees.
5. Patient places one hand on edge of board and other hand on wheelchair seat.
6. Patient leans forward.
7. Patient transfers upper body weight in direction opposite to transfer. Patient should use both arms to push along board. Upper extremity strength and patient's balance are used to scoot along sliding board.
8. Assist by putting hands on patient's waist or scapulae and helping patient shift weight forward and slide across board as needed.

### Bent-Pivot Transfer: Bed to Wheelchair

The **bent-pivot transfer** (Figure 18-9) is used when the patient cannot initiate or maintain a standing position. A clinician often prefers to keep a patient in the bent-knee position to maintain equal weight bearing, to provide optimal trunk and lower extremity support, and to assist in transfer more safely and easily.

#### *Procedure*

1. Assist patient to scoot to edge of bed until both feet are flat on floor. Grasp patient around waist or hips or even under buttocks if a moderate or maximal amount of assistance is required.
2. Guide patient's trunk into a midline position.
3. Shift weight forward from buttocks toward and over patient's feet (Figure 18-9, *A*).
4. Have patient either reach toward transfer surface or push from starting surface (Figure 18-9,

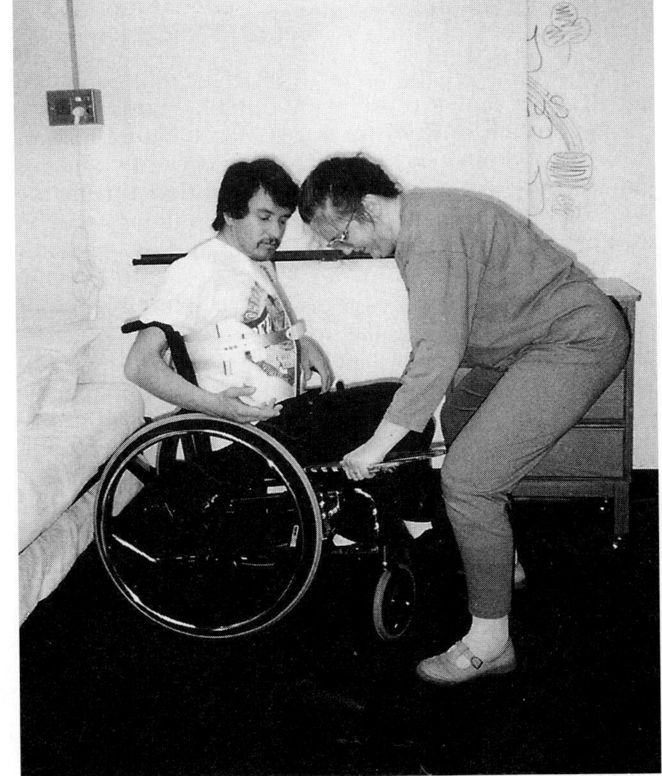

*Figure 18-8* Positioning sliding board. Lift patient's leg closest to transfer surface. Place board at midthigh between buttocks and knee and angled toward opposite hip.

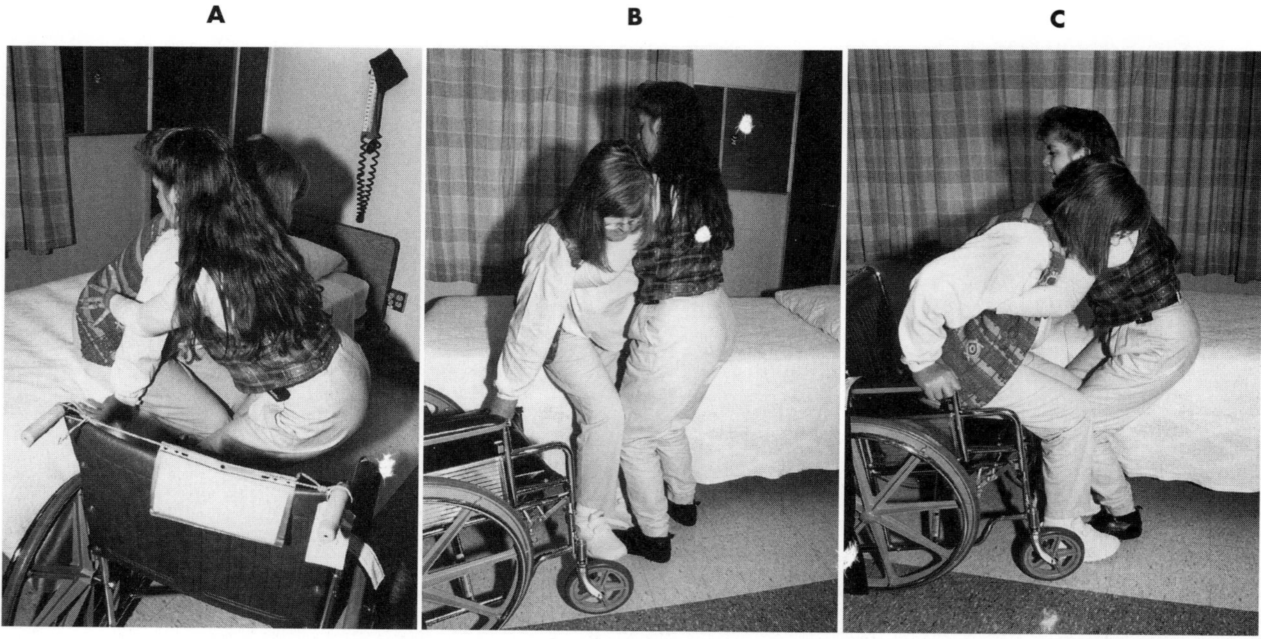


*Figure 18-9* Bent-pivot transfer: bed to wheelchair. **A,** Clinician grasps patient around trunk and assists in shifting patient's weight forward over feet. **B,** Patient reaches toward wheelchair. **C,** Clinician assists patient down to sitting position. (Courtesy Luis Gonzalez, SCVMC.)

5. Assist by guiding and pivoting patient around toward transfer surface (Figure 18-9, *C*).

Depending on the amount of assistance required, the clinician can perform the pivoting portion in two or three steps while repositioning self and patient's lower extremities between steps. The clinician has various choices of where to hold or grasp the patient during the bent-pivot transfer, depending on the patient's weight and height in relation to the clinician and the patient's ability to assist in the transfer. Variations include using both hands and arms at the waist or trunk or one or both hands under the buttocks. When choosing the site, the clinician must consider proper body mechanics. Several attempts, using trial and error, may be needed to achieve the best arrangement for patientindependence, safety, and the clinician's proper body mechanics. One important safety point is that the clinician never grasps under or on the patient's weak arm, because this may cause significant injury from weak musculature and poor stability around the shoulder girdle.

## Dependent Transfers

The **dependent transfer**[2] is designed for use with the patient who has minimal to no functional ability. If this transfer is performed incorrectly, it is potentially hazardous for both the OT practitioner and the patient. This transfer should be practiced with able-bodied persons and used initially with the patient only when another person is available to assist.

The purpose of the dependent transfer is to move the patient from surface to surface. The requirements are that the patient be cooperative and willing to follow instructions. Practitioners should be keenly aware of correct body mechanics and their own physical limitations. With heavy patients, it is always best to use the two-person transfer or at least have a second person available to spot the transfer.

### *Wheelchair-to-Bed Sliding-Board Dependent Transfer*

The procedure for transferring the patient from wheelchair to bed is as follows (Figure 18-10):

1. Set up wheelchair as previously described.
2. Position patient's feet together on floor directly under knees and swing outside footrest away. Grasp patient's legs from behind knees and pull patient slightly forward in wheelchair so that buttocks will clear large wheel when transfer is made (Figure 18-10, *A*).
3. Place sliding board under patient's inside thigh, midway between buttocks and knee, to form a bridge from bed to wheelchair. Angle sliding board toward patient's opposite hip.
4. Stabilize patient's feet by placing own feet laterally around patient's feet.
5. Stabilize patient's knees by placing own knees firmly against anterolateral aspect of patient's knees (Figure 18-10, *B*).
6. Assist patient to lean over knees by pulling pa-

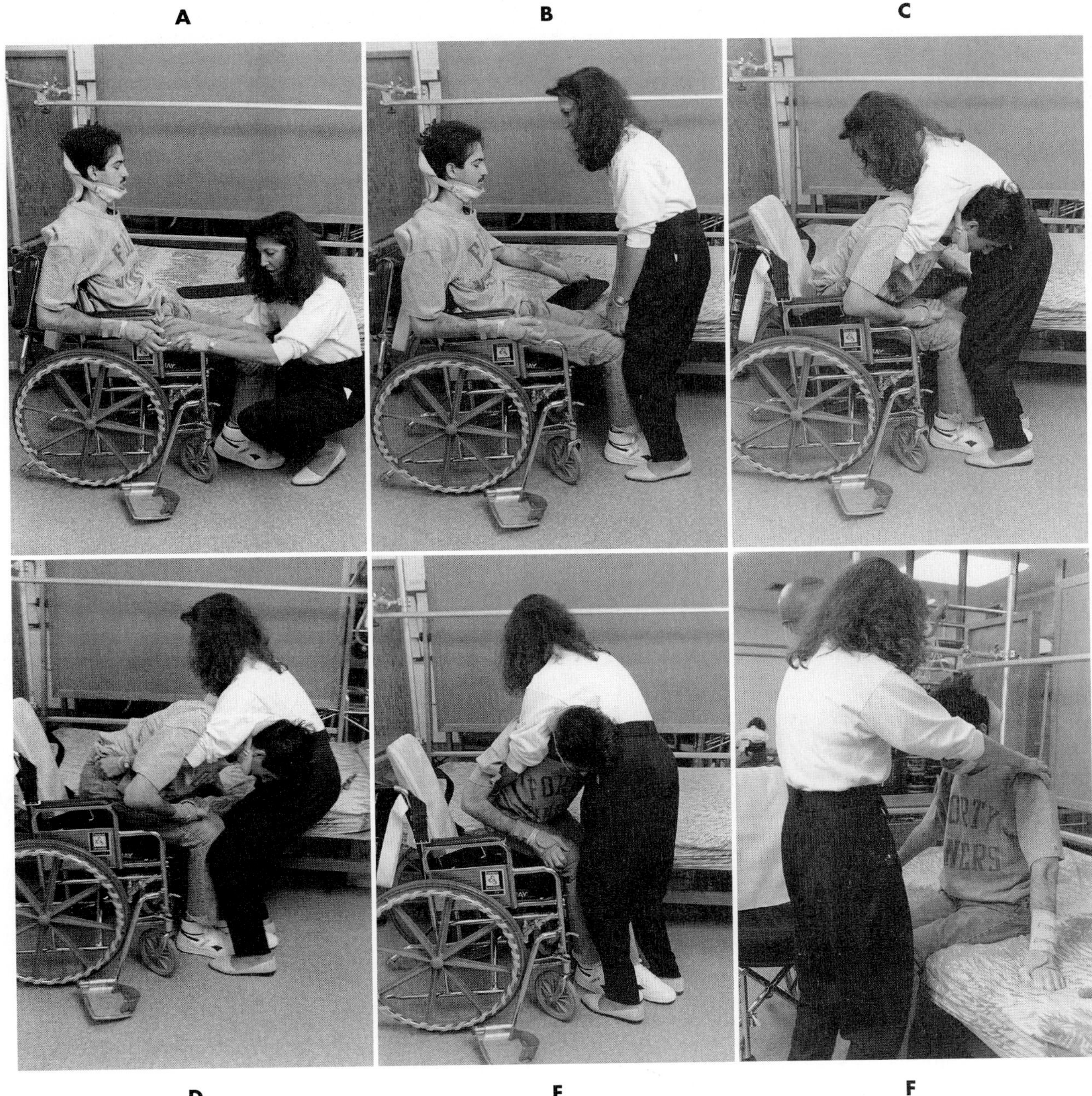


*Figure 18-10* Wheelchair-to-bed, sliding-board transfer. **A,** Clinician positions wheelchair and patient and pulls patient forward in chair. **B,** Clinician stabilizes patient's knees and feet after placing sliding board. **C,** Clinician grasps patient's pants at lowest point of buttocks. **D,** Clinician rocks with patient and shifts patient's weight over clinician's feet, making sure clinician's back remains straight. **E,** Clinician pivots with patient and moves patient onto sliding board. **F,** Patient is stabilized on bed.

tient forward from shoulders. Patient's head and trunk should lean opposite to direction of transfer. Patient's hands can rest on lap.

7. Reach under patient's outside arm and grasp waistband of trousers or under buttock. On other side, reach over patient's back and grasp waistband or under buttock (Figure 18-10, C).
8. After own arms are correctly positioned, lock to stabilize patient's trunk. Keep knees slightly bent and brace them firmly against patient's knees.

A

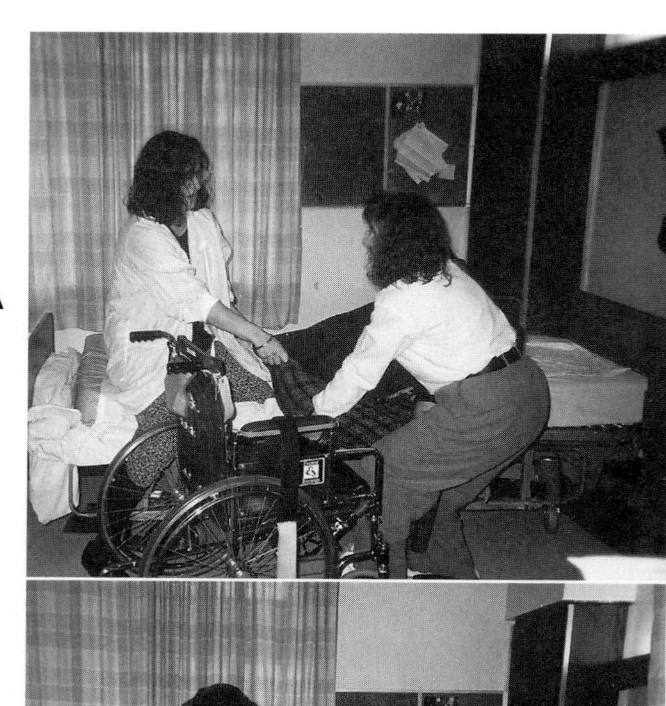

B

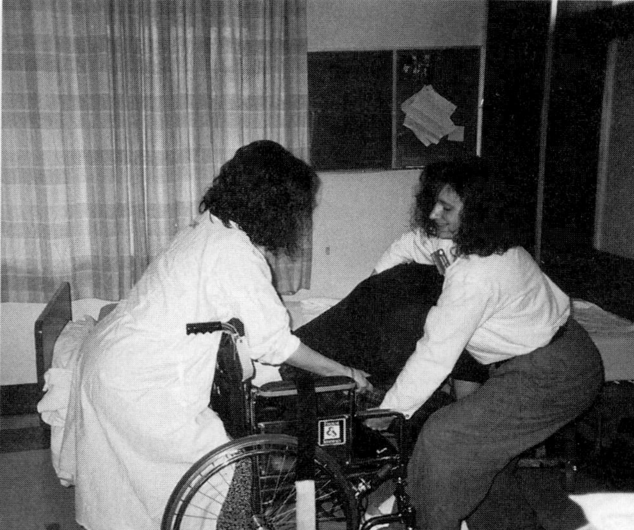

C

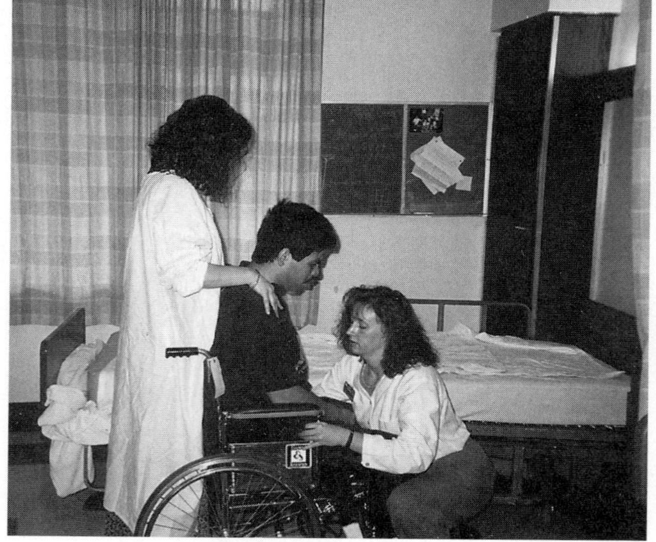

*Figure 18-11* Two-person dependent transfer, bed to wheelchair. **A,** One clinician positions self in front of patient, blocking patient's feet and knees. Clinician in back positions self behind patient's buttocks and assists by lifting. **B,** Clinician in front rocks patient forward and takes weight off buttocks as clinician in back shifts patient's buttocks toward wheelchair. **C,** Both clinicians position patient in upright, midline position in wheelchair. Seat belt is secured and positioning devices added.

9. Gently rock with patient to gain some momentum and prepare to move after count of three. Both clinician and patient count to three aloud. On "three," with knees held tightly against the patient's knees, lift patient's weight over patient's feet. Clinician's back must be kept straight to maintain good body mechanics (Figure 18-10, *D*).
10. Pivot with patient and move patient onto sliding board (Figure 18-10, *E*). Reposition self and patient's feet and repeat pivot until patient is firmly seated on bed surface, perpendicular to edge of mattress and as far back as possible. This usually can be achieved in two or three stages (Figure 18-10, *F*).
11. Secure on bed by easing patient against back of an elevated bed or on mattress in a side-lying position, then lift legs onto bed.

This transfer can be adapted to move the patient to other surfaces. It should be attempted only when clinician and patient feel secure with the wheelchair-to-bed transfer.

### *Two-Person Dependent Transfer: Bent Pivot: With or Without Sliding Board*

A bent-pivot transfer is used to allow increased clinician interaction and support. It gives the clinician greater control of the patient's trunk and buttocks during the transfer. This technique can also be employed during a two-person dependent transfer (Figure 18-11). It is often used with neurologically involved patients, because trunk flexion and equal weight bearing are often desired with this diagnosis. The steps in the two-person, bent-pivot transfer are as follows:

1. Set wheelchair up as described previously.

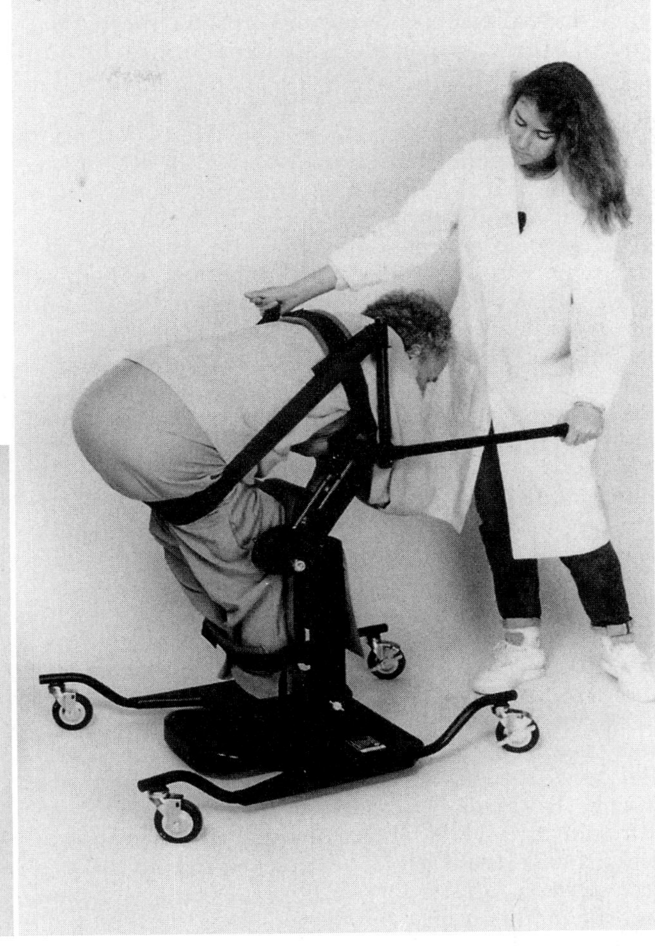

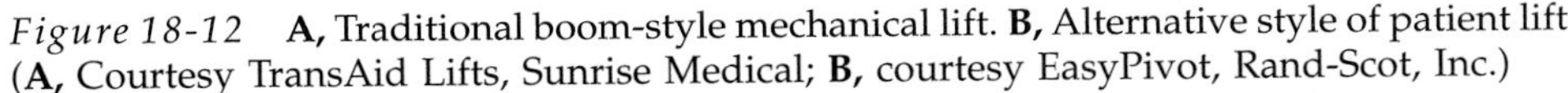

*Figure 18-12* **A,** Traditional boom-style mechanical lift. **B,** Alternative style of patient lift. (**A,** Courtesy TransAid Lifts, Sunrise Medical; **B,** courtesy EasyPivot, Rand-Scot, Inc.)

2. Two clinicians assume positions in front and back of patient.
3. Clinician in front assists in walking patient's hips forward until patient's feet are flat on floor.
4. Same clinician then stabilizes patient's knees and feet by placing own knees and feet lateral to each of patient's feet.
5. Clinician in back positions self squarely behind patient's buttocks, either grasping patient's waistband or placing own hands under patient's buttocks while maintaining proper body mechanics (Figure 18-11, *A*).
6. Clinician in front moves patient's trunk into a midline position, grasps patient around waist or hips, and guides patient to lean forward and shift weight forward over feet and off buttocks. Patient's head and trunk should lean in direction opposite to transfer. Patient's hands can rest on lap (Figure 18-11, *B*).
7. As clinician in front shifts patient's weight forward, clinician in back shifts patient's buttocks in direction of transfer. This can be done in two or three steps, making sure patient's buttocks land on a safe, solid surface. Clinicians reposition themselves and patient to maintain safe and proper body mechanics (Figure 18-11, *C*).
8. Clinicians make sure they coordinate the time of transfer with patient and one another by counting to three aloud and instructing team to initiate transfer on "three."

### *Mechanical Lift Transfer*

Some patients, because of large body size, severe disability, or impaired health and well-being of the caregiver, require the use of a mechanical lift. Mechanical lifting devices can be used to transfer patients of any weight (Figure 18-12). A properly trained caregiver, even one who is considerably smaller than the patient, can learn to use the mechanical lift safely and independently.[8] The patient's physical size, environment in which the lift will be used, and uses to which the lift will be put must be considered when selecting a mechanical lift. The patient and caregiver should demonstrate the ability to use the lift safely before the clinician orders one for their independent use.

### Transfers to Household Surfaces

#### *Sofa and Chair*

Wheelchair-to-sofa/chair transfers (Figure 18-13) are similar to wheelchair-to-bed transfers, with some additional considerations.

The clinician and patient need to be aware that the chair may be light and less stable than a bed or wheelchair. When transferring to the chair, the patient must be instructed to reach for the seat of the chair. Reaching for the armrest or the back of the chair should be avoided because this may cause the chair to tip over. When moving from a chair to the wheelchair, the patient should use a hand to push off from the seat of the chair when standing. Standing from a chair is often more difficult if the chair is low or the seat cushions are soft. Dense cushions may be added to increase height and provide a firm surface for transfer.

#### *Toilet*

Wheelchair-to-toilet transfers are often difficult because of the confined space in most bathrooms. The patient or caregiver should attempt to position the wheelchair next to or at an acute angle to the toilet. Those involved must analyze the space around the toilet and wheelchair to ensure no obstacles are present. To increase independence of the patient during this transfer, adaptive devices such as grab bars or raised toilet seats can be added. The patient can use these devices for support during transfers. A raised seat will maintain an even, level surface to which to transfer.

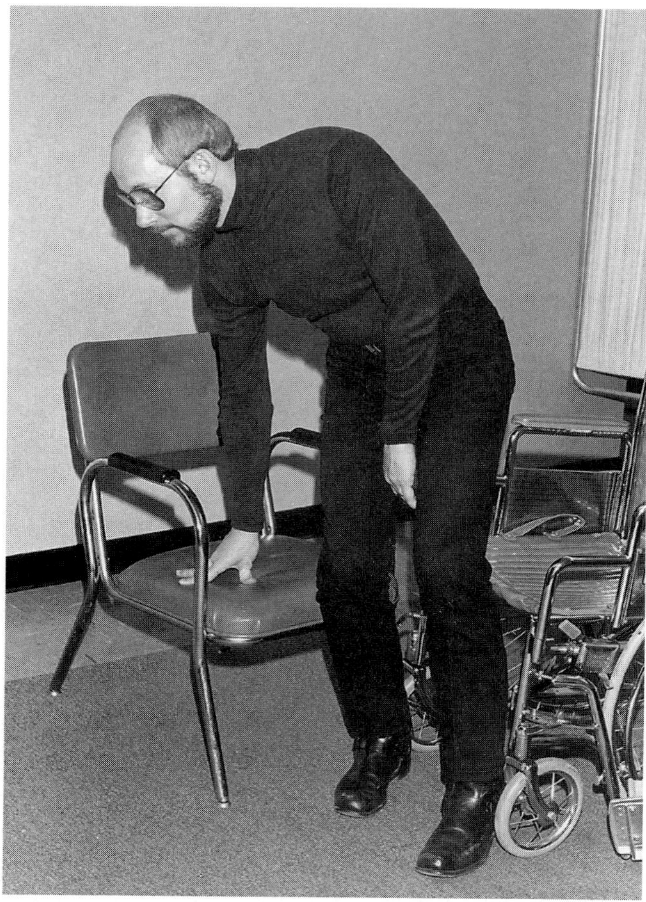

*Figure 18-13* Patient in midtransfer reaches for seat of chair, pivots, and lowers body to sitting.

#### *Bathtub*

The occupational therapist or assistant should be most cautious when assessing or teaching bathtub transfers (Figure 18-14) because the bathtub is one of the most hazardous places in of the home. Wheelchair-to-bottom-of-bathtub transfers are extremely difficult and are used only with patients who have good bilateral strength and motor control of the upper extremities (e.g., paraplegic patients, lower extremity amputees). A commercially produced bath bench, bath chair, or a well-secured straight-back chair is typically used by OT practitioners for seated bathing. Therefore, whether a stand-pivot, bent-pivot, or sliding-board transfer is performed, the technique is similar to a wheelchair-to-chair transfer.

The transfer may be complicated by the confined space, the slick bathtub surfaces, and the bathtub wall between the wheelchair and the bathtub seat.

If a stand-pivot transfer is employed, the locked wheelchair should be placed, if possible, at a 45° angle to the bathtub. The patient should stand, pivot, sit on the bathtub chair, and then place the lower extremities into the bathtub.

If a bent-pivot or sliding-board transfer is used, the wheelchair, with the armrest removed, is placed next to the bathtub. The transfer tub bench alleviates the need for a sliding board, allows the wheelchair to be placed directly next to the bench, and permits a safe, easy transfer of the buttocks to the seat. Then the lower extremities can be assisted into the bathtub.

In general, the patient may exit by first placing the feet securely outside the bathtub on a nonskid floor surface and then performing a standing or seated transfer back to the wheelchair.

### Car Transfers

A car transfer is often the most challenging for clinicians because it involves trial-and-error methods to develop a technique that is not only safe, but also easy for the patient and caregiver to perform. The clinician often uses the patient's existing transfer technique. The patient's size, degree of disability, and vehicle door style (two-door versus four-door) must be considered. These factors will affect level of independence and may necessitate a change in the usual technique to allow for a safe, easy transfer.

In general, it is difficult to move a wheelchair close enough to the car seat, especially with four-door vehicles. Helpful suggestions are as follows:

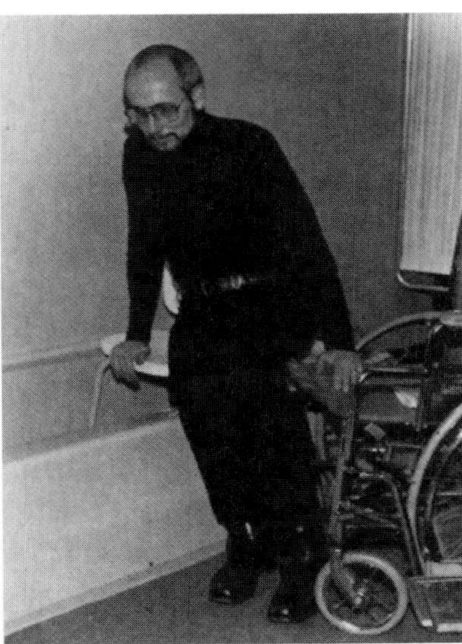

*Figure 18-14* Seated transfer from wheelchair to bathtub chair. Legs are lifted over edge of bathtub once patient is seated on bench.

1. Car seats are often much lower than standard wheelchair seat height, which makes the uneven transfer much more difficult, especially from the car seat to the wheelchair.
2. Occasionally, patients may have orthopedic injuries that require use of a brace such as a halo vest or body jacket (see Figure 36-3) or lower extremity cast or splint. The OT practitioner must alter technique to accommodate for these devices.
3. The practitioner may suggest use of the sliding board for this transfer to accommodate for the large gap between transfer surfaces.
4. Since uphill transfers are difficult, the patient may require a higher level of assistance. The clinician may choose a two-person versus a one-person assist transfer to ensure a safe, smooth technique.

## AMBULATION AIDS

**Ambulation aids** are assistive devices that permit the patient who could not otherwise ambulate safely to do so. Assistive devices for ambulation are indicated for the patient who demonstrates any of the following: decreased ability to bear weight on the lower extremities; lower extremity or trunk paralysis or muscle weakness; pelvic instability; and inadequate balance. Ambulation aids may be alternated with a wheelchair if the patient has poor endurance or cannot ambulate safely for long distances. The most common types of ambulation devices are walkers, crutches, and canes.[4]

### Role of Occupational Therapy

The physical therapist selects the most appropriate ambulation aid and provides ambulation training. Once proficient and safe at the ambulatory level, the patient may attempt functional ambulatory tasks, at which point the occupational therapy practitioner becomes involved. The OT clinician should first observe the patient in physical therapy and work with the physical therapist to ensure safe, correct ambulatory techniques before attempting ambulatory tasks with any patient.

### Impact on Functional Mobility and Functional Ambulatory Tasks

The use of any device during ambulation affects the patient's ability to negotiate the environment. The OT practitioner is most often responsible for training the patient to perform household tasks and ADLs while using the ambulation aid. Some examples of functional ambulatory tasks include negotiating the kitchen, opening and closing the refrigerator, putting away groceries, making beds, doing household chores, performing self-care tasks, and carrying out bathtub, toilet, and car transfers. These activities should be performed in the clinic before the patient's discharge whenever possible. If this is not possible, therapy may be provided at the earliest opportunity in the patient's home.

### Safety Considerations

When first mastering the use of the ambulation device, the patient will necessarily be concentrating on successful ambulation. The occupational therapist or assistant must remember to provide instructions slowly and to guard the patient carefully. Practicing activities on even surfaces in a clutter-free environment increases the safety of the patient and clinician. Working with the physical therapist at this time is highly recommended. As the patient gains in proficiency and confidence with the device, more realistic situations and environmental barriers may be introduced.[4]

## SUMMARY

A wheelchair that fits well and can be managed safely and easily by its user and the caregiver is one of the most significant factors in the patient's ability to perform activities of daily living with maximal independence.[5] Each wheelchair user must learn the capabilities and limitations of the wheelchair and safe methods of performing ADLs. If present, a caregiver needs to be thoroughly familiar with safe, correct techniques of handling the wheelchair and the patient.

Transfer skills are among the most important activities that must be mastered by the wheelchair user. The ability to transfer increases the possibility of mobility and travel. Transfers can be hazardous, however, and safe methods must be learned and followed.[8] Besides the basic transfer techniques outlined in this chapter, additional methods and more detailed training and instructions are available, as cited previously. OT practitioners should recognize that many wheelchair users with exceptional abilities have developed unique methods of wheelchair management. Although such innovative approaches may work well for the patient who has devised and mastered them, they cannot be considered basic procedures that everyone can learn.[8]

Assistive devices for ambulation are used by patients who cannot otherwise ambulate safely. They may be used in combination with a wheelchair if the patient has poor endurance or is unable to ambulate long distances. Training in functional ambulatory tasks while using ambulation aids should occur once the patient is competent and safe while using the device.

## *Selected Reading Guide Questions*

1. List three factors that the occupational therapy practitioner must consider before making specific recommendations for a wheelchair.
2. What is the purpose of measuring seat width?
3. What is the danger in having a wheelchair seat that is too deep?
4. List three types of wheelchair frames and the general uses of each.
5. Describe three types of wheelchair propulsion systems, and identify when each would be used.
6. What are the advantages of detachable desk arms and swing-away footrests?
7. Name at least three general wheelchair safety principles, and describe the rationale for each.
8. Describe or demonstrate how to descend a curb in a wheelchair with the help of a caregiver.
9. List four safety principles for correct moving and lifting technique during wheelchair transfers.
10. Describe or demonstrate the basic stand-pivot transfer from a bed to a wheelchair.
11. Describe or demonstrate the wheelchair-to-bed transfer using a sliding board.
12. Describe the correct placement of a sliding board before a transfer.
13. What possible diagnosis and circumstances would indicate the use of a sliding-board transfer?
14. When would you use the bent-pivot transfer rather than the stand-pivot transfer?
15. List the requirements for the patient and OT practitioner to perform the dependent transfer safely and correctly.
16. List two potential problems and solutions that can occur with the wheelchair-to-car transfer.
17. When is the mechanical lift transfer most appropriate?
18. How does the use of ambulation aids influence the patient's ability to perform functional ambulatory tasks?
19. At what point does the OT practitioner begin to train the patient in functional ambulatory tasks using an ambulation aid?

## *Exercise*

1. Spend a minimum of 4 hours in a wheelchair, and experience as many of the following as possible: transferring to a toilet, opening and going through a door, going up and down a curb, crossing a street, and making a purchase in a store or restaurant. Observe appropriate safety precautions and body mechanics. Write a journal entry describing your experiences.

### *REFERENCES*

1. Adler C: *Wheelchairs and seat cushions: a comprehensive guide for evaluation and ordering,* San Jose, Calif, 1987, Occupational Therapy Department, Santa Clara Valley Medical Center.
2. Adler C, Musik D, Tipton-Burton M: *Body mechanics and transfers: multidisciplinary cross training manual,* San Jose, Calif, 1994, Santa Clara Valley Medical Center.
3. Bromley I: *Tetraplegia and paraplegia: a guide for physiotherapists,* ed 3, London, 1985, Churchill Livingstone.
4. Duesterhaus Minor M, Duesterhaus Minor S: *Patient care skills,* ed 3, East Norwalk, Conn, 1995, Appleton & Lange.
5. *Lifting and moving techniques,* San Jose, Calif, 1985, Physical Therapy Department, Santa Clara Valley Medical Center.
6. Pezenik D, Itoh M, Lee M: *Wheelchair prescription.* In Rusking AP: *Current therapy in physiatry,* Philadelphia, 1984, Saunders.
7. *Wheelchair prescription: measuring the patient,* Booklet no 1, Camarillo, Calif, 1979, Everest and Jennings.
8. *Wheelchair prescription: safety and handling,* Booklet no 3, Camarillo, Calif, 1983, Everest and Jennings.
9. *Wheelchair prescription: wheelchair selection,* Booklet no 2, Camarillo, Calif, 1979, Everest and Jennings.
10. Wilson AB: *Wheelchairs: a prescription guide,* Charlottesville, Va, 1992, Rehabilitation Press.

### *RECOMMENDED READING*

Bergen A, Presperin J, Tallman T: *Positioning for function,* Valhalla, NY, 1990, Valhalla Rehabilitation.

Davies PM: *Steps to follow: a guide to the treatment of adult hemiplegia,* New York, 1985, Springer-Verlag.

Ford JR, Duckworth B: *Physical management for the quadriplegic patient,* Philadelphia, 1974, Davis.

Gee ZL, Passarella PM: *Nursing care of the stroke patient: a therapeutic approach,* Pittsburgh, 1985, AREN.

Hill JP, editor: *Spinal cord injury: a guide to functional outcomes in occupational therapy,* Rockville, Md, 1986, Aspen.

Hockenberry J: *Moving violations,* New York, 1995, Hyperion.

Chapter 19

# Specialized Areas of Activities of Daily Living

*Karen L. Nelson*
*Susan M. Lillie*

## Chapter Objectives

*After studying this chapter, the student or practitioner will be able to:*

1. Define *dysphagia,* and identify disabilities in which dysphagia may be present.
2. Discuss the role of occupational therapy within the context of the interdisciplinary team in dysphagia evaluation and treatment.
3. Contrast the roles of the registered occupational therapist and the certified occupational therapy assistant in dysphagia evaluation and treatment.
4. Identify safety precautions and areas of risk in dysphagia treatment.
5. State the overall goals of dysphagia treatment and training.
6. Name and describe the stages of diet progression.
7. Explain the principles of oral feeding.
8. Identify signs of nutritional deficiency and dehydration.
9. Describe the contribution of occupational therapy to the assessment of the disabled individual's driving.
10. Contrast the roles of the registered occupational therapist and the certified occupational therapy assistant in driving evaluation and treatment.
11. Identify equipment modifications for driving that are recommended for individuals with selected disabilities.

## Key Terms

dysphagia
aspiration
aspiration pneumonia
deglutition
oral preparatory phase
salivation
bolus
oral phase
voluntary swallow
pharyngeal phase
swallow response
esophageal phase
peristaltic wave
tracheostomy
tracheostomy tube
fenestrated tube
videofluoroscopy
diet progression
clinical assessment
stationary assessment
predriving tasks
palmed steering
steering device
hand control
mechanical lift
behind-the-wheel performance testing
driver instructor/educator
driving evaluator/observer

# Section I Treatment of Dysphagia

KAREN L. NELSON

Eating is the most basic activity of daily living (ADL) and is necessary for survival. Eating incorporates the abilities to reach for food, place it in the mouth, chew it, and swallow it. Inability or difficulty in swallowing is termed **dysphagia.**

The registered occupational therapist (OTR) is trained to evaluate and treat all factors contributing to dysphagia, including motor control (muscle tone; positioning of trunk, head, and upper and lower extremities), inhibition of primitive reflexes, oral and pharyngeal function, and the components of sensory, perceptual, and cognitive dysfunction that may interfere with the eating process. The certified occupational therapy assistant (COTA) supports the plan formulated by the OTR by implementing selected aspects of treatment, as directed, under supervision of the OTR. The experienced COTA can be a valuable member of the dysphagia team.

Dysphagia treatment is a complex and potentially dangerous area, because patients may choke or lose the ability to breathe if they cannot swallow. For this reason the COTA requires direct supervision and must not initiate any treatment procedure unless specifically directed by the supervising therapist, and then only when completely service competent. Dysphagia treatment requires knowledge of first aid and the Heimlich maneuver, as well as consistent application of universal precautions for infection control (e.g., use of latex gloves, appropriate handwashing). **Aspiration** (entry of material into the airway) is a significant risk with the dysphagic patient.[16] **Aspiration pneumonia** is a complication that occurs when food enters the lungs. Evaluation of dysphagia is not within the COTA's scope of practice.

This chapter provides the COTA with an overview of the occupational therapy process for the patient with an acquired dysphagia. Some of the conditions that can result in an acquired dysphagia are cerebrovascular accident (CVA, stroke), head injury, brain tumor, anoxia, Guillain-Barré syndrome, multiple sclerosis, amyotrophic lateral sclerosis, Parkinson's disease, myasthenia gravis, poliomyelitis, and quadriplegia.[21]

## ANATOMY AND PHYSIOLOGY OF NORMAL SWALLOWING

**Deglutition,** the normal eating of solids or liquids, involves the brain stem, six cranial nerves, the first three cervical nerve segments, and 48 muscles.[9,24] Figure 19-1 illustrates the oral structures involved in eating, and Figure 19-2 shows the anatomy of a swallow. The swallowing process can be divided into four stages: (1) oral preparatory phase, (2) oral phase, (3) pharyngeal phase, and (4) esophageal phase.[16]

### Oral Preparatory Phase

The **oral preparatory phase** of swallowing begins with the act of looking at and reaching for food.[8] Sight and smell stimulate **salivation,** which helps to trigger the entire swallowing process.[24] As contact is made with the food, the jaw comes forward to open. The lips close around a glass or utensil to remove the food. The muscles of the lips form a seal to prevent any material from leaking out of the oral cavity.

As chewing begins, the mandible moves in a strong, combined, rotary, and lateral direction. The upper and lower teeth shear and crush the food. The tongue moves from side to side to push the food between the teeth. The buccinator muscles of the cheeks contract to prevent food particles from falling into the sulcus (pocket) between the jaw and cheek.[15] The tongue sweeps through the mouth, gathering food particles

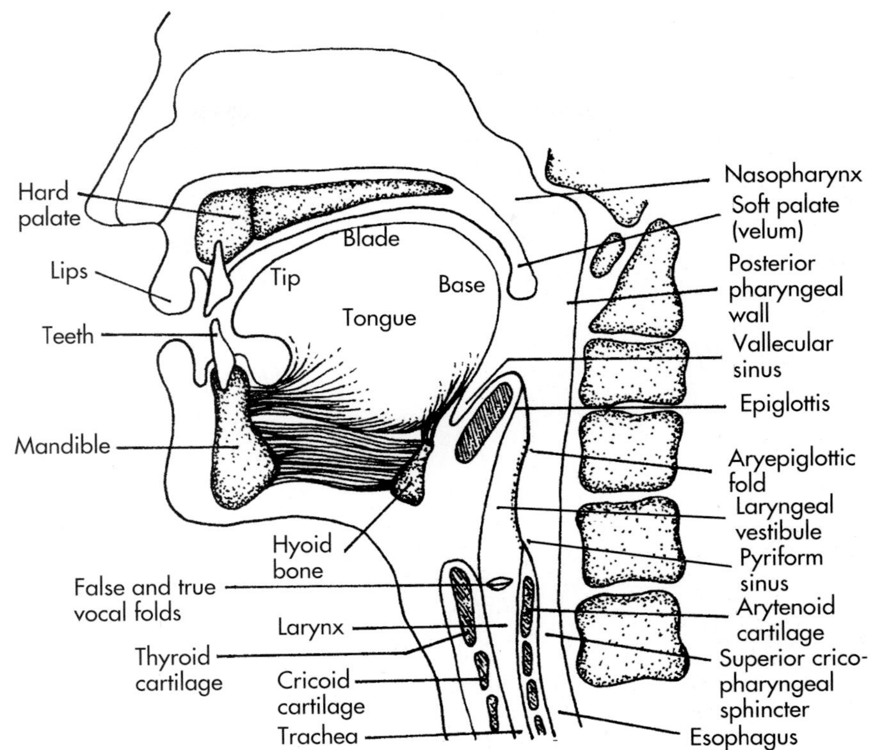


*Figure 19-1* Oral structures, swallowing mechanism at rest. (Courtesy Rene Padilla, MS, OTR, Occupational Therapy Department, Creighton University, 1994.)

and mixing them with saliva to shape a **bolus** (a round lump of chewed food). The tongue carries sensory information about the taste, texture, and temperature of the bolus or liquid through the seventh and ninth cranial nerves (CN VII and IX) to the brain stem. The chewing action of the mandible and tongue is repeated rhythmically until a cohesive bolus is formed. The back of the tongue forms a tight seal against the soft palate to prevent food or liquids from slipping into the pharynx.

When liquids are introduced into the oral cavity, the tongue moves toward the front of the mouth, stopping behind the incisors and forming a groove. The shape of this groove along the dorsal surface of the tongue funnels the liquid toward the pharynx.[11]

In preparation for the next stage, the bolus is held between the front of the tongue and the palate. The tongue cups around the bolus to seal it against the hard palate. The larynx and the pharynx are at rest during this phase of the swallowing process.

### Oral Phase

The **oral phase** of swallowing begins when the tongue moves the bolus toward the back of the mouth.[3] The tongue elevates to squeeze the bolus up against the hard palate. A central groove is formed by the tongue to funnel the food to the back of the mouth. The oral stage is voluntary, so the person must be alert.[20] This normal **voluntary swallow** is essential, or the reflexive part of the swallow in the next stage will not be strong. Overall, the oral sequence takes approximately 1 second to complete with thin liquids.

### Pharyngeal Phase

The **pharyngeal phase** of swallowing begins when the bolus passes into the pharynx. Here the involuntary swallow is triggered. After the **swallow response** begins, it continues without pause until the bolus moves completely through the pharynx into the esophagus. The swallow response is controlled by the medulla oblongata of the brain stem. Speech and respiratory reflexes are temporarily suspended during the swallow response.[20] The movement of the bolus must be rapid and efficient so that respiration is interrupted only briefly. Food is prevented from entering the airway by elevation of the larynx beneath the back of the base of the tongue.

The entire pharyngeal phase of the swallow takes about 1 second to complete. Both voluntary *and* involuntary components are needed in a normal swallow. Neither mechanism alone is sufficient to produce the immediate, consistent swallow necessary for normal feeding.[16]

### Esophageal Phase

The **esophageal phase** of the swallow starts when the bolus enters the esophagus. The esophagus is a straight

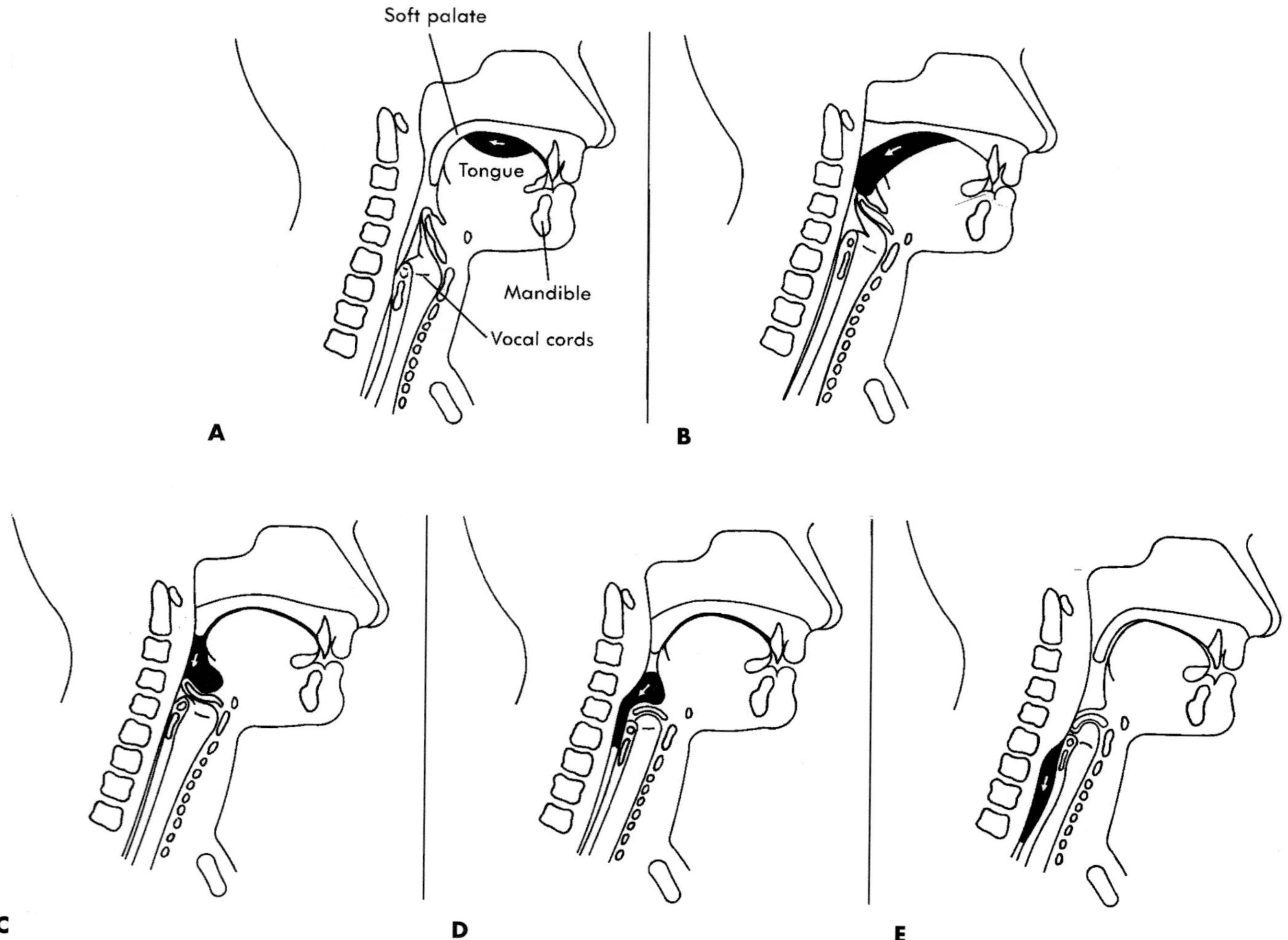


*Figure 19-2* The normal swallow. **A,** Voluntary initiation of swallow. **B,** Swallow response. **C,** Bolus passage through the pharynx. **D,** Bolus begins to enter esophagus. **E,** Completion of pharyngeal stage as entire bolus moves into esophagus. (From Logeman J: *Evaluation and treatment of swallowing disorders,* San Diego, 1983, College-Hill.)

tube, 10 inches (25 cm) in length, which runs from the pharynx to the stomach. The upper third of the esophagus is composed of both striated and smooth muscle. The lower two thirds of the tube is made up of smooth muscle. The food is transported through the esophagus by **peristaltic wave** contractions. The overall transit time needed for the bolus to reach the stomach varies from 8 to 20 seconds.

## TRACHEOSTOMY AND TRACHEOSTOMY TUBES

A **tracheostomy** is a surgical opening through the neck into the trachea that ensures continuity of breathing. A **tracheostomy tube** is inserted to keep the tracheostomy open. The patient breathes through the hole in the neck from which the tube emerges. The patient with a tracheostomy may be a candidate for dysphagia evaluation and treatment. The COTA should have some understanding of the types of tracheostomy tubes.

The two major types of tracheostomy tubes are fenestrated and nonfenestrated.[16,22] A **fenestrated** (from the Latin *fenestra,* meaning "window") **tube** is designed with an opening in the middle of the tube to allow for increased airflow. A fenestrated tube is frequently used for patients being weaned from a tube. The fenestrated opening can be closed off with an inner cannula piece. This allows a patient to breathe nasally for periods while relearning a normal breathing pattern. With the inner cannula in place, a trachea button also may be used to allow the patient to talk. A *nonfenestrated tube* has no opening. A fenestrated tube is used more often when treating a dysphagic patient.

A tracheostomy tube, fenestrated or nonfenestrated, may also be cuffed or uncuffed. A *cuffed tube* has a balloonlike cuff surrounding the bottom of the tube. When inflated, the cuff comes into contact with the trachea wall, preventing the aspiration of secretions into the airway. A cuffed tube is used when aspiration has occurred. The patient with a tracheostomy needs to be suctioned orally and through the tracheostomy to ensure that all secretions have been cleared.[16] This procedure is performed only by the nursing staff or by a therapist who is considered competent in this procedure.

## EVALUATION

On receiving a physician's referral, the OTR will complete a thorough dysphagia evaluation. This includes a review of the patient's medical history and assessment of the patient's mental status; physical control of head, trunk, and extremities; and oral structures. In reviewing the medical history, the therapist seeks out information regarding the onset and duration of the patient's swallowing difficulties and whether previous surgeries have involved the head, neck, and gastrointestinal tract and might affect eating. The OTR pays particular attention to reported episodes of pneumonia or aspiration.[16] Spiking temperatures may indicate that a patient is aspirating.

The OTR obtains information regarding the patient's current nutritional status from the dietary section of the chart or the nursing progress notes. Prescribed medications that may alter the patient's alertness, orientation, and muscle control are noted. The OTR checks whether the patient is receiving food orally or through a nasogastric or gastrostomy tube, is able to take all nutrients orally, or is receiving supplemental tube feedings.

Other areas assessed include the patient's mental status and cognitive ability to participate actively in a feeding evaluation or treatment program. The therapist must know if the patient is alert, oriented to name, day, and date, and able to follow simple directions, either verbally or with guidance. The patient who exhibits confusion, dementia, or a poor level of alertness may not be a good candidate for eating, because chewing and swallowing require voluntary control.[3,4]

Head and trunk control are important components for a safe swallow. To participate in a feeding training program, the patient must maintain an upright position, with head and trunk in midline to provide alignment of the swallowing structures.[6] Poor head control may indicate decreased strength, decreased or increased muscle tone, or decreased awareness. Head control is important because it develops first; jaw movement follows, with quality tongue movement appearing last.

In evaluating the patient's trunk control, the therapist observes whether the patient is sitting in midline with equal weight bearing on both hips. Postural aids such as a wheelchair trunk support or lapboard may be required to assist the patient with trunk control. The COTA should notify the OTR if the patient has difficulty with sitting as described or with returning to midline when balance is disturbed.

The oral evaluation is extremely complex and technical. The face and mouth are sensitive areas to evaluate. Most adults are cautious about or even threatened by having another person touch their face. The OTR is especially careful in using a gentle touch and giving the patient clear descriptions of what will occur when evaluating oral sensation, musculature, and reflexes.

The outer oral area is evaluated first, using specific sensory tests. Signs of poor sensation that may be easily observed are drooling, food on the mouth, or food falling out of the mouth without the patient's awareness. Poor sensory awareness affects the patient's ability to move facial musculature appropriately. The patient's self-esteem also may be affected, especially in social situations, if decreased awareness causes the patient to ignore food or liquids remaining on the face or lips. The COTA should report any observations of such symptoms to the OTR.

A patient with dysfunction in the facial muscles often shows visible asymmetry, facial droop, or peculiar expressions such as frowning or grimacing. A patient with a clearly documented neurological involvement may display primitive oral reflexes that interfere with a dysphagia retraining program. The therapist tests for each reflex separately.

The inner oral status examination follows the outer oral status evaluation, during which the therapist has had time to establish rapport and trust with the patient. This includes an examination of oral structures, the tongue, palatal functions, and swallowing. Each procedure is first explained to the patient. The therapist works within the patient's visual field and gives the patient time to process the instructions. The OTR examines the patient's teeth and gums and, if applicable, checks whether dentures fit adequately for chewing. The tongue is examined for shape, range of motion (ROM), and ability to move normally. The therapist evaluates the patient's ability to swallow safely and protect the airway.

The OTR must assimilate all the information obtained during the entire evaluation process. Clinical judgment plays an important role in the accurate assessment of dysphagia.[3,8] Questions that must be asked include the following:

- Is the patient alert enough to follow through with bolus formation and an immediate swallow when presented with food?
- With assistance, does the patient maintain adequate trunk and head control, normalizing tone and facilitating quality movement?
- Does the patient display adequate tongue control to form a partially cohesive bolus and to regulate the speed in which the bolus enters the pharynx?
- Is the larynx mobile enough to elevate quickly and strongly?

- Can the patient handle saliva with minimal drooling?
- Does the patient have a cough reflex strong enough to expel any material that may enter the airway?

If the answer is "yes" to all these questions, the therapist may evaluate the patient's oral and swallow control with a variety of food consistencies. An evaluation tray of specific solids and liquids is used[1] and includes the following: puréed foods, soft foods, ground foods, thickened liquids, and thin liquids. The OTR gives these to the patient using specific techniques. While performing the feeding evaluation, the therapist observes the patient for signs of fatigue, prolonged swallowing, difficulty chewing, delayed or absent swallow reflex, gurgly voice quality, and any significant coughing.

The patient's performance on the swallowing evaluation determines whether the patient is able to participate in a feeding program and indicates which food and liquid consistencies the patient can handle efficiently. The therapist must decide which consistency is the safest for the patient. The safest consistency is the one the patient is able to chew, move through the oral cavity, and swallow with the smallest risk of aspiration.

The presence of any swallowing dysfunction can lead to aspiration pneumonia. Acute symptoms of aspiration occurring immediately after the swallow are any change in the patient's color (particularly if the airway is obstructed), gurgly voice, and extreme breathiness or loss of voice.[8,12] Over the next 24 hours the medical staff must observe the patient for other signs of aspiration, such as nasal drip, an increase to profuse drooling of a clear liquid, and temperatures of 100° F (37.7° C) or greater, which may not have been evident during the clinical examination.[8,14,16] A patient who develops aspiration pneumonia must be reevaluated for a change in diet levels or taken off the feeding program, if necessary. An alternative feeding method is required.

### Videofluoroscopy

An important technique that can be used to evaluate a patient's swallow is **videofluoroscopy,** a radiographic procedure using a modified barium swallow recorded on videotape. This technique allows the therapist to see the patient's jaw and tongue movement and measure the transit times of the oral and pharyngeal stages, the swallow, any residue in the sinuses, and any aspiration. Videofluoroscopy also may be used to determine which treatment techniques may be effective in assisting the patient to achieve a safe swallow.

Videofluoroscopy is necessary to rule out silent aspiration; 40% of dysphagic patients are silent aspirators during the clinical evaluation.[16,17] The COTA involved in a dysphagia program may ask to observe this procedure to better understand the videofluoroscopic information.

The results of a thorough evaluation determine the course of treatment to increase a patient's ability to eat. The therapist documents the patient's major problems and the treatment recommendations, plan, and goals. The treatment plan should include the type of diet needed, the training and assistance the patient requires, positioning techniques during feeding, and the type of supervision necessary. The COTA is most likely to be involved at the level of following through on treatment recommendations (Figure 19-3). These treatment recommendations are also communicated to the appropriate nursing and medical staff.

## TREATMENT

Because a patient may display one or more problems at each stage of deglutition, the treatment of dysphagia is multifaceted, including trunk and head positioning and control, hand-to-mouth skills, oral motor skills, and swallowing. Perceptual and cognitive deficits that interfere with eating also are addressed. To treat the dysphagic patient, the OTR devotes 35% to 45% of the patient's total daily treatment time to oral motor and swallowing retraining.[14] A patient with severe problems may require up to 6 months of intense intervention before reaching optimal recovery. In preparing a treatment plan for the patient with acquired dysphagia, the therapist must identify the symptoms and causes of the patient's deficits.[8,10,18]

### Goals

The overall goals of occupational therapy in the treatment of dysphagia are as follows[2,8,11,16]:

1. Facilitate appropriate positioning during eating.
2. Improve motor control at each stage of swallowing by normalizing muscle tone and facilitating quality movement.
3. Maintain an adequate nutritional intake.
4. Prevent aspiration.
5. Reestablish oral eating to the safest, optimal level.

### Treatment Team

Dysphagia treatment is complex and is best managed by a team approach. The dysphagia team typically consists of the patient's attending physician, the occupational therapist, the dietitian, the nurse, the physical therapist, the speech-language pathologist, the radiologist, and the patient's family. The leader in evaluation and treatment is often the occupational therapist but in some facilities may be the speech-language pathologist or even the physical therapist. Each professional contributes personal expertise toward patient improvement. All members of the dysphagia team must have a thorough working knowledge of treating patients with dysphagia. This may be supported through interdepartmental in-service training.

## Dysphagia Evaluation and Treatment Plan

Pt: ______

Dx: TBI

Onset: 4-13-94

**Medical hx:** Pt. is a 20 y.o. male who was involved in a single car accident resulting in bihemispheric cerebral damage, brainstem contusion, & subcortical damage to the reticular activating system.

**Current nutritional status:** gastrostomy tube, NPO

| | WNL | Adequate—without assistance | Unable | Comments |
|---|---|---|---|---|
| **Mental status:** | | | | |
| Alert/oriented | | c̄ assist | | oriented to name, max assist for date |
| Direction following | | c̄ assist | | appropriate c̄ guiding |
| **Physical status** (symmetry, control, tone): | | | | |
| Head control | | c̄ assist | | slight ↑'d tone c̄ head turning |
| Trunk control | | c̄ assist | | ataxic, TLR present |
| Endurance | | c̄ assist | | fatigues after 30 min. |
| Respiratory | | | | |
| Suctioning required | ✓ | | | |
| Tracheostomy | ✓ | | | |
| **Outer oral status:** | | | | |
| Facial expressions | | c̄ assist | | flat affect 2° ↑'d tone to moderate degree |
| Jaw movement | | | ✓ | poor rotary chew, poor jaw glide, pt. uses up & down movt. |
| Lip movement | | c̄ assist | | unable to purse & retract, poor lip compression |
| Sensation | | c̄ assist | | delayed 2° ↓'d attention |
| Abnormal reflexes | | c̄ assist | | suck-swallow present, others absent |
| **Inner oral status** (symmetry, control, tone): | | | | |
| Dentition | ✓ | | | good, slightly inflamed gums |
| Tongue | | | | |
| Appearance | | c̄ assist | | slight white coating & mid Ⓡ tongue laceration |
| Tone | | c̄ assist | | ↑'d c̄ retraction |
| Movement: Protrusion | | c̄ assist | | deviated to Ⓡ |
| Lateralization | | c̄ assist | | mild weakness |
| "ng"→"ga" | | | ✓ | poor anterior to posterior |
| **Soft palate/gag reflex:** | ✓ | | | uvula rises symmetrically |
| **Cough (reflexive/voluntary):** | ✓ | | | |
| **Swallow:** | | | | |
| Spontaneous | ✓ | | | intact |
| Voluntary | ✓ | | | delayed 2° to tone |
| Laryngeal movement | | | | |
| Tongue | | c̄ assist | | requires tone reduction |
| Elevation | | c̄ assist | | delayed fatigue factor after serial swallows |
| **Food management:** | | | | Overall pt. shows ↓'d cognitive awareness of food in mouth & requires cueing |
| Puree | | c̄ assist | | pt. uses suck-swallow |
| Mechanical soft | | c̄ assist | } | pocketing assist |
| Chopped/ground | | c̄ assist | } | needed c̄ rotary chew |
| Regular diet | | | N/A | |
| Liquids: Thick | | c̄ assist | | c̄ straw, 5 sec. delay, ∅ cough |
| Semithick | | c̄ assist | | c̄ straw, 5 sec. delay, coughing |
| Thin | | | N/A | |

*Figure 19-3* Dysphagia evaluation and treatment plan.

*Continued.*

**Dysphagia Evaluation and Treatment Plan**

**Major problems:**

① ↓'d cognition for attention and awareness of food in mouth s̄ cueing.
② ↑'d jaw & facial tone resulting in poor rotary chew.
③ Poor isolated tongue movements for lateralization, humping.
④ ↑'d laryngeal tone resulting in delayed swallow.

**Recommendations/treatment plan:**
(positioning, diet level, environment, techniques)

① Positioning-upright on solid seating surface, slight forward lean.
② Tone reduction techniques for jaw, tongue, & larynx before & during meal.
③ Diet level-pureed & mechanical soft foods, thickened liquids 2x daily c̄ therapist only.
④ Therapeutic feeding in quiet setting.
⑤ No food or liquid in pts. room.
⑥ Monitor patient for signs of aspiration.
⑦ Videofluoroscopy for confirmation.

**Long-term goals:**

① Independent trunk and head control.
② ↑ attention and awareness of food in mouth to WFL.
③ ↑ isolated motor control of facial expression to WNL.
④ ↑ isolated motor control of jaw, tongue, & larynx to WFL.
⑤ ↑ oral intake for solids from pureed to regular diet.
⑥ ↑ oral intake for liquids from thick to thin.
⑦ Family education.

*Figure 19-3, cont'd* For legend see p. 303.

When the occupational therapist's role is to evaluate the patient and implement the appropriate course of treatment, the OTR also may be responsible for coordinating the team effort. This includes obtaining physician's orders as needed, selecting the appropriate diet, communicating with all other team members and staff, and educating the family to ensure proper follow-through.[4,24]

The attending physician manages the medical aspect of the patient's health and safety, overseeing all decisions regarding treatment for diet-level selection, oral/nonoral feeding procedures, and the patient's progression. The physician should reinforce the plan of treatment with the patient and family.[12,14,16,24]

The dietitian monitors the patient's caloric intake and makes recommendations to ensure that the patient receives a balanced nutritional diet in accordance with the medical condition. The dietitian is involved in suggesting types of feeding formulas for the nonoral-feeding patient. Diet supplements to augment oral intake may be recommended. Working with the OTR, the dietitian ensures that the proper food and liquid consistencies are served to the patient.

The patient's treating physical therapist is involved in muscle reeducation and tone normalization techniques for the trunk, neck, and face. The patient receives treatment in balance, strength, and control. The physical therapist is involved in increasing the patient's pulmonary status for breath support, chest expansion, and cough.[1]

The role of the speech-language pathologist involves the reeducation of the oral and laryngeal musculature used in speaking and voice production. Because these muscles also are used in swallowing, a speech-language pathologist with dysphagia experience may participate in oral motor and swallowing training during prefeeding and feeding sessions.[14]

The nurse is another key member of the dysphagia team. The nursing staff is responsible for monitoring the patient's medical and nutritional status. The nurse usually is the first to notice changes in the patient's condition, such as an elevated temperature and an increase in secretions indicating swallowing dysfunction. The nurse then informs the physician and occupational therapist of these changes. The patient's oral and fluid intake is recorded in the nursing notes, and the nurse tells the dysphagia team whether the patient's nutritional status is adequate or inadequate. Supplemental tube feedings ordered by the physician are administered by the nursing staff, who also provide oral hygiene, tracheostomy care, and supervision for appropriate patients during meals.[1,12,16,19]

The patient's family is included as a team member to act as a program supporter. The family frequently underestimates the danger of aspiration; therefore the staff must educate the family and the patient from the first day of evaluation. The family and patient should understand which food consistencies are safe to eat and which foods must be avoided.[2,23] Family members may attempt to bring the patient special foods, many of which are inappropriate. The COTA can help by reinforcing with the family that all food must be cleared with the nurse responsible for the patient's intake before it is given to the patient.

Although the roles just described may vary from facility to facility, designated roles must be clearly defined to ensure a coordinated team approach.

### Positioning

Proper positioning is essential for treating the dysphagic patient because the position of the head and trunk influences the swallowing response and the tone of the muscles involved in feeding and eating. The patient should be positioned symmetrically, with normal alignment through the head, neck, trunk, and pelvis. To achieve this goal, the patient is seated on a firm surface (e.g., a chair) with feet flat on the floor, knees at 90° flexion, equal weight bearing on both ischial tuberosities of the hips, trunk flexed slightly forward (100° hip flexion) with a straight back, both arms placed forward on the table, and head erect in midline with chin slightly tucked.[4,5,10]

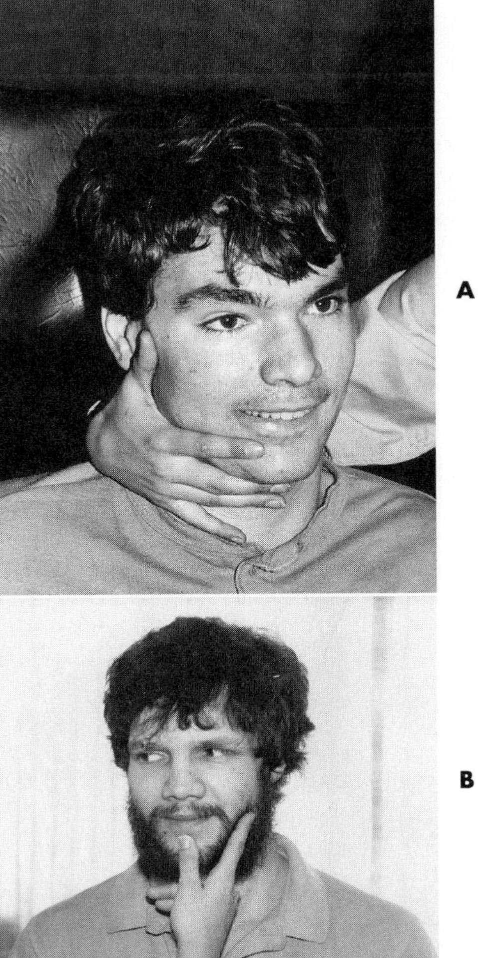


*Figure 19-4* Head control. **A,** Side-hold position for patients requiring moderate to maximal assistance. **B,** Front-hold position for patients requiring minimal assist. (Courtesy Meadowbrook Neurological Care Center, San Jose, Calif, 1988.)

Figure 19-4 illustrates two hand-hold techniques that allow the OT practitioner to assist the patient in maintaining head control. Correct positioning normalizes tone, thereby facilitating quality motor control and function of the facial musculature, jaw and tongue movement, and the swallow process, all of which minimize the risk for aspiration.

A patient who has difficulty moving into the correct position or maintaining the position presents a challenge to the clinician. A more careful analysis of the patient is required to determine the major problem preventing good positioning. Poor positioning may be caused by decreased control or balance from hypertonicity or hypotonicity or poor body awareness in space from perceptual dysfunction (Figure 19-5).[5,8,10] After the cause is identified, the therapist can treat it

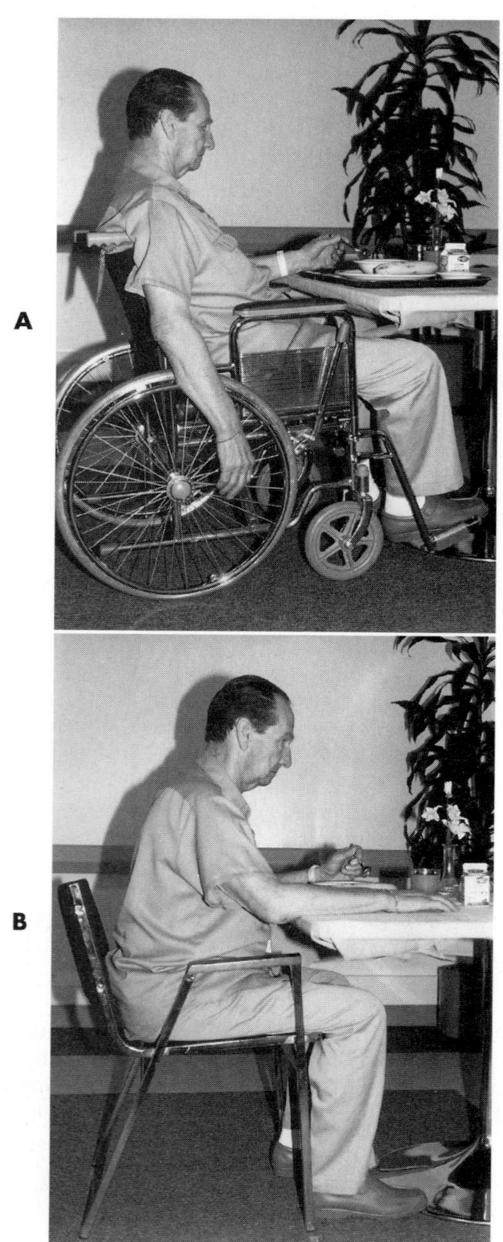


*Figure 19-5* Positioning of dysphagic patient. **A,** Incorrect positioning. **B,** Correct positioning. (Courtesy Meadowbrook Neurological Care Center, San Jose, Calif, 1988.)

accordingly. The OTR instructs the COTA as to the correct position for each patient.

## Oral Hygiene

Oral care by nursing and therapy team members prevents gum disease, the accumulation of secretions, the development of plaque, and the aspiration of food particles that remain after eating. To begin the oral hygiene process, the patient is positioned upright and symmetrically. The patient who is apprehensive or whose oral cavity is hypersensitive may first require preparation by the clinician. Preparation steps may include firmly stroking outside the patient's mouth or lips with the patient's or clinician's gloved finger. Sensitive gums can also be firmly rubbed, preparing the patient for the toothbrush.

For cleaning purposes, the mouth can be divided into four quadrants. A toothbrush with a small head and soft bristles is used to clean each quadrant, starting with the top teeth and moving from front to back. When brushing the bottom teeth, the COTA brushes from back to front. Next, holding the toothbrush at a vertical angle, the inside teeth are brushed in a downward motion from gums to teeth. Finally, the cutting surfaces of the teeth are brushed. An electric toothbrush is more effective if the patient can tolerate it.

After each procedure the patient is allowed to dispose of the secretions. After brushing the patient is carefully assisted in rinsing the mouth. If the patient can tolerate thin liquids, small amounts of water can be given. Having the patient flex the chin slightly toward the chest helps prevent the water from being swallowed. The COTA can assist the patient to expel the water by placing one hand on each cheek and simultaneously pushing inward on the cheeks while the chin remains slightly tucked. If the patient cannot manipulate liquids, a dampened sponge toothette can be used. The COTA and nursing staff also can consider using small amounts of baking soda instead of toothpaste because it is easier to rinse out.[8,10] Baking soda should be used with caution in patients on a restricted salt diet who are also at risk for swallowing the baking soda (e.g., head-injured patients).

Oral hygiene for the nonoral-feeding or oral-feeding patient provides sensory stimulation of touch, texture, temperature, and taste and can be used to facilitate beginning jaw and tongue movement and to encourage an automatic swallow.[8] Lack of oral stimulation over a prolonged period leads to hypersensitivity within the oral cavity. Patients who display poor tongue movement frequently have food remaining on their teeth or dentures or between the cheek and gum. A patient with decreased sensation is unaware of the remaining food. A thorough cleaning should occur each time the patient eats.

## Nonoral Feedings

A patient who is aspirating more than 10% of food or liquid consistencies or whose combined oral and pharyngeal transit time is more than 10 seconds, regardless of positioning or facilitation techniques, is not a candidate for oral eating.[8,16] This patient needs a nonoral nutritional method until again capable of eating or drinking. Patients who lack the endurance to take in sufficient calories also may require nonoral feedings or supplements.

The two most common procedures for nonoral feedings are nasogastric (NG) tube and a gastrostomy

*Table 19-1*

Dysphagia, Stage I Food Level* (Puréed)

| *Food groups* | *Foods allowed* | *Foods to avoid* |
|---|---|---|
| Cereals/breads | Cooked refined cereals, cream of wheat/rice | All others |
| Eggs | Custard, puréed egg salad (without onions or celery) | All others |
| Fruits | Puréed fruit, applesauce | Whole fruits, juicy fruits, all others |
| Potatoes or substitutes | Mashed (white or sweet) potatoes mixed with thick gravy | All others |
| Vegetables | Puréed asparagus, beets, carrots, green beans, peas, spinach, squash | All others |
| Soups | Thickened, strained cream soups with consistency of puréed vegetable | All others |
| Meat, fish, poultry, cheese | Puréed meat, puréed poultry | All others |
| Fats | Butter, margarine, cream mixed with puréed foods | All others |
| Desserts | Plain puddings, smooth yogurt without fruit, custard | Any with nuts, coconut, seeds, all others |
| Sugars/sweets | Honey, sugar, syrup, jelly mixed in with puréed food | All others |

*References 17, 19, 23.

tube feedings[12] (see Chapter 12). The NG tube can desensitize the swallow reflex. The gastrostomy tube allows the therapist to begin a prefeeding or feeding program while the tube is in place, carries less risk of reflux and aspiration, does not irritate or desensitize the swallowing mechanisms, and can be removed when the patient no longer requires supplemental feedings or liquids. A gastrostomy tube is often used for the involved dysphagic patient who may require tube feeding or supplemental feedings for longer than 3 months.[16]

A commercially prepared liquid formula that provides complete nutrition typically is used for tube feedings. While the patient is following a nonoral program, the OTR concentrates efforts on retraining the patient in oral motor control and swallowing. Nelson[21] describes tube feeding in more detail.

### Oral Feedings

To determine whether a patient is an appropriate candidate for oral feeding, several criteria must be met. The same criteria to evaluate a patient's swallow response with foods or liquids can be used. To participate in an oral feeding program, a patient must be alert, able to maintain adequate trunk and head positioning with assistance, have beginning tongue control, manage secretions with minimal drooling, and have a reflexive cough. The OTR needs to identify the food or liquid consistency most appropriate for the patient. The safest consistency with which to initiate the oral program is one that enables the patient to complete the oral and pharyngeal stages combined in less than 10 seconds and to swallow with minimal aspiration (10% or less).[16] The overall goal of an oral feeding program is for the patient to achieve swallowing without aspiration.

#### *Diet Selection*

A diet is carefully selected to reflect the dysphagic patient's needs. Foods chosen for these diets are uniform in consistency and texture, provide sufficient density and volume, remain cohesive, provide pleasant taste and temperature, and are easily removed or suctioned when necessary.[8,12] Inappropriate foods are those with multiple textures, such as vegetable soup and salads, fibrous and stringy vegetables, meats and fruits, crumbly and flaky textures, foods that liquefy (e.g., gelatin, ice cream), and foods with skins and seeds.[7,19] Garnishes, such as lettuce and parsley, are avoided because they may be unsafe for the confused patient.

The OTR works closely with the dietitian to develop diet levels for both solids and liquids. Specific diets for dysphagic patients facilitate ordering appropriate foods and liquids consistently. Once the diets are developed, the medical, nursing, and therapy staff are taught which foods are in each level to ensure the patient's safety. When requesting a diet, the OTR specifies levels desired for both liquids and solids because a dysphagic patient may handle each differently.

#### *Diet Progression*

Information on **diet progression** is provided here so that the COTA can understand the rationale behind it. The COTA who assists in oral feedings also needs to monitor the patient's foods. Tables 19-1 to 19-3 are

*Table 19-2*

**Dysphagia, Stage II Food Level* (Mechanical Soft)**

| *Food groups* | *Foods allowed* | *Foods to avoid* |
|---|---|---|
| Cereals/breads | Cooked refined cereals, cream of wheat/rice, oatmeal; white, wheat, or rye bread (without crust or seeds); graham crackers, soft French toast without crust | Hard rolls, bread with nuts, seeds, coconut, and fruit; bread with cracked-wheat particles; sweet rolls; waffles, Melba toast, English muffins, popcorn, cereals (e.g., corn flakes, crisp/puffed rice) |
| Eggs | Custard; boiled, poached, and scrambled eggs; minced egg salad (without onions or celery) | All others |
| Fruits | Puréed fruit, applesauce, ripe banana and avocado; soft, canned and cooked fruits such as peaches, pears, apricots, pitted plums, stewed prunes, grapefruit, and orange sections (no membrane); baked apple (no skin); cranberry sauce | Fruits with seeds, coarse skins, and fibers; fruits with pits; all raw fruit except those listed as allowed; raisins, grapes, fruit cocktail |
| Potatoes or substitutes | Mashed potatoes (white or sweet), baked potatoes (no skin), soft noodles, spaghetti/macaroni (finely chopped) | Fried potatoes, potato or corn chips, rice |
| Vegetables | Cooked or canned artichoke hearts, asparagus tips, beets, carrots, mushrooms, squash, pumpkin, green beans, tomato purée and paste (no skins or seeds) | All other raw, stringy, fried, and dried vegetables; pickles |
| Soups | Thickened, strained cream soups made with puréed allowed vegetables | All others |
| Meat, fish, poultry, cheese | Finely ground meat; poultry, tuna (without celery or onions); soft casseroles/sandwiches (without crust); cream or cottage cheese, American cheese | Fish (because of bones); meat, any consistency other than finely ground; bacon; all other cheeses |
| Fats | Butter, margarine, cream, mayonnaise mixed with food; thick gravy, thick cream sauce | Nuts, olives; all others |
| Desserts | Plain puddings, custard, tapioca, fruit whip, smooth yogurt, soft cake, cream pie with graham cracker crust | Cookies, cake with nuts, seeds, raisins, dates, coconuts, and fruits not on allowed list; all others |
| Sugars/sweets | Honey, sugar, syrup, jelly, plain soft milk-chocolate bars | Marmalade, coconut; all others |

*References 17, 19, 23.

samples of diets for three dysphagia levels stated in order of progression.[1,7,19] After mastering the stage III food items, the patient may progress to a regular diet.

*Stage I foods* are puréed and are used for patients with little or no jaw or tongue control, a moderately delayed swallow, and a decreased pharyngeal stage.[8,16] Puréed foods move more slowly into the pharynx, allowing time for the swallow reflex to trigger. Because puréed foods cannot be formed into an adequate bolus, they offer the patient little opportunity for increasing oral motor control.[8] Stage I foods are best used only to increase the patient's oral intake, with the patient progressed to the next level as soon as possible.

*Stage II foods* are soft food items that stay together as a cohesive bolus; thus the possibility of particles spilling into the airway is decreased. Stage II foods are

Table 19-3

## Dysphagia, Stage III Food Levels* (Chopped/Ground)

| *Food groups* | *Foods allowed* | *Foods to avoid* |
|---|---|---|
| Cereals/breads | Cooked cereals, ready-to-eat cereals† (e.g., corn flakes, crisp/puffed rice); pancakes, French toast, white, wheat, and rye bread (with crust); salt crackers, soda and graham crackers; sweet rolls, English muffins, Melba toast, donuts | Hard rolls, bread with nuts, seeds, coconut, and fruit; coarse cereals (e.g., granola, Grapenuts), popcorn |
| Eggs | Soft- and hard-boiled, poached, fried, and scrambled eggs; egg salad (without onions and celery) | All others |
| Fruits | Bananas, avocado; soft, canned and cooked fruit, ripe fruit | Fruits with seeds, coarse skins and fibers, pits; fruit cocktail |
| Potatoes or substitutes | Mashed potatoes (white or sweet), creamed potatoes, baked potatoes (without skin), noodles, spaghetti, macaroni | Fried potatoes, potato and corn chips, rice without gravy |
| Vegetables | Cooked and canned vegetables (without skins, seeds, and stringy fibers) | All raw, stringy, fried, and dried vegetables |
| Soups | Thickened creamed soups made with puréed or whole allowed vegetables only | All others |
| Meat, fish, poultry, cheese | Finely diced/minced meat, poultry, tuna (without onions or celery), flaked fish, fish sticks; soft casseroles, sandwiches, and cheeses | Bacon; fish with bones; poultry with skin |
| Fats | Butter, margarine, cream, mayonnaise, gravy, cream sauces | Nuts; all others |
| Desserts | Soft cookies, cakes, pies, puddings, custard, yogurt | Cookies, cake with nuts, seeds, coconut, and fruits not on allowed list; hard pies, crusts/pastries; all others |
| Sugars/sweets | Honey, sugar, syrup, jelly; plain soft milk-chocolate bars | Marmalade, coconut; all others |

*References 2, 7, 19, 23.
†Allowed only if thin liquids are appropriate.

best for patients with a beginning rotary chew, enough tongue control with assistance to propel food back toward the pharynx, and a minimally delayed swallow.[8] Mechanical soft foods reduce the risk of aspiration in patients who have both a motor and a sensory loss affecting the triggering of the swallow response.[3,13] Mechanical soft foods with a density provide increased proprioceptive input throughout the mouth. These foods also stay as a cohesive bolus rather than crumbling and falling uncontrolled into the airway. Because the patient at this diet stage displays improved tongue control, the swallow response is triggered faster as the back of the tongue elevates toward the hard palate. For the patient who is just beginning to chew, mashing the food with a fork enhances the ability to keep it together as a bolus.[8]

*Stage III foods* require chewing, controlled bolus formation, and an adequate swallow. This food group offers a wider variety of consistencies. Meats should be finely cut to facilitate a controlled swallow. Smaller particles are less likely to obstruct the airway and are less of a health risk than large pieces, if minimal aspiration occurs. These foods are safer than items found in a regular diet but require patient effort. Stage III foods are for patients who have minimal problems with jaw or tongue control and an intact swallow response. The patient who has reached a stage III level needs to be concerned with a delayed swallow only when fatigued.

When a patient is ready to progress to the next diet level, the OTR can adjust the meals by requesting one or two items from the higher group, enabling assessment at the new level. This technique is also appropriate for patients who fatigue. The patient is thus able to work with the OT practitioner on the more difficult food item first, then continue the meal with "easier" foods. The OTR might also arrange several small meals throughout the day for the patient who fatigues, rather than three traditional meals.

A patient is progressed to a regular diet when oral motor control is within functional limits, allowing the patient to chew and form any consistency into a bolus and propel it back toward the faucial arches. The patient at this level should be able to swallow any food or liquid consistency with only occasional coughing. The patient with a history of dysphagia should continue dietary precautions for avoiding raw vegetables, stringy foods, and foods containing nuts or seeds.[1,7]

The patient may exhibit a difference in ability to handle liquids; thus the OTR develops a progression of liquid levels separate from the solid levels. The liquid progression is divided into three groups: thin, semithick, and thick liquids.[1,7,19] Box 19-1 provides examples of these levels. Thick liquids are made by adding thickening agents such as banana, puréed fruit, yogurt, dissolved gelatin, baby cereal, and cornstarch. These substances are usually added to the liquids and power-blended for smoothness. The thick drink or soup should stay blended and not be allowed to separate or liquefy. Thick liquids are the appropriate choice for patients with a greatly delayed swallow response. A thick liquid moves more slowly, giving some time for the swallow response to trigger. Semithick liquids such as fruit nectars, buttermilk, tomato juice, and yogurt drinks are used with patients who have a moderate swallow delay of 3 to 5 seconds.[8,16] Thin liquids, the most difficult liquid level, require an intact swallow.

Box 19-1

## Examples of Liquid Levels*

**Thin liquids**
Water
Coffee (regular, decaffeinated), tea
Milk, hot chocolate
All fruit juices
Broth/consommé
Gelatin dessert, ice cream, sherbet

**Semithick liquids**
Extra thick milkshake/eggnog
Strained creamed soup
Tomato juice, V-8 juice
Plain nectars
Yogurt and milk blended

**Thick liquids**
Nectar thickened with banana
Nectar with puréed fruit
Regular applesauce with juice
Eggnog with baby cereal
Creamed soup thickened with mashed potatoes

*References 2, 7, 19, 23.

### *Principles of Oral Feeding*

As stated earlier, dysphagia treatment is complex, with potentially fatal consequences because of the risks of choking and aspiration. The COTA may assist with oral feeding under the OTR's direct supervision. It is essential that the COTA has achieved and proved service competency in this area and in the necessary safety precautions.

While assisting in an oral feeding program, the COTA should follow certain basic principles. First, the patient should be alert and ready and able to eat. The COTA must observe the patient at the beginning of each session because alertness can vary from day to day. Patients should not participate in the dysphagia feeding program when they are sleepy.

Second, an important aspect of the oral preparation stage is looking at and reaching for food. The patient must actively see, look at, and participate in the eating process. Food presented should be within the patient's visual field. For the patient with a severe field deficit or unilateral neglect, the COTA can assist and perhaps even physically cue the patient to turn the head from side to side to scan the plate or tray visually.

Third, when physically possible, the patient should be allowed to perform self-feeding. If the patient does not have a normal hand-to-mouth movement pattern, the COTA must assist the patient to achieve one by guiding the extremity in the correct pattern. The pattern must be as close to normal as possible. Abnormal position and movement of the upper extremity will elicit abnormal movement in the trunk, head, face, tongue, and pharynx. Abnormal movement interferes with normal food transit and the swallowing mechanism.

If the patient is not capable of self-feeding, the COTA can keep the patient actively involved by having the patient choose which food or liquid is preferred for each bite. During feeding of the patient, food is presented from the front of the patient by moving the utensil slowly toward the mouth so that the patient can see the food for the entire time. The COTA may need to remind the patient to look at the food. The utensil should not be brought in from the side because the patient will have less preparation time. The patient should be allowed as much control of the situation as possible.

Fourth, eating should occur in an appropriate context. If possible, the patient should eat in a normal setting while participating in oral feeding training. For adults, eating is a social activity shared with friends and family. The patient can be redirected if distracted, and the COTA can use environmental cuing when the patient is eating in a dining room with others. Adjustments, such as eating in the dining room but at a separate table, can help the distractible patient to concentrate.

Fifth, the COTA needs to be conscious of how the patient appears to others and help the patient to eat in a normal manner. Some dysphagic patients are impulsive and may shovel food into their mouths at an unsafe pace or one that appears rude. The COTA can verbally cue the patient to slow down. If this does not work, the clinician can gently place a restraining hand on the patient's eating arm while repeating the verbal cue. Another technique is for the COTA to precut the food into smaller pieces and require the patient to chew each one separately. Alternately, the COTA can require the patient to wipe the mouth between bites or to place the utensil on the table after each bite and before the next.

Sixth, the COTA providing the feeding must continually observe the patient's positioning, upper extremity movement, muscle tone, oral control, and swallow while the patient is eating, whether it is one food item or an entire meal. The COTA assists the patient to perform the task correctly and does not allow eating while the patient exhibits an abnormal pattern. Problems in head, trunk, and upper extremity position and movement can often be resolved by adjustments in seating, supports, or positioning. It is essential that the patient is erect, with hips level on a flat supporting surface.

If the patient displays poor oral motor skills, the COTA must check for "food pocketing" after every few bites. The rate of the patient's intake is monitored. The COTA should note when too much food is in the mouth and watch that the patient does not put food into the mouth before the previous bite has been cleared. The trained COTA may feel for the swallow with a finger at the hyoid notch if the patient displays abnormal laryngeal tone or a delayed swallow.[8] The COTA also listens for voice quality on completion of the swallow, because this will indicate whether food is pooling in the piriform sinuses, increasing the risk of aspiration.

The frequency with which the clinician must check each component depends on the patient's skill level and performance. The more difficulty that the patient exhibits, the more frequent the assessment. Patients who are having great difficulty should be trained only by the OTR. After completing the feeding process, the patient should remain in an upright position for 30 minutes to reduce the risks of refluxing food back up and aspirating small food particles that may remain in the throat.[3] The COTA also must report any signs or observations of swallowing difficulties to the OTR.

The indicators of swallowing dysfunction include coughing or throat clearing before, during, or after the swallow; gurgly voice quality; changes in breathing pattern; delayed or absent swallow response; poor cough; and reflux of food after meals. The presence of any swallowing dysfunction can lead to aspiration pneumonia (see earlier description).

All persons working with individuals with dysphagia must be able to identify the symptoms of an obstructed or ineffective airway and competently administer the *Heimlich maneuver* for clearing the airway. The signs of an obstructed airway are an inability to breathe or speak. The signs of an ineffective airway are a high-pitched whistling sound as the patient breathes. In both cases, cyanosis and eventual loss of consciousness quickly follow if the airway is not cleared. The Heimlich maneuver is taught in all basic cardiopulmonary resuscitation (CPR) courses. The resuscitator must be prepared to summon assistance if this technique is unsuccessful. All involved persons must be familiar with the emergency procedures or the facility or practice setting.

Patients who develop a gurgling or rasping quality to their speech, without signs of a dangerously compromised airway, can usually clear the airway by coughing. The clinician may need to instruct the patient to cough repeatedly before the airway clears. Slowly taking a deep breath before coughing increases the cough's power and effectiveness. If the rasping quality persists despite repeated coughing attempts, the COTA should seek immediate assistance from a more highly trained clinician.

When a patient is participating in oral feedings, nutritional status must be carefully monitored. The caloric needs for each patient are determined by the dietitian and the physician and depend on height, weight, activity level, and medical condition.[19] A patient's fluid intake is monitored by having the physician order a calorie count. The COTA must remember to report the approximate percentage of each food item or the percentage of the meal consumed by the patient to the person (usually a nurse) responsible for calorie recording. The dietitian converts the percentages into a daily calorie total.

The patient should also be monitored for physical signs of nutritional deficiency and dehydration. These symptoms are weakness, irritability, decreased alertness, change in eating habits, hunger, thirst, decreased turgor (smoothness and fullness of skin tone), and changes in amounts or color of urine.[24] If a patient is not able to take in the necessary calories (50% of the determined total), supplemental feedings are necessary to make up the difference.[7,13] The physician and dietitian determine the number of supplemental feedings.

### Treatment Techniques

A variety of strategies are used with specific problems. Using the wrong technique can cause more harm than good. The COTA will be shown the desired techniques as needed and should use only the techniques specified by the supervising OTR. Treatment of feeding problems requires special training. Ideally the COTA should take a training course and then perform techniques under the immediate supervision of the dysphagia therapist until service competency is well established. The COTA can assist and best support the OTR by following the directions given, asking for and receiving clarification on anything not understood, and developing and using good observational skills while interacting with the patient. This ensures safe, high-quality patient care.

## SUMMARY

Eating is a fundamental human activity essential to survival. Eating is a context for interacting with others and as such is social and pleasurable. Impairment of the ability to eat independently (dysphagia) is distressing to patients. In a dysphagia program the OTR or other professional performs a detailed evaluation and makes specific treatment recommendations. Dysphagia treatment requires advanced training and knowledge of specific techniques. Because of the risks of choking and aspiration, those working with the dysphagic patient must have a thorough understanding of the mechanism of swallowing, the anatomy and reflexes of the head and neck, and emergency measures.

The COTA is a valuable member of the dysphagia team, providing feeding training and treatment to patients under direct or immediate supervision. Helping individuals regain control over the process of eating can be an especially rewarding treatment area in occupational therapy.

# Section II Driving With a Physical Dysfunction

SUSAN M. LILLIE

## DRIVING EVALUATION

### Importance of Driving

Driving is an essential activity of daily living (ADL) in today's society, playing a pivotal role in personal independence, employment, and aging. A driver's license symbolizes a rite of passage to adulthood for the teenager, independence for leisure activities and employment opportunities for the adult, and wellness and competence for the older adult. The ability to drive is seen as instrumental in obtaining and maintaining an independent lifestyle.

Driving requires continuous integration of visual, motor, cognitive, and perceptual skills at a high level of functioning. A complex task, driving carries more risk of harm than other ADLs; consequently, evaluation of the ability to drive is critical for individuals whose disabilities may impair any of the skills involved.

The registered occupational therapist (OTR) plays a vital role in assessing driving potential, using analysis of activity and occupational role performance as a framework. The certified occupational therapy assistant (COTA) may contribute to the evaluation, working as a partner or collaborator with the OTR, under OTR supervision and direction.

### Purpose of Driving Evaluation

The purpose of a driving evaluation is to assess a person's ability to drive. The ability to drive may be disrupted because of a medical condition, disability, or condition of aging. Driver evaluations also help determine the most appropriate vehicle for an individual and the adaptive equipment and training necessary for safe driving.

Driver evaluation programs vary greatly in the types of services offered. Some programs offer clinical assessment or simulator road tests. These programs are valuable in general problem identification, but research shows these results do not predict road performance. A comprehensive driver evaluation program includes clinical, stationary, and behind-the-wheel performance testing in a special evaluation vehicle.[7,13,14]

### Candidates for Driving Assessment

Health care professionals, including physicians, therapists, and case managers, play an important role in identifying those individuals requiring a driver evaluation. The purpose of the referral is most frequently to promote independent driving. Driver assessments are costly[4] and are generally not covered by insurance or Medicaid plans. By thoroughly screening referrals for appropriateness, therapists conserve patient resources and provide cost-effective treatment. A referral to a qualified driver evaluation program should be made if any of the following conditions arises:

- The patient, family, or health care professional expresses concerns about the driver's safety or competence.

- The patient has limitations that preclude use of the standard driving pattern of two-handed steering and right foot on the gas and brake pedals.
- The patient has neuromuscular weakness or disease (e.g., multiple sclerosis, muscular dystrophy, polio).
- The patient has a neurological condition (e.g., traumatic brain injury, cerebrovascular accident, cerebral palsy, peripheral neuropathy, Parkinson's disease, tumor, dementia).
- The patient has impaired or low vision.

### Older Drivers

Older drivers are increasing in numbers with the "graying of America," causing possibly unfounded concern among legislators and public policy makers. To date, research has not identified those skills or qualities that make an older driver incompetent.[6,8,9,10,16] Older adults have different driving habits and patterns, but most are within the continuum of safe driving performance.[9] Older drivers with multiple medical conditions may be most at risk, requiring a screening and evaluation process.

To an older person, loss of a license has significant psychological impact. Some older drivers report they would rather die than not drive again. Evaluation of older drivers with consideration of graded licenses to prolong safe driving will enable more older adults to maintain self-sufficiency and independence.[5]

### Analysis of Driving

Occupational role assessment and activity analysis are necessary steps in providing a thorough driver evaluation. Activity analysis reduces the task of driving to its component parts. Each component skill can be assessed separately in the clinic. The person's ability to coordinate these skills into the integrated task of driving is evaluated during the on-road test.

Occupational role theory is also helpful in driver assessment. Examination of the roles a person performed before the onset of physical dysfunction and the roles the person will resume should influence selection of the appropriate vehicle and driving equipment. Roles held by the driver (e.g., parent, student, homemaker, employee) require activity analysis to provide additional information. A person who travels to multiple job sites, for example, may need to transfer several times each day, which directly threatens fatigue level and joint viability. Use of airports or businesses that have parking structures or covered parking makes vehicle height a critical factor in accessibility. A parent may need to fasten the car seat of a toddler or supervise other children while managing predriving tasks. In each of these examples, vehicle selection and driving equipment may be affected by life roles.

A holistic viewpoint is also integral to the driver evaluation. A person's psychological state, coping strategies, acceptance of disability, tolerance of technology, and chosen lifestyle require evaluation. Recognizing this complexity, the State of California Department of Rehabilitation recommends a minimum of 2 years' experience in physical disabilities, knowledge of adaptive equipment, driving systems, and equipment vendors for therapists conducting driving evaluations.[14]

## SUBASSESSMENTS WITHIN THE DRIVING EVALUATION

### Clinical Assessment

The **clinical assessment,** also referred to as a *prescreening evaluation* or *predriving evaluation,* is primarily a screening process used to identify strengths and problem areas related to driving. This assessment is conducted by the OTR, who may delegate parts to the COTA.

The clinical assessment begins with a review of medical information, medication and side effects, episodes of seizure or loss of consciousness, mobility status, social history, vocational history, driving history, and purpose of the evaluation. Patients with progressive conditions may be able to drive, but additional medical data are usually required. The rate and history of decline are informative for building in safety margins and designing a driving system that can accommodate future changes in condition.

The clinical assessment can be performed solely by occupational therapy practitioners[13,14] or rehabilitation team members from many disciplines.[4] In either case the clinical evaluation includes the same basic components of vision, motor function, cognition, and visual perception.

#### *Vision Screening*

Comprehensive visual testing includes tests of acuity and other components, such as oculomotor pursuit and convergence. Standards for far acuity vary among the states, but 20/40 to 20/50 is generally the cutoff point before the motor vehicle department requires lenses from a vision specialist. *Acuity* is a universal standard applied by motor vehicle departments. The comprehensive vision screening is important because vision is the primary sense used to gather information required for driving-related decision making.

#### *Physical Measurements*

Muscle strength, active range of motion (ROM), grip, and reaction time are frequently cited as the basic areas requiring measurement.[8,14,15,17] Head and trunk control, balance, and endurance are also important. Other areas that provide critical information when neurological disturbances are present include quality of selective movement, muscle tone, and coordination. Specialized measurements, such as steering wheel force readings with a torque wrench or push/pull motions with a Chatillon scale, provide objective data in selecting more complex modifications for driving, such as the level of resistance required for steering or braking.

### *Cognitive and Visual Perceptual Skills*

Driving requires adequate, reliable perception of a rapidly changing environment, blending both cognitive and visual perceptual skills. Cognitive areas requiring assessment include selective and divided attention, decision making, safety judgment, planning ahead, and awareness of how the disability impacts driving safety. Visual perceptual components include visual organization, visual search and scanning, spatial relations, directionality, and visual processing speed.[7,8,14,17] These areas overlap and blur, making problem identification a challenge even to experienced therapists.

## Stationary Assessment

In the **stationary assessment** the driver candidate uses a nonmoving vehicle. This is helpful in evaluating predriving tasks and equipment setup. The vehicle for evaluation must be chosen first because of variations in the driver station, including steering resistance; gas/brake pedal angle, size, and resistance; seating; and overall layout. A stationary assessment worksheet or checklist may be used to ensure that all essential elements of the driving task are routinely included.

### *Predriving Tasks*

**Predriving tasks** include mobility to the vehicle, inserting and turning a key (or keyless entry operation), opening and closing the door, entering and exiting the vehicle, loading and unloading mobility devices (cane, walker, wheelchair), adjusting the driver seat, adjusting the mirrors, and fastening the seat belt (and chest strap when needed). Adaptive devices to facilitate independence in predriving tasks include special key holders, loops for lower extremity management, a wheelchair strap to extend reach for wheelchair loading, and modifications for independent retrieval of the seat belt. Mechanical devices enable some patients to manage mobility equipment independently and to continue using a car, truck, or minivan without expensive modifications. Since the effectiveness of adaptive devices can vary with different products, a trial-and-error approach is appropriate for selecting the proper adaptive device or equipment for a patient.

### *Steps in Equipment Selection*

The first step is to achieve optimal positioning of the driver, either from the vehicle's driver seat or from a wheelchair. Positioning is important for optimal upper extremity function and safety. Poor trunk stability may require special positioning devices or the use of an upper torso or chest strap.[1,2] All restraint devices (seat belts, chest straps) should be in place before proceeding with the assessment, because these stability devices can inhibit reach or alter substitution patterns used by a patient.

Equipment setups proceed in a logical progression, starting with the primary controls. *Primary controls* are those devices that control the steering, accelerator, and braking of a vehicle. Steering is the first primary control assessed, followed by the gas and brake controls. All other controls, such as turn signals, horn, and headlights, are secondary controls. It is vital to safety that the driver be able to access the horn, windshield wiper, turn signals, and dimmer switch quickly and efficiently with the vehicle in motion.[12] Adaptive equipment should be recommended only when a driver can demonstrate the ability to use the "same general type of device" in a behind-the-wheel assessment.[14]

### *Steering Options*

Smooth, controlled steering is the goal whether the driver uses two-handed steering techniques (i.e., hand over hand, shuffling or feeding the wheel) or one-handed steering with a steering device. When steering is done single-handedly, a steering device is recommended for safety to maintain control of the wheel at all times. Without such a device, driving with one hand requires "palming" of the steering wheel during turns. In **palmed steering** the driver rests the palm on the rim of the wheel rather than locking the wheel with a grip or pinch.

One-handed steering by palming the wheel is not recommended. When palming the wheel, a driver generally must turn more slowly to maintain control, sometimes at a speed well below the flow of traffic. Use of a **steering device** (spinner knob, v-grip, tri-pin, palmar cuff, or amputee ring) provides constant control of the steering wheel and gives the driver the ability to make turns quickly and efficiently. Additional modifications, including smaller diameter steering wheels and reduced levels of steering resistance, are available but require meticulous evaluation for safety. Smaller diameter steering wheels are more difficult to turn and require low-effort or zero-effort modifications to enable a patient to turn the steering wheel efficiently. Veterans Administration (VA) or each state's department of rehabilitation regulations can assist in the selection process for the steering setup. Only after the steering setup is determined does the process move to the accelerator and brake controls.

### *Accelerator and Brake Controls*

Modified accelerator and brake controls can be installed in most vehicles. Simple modifications such as pedal extensions can be installed on both the accelerator and the brake pedals to compensate for limited reach. If the person has significant right hemiplegia, however, the right foot is unable to operate the standard pedals. A left-sided accelerator pedal can be placed to the left of the standard gas pedal; the left foot can then operate gas and brakes safely. When the lower extremities lack adequate motor control or are paralyzed, a device called a **hand control** allows operation of the accelerator and brake pedal with an upper extremity (Figure 19-6).

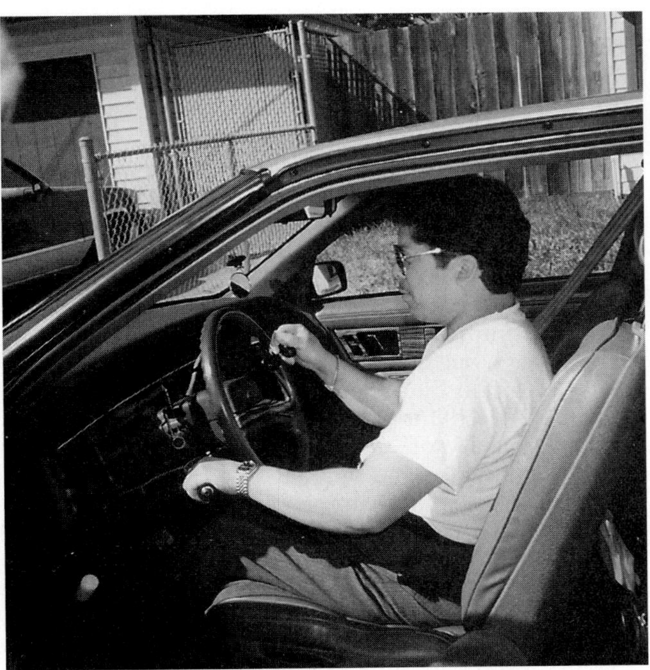

*Figure 19-6* Basic setup for paraplegic patient includes spinner-knob steering device for right-handed steering, push-right-angle-pull hand control to operate gas and brake, and extended brake handle to set parking brake.

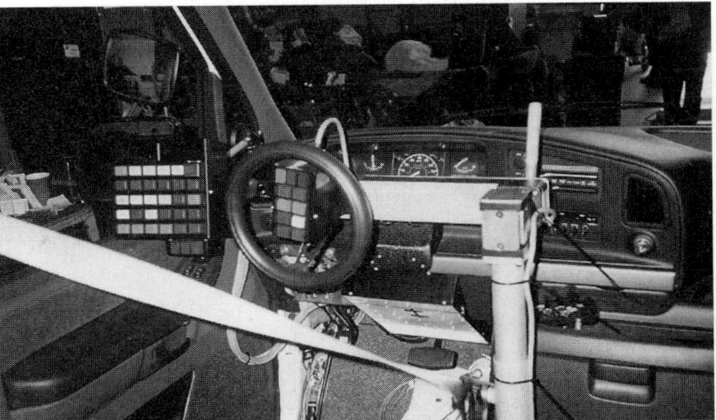

*Figure 19-7* Driving Systems Incorporated (dSi) and joystick systems combine gas, brake, and steering functions on one lever. These sophisticated unilever systems enable many persons with severe disabilities (e.g., arthrogryposis, fifth cervical quadriplegia, muscle diseases) to drive.

Hand controls can use rotary, push/pull, push/pull down, or side-to-side motions to apply pressure to the accelerator and the brake. Selection is determined by the patient's medical condition and potential problems with motion specific to the hand control. For example, for a person with severe arthritis in the hand or carpal tunnel syndrome, the rotary-style hand control could exacerbate the symptoms.

High-technology gas/brake controls, operated by vacuum, pneumatics, or computer, allow more disabled persons to drive than ever before by requiring less ROM to activate the device (Figure 19-7).

## Vehicle Selection

### *Cars*

A car is generally appropriate if a person can enter and exit the vehicle and load mobility equipment devices independently. Transfer methods include the stand pivot, bent pivot, sliding board, and upper extremity depression. A person using the sliding board or upper extremity depression method must be able to transfer up inclines because transferring from a wheelchair to a car is generally uphill. When loading equipment manually is not feasible, independence can sometimes be obtained by using a mechanical device to perform the task. Vehicles and mechanical aids are not universally compatible; compact and subcompact vehicles are usually too small to accommodate mechanical wheelchair-loading aids.

The standard car recommendation is a two-door vehicle with power steering, power brakes, and automatic transmission. Bench seats are easiest to transfer into but may not be available from the manufacturer. Bucket or semibucket seats are more common and becoming the standard.

Gear shift levers positioned in a central console between the driver and passenger seats may present problems with transfers. In addition, dexterity is required to depress the gear shift release button to shift gears. Patients with hand impairments may operate better with a gear shift lever mounted on the steering column.

### *Vans*

Two types of drivers use vans: those transferring to a driver seat and those driving from their wheelchairs. Drivers must choose between full-size vans and minivans. Evaluations for patients driving from their wheelchairs are more complex and require greater skill because of increased variables that affect driving performance and equipment selection.

Entry into a van requires a **mechanical lift** for most people using a wheelchair or scooter. Mechanical lifts can be mounted on the rear or side of a full-size van or the side of a minivan. Lifts fall into two basic categories: rotary- or "swing-in"-style lifts and platform-style lifts (Figure 19-8). Each lift has unique characteristics, strengths, and drawbacks.[11] Minivans also have fully automatic mechanical ramps for independent entry and exit (Figure 19-9). The clinician must provide a safe, compatible match among lift choice, parking needs, and chosen lifestyle. Restrictions by each state's department of vocational rehabilitation can also influence vehicle and equipment selections for those patients funded by these agencies.

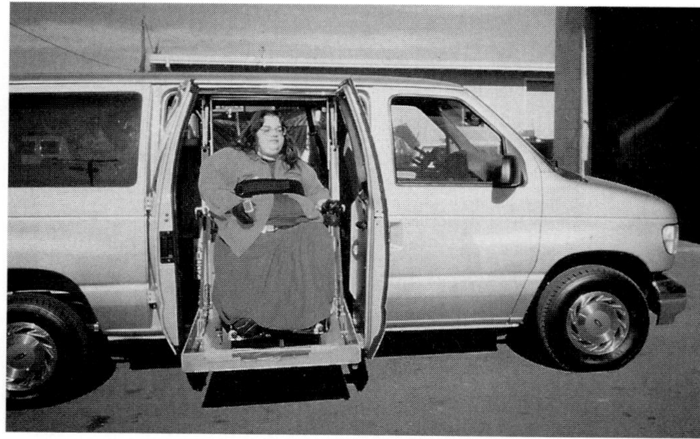

*Figure 19-8* Platform-style lift can be located at side or rear of van. Additional entry headroom, obtained through lowering floor, allows this patient to see out windshield when driving from a power wheelchair.

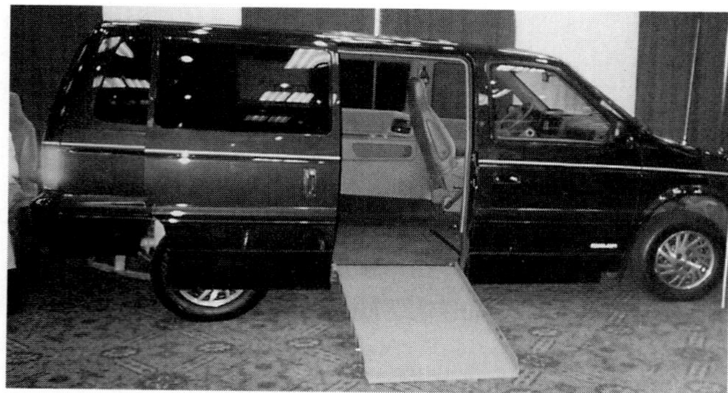

*Figure 19-9* Minivan conversions have access ramp instead of lift, along with 10-inch (25 cm) floor drop. Airbag system lowers van to decrease ramp angle for easier entry and exit.

## Behind-the-Wheel or On-Road Assessment

Once the primary controls in the evaluation vehicle have been selected and set up, the driver's ability to use these controls must be verified through actual driving, usually called **behind-the-wheel performance testing** or the on-road portion of the evaluation. Sometimes several driving equipment setups are attempted during the behind-the-wheel session before the right combination for safe driving is determined.

### *Road Test Components*

The industry standard is to accept the on-road driving test as the optimal measure of driving competence.[3,6,9,10,14] Therefore a decision made on a person's license, when based on an actual road test, is considered a sound decision. Efforts are being made to standardize the behind-the-wheel test and scoring system to improve validity and interrater reliability. For safety and comprehensive testing, it is recommended that the moving-vehicle portions of a driver evaluation employ two staff members, the **driver instructor/educator** and the **driving evaluator/observer.** The driving instructor, a state-licensed instructor or a therapist with special training, sits in the front passenger seat,[2,15] and the driving evaluator sits in the back seat. The driving instructor tells the patient where to drive, instructs in the use of adaptive driving equipment, maintains vehicle control by intervening when necessary, and keeps the vehicle occupants safe by adhering to laws and rules of the road. The evaluator observes the task of driving, takes written notes, and completes a scoring sheet. The driving instructor and evaluator work as a team, and both must be able to implement driving and equipment modification recommendations. A standardized or consistent score sheet to rate drivers is recommended for objectivity and data comparison.

### *Driving Route*

Driving routes should include a sampling of road conditions, traffic patterns, and unusual settings common to the region. The assessment route needs to progress through faster and more congested traffic and various traffic conditions to obtain information on the driver's skills in various conditions. The driving route should be graded and should allow the patient time to become familiar with the evaluation vehicle and adaptive equipment. This period of learning and accommodation will be longer for novice or apprehensive drivers. Driving performance scores should reflect physical handling of the vehicle, ability to use the adaptive equipment,[1] interaction with other traffic, adherence to rules of the road, and safety judgment.[6,13,16]

### *Recommendations for Driving*

After the drive test is completed, the driving team reviews the results with the patient. Asking the patient for feedback first provides valuable perspective on the patient's insight. All recommendations for driving should be made in writing to the patient and submitted for inclusion in the medical record. The comprehensive driving report[14]:

> . . . shall contain a summary of the clinical assessment and a statement of the client's potential to be a safe and independent driver. The report should specify the type of vehicle which is necessary, the modifications required, other adaptive equipment required, vendor sources, and special instructions or problems. The report shall make recommendations on the type of follow-up required, what to look for, and who is best suited to provide the follow-up services. The report should also estimate the amount of driver's training needed, what specific areas of training should be emphasized, and where the training is available.

### *Unsafe Driver*

One of the most difficult tasks facing a driver evaluator is notifying a driver candidate and the family that the person is not safe to drive. The decision to rate a driver as unsafe immediately raises dependency and transportation issues that have no easy solution. Clinicians must develop the skill of listening to the driver's response and frustration while remaining united in the decision. Referring the driver to the motor vehicle department for a photo identification card and providing materials on alternative transportation, such as mass transit or paratransit systems, are other means of assisting the patient at the current level of functioning.

## LEGAL ISSUES AND PUBLIC POLICY

### State Laws Pertaining to Occupational Therapy

Occupational therapy practitioners and physicians need to be aware of their state's laws concerning medical conditions and driving. Most states do not require the reporting of medical conditions, seizures, or loss of consciousness to the motor vehicle department.[8,10,16] Instead, most states rely on voluntary reporting of medical conditions by the driver. Although some states advocate reporting by family, physician, or law enforcement, not all states provide immunity for such reporting. Once identified to the motor vehicle department, the patient undergoes a license review that varies from state to state.

Laws affecting the legality of the OTR or COTA in the driver instructor role also vary by state. Some states allow the clinician to conduct training without being a licensed driver trainer. Other states allow OTRs to perform the driver instructor role legally for evaluations only, whereas ongoing driver instructor training requires the state driver instructor license. Practitioners must know their state's regulations and not exceed them. All clinicians involved in such programs should seek additional education and training to minimize liability and ensure skills that meet industry standards.

### Public Policy Development

Department of motor vehicle medical advisory boards have been reactivated across the United States in response to public safety concerns and policy needs. As occupational therapy practitioners start to be recognized for their expertise and contributions in driver safety, more OTRs are being appointed to medical advisory boards in the 50 states. Therapists add a valuable functionally based perspective to driver evaluation that aids sound development of public policy and licensing decisions.

## SUMMARY

Driving is a valued and necessary ADL for most adults in the United States and other industrialized countries. Occupational therapy practitioners may provide driver evaluation and training and equipment recommendations to enable persons with physical disabilities to resume or acquire the ability to drive.

## *Selected Reading Guide Questions*

1. List the four stages of swallowing and the characteristics of each.
2. Describe the voluntary and reflex aspects of the swallow.
3. List the physiological functions that occur when the swallow reflex triggers, and explain why these functions are necessary.
4. Why is it necessary for the OTR to assess a patient's mental status during a dysphagia evaluation?
5. List signs of poor oral sensory awareness that can be easily observed.
6. Why does the evaluating OTR listen for voice quality after a swallow?
7. List the acute symptoms of aspiration.
8. Describe the position in which the dysphagic patient should be treated, and give the rationale for this position.
9. Describe how to perform oral hygiene with a dysphagic patient.
10. Why is oral hygiene so important for the dysphagic patient?
11. Name five important criteria that a patient must meet to participate in an oral feeding program.
12. List the properties of food preferred for dysphagic patients' diets. List properties of food that would be inappropriate.
13. If a patient has no difficulty handling solids, does this mean that the patient can handle liquids easily as well? Explain.
14. Describe how poor hand-to-mouth movements affect the patient's swallow.
15. Why is it important to involve the patient in the eating process?
16. Discuss ways to reduce impulsivity during eating in the dysphagic patient.
17. Explain why universal precautions are required in dysphagia treatment.
18. Explain why those involved in dysphagia treatment should know basic first aid.
19. Describe how food intake of the dysphagic patient should be reported.
20. What are the symptoms of nutritional deficiency?
21. Explain why driving is an important activity.
22. Describe some situations (disabilities, conditions) in which a driving evaluation might be recommended.
23. Describe some of the skills assessed during the driving evaluation.
24. What is meant by a *predriving task?* Give several examples.

25. For what conditions might a hand control for accelerator and brake be used?
26. What is the ideal staffing for the road test portion of the driving evaluation?
27. List six physical and performance skills that can help to determine driving potential.

## REFERENCES


**Section I**

1. Alta Bates Hospital, Rehabilitation Services: *Dysphagia evaluation and treatment protocol,* Berkeley, Calif, 1990, The Hospital.
2. American Occupational Therapy Association: *AOTA resource guide: feeding and dysphagia,* Rockville, Md, 1994, The Association.
3. Avery-Smith W: Management of neurologic disorders: the first feeding session. In Groher M, editor: *Dysphagia: diagnosis and management,* ed 2, Stoneham, Mass, 1992, Butterworth-Heinemann.
4. Avery-Smith W, Dellaosa D: Approaches to treating dysphagia in patients with brain injury, *Am J Occup Ther* 48:236, 1994.
5. Bobath B: *Adult hemiplegia: evaluation and treatment,* ed 2, London, 1978, Heinemann.
6. Buchholz D, Bosma J, Donner M: Adaption, compensation, and decompensation of the pharyngeal swallow, *Gastrointest Radiol* 10:235, 1985.
7. Community Hospital Los Gatos–Saratoga: *Rehabilitation Services dysphagia protocol,* Los Gatos, Calif, 1992, The Hospital.
8. Coombes K: *Swallowing dysfunction in hemiplegia and head injury.* Four-day course presented by International Clinical Educators, 1986/1987, Los Gatos, Calif.
9. Daniels L, Worthington C: *Muscle testing,* ed 5, Philadelphia, 1986, Saunders.
10. Davies P: *Steps to follow,* New York, 1985, Springer-Verlag.
11. Farber S: *Neurorehabilitation: a multisensory approach,* Philadelphia, 1982, Saunders.
12. Griggs B: Nursing management of swallowing disorders. In Groher M, editor: *Dysphagia: diagnosis and management,* ed 2, Stoneham, Mass, 1992, Butterworth-Heinemann.
13. Groher M: Bolus management and aspiration pneumonia with pseudobulbar dysphagia, *Dysphagia* 1:215, 1987.
14. Groher M, Asher I: Establishing a swallowing program. In Groher M, editor: *Dysphagia: diagnosis and management,* Stoneham, Mass, 1984, Butterworth.
15. Kendall H, Kendall F, Wadsworth G: *Muscles: testing and function,* Baltimore, 1971, Williams & Wilkins.
16. Logemann J: *Evaluation and treatment of swallowing disorders,* San Diego, 1983, College-Hill.
17. Logemann J: *Manual for the videofluorographic study of swallowing,* ed 2, Austin, Tex, 1993, Pro-Ed.
18. Martin BJW: Treatment of dysphagia in adults. In Cherney L, editor: *Clinical management of dysphagia in adults and children,* Gaithersburg, Md, 1994, Aspen.
19. Meadowbrook Neurologic Care Center, Rehabilitation Services: *Dysphagia protocol,* San Jose, Calif, 1986, The Center (unpublished).
20. Miller A: The search for the central swallowing pathway: the quest for clarity, *Dysphagia* 8:189, 1993.
21. Nelson K: Dysphagia: evaluation and treatment. In Pedretti LW, editor: *Occupational therapy: practice skills for physical dysfunction,* ed 4, St Louis, 1995, Mosby.
22. Pillsbury H, Buckwalter J: Surgical intervention in dysphagia. In Groher M, editor: *Dysphagia: diagnosis and management,* Stoneham, Mass, 1984, Butterworth.
23. Rader T, Rende B: *Swallowing disorders: what families should know,* Tucson, Ariz, 1993, Communication Skill Builders.
24. Silverman EH, Elfant IL: Dysphagia: an evaluation and treatment program for the adult, *Am J Occup Ther* 33:382, 1979.

**Section II**

1. Babirad J: Considerations in seating and positioning severely disabled drivers, *Assist Technol* 1:31-37, 1989.
2. Blanc C, Hunt JT: Getting in gear, *Team Rehabil Rep,* August 1994, pp 33-39.
3. Bouska MJ, Gallaway M: Primary visual deficits in adults with brain damage: management in occupational therapy, *Occup Ther Pract* 3:1-11, 1991.
4. Breske S: The drive for independence, *Adv Rehabil* 3:10-19, 1994.
5. *Graduated driver licensing creating mobility choices,* PF5078 (793)·cdD15109, Washington, DC, 1993, American Association of Retired Persons.
6. Janke MK: *Age-related disabilities that may impair driving and their assessment,* Sacramento, Calif, 1994, State of California Department of Motor Vehicles.
7. Latson LF: Overview of disabled drivers' evaluation process, *Phys Disabil Special Interest Sect Newslett* 10(4), 1987.
8. Lillie SM: Evaluation for driving. In Yoshikawa TT, Cobbs EL, Brummel-Smith K, editors: *Ambulatory geriatric care,* St Louis, 1993, Mosby.
9. Odenheimer GL: *Cognitive dysfunction and driving abilities.* Presentation to the Annual Meeting of the American Geriatrics Society, Atlanta, May 18, 1990.
10. Odenheimer GL et al: Performance-based driving evaluation of the elderly driver: safety, reliability, and validity, *J Gerontol Med Sci* 49:M153-M159, 1994.
11. Perr A, Barnicle K: Van lifts the ups and downs and ins and outs, *Team Rehabil Rep,* June 1993, pp 49-53.
12. Roush L, Koppa R: *A survey of activation: importance of individual secondary controls in modified vehicles,* College Station, Tex, 1992, Human Factors Program, Safety Division, Texas Transportation Institute, Texas A&M University.
13. Sabo S, Shipp M: *Disabilities and their implications for driving,* Ruston, La, 1989, Center for Rehabilitation Sciences and Biomedical Engineering, Louisiana Tech University.
14. *Statement of assurances for providers of driver evaluation services,* Downey, Calif, 1990, State of California Department of Rehabilitation Mobility Evaluation Program.
15. Strano CM: Driver evaluation and training of the physically disabled driver: additional comments, *Phys Disabil Special Interest Sect Newslett* 10(4), 1987.
16. Summary of Proceedings of the Conference on Driver Competency Assessment, CAL-DMV-RSS-91-132, Sacramento, 1993, Program and Policy Administration, Research and Development Section, State of California Department of Motor Vehicles.
17. Taira ED, editor: *Assessing the driving ability of the elderly,* Binghamton, NY, 1989, Hayworth.

Chapter 20

# Balanced Forearm Orthosis and Suspension Sling

*Carole Adler*
*Lorraine Williams Pedretti*

## Chapter Objectives

*After studying this chapter, the student or practitioner will be able to:*

1. Describe the purposes and applications of the balanced forearm orthosis (BFO).
2. Describe the necessary range of motion and other functions needed for a patient to operate the BFO.
3. Describe the parts of the BFO and their interrelationships.
4. Explain how the BFO works to extend the power of a patient's movements.
5. Recognize the proper positioning and checkout procedure for the BFO.
6. Sequence the training activities for using the BFO.
7. Describe the purposes and applications of the suspension sling.
8. Describe the parts of the suspension sling and their interrelationships.

## Key Terms

balanced forearm orthosis
bracket assembly
proximal swivel arm
distal swivel arm
rocker arm assembly
forearm trough
suspension sling
suspension spring or strap
cuffs

Some patients want to perform activities of daily living (ADLs), such as feeding or brushing teeth, but do not have sufficient strength to lift their hands to their mouths. Two devices, the balanced forearm orthosis and the suspension sling, can be used to amplify or increase the limited strength and motion of such patients and enable them to do these and other table-top activities. Both devices support the upper extremity in a plane parallel to the floor. They facilitate useful upper extremity motion in patients with significant muscle weakness.

## BALANCED FOREARM ORTHOSES

The **balanced forearm orthosis** (BFO) is sometimes called a *mobile arm support* or a *ball-bearing feeder.*[5] Usually mounted on the wheelchair, it can also be mounted on a table or working surface. The BFO consists of a trough that supports the user's forearm and a pivot-and-linkage system under the trough. This system can be preset and adjusted for the user to produce elbow and shoulder motion with only slight motions of the trunk or shoulder girdle[1] (Figure 20-1).

The BFO must be adjusted so that gravity can assist weak muscles. Various adjustments are possible and are individualized to suit the patient's needs. The BFO provides assistance for shoulder and elbow movement by using gravity to aid lost muscle power. It provides a large, usable arm range of motion (ROM) that would otherwise not be available to the patient. The BFO helps support, assist, and strengthen weakened musculature and enables patients to perform simple ADLs and leisure activities that they normally could not perform.[5]

### Candidates for Use

Generally, those patients with disabilities that result in muscle weakness, such as poliomyelitis, cervical spinal cord injuries, Guillain-Barré syndrome, muscular dystrophy, and amyotrophic lateral sclerosis, are candidates for BFOs. The BFO is used to increase function in patients who have moderate to severe muscle weakness in the upper extremities (muscle grades trace [1] to fair [3] at the elbow and the shoulder) and limited endurance for sustained movement.[6]

The patient must have a source of muscle power to initiate movement of the BFO. This may be at the trunk or shoulder. The patient should have adequate, pain-free ROM as follows[6]:

1. Shoulder flexion to 90°, abduction to 90°, external rotation to 30°, and internal rotation to 80°
2. Elbow flexion from 0° to 140°
3. Full forearm pronation from midposition and supination to midposition
4. Hip flexion from 0° to 95°, required for the upright sitting position

The patient must have sufficient coordination to control and cope with movement of the freely swinging arms of the BFO. Involuntary movement, such as spasticity, significantly interferes with voluntary control of the upper extremity. The relatively free movement of the BFO can actually increase involuntary movement.[6] An involuntary spasm in a trunk muscle, for example, may send the arm swinging wildly.

A consistently stable sitting posture and good body alignment are key factors in the successful use of the BFO. Adequate trunk and neck stability must be provided by the patient's own muscle power or by outside support. The BFO works best when the patient is sitting in an upright position with the trunk in midline. Ease and effectiveness of use decrease as the patient reclines.[6] The patient must have adequate balance and sitting tolerance and sufficient "gadget tolerance"[5] to engage in the training program and make use of the BFO worthwhile.[2] Because the BFO increases the overall width of a wheelchair, it is not functional for passing through standard-width doors.

The patient must possess sufficient motivation and adequate frustration tolerance to persevere at the BFO training program until use is mastered.[2] It is important that the patient know the purpose in using the BFO. Motivation to take care of personal needs, eat independently, enjoy avocational activities, or operate a power wheelchair (tasks that would otherwise be impossible) can help the patient to accept and master the BFO. Successful experience with the BFO can also be a motivating factor.[5,6] The patient and occupational therapy practitioner should be aware that the BFO elicits active motion that will strengthen muscles and that the device may not be required for long-term or permanent use.[6]

### Parts and Their Functions

There are several types of BFOs. Figure 20-2 shows the most frequently used parts of a standard BFO. Addi-

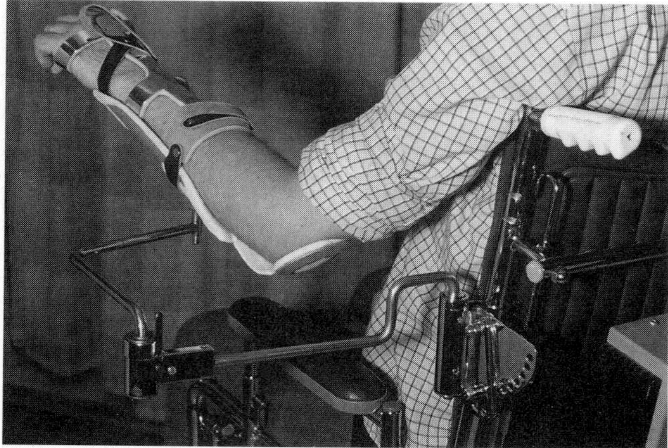

*Figure 20-1* Balanced forearm orthosis (BFO) mounted on wheelchair with patient's arm positioned in forearm trough.

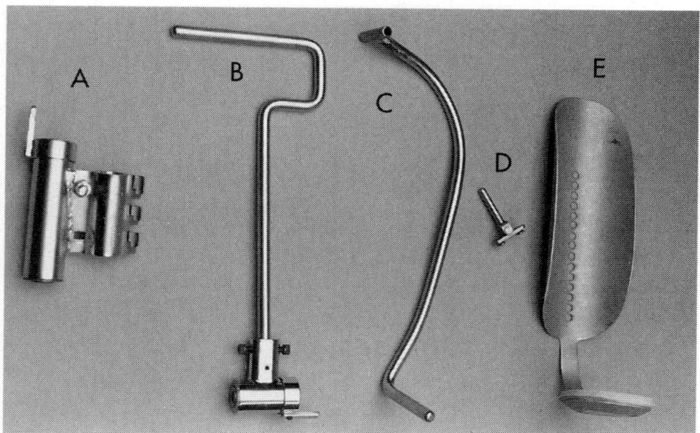


*Figure 20-2* Parts of BFO. **A,** Bracket assembly with stop; **B,** proximal swivel arm and proximal ball-bearing housing with stop; **C,** distal swivel arm; **D,** rocker arm assembly; **E,** forearm trough.

tional attachments and assisting devices are available to suit individual needs.[5,6] The semireclining, adjustable **bracket assembly** holds the BFO to the wheelchair. It supports the proximal (nearest to patient's shoulder and to wheelchair) arm. The bracket can be positioned to control the height of the BFO. It can be adjusted to assist horizontal movement at the shoulder and elbow. It may be adapted for use by a patient in the reclining position, but the upright position is most desired.[2,6]

The standard **proximal swivel arm** permits horizontal abduction and horizontal adduction at the shoulder and contains the distal ball bearings. Both the bracket assembly and the proximal ball-bearing housing have stops that can be set at any position on the circumference of the housing unit to limit horizontal motion. The proximal ball-bearing housing on the proximal swivel arm can also be tilted so that gravity assists elbow flexion or extension.[6] An additional option, the *proximal elevating arm* (Figure 20-3), is used for active assistance with shoulder abduction and flexion in the patient with anterior or middle deltoids with a strength grade of fair or 3. A rubber band assist facilitates this action.

The **distal swivel arm,** which can be used with either the standard proximal or the proximal elevating arm, permits forearm motion in the horizontal plane. It supports the rocker arm assembly and forearm trough.

The **rocker arm assembly** is attached to the forearm trough. It is positioned on the distal swivel arm and permits vertical (hand-to-mouth) motions. It swivels to produce added horizontal motion.

The **forearm trough** supports the forearm. It provides stable elbow support but may limit elbow extension. The elbow dial can be bent to produce adjustments for comfort and vertical motion.[6] Figure 20-4 shows the assembled BFO.

### How the Balanced Forearm Orthosis Works

The patient must have adequate voluntary muscle power to activate the BFO. Some source of power at the neck, trunk, shoulder girdle, shoulder, or elbow may serve alone or in combination to operate the BFO. Some controlling muscle in both elbow and shoulder is necessary if the user is to have control of motions in the horizontal plane across the midline of the body.[6]

The BFO allows horizontal and vertical motions. The device assists horizontal motions across the table top (e.g., assembling a jigsaw puzzle, playing chess). To assist horizontal motion, the bracket assembly and the proximal ball-bearing housing on the proximal swivel arm can be adjusted to produce an inclined plane in the direction of horizontal abduction or horizontal adduction, according to need. Gravity assists motion to the low point in the plane. Muscular effort must be exerted to return the arm to the high point of the plane.[6]

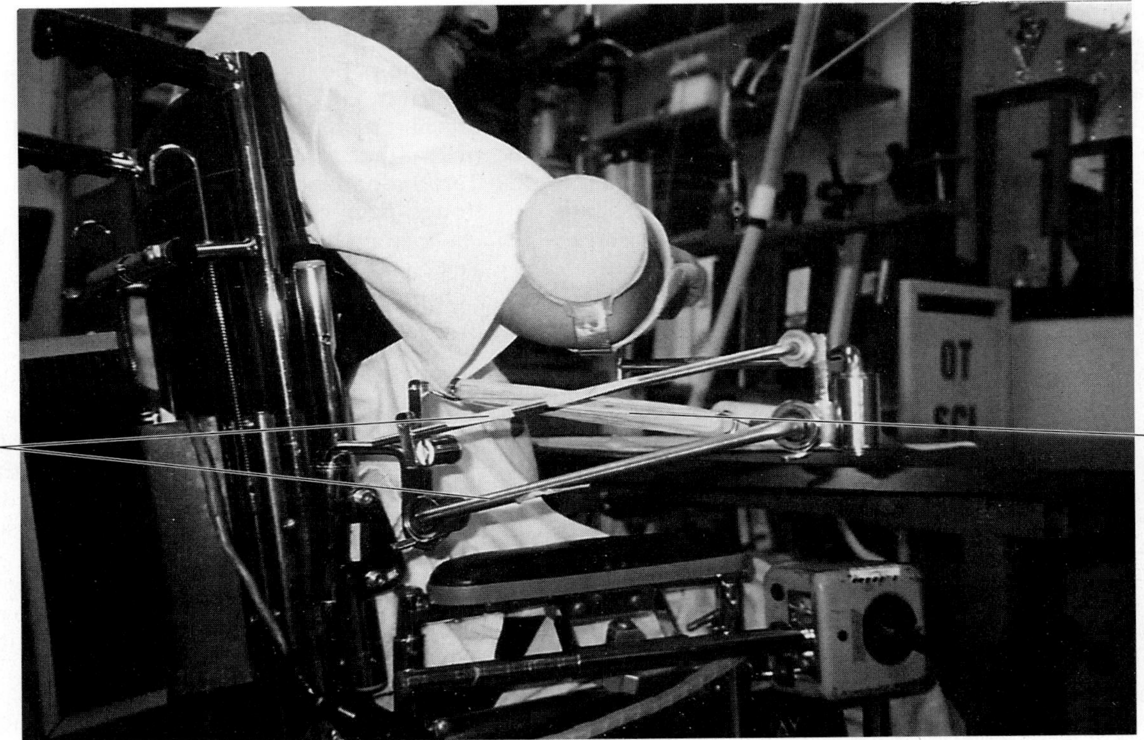


*Figure 20-3* Proximal elevating arm for BFO.

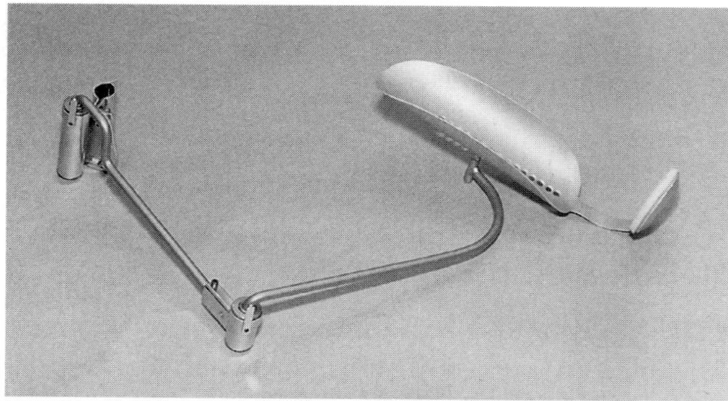

*Figure 20-4* Assembled BFO arm support.

Vertical movement allows table-top-to-face activity (e.g., feeding). Adjustments for vertical motions are somewhat more complex. Several holes along the underside of the forearm trough allow the rocker arm to be positioned toward or away from the elbow. The rocker arm assembly acts as a fulcrum for the forearm trough, which acts as a lever. The rocker arm assembly (fulcrum) can be adjusted to the most effective position for the patient. Any force applied by the user proximal to the fulcrum lifts the weight of the hand and anything in the hand toward the face. The distance of the fulcrum from the elbow will determine whether the mechanical advantage is on the load side (hand) or force side (elbow) of the lever.[6] Shoulder elevation and depression are used to carry out the vertical motions of the forearm trough.

### Adjustment and Checkout

Before adjusting the BFO, the occupational therapy practitioner must find the best position for the patient in the wheelchair, choose the correct bracket assembly for the arm being fitted (because the right and left are not interchangeable), and set the bracket's height. The bracket is positioned so that the forearm trough rides at a height that allows the patient to accomplish the desired motions, bringing the hand as close as possible to the mouth, without pushing the shoulders into elevation. The bracket must be tightened to the wheelchair so that it will not slip down under the weight of the assembly and the patient's arm.

The forearm trough is then fitted to the patient. It is balanced so that it permits maximal range and force in vertical motion. The bracket is adjusted to allow maximal range and force in horizontal motion at the glenohumeral joint. The OT practitioner must then tilt the distal bearing, if necessary, to produce the maximal range and force in horizontal motion at the elbow joint. The therapist or assistant should then reevaluate range and force of combined horizontal motions of the glenohumeral and elbow joints and reevaluate the vertical motion of the trough. Some patients may require special attachments, such as straps, to stabilize the forearm in the trough.[6]

Specific questions can serve as a guide for the OT practitioner to determine the correctness of fit and adjustments of the BFO and include the following[3]:

1. Are the hips set back in the chair?
2. Is the spine in good vertical alignment?
3. Is there good lateral trunk stability?
4. Are the chair seat and back adequate for comfort and stability?
5. Is the patient able to sit upright?
6. If the patient wears hand splints, are they on? (Splints add weight and change the balance of the forearm trough.)
7. Does the patient have adequate passive ROM?
8. Is the bracket tight on the wheelchair and positioned perpendicular to the floor?
9. Is the bracket at the proper height so that the shoulders are not forced into elevation?
10. Is the proximal arm all the way down in the bracket?
11. Does the elbow dial clear the lap or lapboard surface when the trough is in the up position?
12. When the trough is in the up position, is the hand as close to the mouth as possible?
13. Can the patient obtain maximal active reach?
14. Is the trough the correct length? Does the distal end of the trough stop at the wrist joint?
15. Are the trough edges rolled so that they do not contact the forearm?
16. Is the elbow secure and comfortable in the elbow support?
17. Is the trough balanced correctly?
18. In vertical motion, is the dial free of the distal arm?
19. Can the patient control motion of the proximal arm from either extreme?
20. Can the patient control motion of the distal arm from either extreme?
21. Can the patient control vertical motion of the trough from either extreme?
22. Have stops been applied to limit ROM, if necessary?
23. Can the patient lift a sufficient amount of weight to perform appropriate functional tasks?

### Training in Use

The clinician should ensure that the BFO fits well and is correctly adjusted before attempting to instruct the patient in its use. If bilateral BFOs are used, the patient should practice with one at a time until each is mastered separately. Coordinated bilateral use of BFOs requires considerable practice.

Training in vertical motions (achieved by external and internal rotation of the shoulder) is usually given first. The patient may initiate external rotation by performing any of the following actions:

- Depressing the shoulder to elevate the hand
- Shifting the body weight to the side of the BFO
- Rolling the shoulder back

- Tilting or turning the head toward the side of the device
- Leaning backward

Internal rotation is accomplished by gravity or by the following:

- Elevating the shoulder on the same side as the BFO
- Shifting the body weight to the opposite side from the device
- Rolling the shoulder forward
- Tilting and turning the head to the opposite side from the BFO
- Leaning forward

Horizontal adduction and abduction are taught next, with the trough balanced at midposition. Then the patient can proceed to practice these motions with the trough at various heights between table top and head. Practice progresses to include elbow flexion and extension with the trough at various heights. Activities that may be practiced with BFOs include arm-driven power wheelchair propulsion, typing or computer work, turning book pages, using the phone, grooming, performing hygiene activities at the sink, and playing games (e.g., checkers, cards, puzzles).

The BFO helps the patient with upper extremity weakness make maximal use of minimal muscle power. Once assembled, fitted, and adjusted, the BFO enables the patient to perform a variety of self-care and leisure activities that promote self-esteem and independence. (See References for more comprehensive discussion of BFOs and their use.[2,5,6])

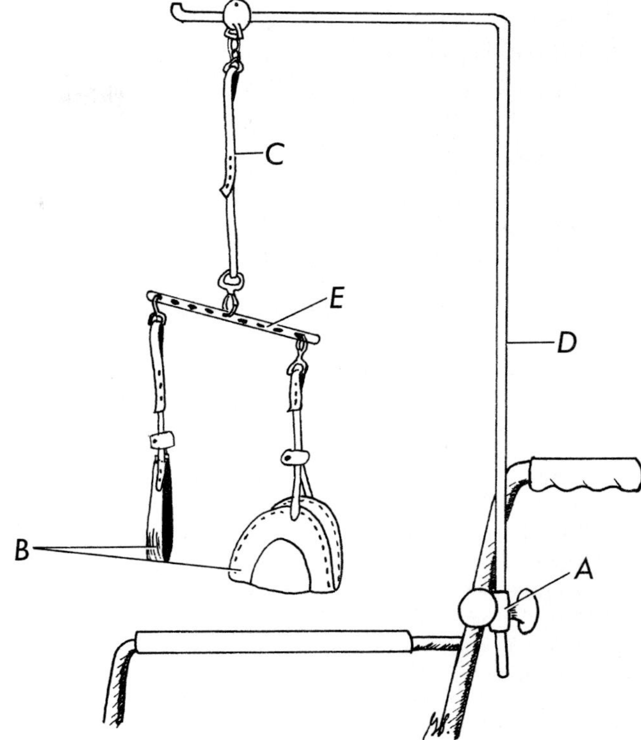


*Figure 20-5* Parts of suspension sling. **A,** Bracket; **B,** arm cuff; **C,** suspension strap; **D,** suspension rod; **E,** horizontal supporting device for cuffs. (Modified from Occupational Therapy Department, Rancho Los Amigos Hospital, Downey, Calif.)

## SUSPENSION SLINGS

The **suspension sling** reduces the effect of gravity by supporting the forearm in a plane parallel to the floor. The suspension sling is used to facilitate horizontal movement during activity or exercise (Figure 20-5).[4]

### Parts and Their Functions

A bracket holds the suspension rod to the back of the wheelchair. The bracket must be adjusted to keep the top of the suspension rod parallel to the floor. The height is also adjustable. The suspension sling is hung from the suspension rod with a spring or a strap. The length of the **suspension spring or strap** determines the height of the sling in relation to the patient's body. The suspension spring or strap also swivels to eliminate friction or twisting and to allow maximal mobility. If a spring suspension is used, it adds to the amount of motion that the patient can produce in the sling but may decrease coordination.

The **cuffs** of the suspension sling are fastened to a horizontal bar that has holes along its entire length. These allow the cuffs of the sling to be placed for optimal balance to assist vertical or horizontal motions of the arm. A *forearm trough,* as used on the balanced forearm orthosis, is sometimes substituted for the arm cuffs shown in Figure 20-5, in which case the assembly is referred to as a *suspension feeder.*[4]

### Applications

In many instances the suspension sling can be used with patients who have the same diagnoses as previously cited, although somewhat greater muscle power and control are required for effective use. Training in the use of the suspension sling may begin with enabling exercises to establish patterns of horizontal abduction and adduction, hand-to-body movements, and hand-to-face movements. Use may then progress to activities, such as eating, performing hygiene activities at the sink, table-top communication skills, and leisure activities.

## SUMMARY

The balanced forearm orthosis (BFO) and the suspension sling are devices that assist movements of the upper extremity. Properly fitted and positioned, these devices increase functional capacities of patients who have weakness in the shoulder. Given adequate training, the COTA may be expected to position, adjust, and fit these devices.

## Selected Reading Guide Questions

1. Which patients are good candidates for use of the BFO in terms of disability or muscle grades?
2. Which patients are poor candidates for use of the BFO? Why?
3. List the five criteria a patient must meet to use the BFO successfully.
4. What activities can be performed with the BFO?
5. List the three major steps in training the patient to use the BFO.
6. List two ways shoulder external rotation motion can be accomplished.
7. List two ways shoulder internal rotation motion can be accomplished.
8. What are some suitable activities for practicing use of the BFO?
9. What is the primary purpose of the suspension sling?
10. List three purposeful activities that may be performed by patients with significant upper extremity dysfunction while using a suspension sling. Think of others not listed in the text.
11. When is a proximal elevating arm the appropriate choice for a patient?

### REFERENCES


1. Bender LF: Upper extremity orthotics. In Kottke FJ, Lehmann JF: *Krusen's handbook of physical medicine and rehabilitation,* ed 4, Philadelphia, 1990, Saunders.
2. Dicus RG: *Mobile arm supports.* Part 1 (film), Downey, Calif, 1970, SRS Service Department, Rancho Los Amigos Hospital. (Available from the Instructional Resources Center, San Jose State University.)
3. Rancho Los Amigos Hospital: Check-out sheet for feeders. In Marshall E: *Occupational therapy management of physical dysfunction,* Loma Linda, Calif, 1981, Department of Occupational Therapy, School of Allied Health Professions, Loma Linda University.
4. Rancho Los Amigos Hospital: Suspension feeders and slings: parts and their functions. In Marshall E: *Occupational therapy management of physical dysfunction,* Loma Linda, Calif, 1981, Department of Occupational Therapy, School of Allied Health Professions, Loma Linda University.
5. Thenn JE: *Mobile arm support: installation and use,* San Jose, Calif, 1975 (self-published).
6. Wilson DJ, McKenzie MW, Barber LM: *Spinal cord injury: a treatment guide for occupational therapists,* rev ed, Thorofare, NJ, 1984, Slack.

# Chapter 21

# Electronic Assistive Technologies

*Albert M. Cook*
*Susan M. Hussey*

## Chapter Objectives

*After studying this chapter, the student or practitioner will be able to:*

1. Define *assistive technology.*
2. Describe the human activity assistive technology (HAAT) model.
3. Understand the transdisciplinary nature of assistive technology service delivery.
4. List and describe steps in the assistive technology service delivery process.
5. Describe the characteristics of control interfaces.
6. Identify and define the basic selection methods.
7. Identify technologies for direct selection and indirect selection.
8. List the major components of a personal computer system, and give the functions of each.
9. Describe standard adaptations of both input and output to enable computer operation by patients with a variety of disabilities.
10. Describe a variety of augmentative and alternative communication methods.
11. Describe the functions, components, and possible configurations of an environmental control system.

## Key Terms

assistive technology device
human activity assistive technology (HAAT) model
human/technology interface
environmental interface
control interface
selection set
direct selection
indirect selection
command line interface (CLI)
graphical user interface (GUI)
general input device emulating interface (GIDEI)
screen reader
augmentative and alternative communication (AAC)
rate enhancement
semantic encoding
environmental control unit (ECU)

This chapter discusses electronic assistive devices and the role they play in the lives of persons with disabilities. The key to successful application of electronic assistive devices for disabled persons is a thorough understanding of the individual's needs, the context in which the technology will be used, and the skills the person brings to the task.

## WORKING DEFINITION OF ASSISTIVE TECHNOLOGIES

One widely used definition of assistive technologies is provided in Public Law (PL) 100-407, the Technical Assistance to the States Act in the United States. The definition of an **assistive technology device** follows:

> Any item, piece of equipment or product system, whether acquired commercially off the shelf, modified, or customized, that is used to increase or improve functional capabilities of individuals with disabilities.

This definition has also been incorporated into other U.S. legislation and is used in other countries as well. Note that the definition includes commercial, modified, and customized devices. Products made for the general population are covered. The definition also emphasizes *functional* capabilities of *individuals* with disabilities.

## FRAMEWORK FOR APPLYING ASSISTIVE TECHNOLOGIES

A person with a disability who is faced with an activity in a given context may require assistive technologies to facilitate performance. The model shown in Figure 21-1 illustrates the **human activity assistive technology (HAAT) model.**[12] In this model, assistive technology (AT) interacts with the human (H) and the chosen activity (A) within a specific context. The HAAT model and its four interacting elements form the framework for this discussion of electronic assistive technologies.

Each of the elements shown in Figure 21-1 plays a unique part in the total assistive technology system. The development of a system begins with a need by the person to perform an *activity* (e.g., cooking, writing, playing tennis). This defines the goal of the assistive technology system. Each activity is carried out within a *context.* The context includes social and cultural aspects as well as environments and physical conditions (e.g., temperature, noise level, lighting). The combination of the activity and the context determines which *human* skills are required to achieve the specified needs and goals. When human skills to complete a task are lacking, the occupational therapy practitioner determines ways to make adaptations so that the desired goal is achieved. Electronic assistive technologies may be used as part of this adaptation, matched to the person's individual capabilities and then used to accomplish the desired activity.

Figure 21-2 illustrates the forces and flow of information between the assistive technology and the other elements of the HAAT model. The **human/technology interface** represents the relationship between the human and the assistive technology and is the boundary between these two parts of the HAAT model. The human/technology interface is two-way; that is, information may be directed from the human to the technology, or vice versa. Through the human/technology interface the person sends information to the *processor,* then to the *activity output* component. The processor translates this information into signals that

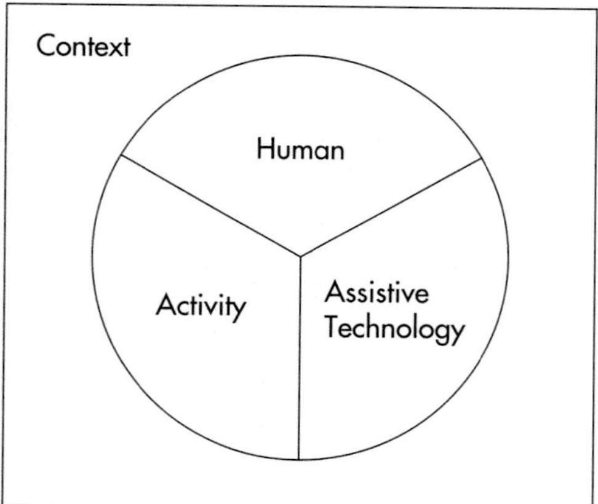


*Figure 21-1* The Human Activity Assistive Technology (HAAT) Model. (From Cook AM, Hussey SM: *Assistive technologies: principles and practice,* St Louis, 1995, Mosby.)

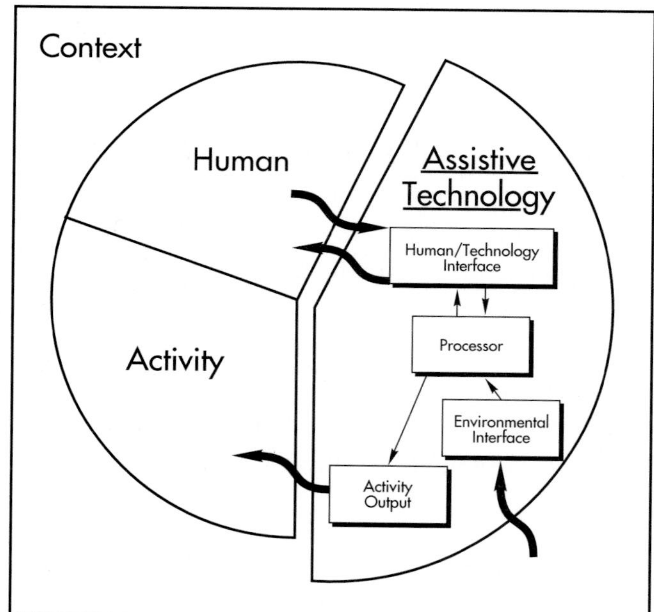


*Figure 21-2* Flow of information between assistive technologies and other elements of HAAT model. (From Cook AM, Hussey SM: *Assistive technologies: principles and practice,* St Louis, 1995, Mosby.)

control the activity output. Assistive technologies such as sensory aids must also be capable of detecting external environmental data through an **environmental interface.** The external data are interpreted and formatted by the processor and communicated to the user through the human/technology interface. Not all assistive technologies have all the components shown in Figure 21-2. However, all electronic assistive technologies have three, and usually they have either the activity output or the environmental sensor.

The following example illustrates the interaction among the components of the HAAT model.[12] Tony needs to write reports. Writing is the *activity.* He is required to accomplish this as part of his work, and this specifies part of the *context.* Because of a spinal cord injury, Tony is unable to use his hands, but he is able to speak clearly. A voice recognition system (the assistive technology) is obtained for him. This system allows Tony to use his skills (speaking) to accomplish the activity (writing) by translating what Tony says into computer-recognizable characters. As Tony speaks, the assistive technology recognizes what is said and sends it to the computer as if it had been typed. Since there are other workers in the office, Tony uses a noise-canceling microphone to avoid errors in voice recognition, and he works in a cubicle to avoid bothering other workers. These further define the context of this system. Tony's assistive technology system consists of the activity (writing), the context (at work in a noisy office), the human skills (speaking), and the assistive technology (voice recognition). For any other individual, one or more parts of this system may be different. For example, another person may be able to type, but only with an enlarged keyboard. Another person may need to write at home rather than at work. Thus each assistive technology system is unique.

## SERVICE DELIVERY IN ASSISTIVE TECHNOLOGY

Assistive technology delivery involves many different professionals, including occupational and physical therapy practitioners, speech-language pathologists, special educators, and rehabilitation engineers. Collectively, these professionals are referred to as *assistive technology practitioners* (ATPs). The ATP role could easily be assumed by a certified occupational therapy assistant (COTA) with an interest in electronics and a willingness to acquire the specific technical expertise and network resources required for effective practice in this area.

Figure 21-3 shows the basic process by which assistive technology devices and services are delivered to the consumer.[12] The first step in the service delivery process is *referral and intake.* The consumer has identified a need and contacts an ATP (referral). The ATP then gathers basic information and determines whether a match exists between the type of services provided and the identified needs of the consumer (intake). Funding for the services to be provided is then sought.

If the criteria for intake are met, the *evaluation* phase begins. This differs from the usual occupational therapy evaluation. One of the most important steps in the evaluation process is *needs identification.* It is particularly important that the needs identified be related to the capabilities of potential assistive technologies. The evaluation continues with an assessment of the consumer's sensory, physical, and central-processing skills as they relate to the use of assistive technologies. The primary purpose of assistive tech-

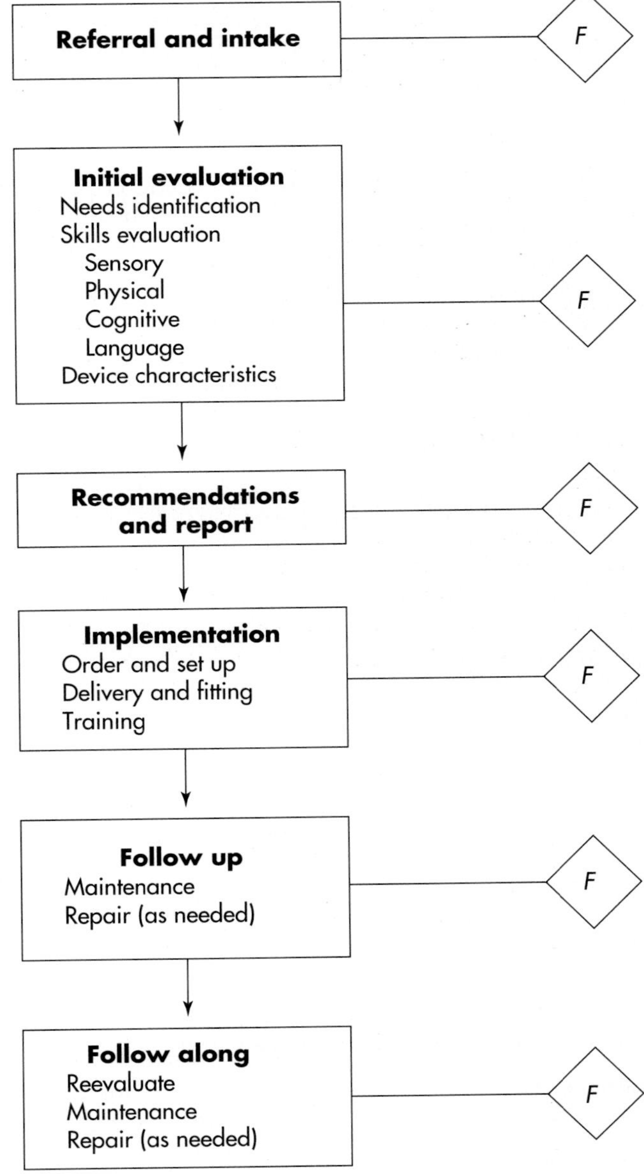


*Figure 21-3* Steps in the assistive technology service delivery process. *F,* At this stage, funding usually requested to continue process. (From Cook AM, Hussey SM: *Assistive technologies: principles and practice,* St Louis, 1995, Mosby.)

nology intervention is not to remediate an impairment, but to *enable* an individual with a disability to be functional in activities of daily living (ADLs) through the provision of hard and soft technologies.

The needs identification and skills evaluation define the activity and human operator portions of the HAAT model. Once these are clearly known, it is possible to match assistive technologies to the consumer's needs and skills. Generally, a trial evaluation of "matched" technologies takes place to ensure that a "match" will lead to effective functional outcomes. This matching process is another distinguishing feature of assistive technology service delivery, and it requires that the assistive technology team be aware of available devices and their characteristics. The evaluation results are summarized, and *recommendations* for technologies are made based on consensus among those involved. A written report is generally prepared for the funding source, school or work site, residence staff or family, and other professionals working with the consumer.

An important part of the report is a description of the plan for acquiring the technologies, installing or setting them up, and training the consumer and care providers. This portion of the service delivery process is often referred to as the *implementation phase.* At this phase the recommended equipment is ordered, modified and fabricated as necessary, then set up and delivered to the consumer. Training for mastery of complex electronic assistive technologies can take many hours of practice and tutoring. The user must come to understand basic operation of the device and to develop strategies for using it effectively.

After completion of training the effectiveness of the system as a whole is evaluated during the *follow-up phase.* This phase focuses on outcomes: to what extent have the established goals (of facilitating or enabling a particular activity) been met through the assistive technology intervention?

In the *follow-along phase* the ATP periodically contacts the consumer to see if further assistive technology intervention is necessary. Over time the consumer's skills, needs, or contexts of use may change, and further assistive technology intervention may be needed. Changes in the technology may also create new opportunities for independence by the consumer. In either case the consumer is brought back to the referral and intake phase, and the process (wholly or partially) is repeated.

## CONTROL INTERFACES FOR ELECTRONIC ASSISTIVE TECHNOLOGIES

Three elements make up the human/technology interface: the control interface, the selection set, and the selection method.[12] The **control interface** communicates from the user to an electronic or mechanical assistive technology device. This is what allows the individual to operate, or control, the device. Control interfaces include joysticks for powered wheelchairs, keyboards for computers and communication devices, and single switches used to control household devices such as lights or radios.

The **selection set** presents items from which the user makes choices. Selection sets may consist of written letters, words and sentences, symbols used to represent ideas, computer icons, or line drawings and pictures. They may be presented in visual (e.g., letters on keys), tactile (e.g., Braille), or auditory (e.g., voice synthesis) form. Selection methods may be either direct or indirect. For any particular application the control interface, selection set, and selection methods should be matched to the consumer's skills (motor, sensory, linguistic, and cognitive).[12]

The fastest and easiest selection method to understand and use is **direct selection.** In this method, each possible choice in the selection set is available at all times, and the user merely chooses the one desired. **Indirect selection** methods were developed to provide access for individuals who lacked the motor skills to use direct selection. Indirect selection methods are scanning, directed scanning, and coded access. Each of the indirect selection methods involves one or more intermediate steps between the consumer's action and the actual selection.

One of the most frequently used methods is *scanning.* In scanning the selection set choices are presented to the user sequentially, and the user indicates a choice when it is presented, usually by a single movement of any body part.

Since sequential scanning is slow, various methods are used to increase the rate of selection. The most common is *group item scanning.* Groups of selection set items are presented first, and the user chooses the group in which the choice appears. The device then presents the items from that group, and the user makes a final choice of the desired item. The scanned items may be arranged in a circle (rotary) or straight line (linear). They also may be placed in a rectangular matrix, which provides a row/column scan. Vanderheiden and Lloyd[25] describe a variety of other scanning strategies. Single-switch scanning depends on good visual tracking skills and the ability to attend and sequence. On the other hand, this type of scanning requires very little motor control to make a selection.

In a combined approach, called *directed scanning,* the user first activates the control interface to select the direction (vertically or horizontally) in which the selection set is scanned by the device. The user then sends a signal to the *processor* to make the selection when the desired choice is reached. This signal may be generated by pausing at the choice (an *acceptance time*) or by activating another control interface to indicate the choice. Joysticks or other switch arrays (two to eight switches) are typically used with directed scanning. This selection approach takes advantage of greater user motor skills (i.e., the ability to move a joystick in one of four directions or activate one of four switches) to increase selection rate.

In *coded access* the individual executes a unique sequence of movements to select a code corresponding to a single item in the selection set. There are several examples of coded access used in assistive technologies. One is Morse code, in which the selection set is the alphabet. An intermediate step (e.g., holding longer "dash" or shorter "dot", or hitting one switch for short and one for long) is necessary to make a selection. Efficiency was a major goal in the development of Morse code for telegraphy. Therefore the shortest codes were assigned to the most frequently used letters (e.g., "e" is one dot, "t" is one dash). This efficiency can be very useful in augmentative communication and computer access.

A second example of coded access applied for computer input is Darci code,* which is based on an eight-way switch code. The eight-way switch is similar to a four-position-switched joystick, with the diagonal positions used as additional switch positions. In this code, letters are generated by moving the switch to specific locations (e.g., to position 2, then to position 1, then to the center) to select a specific letter. This sequence of movements tells the processor what letter has been selected. Since codes are usually memorized, this method does not require that a selection set be visually displayed. This has advantages for persons who have visual limitations. Coded access also requires less physical skill than direct selection, and the timing of the input is under the control of the user rather than the device. However, coded access requires more cognitive skill, especially memory and sequencing, than other methods.

*WesTest Engineering, Bountiful, Ut.

*Control enhancers* extend the person's motor capabilities to allow activation of a control interface. Examples of control enhancers are arm supports, mouthsticks, and head or hand pointers. For example, if a consumer lacks sufficient fine hand control to press the keys on a keyboard, a control enhancer such as a hand pointer may make it possible for the consumer to use the keyboard for direct selection. In other cases a control enhancer such as a mobile arm support may be used to reduce fatigue by making the task physically easier.

### Methods of Activation Used for Control Interfaces

Control interfaces may be classified by the way in which the consumer activates them.[12] Three types of activation are possible: movement, respiration, and phonation (Table 21-1).

*Mechanical control* interfaces (e.g., switches, keyboard keys, joysticks, mouse, trackball) operate the switch directly and represent the largest category of control interfaces. Such switches vary in the anatomical site to be used (some are very specific, others more general), the amount of force required, the sensory feedback provided, and the flexibility with which they can be mounted for easy access by the consumer.

*Electromagnetic control* interfaces operate indirectly, detecting movement at a distance through either light or radio frequency (RF) energy. These interfaces

*Table 21-1*

**Methods of Activation**

| *Signal sent, user action (what the body does)* | *Signal detected* | *Examples* |
|---|---|---|
| 1. Movement (eye, head, tongue, arms, legs) | 1a. Mechanical control interface: activation by the application of a force | 1a. Joystick, keyboard, tread switch |
| | 1b. Electromagnetic control interface: activation by the receipt of electromagnetic energy such as light or radio waves | 1b. Light pointer, light detector, remote radio transmitter |
| | 1c. Electrical control interface: activation by detection of electrical signals from the surface of the body | 1c. Electromyograpic (EMG), electroculographic (EOG), capacitive, or contact switch |
| | 1d. Proximity control interface: activation by a movement close to the detector, but without contact | 1d. Heat-sensitive switches |
| 2. Respiration (inhalation/expiration) | 2. Pneumatic control interface: activation by detection of respiratory airflow or air pressure | 2. Puff and sip |
| 3. Phonation | 3. Sound or voice control interface: activation by the detection of articulated sounds or speech | 3. Sound switch, whistle switch, speech recognition |

From Cook AM, Hussey SM: *Assistive technologies: principles and practice*, St Louis, 1995, Mosby.

include head-mounted light sources or detectors and transmitters used with environmental control systems for remote control.

A third type of movement detection is *electrical.* These detectors are sensitive to electricity generated by the body. Switches of this type require no force; a common example of this type of interface is buttons on some elevators.

Another type of body-generated signal is *respiration* or *ventilation,* which is detected by measuring either airflow or air pressure using what is called a *sip-and-puff switch.* This pneumatic control interface is essentially a mechanical control type of switch, with the air movement providing the force.

Two types of switch arrays are possible. The first is a special construction that allows multiple outputs, such as the eight-way switch described for use with Darci code. The second is a group of single switches mounted to one plate (e.g., two puff-and-sip switches mounted side by side for wheelchair control).

### Control Interfaces for Direct Selection

The most common control interface for direct selection is the *keyboard.* Many different types of keyboards are available, each requiring unique skills. For consumers with limited range of movement and good fine motor control, a contracted keyboard can be more useful than the standard keyboard. Individuals who have difficulty accessing small targets but who have good range of movement may benefit from an expanded keyboard, in which the size of each key can be enlarged up to several inches. Keys can be used individually or redefined to form larger keys. Different keyboard layouts can also be used (e.g., for left-hand-only or right-hand-only typing). The keys can also be made in different sizes and different shapes on the same keyboard.

Touch screens are available on both desk-top and portable computers. The user makes a choice from the selection set by pointing directly to the item on the screen. Because the item is chosen directly by pointing, this method requires less abstract reasoning and may be easier for some consumers.

The other frequently used control interface for direct selection in general-purpose computers is a *mouse.* Alternative pointing interfaces are often used in assistive technologies to replace the mouse. These include the trackball, the head-controlled mouse, the continuous joystick, and the arrow keys on the keypad (called "mouse keys"). In each case a pointer on the screen is moved by changing the position of the pointing device. Once the pointer is moved to the desired item, the user can make a selection either by pausing for a preset time (acceptance time selection) or by pressing a switch (manual selection).

The intensity and clarity of sensory feedback provided by the different pointing devices varies widely and may affect user performance. Successful use of pointing devices requires the user to coordinate eye tracking of the pointer on the screen, with the body site movement operating the screen pointer.

Another alternative to keyboard input is *voice recognition,* in which the individual uses sounds, letters, or words as a selection method. In most systems the voice recognition is *speaker dependent,* and users either "train" the system to recognize their voice by producing several samples of the same sound or word element, or the system adapts to consumers through use.[6] *Speaker-independent* systems recognize speech patterns of different individuals without training.[14] These systems are developed using samples of speech from hundreds of people and information provided by phonologists on the various pronunciations of words. The total recognition vocabulary for such systems is generally small because of the memory required to store speech variations.[6] Voice recognition is used in assistive technology applications for computer access, wheelchair control, and environmental control systems.

### Control Interfaces for Indirect Access

Indirect methods of selection use a single switch or an array of switches and require less motor skill. Most of these switches require mechanical activation. Most often, single switches are activated by the hand, head, arm, leg, or foot. Switch arrays, including some joysticks, are generally activated by hand, foot, or head movement (e.g., chin). Pneumatic switches include puff-and-sip or pillow switches. *Puff-and-sip switches* are activated by blowing air into the switch or sucking air out of it. In some cases the person can vary the amount of air pressure to the switch and generate different commands. *Pillow switches* are activated by squeezing (e.g., with a hand bulb). Some electrical switches detect muscle electrical activity (electromyographic [EMG]) or eye movement (electroculographic [EOG]) through electrodes attached to the skin. Cook and Hussey[12] and Bergen, Presperin, and Tallman[7] describe a variety of interfaces used for indirect selection.

Several selection techniques are employed for scanning. These include *automatic* (user stops cursor at desired element), *step* (user moves cursor one element at a time), and *inverse* (user holds a switch to move cursor and releases it to stop cursor). Each of these places different motor demands on the user, and it is important to match the selection technique to the user's skills.

## COMPUTER ACCESS BY PERSONS WITH DISABILITIES

Computer use by persons with disabilities has opened up new opportunities for education, employment, and recreation. Persons with disabilities use both stand-alone computers (e.g., those used in general business and educational applications) and special-purpose computers built into assistive devices. In both cases the computer offers (1) flexibility (multiple options with the same hardware), (2) adaptability (e.g., as user's skills change over time), (3) customization to a specific user and need (e.g., settings of scanning rate in augmentative communication, acceleration rate on powered wheelchair), (4) specific applications and upgrades can be based on software rather than hardware (e.g., augmentative communication application software and upgrades, specific user profile of speed and acceleration parameters in a powered wheelchair controller).[12]

Despite these advantages, people who have motor and/or sensory impairments often have difficulty using standard stand-alone computers. To use a computer successfully, an individual must have sensory and perceptual abilities for processing computer outputs, motor control for generating input to the computer, and cognitive skills (e.g., problem solving, decision making, memory, language) for understanding the computer functions. When a person with one or more disabilities has difficulty carrying out these functions, the computer can be adapted to facilitate use.

### Personal Computer Basics

Figure 21-4 shows the major functional components of a standard (nonadapted) computer system. The *central processing unit* (CPU) portion of the computer contains the brains of the computer. Through a combination of hardware (electronic circuitry) and software (coded instructions) the CPU can carry out instructions, accept input and send output, and transfer information among the components.

Information, data, and instructions are stored in computers in several ways. Electronic circuits are used for temporary storage (i.e., only as long as the power is on) in *random access memory* (RAM) and permanently in *read-only memory* (ROM). Contained within ROM are the computer's instructions to itself: how to turn itself on, how to power up the video screen, how to recognize input and output devices and commands, and so on.

RAM is a type of temporary memory-holding area. When the computer is turned on, RAM memory is available for use by a word-processing program, for example, and a document or series of documents that the user is working on. The more RAM a computer has, the more types and amount of information that can be available simultaneously (e.g., word-processing program and document, library data base, list of telephone numbers).

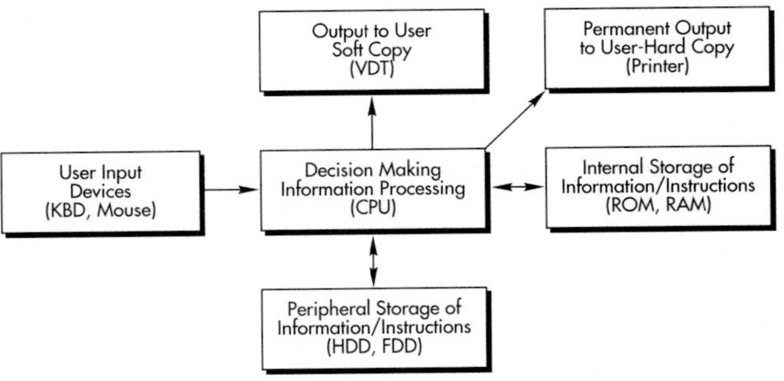


*Figure 21-4* Major functional components of standard (nonadapted) computer system. (From Cook AM, Hussey SM: *Assistive technologies: principles and practice,* St Louis, 1995, Mosby.)

Computers also use storage in magnetic media form in either *floppy disk* (removable) or *hard disk* (permanently mounted in the computer or in a separate hard drive) form. *Compact disk read-only memory* (CD-ROM) uses optical rather than magnetic means to store data. These disks, similar to the CDs used for audio recording, can store music and pictures in addition to very large amounts of data.

Computers do not "know" how to do anything by themselves. They require instructions in the form of *application programs.* These programs may be for word processing, playing a game, performing statistical operations, and so forth. Application programs may be stored on floppy disks or on CD-ROM and generally can be copied onto a hard drive.

The most common user *input* to general-purpose computers is provided through either a keyboard or a mouse. As discussed earlier, many alternatives exist to both these input devices.

User *output* from the computer is typically provided by either a *video display terminal* (VDT), referred to as "soft copy," or *printers,* called "hard copy." Output may also be by network or by modem to another computer or to a fax machine.

A human operator interacts with a computer through a *computer user interface.* A **command line interface (CLI)** uses a marker called a *cursor* (which appears on the VDT) to show where the input information will appear. This interface is ideally suited to short commands and the use of text rather than graphics.[17] The CLI can be slow for individuals who have difficulty with keyboard entry but is easier for individuals who have visual limitations, because all text can be spoken with a voice synthesizer. The CLI is used in the MS-DOS operating system.*

The other common user interface is the **graphical user interface (GUI),** which employs symbols or icons (e.g., a trash can for things to be thrown away), a mouse pointer (instead of the CLI cursor), a menu bar containing tiered choices, and one or more windows from which to select.[17] Entries are made by moving the pointer to a desired item by a mouse or equivalent device and then pressing a button to choose the item. The GUI reduces the number of keyboard entries required because it uses a menu approach from which items are selected as a whole. For persons with limited motor skills, this reduces effort and increases accuracy. The use of icons generally helps with recall and ease of use because the operator does not need to remember as many commands. Icons make it possible for persons who cannot read to use the interface. These features can be very helpful to persons who have difficulty with keyboard entry. However, the GUI environment is not easily converted to voice or tactile output for persons with visual impairments.

*Microsoft, Redmond, Wash.

A *virtual keyboard* is a special-purpose GUI that consists of an image of the keyboard on the video screen. Each screen image "key" is labeled with an alphanumerical character, special character, or function. The user selects a character or function by positioning the cursor inside the desired "key" using a pointing device. Once the cursor is located inside the targeted key, the user makes the selection either by activating another switch or holding the cursor on the choice until it is accepted by the device. A variety of virtual keyboard programs can be used with the Apple IIGS, Macintosh, or IBM-compatible personal computer (PCs).[3,4]

### Adaptations of Computer Inputs

Adapted computer input can be provided in many ways depending on the consumer's needs. Table 21-2 lists the most common problems experienced by patients with disabilities when using a standard keyboard and typical hardware and software solutions. For the IBM and compatible PCs, these software adaptations are included in AccessDOS* and Access Pack for Windows.† For the Apple Macintosh the software adaptations are built into the operating system. Commercial keyboard alternatives, often called *emulators,* use an assisted-keyboard method to accomplish the minimal need shown in Table 21-2.

*IBM, Armonk, NY.
†Microsoft, Redmond, Wash.

The most common alternatives to the standard keyboard are expanded or contracted keyboards and voice recognition. A common alternative to the standard mouse is the use of the arrow keys on the keyboard to move the on-screen pointer. This is listed in Table 21-2 as MouseKeys. Alternative pointing devices such as a trackball, joystick, or head pointer can also be used.

Access for persons who have cognitive difficulties can be increased by using concept keyboards. These keyboards replace the letters and numbers of the keyboard with pictures, symbols, or words that represent the concepts required by the software program. For example, a program designed to teach monetary concepts might use a concept keyboard in which each key is a coin rather than a number or letter. The user can push on the coin to enter that amount.

To use many of the alternative control interfaces for computers (e.g., expanded keyboard or a single switch), a **general input device emulating interface (GIDEI)** is employed. This is a special-purpose processor that translates signals from the control interface into those required for input to the computer. For example, if the computer application requires the use of [ESC] or [DEL] keys, the GIDEI allows the control interface to generate these key commands. Each commercially available GIDEI provides a *setup* that allows the computer to be altered for a given application to match the needs of a specific consumer. The

*Table 21-2*

**Minimal Adaptations to the Standard Keyboard and Mouse**

| *Need addressed* | *Software approach** | *Hardware approach* |
|---|---|---|
| User is not able to "chord" or hold one key while pressing another. | StickeyKeys | Mechanical latch |
| User cannot release key before it starts to repeat. | RepeatKeys | Keyguard |
| User accidentally hits wrong keys. | SlowKeys<br>BounceKeys | Keyguard, template, shield |
| User cannot easily point with hand or finger. | NONE | Typing aid, mouthstick, head pointer |
| User cannot manipulate mouse. | MouseKeys | Trackball, head sensor, joystick |
| User wants to use augmentative communication device as input. | SerialKeys | General input device emulating interface (GIDEI) |

Modified from Cook AM, Hussey SM: *Assistive technologies: principles and practice,* St Louis, 1995, Mosby.
*Software modifications developed at the Trace Center University of Wisconsin, Madison. These are included as before-market modifications to DOS, OS/2, or Windows in some personal computers and are available as after-market versions in others (Macintosh, Apple Computer, Cupertino, Calif; AccessDOS, IBM, Armonk, NY; AccessWindows and AccessDOS, Microsoft, Seattle, Wash. Visual features also included). The functions of StickyKeys, RepeatKeys, and MouseKeys are also built into several GIDEIs. The functions of each program are as follows:

*StickeyKeys:* user can press modifier key, then press second key without holding both down simultaneously.
*RepeatKeys:* user can adjust how long key must be held before it begins to repeat.
*SlowKeys:* delay can be added before the character selected by hitting a key is entered into the computer; thus user can release an incorrect key before it is entered.
*BounceKeys:* prevents double characters from being entered if user bounces on the key when pressing and releasing.
*MouseKeys:* substitutes arrow keys for mouse movements.
*SerialKeys:* allows any serial input to replace mouse and keyboard.

setup consists of three basic elements: (1) an input method, (2) overlays, and (3) a set of options.

As shown in Figure 21-5, each setup is used with an application program.[12] The first example (Figure 21-5, *A*) is intended to be used for text entry in a business environment with word processor, spreadsheet and data base applications. For a single-switch user, the overlay on the screen would be a scanning array with special characters included (Figure 21-5, *B*). The second example setup (Figure 21-5, *C* and *D*) is for a young child who is using any of a wide range of software programs that require selection of an answer by matching a pointer with the correct numbers, letters, shapes, words, or pictures. Often one key (e.g., [RIGHT ARROW]) is used to move the cursor, and another key (e.g., [RETURN]) selects the student's choice. Since the user is likely to be a prereader, the speech overlay helps to identify the possible choices. Speech is also used as a reinforcer when the choice is made. Cook and Hussey[12] describe several commercially available GIDEIs.

### Adaptations of Computer Outputs

Standard visual display devices and printers are often not suitable for persons with visual impairments because the standard size, contrast, and spacing of the displayed information are inadequate. For blind individuals, alternative computer outputs based on audition (hearing) or tactile (feeling) modes are used.

Persons who are deaf or hard of hearing may experience difficulties in recognizing auditory computer outputs such as beeps. Table 21-3 shows adaptations that replace or augment some of these functions and that are included in AccessDOS and AccessWindows.* ToggleKeys uses a beep to replace light indicators on keys such as "CAPS LOCK." SoundSentry replaces auditory tones with flashing lights or cursors. These adaptations are also required by Section 508 of the Rehabilitation Act.

#### *Low Vision Adaptations*

The major problem with visual computer displays for individuals with low (poor) vision is that the text characters and icons are not easily readable. The three factors that affect the readability of text characters are (1) size (vertical height), (2) spacing (horizontal distance between letters and width of letters), and (3) contrast (the relationship of background and foreground color). Brown[10] has identified the capabilities of an ideal low vision system for computer output. The most important of these are compatibility with all commercial software programs, adjustability for degree of magnification, inclusion of both text and graphics, and compatibility with different types of video display terminals.

Goodrich and McKinley[15] describe several commercial adaptations that allow persons with low vision to access the computer screen. Software programs that are built into the computer operating system, such as Closeview† for the Apple Macintosh, are the most cost-effective. Magnifiers and filters attached in front of the VDT screen also provide enlargement of text and graphics, but limited magnification (about 2×) and distortion are major problems. Software programs may also be purchased separately from the computer. These offer a wider range of magnification and have more features than built-in software programs. Cook and Hussey[12] discuss several commercial products. Some of these adaptations include both hardware and software, which generally provides the greatest compatibility but at the highest cost.

*Microsoft, Redmond, Wash.

†Berkeley Systems, Berkeley, Calif.

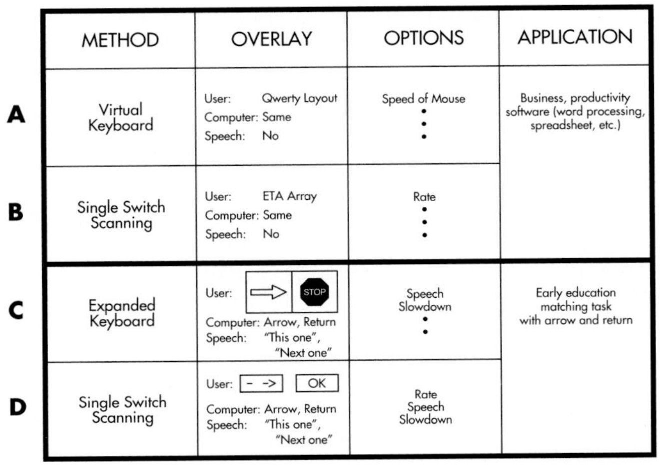

| | METHOD | OVERLAY | OPTIONS | APPLICATION |
|---|---|---|---|---|
| **A** | Virtual Keyboard | User: Qwerty Layout<br>Computer: Same<br>Speech: No | Speed of Mouse<br>•<br>•<br>• | Business, productivity software (word processing, spreadsheet, etc.) |
| **B** | Single Switch Scanning | User: ETA Array<br>Computer: Same<br>Speech: No | Rate<br>•<br>•<br>• | |
| **C** | Expanded Keyboard | User: ⇨ STOP<br>Computer: Arrow, Return<br>Speech: "This one", "Next one" | Speech Slowdown<br>•<br>• | Early education matching task with arrow and return |
| **D** | Single Switch Scanning | User: --> OK<br>Computer: Arrow, Return<br>Speech: "This one", "Next one" | Rate<br>Speech<br>Slowdown | |

*Figure 21-5* Elements of a general input device emulating interface (GIDEI). (From Cook AM, Hussey SM: *Assistive technologies: principles and practice,* St Louis, 1995, Mosby.)

*Table 21-3*

**Simple Adaptations for Sensory Impairment**

| *Need addressed* | *Software approach** |
|---|---|
| User cannot see toggle keys' lights (for showing status of CAPS LOCK, NUM LOCK, etc.) | ToggleKeys |
| User cannot hear beeps used to signal user of change of operation or error during program operation. | SoundSentry |

Modified from Cook AM, Hussey SM: *Assistive technologies: principles and practice,* St Louis, 1995, Mosby.
*Software modifications developed at the Trace Center University of Wisconsin, Madison. These are included as before-market modifications to DOS, OS/2, or Windows in some personal computers and are available as after-market versions in others.

Hard copy (printer) output may also need to be altered for persons with low vision. For enlarged print the most common approach uses a large font on a printer. The formatting (e.g., to avoid breaking words at the end of a line) is accomplished by special large-print software programs.

### *Alternatives to Visual Output for Blind Individuals*

For blind patients, computer outputs must be provided in either auditory or tactile form, or both. Auditory output is typically through voice synthesis, generally referred to as **screen readers.** Brown[10] lists the capabilities of an ideal screen reader: compatibility with all commercial software, capability of accessing both text and graphics, and hardware compatibility with a range of voice synthesizers.

Several commercial screen reader systems are available.[12] Screen readers are ideally suited for text applications in CLI. The use of graphics, such as with the GUI, adds considerable complexity to the screen reader system. In this case it is necessary to speak the names of icons, to locate which screen window is open, and to provide a spatial representation of the entire screen using auditory information only. Boyd, Boyd, and Vanderheiden[9] describe the fundamental screen reader approaches used for access to the GUI.

Tactile presentation of information is the other major alternative to visual output for blind persons. This tactile information can be presented in one of two ways: (1) tactile facsimile and (2) Braille.[12] Tactile facsimile provides a tactile image of the letter using vibrating pins incorporated into the Optacon II.* Braille output is based on a pattern of six-dot or eight-dot cells. Both paper and electromechanical (often called "paperless") formats are available for Braille. To use the Optacon II or a Braille cell array with a computer, interface software is required. A combination of Braille or tactile facsimile can also be used with speech synthesis to increase the information provided to the user who is blind (see Vanderheiden and Kunz[24]).

## AUGMENTATIVE AND ALTERNATIVE COMMUNICATION

The term **augmentative and alternative communication (AAC)** is used to describe any communication that requires something beyond the person's own body. Pens or pencils, letter or picture communication boards, typewriters, or electronic communication devices are all AACs. Two basic communication needs lead to the use of AAC systems: *conversation* and *graphics.*[11]

Conversational needs would typically be accomplished using speech, if it were available. Conversational use typically focuses on interaction between two or more people. Light[19] describes four types of communicative interaction: (1) expression of needs and wants, (2) information transfer, (3) social closeness, and (4) social etiquette. Each of these has unique features that dictate the AAC characteristics required. Since speech allows communication at a rapid rate, between 150 and 175 words per minute,[20] an AAC system output must be as rapid as possible. In all AAC systems, some form of letter or symbol selection is required, and in many cases persons who are unable to speak use a keyboard to type their messages, which are then spoken by an AAC device. If the person has limited motor skills, rate of communication will be significantly slower than for speech (as low as a few words per minute).

Graphic communication describes all the things that are normally done using a pencil and paper, typewriter, word processor, calculator, and other similar tools and includes writing, mathematics, and drawing or plotting. Each of these serves a different need, and therefore AAC devices designed to meet each type of need have different characteristics.[12] For example, all AAC systems for writing must be capable of providing output in a hard copy or printed format using either normal text (letters, numbers, special characters) or special symbols. If spelling is difficult for the user, some devices allow the selection of whole words.

Although a person can learn basic arithmetic without being able to write the numbers down, it is rather difficult. AAC systems used for mathematics allow the cursor to move from left to right as numbers to be added are entered. Once a column of numbers is prepared, the cursor moves right to left as the user enters the sum. Special symbols (e.g., Greek letters) and superscripts and subscripts required for algebra must also be possible in AAC systems for mathematics.

AAC device characteristics required for drawing include cursor movement in all four directions, choice of colors, line widths, and other features and the ability to save a drawing for later editing.

Table 21-4 shows three major groupings of AAC device characteristics that correspond to the assistive technology component of the HAAT (see Figure 21-2): (1) human/technology interface, (2) processor, and (3) activity output. The human/technology interface includes a user control interface, selection method and selection set, and an optional user display to provide feedback for self-correction. For AAC systems the processor has several specific functions: (1) selection technique, (2) rate enhancement and vocabulary expansion, (3) vocabulary storage, (4) text editing, and (5) output control. The activity output may be conversational and graphic communication in many different settings.

The human/technology interface for AAC devices may use special symbols in the selection set. Figure 21-6 shows examples of symbols typically used in AAC systems. In addition to those shown in this figure, text characters and multimeaning icons† are frequently

*Telesensory, Mountain View, Calif.

†Minsymbols, Prentke Romich, Wooster, Ohio.

Table 21-4

## Characteristics of Augmentative Communication Systems

| *Human/technology interface* | *Processor* | *Activity outputs* |
|---|---|---|
| Control interface | 1. Selection technique | To partner: |
| Selection method | 2. Rate enhancement and vocabulary expansion: | Visual |
| Selection set | a. Codes | Voice |
| User visual display | b. Prediction | Print |
| | c. Levels | To external device: |
| | 3. Vocabulary storage | Serial |
| | 4. Text editing | Parallel |
| | 5. Output control | |

From Cook AM, Hussey SM: *Assistive technologies: principles and practice,* St Louis, 1995, Mosby.

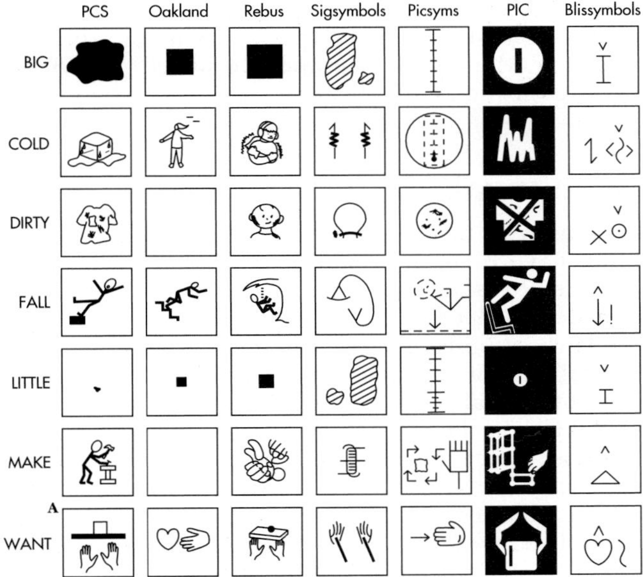


*Figure 21-6* Examples of symbols typically used in AAC systems. (From Blackstone S: *Augmentative communication,* Rockville, Md, 1986, American Speech-Language and Hearing Association. In Cook AM, Hussey SM: *Assistive technologies: principles and practice,* St Louis, 1995, Mosby.)

used. All the selection methods discussed earlier are available in AAC devices.

To increase the rate of output, AAC devices use techniques of **rate enhancement** to generate characters at a greater rate than the individual's selection rate. Rate enhancement may be achieved by encoding techniques or prediction techniques. For encoding, numbers (numerical code) can be related to words or complete phrases or sentences. When the user enters one or more numbers, the device outputs the complete stored vocabulary item. This can save many entries by the user.

Abbreviation expansion is another encoding technique in which a shortened form of a word or phrase (the abbreviation) stands for the entire word or phrase (the expansion). When an abbreviation is entered, it is automatically expanded by the device into the desired word or phrase. For example, the abbreviation ASAP would be typed by the user, and the device would expand it to be "as soon as possible."[23]

**Semantic encoding** codes words, sentences, and phrases based on their meaning.[5] In this approach, pictorial representations, called *icons,* are used in place of numerical or letter codes. If the icons are carefully chosen, they can make recall much easier. For example, a picture of an apple for "food" and a sun rising for "morning" may be combined in "apple sunrise" as a code for "What's for breakfast?" This is easier to remember than an arbitrary numerical or letter code for the same phrase.

Rate may also be increased by using word prediction or word completion techniques with any selection method.[22] Devices that use these techniques typically display on the screen a list of the most likely words based on the letters that have previously been entered. The user selects the desired word, if it is listed, by entering the number shown next to the word. If the desired word is not displayed, the user continues to enter letters, and the listed words change to correspond to the entered letters. In an *adaptive system* the presented list for word prediction or word completion changes based on the person's frequency of use. Newell et al.[21] demonstrated that the long-term use of word completion and word prediction devices resulted in improvements in spelling and the intelligibility of written work for children and adults.

Some AAC devices include both abbreviation expansion and word prediction, allowing the user access to the strengths of each approach. Abbreviations are more direct because the user enters the code and immediately obtains the desired word or phrase or sentence. Predictions are easier to use because they do not require memorization of codes.

A very different approach is to model conversational acts and build typical sequences of such acts into the AAC system. One approach, called CHAT (for

Conversation Helped by Automatic Talk), is based on the premise that each keystroke should produce a complete "speech act" (an utterance with a purpose).[1,2] CHAT breaks the conversation into five discrete sections: (1) greetings, (2) small talk, (3) main section, (4) wrap-up remarks, and (5) farewells. CHAT also allows the superimposition of mood on the other features: polite, informal, humorous, or angry. The user of CHAT is presented with the conversational sections in the order listed. Pressing one key generates a complete phrase for each section of the conversation. The user can also override the automatic choice with either a "filler" (e.g., "That's nice", "I don't think so") or a typed message. Alm, Arnott, and Newell[2] present the details of the CHAT software program. The essential features of CHAT are available for the IBM PC or compatible computers and as Talk About for the Macintosh computer.*

The term *vocabulary expansion* is used here to refer to methods by which the available vocabulary can be increased through the use of codes or levels. Using levels, multiple language items can be stored and retrieved from one location.[18] Storage or retrieval is accomplished by selecting the level and then selecting the location. If the device has more than a few levels, it can be difficult to display on screen all the items represented by that location. This problem can be addressed by using dynamic communication displays that change the displayed selection set when a new level is selected. The displayed information is changed based on previous entries. For example, a general selection set might consist of categories such as work, home, food, clothing, greetings, or similar classifications. If one of these is chosen, either by touching the display surface directly or using scanning, a new selection set is displayed. For example, a variety of food-related items and activities (e.g., eat, drink, ice cream, pasta) would follow the choice of "foods" from the general selection set. Thus the user does not have to remember what is on each level. Vocabulary expansion can also be achieved by vocabulary storage.[8]

Augmentative communication devices can be grouped in five categories: (1) simple scanners, (2) simple voice output, (3) direct selection, spelling, (4) direct selection with rate enhancement, and (5) multiple selection method with rate enhancement. Simple scanners are generally operated by a single switch (although some can have multiswitch-directed scanning) and use a light to indicate the output selection. Devices in this category generally do not have voice output as a standard feature.

Simple voice output devices were all developed to provide a limited-vocabulary, easy-to-use output generated using direct selection. Speech is typically stored using digital recording. Some devices in this category have rate enhancement (e.g., levels, simple codes, key sequences), and vocabulary storage varies from a low of 8 or 16 utterances to more than 100.

Direct-selection, spelling-only devices are distinguished by their small size, built-in printer, and lack of any significant rate enhancement or vocabulary expansion.

The last two categories represent the electronically most sophisticated devices currently available. These devices include all the rate enhancement and vocabulary expansion techniques discussed. They provide flexibility in control interfaces and selection methods. Some of these are commercially available software programs written for general-purpose computers such as lap-top or notebook types, and others have specially designed computer hardware and software programs.

The multiple selection method devices in the last category allow many different types of control interfaces and selection methods. Selection methods available on these devices include scanning, directed scanning, Morse code (one and two switch), and direct selection using light pointers (typically attached to the user's head).[12]

## ENVIRONMENTAL CONTROL UNITS

Persons with severe upper extremity (UE) limitations often have difficulty manipulating electrically powered devices such as appliances (e.g., television, room lights, fans, kitchen appliances such as blenders or food processors) powered from standard house wiring. These may be controlled by assistive devices called **environmental control units (ECUs).** Figure 21-7 shows a typical ECU for turning appliances on and off. The user control interface may be a keypad (as shown) or a single switch with an indirect selection method. The appliances are plugged into modules that are controlled by the ECU. The most common type of on/off module is the X-10.†

ECUs can be remotely controlled using one of three methods. The most common is *infrared* (IR) transmission such as that used in most TV remote units. A second method, also sometimes used for TV control, is *ultrasound* transmission. The third method, often used in garage door openers, is *radio frequency* (RF) transmission. IR and ultrasound require that the user control interface shown in Figure 21-7 be aimed directly at the distribution and control unit. This is often called *line of sight.* RF transmission does not have this requirement.

The ECU system may be modified to give the user remote control over TV or VCR functions such as volume control, channel selection, play, fast forward, and reverse. Standard TV or VCR remote controls may be modified by adding a single switch to the remote control or by more elaborate adaptations that allow indirect selection. Universal remote controls that can

*Don Johnston Developmental Equipment, Wauconda, Ill.

†X-10 Powerhouse System, Northvale, NJ.

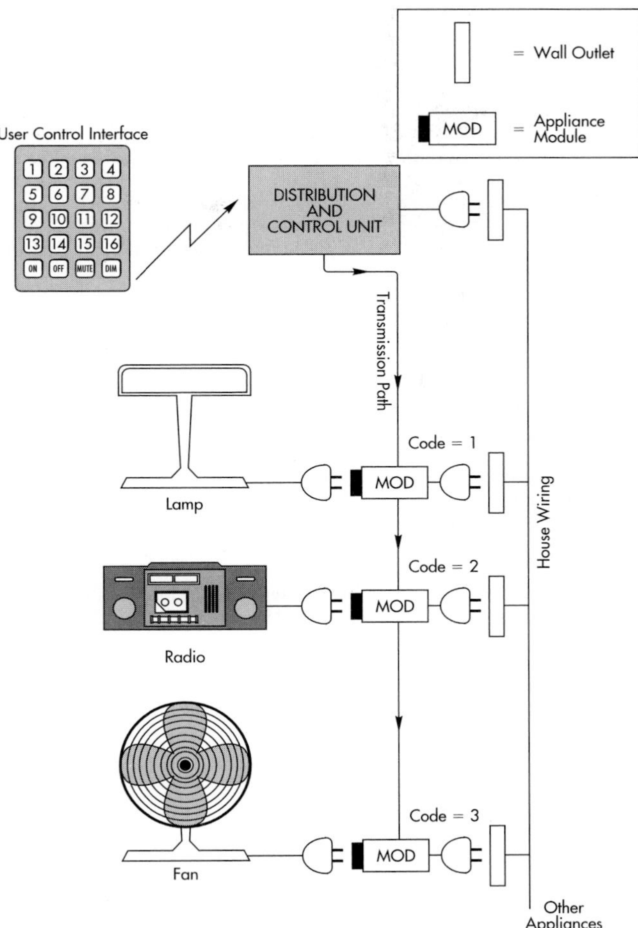


*Figure 21-7* Environmental control unit (ECU) that uses individual appliance control modules plugged into house wiring, with remote control from user control interface to ECU. (From Cook AM, Hussey SM: *Assistive technologies: principles and practice,* St Louis, 1995, Mosby.)

"learn" the signal for a particular TV or VCR can also be used. This allows several appliances to be controlled from the same ECU.

Persons with UE physical disabilities often have difficulty in carrying out the actions associated with telephone use: lifting the handset, dialing, holding the handset while talking, and replacing the handset in its cradle. Several options exist for accomplishing these tasks. Nonelectronic methods such as mouthsticks or head pointers can be used to press a button to open a line on a speaker phone, to dial, and to hang up. ECUs perform these same telephone tasks electronically.

For persons who require single-switch access to the system, the control interface is connected to a control unit, which also interfaces with a display and with standard telephone electronics. A typical approach is for the device to present numbers sequentially on the display. The user presses a switch when the desired number appears on the display. By repeating this process, any phone number can be entered and then sent through the standard telephone electronics for automatic dialing. Because many persons with disabilities respond slowly, all practical systems use stored numbers and automatic dialing. Most systems have a capacity of 50 to 100 stored numbers and include a "help" or emergency phone number that can be dialed quickly. Some telephones are IR controlled and can be included with ECUs that learn device codes.

Dickey and Shealy[13] described the evaluation of consumers for the specification of ECUs. Gross[16] presents a detailed case study of the process of selecting and implementing an ECU for a person who had a high-level spinal cord injury.

## SUMMARY

A basic framework for viewing assistive technologies is the HAAT model. Assistive technology is becoming increasingly integrated into occupational therapy practice. This trend is expected to continue, with many of the advancements in the application of assistive technologies coming from OT practitioners.

## *Selected Reading Guide Questions*

1. What is the definition of *assistive technology devices* according to PL 100-407?
2. What is the purpose of assistive technologies in the rehabilitation of persons with disabilities? How is occupational therapy concerned with the assessment and delivery of assistive technologies?
3. What are the components of the HAAT model? Describe and give an example of the interaction between the components of the HAAT model.
4. Which professional disciplines might be involved in assistive technology delivery to the client or patient?
5. List the steps in the process of service delivery, and describe the components of each step.
6. What is meant by *control interface?*
7. Describe several examples of control interfaces.
8. What is the *selection set?* Give some examples of different types of selection sets.
9. List and compare selection methods. What are the advantages and disadvantages of each in relation to the user's capabilities?
10. How are control interfaces activated? Give some examples of each method.
11. Discuss the types of disabilities for which each type of control interface is most appropriate.
12. What is a *virtual keyboard?* How does it work?
13. List two alternatives to the standard computer keyboard.
14. What is a GIDEI? Why is it necessary?
15. List and describe at least two types of computer outputs.

16. Define *augmentative and alternative communication.*
17. How is vocabulary expansion accomplished?
18. What is an *environmental control unit (ECU)?*
19. What types of household devices can be operated by an ECU?
20. How are ECUs controlled?

## REFERENCES


1. Alm N, Newell AF, Arnott JL: A communication aid which models conversational patterns, *Proceedings of the 10th Annual Conference on Rehabilitation Engineering,* 1987, pp 127-129.
2. Alm N, Arnott JL, Newell AF: Prediction of conversational momentum in an augmentative communication system, *Communications ACM* 35:46-57, 1992.
3. Anson D: Presentation to RESNA Workshop on Instructional Materials Development, RESNA 13th Annual Conference, Washington, DC, 1990.
4. Anson D: Virtual keyboard techniques, *Occup Ther Forum* 6:1-7, 1991.
5. Baker B: Minspeak, *Byte* 7:186-202, 1982.
6. Baker JM: How to achieve recognition: a tutorial/status report on automatic speech recognition, *Speech Technol* Fall 1981, pp 30-31, 36-43.
7. Bergen AF, Presperin J, Tallman T: *Positioning for function: wheelchairs and other assistive technologies,* Valhalla, NY, 1990, Valhalla Rehabilitation.
8. Beukelman DR, Mirenda P: *Augmentative and alternative communication: management of severe communication disorders in children and adults,* Baltimore, 1992, Brooks.
9. Boyd LH, Boyd WL, Vanderheiden GC: The graphical user interface: crisis, danger, and opportunity, *J Vis Impair Blind* 84:496-502, 1990.
10. Brown C: *Computer access in higher education for students with disabilities,* ed 2, Monterey, Calif, 1989, US Department of Education.
11. Cook AM: Communication devices. In Webster JG, editor: *Encyclopedia of medical devices and instrumentation,* New York, 1988, Wiley and Sons.
12. Cook AM, Hussey SM: *Assistive technologies: principles and practice,* St Louis, 1995, Mosby.
13. Dickey R, Shealey SH: Using technology to control the environment, *Am J Occup Ther* 41:717-721, 1987.
14. Gallant JA: Speech-recognition products, *EDN* Jan 19, 1989, pp 112-122.
15. Goodrich GL, McKinley JL: A guide to large print computer access, *J Vis Rehabil* 1:29-40, 1987.
16. Gross K: Controlling the environment, *Team Rehabil Rep* 3:14-16, 1992.
17. Hayes F: From TTY to VDT, *Byte* 15:205-211, 1990.
18. Kraat A, Stiver-Kogut M: *Features of portable communication devices,* Wilmington, Del, 1991, Applied Science and Engineering Laboratories, University of Delaware.
19. Light J: Interaction involving individuals using augmentative and alternative communication systems: state of the art and future directions, *Augment Altern Communication* 4:66-82, 1988.
20. Miller GA: *Language and Speech,* San Francisco, 1981, Freeman.
21. Newell AF et al: Effect of the "PAL" word prediction system on the quality and quantity of text generation, *Augment Altern Communication* 8:304-311, 1992.
22. Swiffin AL et al: Adaptive and predictive techniques in a communication prosthesis, *Augment Altern Communication* 3:181-191, 1987.
23. Vanderheiden GC, Kelso DP: Comparative analysis of fixed-vocabulary communication acceleration techniques, *Augment Altern Communication* 3:196-206, 1987.
24. Vanderheiden GC, Kunz DC: Systems 3—an interface to graphic computers for blind users, RESNA 13th Annual Conference, Washington, DC, 1990, pp 259-260.
25. Vanderheiden GC, Lloyd LL: Communication systems and their components. In Blackstone S, Bruskin D: *Augmentative communication: an introduction,* Rockville, Md, 1986, American Speech-Language and Hearing Association.


## RECOMMENDED READING


Gookin D: *DOS for dummies,* ed 2, Foster City, Calif, 1993, IDG Worldwide.

Pogue D: *MACs for dummies,* ed 3, Foster City, Calif, 1994, IDG Worldwide.

Chapter 22

# Hand Splinting

*Serena Berger*
*Lorraine Williams Pedretti*

## Chapter Objectives

*After studying this chapter, the student or practitioner will be able to:*

1. Locate important landmarks in the anatomy of the hand.
2. Recognize arches and other structural elements that contribute to hand function.
3. Identify normal prehension and grasp patterns.
4. Describe the three basic positions of the hand.
5. Understand the basic purposes of splinting an extremity.
6. Understand the biomechanical considerations involved in splint selection and fabrication.
7. Determine what low-temperature thermoplastic handling and performance characteristics are useful when fabricating different splints.
8. Recognize indications for soft splinting.
9. Explain basic pattern-making, fabrication, and strapping principles and techniques.
10. Draw patterns for and fabricate three basic upper extremity splints.

## Key Terms

splint
arch
metacarpal
radial
ulnar
crease
distal
proximal
dorsal
volar
thenar
hypothenar
extrinsic muscle
intrinsic muscle
phalanx
tenodesis action
low-temperature thermoplastic
handling characteristics
performance characteristics
circumferential

The hand serves to obtain information, execute motor activities, and express emotions. The hand requires sensation, mobility, and stability to interact effectively with the environment. Any defect in sensory, neuromuscular, skeletal, articular, vascular, or soft tissue structures affects the functioning of the hand and its appearance.[3,5] The function of the proximal joints (shoulder, elbow, forearm) is to place and stabilize the hand for functional activities. Thus the hand must be assessed in relation to function of the entire arm.

Because of its primary role in daily activities and interaction, the appearance of the hand is important. Use of skin softeners, manicures, and jewelry testify to the importance of its attractiveness in interpersonal contact. The exquisite sensibility of the hand permits an amazing level of coordinated activity, and it transmits enormous amounts of information about the environment to the brain. People use their hands to prepare for and perform all activities of daily living (ADLs) and to express themselves. The hand may caress or may slap. The hearing-impaired person uses the hand to speak and the blind person uses it to see.

Psychosocial problems may be associated with dysfunction or injury that disrupts the hand's primary role in daily interactions with both the physical world and other people.[13] Splinting is one of several treatment modalities used to restore normal function and appearance of the hand. The certified occupational therapy assistant (COTA) is often called on to fabricate **splints** (orthopedic devices used to immobilize or protect a body part) and to assist with the assessment of patient positioning. This chapter (1) briefly reviews the structures and function of the hand, (2) introduces basic principles and goals of hand splinting, and (3) provides basic instruction on fabrication of three common hand splints.

## STRUCTURES OF THE HAND

### Bones

The wrist and hand are composed of 27 bones: 8 carpals (wrist), 5 metacarpals (palm), and 14 phalanges (fingers). The proximal row of carpals articulate with the radius and ulna of the forearm. Combined movements of hand, wrist, and forearm permit an amazing variety of positions during activity.

### Alignment

The precise relationship of length, mobility, and position of each finger and between the thumb and fingers is the key to functional use. The fingertips converge toward the pad of the thumb during palmar prehension. When individually flexed, they converge toward the center of the wrist (capitate bone), but when simultaneously flexed, they contact the palm parallel to each other. Alignment of the digits must be respected during splint design and fabrication.

### Arches

Three **arches** (curves) are present in the hand: the longitudinal, the proximal transverse, and the distal transverse. The longitudinal arch follows the lines of the carpal and **metacarpal** bones down along the third finger. The ability to flex and extend the digits occurs along this arch. The proximal transverse arch is a bony, fixed arch formed by the proximal row of carpal bones and annular ligaments. This arch is deep, and through it pass all the nerves, blood supply, and tendons of the extrinsic hand muscles. This arch also acts as a fulcrum for the finger flexors, preventing them from bowing during flexion. The distal transverse arch (also called the metacarpal arch) lies across the metacarpal heads (knuckles). The dexterity and functional use of the hand rely on the mobility of this arch.

Place your left thumb on the palm side of the fourth and fifth metacarpal heads of your right hand and push them back to where they are flat across with the second and third metacarpal heads. When you attempt to make a fist with your right hand, you will see that it is not possible. Flattening of the distal transverse arch is not a functional position. Flattening may be caused by many conditions, including intrinsic muscle paralysis, edema, scarring, contractures, or poor positioning in a splint. A splint must be formed to the distal transverse arch to ensure maximal functional use of the hand while the splint is on or off.

### Dual Obliquity

The dual obliquity (or two nonparallel lines) (Figure 22-1) in the hand occurs because the length of the second to fifth metacarpals gradually decreases from the radial (thumb) side of the hand to the ulnar side of the hand. A line drawn through the metacarpal heads

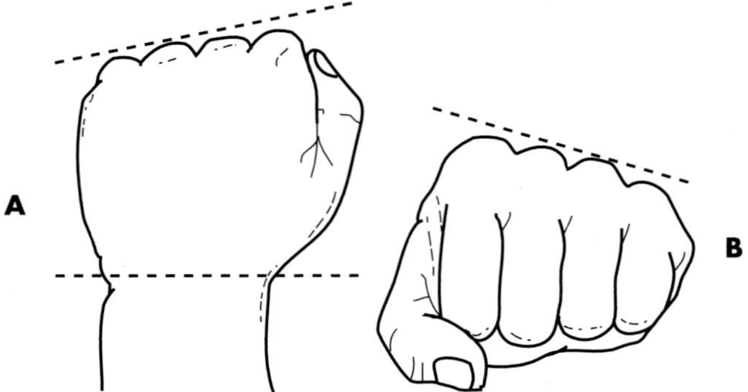


*Figure 22-1* Dual obliquity of hand. **A,** Oblique angle of metacarpal heads in relation to axis of wrist joint. **B,** Oblique angle of metacarpal heads from radial to ulnar side of hand. (From Fess EE, Philips CA: *Hand splinting: principles and methods,* ed 2, St Louis, 1987, Mosby.)

The first author would like to acknowledge the assistance of the occupational therapists at Smith and Nephew Rolyan for their enthusiasm, practical information, and technical tips. I would also like to thank the therapists and students I work with who have taught me so much. Lastly, I would like to thank my father for his invaluable editorial assistance.

forms an oblique angle with a line drawn through the wrist. A second oblique angle occurs at the distal transverse arch. The second and third metacarpals are relatively fixed, stable bones, whereas the fourth and fifth move more freely. Functionally, this means that an object, when grasped cylindrically, is higher on the radial side of the hand and not parallel to the floor when the hand is in full pronation. An easy way to remember this is simply that the **radial** (thumb) side of the hand is longer and higher than the **ulnar** (small finger) side. Any hand or forearm-based splint must respect this anatomy.

### Creases

The skin **creases** (folds) (Figure 22-2) can act as guides when designing and fitting splints. The creases indicate where the axis of motion for the joint occurs. The wrist, palmar, thenar, and proximal, middle, and distal finger creases deepen when the associated joint is moved. For the palmar creases the **distal** crease is associated with metacarpophalangeal (MP) flexion of digits III, IV, and V and the **proximal** crease with digits II and III. **Dorsal** (on the back of the hand) splints should be constructed so that the splint extends to the midpoint of the next proximal joint. For **volar** (on the palm side) splints the splint extends up to but does not include the next distal crease. The splint pattern is drawn to the crease and then shortened approximately ⅛ inch (0.3 cm) to accommodate skin folds.

### Skin

The dorsal skin of the hand on the extensor surface is fine, supple, and mobile to allow it to move freely during flexion and extension of the fingers. Scarring or edema limit hand function by destroying skin mobility.

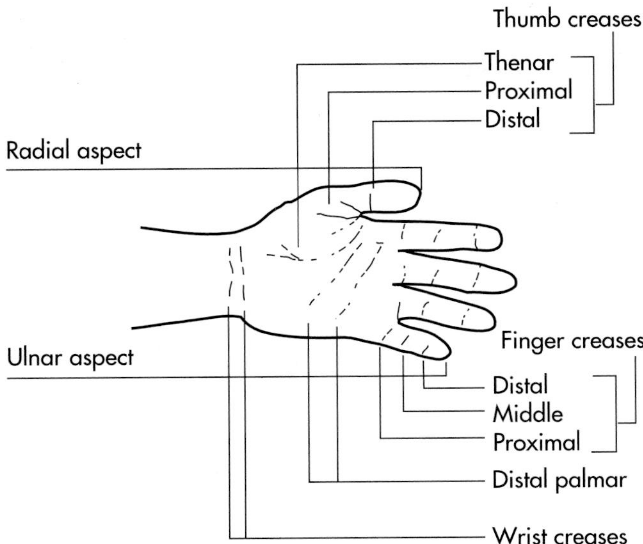


*Figure 22-2* Palmar creases of hand. (From Malick MH: *Manual on static hand splinting*, rev ed, Pittsburgh, 1972, Harmarville Rehabilitation Center.)

The palmar skin (on the flexor surface) by comparison is tough, thick, and inelastic. It protects and supports the underlying structures and prevents slippage between the skeleton and an object grasped.[13] The integrity of the skin is affected by many factors, including medical and neurological conditions, hydration, and job tasks.

### Muscles

The movements of the hand and wrist involve 39 muscles: 20 extrinsic (outside the hand) muscles and 19 intrinsic (inside the hand) muscles.[13] The 20 **extrinsic muscles** include the long flexors and extensors of the wrist and fingers, the pronators, and the supinator and are located in the forearm. The 19 **intrinsic muscles** include those of the **thenar** (thumb side) and **hypothenar** (little finger side) eminences, the lumbricals, and the interossei.[3] An elaborate ligamentous system in the hand and wrist helps bony alignment by providing both stability and mobility. A pulley system improves the mechanical advantage of the long finger muscles by keeping the tendons close to the bones as they glide.

### Nerve Supply

Three peripheral nerves supply the hand: the radial, median, and ulnar. In general the radial nerve supplies the extensor/supinator muscle group and sensation to the dorsal surface of the radial side of the hand. The median nerve supplies the flexor/pronator muscles, the thenar group, and the first and second lumbricals. This nerve provides sensation to the radial side of the palm and thumb. The median nerve therefore is crucial in grasp, prehension, and tactile discrimination functions. The ulnar nerve innervates most of the intrinsic muscles and supplies sensory fibers to the ulnar side of the hand and digits. Figure 22-3 shows the sensory distribution.

## NORMAL HAND FUNCTION

Understanding the normal functions of the hand is fundamental in designing and fabricating effective

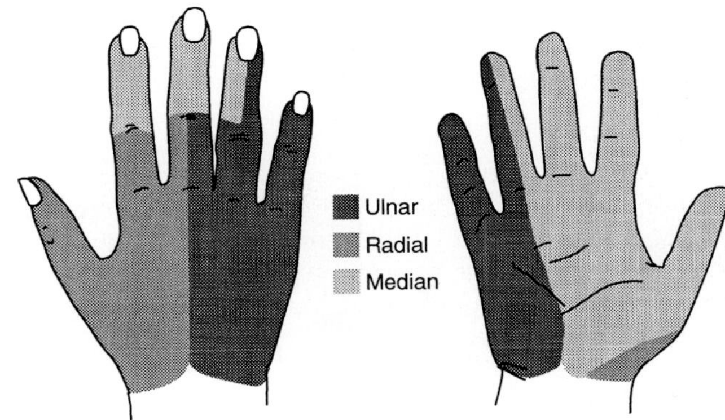


*Figure 22-3* Sensory distribution in hand. Median nerve distribution includes most of prehensile surface of palm.

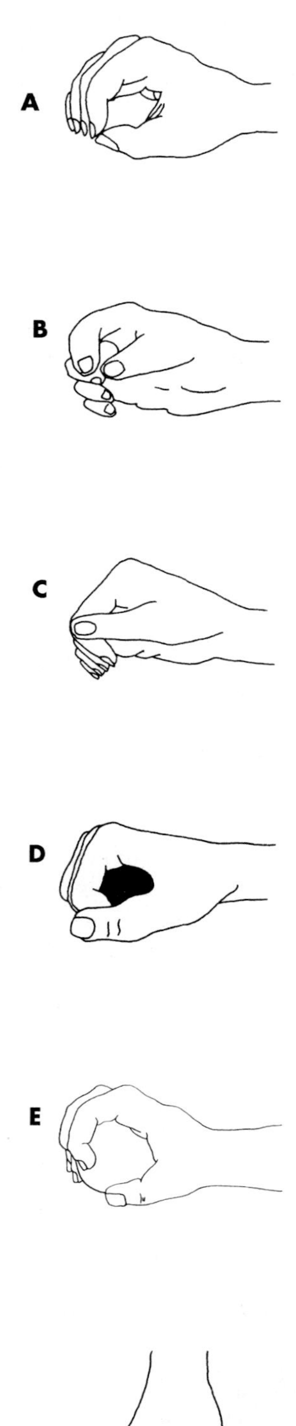


*Figure 22-4* Basic types of prehension and grasp. **A,** Fingertip prehension. **B,** Palmar prehension. **C,** Lateral prehension. **D,** Cylindrical grasp. **E,** Spherical grasp. **F,** Hook grasp.

splints. The hand is the terminal point of the arm. Adequate range of motion (ROM) and sufficient muscle strength in the upper extremity joints are necessary for full use of the hand. Shoulder motions are critical for reaching and for such hand-to-body activities as toileting and combing hair. Elbow motion and supination/pronation of the forearm permit hand-to-face activities. The wrist, used chiefly to stabilize the hand during activity, contributes significantly to functional grip strength (see later section on tenodesis).

MP joint flexion and stabilization are critical to grasp and prehension, and MP joint extension is needed for release. The distal palmar arch formed by the metacarpals ensures the motion and opposition of the thumb and little finger, the ability to grasp round or large objects, convergence of the fingers during flexion, and the ability to press with the palm against resistance.

Opposition of the thumb is the basis of all prehension patterns. Thumb rotation at the carpometacarpal (CMC) joint is necessary to perform pad-to-pad prehension. Splints are typically fabricated to stabilize and position the thumb so that grasp and prehension can occur.

The normal hand is capable of mobility and stability at all joints. A splint can provide one or the other, but rarely both.[6,10] The use of a splint ultimately may aid in the recovery of dexterity, but while it is being worn, hand function is hindered.

The normal hand can perform a variety of prehension and grasp patterns. These patterns may be assisted by splinting when muscle function is impaired or deformity is present.[10]

### Prehension and Grasp Patterns

Hand movements are complex and occur in smooth sequence and combinations but may be reduced to six basic patterns.[6,7,10]

#### *Fingertip Prehension*

Fingertip prehension (Figure 22-4, *A*), or *tip-to-tip pinch,* is the contact of the thumb pad with the pad of the index or middle finger. Using fine, coordinated movement allows the fingertips to pick up small objects, fasten snaps and buttons, or hold a needle for sewing.

#### *Palmar Prehension*

Palmar prehension (Figure 22-4, *B*), also known as *three jaw chuck,* is contact of the thumb, middle, and index fingers. It is the most common prehension pattern and requires a high degree of coordination. It is the prehension pattern used for holding a pen, utensil, or small object of any shape (e.g., marble, cookie).

#### *Lateral Prehension*

Lateral prehension (Figure 22-4, *C*) is contact of the thumb pad with the lateral surface of the distal or middle **phalanx** of the index finger. The other digits may support the index finger, but the stability provided by the contraction of the first dorsal interossei is essential. This pattern requires less coordination than the others but is stronger. Examples include turning a key or carrying a mug by its handle.

### *Cylindrical Grasp*

Cylindrical grasp (Figure 22-4, *D*) occurs when an object is stabilized against the palm by finger flexion. Intrinsic and thenar muscles are essential to the power of this grasp. Examples include holding a drinking glass, hammer, or pot handle.

### *Spherical Grasp*

Spherical grasp (Figure 22-4, *E*), or *ball grasp,* is used to hold round objects against an arched palm. Wrist stability and intrinsic and extrinsic hand muscle strength contribute to the ability to hold an apple, a ball, or a round doorknob.

### *Hook Grasp*

Hook grasp (Figure 22-4, *F*) can be accomplished using the fingers only. It requires flexor strength and stability of the interphalangeal (IP) joints, MPs, and wrist remaining in neutral. Examples include carrying a briefcase or shopping bag or pulling open a drawer.

## Tenodesis

The tendons of the intrinsic hand muscles are held close to the bones of the wrist and hand by connective tissue. This close association between tendon and bone results in **tenodesis action.** In the normal hand when the wrist is flexed, the fingers are passively pulled into extension (Figure 22-5). The tendons of finger extensors are too short to permit simultaneous flexion of all the joints that the finger extensors cross: wrist, MP, proximal IP, and distal IP. The opposite is also true. With wrist extension the fingers are slightly pulled into flexion (Figure 22-5, *A*). This tenodesis action (wrist flexion with finger extension, wrist extension with finger flexion) is easily seen if you relax your fingers and move your wrist into flexion and extension rapidly. Tenodesis action results in a passive prehension pattern.

For a patient with radial nerve palsy, a dynamic splint may take advantage of tenodesis to increase wrist extension passively during active finger flexion. For a patient with quadraparesis, a tenodesis splint may cause passive finger flexion through active wrist extension. Release is effected by relaxation of wrist extension.

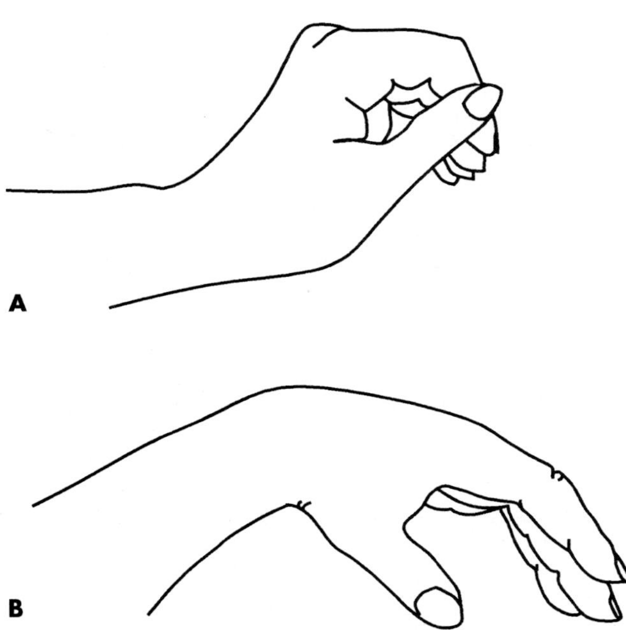


*Figure 22-5* Tenodesis. **A,** Active wrist extension results in passive finger flexion. **B,** Active wrist flexion results in passive finger extension.

## Basic Positions of Hand

### *Functional*

The functional position (Figure 22-6) is the hand position most often used during activity. It is similar to holding a soda can or ball. The wrist is in 20° to 30° of extension; the thumb is abducted and opposed to the pad of the middle finger; metacarpals are flexed to approximately 30° and IPs to 45°. In this position there is equal tension of all muscles; the hand is in its most mechanically efficient posture.

### *Resting*

Resting position (Figure 22-7) is the position a normal hand assumes when resting passively. In this position the wrist is in 10° to 20° of extension; all finger joints are slightly flexed; the thumb is midway between opposition and abduction, with the thumb's pad facing the side of the index finger. The proximal, distal, and longitudinal arches are maintained in this position. Splints are often fabricated in this position to rest joints or to prevent deformity.

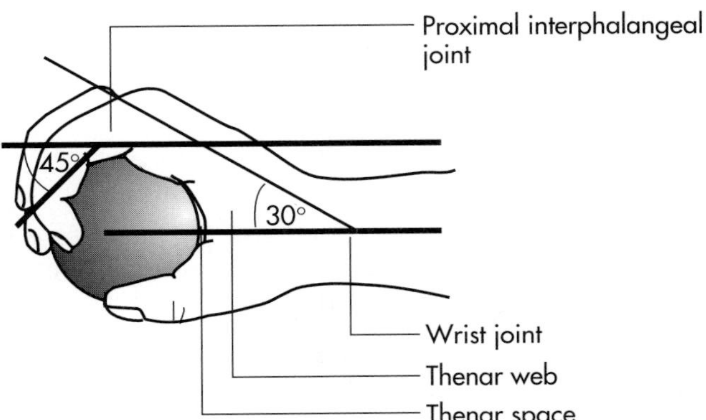


*Figure 22-6* Functional position, lateral view, right hand. (From Malick MH: *Manual on static hand splinting,* rev ed, Pittsburgh, 1972, Harmarville Rehabilitation Center.)

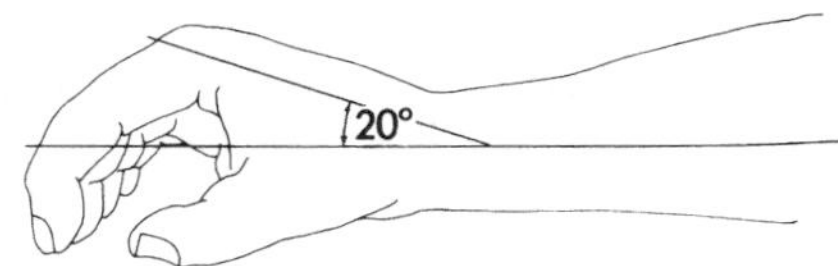


*Figure 22-7* Resting position. (From Malick MH: *Manual on static hand splinting,* rev ed, Pittsburgh, Harmarville Rehabilitation Center.)

### *Safe*

The safe position maintains optimal stress on metacarpal, phalangeal, and interphalangeal collateral ligaments,[3] thereby "saving" the hand for eventual motion. In this position the MPs are flexed, IPs are in full extension, and the wrist is in 10° to 30° of extension. This position is common after thermal injuries, trauma, and invasive surgery.

## PRINCIPLES OF HAND SPLINTING

### Types of Splints

The three basic types of splints are static, dynamic, and static progressive.

#### *Static Splints*

Static splints, by definition, have no moving parts and can be made for different purposes. They are primarily used to protect, support, or immobilize. Burn splints, in the safe position, are used to maintain orthopedic and soft tissue integrity of the structures of the hand. Resting splints place painful wrist and MP joints at rest. In an arthritis resting mitt splint, the inflammation is given a chance to subside. Cock-up splints, with the wrist set at neutral to 10° of extension, are used to limit motion to a range that will not aggravate the symptoms of carpal tunnel syndrome.

#### *Dynamic Splints*

Dynamic splints have movable parts and are used to substitute for or to increase ROM as well as to maintain alignment during active ROM. They employ forces that may be *internal,* as in muscle power, or *external,* as in a spring wire or rubber band.[2] Dynamic splints are beyond the scope of this chapter.

#### *Static Progressive Splints*

Static progressive or serial splints apply low-load, prolonged stretch to soft tissue by means of a series of advancing positions intended to increase ROM. Serial casting is probably the most common application of this type of splinting. The Rolyan PIP joint extension splint (Figure 22-8) applies a constant force to help correct flexion contractures. As the patient gains PIP extension, the OT practitioner adjusts the length of the bolt to accommodate the increased ROM at the joint and to stretch the joint further to its end range.

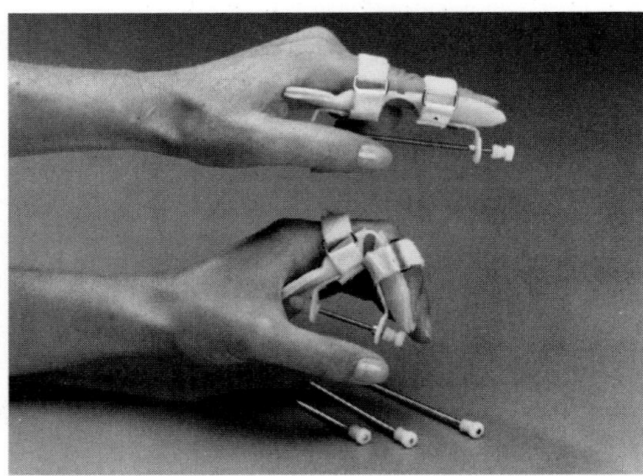

*Figure 22-8* Rolyan PIP joint extension splint for static progressive splinting. (Courtesy Smith and Nephew Rolyan.)

### Purposes of Splinting

The goal of all splinting is to enable the patient to perform daily life tasks as easily as possible. Static, dynamic, and static progressive splints may be used to achieve any combination of the following[3,12]:

1. *To protect, support, or immobilize joints* to permit healing after inflammation or injury to the tendons, joint, soft tissue, or vascular/nerve supply. An arthritis resting mitt, which immobilizes the MP and wrist joints (of an inflamed arthritic hand), permits IP movement to allow for function (Figure 22-9).
2. *To position and maintain alignment* to keep the integrity of the arches, the ligamentous structures, and joint relationships. This can be accomplished using resting, functional, and safe positions and footdrop splints. An adjustable outrigger is used to ensure alignment of the MPs after surgical replacement.
3. *To correct deformity or to prevent further deformity.* An ulnar deviation splint (Figure 26-15) is used to align the fingers of a patient with rheumatoid arthritis in a neutral position. In the early stages of the disease the splint acts to prevent the rapid progression of the deformity. Later on, it acts to position the digits for more effective functional use.
4. *To substitute for weak or absent muscle function* caused by neuromuscular disease and spinal cord or peripheral nerve injury. A radial nerve splint (Figure 22-10) amplifies the strength of the tenodesis action for the patient who is unable to actively extend the wrist or fingers. With active finger flexion the wrist is passively extended, thus functionally increasing prehensile strength.
5. *To maximize ROM* by preventing contractures caused by adhesion formation. A dorsal blocking splint assists flexion yet blocks extension to decrease stress and stretch on the surgical repair side while permitting tendon excursion. Increases

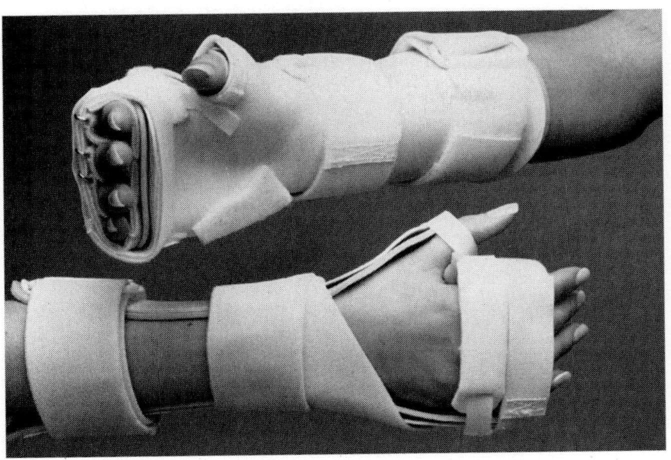

*Figure 22-9* Arthritis resting mitt splint. (Courtesy Smith and Nephew Rolyan.)

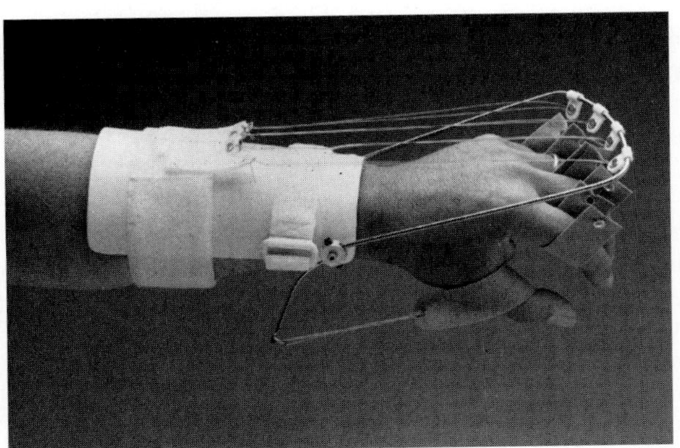

*Figure 22-10* Rolyan static radial nerve splint. (Courtesy Smith and Nephew Rolyan.)

in ROM can be accomplished through dynamic and static serial splinting.

6. *To increase ADL independence* by acting as a base for the attachment of devices or compensating for decreased hand function. It is easier for the patient, for example, to have a splint attached to his razor to allow him to hold it or use a walker splint (Figure 22-11) to compensate for weakness or sensory loss.
7. *To exercise,* which can be accomplished using dynamic splints when the patient actively moves in the direction opposite the pull of the splint.
8. *To inhibit tone* through the use of positioning in a reflex-inhibiting posture (Figure 22-12). The fingers are abducted. Sensory input to the hypertonic muscle bellies is limited, and there is a prolonged stretch to the hypertonic muscles and tendons.

## Biomechanical Considerations

The occupational therapy practitioner must bear in mind the following when constructing a splint.

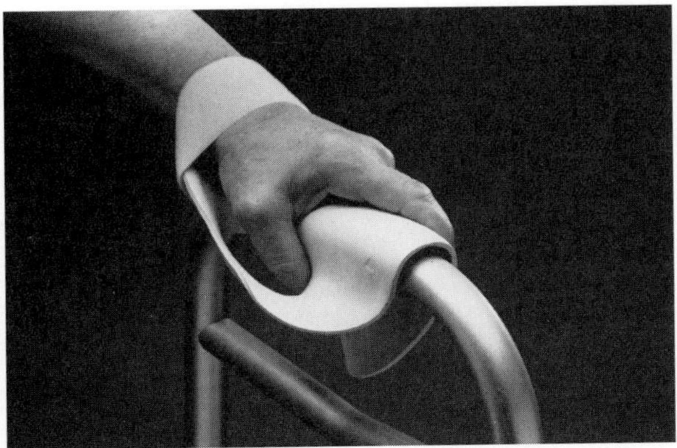

*Figure 22-11* Rolyan walker splint. (Courtesy Smith and Nephew Rolyan.)

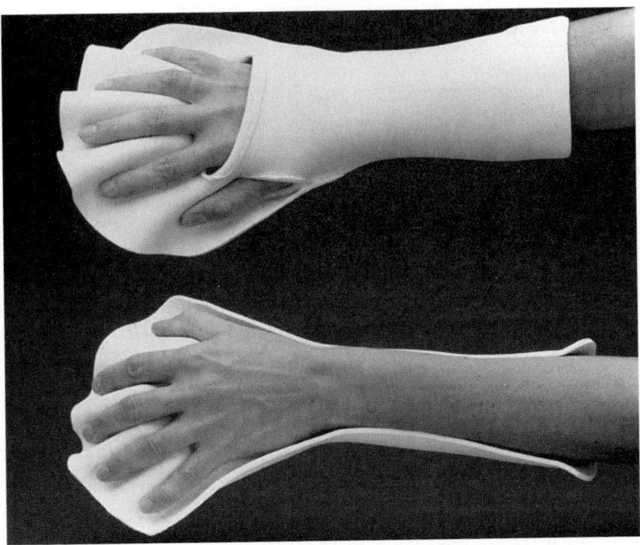

*Figure 22-12* Antispasticity ball splint—dorsal (top) and volar (bottom) versions. (Courtesy Smith and Nephew Rolyan.)

### *Bony Prominences*

Soft tissue is particularly thin over bony prominences such as the radial and ulnar styloids, the pisiform, the metacarpal heads, and the base of the thumb's metacarpal. Because of the lack of natural padding over these areas, significant potential exists for skin breakdown caused by pressure. If possible, the practitioner should avoid splint contact with bony prominences by trimming and flaring the thermoplastic. If the COTA chooses to pad an area, a self-stick circle of closed-cell padding is placed on the bone before molding the thermoplastic so that the COTA can either put the padding back onto the thermoplastic to ensure consistent pressure or leave a "bubble" where the thermoplastic will be flared out to avoid the prominence. A small wad of exercise putty may be used for the "bubble" technique. A circle of sticky-back foam may

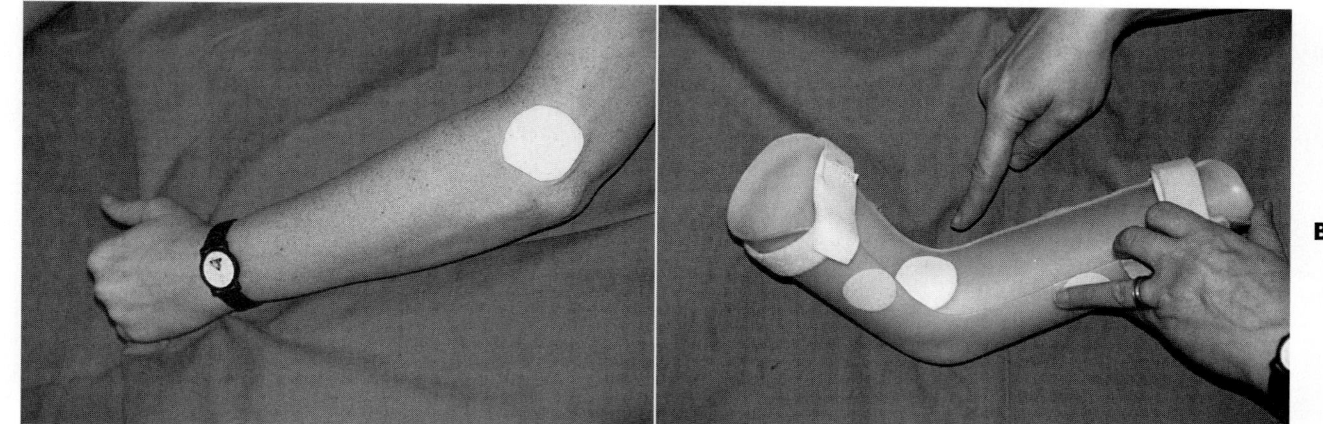

*Figure 22-13* Prepadding technique for bony prominence. **A,** Circle of self-adhesive foam applied to patient before application of thermoplastic. **B,** Self-adhesive foam pad in splint ensures consistent pressure.

be used when padded consistent contact is indicated (Figure 22-13).

### *Alignment*

The normal alignment of the digits should be maintained in the splint. The digits, when flexed, are parallel across the palm. At the wrist, 10° of ulnar deviation is the normal resting posture.

### *Dual Obliquity*

The radial side of the splint is longer and higher than the ulnar side to match the hand's anatomy (Figure 22-14).

### *Joints*

Exact positioning of the joints varies and depends on the patient's diagnosis and the purpose for which the splint is used. For example, the wrist is usually placed at 0° to 10° of extension for carpal tunnel syndrome, 30° of extension for functional position, or at 20° extension for resting. For the patient with increased flexor tone, wrist extension is sometimes compromised to permit adequate finger extension. Diagnosis, common sense, and physician preference all enter into the decision-making process. The COTA should consult the supervising registered occupational therapist (OTR) to ensure that positioning is as desired.

The prevention of adverse effects of immobilization is extremely important. To a joint, motion is lotion. Static splinting can cause joint stiffness with a resulting decrease in ROM. This leads to two actions. First, static splints must be removed periodically for active or passive exercise unless contraindicated by surgery, infection, or trauma. Second, unless absolutely necessary, joints that do not require immobilization should not be included in or restricted by the splint.

### *Creases*

The skin creases must be acknowledged as described earlier. Exceptions to this rule are (1) when including a joint because a muscle or tendon passes over it (e.g., immobilization of the wrist after flexor tendon repair in the digit) and (2) when the splint physically needs to be made longer to counterbalance the distal force (as in some dynamic splints).

In the normal hand, joints have an amazing capacity for stability or mobility. A splint cannot provide both; therefore the supervising OTR must choose between stability and mobility based on the patient's dysfunction, purpose of splinting, potential deformity, and the functional use of the hand. The patient may be given both dynamic and static splints for the same diagnosis.

### *Collateral Ligaments*

It is important to maintain the maximal length of collateral ligaments whenever possible. IP extension and MP flexion preserve this length. If the ligaments are allowed to shorten, restrictions in ROM may result.

### *Skin*

As discussed earlier, more padding exists on the volar surface of the hand and forearm than on the dorsal surface; therefore it is the preferred splinting surface if skin condition and function needs can be met. The sensory input received through cutaneous receptors is the key to functional use of the hand. A secretary might prefer a dorsal cock-up splint for carpal tunnel syndrome so that writing is not inhibited by decreased sensory input from the wrist and the ulnar border of the hand.

Open wounds and incision sites should be avoided whenever possible. Pressure or friction results in microtrauma to underlying structures. This trauma causes an increase in circulation to the area, and a red spot is seen after wearing the splint for approximately 20 minutes. All splints should be checked for fit after 20 minutes of wear in the clinic to assess potential pressure areas. For patients with darker pigmentation, the COTA runs a finger over the bony prominences to

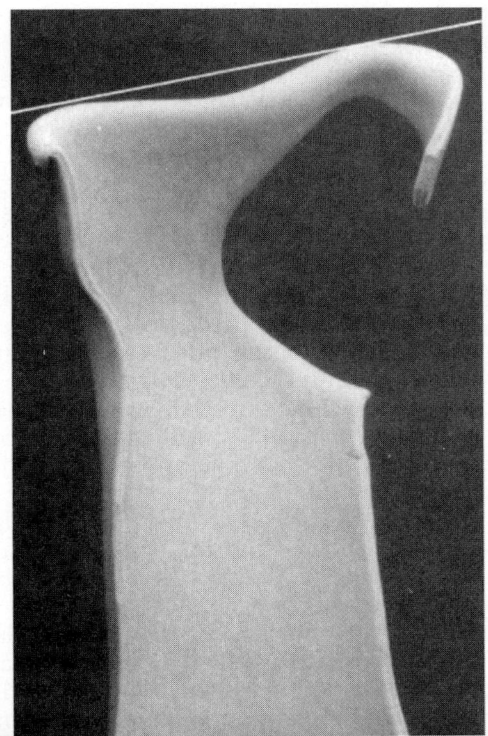

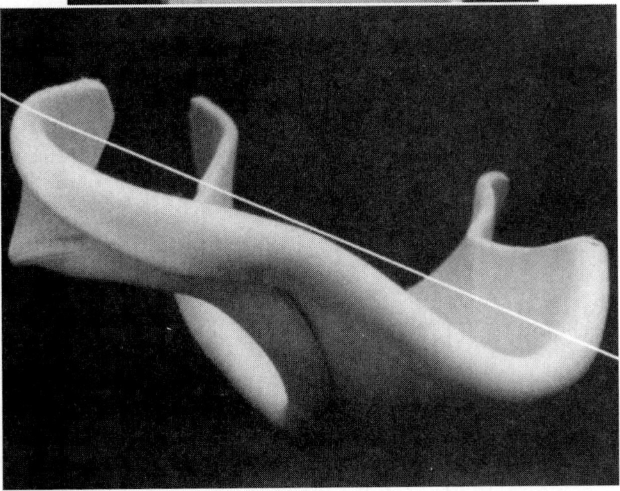

*Figure 22-14* Distal end of cock-up splint demonstrates dual obliquity.

check for "hot spots," then makes modifications as necessary.

Generally, the patient's arm is warm from wearing the splint or may look pinker in appearance. This is normal after several minutes; it is warm under the plastic. Usually the COTA or OTR provides the patient with some stockinette to wear under the splint to absorb perspiration. Thermoplastic materials do not breathe; however, perforated material does permit some air exchange.

Pressure is probably the greatest overall problem with fabricating a splint. In addition to potential spots over bony prominences, pressure may also be caused by poor fit and design. Wider, longer splints fit better than short, narrow ones.

General rules for avoiding pressure areas during splint fabrication are as follows:

1. The splint should be two-thirds the length of the forearm.
2. The splint should cover approximately half the circumference of the extremity (midbone trim marks work well).
3. Splint up to but do not include the next skin crease in the wrist/hand area in order to leave room for skin folds during ROM.
4. Fold or flare proximal and distal edges so they are rounded.
5. Round all internal and external corners. (Sharp corners wear poorly and will dig into the patient's skin.)
6. Reduce unequal pressure by means of a more conforming fit. The more conforming the splint, the better the pressure is distributed. What is more comfortable, a brand new pair of stiff, leather dress shoes or a pair of soft, conforming sneakers?

### *Sensorimotor Function*

Sensory information and feedback are essential components of normal movement. Splinting reduces sensory input from the area covered with thermoplastic and therefore may contribute to the patient's discomfort. Many patients requiring a splint have decreased sensation because of central or peripheral nerve deficits, and their risk of developing pressure areas with resulting skin breakdown is greater. Because their sensation is diminished, they may not complain that the splint is uncomfortable. These patients must be taught to compensate visually and to use their other hand to check for hot spots.

### Precautions

Significant precautionary measures have already been covered in this chapter, especially the risks involved with a poorly fitting splint. In addition, the skin's integrity is influenced by general medical conditions such as diabetes (sensory loss and atrophy), dehydration, and congestive heart failure (vascular compromise and edema).

Edema occurs, to a slight degree, whenever an extremity is immobilized, because the splint prohibits active ROM. Active motion is the muscle pump to keep fluids moving. Often therapists are required to splint an edematous extremity. Significant edema can occur after trauma and may also be seen in patients with compromised cardiac status. The splint must be large enough to accommodate the edema. If the patient swells during the course of the day, the OT practitioner should fabricate the splint later in the day. If this is not possible, the practitioner can allow for the anticipated swelling by using multiple layers of stockinette on the arm during fabrication. The patient is instructed to keep the arm elevated whenever possible by placing it up on a pillow when watching television or using a sling when standing for extended periods.

Patient compliance is essential, but many reasons exist why a patient may be noncompliant. The COTA should address these from the start. First, the splint must fit well; no one wants to wear something uncomfortable. Second, it must be cosmetically acceptable. Splints should be clean and neat, not marred by ragged edges and fingerprints. The patient pays a significant sum of money for the splint, and the splint is a reflection of the practitioner and the clinic. Third, splints are generally an inconvenience to the patient. They limit motion and sensation, are warm, and often seem "in the way." The COTA must explain that the temporary inconvenience is necessary for long-term gain in function. A carpal tunnel splint that sits atop a computer does no one any good.

### Material Selection

A tremendous variety of splinting material is available in the market today. Low-temperature thermoplastics are generally used for rigid splints. Flexible materials such as heavy fabric, neoprene, knitted elastics, and foam laminates may be used alone or in combination with rigid metal or thermoplastic stays. A quick overview of these "soft splints" follows later in this chapter.

#### *Low-Temperature Thermoplastics*

**Low-temperature thermoplastics** are generally heated in a water bath (splint pan, hydrocollator, electric frypan) to approximately 160° F (71.1° C), their molding temperature. The heated thermoplastic is applied to the patient dry. Low-temperature thermoplastic selection is based on two primary criteria: (1) how it handles during the forming (fabrication) process and (2) how it performs as a finished product.

**Handling characteristics** when the material has been heated to the recommended molding temperature include the following:

1. *Moldability* refers to how the material shapes around contours, or how easy it is to form. Moldability allows the OT practitioner to have the material take a specific shape.
2. *Drapability* refers to how easily the warm material forms to the patient with only gravity to mold it down. The drapier a material, the gentler the clinician's touch must be. These materials must be stroked, not poked or pushed into place. By keeping the hands moving during the forming process, the clinician will not leave fingerprint marks behind.

   The more drapey the material, the less appropriate it is for large splints. Generally the less experienced splinter prefers a low to moderate drape material. Very drapey materials should only be used on "cooperative" patients, those who are capable of holding their extremity in the appropriate position so that gravity can assist the practitioner during forming. *Rebound* is the term used when a nondrapey material springs back slightly during molding.
3. *Elasticity* refers to how much the material resists stretch. When pulled or tugged, does it follow easily or does it resist?
4. *Memory materials,* when reheated, return to their original size and shape. They are more elastic than nonmemory materials.
5. *Consistency* relates to the material handling the same way every time it is used. The practitioner wants it to have the same drape every time it is heated to the recommended molding temperature.
6. *Heating* is how much time is required in the water bath to reach molding temperature. Usually, 1 minute will heat material ⅛-inch (0.3 cm) thick.
7. *Edge finishing* is the ease of finishing the edges in a smooth manner. Generally, synthetic (all-plastic) materials edge more easily than rubber-based thermoplastics.
8. *Self-bonding materials* bond to each other when they are warm and dry. Coated materials tack together at the edges, but once the material hardens, they can be popped apart. For a more permanent bond, the coating must be scraped off or removed with a solvent before bonding. A coated material, once stretched, is tackier and more likely to self-bond.
9. *Shrinkage* may occur in some materials during the cooling process. This must be compensated for in the final adjustments.
10. *Working time* averages 3 to 5 minutes for solid ⅛-inch thick material. The thinner or more perforated the material, the faster it cools. In some materials the conformability during cooling may slowly ease off; in others it cuts off quickly.

**Performance characteristics** relate to the end results, or how the splint works once it has hardened, and include the following:

1. *Conformability* is how intimately the splint fits into contoured areas. The COTA may see the imprint of the patient's fingerprints and hand creases when using a very drapey material. More conforming splints are usually more comfortable and less likely to migrate during use.
2. *Rigidity* is the strength of the splint. Will it bend under stress (from the patient's weight, muscle tone, or strength)? Rigidity of the splint also increases with the number of arches and contours built into the splint. Note that rigidity and drape are not related, although OT practitioners often use these terms interchangeably. A very drapey material may produce a very rigid end product, and vice versa.
3. *Flexibility* relates to how much repeated stress a splint can take. This is an important function in

a **circumferential** (going around the arm) splint design, in which the splint is pulled open for application or removal.
4. *Durability* is how long the splint will last. Natural rubber-based materials are more likely to become brittle with age and use than all-plastic materials.
5. *Finish* on the material may be smooth or slightly textured. Coated materials are slightly easier to keep clean.
6. *Moisture permeability* (air exchange) is affected solely by the amount of perforation (if any). Memory materials are available in superperforated versions for maximum air exchange.
7. *Colors* have an effect on patient compliance, especially with children. The darker thermoplastic colors are less likely to become lost in institutional bedsheets.
8. *Thickness*. The thinner the material, the more responsive it is to handling during the forming process and the lighter it is in weight. Thicker materials are usually stronger than thinner ones. Generally, ⅛-inch material is used for most splints.

Manufacturers' catalogs and their representatives assist the clinician in selecting appropriate materials for specific splint types and for the fabricator's level of skill. Materials change, new ones appear, former ones are retired, and a clinician must keep up to date. The practitioner should mold a sample of material before using it to fabricate a splint to acquire some experience with its handling characteristics.

### *Soft Splints*

Soft splints, because they are fabricated from more flexible materials, may permit partial motion at a joint. These semiflexible splints are used to limit motion or protect an area. They may be used for patients who "just won't tolerate" rigid immobilization. Other uses are for joint protection to ease chronic pain syndromes and for patients with arthritis in whom total immobilization would cause painful joint stiffness.

Soft splints are often fabricated for geriatric patients who have an increased potential for skin breakdown because of fragile skin or poor carry-over of the wearing regimen. Figure 22-15 provides examples of soft splints.

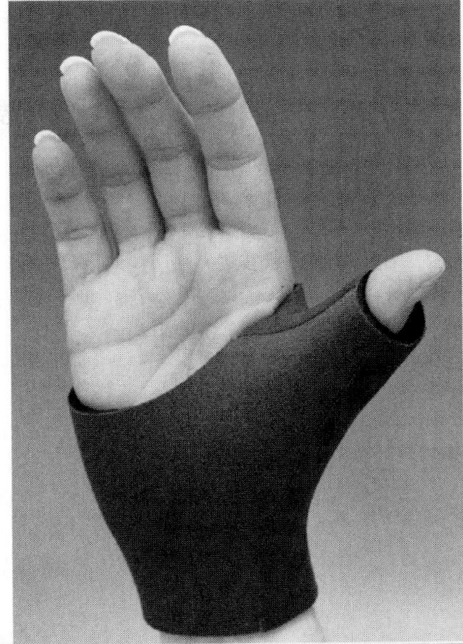


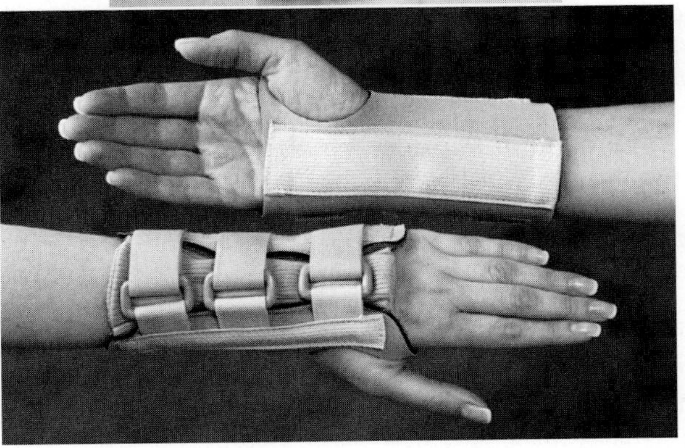


*Figure 22-15* **A,** Rolyan neoprene pull-on-thumb support. Warmth and compression of neoprene help reduce pain resulting from overuse of thumb and wrist. **B,** Rolyan D-ring wrist brace with metal support bar in a sleeve on flexor surface. (Courtesy Smith and Nephew Rolyan.)

## Strapping and Padding Principles

Straps are used to hold the splint in place and are fastened down with rivets, hook and loop material, or adhesive. Most splints are fastened with a hook and loop at three points to ensure that they do not migrate or rotate on the extremity. Hook fasteners and loop strapping are available with and without self-adhesive backing. The loop strapping is always applied facing the skin to prevent abrasion. Soft straps such as Durable are also compatible with Velcro hook fasteners. Straps with foam laminate (Velfoam, SoftStrap) are used when increased softness is needed. They can collapse somewhat to accommodate edema. Stretchy strapping (neoprene, Velfoam-2) is often used to reduce constriction.

D-ring straps may be used for a more secure fit or for a patient with decreased coordination. Straps where a self-adhesive hook is sewn onto the loop strap decrease the risk of losing the strap, which is beneficial in institutional settings. A variety of colors and widths is available in strapping materials.

Padding is available in two basic types: closed cell or open cell. Closed-cell paddings are nonabsorbent and can be wiped clean and dry. They do not absorb moisture or bacteria. Closed-cell foams may be applied directly to the thermoplastic before heating (the material floats in the heat pan, foam side up). This technique is desirable when additional insulation from heat is needed, as for burn patients or babies. Polycushion padding is soft and stretchable, easily molded around contours, whereas Kushionflex, Quickstick, and Plastazote paddings are less stretchable. The clinician should use padding that resists bottoming out (completely compressing) under pressure.

Open-cell cushioning is absorbent, similar to a sponge, and therefore needs to be changed frequently to ensure adequate hygiene. Rolyan Contour Foam is a slow-recovery foam often used to compensate for lack of splint contour. Moleskin and Molestick are thin paddings often used to reduce the risk of migration when a noncontouring thermoplastic is used. PPT foam padding is a very durable, shock-absorbing padding. Although open-cell, it has a nylon top skin that allows for easy washing.

Most padding materials are available in 1/16-, 1/8-, 1/4-, and 1/2-inch (0.15 to 1.25 cm) thicknesses, with or without self-adhesive backing. The 1/16- and 1/8-inch sticky-back paddings are the most frequently used. To ensure a firm purchase on the splinting material around the edges of the padding (and self-adhesive Velcro), the glue surface is heated with a heat gun before applying to the splint. When applying sticky-back foam directly to a bony prominence, it is helpful to use a circular shape; it is easier to replace the foam in the indentation left in the thermoplastic. Also, before applying padding directly to the patient's skin, the OT practitioner should stick and unstick the glued side on a towel to decrease its adhesive power so it will not stick too firmly to the patient's skin and so it can be easily removed.

### Patient Instruction

The patient instruction handout should always include wearing schedules, care instructions, and a precaution statement. When possible, wearing time should be built up over a few days so that the patient can become accustomed to the splint. The clinician must perform frequent skin checks and make sure the patient knows how to clean the splint with mild soap and warm, not hot, water and to dry the splint thoroughly before reapplying. The patient cannot put splints in the washing machine or dishwasher or leave them in a hot car in the summer or on a radiator. The splint will begin to melt at 135° F (57.2° C).

Straps should be snug, not tight. The patient should be able to insert a finger under the strap once it is fastened. (Tight fit cuts off the vascular supply and can increase edema.)

## SPLINT FABRICATION

Specific pattern-making techniques, material suggestions, fabrication instructions, and strapping patterns are provided for each of the three splints discussed in this chapter. To start, the following supplies are needed: (1) a heat pan, (2) a plastic spatula, (3) a towel, (4) sharp, clean scissors, (5) paper toweling, (6) a grease marker or awl, and (7) a heat gun. The heat pan needs a minimum of 2 inches of water heated to 160° F (71.1° C) (just beyond the simmer setting). It should have an unscratched, nonstick coating. If it does not, line the bottom of the pan with a pillowcase or paper toweling.

The following general technical tips will aid the reader in cutting, molding, and finishing various types of splints.

### Pattern Making

Patterns are usually made on a paper towel. The COTA or OTR cuts out and checks the fit on the patient, then traces the pattern onto the thermoplastic. If it is difficult to position the extremity because of the patient's muscle weakness, abnormal muscle tone, or pain, the pattern may be made on the opposite extremity and then inverted. Precut splint blanks are becoming more popular because they significantly decrease fabrication time and cost.

### Cutting

1. Place the pattern on the thermoplastic. Trace it with an awl or marker.
2. Using a utility knife, score a rectangular shape around the pattern and snap off the piece.
3. Heat the thermoplastic to the correct temperature by leaving it in the heat pan until it is uniformly flexible.
4. Remove the thermoplastic from the heat pan using the spatula. A plastic spatula will help prevent marring the nonstick coating of the pan.
5. Place the material promptly on the towel and gently pat it dry. Repeatedly flip the stickier materials over during drying so that they do not adhere to the towel. Do not hold the material vertically to allow the excess water to drip off because some materials may stretch in this position.
6. Support the excess material with one hand *and* the working surface to prevent stretching. Cut out the marked splint. Use the scissors as if you were cutting paper, leaving the blades slightly open between cuts. Round all the corners (Figure 22-16).

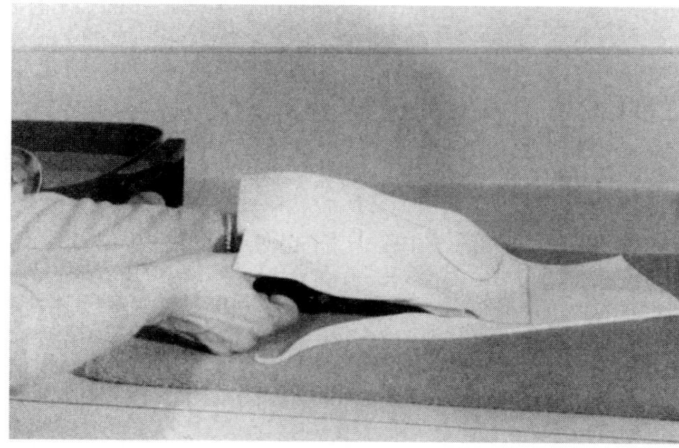

*Figure 22-16* Cutting splint out of heated thermoplastic.

Never cut the material when it is cool because this may strain the clinician's thumb and cause the splint edges to be jagged.

**Molding**

1. Heat a thermoplastic precut splint blank (or reheat the custom-cut splint) to the appropriate temperature. Remove the material from the heat pan, dry it, and let it cool for several seconds until it is comfortable to touch.
2. Position the patient, preferably so that the thermoplastic will be draping in a gravity-assisted manner.
3. Place the thermoplastic material on the arm/hand. Be sure to align the pattern properly. Stroke it into place. Use firm strokes with the pads of the fingers or the side of the hand to mold the plastic. Do not poke at the material or grasp it once it is in place because this may leave behind fingerprints and may affect the contour of the splint. Keep your hands moving when they are on the thermoplastic to prevent imprinting. Make sure to acknowledge the arches and to contour them into the splint carefully.
4. Flare the proximal edges of the splint and any other edges where pressure might occur. Flared or folded edges are more comfortable and increase the splint's strength.
5. Allow the splint to set until it is fairly rigid. Total working time is usually 3 to 5 minutes. Make sure to maintain the patient's position while the material sets. Thermoplastics with memory need to be molded until the material is firm.
6. If the splint was molded in supination, pronate the patient's forearm and check the fit. If the forearm trough is not centered, grasp the dorsal end and twist it to center the trough. ("Off-centering" occurs because the contour of the forearm changes as gravity pulls on the flexor muscles.)
7. Mark any trim lines that are indicated (e.g., midbone on the forearm, crease clearance, two-thirds length of the forearm).

**Finishing**

1. Hold the splint up vertically and dip area to be trimmed repeatedly in and out of the heat pan. When slightly softened, trim to the marked length and gently flare the end out with a sweeping stroke using the palm of the hand. This flare prevents the proximal end from digging into the forearm musculature.
2. To trim the sides or top, heat the side or top edge either by dipping the material in and out of the heat pan, pouring warm water over the spot to be trimmed, or using a heat gun. Once the material is slightly warm, cut along the trim lines. Do not heat the material to full molding temperature to do this; it may result in disfiguring the edge.
3. If necessary, smooth rough or jagged edges, again by dipping in and out of the water to slightly heat the material. Polish carefully with the fingertip or palm.

If major fit changes are required, reheat the entire splint and remold it. Do not attempt to spot-heat large areas such as the wrist or thumb.

**Strapping**

Straps are applied last. Refer to strapping methods and technical information discussed earlier in this chapter. Remember that three points of control are usually necessary to hold a splint in place, so three straps are used (see Figure 22-26).

**Evaluation**

On completion the splint must be analyzed for function, fit, and appearance.

***Function***

1. Are the arches of the hand maintained? Looking at the splint directly on, is the metacarpal area properly arched? Is the radial side of the palm higher than the ulnar side? Looking at the splint from the side, is the longitudinal arch obvious?
2. Is the hand splinted in the proper position? Use a goniometer to check joint angles.

***Fit***

1. Are the straps correctly placed to promote stability and to avoid pressure points?
2. Do the sides of the splint extend at least to midbone?
3. Is the splint long enough to support effectively the body parts involved? Are the appropriate joint creases visible to permit full joint ROM?
4. Are there any edges or corners that could press into the patient's skin? Any potential pressure sites over bony prominences such as the ulnar styloid? Check for reddened or warmer areas on the skin after 20 minutes of wearing time.

***Appearance***

1. Is the splint surface smooth and free of marks, dents, and rough edges?
2. Are all the corners rounded, edges smooth, and proximal and distal ends flared where appropriate?
3. Are the straps neat and aligned correctly? Is the self-adhesive hook fully covered by the strap?
4. Is it cosmetically acceptable to the clinician and the patient?

**Directions**

***Radial Bar Wrist Cock-Up Splint***

A cock-up splint is used to support and/or position the wrist. For functional positioning the wrist is aligned at 20° to 30° of extension. In patients with carpal tunnel syndrome the wrist is positioned at 0° to 10°. Use a drapey material such as Polyform, Polyflex II, Aquaplast-T, or Aquaplast ProDrape-T splinting material.

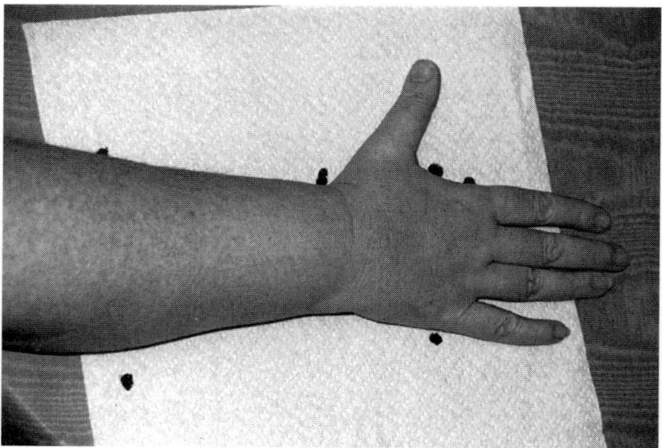

*Figure 22-17* Marking bony landmarks for radial bar cock-up splint on paper towel.

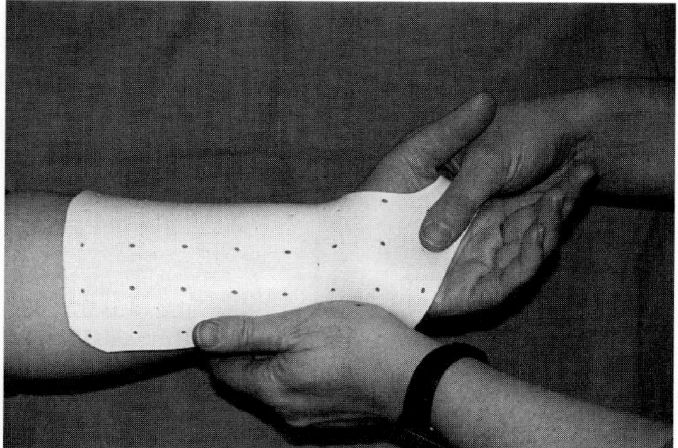

*Figure 22-19* Align splint with palmar arch and begin to mold in contours.

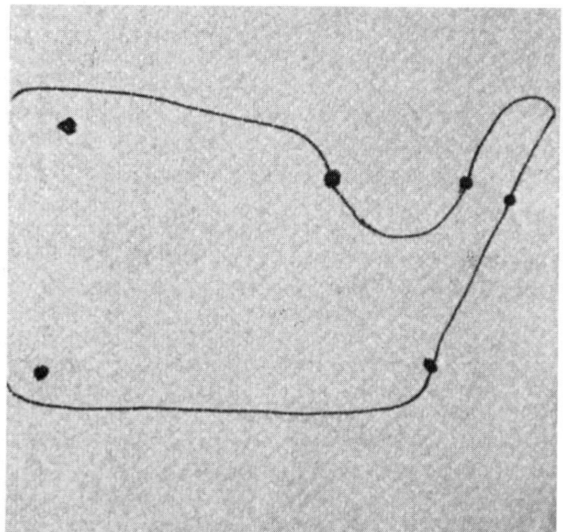

*Figure 22-18* Radial bar cock-up splint pattern.

*Pattern*

1. Mark the following landmarks: the MP heads on the radial and ulnar sides of the hand, the base of the web space, the wrist joint on the radial side, and two-thirds the length of the forearm.
2. Draw the pattern as shown in Figure 22-17, allowing sufficient excess for the width of the splint to wrap halfway around the forearm.
3. Remove the patient's arm and connect, with a circular arc, the web space and wrist markings as seen in Figure 22-18.
4. Cut out the pattern and check the fit on the patient. Make adjustments as needed.

*Fabrication*

1. Trace the pattern onto the thermoplastic and heat it. Cut out the splint blank and reheat to molding temperature if needed.
2. With the patient's forearm supinated, position the wrist at the appropriate angle of extension and ulnar deviation. Drape the material over the hand/forearm, taking care to line up the distal end with the palmar crease. Wrap the radial bar through the web space around to the dorsum of the hand.
3. Smooth the wrist area of the material by stroking it into place laterally and continue proximally up the forearm, taking care not to twist the trough to either side (Figure 22-19).
4. Place the thumb gently in the palmar arch area to ensure contour and stroke into place. Flare or fold the distal edge so that the palmar crease (proximal crease at the second MP, distal crease for third to fifth MP) is visible and continues through the web space. Have the patient oppose the thumb to tip of the index or middle finger. This will cause a fold at the thenar eminence. Flatten this fold down and continue along the radial bar into the web space area as seen in Figure 22-20.
5. Allow the splint to set.
6. Apply straps (Figure 22-21) to the splint proximally, across the wrist and across the dorsum of the hand to the radial bar tab.

### *Resting Hand Splint*

Resting hand splints are used for positioning the wrist and fingers. Common goals for using resting splints are to decrease joint inflammation or prevent joint contractures. Use a material with moderate drape and rigid performance, such as Ezeform, Aquaplast-T, or San-Splint splinting material.

*Pattern*

1. Trace the hand, leaving approximately ½-inch excess width around the hand area and 1½ inches in the forearm area. Mark two-thirds the length of the forearm. Your pattern should resemble a mitten (Figure 22-22).

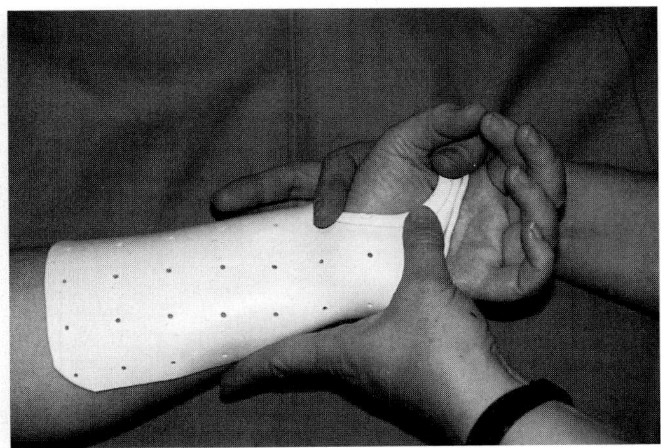

*Figure 22-20* With patient in opposition, fold splint at palmar and thenar creases.

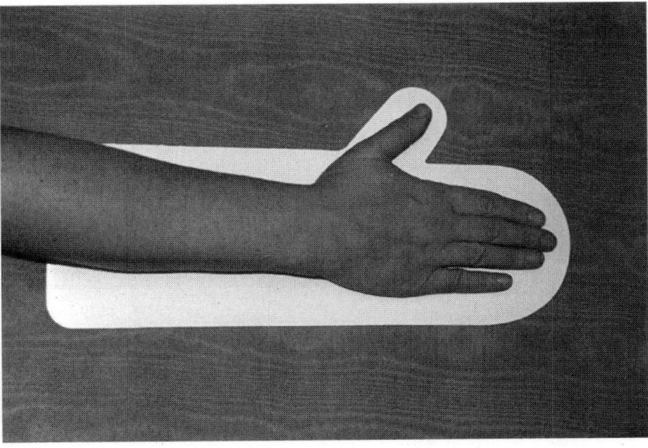

*Figure 22-22* Resting mitt splint with precut splint blank/pattern.

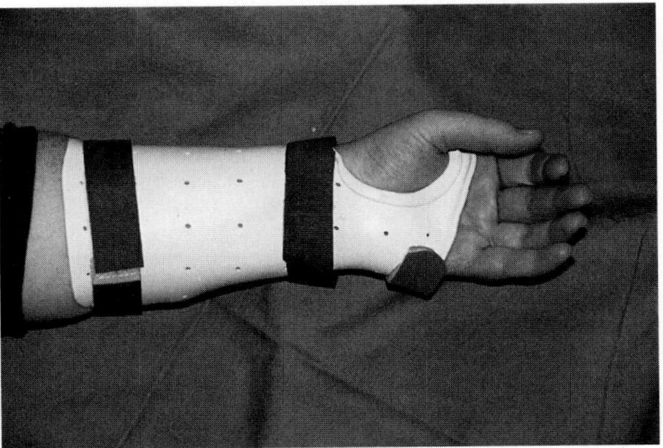

*Figure 22-21* Completed radial bar cock-up splint.

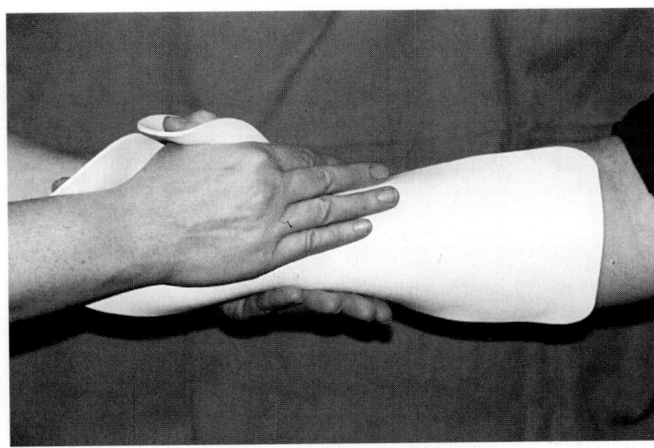

*Figure 22-23* Place warm thermoplastic on patient, making sure thumb/web space area is properly seated and trough is aligned with forearm.

2. Cut it out of the paper toweling and check the fit on the patient before transferring the pattern to the thermoplastic. Once the splint blank is cut out of the thermoplastic, reheat to molding temperature if necessary.

*Fabrication*

1. Place the warm splinting material on the patient as seen in Figure 22-23, preferably with the patient's forearm in a supinated position so that gravity assists in holding the material in place. Make sure the thumb/web space area is seated properly, and flare the thermoplastic to create the flange on the splint in the thumb/web area.
2. Stroke the material into position at the wrist. This creates a waist in the material and helps keep it from sliding. Continue molding up the forearm.
3. Using two hands, one to ensure correct anatomical position of the wrist/hand and the other to mold, gently form the material. Create a flange along the sides of the fingers to increase material strength in the hand area as seen in Figure 22-24. Use alternate hands: one to position, the other to mold. Use your thumb to ensure proper forming in the palmar arch area.
4. Once the material is semirigid, pronate the forearm (Figure 22-25) and proceed as previously described to trim and finish.
5. Apply straps proximally, at the wrist, across the dorsum of the hand or proximal phalanges, and at the thumb (Figure 22-26).

### Short Opponens Splint

A short opponens splint is used to support the CMC (knuckle) joint of the thumb when it is inflamed from overuse or arthritic changes. Use a drapey material with a high degree of contour. In some cases, because of an enlarged IP joint or a bulbous distal phalanx, it may be necessary to open the thumb spica area to be able to don and remove the splint. For such patients, Aquaplast-T or Polyflex II splinting material would be

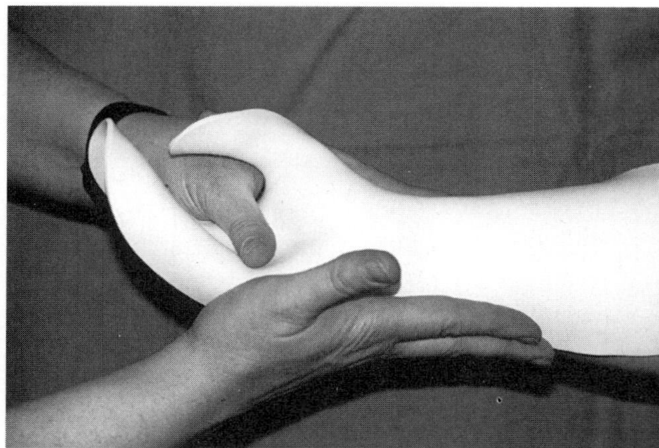

*Figure 22-24* Stroke material into place. Create flanges in hand/thumb/wrist areas. Practitioner's thumb is used to help form palmar arch.

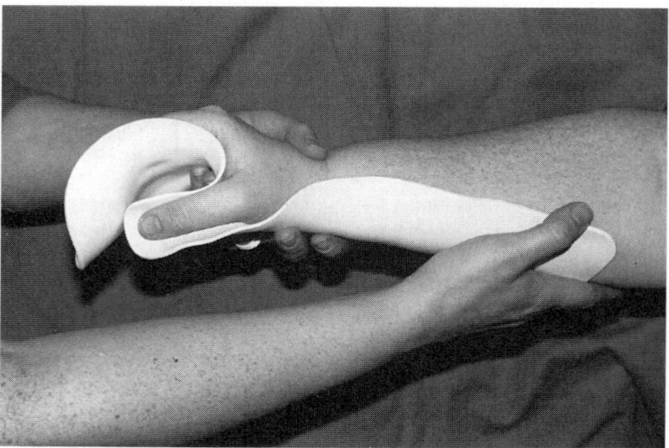

*Figure 22-25* With forearm in pronation, grasp proximal end of splint and twist it to center the trough.

good choices. They are slightly flexible and hold up well under the repeated stress of being pulled open.

*Pattern*

1. Mark the following landmarks on the paper toweling: the MP heads on the radial and ulnar sides of the hand, the radial and ulnar sides of the wrist, and the IP crease of the thumb (Figure 22-27).
2. Draw the pattern as shown in Figure 22-28 and cut out the pattern. Check the fit on the patient. The bulbous end of the pattern wraps circumferentially around the thumb. Trace the pattern onto the splinting material and proceed as described earlier.

*Fabrication*

1. Reheat the splint to molding temperature. Position the patient's elbow on the table with the forearm straight up. Align the edge of the splinting material with the IP crease and wrap the splinting material snugly around the thumb as seen in Figure 22-29.
2. Wrap the narrow end of the splint around the ulnar border of the hand (Figure 22-30). Keep this part centered. Ask the patient to oppose the thumb to the second digit while you smooth the material into place. Make sure the splint contours well into the web space. (NOTE: Give the patient a quarter to pinch. This prevents the thumb from moving out of alignment while the splint hardens.)
3. Have the patient flex and extend the wrist as the fit is checked. Wrist motion should not be restricted. Trim if necessary to allow full ROM.

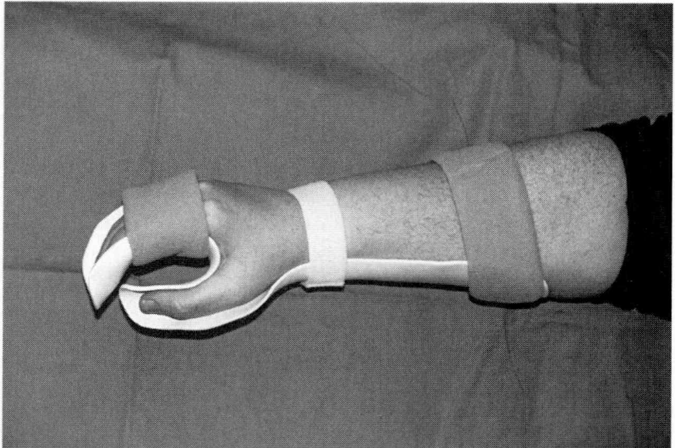

*Figure 22-26* Completed resting splint.

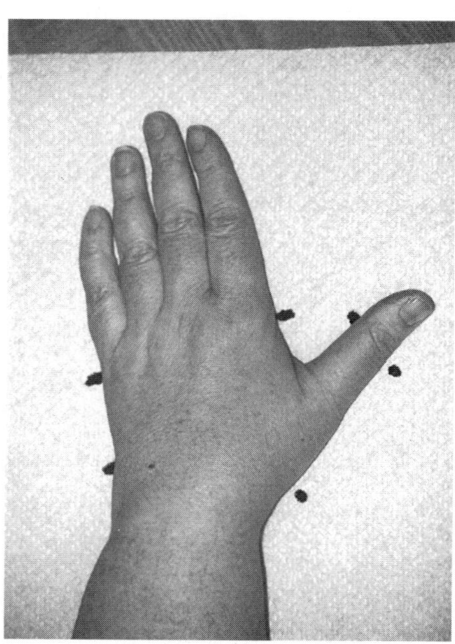

*Figure 22-27* Mark bony landmarks for short opponens splint on paper towel.

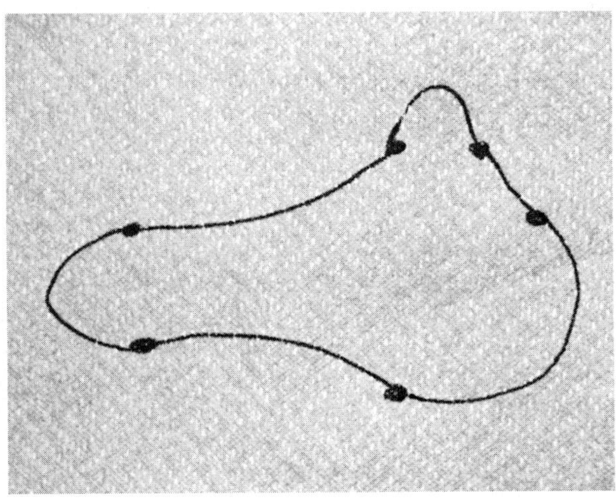

*Figure 22-28* Draw pattern for short opponens splint.

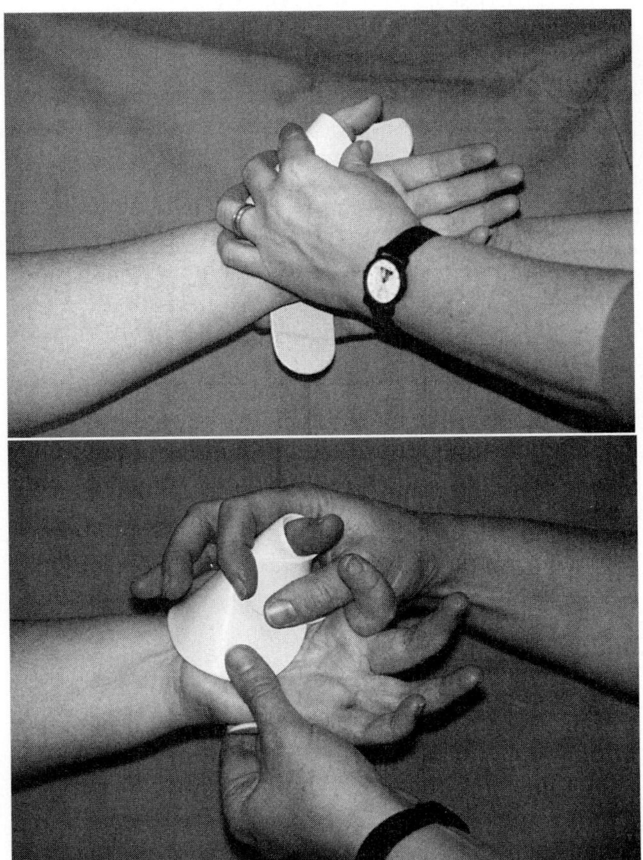

*Figure 22-29* Align edge of splint with IP crease and wrap snugly around thumb.

4. Once the splint is set, trim if needed around the thenar crease.
5. Apply a strap to secure the ulnar border to the thenar area (Figure 22-31). If the patient has difficulty inserting and removing the thumb through the splint, pop the overlapped area open by twisting it once the material is completely cool. Secure with hook-and-loop strapping material.

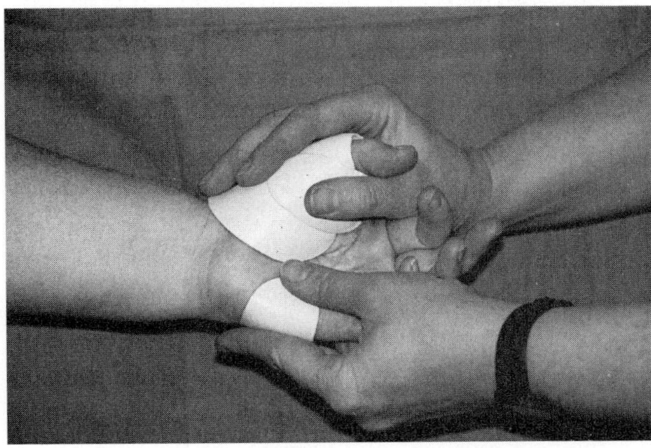

*Figure 22-30* Wrap narrow end of splint dorsally around hand, over ulnar border.

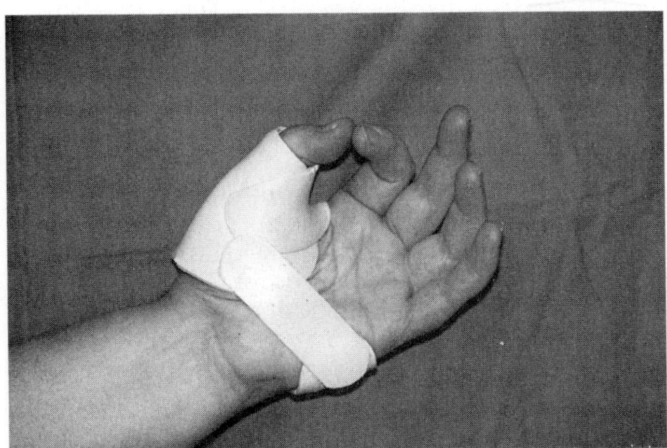

*Figure 22-31* Completed short opponens splint.

## SUMMARY

The purpose of splinting is to preserve or enhance the use of the hand. Thus the construction of every splint must respect the hand's natural arches, contours, and mechanics.

The COTA who has achieved service competency may independently construct resting splints and other static (non-moving) splints. Effective splint construction requires an understanding of the performance and handling characteristics of the materials, an awareness of precautions, and expertise in pattern making and use of materials.

The splint affects the appearance of the hand and should be as neat and attractive as possible.

## *Selected Reading Guide Questions*

1. What is the role of the occupational therapy assistant in hand splinting?
2. List five functions of the normal hand.
3. Describe the relationship of shoulder, elbow, and wrist function to hand use.
4. Which type of prehension is used to pick up a straight pin?
5. Which type of prehension is used to turn a key in a lock?
6. Which type of grasp is used to hold a soda can?
7. What happens to the hand if the metacarpal transverse arch is flattened?
8. In which position are the muscles of the hand at the best mechanical advantage to function efficiently?
9. Describe and demonstrate the dual obliquity of the hand. Why is it an important consideration in hand splinting?
10. Name the three nerves that supply sensation and motion to the hand. Which one is most critical to tactile discriminative function?
11. Name the three major classifications of splints. Give one example of each.
12. How are the adverse effects of immobilization by splinting best prevented?
13. What is the optimal position for splinting the wrist for function?
14. What is the optimal position for splinting the wrist for carpal tunnel syndrome?
15. What effect does wrist flexion have on hand function?
16. Why is it important to splint the MP joints in some flexion if these joints are to be splinted?
17. State six purposes of splinting.
18. List and describe three limitations of splints.
19. What are the two main characteristics that influence selection of thermoplastic material? Give several examples of each.
20. List six general guidelines for achieving optimal fit and function of the splint.

### *REFERENCES*


1. Bender LF: Upper extremity orthotics. In Kottke FJ, Stillwell GK, Lehmann JF: *Krusen's handbook of physical medicine and rehabilitation,* ed 3, Philadelphia, 1982, Saunders.
2. Brand P: The forces of dynamic splinting: ten questions before applying a dynamic splint to the hand. In Hunter JM, Mackin EJ, Callahan AD, editors: *Rehabilitation of the hand,* ed 4, St Louis, 1995, Mosby.
3. Fess EE, Gettle KS, Strickland JW: *Hand splinting: principles and methods,* St Louis, 1987, Mosby.
4. Gribben M: Splinting principles for hand injuries. In Moran CA, editor: *Hand rehabilitation,* New York, 1986, Churchill Livingstone.
5. Hardy MA: Preserving function in the inflamed and acutely injured hand. In Moran CA, editor: *Hand rehabilitation,* New York, 1986, Churchill Livingstone.
6. Kiel JH: *Basic hand splinting: a pattern designing approach,* Boston, 1983, Little, Brown.
7. Malick M: *Manual on static hand splinting,* rev ed, Pittsburgh, 1972, Harmarville Rehabilitation Center.
8. Malick M: *Manual on dynamic hand splinting with thermoplastic materials,* Pittsburgh, 1982, Harmarville Rehabilitation Center.
9. Melvin JL: *Rheumatic disease: occupational therapy and rehabilitation,* Philadelphia, 1977, Davis.
10. *Principles of hand splinting,* Downey, Calif, 1962, Occupational Therapy Department, Ranchos Los Amigos Hospital (unpublished).
11. Smith and Nephew Rolyan: *1996 rehabilitation products catalog,* Germantown, Wis, 1996, Rolyan.
12. *Static splinting workshop,* Germantown, Wis, 1995, Smith and Nephew Rolyan (unpublished).
13. Tubiana R: Architecture and functions of the hand. In Tubiana R, Thomine J, Mackin E: *Examination of the hand and upper limb,* Philadelphia, 1984, Saunders.


### *RECOMMENDED READING*


Coppard BM, Lohman HL: *Introduction to splinting: a critical-thinking and problem-solving approach,* St Louis, 1996, Mosby.

Chapter 23

# Sensorimotor Approaches to Treatment

*Patricia A. Gentile*
*Jan Zaret Davis*
*Fred Feuchter*
*Guy L. McCormack*
*Lorraine Williams Pedretti*
*Sara A. Pope-Davis*

## *Chapter Objectives*

*After studying this chapter, the student or practitioner will be able to:*

1. Describe in general terms what is meant by a sensorimotor treatment approach.
2. Name the four traditional sensorimotor treatment approaches.
3. Describe the basic goals and focus of each of the four sensorimotor treatment approaches.
4. Discuss common sensorimotor deficits seen in patients with neurological dysfunction, and provide examples of how these problems can interfere with function.
5. Provide an example of how each of the sensorimotor treatment approaches can be incorporated into activities of daily living (ADLs) training.

## *Key Terms*

muscle tone
spasticity
flaccidity
proprioceptive stimulation
cutaneous stimulation
cerebrovascular accident (CVA)
Rood approach
Brunnstrom approach (movement therapy)
proprioceptive neuromuscular facilitation (PNF)
manual contact
stretch
traction

### Key Terms—cont'd

approximation
maximal resistance
repeated contraction
rhythmical initiation
reversal of movement
rhythmical stabilization
relaxation techniques
neurodevelopmental (Bobath) treatment (NDT) approach
facilitation techniques
inhibition techniques

Sensorimotor treatment approaches are used with patients who have central nervous system (CNS) dysfunction. The CNS consists of the brain and spinal cord. When damage to these structures occurs, the ability to produce controlled, coordinated movement is frequently lost, resulting in abnormal changes in muscle tone, balance, posture, and reflexive movement. **Muscle tone,** which refers to the natural tension within a muscle, can become either too high **(spasticity)** or too low **(flaccidity).**

Changes in muscle tone can affect the ability to move. Patients with spasticity may decrease their movement or be unable to initiate movement. This may result in joint contractures. Flaccidity can have the opposite effect. If muscle tone is too low, a patient may have difficulty maintaining an upright position or lifting an arm or leg against gravity.

Balance and posture are typically affected in patients with CNS dysfunction. A patient's posture may appear asymmetrical or uneven because of low tone of the trunk muscles, giving the person the appearance of leaning toward one side. Balance, which depends on the ability to shift weight and react to changes in positioning, may also become impaired. Because of the inability to maintain balance while sitting or standing, patients may experience difficulty performing self-care activities. Poor balance may also put patients at risk for falling.

The reappearance of reflexes after CNS dysfunction is common. Reflexes are stereotypical, automatic movements present in all individuals. During normal motor development, reflexes become integrated, allowing an individual to perform controlled movements. When damage to the CNS occurs, reflexes may reappear, limiting the types of movement available. For example, the placement of an object in the palm of the hand may result in automatic closing of the fingers and the inability to open the hand. This can affect function.

Finally, CNS damage can adversely affect a patient's sensation. Some patients may report "not feeling" the affected limbs or may describe the arm or leg as feeling heavy and clumsy. Others may not be able to distinguish where the arm is in relationship to objects or other body parts, resulting in decreased coordination.

Sensorimotor treatment approaches are geared toward reducing the abnormal changes just described. These approaches are based on the idea that abnormal motor responses can be reduced, and more normal motor responses can be learned by the CNS. This is the ultimate goal of all the sensorimotor approaches.

Many sensorimotor treatment approaches use sensory stimuli to influence motor responses. Frequently used stimuli include proprioceptive and cutaneous. **Proprioceptive stimulation** refers to stimulation that affects joint and muscle receptors and includes techniques such as stretching, weight bearing, and resistance.[40] **Cutaneous stimulation** affects the exteroceptors of the skin.[1,4,36] *Exteroceptors,* located immediately under the skin, respond to stimuli such as touch, temperature, and pain.[28,41] Cutaneous stimuli can be used to facilitate or inhibit muscle responses. Combined with proprioceptive stimulation, cutaneous stimulation may be used to elicit voluntary control of specific muscles.

Reflex mechanisms may also be used in some treatment approaches. As described earlier, reflexes are automatic, stereotypical motor responses. In some approaches, reflexes may be used early in treatment to elicit movement. For instance, when a patient with poor balance is encouraged to lean toward the weak side, the person may demonstrate a reflexive extension of the affected arm to prevent falling. This is an example of a specific reflexive response known as a *protective reaction.*

Sensorimotor treatment approaches are used with individuals who have sustained injury to the CNS. This injury could be the result of a disease process, a structural or genetic defect, or a traumatic event. Such CNS injuries include **cerebrovascular accident (CVA),** head injury, and cerebral palsy. Sensorimotor treatment approaches work to normalize muscle tone, to facilitate symmetrical posture, and to improve balance. The successful achievement of these objectives can help to restore coordinated and purposeful movements.

When treating patients with CNS dysfunction, the registered occupational therapist (OTR) begins by selecting a specific sensorimotor approach. Selection depends on several factors, including the patient's strengths and weaknesses, the therapist's preference, and the philosophy of a particular treatment setting. Using the evaluation procedures for the approach selected, the OTR performs a comprehensive evaluation. The evaluation establishes a baseline for the patient, and this baseline is the starting point for treatment. When working together with the certified occupational therapist assistant (COTA), the OTR directs and oversees the COTA in using aspects of the selected approach in treatment. Both OTR and COTA must recognize that many sensorimotor techniques have the potential to affect the patient adversely; therefore all clinicians using these techniques must demonstrate sufficient knowledge and skills for safe application.

To implement treatment plans effectively for persons with neurological dysfunctions, the COTA should be familiar with the various sensorimotor approaches, their basic principles, and the specific techniques used in each. The COTA who treats patients with CNS damage and intends to use any of these techniques can do so only with specific directions from the OTR. The COTA must always be thoroughly trained and properly supervised when using these techniques. Instruction about the nature of the technique, the specific procedure for application, the expected response, and possible risks and contraindications must be provided to the COTA by the OTR.

The purpose of this chapter is to provide the COTA with an introduction to and practical information about the sensorimotor approaches used in occupational therapy treatment. This chapter discusses the following approaches: the Rood approach, the Brunnstrom (movement therapy) approach, the proprioceptive neuromuscular approach, and the neurodevelopmental (Bobath) approach.

## THE ROOD APPROACH

Margaret S. Rood was both an occupational therapist and a physical therapist. Her theory originated in the 1940s and evolved from the developmental and neurophysiological literature of the previous decade.[41] Rood integrated this literature with her own clinical observations to create an approach based on the use of sensory stimulation to effect motor responses.

Rood did not write extensively, seeming to prefer clinical teaching to disseminate her ideas. Most of the literature that describes the **Rood approach** is based on interpretations by accomplished physical and occupational therapists, such as Ayres,[2,3] Farber,[13,14] Heininger and Randolph,[16] Huss,[18] and Stockmeyer.[35] Despite some controversy about the efficacy of Rood's techniques, current neuroscience research continues to support the importance of sensory stimulation.

The basic assumption of Rood's theory is the belief that appropriate sensory stimulation can elicit specific motor responses. Rood combined controlled sensory stimulation with a sequence of positions and activities that replicate normal ontogenic motor development (i.e., the normal progression of motor skills) to achieve purposeful muscular responses.[18]

### Basic Assumptions

The basic assumptions of Rood's theory are summarized as follows:

*Normal muscle tone is a prerequisite to movement.*

Patients with CNS dysfunction may exhibit changes in muscle tone, ranging from *hypertonicity* (too much tone) to *hypotonicity* (too little tone). This abnormal tone interferes with movement, and the achievement of normalized muscle tone is essential for controlled movement.

Normal muscle tone flows smoothly and is constantly changing depending on the demands of a motor act. For example, to turn on the ignition of a car, a person must have good eye-hand coordination, postural control of the trunk muscles, co-innervation of the proximal arm muscles, forearm pronation and supination, and moderately fine prehension and dexterity in the hands.

In addition, the demands placed on the various muscle groups are different. Rood recognized this when she stated, "Muscles have different duties," with some muscles predominantly used for heavy work and others for light work. *Light-work muscles* are referred to as *mobilizers* and are primarily the flexors and adductors. The primary function of the light-work muscles is directed toward skilled movement patterns. *Heavy-work muscles*, however, act as *stabilizers* and consist of the extensors and abductors.[15] The primary function of heavy-work muscles is to allow maintenance of posture and holding patterns of movement. Heavy-work and light-work muscles act together to allow coordinated movements to occur. For example, when putting on a necklace, the heavy-work muscles are responsible for co-contraction proximally at the trunk, shoulder, and forearm, thereby maintaining the arm up against gravity. The light-work muscles, located more distally, are responsible for the coordination and dexterity needed to manipulate the clasp.

Rood[30] also believed that reflexes are the foundation of any voluntary motor act. These reflexes are modified, controlled, and integrated by the CNS. Rood began therapy by eliciting motor responses on a reflex level and using developmental patterns to improve the motor response.

*Treatment begins at the developmental level of functioning.*

Rood believed that movement occurs in a developmental sequence. Patients are evaluated developmentally, and treatment follows a developmental sequence. Because one skill builds on the other, patients do not proceed to the next level of sensorimotor development until some degree of voluntary control is achieved. This principle follows the *cephalocaudal rule*. Treatment begins from the head and proceeds downward segment by segment, from proximal to distal, to the sacral area. The flexors are stimulated first, the extensors second, the adductors third, and the abductors last.[35]

- *Motivation enhances purposeful movement.*

Rood realized that motivation plays an important role in rehabilitation. Activities that are meaningful for the patient encourage practice of desired movements. This results in greater patient participation in treatment.

- *Repetition is necessary for the reeducation of muscular responses.*

Repetition helps develop coordination.[20,21] Repetition assists the brain to develop an internal "memory" of a specific motor activity. Repetition, however, can be monotonous. To avoid boredom, various activities that incorporate similar motor patterns should be provided.

### Principles of Treatment

Rood suggested four general principles in the treatment of neuromuscular dysfunction, as follows[31]:

- *Reflexes can be used to assist or retard the effects of sensory stimulation.*

According to Rood, reflexes can be used to influence muscle tone. Two mechanisms frequently mentioned are the *tonic neck reflexes* (TNRs) and *tonic labyrinthine reflexes* (TLRs). The TNRs are triggered by changes in the relationship of the head to the neck; TLRs occur with changes in the relationship of the head to gravity. Consequently, any changes in the position of the head to the neck, or in relationship of the head to gravity, can result in increases or decreases in muscle tone. Clinicians must therefore be aware of the position of the head and neck and the potential effects of gravity on the body.

- *Sensory stimulation of receptors can produce predictable responses.*

Responses following sensory stimulation to specific receptors are predictable. Clinicians using sensory stimulation can use this predictability to achieve a desired outcome. For example, a slow rocking stimuli produces a calming effect and may be beneficial for patients with high tone or agitation.

- *Muscles have different duties.*

As discussed earlier, some muscles predominate as stabilizers (heavy-work muscles), whereas others undertake the duties of mobilization (light-work muscles). According to Rood, each group has distinct functions and characteristics.

- *Heavy-work muscles should be integrated before light-work muscles.*

The principle of integrating heavy-work muscles before light-work muscles primarily refers to the use of the upper extremities (UEs). For example, fine fingertip manipulation is not functional if the proximal muscles are not strong enough to lift or stabilize the position of the arms.

### Sequence of Motor Development

Rood proposed four sequential phases related to the development of motor control, as follows[3,31,32]:

1. *Reciprocal inhibition (innervation).* Reciprocal inhibition is an early mobility phase that serves a protective function. The muscle acting on one side of a joint *(agonist)* quickly contracts while its opposite *(antagonist)* relaxes. An example of reciprocal innervation is seen in infants who randomly flex and extend their arms and legs.
2. *Co-contraction.* Co-contraction occurs when opposing muscles (usually those surrounding a joint) contract simultaneously, resulting in stabilization of the joint. The co-contraction phase allows an individual to hold a position or an object for a longer time. Standing upright is a result of co-contraction of the trunk muscles.
3. *Heavy work.* The heavy-work phase as been defined as "mobility on stability."[35] In this phase the proximal muscles move and the distal segments are fixed. An example of this phase is creeping. During creeping the infant is in a quadruped (all-fours) position. The hands and feet are in a fixed position, but the shoulders and hips move.
4. *Skill.* Skill is the highest level of control and combines the efforts of mobility and stability. In a skilled movement pattern the proximal segment is stabilized while the distal segment moves freely. Reaching overhead to unscrew a light bulb is an example of this pattern.

### Ontogenic Movement Patterns

The sequence of motor development described previously occurs as the patient is put through a specific sequence that Rood called *ontogenic motor patterns.*[15] Figure 23-1 illustrates the eight ontogenic motor patterns.

#### *Supine Withdrawal (Supine Flexion)*

Supine withdrawal is a total flexion response toward the navel. This is a protective position. Supine withdrawal is a mobility posture requiring reciprocal innervation; it also requires heavy work of the proximal muscles and trunk.[31] Rood recommended this pattern for patients who do not have the reciprocal flexion pattern and for those dominated by extensor tone (Figure 23-1, *A*).

#### *Roll Over (Toward Side Lying)*

When rolling over, the arm and leg flex on the same side of the body (Figure 23-1, *B*). Rolling over is a mobility pattern for the UEs and lower extremities (LEs) and activates the lateral trunk musculature.[35]

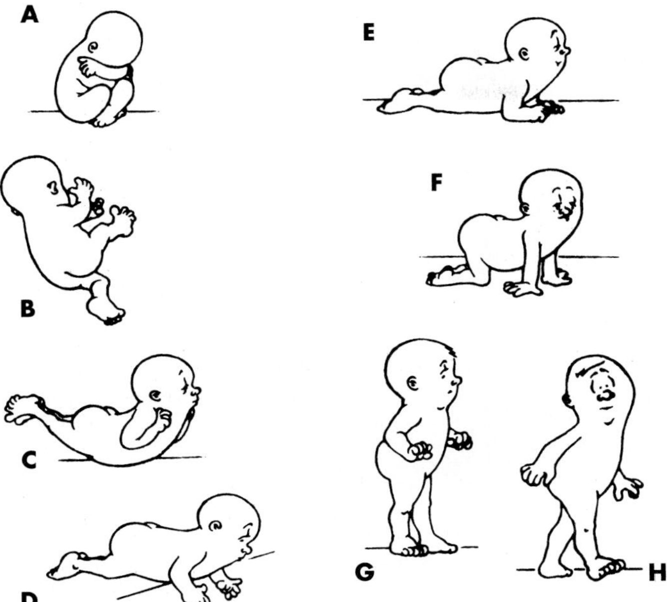


*Figure 23-1* Ontogenic motor patterns. **A,** Supine withdrawal. **B,** Roll over toward side lying. **C,** Pivot prone. **D,** Neck contraction. **E,** Prone on elbows. **F,** Quadraped pattern. **G,** Static standing. **H,** Walking.

This pattern is encouraged for patients who are dominated by reflexes or need segmental movements of the extremities.

### *Pivot Prone (Prone Extension)*

The pivot-prone position demands a full range of extension of the neck, shoulders, trunk, and LEs (Figure 23-1, *C*). This pattern has been called both a mobility pattern and a stability pattern. The position is difficult to assume and hold. It plays an important role in preparation for stability in the upright position.

### *Neck Co-Contraction (Co-Innervation)*

Neck co-contraction is the first real stability pattern. It is used to develop head control and stability of the neck (Figure 23-1, *D*). This pattern is needed to raise the head against gravity.

### *On Elbows (Prone on Elbow)*

Following co-contraction of the neck and prone extension, weight bearing on the elbows is the next pattern to achieve. This pattern helps develop stability in the scapular and glenohumeral (shoulder) regions. This position gives the patient a better view of the environment and an opportunity to shift weight from side to side (Figure 23-1, *E*).

### *All Fours (Quadruped Position)*

The quadruped position develops stability of the lower trunk and legs. Initially the patient holds the position. Eventually, weight shifting forward, backward, side to side, and diagonally is added. The weight shifting may be preparatory for balance responses (Figure 23-1, *F*).

### *Static Standing*

Static standing is thought to be a skill of the upper trunk because it frees the UEs for prehension and manipulation.[35] At first, weight is equally distributed on both legs, then weight shifting begins. This position requires higher level integration, such as maintaining and achieving balance (Figure 23-1, *G*).

### *Walking*

Walking unites skill, mobility, and stability. Walking is a complicated process requiring coordinated movement patterns of the various parts of the body (Figure 23-1, *H*).

## Specific Techniques Used in Treatment

Rood described in detail the use of cutaneous and proprioceptive stimulation in treatment. Stimuli typically used in clinical practice are briefly described next. Before using any of these techniques with patients, the COTA must be properly trained and demonstrate service competency. During the actual use of these techniques, the OTR is responsible for providing proper supervision to the COTA. Emphasis during supervision should be on safe application, precautions, and awareness of the expected outcome of the technique.

When applying any of the cutaneous or proprioceptive techniques, the COTA should always remember that these techniques are preparatory to functional activity. Whenever possible, the application should be followed immediately by the patient's involvement in a functional activity. For example, applying deep pressure to the tendon of the biceps may help relax the elbow so the patient can place the arm in the sleeve of a shirt with less difficulty.

### *Cutaneous Stimulation*

Cutaneous stimulation is applied to the skin. Light-moving touch, fast brushing, and icing are examples of cutaneous stimulation. *Light-moving touch,* or slow stroking of the skin, has been used to activate superficial muscles. Clinically this results in a reflexive withdrawal response. *Fast brushing,* applied through a battery-operated brush, can be performed over the muscle belly of these muscles to be facilitated.[15,35] The results of fast brushing are delayed and do not have a maximal effect until 30 minutes after application.

*Icing,* a thermal stimulus, has also been used for facilitation of muscle activity.[30] Icing is a powerful stimulus, and the results can be unpredictable. Icing can be used to facilitate a flexor withdrawal response in superficial muscles.[35] Icing can also be used to facilitate opening and closing of the mouth and to induce swallowing.[18]

Strict precautions must be followed when applying icing or fast brushing; improper use can adversely

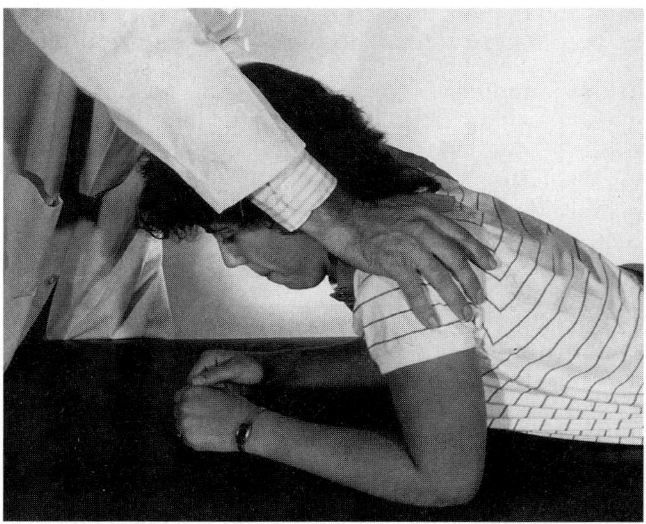

*Figure 23-2* Heavy joint compression.

affect the patient. All clinicians using these techniques must be familiar with and strictly adhere to these precautions.

### *Proprioceptive Stimulation*

Proprioceptive stimulation refers to the facilitation of joint and muscle receptors and the vestibular system.[22,25,33] In general, proprioceptive stimulation gives the clinician more control over the motor response. The motor response lasts as long as the stimulus is applied.[12,33] Several proprioceptive stimulation techniques are used.

*Heavy joint compression* (Figure 23-2) is used to facilitate contraction at the joint undergoing compression. This can be combined with developmental patterns, such as prone on elbows, quadruped (Figure 23-3), sitting, and standing. Clinically, joint compression is most effective when applied through the longitudinal axis of long bones such as the humerus (glenohumeral joint) and the femur (acetabulum).

*Quick stretch* is applied by holding the proximal bony prominences of the limb to be stretched while moving the distal joint in one direction. For example, to stretch the triceps, the elbow joint is secured while the forearm is pushed into flexion. The response is immediate and short-lived.

The *tapping* technique is done by tapping over the belly of a muscle with the fingertips. The OTR or COTA percusses (taps) three to five times over the muscle to be facilitated. This may be done before or during the time a patient is voluntarily contracting the muscle. Tapping on spastic muscles, or muscles that are likely to develop spasticity, should be avoided.

*Vestibular stimulation* is another type of proprioceptive input.[8] Extreme caution should be taken when using vestibular stimulation because it can have a profound effect on the body. Any clinician planning to use this form of stimulation must be adequately trained. The COTA who has been instructed in vestibular stimulation by the OTR must receive close supervision to ensure the patient's safety.

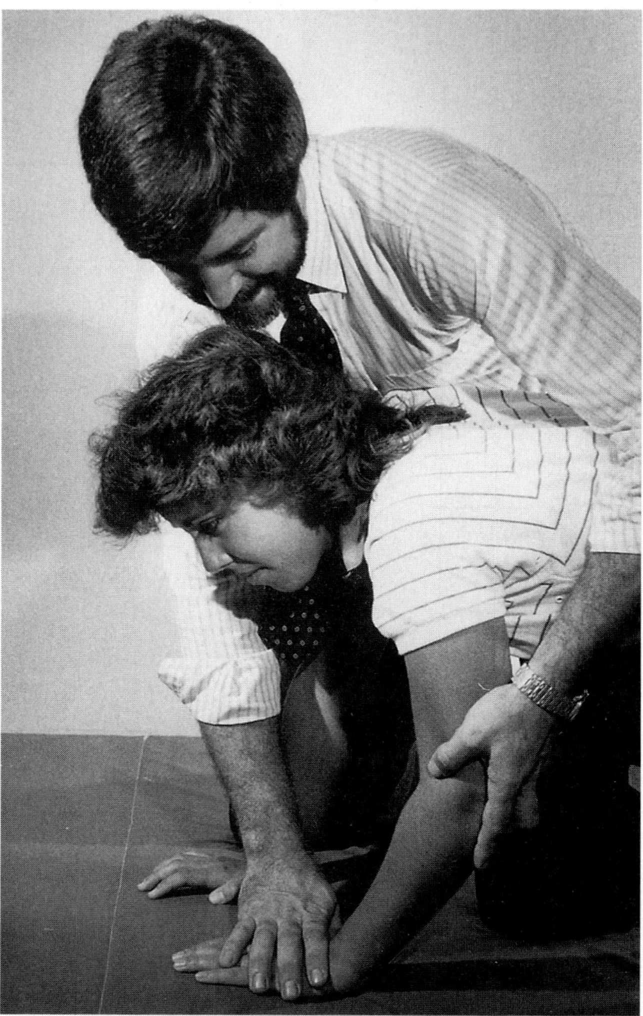

*Figure 23-3* Joint compression in quadraped position.

*Vibration,* applied with a hand-held vibrator, has been used to produce tonal changes in muscles.[14,16,18] Vibration over spastic muscles, or muscles prone to developing spasticity, should be avoided. The patient's age may be a factor in using vibration. For example, vibration should not be used with children less than 3 years of age and must be used with caution in elderly persons over age 65. COTAs using vibration in treatment must be properly trained and supervised.

*Neutral warmth,* an inhibitory technique, has been successful for general relaxation and to reduce muscle tone. It may also be helpful for children with attention deficit disorders.[14]

To inhibit spastic or tight muscles groups in which the tendons are accessible, *manual pressure* can be applied to the tendinous insertion of a muscle or across long tendons.[3,16] Pressure provided by hard surfaces is more effective than that provided by soft surfaces.[10] In the hand a hard cone with the tapered end toward the thumb side to inhibit the flexors can be used.[14] This principle has been used in various orthotic devices to manage muscle imbalance and contracture resulting from spasticity.

To inhibit spastic muscles around a joint, *light joint compression* (approximation) can be used. This technique may be used with hemiplegic patients to alleviate pain and to offset muscle imbalance temporarily around the shoulder joint.[14]

Rood also recommended positioning hypertonic extremities in the *elongated position* for various periods.[24,32] Maintaining stretch in this position has an inhibitory effect. This principle is the basis for inhibitory casting, which is frequently used with patients who demonstrate severe spasticity of the extremities.

Finally, Rood suggested the use of olfactory and gustatory stimuli to facilitate cranial nerves and to influence the autonomic nervous system.[32,39] Odors could be used to facilitate a response. Pleasant odors, such as vanilla, may have a calming effect. Unpleasant and noxious substances, such as sulfa and ammonia, could trigger protective responses, including coughing and sneezing.[15] Rood did not provide specific guidelines for the stimulation of special senses.

Sensory stimulation in patients with neurological dysfunction can have a powerful effect. COTAs must be properly trained and appropriately supervised when using any of the cutaneous or proprioceptive modalities described in this chapter.

### Occupational Therapy Application

The occupational therapy treatment process begins with the OTR's evaluation. The evaluation identifies the patient's level of motor development. Treatment starts at this level and is directed toward progressing the individual along the developmental continuum. Initially, if severe neurological damage is present, the patient may have to begin with reflexive movements. The OTR then progresses the patient along the ontogenic development patterns. Sensory stimulation can reinforce these patterns and can be used to inhibit or facilitate specific muscle activity as needed. The sensory stimulation techniques described are used primarily to prepare the patient for purposeful activities.

In treatment the COTA should consider ontogenic patterns when positioning patients for activities. For example, the roll-over pattern can be reinforced by having the patient turn in bed to reach bed controls. Prone-on-elbows positioning can be adapted for tabletop use by having the patient sit at a table and lean on elbow and forearm while playing a recreational game. Grooming activities, such as shaving or makeup application, can also be positioned so that the patient must lean on the affected elbow and forearm while reaching for object. The standing position often provides the best position for activities of daily living (ADLs) and purposeful activities. While standing, the patient can use arms to explore and manipulate the environment. For example, while performing a homemaking activity, the individual can reach up to place objects in a cabinet. As the patient develops stability in standing, activities that require more weight shifting and balance reactions can be provided.

## MOVEMENT THERAPY: THE BRUNNSTROM APPROACH TO TREATMENT OF HEMIPLEGIA

Signe Brunnstrom was a physical therapist from Sweden. Her practice, teaching, and theory development in the United States extended from the World War II years through the 1970s. Her clinical observations and research led to the development of the treatment approach she called **movement therapy.** Her book, *Movement Therapy in Hemiplegia*[6] was published in 1970 and applied movement therapy, also known as the **Brunnstrom approach,** to the treatment of hemiplegia.

### Theoretical Foundations

Brunnstrom evolved her treatment approach after study of the literature in neurophysiology, CNS mechanisms, effects of CNS damage, sensory systems and related topics, and clinical observations and application of training procedures.[6] Brunnstrom based her intervention on the concept that the damaged CNS has undergone an "evolution in reverse" and regressed to former patterns of movement. These patterns include the *limb synergies,* which are gross patterns of limb flexion and extension that are primitive spinal cord patterns and primitive reflexes.[6] In the normal individual these primitive movement patterns are thought to be modified through the influence of higher centers of CNS control. After a CVA, because the influence of higher centers is disturbed or destroyed, motor function reverts to this primitive state.[6] Reflexes present in early life reappear, and normal reflexes become exaggerated.

The Brunnstrom approach to the treatment of hemiplegia uses the motor patterns available to the patient at any point in the recovery process. The goal is to allow progress through the stages of recovery toward more normal and complex movement patterns. Brunnstrom saw synergies, reflexes, and other abnormal movement patterns as a normal part of the process an individual with CNS dysfunction must go through before normal voluntary movement can occur. Brunnstrom noted that synergistic movements are used by normal persons all the time, but they are controlled, can occur in a variety of patterns, and can be modified or stopped at will. Brunnstrom maintained that the synergies appear to constitute a necessary intermediate stage for further recovery. She believed that the gross movement synergies of flexion and extension always precede the restoration of advanced motor functioning after hemiplegia.[6] During the early stage of recovery, Brunnstrom recommended that the patient should be aided to gain control of the limb synergies and that selected sensory stimuli can help the patient initiate and gain control of movement. Once the synergies can be performed voluntarily, they are modified, and movement combinations that deviate from the synergy pattern can be performed.[6]

### *Limb Synergies*

A limb synergy of flexion or extension, seen in hemiplegia, is a group of muscles acting as a bound unit in a primitive and stereotypical manner.[6] The muscles acting in synergy are linked and cannot act alone. If one muscle in the synergy is activated, each muscle in the synergy responds partially or completely. As a result, the patient cannot perform isolated movements when bound by these synergies.

The *flexor synergy* of the UE consists of scapular adduction and elevation, shoulder abduction and external rotation, elbow flexion, forearm supination, wrist flexion, and finger flexion. Hypertonicity (spasticity) is usually greatest in the elbow flexion component and least in shoulder abduction and external rotation (Figure 23-4). The *extensor synergy* consists of scapular abduction and depression, shoulder adduction and internal rotation, elbow extension, forearm pronation, and wrist and finger flexion or extension. Shoulder adduction and internal rotation are usually the most hypertonic components of the extensor synergy, with much less tone in the elbow extension component (Figure 23-5).

In the LE the flexor synergy consists of hip flexion and abduction and external rotation, knee flexion, ankle dorsiflexion and inversion, and toe extension. Hip flexion is usually the component with the highest tone, and hip abduction and external rotation are the components with the least tone. The extensor synergy is composed of hip abduction, extension, and internal rotation; knee extension; ankle plantar flexion and inversion; and toe flexion. Hip abduction, knee extension, and ankle plantar flexion are usually the most hypertonic components, whereas hip extension and internal rotation are usually less hypertonic.

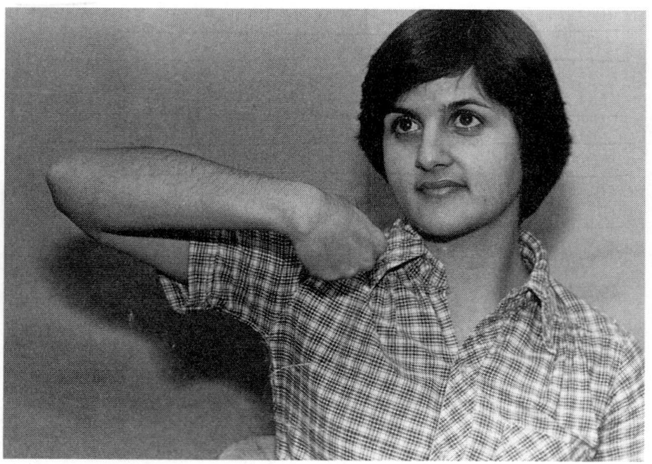

*Figure 23-4* Flexor synergy of upper extremity (UE) in hemiplegia.

### *Characteristics of Synergistic Movement*

The flexor synergy is more often seen in the arm and the extensor synergy in the leg. When the patient performs the synergy, the components with the greatest degree of hypertonicity are often most apparent, rather than the entire classical patterns just described. Also, the resting posture of the limb, particularly the arm, is usually characterized by a position that represents the most hypertonic components of both flexor and extensor synergies, that is, shoulder abduction, elbow flexion, forearm pronation, and wrist and finger flexion. With facilitation or voluntary effort, however, the more classical synergy pattern can usually be evoked.[6]

### *Motor Recovery Process*

After a CVA resulting in hemiplegia, Brunnstrom observed that the patient progresses through a series of *recovery steps* or *stages* in fairly stereotypical fashion (Table 23-1). The progress through these stages may be rapid or slow.

The recovery follows an ontogenic process, usually proximal to distal, so that shoulder movement can be expected before hand movement. Flexion patterns occur before controlled, volitional movement, and gross movement patterns can be performed before isolated, selective movement.[6]

Recovery may cease at any stage and is influenced by factors such as sensation, perception, cognition, motivation, and mood. Few patients make a very good recovery of arm function, and the greatest loss is usually in the wrist and hand. Also, no two patients are exactly alike; much individual variation occurs in the recovery process. The motor behavior and recovery

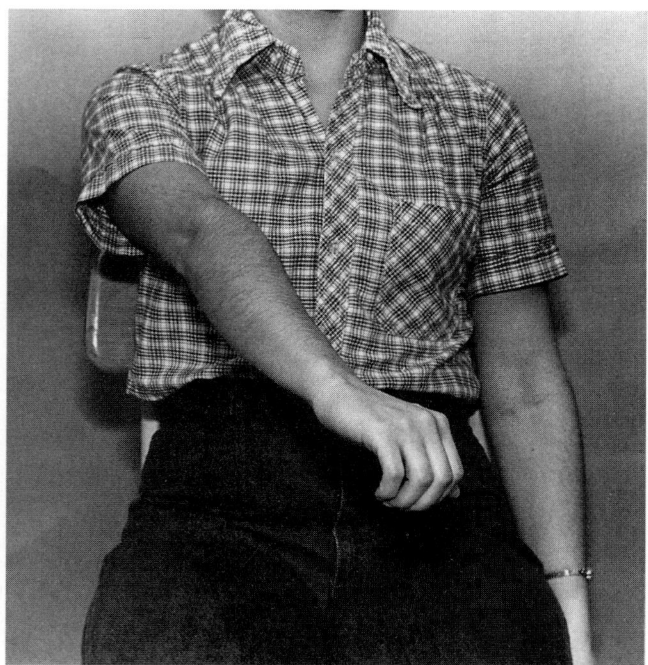

*Figure 23-5* Extensor synergy of UE in hemiplegia.

process described represents common characteristics that may be observed in most persons after CVA occurs.[6]

## Principles of Treatment

The goal of Brunnstrom's movement therapy is to facilitate progress through the recovery stages that occur after the onset of hemiplegia (see Table 23-1). This could be facilitated by the patient's position and the use of associated reactions. Changes in head and body position can influence muscle tone. *Associated reactions,* which are movements seen on the hemiplegic side in response to forceful movements on the sound side, may be used to initiate or elicit synergies. This can be done by giving resistance to the contralateral (opposite-side) muscle group on the normal side.

To facilitate a synergy pattern, the skin over the muscle belly can be rubbed with the fingertips. This produces a contraction of the muscle and elicits the synergy pattern to which the muscle belongs. For example, briskly rubbing the triceps muscle while the patient attempts to push the arm through the sleeve of a shirt can promote the appearance of the extensor synergy.

Synergistic movement may be reinforced by the patient's voluntary efforts. This can be done through the use of visual feedback using mirrors or videotapes, or auditory stimuli in the forms of loud and repetitive commands.

## General Treatment Goals and Methods

Before initiating any intervention strategies, the OTR performs a thorough evaluation of the patient's motor, sensory, perceptual, and cognitive functions. The motor evaluation yields information about stage of recovery, muscle tone, passive motion sense, hand function, and sitting and standing balance.[6]

Based on the results of this evaluation, the OTR outlines a treatment plan. The COTA can easily incorporate many of Brunnstrom's techniques into this plan. The treatment goals and methods summarized in this chapter are directed primarily to the rehabilitation of the UE. The treatment goals and techniques chosen depend on the stage of recovery and muscle tone of the individual patient.

### *Bed Positioning*

The COTA frequently instructs the patient and caregivers on positioning strategies. Proper bed positioning begins immediately when the patient is in the flaccid stage.[6] Proper positioning promotes normal alignment and can decrease the influence of hypertonic muscles.

*Table 23-1*

**Motor Recovery After Cerebrovascular Accident (CVA)**

| Stage | Characteristics: Leg | Arm | Hand* |
|---|---|---|---|
| 1 | Flaccidity | Flaccidity; inability to perform any movements | No hand function |
| 2 | Spasticity develops; minimal voluntary movements | Beginning development of spasticity; limb synergies or some of their components begin to appear as associated reactions | Gross grasp beginning; minimal finger flexion possible |
| 3 | Spasticity peaks; flexion and extension synergy present; hip-knee-ankle flexion in sitting and standing | Spasticity increasing; synergy patterns or some of their components can be performed voluntarily | Gross grasp, hook grasp possible; no release |
| 4 | Knee flexion past 90° in sitting, with foot sliding backward on floor; dorsiflexion with heel on floor and knee flexed to 90° | Spasticity declining; movement combinations deviating from synergies are now possible | Gross grasp present; lateral prehension developing; small amount of finger extension and some thumb movement possible |
| 5 | Knee flexion with hip extended in standing; ankle dorsiflexion with hip and knee extended | Synergies no longer dominant; more movement combinations deviating from synergies performed with greater ease | Palmar prehension, spherical and cylindrical grasp and release possible |
| 6 | Hip abduction in sitting or standing; reciprocal internal and external rotation of hip combined with inversion and eversion of ankle in sitting | Spasticity absent except when performing rapid movements; isolated joint movements performed with ease | All types of prehension, individual finger motion, and full range of voluntary extension possible |

From Brunnstrom S: *Movement therapy in hemiplegia,* New York, 1970, Harper & Row.
*Recovery of hand function is variable and may not parallel six recovery stages of arm.

This is important in the prevention of contractures and deformity. For example, the LE often tends to assume a position of hip external rotation and abduction and knee flexion. This position mimics the LE's flexor synergy. If the extensor synergy is developed in the LE, a different position may be present. In this case the LE's posture is characterized by extension and adduction at the hip, knee extension, and ankle plantar flexion.

If the extensor synergy dominates in the LE, the recommended bed position in the supine position is slight hip and knee flexion maintained by a small pillow under the knee. Lateral support of the leg at the knee with pillows or a rolled blanket or bolster should be provided to prevent abduction and external rotation.

If the flexor synergy dominates in the LE, the knee must be maintained in extension. Hip external rotation can be prevented with supports as described.

To position the affected UE, the arm is supported on a pillow in a position comfortable for the patient. Abduction of the UE should be avoided because this position can contribute to shoulder subluxation. While moving the patient, the COTA avoids pulling on the affected UE. The patient is instructed to use the unaffected hand to support the affected arm when moving about in bed.

### *Bed Mobility*

Turning toward the affected side is easier than turning toward the unaffected side. For turning in bed, the COTA can instruct the patient to raise the affected arm to a position of forward shoulder flexion with the elbow in extension. The affected LE is then positioned in partial flexion at the knee and hip; the clinician may need to stabilize it in this position. The patient turns by swinging the arms and the affected knee across the body toward the unaffected side. As control improves, the patient may perform this technique independently to roll toward both sides of the bed.

### *Balance and Trunk Control*

Early in treatment the patient needs to develop balance, a prerequisite for functional activities. Many patients with hemiplegia demonstrate a "listing" (leaning) toward the affected side, which may result in a fall. To improve balance, treatment should involve altering the patient's sitting posture in a variety of directions, including forward to backward and side to side. The patient should support the affected arm to protect the shoulder during these balance-challenging activities. This also prevents the patient from grasping the supporting surface during the activity. As trunk control improves, the clinician initiates and assists the patient to bend the trunk in various directions. If balance is poor, the clinician can stabilize the patient's knees. In this position the clinician can guide the patient while moving the trunk in various directions. Passive range of motion (ROM) at the shoulder may also be incorporated by raising the patient's arms up as the trunk bends forward.

### *Shoulder Range of Motion*

The maintenance of pain-free shoulder ROM is important in hemiplegic patients. Brunnstrom believed that traditional passive exercises may actually contribute to pain in these patients.[6] Instead, the shoulder joint should be mobilized through guided trunk motion without forceful stretching.

To accomplish this, the patient sits erect, cradling the affected arm. The clinician supports the arm under the elbows while the patient leans forward. The more the patient leans, the greater the range of shoulder flexion that can be obtained. The clinician guides the arm gently and passively into shoulder flexion while the patient's attention is focused on the trunk motion. In a similar manner the clinician can guide the arms into abduction and adduction while the patient rotates the trunk from side to side. Later, active-assistive movements of the arm in relation to the trunk can begin.

When performing passive ROM of the UE, the clinician can replicate synergies. This reinforces these early patterns of movement.

### *Shoulder Subluxation*

Glenohumeral subluxation appears to be a result of dysfunction of the rotator cuff muscles. These muscles maintain the humeral head in the glenoid fossa. Activation of the rotator cuff muscles is necessary if subluxation is to be minimized or prevented. Slings have been used in an effort to hold the humeral head in the glenoid fossa, but they do not activate the muscles needed to protect the integrity of the shoulder joint.[6] The use of slings has been found to be of little value and may be harmful.[7]

### *Methods of Treatment*

The training procedures for improving arm function are geared to the patient's recovery stage. These procedures are performed primarily by the OTR. During stages 1 and 2, when the arm is essentially flaccid or some components of the synergy patterns are beginning to appear, the aim is to elicit muscle tone and the synergy patterns on a reflex basis. This is accomplished through a variety of facilitation procedures.

Treatment methods are not employed by the OTR in any set order but vary depending on the patient's needs. Because the flexor synergy usually appears first, it may be useful to begin trying to elicit the flexor patterns. This attempt should be followed immediately with facilitation of the extensor synergy components, which tend to be weaker and more difficult to perform in later stages of recovery.[6,29]

When the patient has recovered to stages 2 and 3, the synergies are present and components may be performed voluntarily. During this period the goal is for the patient to achieve voluntary control of the synergy patterns.

The treatment aim during stages 4 and 5 is to move away from the synergies. This is achieved by mixing components from both synergies to perform new and complex patterns of movement.

In the final recovery period, stage 6, the goal of treatment is to achieve ease in performance of movement combinations, to increase isolated motions, and to increase speed of movement. Activities that encourage varying motions and increasing speed of performance can be introduced during this stage.

For retraining hand function, Brunnstrom described separate techniques. As in treatment of the rest of the UE, the concept of helping the patient progress through the stages of hand recovery is the same. For example, patients are first provided with activities to promote gross grasp, followed by wrist fixation for grasp, then active release.[6]

### Occupational Therapy Application

The focus of occupational therapy using the Brunnstrom technique is to help the patient use newly learned movement patterns for functional and purposeful activities. Using this principle, the COTA can consider incorporating whatever movement the patient demonstrates into treatment activities. For instance, during stage 3, when the patient can perform synergy voluntarily, the extensor synergy may be used to stabilize an object on a table while the unaffected arm is performing a task.

During stage 4 the COTA can provide activities that encourage movements deviating from synergy. These could include skateboard activities (Figure 23-6), sponging off table tops, or finger painting.

Practice in functional movement patterns for self-care can also be performed. These can include hand-to-mouth motions used in eating finger foods, combing hair, washing the face, washing the unaffected arm, and reaching the opposite axilla for washing or application of deodorant.[6] The clinician's role is to analyze activities for movement patterns the patient can perform and to select meaningful and interesting activities with the patient.

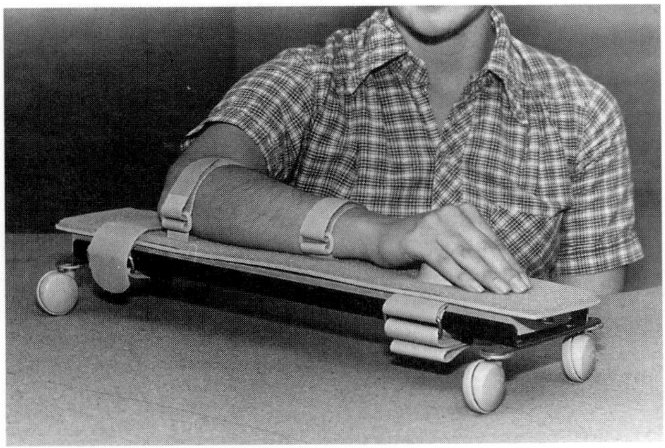

*Figure 23-6* Skateboard activities for synergy or combined movement patterns.

The COTA should reinforce any voluntary movement of the affected limb during the performance of self-care activities. Using the arm for dressing and hygiene skills translates the movements to purposeful use. If the patient moves beyond stage 4, the number of activities that can be performed increases, and more movement combinations are possible. The involvement of the affected limbs in ADLs should be encouraged. Gardening, rolling out dough, sweeping, dusting, and washing dishes are a few of the activities that may enlist the use of the affected arm purposefully if hand recovery is adequate.

## PROPRIOCEPTIVE NEUROMUSCULAR FACILITATION

**Proprioceptive neuromuscular facilitation (PNF)** originated with Dr. Herman Kabat, a physician and neurophysiologist, in the 1940s. He applied neurophysiological principles to the treatment of paralysis resulting from poliomyelitis and multiple sclerosis. In 1948 Kabat and Henry Kaiser founded the Kabat-Kaiser Institute in Vallejo, Calif. At the institute Kabat worked with physical therapist Margaret Knott to develop the PNF method of treatment. By 1951 the diagonal patterns and several PNF techniques were established. In 1952 Dorothy Voss, a physical therapist, joined the staff at Kabat-Kaiser Institute. She and Knott undertook the teaching and supervision of staff therapists. In 1956 the first edition of *Proprioceptive Neuromuscular Facilitation* by Knott and Voss was published.[37,38]

PNF is based on normal movement and motor development. In normal motor activity the brain registers total movement and not individual muscle action.[19] The PNF approaches use mass movement patterns that resemble normal movement during functional activities. Facilitation techniques are superimposed on these movement patterns and postures through manual contacts, verbal commands, and visual cues.

### Principles of Treatment

Voss presented 11 principles of treatment at the Northwestern University Special Therapeutic Exercise Project in 1966. These principles were developed from concepts in the fields of neurophysiology, motor learning, and motor behavior and are as follows[32]:

1. *All humans have potentials that have not been fully developed.* This is the underlying philosophy of PNF. During the PNF evaluation the patient's abilities and potentials are identified. These abilities are emphasized in the treatment process. For example, the patient who has weakness on one side of the body can use the intact side to assist the weaker part.
2. *Normal motor development proceeds in a cervicocaudal and proximodistal direction.* During evaluation and treatment the cervicocaudal (head to "tail

bone") and proximodistal (body center to extremities) directions are followed. Attention is given first to the head, followed by the neck, trunk, and finally the extremities. This is of particular importance in treatment that facilitates fine motor coordination in the UEs. Without adequate control of the head, neck, and trunk region, fine motor skills cannot be developed effectively.

3. *Early motor behavior is dominated by reflex activity.* Mature motor behavior is supported or reinforced by postural reflexes. As a person matures, primitive reflexes are integrated and available for reinforcement to allow for progressive development such as rolling, crawling, and sitting. Reflexes also affect tone and movement in the extremities, and head and neck movement affect arm and leg movement.[17] For example, reaching for an object can be reinforced by having the head turned toward the object.
4. *Early motor behavior is characterized by spontaneous movement that oscillates between extremes of flexion and extension.* These movements are rhythmical and reversing in character. In treatment the OT practitioner must attend to all directions of movement. For example, when working with a patient on arising from a chair, the COTA also must attend to sitting back down.
5. *Developing motor behavior is expressed in an orderly sequence of total patterns of movements and posture.* Motor skills develop progressively. For example, an infant learns to roll, to crawl, to creep, and finally to stand and walk. Throughout these stages the infant also learns to use the extremities in different patterns and postures. Initially the hands are used for reaching and grasping within the most supported postures, such as supine and prone. As control in these postures develops, the infant begins to use the hands in side lying, sitting, and standing. Coordination develops as a result.
6. *The growth of motor behavior has cyclical trends, as evidenced by shifts between flexor and extensor dominance.* These shifts help to develop muscle balance and control. One of the main goals of the PNF treatment approach is to establish a balance among opposing (antagonistic) muscle groups. In treatment the clinician must establish a balance between muscles by first observing where imbalance exists and then facilitating the weaker component. For example, if a patient demonstrates a flexor synergy, extension should be facilitated.
7. *Normal motor development has an orderly sequence but lacks a step-by-step quality.* Overlapping occurs; the child does not perfect performance of one activity before beginning another, more advanced activity. Normal motor development follows a predictable pattern, which the practitioner must consider when positioning a patient. If one posture technique is not effective in obtaining a desired result, the COTA may need to attempt the activity in another developmental posture. For example, if a patient with ataxia is unable to write while sitting, the person may practice writing in a more supported posture, such as prone on elbows. If the patient has not perfected a motor activity such as walking on level surfaces, however, the person may benefit from attempting a higher level activity such as walking up or down stairs. This in turn can improve ambulation on level surfaces. Moving up and down the developmental sequence is a natural occurrence and allows for multiple, varied opportunities for practicing motor activities.
8. *Establishing a balance between antagonists is a main objective of PNF.* As movement and posture change, continuous adjustments in balance are made. When these adjustments are not made, an imbalance in muscles occurs, such as seen in the patient with a head injury who is unable to maintain adequate sitting balance during a tabletop activity because of a dominance of trunk extensor tone. In treatment, emphasis would be placed on correcting the imbalance. In the presence of spasticity, this may have to be done by first inhibiting (reducing) the spasticity, then facilitating the antagonistic muscles, reflexes, and postures.
9. *Improvement in motor ability depends on motor learning.* Multisensory input facilitates the patient's motor learning and is an integral part of the PNF approach. For example, when working with a patient on a shoulder flexion activity, such as reaching into the cabinet for a cup, the clinician may say "reach for the cup." This verbal input encourages the patient to look in the direction of the movement to allow vision to enhance the motor response. Thus tactile, auditory, and visual inputs are used. Motor learning has occurred when these external cues are no longer needed for adequate performance.
10. *Frequency of stimulation and repetitive activity are used in promotion and retention of motor learning and for the development of strength and endurance.* Patients must be allowed to practice in various positions and patterns. This repetition builds skill and coordination.
11. *Goal-directed activities coupled with techniques of facilitation are used to hasten learning of total patterns of walking and self-care activities.* When applying facilitation techniques to ADLs, the objective is improved functional ability. This improvement requires more than instruction and practice alone. Correction of deficiencies is accomplished by directly applying manual contacts and techniques to facilitate the desired response.[39] In treatment this may mean applying stretch to finger extensors to facilitate release of an object

or providing joint approximation through the shoulders and pelvis of a patient with ataxia to provide stability while standing to wash dishes.

### Motor Learning

Motor learning requires a *multisensory* approach; auditory, visual, and tactile systems all are used to achieve the desired response. The correct combination of sensory input for each patient should be identified and altered as the person progresses.

*Verbal commands* should be brief and clear. Timing of the command is important so that it does not come too early or too late in relation to the motor act. Tone of voice may influence the quality of the patient's response. Strong, sharp commands are used when maximal stimulation of motor response is desired. A soft tone of voice is used to encourage a smooth movement (e.g., in the presence of pain).

Loomis and Boersma[23] studied another effect of auditory feedback on motor performance, using a *verbal mediation* strategy to teach wheelchair safety to patients with right-sided CVA. Patients were taught to say aloud the steps required to leave the wheelchair safely and independently. The authors found that only those patients who used verbal mediation learned sufficiently to perform safe, independent transfers. Their retention of the sequence was better, suggesting that verbal mediation is beneficial in reaching independence, with better sequencing and fewer errors.

*Visual stimuli* help to initiate and coordinate movement. Visual input should be monitored to ensure that the patient is tracking in the direction of movement. The clinician's position and the treatment activity must be considered. For example, if the treatment goal is to increase head, neck, and trunk rotation to the left, the OT practitioner and activity should be located in front and to the left of the patient.

The use of *tactile input* is essential to guide and reinforce the desired patterns of movement. Manual contacts by the clinician provide this input.

Finally, to increase speed and accuracy in motor performance, the patient needs the opportunity to *practice.* The PNF approach uses the concepts of part-task and whole-task practice. In part task, emphasis is placed on the parts of the task that the patient is unable to perform independently. Performance of each part of the task is improved by practice. For example, the patient learning to transfer from a wheelchair to a tub bench may have difficulty lifting the leg over the tub rim. This part of the task should be practiced with repetition and facilitation techniques to the hip flexors during performance of the transfer. When the transfer becomes smooth and coordinated, it is no longer necessary to practice each part individually.

### Evaluation

Evaluation of the patient requires keen observational skills and knowledge of normal movement. The OTR completes an initial evaluation to identify the patient's abilities, deficiencies, and potential. After the treatment plan is established, ongoing patient assessment is necessary to determine the effectiveness of treatment. Modifications are made as the patient changes. The PNF evaluation follows a sequence from proximal to distal. Special attention is given to muscle tone, alignment (midline or a shift to one side), and stability/mobility.[26]

When examining the trunk and extremities, the clinician evaluates each segment individually in specific movement patterns as well as in developmental activities using interaction of body segments. For example, shoulder flexion can be observed in an individual UE movement pattern as well as during a total developmental pattern such as rolling.

During the evaluation the OTR should note which facilitation techniques and sensory inputs (auditory, visual, tactile) the patient responds to most effectively. Once identified, these techniques and sensory inputs are used to promote controlled movements.

Finally, the patient is observed during self-care and other ADLs to determine whether performance patterns are adequate within the context of a functional activity. Because performance may vary from one setting to another, the treatment plan must allow for practice of motor skills in a variety of settings and in locations appropriate to the specific activity.

### Treatment

Once the evaluation is completed, a treatment plan is developed, including goals the patient hopes to accomplish. The clinician uses the techniques and procedures identified in the evaluation as having favorably influenced movement and posture. Similarly, appropriate total patterns and patterns of facilitation are selected to enhance performance.

The treatment techniques used in the PNF approach are diagonal patterns, total patterns, and facilitation techniques.

#### *Diagonal Patterns*

The diagonal patterns used in the PNF approach are mass movement patterns observed in most functional activities. Part of the challenge in using this approach is recognizing the diagonal patterns in ADLs. Two diagonal motions ($D_1$, $D_2$) are present for each major part of the body: head and neck, upper and lower trunk, and extremities. Each diagonal pattern has a flexion and extension component together with rotation and movement away from or toward the midline. Unilateral and bilateral diagonal patterns are described for the extremities.

The movements associated with each diagonal pattern and examples of these patterns seen in ADLs are described next. Not all components of the pattern or full ROM are necessarily seen during functional activities. Furthermore, the diagonals interact during functional movement, changing from one pattern or combination to another.[27]

*Unilateral patterns*

1. *UE (upper extremity) $D_1$ flexion (antagonist of $D_1$ extension).* Scapular elevation, abduction, and rotation; shoulder flexion, adduction, and external rotation; elbow in flexion or extension; forearm supination; wrist flexion to the radial side; finger flexion and adduction; thumb adduction (Figure 23-7, *A*). Examples in functional activity: hand-to-mouth motion in feeding; combing hair on left side of head with right hand (Figure 23-8, *A*).
2. *UE $D_1$ extension (antagonist of $D_1$ flexion).* Scapular depression, adduction, and rotation; shoulder extension, abduction, and internal rotation; elbow in flexion or extension; forearm pronation; wrist extension to the ulnar side; finger extension and abduction; thumb in palmar abduction (Figure 23-7, *B*). Examples in functional activity: pushing car door open from inside (Figure 23-8, *B*); rolling from prone to supine.
3. *UE $D_2$ flexion (antagonist of $D_2$ extension).* Scapular elevation, adduction, and rotation; shoulder flexion, abduction, and external rotation; elbow in flexion or extension; forearm supination; wrist extension to radial side; finger extension and abduction; thumb extension (Figure 23-9, *A*). Examples in functional activity: combing hair on right side of head with right hand (Figure 23-10, *A*); backstroke in swimming.
4. *UE $D_2$ extension (antagonist of $D_2$ flexion).* Scapular depression, abduction, and rotation; shoulder extension, adduction, and internal rotation; elbow in flexion or extension; forearm pronation; wrist flexion to the ulnar side; finger flexion and adduction; thumb opposition (Figure 23-9, *B*). Examples in functional activity: pitching baseball; buttoning pants on left side with right hand (Figure 23-10, *B*).

The rotational component in LE $D_1$ flexion and extension parallels the UE patterns.

5. *LE (lower extremity) $D_1$ flexion (antagonist of $D_1$ extension).* Hip flexion, adduction, and external rotation; knee in flexion or extension; ankle and foot dorsiflexion with inversion and toe extension. Examples in functional activity: rolling from supine to prone; putting on shoe with leg crossed (Figure 23-11, *A*).
6. *LE $D_1$ extension (antagonist of $D_1$ flexion).* Hip extension, abduction, and internal rotation; knee in flexion or extension; ankle and foot plantar flexion with eversion and toe flexion. Examples in functional activity: putting leg into pants (Figure 23-11, *B*); rolling from prone to supine.

The rotational component of LE $D_2$ flexion and extension is opposite to the UE patterns.

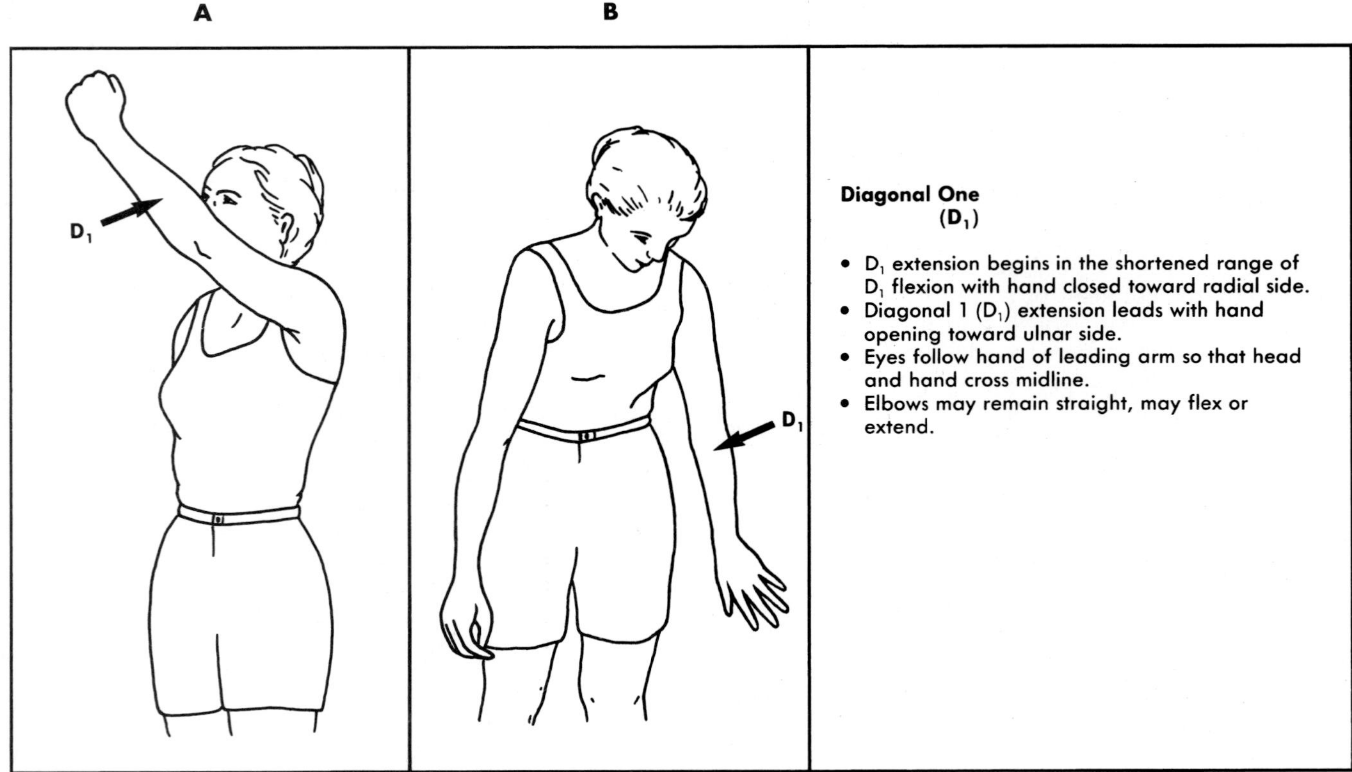


*Figure 23-7* **A,** UE $D_1$ flexion pattern. **B,** UE $D_1$ extension pattern. (From Myers BJ: *PNF: diagonal patterns and their application to functional activities,* Chicago, 1982, Rehabilitation Institute of Chicago [videotape].)

7. *LE $D_2$ flexion (antagonist to $D_2$ extension).* Hip flexion, abduction, and internal rotation; knee in flexion or extension; ankle and foot dorsiflexion with eversion and toe extension. Examples in functional activity: karate kick (Figure 23-12, *A*); drawing heels up during breaststroke in swimming.
8. *LE $D_2$ extension (antagonist of $D_2$ flexion).* Hip extension, adduction, and external rotation; knee in flexion or extension; ankle and foot plantar

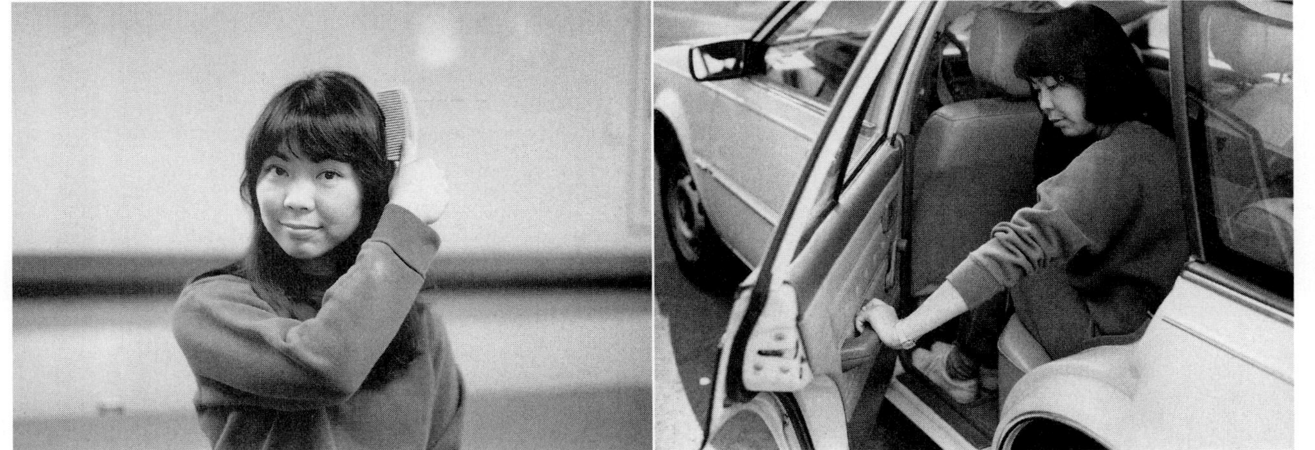


*Figure 23-8* **A,** UE $D_1$ flexion pattern used in combing hair, opposite side. **B,** UE $D_1$ extension pattern used in pushing car door open.

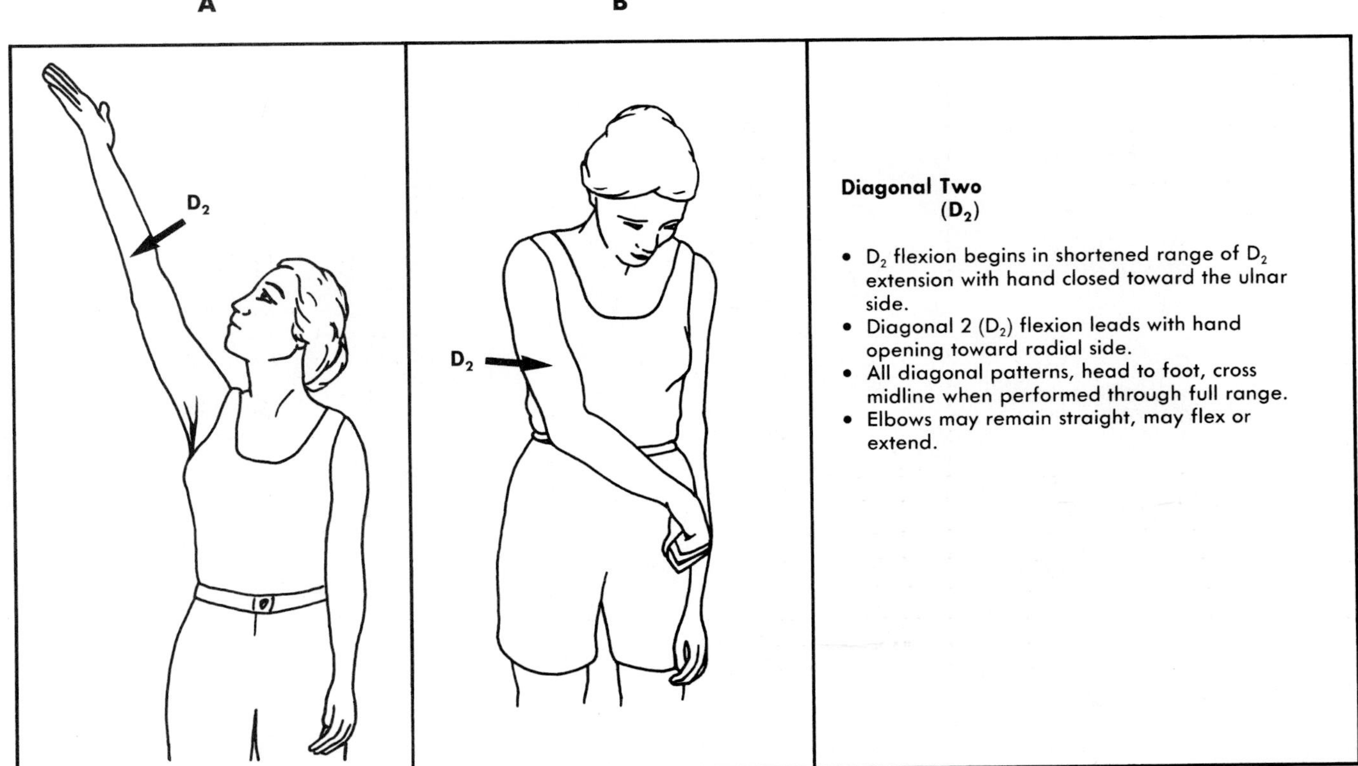


*Figure 23-9* **A,** UE $D_2$ flexion pattern. **B,** UE $D_2$ extension pattern. (From Myers BJ: *PNF: diagonal patterns and their application to functional activities,* Chicago, 1982, Rehabilitation Institute of Chicago [videotape].)

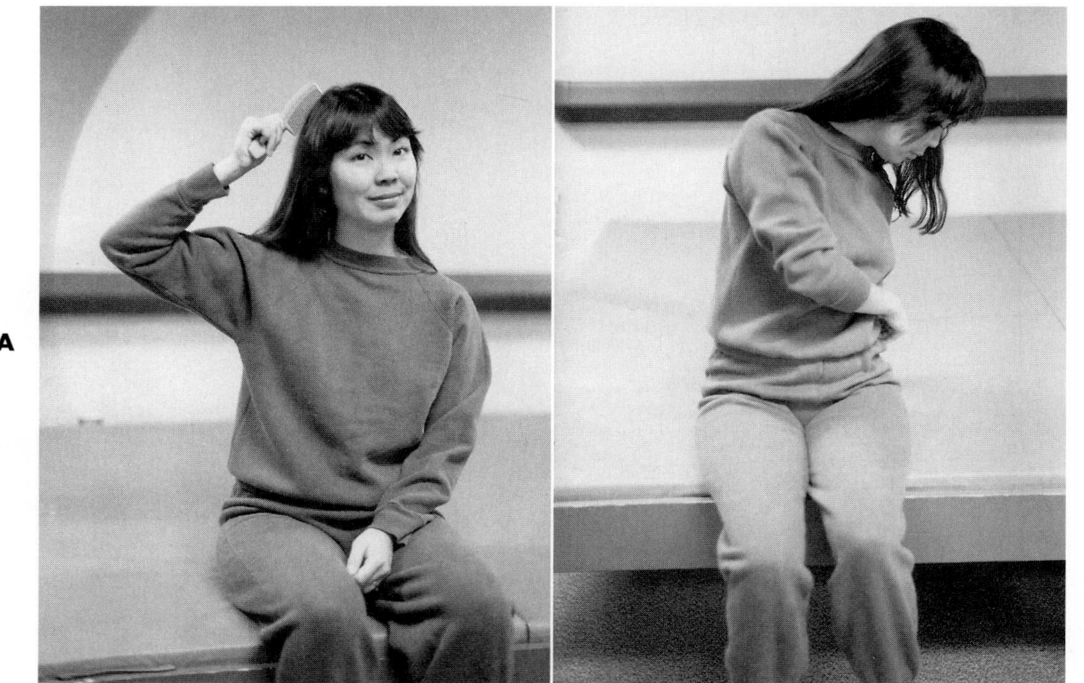

*Figure 23-10* **A,** UE $D_2$ flexion pattern used in combing hair, same side. **B,** UE $D_2$ extension pattern used in buttoning trousers, opposite side.

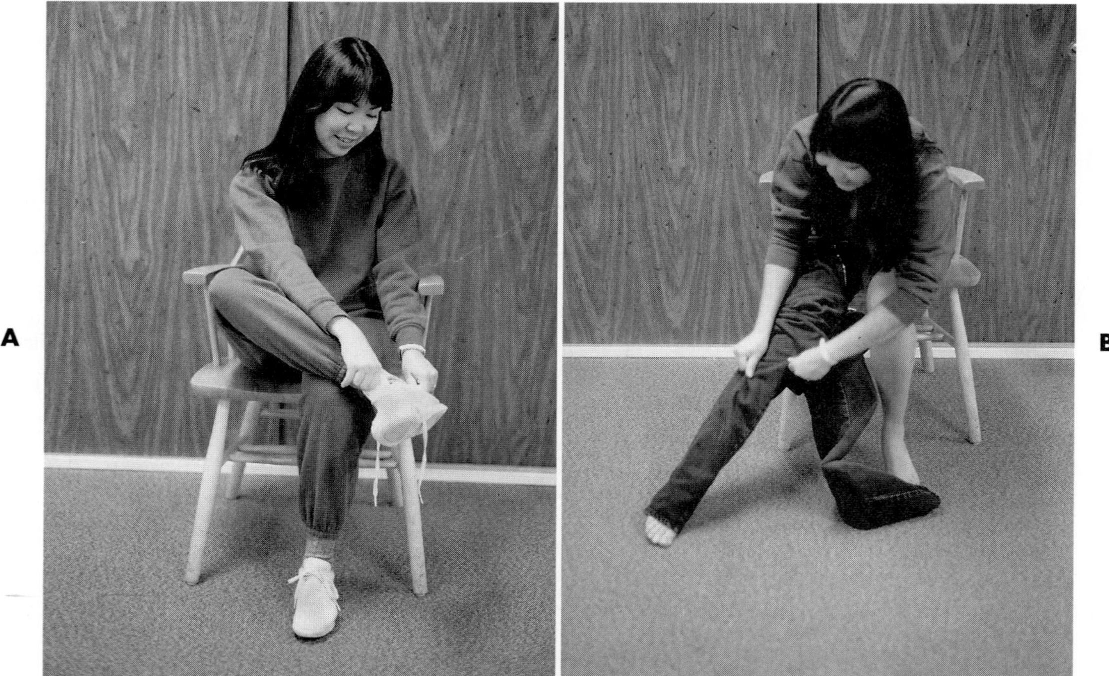

*Figure 23-11* **A,** LE $D_1$ flexion pattern used in putting on shoe with leg crossed. **B,** LE $D_1$ extension pattern used in pulling on trousers.

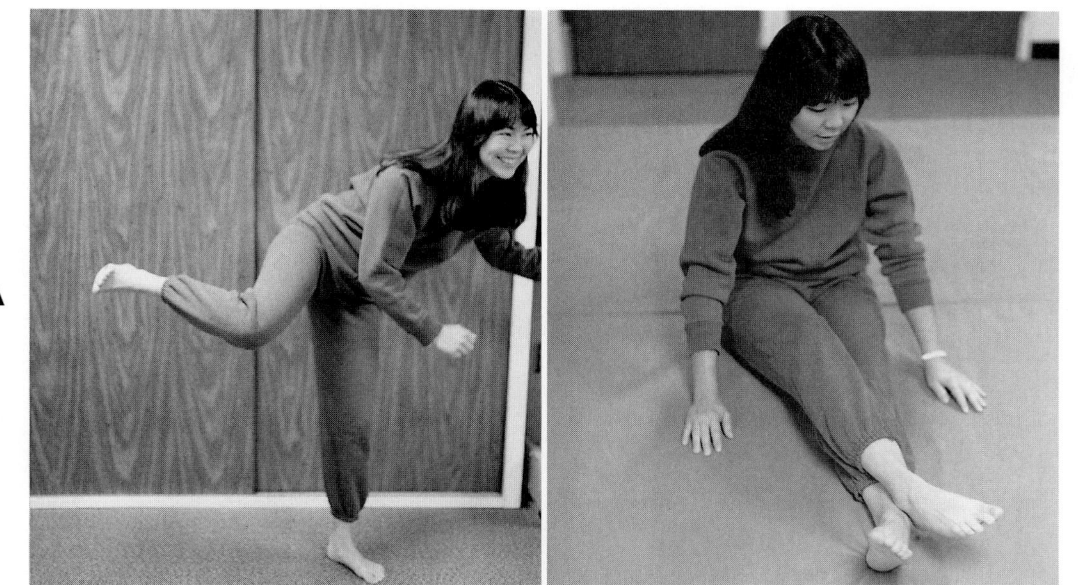

*Figure 23-12* **A,** LE $D_2$ flexion used in karate kick. **B,** LE $D_2$ extension used in long sitting with legs crossed.

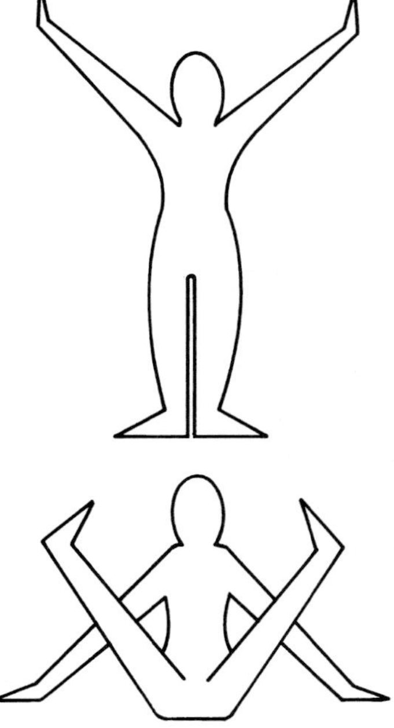

*Figure 23-13* Symmetrical patterns.

flexion with inversion and toe flexion. Examples of functional activity: push off in gait; long sitting with legs crossed (Figure 23-12, *B*).

*Bilateral patterns* Movements in the extremities may be reinforced by combining diagonals in bilateral patterns as follows:

1. *Symmetrical patterns.* Paired extremities perform like movements at the same time (Figure 23-13): bilateral symmetrical $D_2$ extension, such as starting to take off pullover sweater (Figure 23-14, *A*); bilateral symmetrical $D_2$ flexion, such as reaching to lift large item off high shelf (Figure 23-14, *B*).

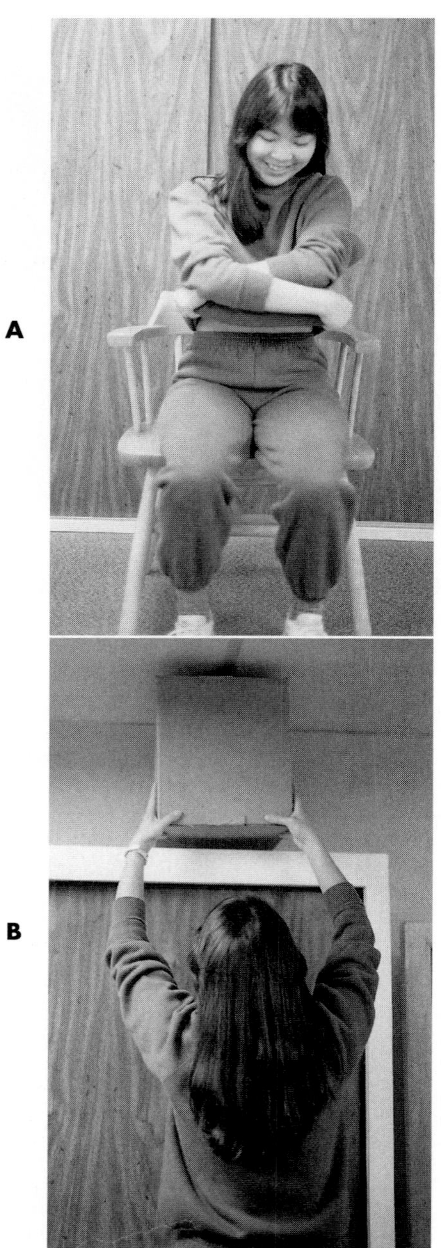


*Figure 23-14* **A,** UE bilateral symmetrical pattern used when starting to take off pullover shirt. **B,** UE bilateral symmetrical pattern used when reaching to lift box off high shelf.

2. *Asymmetrical patterns.* Paired extremities perform movements toward one side of the body at the same time. This facilitates trunk rotation. The asymmetrical patterns can be performed with the arms in contact, such as chopping and lifting patterns in which greater trunk rotation is seen (Figure 23-15 and 23-16). Examples are bilateral asymmetrical flexion to left, with left arm in $D_2$ flexion and right arm in $D_1$ flexion, such as putting on left earring (Figure 23-17); bilateral asymmetrical extension to left, with right arm in $D_2$ extension and left arm in $D_1$ extension, such as zipping a left-sided skirt zipper.
3. *Reciprocal patterns.* Paired extremities perform movements in opposite directions at the same time. Reciprocal patterns have a stabilizing ef-

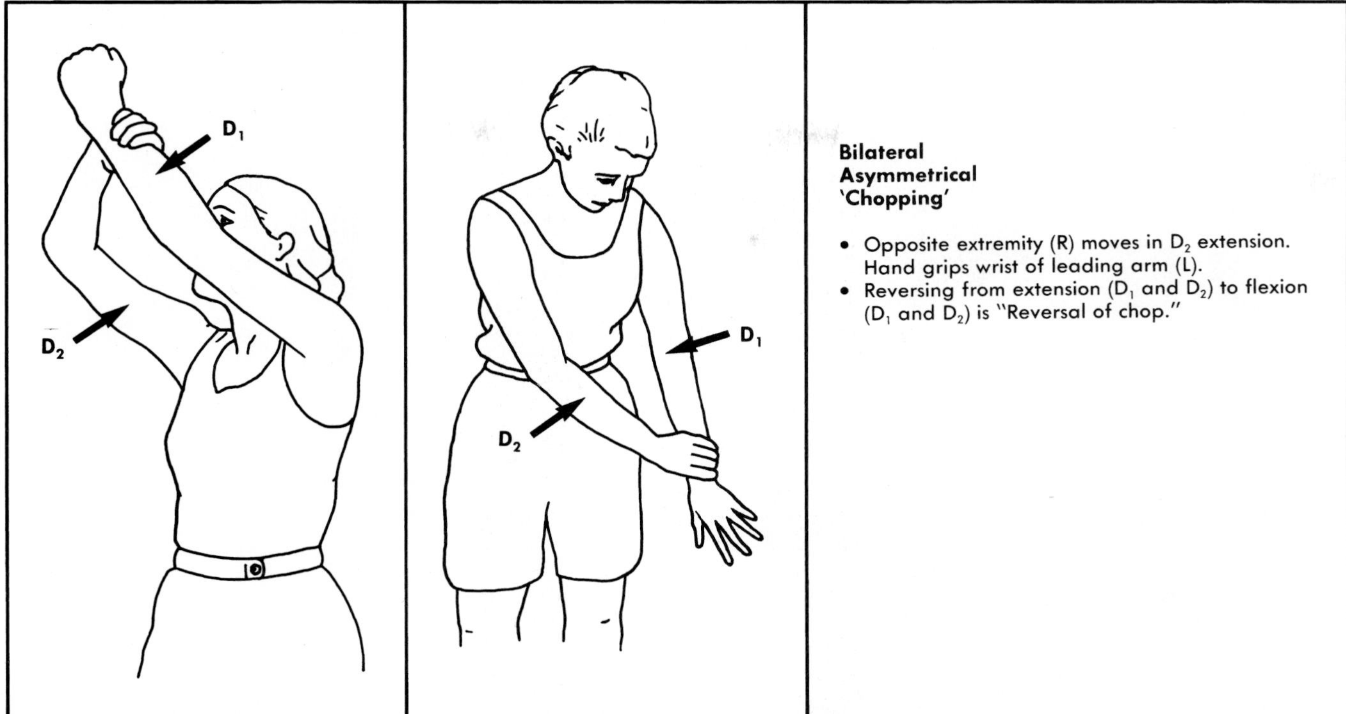


*Figure 23-15* Bilateral asymmetrical chopping. (From Myers BJ: *PNF: diagonal patterns and their application to functional activities,* Chicago, 1982, Rehabilitation Institute of Chicago [videotape].)

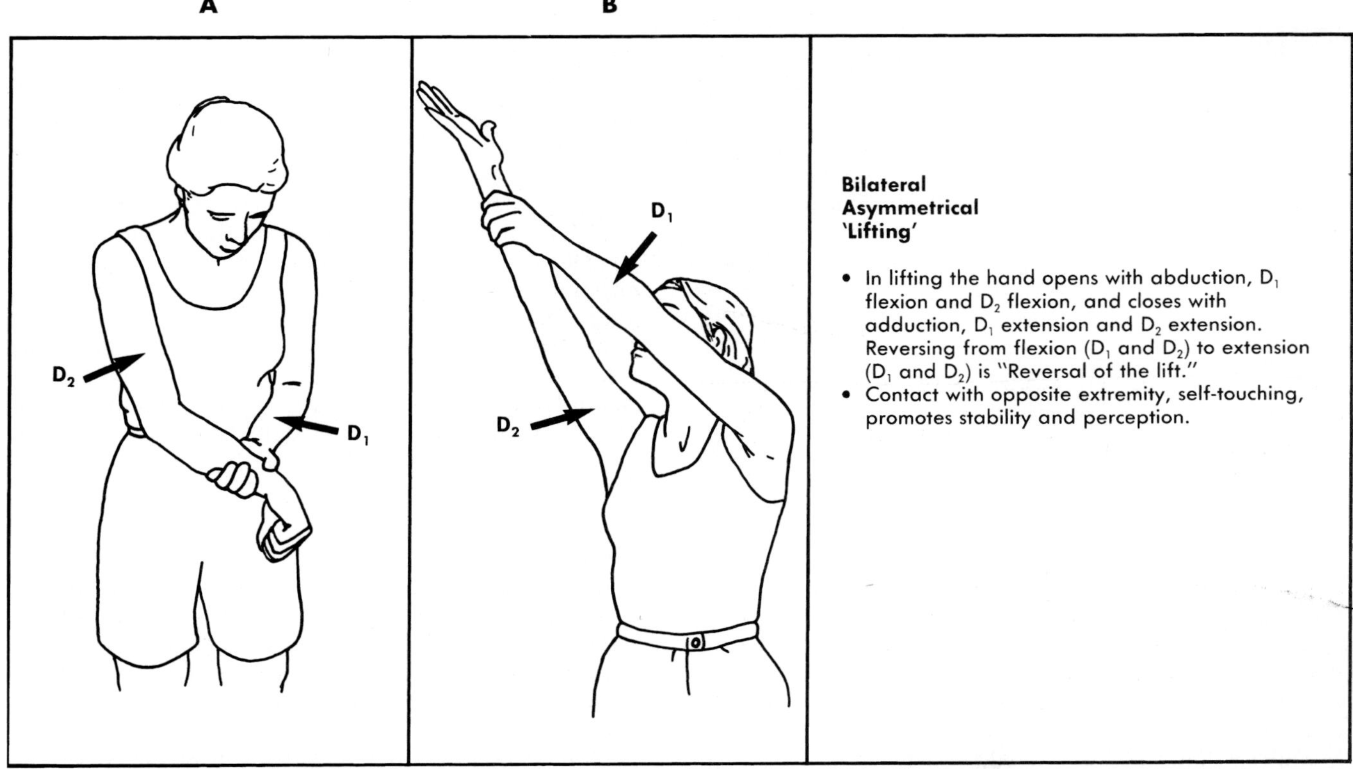


*Figure 23-16* Bilateral asymmetrical lifting. (From Myers BJ: *PNF: diagonal patterns and their application to functional activities,* Chicago, 1982, Rehabilitation Institute of Chicago [videotape].)

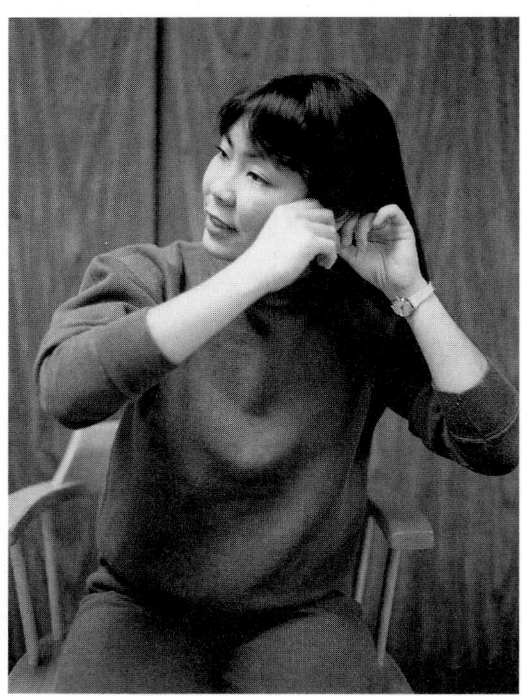

*Figure 23-17* Putting on earring requires use of UE bilateral asymmetrical flexion pattern.

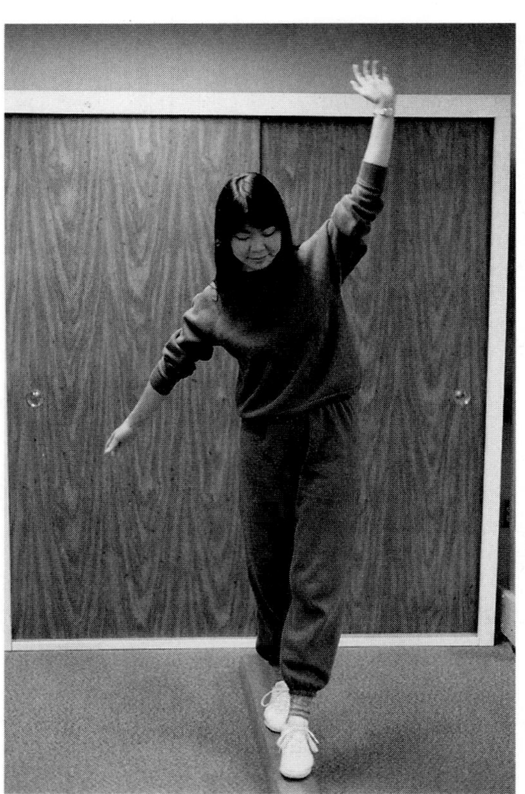

*Figure 23-18* Bilateral reciprocal pattern of UEs used to walk balance beam.

fect on the head, neck, and trunk. Examples are pitching in baseball; walking balance beam with one extremity in diagonal flexion pattern and other in diagonal extension pattern (Figure 23-18). During activities requiring high-level balance, reciprocal patterns come into play, with one extremity in $D_1$ extension and other extremity in $D_2$ flexion.

*Combined movements of upper and lower extremities* Interactions of the UEs and LEs are also important considerations in the PNF approach. The combinations of UE and LE movements are observed during activities such as crawling and walking. Awareness of these patterns is important in the evaluation of the patient's motor skills.

Several advantages exist to using the diagonal patterns in treatment. First, crossing of the midline of the body occurs. Most functional activities require crossing the midline, which can also be important in the remediation of perceptual motor deficits such as unilateral neglect, in which integration of both sides of the body and awareness of the neglected side are treatment goals. Second, because each muscle has an optimal pattern in which it functions, the total pattern can be used to strengthen weaker ones. Third, the diagonal patterns use groups of muscles; this is typical of movement seen in functional activities. Finally, rotation is always a component in the diagonals. With an injury or the aging process, rotation frequently is impaired and can be facilitated with movement in the diagonals.

In treatment the OTR or COTA should place activities so that movement occurs in the diagonal. For example, if the patient is working on a wood-sanding project, trunk rotation with extension can be facilitated by placing the project on an inclined plane in a diagonal.

### Total Patterns

In PNF, developmental postures are called *total patterns of movement* and posture.[26] Total patterns require interaction between proximal (head, neck, trunk) and distal (extremity) components. Maintenance of postures is important. When posture is unable to be maintained, emphasis is placed on the assumption of posture.[38] Before sustaining a sitting posture, for example, the patient must have ability in lower developmental total patterns of movement, such as rolling and moving from side-lying to side-sitting positions. The active assumption of postures can be incorporated into functional activities. For example, a reaching and placing activity could be set up so that the patient must reach for the object in the supine posture and place the object in the side-lying posture. The use of total patterns also can reinforce individual extremity movements. For example, in an activity such as wiping a table top, wrist extension is reinforced while the patient leans forward over the supporting arm.

### *Procedures*

PNF techniques are superimposed on diagonal movements and posture. Two procedures, verbal commands and visual cues, have been discussed previously. Other procedures are described next.

**Manual contact** refers to the placement of the clinician's hands on the patient. Pressure from the clinician's touch is used as a facilitating mechanism and serves as a sensory cue to help the patient understand the direction of the anticipated movement.[38] The amount of pressure applied depends on the specific technique being used and the desired response. Location of manual contacts is chosen according to the groups of muscles, tendons, and joints responsible for the desired movement patterns. For example, if a patient is having difficulty reaching to comb the back of the hair because of scapular weakness, the desired movement pattern would be $D_2$ flexion. Manual contacts would be on the posterior surface of the scapula to reinforce the muscles that elevate, adduct, and rotate the scapula.

**Stretch** is used to initiate voluntary movement and enhance speed of response and strength in weak muscles. When stretch is used in this approach, the part to be facilitated is placed in the extreme lengthened range of the desired pattern (or where tension is felt on all muscle components of a given pattern). After the correct position for the stretch stimulus has been achieved, stretch is superimposed on the pattern. The patient should attempt the movement at the exact time that the stretch reflex is elicited. Verbal commands should coincide with the application of stretch to reinforce the movement. The COTA must take care when using stretch to prevent increasing pain or muscle imbalances. The COTA who plans to use the stretch technique must be thoroughly trained on proper application and precautions.

**Traction** facilitates the joint receptors by creating a separation of the joint surfaces. Traction promotes movement and is used for pulling motion.[39] In an activity such as carrying a heavy suitcase, traction can be felt on joint surfaces. Traction may be contraindicated in patients after surgery or a fracture.

**Approximation** facilitates joint receptors by creating a compression of joint surfaces. It promotes stability and postural control and is used for pushing motion.[39] Approximation is usually superimposed on a weight-bearing posture. For example, to enhance postural control in the prone-on-elbow position, approximation may be given through the shoulders in a downward direction.

**Maximal resistance** applies the concept that stronger muscles and patterns reinforce weaker components.[34] Maximal resistance is defined as the greatest amount of resistance than can be applied to an active contraction while still allowing full ROM. Maximal resistance is also applied to an isometric (holding) contraction without defeating or breaking the patient's hold.[39]

If the resistance applied by the clinician results in uncoordinated or jerky movement or if it breaks the patient's hold, too much resistance is being given. Movement against maximal resistance should be slow and smooth. For patients with neurological impairment or pain, the resistance applied should be very light. In the presence of spasticity, resistance may increase existing muscle imbalance and needs to be closely monitored. Therefore the COTA using this technique must have a thorough understanding of the outcome of resistance and the expected effects of the procedure before application.

### *Techniques*

Specific techniques are used with these basic procedures; a few have been selected for mention here. Before incorporating any of these techniques into treatment, both OTR and COTA must be properly trained in safe applications and precautions. Improper application can result in spasticity, pain, and abnormal movement patterns.

**Repeated contraction** is a technique based on the assumption that repetition of an activity is necessary for motor learning and helps develop strength, ROM, and endurance.

**Rhythmical initiation** is used to improve the ability to initiate movement, a problem that may be seen in patients with Parkinson's disease or apraxia.

**Reversal of movement** employs a characteristic of normal development: movement is reversing and changes direction. *Slow reversal* is an isotonic contraction (against resistance) of the antagonist followed by an isotonic contraction (against resistance) of the agonist. Slow reversal–hold is the same sequence, with an isometric (holding) contraction at the end of the ROM.

**Rhythmical stabilization** is used to increase stability by eliciting co-contractions of opposing groups. Because this technique requires repeated isometric contractions of both agonist and antagonist muscles, increased circulation or the tendency to hold one's breath (or both) occurs. Therefore rhythmical stabilization may be contraindicated for patients with cardiac involvement, and no more than three or four repetitions should be done at a time.

**Relaxation techniques** are an effective means of increasing ROM, particularly when pain or spasticity increases with passive stretch. Two examples of PNF relaxation techniques are contract-relax and hold-relax.

*Contract-relax techniques* involve a holding contraction of the antagonistic pattern against maximal resistance, followed by relaxation, then passive movement into the agonistic pattern. This procedure is repeated at each point during the ROM in which limitation is felt to occur.[39] Contract-relax is used when no active ROM in the agonistic pattern is present.

*Hold-relax techniques* are performed in the same sequence as contract-relax techniques but involve an isometric contraction of the antagonist, followed by relaxation, then active movement into the agonistic pattern. This technique may be beneficial for patients with pain.

### Occupational Therapy Applications

The PNF approach can be incorporated into occupational therapy practice in a variety of ways. The OTR or COTA should learn the diagonal patterns and how they are used in ADLs. Activities can be positioned so that a patient can perform a particular diagonal needed for function. During homemaking, for example, the process of reaching into a bag to retrieve items that are placed on a kitchen shelf could be set up to incorporate the $D_1$ flexion and $D_2$ extension patterns. Specific treatment techniques and procedures could be used with these functional activities.

## NEURODEVELOPMENTAL TREATMENT OF ADULT HEMIPLEGIA: THE BOBATH APPROACH

The **neurodevelopmental (Bobath) treatment (NDT) approach** was first developed in the 1940s by Bertha Bobath, a physical therapist, and her husband, Dr. Karel Bobath, a neurologist.[5] The term *neurodevelopmental treatment* was first coined by the Bobaths to describe their work with children with cerebral palsy. Also known as the *Bobath approach,* NDT has been used successfully by both occupational and physical therapists in the treatment of adult hemiplegia. The Bobath approach is described in detail in Bertha Bobath's book, *Adult Hemiplegia: Evaluation and Treatment.*[5]

The Bobaths believed strongly in the potential of the hemiplegic side for normal function. Based on this belief, they established a treatment program that focused on relearning normal movement. NDT is geared toward encouraging the use of both sides of the body. Development of alignment and symmetry of the trunk and pelvis is emphasized; this is thought to be necessary for normal function of the extremities. In NDT, patients should not be trained solely in compensatory techniques because this will interfere with functional recovery of the hemiplegic side. Adaptive equipment is used only when necessary for safety, and compensatory techniques are avoided.

### Typical Problems of Hemiplegia

The Bobaths believe that the major motor problem in hemiplegia is the lack of motor control affecting voluntary movement.

*Flaccidity* is most common at the onset of a CVA. During this time the patient demonstrates low endurance and low activity tolerance. The period may last a few days or several months. Although no movement in the affected extremities is displayed at this time, a proper treatment program can strongly impact the eventual functional outcome.[5]

After the flaccid stage the patient enters a stage of *mixed tone,* displaying a combination of flaccidity and spasticity. For example, the UE might have an increase in tone proximally at the scapula, but a decrease in tone distally at the wrist and hand. If treatment does not address the problems of high tone at this stage, the patient progresses to the next stage of spasticity.

*Spasticity* is the most frequently identified problem and often the most difficult motor problem to treat after a CVA. If not treated correctly, spasticity can severely compromise the ability to move and perform ADLs. Spasticity produces abnormal sensory feedback and contributes to weakness of antagonist muscles. It can cause contractures, pain, and an all-consuming fear in many patients. Fear, pain, and spasticity are often so intertwined that a vicious cycle appears. The spasticity can cause an increase in pain, which can cause an increase in fear, which in turn increases the amount of spasticity.[9] Conversely, a reduction in pain and fear can result in a reduction in spasticity. Other factors that may influence the amount of spasticity are emotional stress, physical effort, temperature, and the rate at which an activity is done.

The typical posture in the adult hemiplegic patient (Figure 23-19) can be described as follows:

- Head—lateral flexion is toward the involved side with rotation away from the involved side.
- In the UE a combination of the strongest components of the flexion and extension synergies appears:

  1. Scapula—depression, retraction
  2. Shoulder—adduction, internal rotation
  3. Elbow—flexion
  4. Forearm—pronation
  5. Wrist—flexion, ulnar deviation
  6. Finger—flexion

- Trunk—lateral flexion is toward the involved side.
- In the LE the extension synergy dominates:

  1. Pelvis—posterior elevation, retraction
  2. Hip—internal rotation, adduction, extension
  3. Knee—extension
  4. Ankle—plantar flexion, supination, inversion
  5. Toes—flexion

In addition to motor problems, patients often may have other deficits that can affect function, including

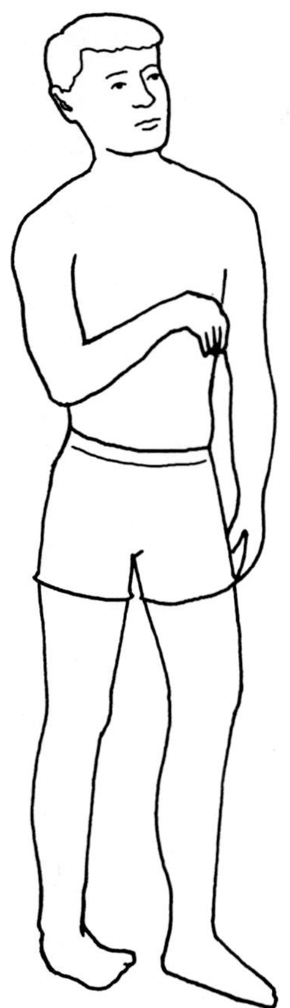

*Figure 23-19* Typical posture of adult with hemiplegia in standing position.

diminished weight bearing on the hemiplegic side, sensory loss, neglect, and fear.

Non–weight bearing on the affected side is common in hemiplegic patients. When sitting or standing, weight is shifted to the nonhemiplegic side, resulting in an asymmetrical posture.

Sensory loss may include the loss of stereognosis (ability to identify an object by touch), kinesthetic awareness (ability to detect movement in an extremity), light touch, and light pressure. Abnormal sensation in an extremity, even with good motor control, can render that extremity useless.[5,9]

Unilateral neglect often occurs after a CVA. *Unilateral neglect* refers to a decreased awareness of the body's affected side. Unilateral neglect can be a combination of one or more factors, including sensory loss, perceptual or cognitive dysfunction, or visual field deficits. Unilateral neglect can result in a nonfunctional extremity despite good motor control.

Fear can also limit function for many patients. Fear can be related to loss of sensory awareness, poor balance reactions, lack of protective extension resulting in a fear of falling, and perceptual or cognitive problems.[9]

Many other problems related to CVA, including aphasia, apraxia, and a variety of perceptual motor problems, also may occur and affect a patient's functional abilities.

### Evaluation

When evaluating a patient, the OTR emphasizes the *quality of movement*, or how the patient moves. During evaluation coordination, tonal changes and postural reactions are observed rather than specific muscles and joints.[5] During the evaluation and treatment the clinician must have a knowledge of normal posture and movement to identify abnormal patterns. Each patient may have a different clinical picture based on age, premorbid physical condition, and normal degenerative changes.

*Observation* is a key component in an NDT evaluation. The patient is observed from the front, back, and both sides. Comparison of the body's hemiplegic and nonhemiplegic sides provides information about the patient's symmetry. The clinician should observe the patient at rest; during sitting, standing, and lying; and while performing activities. During movement any changes in posture and muscle tone of the head, neck, trunk, and extremities should be noted.

When asymmetries are noted, the OTR begins to identify possible underlying causes. The practitioner moves the body part through the normal ROM, noting pain and deviations from movement. If resistance is felt, it is likely the result of abnormally high tone. If no resistance is felt but the arm feels heavy, this probably results from abnormally low tone.

The clinician also observes any movement initiated by the patient on the weak side. *Associated movements*, which are normal, may occur when the patient attempts to move the weak side, and the strong side responds by making the same movement. *Associated reactions*, in which the patient moves using compensatory movements or movements influenced by abnormal synergy patterns, should be avoided. The patient should also avoid excessive effort because it can trigger these abnormal reactions.

By comparing the patient's movement pattern to the normal movement required for the same task, problem areas can be seen. For example, when a patient reaches for an object, the OTR may note that the hemiplegic arm elevates and retracts at the shoulder, flexes at elbow, supinates at forearm, and flexes at wrist and fingers. The trunk may also flex forward to position the hand nearer the object (Figure 23-20). In comparison, a normal pattern of movement might include trunk stability with scapular protraction, selective elbow extension with pronation, wrist extension, and finger flexion (Figure 23-21). When comparing the two sides, the OT practitioner can identify elements of abnormal patterns of movement. Understanding the components of normal movement, both in isolation and within the context of an activity, is essential to identify abnormal patterns.

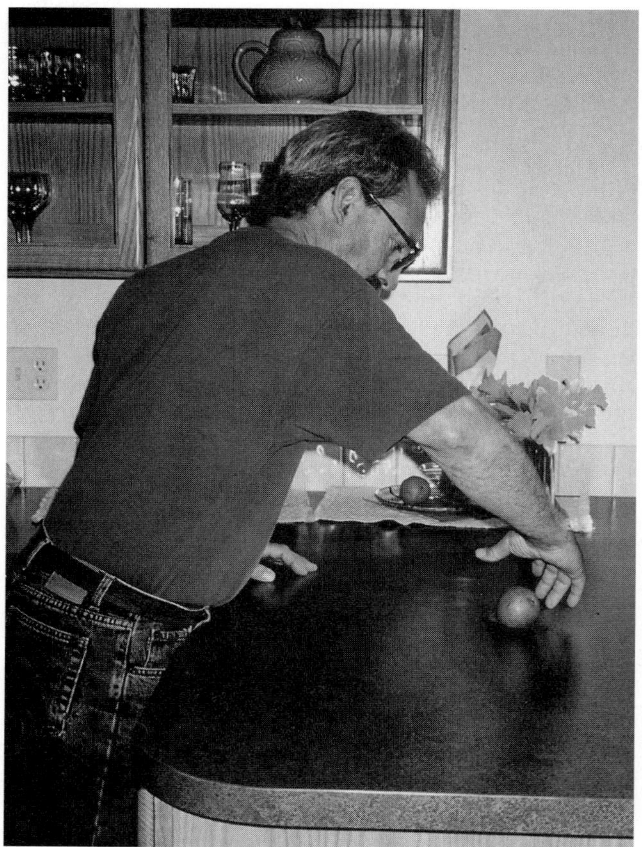

*Figure 23-20* Patient reaching forward using abnormal movement patterns.

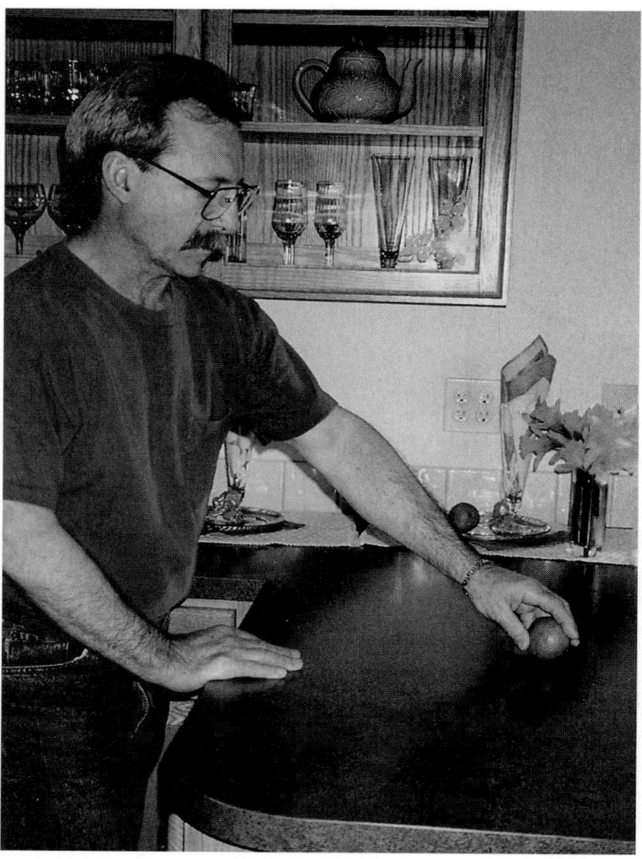

*Figure 23-21* Patient using normal movement patterns while reaching forward with uninvolved side.

In NDT the evaluation and treatment processes are intertwined. While evaluating the patient's movement patterns, the clinician performs techniques to promote normal tone and facilitate controlled patterns of movement. The OTR continuously assesses the effectiveness of these techniques on the patient's movement pattern. This information is communicated to the COTA so that activities reinforcing normal movement patterns can be provided in treatment.

### Treatment Principles

The goal of the NDT approach is to help a patient relearn normal movements. Treatment emphasizes helping the patient experience normal movement patterns. Therefore the amount of movement a patient demonstrates is not as important as the *quality* of movement performed. When examining the quality of movement, the primary concern is whether the patient exhibits good trunk control while moving, whether the movement is free from abnormal muscle tone and synergies, and whether the movement is coordinated.

**Facilitation techniques** or **inhibition techniques** are an important tool in NDT. These techniques are used to normalize, or balance, tone. When tone is normalized, abnormally high tone is reduced (inhibited), and abnormally low tone is increased (facilitated). Once normalized, patterns of movement opposite to spastic patterns are used to allow the patient to experience the normal sensation of normal movement. These normal movement patterns are guided from proximal points of the body, primarily at the shoulder and pelvis.

The reduction of abnormal patterns of movement must be accomplished before normal, selective isolated movements can take place. It is impossible to perform normal movement in the presence of abnormal tone.[6]

According to the Bobaths, normalization of muscle tone may be accomplished by using one or more of the following techniques[5,9,11]:

- Weight bearing over the affected side
- Trunk rotation
- Scapular protraction
- Anterior pelvic tilt/position pelvis forward
- Facilitation of slow, controlled movements
- Proper positioning

These six techniques provide the foundation for NDT treatment. The techniques are most effective in rehabilitation when initiated in the acute phase but can be used at any time in the treatment program.

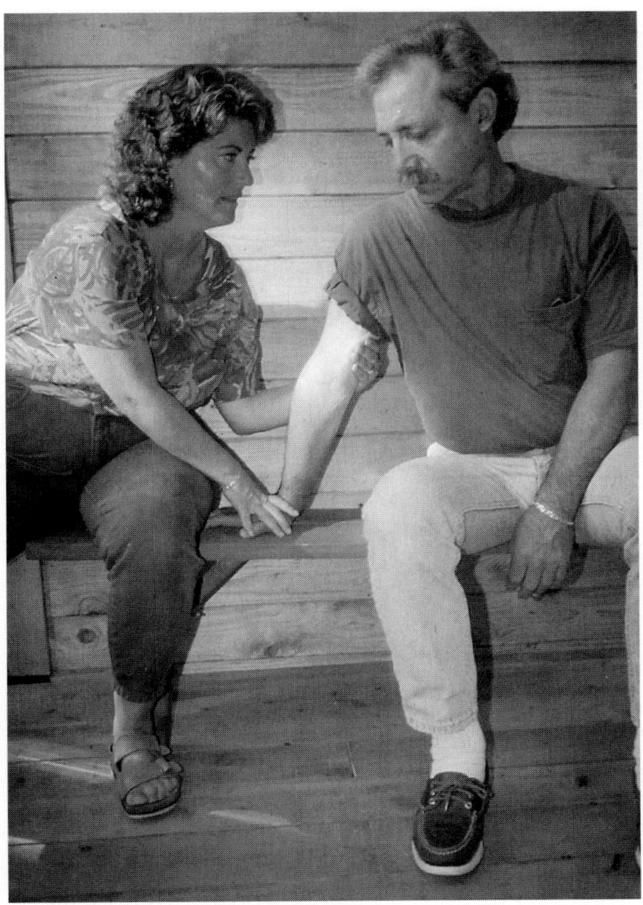

*Figure 23-22* Proper position for weight bearing over hemiplegic side during functional activity.

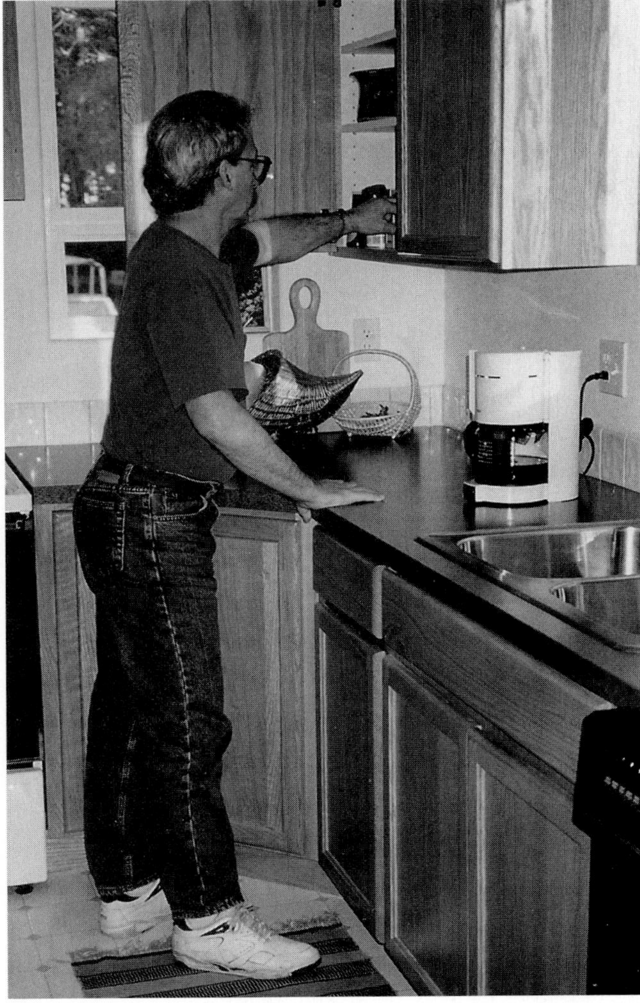

*Figure 23-23* Trunk rotation, side to side, to high surface.

*Weight bearing* over the hemiplegic side is the most effective way to normalize tone. Weight bearing can be either facilitory or inhibitory. Weight bearing also provides sensory input to the hemiplegic side, which can increase the patient's awareness of the hemiplegic side and decrease neglect.

Weight bearing through the UE while sitting or standing helps to normalize tone throughout the arm. Weight bearing is most effective with patients who display a flexor synergy of the UE. The patient can be brought into a weight-bearing position before function, in preparation for function, or during treatment in functional ADLs.

Before weight bearing through the UE, the OTR or COTA must prepare the UE and shoulder girdle by gliding the scapula into forward protraction, elevation, and upward rotation. During weight bearing the patient's hand should be placed on a mat or bench several inches away from the hip to prevent wrist hyperextension. The humerus is placed in external rotation with the elbow in extension. As the patient shifts weight over the hemiplegic side, the clinician should not allow the UE to rotate internally or the elbow to collapse. The patient should not hang on the arm during weight bearing, but instead should move the body over the arm. This will avoid undue stress on the elbow joint (Figure 23-22). Weight bearing should be avoided when hand pain or edema is present.

*Trunk rotation,* or the disassociation of upper and lower trunk, is another effective way of normalizing tone and facilitating normal movement. Hemiplegic patients often move in a blocklike pattern, with little separation of shoulder and pelvic girdles. To promote disassociation, the clinician should introduce activities that incorporate or facilitate trunk rotation. This activates trunk musculature and aids in trunk stability, which will enhance UE movement.

Trunk rotation performed in the sitting or standing position promotes weight shifting to the hemiplegic side. Additional benefits from trunk rotation activities include increased sensory input and improved awareness of the hemiplegic side and trained compensation for visual field deficits (Figures 23-23 to 23-25). Often the easiest and most effective way to facilitate trunk rotation is during ADLs.

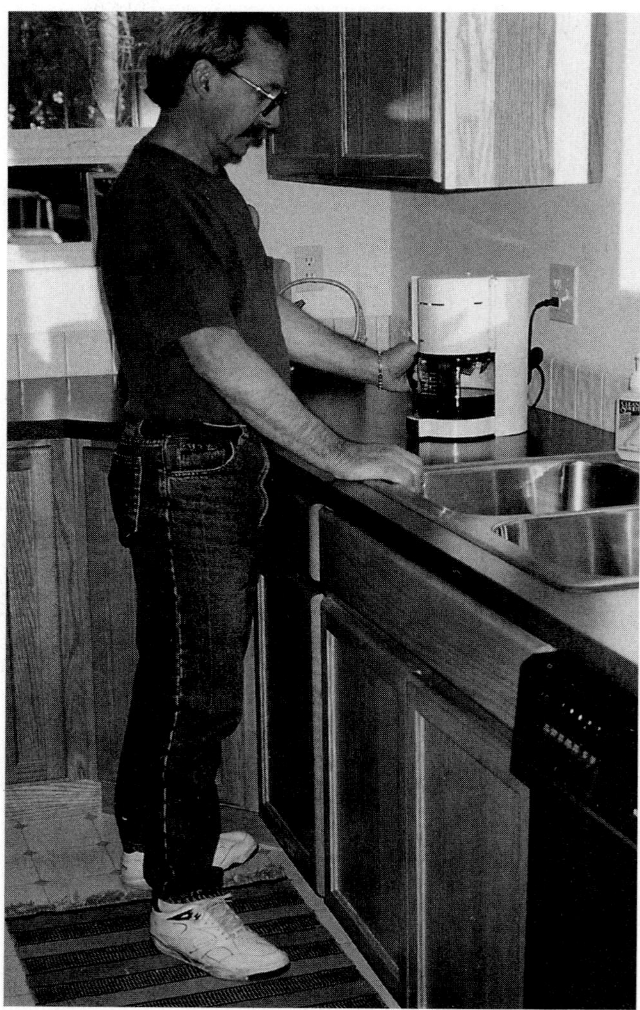

*Figure 23-24* Trunk rotation, side to side, to counter height.

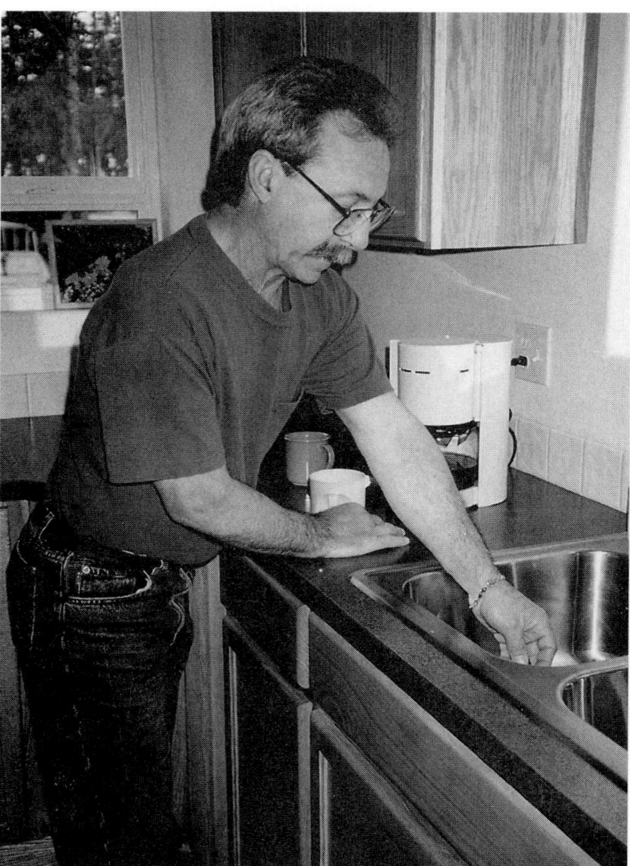

*Figure 23-25* Trunk rotation, side to side, to lower surface.

*Scapular protraction* benefits patients who display a flexor synergy of the UE. Following the rule of working proximal to distal, the scapula should always be guided into forward protraction before attempting to raise the hemiplegic arm or open the hand. The scapula can be protracted by having the clinician cradle the arm with one hand while placing the other hand along the scapula's medial border, then bringing the arm forward. Once forward, this position should be maintained for a few seconds before returning to the starting position. Care should be taken not to glide the scapula back into retraction.

*Anterior pelvic tilt position* forward is the preferred sitting position for patients with hemiplegia. This position provides proper alignment of the pelvis, shoulder, and head. The posterior pelvic tilt position is abnormal and should be avoided; patients who assume this position appear to be sliding out of the chair. This posture has an adverse effect on swallowing, promotes misalignment of the shoulder girdle, and encourages the flexor synergy of the UE.

*Slow, controlled movements* should be facilitated in patients with high tone. Quick movements increase tone and tend to trigger an associated reaction, resulting in a flexor synergy of the UE; they should be avoided. Patients with high muscle tone should be instructed to perform activities slowly and in a controlled manner. The OTR or COTA can accomplish this by providing feedback to help the patient recognize when an activity is performed well.

*Proper positioning* of the patient in bed, sitting, or standing facilitates the development of normal movement throughout the recovery process. It also helps to normalize muscle tone and provide normal sensory input to the body. For example, the preferred position for lying in bed is on the hemiplegic side[6,12] (Figure 23-26), with the patient's back positioned parallel with the edge of the bed; head placed on a pillow, avoiding extreme flexion; shoulder fully protracted with at least 90° of shoulder flexion; forearm supinated and elbow flexed; and hand placed under the pillow. An alternate position is with the elbow extended and the wrist either supported on the bed or slightly off the bed. The nonaffected leg should be placed on a pillow. The affected leg is slightly flexed at the knee with hip

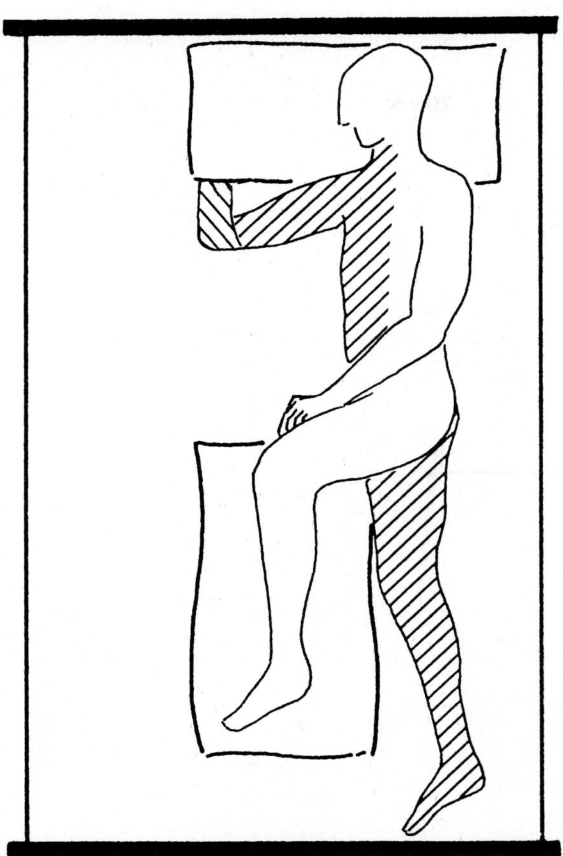

*Figure 23-26* Bed position when lying on affected side.

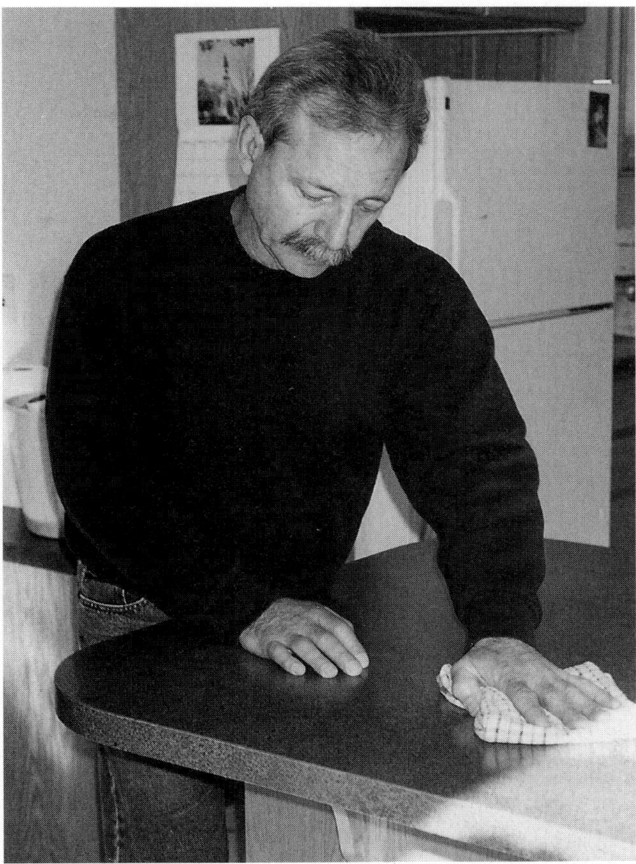

*Figure 23-27* Proper position for weight bearing over hemiplegic side during functional activities.

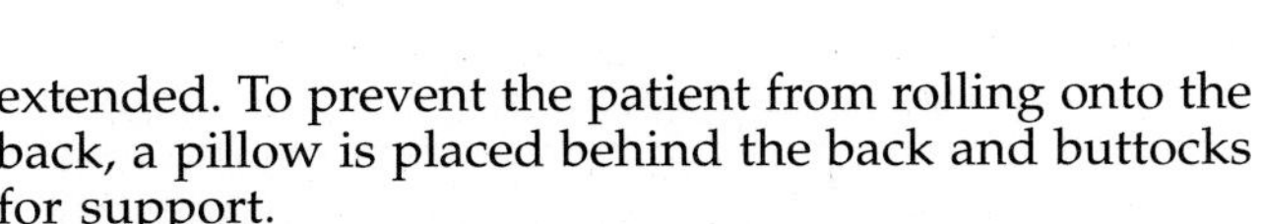

extended. To prevent the patient from rolling onto the back, a pillow is placed behind the back and buttocks for support.

The proper position for sitting is to have the patient place both feet flat on the floor, the hips near 90° flexion, the knees and ankles at less than 90° flexion, and the trunk extended. The head should be in midline and the affected arm fully supported when working at a table. During standing the weight should be equally distributed on both lower extremities, the trunk symmetrical, and the head in midline.[6]

### Occupational Therapy Application

In the NDT approach the COTA must design activities that can incorporate the hemiplegic UE into routine ADLs. This helps to reinforce techniques and interventions used by the OTR in designing the treatment plan. The COTA can incorporate the hemiplegic UE into activities in three ways: (1) weight bearing through the involved UE during functional activities (Figure 23-27), (2) bilateral activities with hand over hand, and (3) the clasped-hands (prayer) position.

Bilateral activity (Figure 23-28) and guiding the affected UE (Figure 23-29) help to discourage the flexion synergy and allow the hemiplegic arm to participate in purposeful activities. In addition, when performing bilateral activities, the patient experiences sensory input to the hemiplegic side, and the hemiplegic UE is brought into the visual field. This can be beneficial to patients who have unilateral neglect or visual inattention. Guiding the affected UE is another way to incorporate the hemiplegic UE into activities and can help the patient experience normal movement patterns during purposeful activities.

When engaging patients in treatment activities using the NDT approach, the COTA should offer meaningful and practical tasks to enhance carry-over from selected normal movement patterns to functional performance. Patients can more easily attend to and be motivated by activities that relate to real-life situations.

#### *Dressing Activities*

Dressing and grooming activities are a part of almost every occupational therapy program. These activities are familiar, purposeful, and necessary for independent functioning. The following methods illustrate how NDT principles can be used in ADL training.

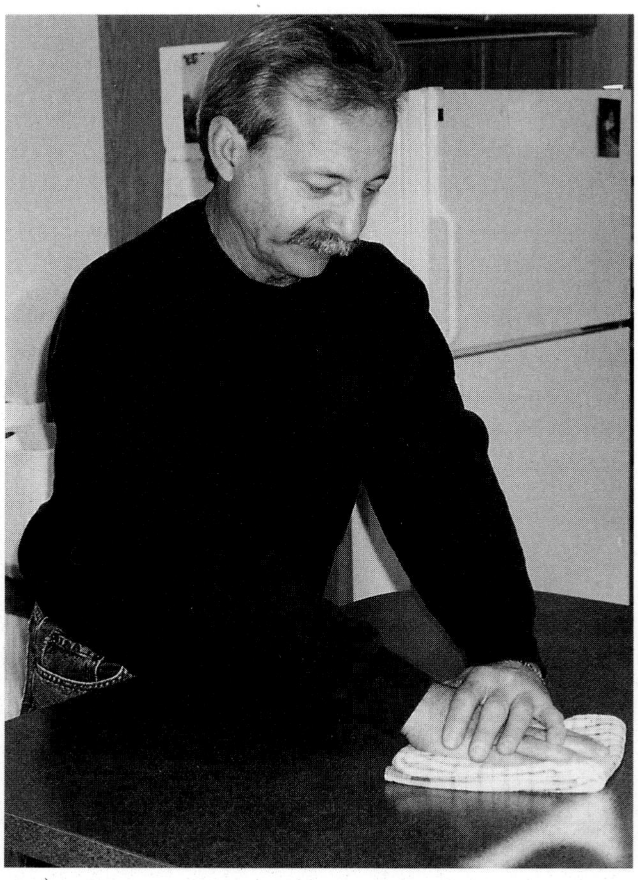

*Figure 23-28* Bilateral use of UE during functional activities.

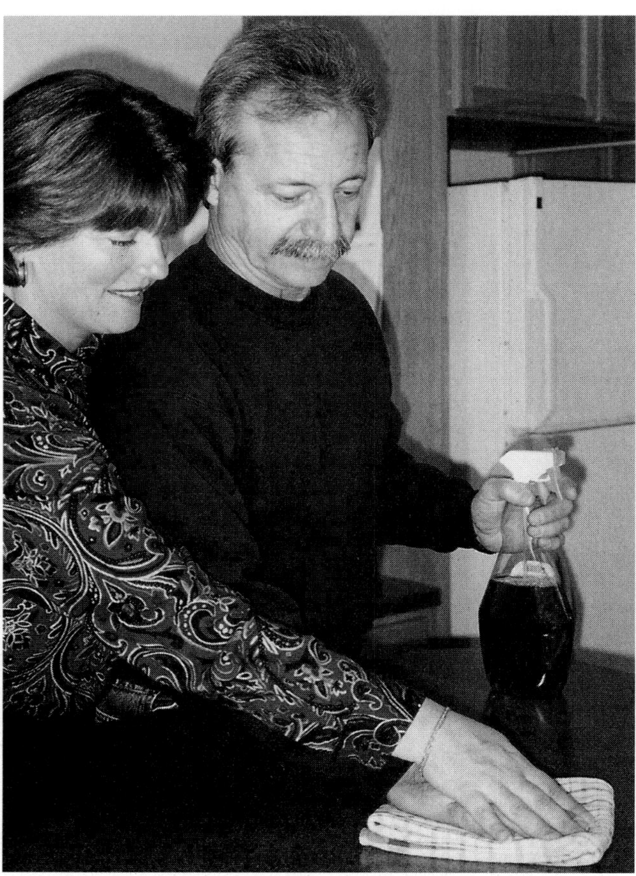

*Figure 23-29* Guiding UE during functional activities.

The patient should sit in a chair with a firm back when performing dressing activities. This provides stability and can improve balance. The same sequence should be followed to enhance learning.

*Donning shirt*

1. Position shirt across patient's knees with armhole visible and sleeve between knees (Figure 23-30).
2. Patient bends forward at hips (inhibiting extensor synergy of LE), placing affected hand in sleeve (Figure 23-31).
3. Arm drops into sleeve; shoulder protraction and gravity inhibit UE flexor synergy.
4. Bring collar to neck.
5. Sit upright; dress nonhemiplegic side.
6. Button shirt from bottom to top.

*Donning underclothes and pants*

1. Clasp hands and cross affected leg over nonhemiplegic leg (Figure 23-32). (Clinician helps when needed.)
2. Release hands. Hemiplegic arm can dangle and should not be trapped in lap. When able, patient can use affected hand as needed.
3. Pull pant leg over hemiplegic foot.
4. Clasp hands to uncross leg.
5. Place nonhemiplegic foot in pant leg (no need to cross legs). This step is difficult because patient must bear weight on hemiplegic side.
6. Pull pants to knees.
7. While holding onto waistband, patient stands with clinician's help.
8. Zip and snap pants.
9. Clinician helps patient return to sitting position.

*Donning socks and shoes*

1. Clasp hands and cross legs (as before) (Figure 23-33).
2. Put sock and shoe on hemiplegic foot.
3. Cross nonhemiplegic leg; put on sock and shoe.

## SUMMARY

Central nervous system dysfunction, such as from a cerebrovascular accident (CVA) or traumatic brain injury, can result in muscle imbalance and abnormal muscle tone, poor posture, decreased balance, and a loss of controlled movements.

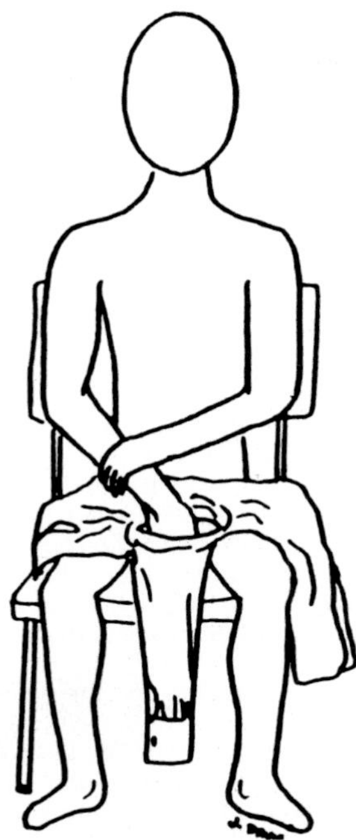

*Figure 23-30* Dressing training. Shirt positioned across patient's knees; armhole visible; sleeve dropped between knees.

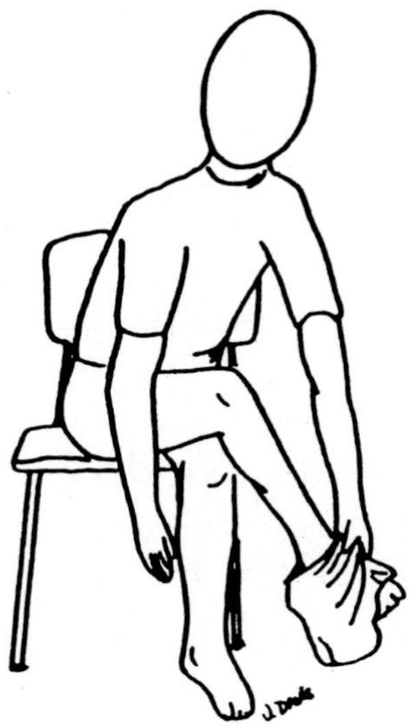

*Figure 23-32* Proper position while putting on undergarments and pants.

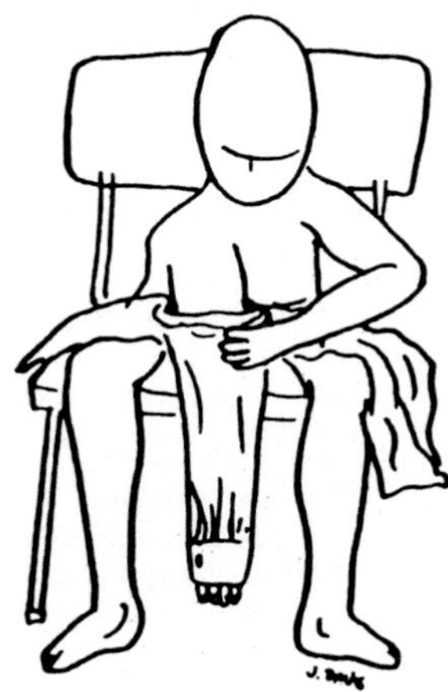

*Figure 23-31* Patient bends forward at hips (inhibiting extension synergy of LE) and places affected hand into sleeve.

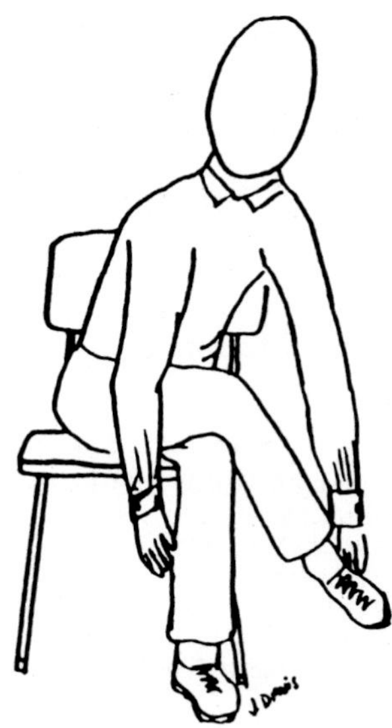

*Figure 23-33* Proper position while putting on socks and shoes.

Sensorimotor treatment approaches are used with patients who exhibit these deficits. The four traditional sensorimotor approaches are the Rood, the Brunnstrom (movement therapy), proprioceptive neuromuscular facilitation, and neurodevelopmental (Bobath).

The Rood approach emphasizes the use of controlled sensory stimulation to achieve purposeful motor responses.[18] Rood's work laid the foundation for the use of sensory stimulation in clinical practice.

The Brunnstrom (movement therapy) approach describes stages of motor recovery after a CVA and applies treatment methods that help a patient progress through the recovery stages.

Proprioceptive neuromuscular facilitation uses a multisensory approach in which mass patterns of movement, usually performed in diagonals, are used to help strengthen weak components of movements.

The neurodevelopmental treatment (Bobath) approach emphasizes relearning normal movement while avoiding abnormal movement patterns. Principles include the normalization of muscle tone, avoidance of synergistic movement, and incorporation of the affected side into purposeful activities.

These sensorimotor treatment approaches are valuable tools for the OTR and COTA. COTAs planning to use these approaches during functional activities should be trained and supervised until competency is achieved. The challenge for all clinicians who use these approaches is to apply them in contexts that are meaningful and purposeful for the patient and that will promote independent functioning.

## Selected Reading Guide Questions

1. Give two examples of patients for whom sensorimotor approaches are used.
2. List two basic goals of the Rood approach.
3. Describe how heavy joint compression is used as a facilitating technique.
4. List the stages of recovery of arm function after a cerebrovascular accident (CVA), as described by Brunnstrom.
5. Describe the upper extremity (UE) flexor and extensor synergy patterns.
6. Describe how tone of voice can be used in proprioceptive neuromuscular facilitation (PNF) treatment.
7. Identify the UE PNF diagonal used to bring the hand to the mouth during feeding.
8. Identify the primary goal of the neurodevelopmental treatment (NDT) approach.
9. Based on the NDT approach, identify the recommended position in bed for a patient with hemiplegia.
10. Describe the NDT technique for donning a shirt.

### REFERENCES


1. Alpern M, Lawrence N, Wolsk D: *Sensory processes,* Belmont, Calif, 1976, Brooks/Cole.
2. Ayres J: *Sensory integration and learning disorders,* Los Angeles, 1972, Western Psychological Services.
3. Ayres J: *The development of sensory integration theory and practice,* Dubuque, Ia, 1974, Kendall/Hunt.
4. Barr ML: *The human nervous system,* ed 2, New York, 1974, Harper & Row.
5. Bobath B: *Adult hemiplegia: evaluation and treatment,* London, 1978, Heinemann.
6. Brunnstrom S: *Movement therapy in hemiplegia,* New York, 1970, Harper & Row.
7. Calliet R: *The shoulder in hemiplegia,* Philadelphia, 1980, Davis.
8. Clark B: The vestibular system. In Mussen PH, Rosenweig MR, editors: *Annual review of psychology,* New York, 1970, Harper & Row.
9. Davis P: *Steps to follow,* Berlin, 1985, Springer-Verlag.
10. Dayhoof N: Re-thinking stroke: soft or hard devices to position hands? *Am J Nurs* 7:1142, 1975.
11. Eggars O: *Occupational therapy in the treatment of adult hemiplegia,* Rockville, Md, 1984, Aspen.
12. Eldred E: Peripheral receptors: their excitation and relation to reflex patterns, *Am J Phys Med* 46:69, 1967.
13. Farber S: *Sensorimotor evaluation and treatment procedures for allied health personnel,* Indianapolis, 1974, Indiana University and Purdue University Medical Center.
14. Farber S: *Neurorehabilitation: a multisensory approach,* Philadelphia, 1982, Saunders.
15. Goff B: The Rood approach. In *Cash's textbook of neurology for physiotherapists,* ed 4, Philadelphia, 1986, Lippincott.
16. Heininger M, Randolph S: *Neurophysiological concepts in human behavior,* St Louis, 1981, Mosby.
17. Hellebrandt FA, Schacle M, Carns ML: Methods of evoking the tonic neck reflexes in normal human subjects, *Am J Phys Med* 4:139, 1962.
18. Huss J: Sensorimotor treatment approaches. In Hopkins HL, Smith HD, editors: *Willard and Spackman's occupational therapy,* ed 6, Philadelphia, 1983, Lippincott.
19. Jackson JH: *Selected writings,* vol 1, London, 1931, Hodder & Staughton (edited by J Taylor).
20. Kotte F: From reflex to skill: the training of coordination, *Arch Phys Med Rehabil* 61:551, 1980.
21. Kotte F, Stillwell K, Lehmann J: *Krusen's handbook of physical medicine and rehabilitation,* ed 3, Philadelphia, 1982, Saunders.
22. Loeb GE, Hoffer JA: *Muscle spindle function in muscle receptors in movement control,* London, 1981, Macmillan.
23. Loomis JE, Boersma FJ: Training right brain damaged patients in a wheelchair task: case studies using verbal mediation, *Physiother Can* 34:204, 1982.
24. Matthews PBC: Muscle spindles and their motor control, *Physiol Rev* 58:763, 1978.
25. McCloskey DI: Kinesthetic sensibility, *Physiol Rev* 58:764, 1978.
26. Myers BJ: Proprioceptive neuromuscular facilitation: concepts and application in occupational therapy as taught by Voss, Chicago, Sept 8-12, 1980, Rehabilitation Institute of Chicago (course notes).
27. Myers BJ: *PNF: patterns and application in occupational therapy,* Chicago, 1981, Rehabilitation Institute of Chicago (videotape).
28. Nolte J: *The human brain: an introduction to its functional anatomy,* St Louis, 1981, Mosby.
29. Perry C: Principles and techniques of the Brunnstrom approach to the treatment of hemiplegia, *Am J Phys Med* 46:789, 1967.
30. Rood M: Neurophysiological reactions as a basis for physical therapy, *Phys Ther Rev* 34:444, 1954.
31. Rood M: Neurophysiological mechanisms utilized in the treatment of neuromuscular dysfunction, *Am J Occup Ther* 10:4, 1956.
32. Rood M: The use of sensory receptors to activate, facilitate and inhibit motor response, automatic and somatic, in developmental sequence. In Sattely C, editor: *Approaches to the treatment of patients with neuromuscular dysfunction,* Dubuque, Ia, 1962, Brown.
33. Schmidt RA: Motor learning principles for physical therapy. In Lister MJ, editor: *Contemporary management of motor control problems,* Proceedings of the 11 Step Conference, Alexandria, Va, 1991, Foundation for Physical Therapy.
34. Sherrington C: *The integrative action of the nervous system,* New Haven, Conn, 1961, Yale University Press.
35. Stockmeyer SA: An interpretation of the approach of Rood to the treatment of neuromuscular dysfunction, *Am J Phys Med* 46:900, 1967.
36. Vallbo A, Hagbarth H, Torebjard H: Somatosensory, proprioception sympathetic activity in human peripheral nerves, *Physiol Rev* 59:919, 1979.
37. Voss DE: Application of patterns and techniques in occupational therapy, *Am J Occup Ther* 8:191, 1959.
38. Voss DE: Proprioceptive neuromuscular facilitation: the PNF method. In Pearson PH, Williams LE, editors: *Physical therapy services in the developmental disabilities,* Springfield, Ill, 1972, Thomas.
39. Voss DE, Ionta MK, Myers BJ: *Proprioceptive neuromuscular facilitation,* ed 3, Philadelphia, 1985, Harper & Row.
40. Willard HL, Spackman CS, editors: *Occupational therapy,* ed 4, Philadelphia, 1971, Lippincott.
41. Williams P, Warwick R: *Functional neuroanatomy of man,* Philadelphia, 1975, Saunders.

# Chapter 24

# Treatment of Disturbances in Tactile Sensation, Perception, Cognition, and Vision

*Lorraine Williams Pedretti*
*Barbara Zoltan*
*Carol J. Wheatley*
*Mary Warren*
*Sherrell Powell*

## Chapter Objectives

*After studying this chapter, the student or practitioner will be able to:*

1. Discuss the functional effects of sensory loss or disturbance.
2. Describe the complementary roles of the OTR and the COTA in the treatment of sensory disturbances.
3. Give examples of strategies taught in a program of compensation for sensory loss for patients with central nervous system (CNS) lesions and peripheral nervous system (PNS) lesions.
4. List guidelines for patients with PNS dysfunction who lack protective sensation.
5. Describe some remedial techniques used for patients with PNS dysfunction.
6. Contrast the adaptive and the remedial approaches in treatment of perceptual dysfunction.
7. Identify appropriate compensatory and adaptive treatment techniques for specific sensory disorders.
8. Contrast the remedial and the compensatory approaches in the treatment of cognitive dysfunction.
9. Identify compensatory strategies for specific cognitive deficits.
10. Contrast internal and external memory strategies.

## Chapter Objectives—cont'd

11. Identify strategies for helping the patient who experiences deficits in executive functions, such as reasoning, judgment, awareness, and behavioral control.
12. Discuss in general terms the complexity of organizing and processing visual perception.
13. Place visual functions within a hierarchy.
14. Identify some remedial strategies used for treatment of visual deficits.
15. Identify and describe compensatory strategies for patients with visual deficits.

## Key Terms

anesthesia
paresthesia
hypoesthesia
hyperesthesia
analgesia
hypalgesia
remedial treatment
compensatory treatment
adaptive treatment
sensory-integrative approach
neurodevelopmental (Bobath) approach
transfer-of-training approach
functional approach
astereognosis
body scheme
ideomotor apraxia
ideational apraxia
constructional apraxia
dressing apraxia
orientation
attention
memory
transfer of learning
generalization
domain-specific learning
executive functioning
vision
visual perception
oculomotor control
visual fields
visual acuity
visual attention
visual scanning
pattern recognition
visual memory
visual cognition
myopia
hyperopia
presbyopia
astigmatism
cataracts
glaucoma
macular area
homonymous hemianopsia
scanning
hand trailing
sighted guiding
punt watch or clock

Performance components are the building blocks of occupation. The abilities to sense, to organize sensations into meaningful representations of the world, and to plan and sequence responses support every action in activities of daily living (ADLs), in work, and in play and leisure. Although the registered occupational therapist (OTR) is the expert on the evaluation and treatment of performance components, the certified occupational therapy assistant (COTA) has a role as well. The extent of this role depends on many factors: the COTA's experience and service competencies, the practice area, the treatment setting, and the geographical location. In rural communities and general medical settings the COTA may find many opportunities to treat disorders in the performance components, often because of a shortage of other trained personnel. Even in the most sophisticated rehabilitation medicine setting, however, the COTA may provide specific treatments for performance components within the context of other treatment. An example is using cueing when teaching a cognitively impaired patient self-dressing.

Recognizing the COTA's important and variable role in the treatment of performance components, this chapter presents some of the techniques the COTA might use. We include treatments that would only be provided by the more advanced COTA practitioner, assuming that the assistant will acquire service competency under qualified supervision before attempting these techniques.

This chapter has four sections: sensation, perception, cognition, and vision. Each section examines the treatment of that performance component, and each may be studied separately.

# Section I Treatment of Sensory Dysfunction

LORRAINE WILLIAMS PEDRETTI

Persons are rarely conscious of the importance of sensation until it is lost or disturbed. Sensation conveys information about the world that individuals process and use so quickly that much is not consciously registered. When sensation is normal, this process works smoothly. When sensation is abnormal, the process of finding and using information is chaotic, as in a library with half the catalog missing and the shelves in disarray. Misplacing eyeglasses, having a limb "fall asleep," and having impaired hearing after an airplane ride give persons with normal sensation a glimpse of life with sensory dysfunction.

Sensory disturbance severe enough to require treatment is disabling. The absence of tactile sensation makes simple tasks such as tying shoes arduous. Finding keys in a purse or pocket requires visual assistance; touch alone is insufficient. Occupational therapy can improve the functioning of persons with sensory loss by teaching techniques to compensate for the absence of sensation and even by restoring lost sensory function in some patients. The roles of the registered occupational therapist (OTR) and the certified occupational therapy assistant (COTA) in this area are complementary. The OTR evaluates, plans treatment, and carries out remedial programs; the COTA teaches compensatory techniques and may assist in remedial treatment.

Sensory disturbances can result from central nervous system (CNS) or peripheral nervous system (PNS) dysfunction or from cranial nerve disorders. In PNS and cranial nerve lesions, the sensory disturbance is experienced in the area supplied by the affected nerve. Sensory disorders of nerve root origin are experienced in the dermatome supplied by the affected nerve root. Sensory dysfunction of CNS origin is more generalized and affects the contralateral side of the body after cerebrovascular accident (CVA, stroke) or head injury, resulting in hemiplegia.

Some of the terms associated with sensory disturbances are **anesthesia** (complete loss of sensation), **paresthesia** (abnormal sensation such as tingling or crawling), **hypoesthesia** (or hypesthesia, decreased sensation), **hyperesthesia** (increased tactile sensitivity), **analgesia** (complete loss of pain sensation), and **hypalgesia** (or hypoalgesia, diminished pain sensation).[3]

Because sensory loss may have a profound effect on the patient's ability to function in everyday activities, the OTR and COTA must promote sensory recovery or reeducation to the extent possible or teach compensatory techniques and safety precautions.

## TREATMENT GUIDELINES

Before treatment of sensory dysfunction can begin, the OTR must complete a sensory evaluation and an evaluation of functional use of the affected part. The therapist must have knowledge of the diagnosis, the cause of the sensory dysfunction, the prognosis for return of sensation, and the current progression of recovery. This information may help to determine whether the treatment approach should be remedial, compensatory, or both.

**Remedial treatment** attempts to change the sensory response itself, restoring more normal sensory function. This is only possible with certain patients with conditions (usually PNS) that are reversible. **Compensatory treatment** teaches strategies for adapting to sensory losses. Such strategies include precautions to avoid injury and the use of other senses to obtain information. For example, a patient who lacks tactile sensation must learn to use the eyes to look for objects that might otherwise have been found by searching through touch.

The patient who is to begin a sensory reeducation program should be motivated and able to concentrate. Cognitive ability should be adequate to understand the purpose of the training. Motivation to persevere in daily sessions and to make every effort to use the affected part in activities of daily living (ADLs) is important.[2,5]

This section now considers treatment approaches for the two major categories of sensory loss, CNS and PNS.

## Central Nervous System Dysfunction

### *Effects of Sensory Loss*

After a CVA and other CNS disorders such as head injury, sensory loss can be a significant problem. Sensory loss inhibits movement, even when good motor return exists. The inclination to move is based on sensory input and feedback. Persons with poor sensation have little urge to move; attempted movement may be clumsy or incoordinated.

Sensory loss may contribute to (but is not the only cause of) neglect of the affected extremity so often seen in patients with CVA. The possibility of injury is a serious concern. Reliance on visual control makes many activities impossible, such as reaching into a purse or pocket to retrieve an item or fastening clothing at the side or back.[5]

### *Compensatory Treatment*

A first concern is safety and ensuring that the patient is not injured by bumping, burning, or becoming snagged in furniture or equipment during performance of ADLs. Examples of compensation are (1) using the less affected hand to perform activities such as cooking, eating, and ironing; (2) using vision to observe motion and location of body parts; (3) testing bath water with the less affected hand or a bath thermometer; and (4) using adaptive devices such as the one-handed cutting board to avoid cutting the affected hand.[9]

The stroke (CVA) patient needs to be made aware of sensory deficits. Safety factors during performance of ADLs must be continuously brought to the patient's attention and reinforced. The patient must learn to check the position of the limbs by looking at them. Patients must be evaluated for safety awareness and trained to consider safety in hazardous activities. The patient who wants to return to home management should demonstrate good judgment, safety awareness, and the ability to use visual compensation for sensory loss.[7] Frequent repetition of instructions and cueing by the OT practitioner are often necessary.

Cognitive disturbances such as poor memory, perseveration, poor judgment, and inability to see cause-and-effect relationships make it difficult for some patients to learn and attend effectively to compensatory techniques. Such patients require supervision.

### *Remedial Treatment*

Sensory bombardment involving as many of the senses as possible has been effective for sensory retraining in some CVA patients. Design and application of sensory reeducation programs are the province of the OTR. The COTA might assist by providing specific sensory input as instructed, under close supervision until service competency is well established. Some input might include (1) touching or stroking the affected parts, (2) encouraging the patient to look at affected parts and see the movement and touch stimulation, and (3) weight bearing on legs, arms, and trunk, which increases proprioceptive feedback.[9]

One remedial approach focuses primarily on tactile and kinesthetic reeducation.[5] The OTR must first normalize the patient's muscle tone and find the best position for the sensory reeducation activities. The therapist must find ways to stimulate sensation without increasing spasticity and must consider other deficits, such as hemianopsia, aphasia, and visual perceptual deficits. Many patients may need additional time to respond because of delayed processing of sensory information. Sensory stimuli must be repeated and varied for patients with CNS dysfunction if they are to relearn sensation.[5]

Eggers[5] describes a graded treatment program for patients with sensory deficits. Initially the patient is allowed to see and hear an object as it is being felt; this allows all the senses to be used together. Next, vision is occluded during the tactile exploration. Finally, a pad is placed on the table top so that both auditory and visual clues are eliminated and the patient relies on tactile-kinesthetic input alone. The program for tactile-kinesthetic reeducation begins with gross discrimination of objects that are very dissimilar (e.g., smooth and rough textures, round and square shapes). Next the patient is asked to estimate quantities through touch (e.g., number of marbles in a box). Then the patient must discriminate between large and small objects hidden in sand, progressing to two-dimensional and three-dimensional objects. Finally, the patient is required to pick a specific small object from among several objects.

## Peripheral Nervous System Dysfunction

### *Treatment of Hypersensitivity*

Patients recovering from peripheral nerve injury often experience heightened, uncomfortable, or irritable responses to nonnoxious stimuli.[1,8] If the patient has no open wounds or infection, treatment of hypersensitivity is best done early, before sensory reeducation begins.[8]

Desensitization is most often done in hand rehabilitation and burn rehabilitation, which require advanced education and experience. Specific details of desensitization programs are beyond the scope of this chapter and the COTA's usual service competencies.

Desensitization includes massage, tapping, or rolling over hypersensitive areas with different textures. Treatment begins at the patient's level of tolerance, then textures are graded to coarser and rougher, with increases in force, duration, and frequency of application. Vibration and immersion in materials (e.g., styrofoam balls, rice, beans, popcorn, buckshot, plastic squares) are also used. This method of treatment is based on increasing the nerve's pain threshold.[1,8] A service-competent OTR would administer these treatments.

Many patients with hypersensitivity tend to protect sensitive areas and avoid using the affected part in bilateral ADLs. The COTA, who is often the primary ADL trainer, must reassure the patient that touching hypersensitive areas is beneficial.[1]

### *Compensatory Treatment*

A compensatory approach for patients with PNS dysfunction is similar to that described earlier for patients with CNS dysfunction. The patient must be made aware of the specific sensory deficits and taught safety awareness for ADLs. The patient may need to avoid using the affected limb during bilateral activities that are potentially hazardous.

Writing about the hand, Callahan[2] proposed the following guidelines for patients with PNS dysfunction who lack protective sensation:

1. Avoid exposure of the involved area to heat, cold, and sharp objects.
2. When gripping a tool or object, be conscious not to apply more force than necessary.
3. Be aware of the fact that the smaller the handle, the less distribution of pressure over gripping surfaces. Avoid small handles by building up the handle or using a different tool whenever possible.
4. Avoid tasks that require use of one tool for extended periods, especially if the hand is unable to adapt by changing the manner of grip.
5. Change tools frequently at work to rest tissue areas.
6. Observe the skin for signs of stress (redness, edema, warmth) from excessive force or repetitive pressure, and rest the hand if these signs occur.
7. If blisters, lacerations, or other wounds occur, treat them with the utmost care to avoid further injury to the skin and possible infection.
8. To keep skin soft and pliant, follow a daily routine of skin care, including soaking and oil massage to lock in moisture.

The patient with simple PNS dysfunction (in whom perceptual and cognitive skills are presumed to be intact) may be more capable of learning and attending to the compensatory techniques than the patient with CNS dysfunction (who may have cognitive or perceptual problems in addition to the deficit in sensation).

### *Remedial Treatment*

As a sensory organ, the hand is an extension of the brain. When nerves in the hand are repaired or recover after injury, the messages to the brain are altered. The new pattern of neural impulses may be so different that the stimulus cannot be identified. The sensory information received cannot be interpreted correctly. Sensory reeducation assists the patient to reinterpret the sensory impulses reaching the consciousness. Sensory reeducation enhances the patient's potential for functional recovery after nerve repair.[4] The following descriptions of sensory reeducation are meant as background for the COTA who might assist in such a program under direct supervision of the OTR.

Dellon's sensory reeducation program is divided into early and late phases.[4] In the early phase the focus is on reeducating moving touch, constant touch, pressure, and touch localization. For moving touch a pencil eraser or fingertip is used to move up and down the area being treated. The patient observes the stimulus. Next, vision is occluded as the patient concentrates on the stimulus, then opens the eyes to verify what is happening. The patient verbalizes what is being felt, such as, "I feel a soft object moving down the palm of my hand."

A similar procedure is followed for constant touch. A pencil eraser is used to press down on one place on the finger or palm in an area where constant touch is recovered. The patient is encouraged to practice these reeducation techniques four times a day for at least 5 minutes each but is directed not to stimulate one hand with the other because this would send two sets of sensory stimuli to the brain.[2,4]

Late-phase sensory reeducation is initiated as soon as moving touch and constant touch are perceived at the fingertips and good localization is present. This is often 6 to 8 months after nerve repair at the wrist. The goal in this phase is to facilitate the recovery of tactile gnosis (knowledge). The exercises involve a series of tactile discrimination tasks. These begin with identification of large objects that are significantly different from one another and progress to objects with finer and more subtle differences. Familiar household objects are used first. The process is to grasp the object while looking at it, then to occlude the vision and concentrate on the perception, and finally to look again at the object for reinforcement. The next objects differ in texture and then are smaller and require more discrete discrimination. Manipulation of the training objects also contributes to motor recovery. Ultimately, the OT practitioner can incorporate activities that simulate those of the patient's occupational roles.[2,4] This type of sensory reeducation program can be integrated with ADL training.

Wynn Parry's sensory retraining program helps patients with PNS injuries affecting the hand to "lay down a new code" in the CNS.[10] The goal is to reprogram the cortical (CNS) representation of sensory nerve fibers in the hand. This training program works best with patients who are cooperative and well motivated and need to use their sensation for ADLs.[10]

The training program begins when the patient has sensation in the fingers, about 6 to 8 months after a nerve suture at the wrist. Large wood blocks of different shapes are used. The patient's vision is occluded, and a block is placed in the affected hand. The patient is asked to feel it, describe its shape, and compare its weight with a block placed in the unaffected hand. If an incorrect response is given, the patient is allowed to look at the blocks and repeat the manipulation, integrating visual and tactile information. The patient then compares the sensory experience with that of the normal hand. The procedure continues with various-shaped blocks, and when these have been mastered, blocks with textures (e.g., sandpaper, velvet) on some surfaces are used. The patient is asked to differentiate textured surfaces from wood surfaces.[10]

In the next phase of training, the patient is asked to identify several textures (e.g., sheepskin, leather, silk, canvas, rubber, plastic, wool, carpet, sandpaper) with the vision occluded. Finally, common objects are used in training, and the patient is asked to identify them without the aid of vision. If incorrect responses are given for texture and object identification, the patient is allowed to perform the manipulations while looking at the training objects and to relate what is felt to what is seen. Objects are graded from large to small. Training sessions may be varied by burying objects in a bowl of sand and asking the patient to retrieve a specific object, using a form board in which to place specific forms, or identifying wooden letters for spelling out words. Training is done in two to four 10-minute sessions a day.[10]

To train touch localization, Wynn Parry[10] recommended the following procedure. Vision is occluded, and the clinician touches several places on the hand's volar surface. The patient is asked to locate each stimulus with the index finger of the unaffected hand. If the response is incorrect, the patient is directed to look at the place where the hand was touched and to relate where the touch was felt to where the stimulus was actually applied.[10]

Turner[9] described a sensory reeducation program for patients with PNS lesions. Retraining can begin when the patient's protective sensation (deep pressure, pinprick) and touch perception return. Activities consist of having the patient identify objects, shapes, and textures with the vision occluded. If the response is incorrect, the patient is allowed to look at the object and compare its sensation in the normal hand; this allows the integration of tactile sensation and vision. Objects such as textured dominoes or checkers, cut-out shapes, and large to small common objects that may be hidden in rice or lentils may be used. Training with these objects is carried out three or four times a day for 45 minutes. The training periods are alternated with periods of general bilateral activity such as pottery making, bread kneading, weaving, and macramé. The patient is encouraged to use the affected hand in bilateral activities and to compare the feelings of the tools and materials in the affected hand with those in the unaffected hand.[9]

La Croix and Helman[6] described a program of sensory reeducation after nerve injury. The purpose is to help the patient correctly interpret different sensory impulses. The patient is exposed to a series of graded stimuli of constant pressure, movement, light touch, and vibration. The least stressful stimuli are presented first. The patient does the training exercises several times a day for short periods. The exercises are done on the unaffected side and then on the affected side, with the aid of vision and then with vision occluded. Areas of hypersensitivity are noted. Sensory stimulation, such as stroking, deep pressure, rubbing, and maintained touch, using different textures and shapes, is used to reduce hypersensitivity.[6]

Sensory reeducation for patients with PNS disorders focuses on applying graded stimuli according to the progression of nerve recovery. Stimuli for touch localization, moving touch, and constant touch are followed by exercises for tactile discrimination of shape, size, texture, and object identification. Integration of tactile impressions with visual, auditory, and tactile senses is an important part of the reeducation program.

## SUMMARY

Sensory information is conveyed from the environment to the brain from receptors in the skin and sense organs by way of peripheral and spinal nerves and the spinal cord. Sensation presents the external environment to the brain and provides information necessary to guide purposeful and effective movement responses. Defects in sensation are disabling because they disrupt the customary flow of sensory information to motor output. Occupational therapy practitioners can help improve the daily lives of persons with sensory impairments by providing both remedial and compensatory treatments. Unless service competent through continuing education, the COTA may provide remedial treatment only under close, direct supervision of the OTR.

# Section II Treatment of Perceptual and Perceptual Motor Deficits

LORRAINE WILLIAMS PEDRETTI, BARBARA ZOLTAN, CAROL J. WHEATLEY

Performance of functional activities depends on perceptual skills as well as motor skills. Therefore remediation of or compensation for perceptual deficits should improve functional performance.[10] Occupational therapy practitioners have used perceptual retraining since the 1950s, focusing on retraining specific perceptual skills and incorporating perceptual retraining into functional tasks such as activities of daily living (ADLs).

## APPROACHES TO TREATMENT

Treatment is classified into two main approaches: adaptive and remedial.[10] **Adaptive treatment** provides training in ADL behaviors with the goal of improving adaptation to the environment to promote maximal functioning of the patient; these approaches are similar to the compensatory treatments addressed in Section I. An example is teaching one-handed self-dressing to the patient who had a cerebrovascular accident (CVA, stroke). Today the certified occupational therapy assistant (COTA) routinely carries out adaptive treatment in many settings.

In contrast, the *remedial* approaches seek to change central nervous system (CNS) functions.[10] In this approach the registered occupational therapist (OTR) might use slow rocking, spinning, or other sensory input to attempt to restore sensation, perception, and motor response in the affected part. These techniques are reserved for the OTR except when the COTA (beyond entry level) has extensive training and proven service competency.

The OTR designs the program for treatment of perceptual deficits, which may use one approach or a combination of approaches. The OTR must rely on experience and clinical judgment to measure and report improvement, because guidelines, protocols, and methods for perceptual training are sketchy in the literature and the results may not be objectively measurable.[9,13]

Treatment of perceptual problems can be difficult and complex. The best results are obtained from consistent daily treatment. Zoltan, Siev, and Freishtat[13] described four approaches that are used for perceptual training of the hemiplegic patient. Three would be classified as remedial: the sensory-integrative approach, the neurodevelopmental (Bobath) approach, and the transfer-of-training approach. The functional approach is considered adaptive.[10] Treatment assigned to a COTA typically involves the functional or transfer-of-training approach because the other two require additional academic and clinical preparation.

### Remedial Approaches

The **sensory-integrative approach** is based on neurophysiological and developmental principles. Ayres[1] described it as a treatment approach for children with sensory-integrative dysfunction.[10] It assumes that controlled sensory input can be used to elicit specific motor responses. This approach may be impractical for adults because it takes much treatment time to be effective. Also, the adult's CNS does not have the same capacity for learning as the child's CNS. Some OT practitioners use modifications and selected techniques from this approach with adults and report some success.[13]

The **neurodevelopmental (Bobath) approach** attempts to retrain perceptual functions by enabling the patient to experience the sensation of normal movement and the sensory feedback from correct performance. Bilateral activities used in the motor retraining program stimulate total body awareness and help to remediate problems of unilateral neglect and homonymous hemianopsia (a visual deficit of the right or left visual field). Weight-bearing activities, an important part of the motor retraining program, enhance proprioception[13] (see Chapter 23).

The **transfer-of-training approach** assumes that practice in a particular perceptual task generalizes to performance of similar tasks or practical activities requiring the same perceptual skills. For example, practice in reproducing pegboard designs for spatial relations training might carry over to dressing skills that require spatial judgment (e.g., matching blouse to body, discriminating right from left shoe). This is a common approach to the treatment of perceptual problems in occupational therapy clinics. Conflicting reports of its effectiveness suggest that more research is needed.[13]

### Adaptive Approach

The **functional approach** is characterized by the repetitive practice of particular tasks that help the patient become more independent in the performance of ADLs. This is probably the most common approach in dealing with perceptual problems. The OT practitioner does not train the patient in specific perceptual functions. Rather, the practitioner helps the patient adapt to or compensate for the perceptual deficits. The patient is made aware of the problem and taught to compensate for it. For example, if the patient has trouble dressing because of a body scheme deficit, the OTR or COTA may set up a regular dressing pattern and routine and provide cues with repetitive practice. With these adaptations the patient may learn to dress.

Adaptation of the environment, methods, or materials is another way to compensate for a perceptual deficit. For example, if the patient is distractible because of visual or auditory figure-ground deficits, the clinician may arrange for treatment to occur in a quiet, uncluttered room to minimize distractions and create the best environment for learning. If the patient has dressing apraxia, colored tabs can be sewn into clothing to provide cues for top and bottom and inside and outside.[13]

## TREATMENT OF SELECTED PERCEPTUAL DEFICITS

### Astereognosis

*Stereognosis* is the perceptual skill that enables an individual to identify common objects and geometric shapes through touch without the aid of vision. Stereognosis is "seeing with the hands" and is basic to the performance of everyday activities, such as finding a key in a pocket.

One treatment approach for **astereognosis** described by Eggers[3] is discussed in Section I. Farber[5] described a treatment approach to retrain stereognosis in adults and children with CNS dysfunction. First, the patient is allowed to examine the training object visually as it is rotated by the clinician. The patient is then allowed to handle the object in the less affected (or unaffected) hand while observing the hand. In the next step the patient is allowed to manipulate the object with both hands while looking. Then the object is placed in the affected hand to be manipulated while looking at it. The patient may place the hand in a mirror-lined, three-sided box during these manipulations to increase visual input. This sequence is then repeated with the vision occluded. Once several objects can be identified consistently, two of the objects may be hidden in a tub of sand or rice. The patient is then asked to reach into the tub and retrieve a specific object. If the sensation of the sand or rice is overstimulating or disturbing, the objects can be placed in a bag.[5]

Vinograd, Taylor, and Grossman[11] described a similar program. However, objects for discrimination of shape, size, weight, and texture, as well as common objects, are included in the training. Wooden blocks are used for shape recognition, sandbags and cotton bags for weight recognition, and different grades of sandpaper and smooth leather for texture discrimination.[11]

Ferreri's approach to intensive stereognostic training of spastic, cerebral palsied adults indicates some favorable results for improving stereognosis.[6] Training sessions of 20 minutes, three to four times a week for 5 weeks, are held. The training program consists of comparing two different objects or forms using the uninvolved hand, then the involved hand. The patients with motor paralysis are assisted with manipulation of the objects. The examiner discusses the qualities of the objects or forms and emphasizes the hand and finger positions. A particular training item is used for each session until five consecutive correct responses are given in the testing portion of the session before a new training item is introduced.[6]

### Body Scheme Disorders

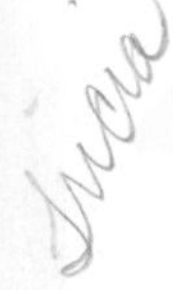

**Body scheme** is a postural model based on a person's perception of the body's position and the relationship of the body parts.[7] The individual's body scheme is considered the foundation for development of future skills in the perception of environmental space.[14]

The treatment of body scheme disorders can include the sensory-integrative, transfer-of-training, functional, or neurodevelopmental approach or a combination of these. Using the transfer-of-training approach, the OTR or COTA may touch the patient's body parts and have the patient identify them as they are touched. Practice in assembling human figure puzzles and quizzing the patient on body parts are other methods in this approach.[13]

Using a remedial approach, unilateral body neglect can be treated by applying sensory input (rubbing the patient's arm or leg) before dressing, using precautions to prevent increased spasticity. These techniques are used only by a qualified OTR.

The therapist or assistant may also engage the patient in activities that focus attention to the neglected side. Examples are placing work materials on the affected side and approaching the patient from the affected side for treatment or conversation. Conversely, using an adaptive or compensatory approach, the clinician may place food, utensils, and work materials on the unaffected side and give all instructions from that side. Repetitive practice and cuing may also be effective. Bilateral weight bearing with handling techniques of the neurodevelopmental approach can be used to facilitate total body awareness.[13]

### Ideomotor and Ideational Apraxia

**Ideomotor apraxia** is an inability to carry out a motor act on command, although the patient is able to perform the act automatically. The patient may be able to describe the intended motion in words but is unable to execute the motor act at will. **Ideational apraxia** is an inability to form the concept of the movement or to execute the act in response to a command or automatically.[7] The distinction between ideational and ideomotor apraxia is often unclear in an individual patient.

Treatment of ideational and ideomotor apraxia is difficult. Use of short, clear, concise, and concrete instructions is necessary, because this apraxia is usually the result of a dominant hemisphere lesion, and often aphasia is present as well. The task should be broken down into its component steps, and each step should be taught separately. Verbal and demonstrated instructions may be ineffective, and it may be helpful to guide the patient through the correct movements, giving tactile and proprioceptive input to the instruction. This can be done while also giving brief verbal instruction. After the patient has performed each step of the task separately, the clinician can begin to combine the steps, grading to the complete task.[13] An example of a complete task is hair combing. The therapist or assistant can break the task into steps: lift comb; bring comb to hair; move comb across top of head, down left side, down right side, and down back; and replace comb on table. Much repetition is necessary for effective results.

### Constructional Apraxia

**Constructional apraxia** is a deficit in the ability to copy, draw, or construct a design, whether on command or spontaneously.[7] Constructional apraxia causes significant dysfunction in ADLs that require constructional ability, such as dressing and food preparation.[4]

Using a transfer-of-training approach, the patient may practice simple copying and constructional tasks. Guidance, demonstration, and three-dimensional models may be necessary. The use of landmarks in simple designs may be helpful. Tasks can be graded in complexity (e.g., number of pieces to assemble). The patient can draw on a clay board or in sand rather than on paper to receive additional proprioceptive input.[13]

### Dressing Apraxia

**Dressing apraxia** is the inability to plan and perform the motor acts necessary to dress oneself. The OTR or COTA teaches a set pattern for dressing and gives cues that help the patient to distinguish right from left or front from back. A helpful method is to have the patient position the garment the same way each time, such as a shirt with the buttons face up and pants with the zipper face up. Labels can be used as cues to differentiate the front from the back of the garment. The garment may be color-coded with small buttons or ribbons for front and back or right side and left side.[13]

## SUMMARY

Understanding the underlying mechanisms and identifying the point of breakdown in a particular action or task are crucial to the effective treatment of apraxia and other perceptual disorders.[8] Activity analysis identifies not only that a patient is unable to put on a shirt, but also when and how performance breaks down.[12] The remedial or transfer-of-training approach is widely used for constructional apraxia. A functional or adaptive approach combined with the neurodevelopmental approach is effective for the patient with dressing apraxia. Although at times a single approach may be indicated, more often a combination of techniques or approaches is most effective.[2] The COTA typically uses the functional or adaptive approach but may carry out other aspects of perceptual training as directed and supervised by the OTR.

# Section III Treatment of Cognitive Dysfunction

CAROL J. WHEATLEY

This section outlines basic treatment for deficits in cognitive function. The certified occupational therapy assistant (COTA) would not be asked to design a cognitive retraining program. The COTA may assist in carrying one out, however, and thus should have some understanding of the basic methods. The principles given in Section III of Chapter 11 should be applied during treatment.

## TREATMENT APPROACHES

Various approaches to the treatment of patients with cognitive dysfunction have been proposed in the literature. The *adaptive approach* focuses on skills that are relatively intact, using these skills to compensate for skills that are deficient. Treatment activities are functional, real-life tasks.[21,22]

The *remedial,* or *transfer-of-training, approach* uses practice with activities in the deficient areas. Typically these are table-top, pencil-and-paper tasks that involve skills found to be insufficient.[38]

Other methodologies include the *process approach*,[1,2] the *multicontext approach*,[31] *applied behavioral analysis*,[13] *sensory integration*,[6,38] and the *cognitive disability approach*.[3,4] Registered occupational therapists (OTRs) may choose to follow a given treatment philosophy or may adopt a more eclectic approach, blending treatment models based on the patient's response.

A treatment task can be analyzed and modified in several ways to improve a patient's performance.[29] This is usually referred to as "providing structure." Many different types of structure can be provided. A treatment activity can be graded by changing the parameters of the task, which include the environment, familiarity with the task, directions given for completion of the task, number of items, spatial arrangement of the items, and the response rate required.

Examples of task grading are the treatment of an inattentive patient in a quiet, uncluttered environment or the treatment of the patient with poor memory in the same environment every day. Various environmental cues can be set up in the person's work area to stimulate recall.

Cues are provided systematically through interpersonal interaction with the OT practitioner or others and modified according to the patient's response. Cues can be used to direct a patient's attention to a particular aspect of a task, to guide problem solving, and to facilitate recall. Examples of cues are repetition ("try again"), analysis ("what do these objects have in common?"), and direction of attention ("look here on your left").[29] Whenever possible, the patient should be involved in the development of the cuing system to select the most meaningful cues. The OTR or COTA must always be aware that the ultimate goals of treatment are for the patient to internalize the cues, thus reducing the need for environmental cuing for successful performance.[38]

The aging process affects an individual's cognitive abilities, although treatment has been shown to improve performance.[7] The OT practitioner must remember this when treating the elderly patient with brain damage. Repetition and practice are important, as is limiting distractions and extraneous information.[5,26] In addition, the therapist or assistant should always allow enough time for the patient to respond and should use appropriate sensory cueing whenever possible.

Several resources are available and offer a variety of treatment tasks and ideas.[10,12,32,38]

## USE OF COMPUTERS IN COGNITIVE RETRAINING

Computers are viewed as a valuable tool for rehabilitation because they provide a means to practice cognitive skills taught by the OT practitioner.[14] Documented research studies are beginning to support the value of computers in reinforcing a cognitive rehabilitation program.[16,19] Available software includes games, educational programs, and packages specifically designed for cognitive rehabilitation.[14] Specific programs can be purchased for remediation of arithmetic, attention and concentration, concept formation, nonverbal memory, reasoning, association, categorization, cause and effect, problem-solving, organization, generalization, level of abstraction, judgment of safety, spatial orientation, sequencing, and verbal memory.

Varied input devices may be used in computer-assisted cognitive rehabilitation. Patients with brain damage may require a mouse, an inverted trackball, an oversized joystick, a light pen, or a touch screen to compensate for specific motor deficits. These and other adaptive input devices may also require additional custom adaptations by the OTR or COTA.[14,20]

For additional information on computer resources for individuals with disabilities and specific software used to treat these and other related areas, the reader is referred to Chapter 21 and specific references for this section.[11,14,15,16,20]

## TREATMENT OF SPECIFIC DEFICIT AREAS

### Orientation

**Orientation** to time and place can be aided by all staff and family members who come into contact with the patient. They should attempt to reestablish orientation as frequently as possible. External aids, such as calendars, bulletin boards, and "orientation boards" with pertinent information such as the facility's name, the date, season, and current events, are often used in rehabilitation centers. An orientation group can be scheduled to meet at the start of each day to review the day's upcoming events and the previous day's occurrences.[18]

### Attention

The initial goal of treatment for the patient with **attention** dysfunction is to identify the optimal environment for enabling the patient to attend for the longest time. As attention and concentration improve, the span of time and complexity of the activity should be increased. Finally, the patient should be gradually weaned from the low-stimulus environment as tolerance increases. Formalized attention training models are available.[8,23,28]

### Memory

Often a person's flexibility in adapting to various teaching approaches is lost or diminished after cognitive deficits, and thus clinicians try to present new information in the most efficient way for the patient. Before treating **memory** deficits, the clinical team (psychologist, speech-language pathologist, other team members) attempts to identify the patient's optimal learning style.[25,34] A person's learning style can be identified by observing responses to instructions (e.g., verbal, written, demonstrated, diagrammatic) given for various standardized tests and functional activities, as well as evaluating data obtained from standardized memory tests.

As the characteristics of the optimal teaching methods become apparent, this information can be communicated to the patient, the team, and the patient's family so that the patient can learn to request that the new information be provided in the most effective manner. The COTA may contribute to the identification of learning style by carefully observing the patient's response during activities of daily living (ADLs) and other training.

The patient's learning style will suggest which strategies are most likely to help the patient remember. Memory strategies fall into two groups. *Internal* methods refer to those techniques carried out using the patient's mental effort. Internal mnemonic strategies include rehearsal, chunking, association, and imagery.[23,35] *External* strategies are provided by the clinician or positioned in the environment to cue the patient's recall. External cues include verbal reminders, signs, cue cards, notebooks, and written instructions, electronic memory aids (e.g., alarm watches), and computer data storage units.[23,36]

A patient who has limited attention and concentration may not be able to use internal strategies but may benefit from strategically placed environmental cues. The goal of therapy is to progress from the use of external cues designed by the clinician to internal and external cues established and maintained by the patient independently. A group approach that empowers the patient to guide the treatment process has also been shown to be effective.[24]

The concepts of generalization and transfer are also critical to the learning of new skills. **Transfer of learning** refers to the application of information learned in one situation to another, similar situation. **Generalization** refers to the ability to apply learned knowledge and skills to a variety of similar but novel situations.[23] Individuals with cognitive deficits frequently have difficulty with transfer of learning and may be unable to generalize skills to novel situations. Opportunity to practice transfer of new skills must be built into treatment planning.

**Domain-specific learning** is used with the patient with global memory deficits who still may be able to learn specific skills in a particular situation and to continue to apply these skills in that situation.[27] Such a patient is unable to transfer learning to a new environment. An example is the patient who is taught one-handed cooking skills in the occupational therapy department kitchen but is unable to generalize those skills to the kitchen at home. This patient may be better served by instruction provided in the home environment.

Job coaching, a type of supported employment, is also based on this premise. The skills needed for the job are taught on the job site, in contrast to the usual approach of training in a specialized school or simulated training setting.[33]

Joli

### Executive Functions

**Executive functioning** includes cognitive abilities in the areas of planning, organizing, setting goals, carrying out a plan, and abstracting.[17] The patient's level of awareness of the executive deficits will determine the treatment approach. At one extreme is the patient who is aware of the problem and who can recognize, comprehend, and appreciate the implications of inactivity. This patient may respond to self-monitoring strategies or environmental cues. For example, the patient may keep a notebook, calendar, lists, and other reminders to stimulate activity.

At the other extreme is the more severely impaired patient who denies or devalues the deficit. Such a patient may require supervision by another individual. A family member or significant other may be trained to set up a daily routine, provide the verbal prompting needed, and maintain the system of environmental cues established.

#### *Reasoning and Problem Solving*

The steps in the problem-solving process are as follows:

1. Define the problem.
2. Develop possible solutions.
3. Choose the best solution.
4. Execute the solution.
5. Evaluate the outcome.

This sequence can be taught to the patient, with instructions to use the steps when a problem is encountered in therapy or in functional tasks.[9,37] The OT practitioner can assist the patient in transferring this technique to a variety of situations.

#### *Awareness*

Awareness can be further addressed in treatment using the following approaches.[30] *Self-estimation* can be encouraged by asking questions requiring the patient to predict performance on a given task. The practitioner and patient also can reverse roles to increase awareness. Patients can be taught to question themselves during activity and evaluate themselves after completing the task.

#### *Behavioral Problems*

Defects in executive functioning often result in problem behavior because the individual lacks normal judgment and self-control. Behavioral management strategies are used to restrict such a patient's behavior. Staff members should give the patient specific, direct feedback regarding the inappropriateness of the behavior. If the person's level of insight and control warrants, internal strategies can be taught, such as *time out* (when persons voluntarily remove themselves from the situation). If this approach fails, external controls may be used, and a staff person may escort the patient to a quiet area until behavioral control is once again established. The staff member must remain calm because a strong emotional response from the staff can exacerbate the situation.

A group approach can also be useful in providing feedback from peers.[18] Videotaping can provide a visual record of behavior that can be discussed with the patient.

## SUMMARY

The area of cognitive dysfunction is complex and requires the COTA to develop astute observational skills and attain knowledge and understanding of underlying principles. Evaluation and design of treatment for cognitive deficits is the OTR's responsibility. The COTA can contribute in this area by carefully observing patient behavior and by applying the general treatment principles and techniques discussed. The COTA is encouraged to seek additional sources and experiences as needed to refine therapeutic skill in dealing with patients with cognitive dysfunction.

# Section IV Treatment of Visual Deficits

MARY WARREN, SHERRELL POWELL

Making use of visual stimuli requires both vision and visual perception. **Vision** refers to the reception of sensory information through the visual receptors. **Visual perception** is a process used by the central nervous system (CNS) to integrate vision with other sensory input in order to adapt and survive. Eye injury or disease and brain injury may alter a person's ability to process visual information. How much function is lost depends on the vision and visual perception required by that person for necessary activities of daily living (ADLs).

## ROLE OF VISION IN ADAPTATION PROCESS

According to Ayres,[2] "The overall function of the brain is to filter, organize and integrate sensory information to make an adaptive response to the environment." The brain receives visual, proprioceptive, tactile, vestibular, and auditory information. In adapting to the environment, the brain puts together the isolated pieces of sensory information it receives, integrating them to form a picture of the environment. Because sensory input into the CNS is constantly changing, the picture created is dynamic and constantly changing as well. A person's decision on how to respond to a situation changes moment by moment with alterations in the person's sensory context.

Given the importance of the sensory context, what role does vision play in the adaptation process? Vision is our most far-reaching sensory system. It takes us out into our environment; it alerts us to danger (e.g., seeing a threatening storm approach) and to pleasure (e.g., seeing a friend waiting by the door). Because of its far-reaching nature, visual input strongly dominates the construction of the environmental picture we use to adapt. We rely on vision to "size up situations." We say to ourselves, "He looks harmless" or "That looks delicious." Our language is peppered with phrases that reflect the importance of vision in decision making (e.g., "I'll believe it when I see it," "I'll keep an eye out for it," "I can see what you mean"). How we "see" a situation triggers the planning and decision-making processes.

## HOW VISUAL PERCEPTION IS ORGANIZED AND PROCESSED

Visual perceptual skills are organized in a hierarchy of levels that interact with and support each other (Figure 24-1).[32] The ability to use visual perceptual skill to adapt to the environment reflects the interaction of all these skills at all the levels shown.

First, at the foundation level, the brain must receive clear, concise visual information from the environment. The three *primary sensory functions* at this level are oculomotor control, the visual fields, and visual acuity.

**Oculomotor control** ensures that eye movements are quickly and accurately completed. The **visual fields** register the entire visual scene and ensure that the CNS receives complete visual information. **Visual acuity** ensures that the visual information sent to the CNS is sharp, clear, and accurate. Acting together, oculomotor control, the visual fields, and visual acuity ensure that an adequate image is generated.

**Visual attention** is the next level in the hierarchy and may shift from object to object of the visual scene. **Visual scanning**, the next level, focuses a selected object on the area of the retina with the greatest ability to process detail.

**Pattern recognition** identifies the salient features of objects and uses these features to distinguish an object from its surroundings.[16] A *salient feature* distinguishes one object from another. For example, the salient feature that differentiates an upper-case "E" from an upper-case "F" is the lower horizontal line on the E.

**Visual memory** is the next skill level in the hierarchy. The brain must be able to create and retain a picture of the object in the mind's eye and store a visual image temporarily in short-term memory. The brain also must be able to store the image in long-term

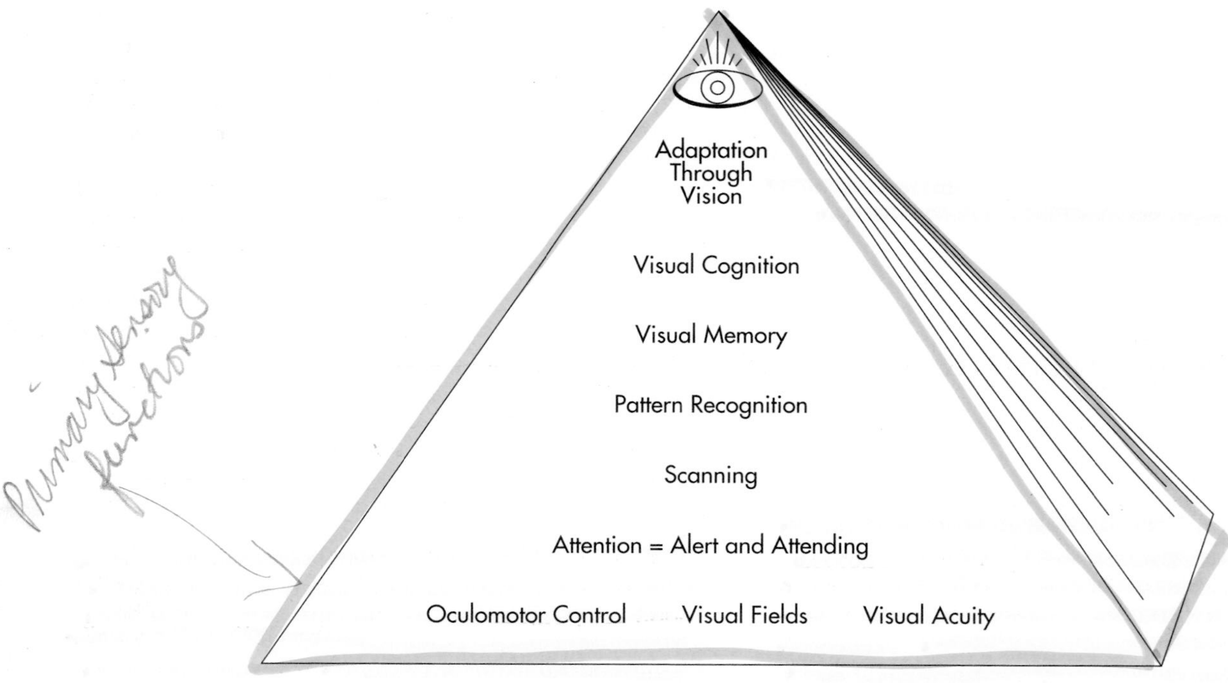


*Figure 24-1* Hierarchy of visual perceptual skill development in the central nervous system. (Courtesy Josephine C Moore, PhD, OTR. From Warren M: A hierarchical model for evaluation and treatment of visual perceptual dysfunction in adult acquired brain injury. Part I, *Am J Occup Ther* 47:42, 1993, American Occupational Therapy Association.)

memory and then retrieve it from memory later when appropriate.

The highest skill in the hierarchy is **visual cognition,** the ability to manipulate visual information mentally and integrate it with other sensory information to gain knowledge and to solve problems, formulate plans, and make decisions. Visual cognition serves as a foundation for all academic endeavors: reading, writing, mathematics, and many vocations (e.g., artist, engineer, surgeon, architect, scientist).

Different areas of the brain have different responsibilities in processing visual information, but all areas must work together to make sense of what is seen.[18,19] As with a car, in which the carburetor is as critical to performance as the spark plugs, the brain runs efficiently only when all systems are working together. Brain injury or disease disrupts the system, and the organization of visual processing breaks down. Warren[33] provides the particulars of this process and a table of brain lesions related to visual perceptual deficits.

Brain injury or disease can disrupt visual processing at any one of the skill levels in the hierarchy. Eye disease or injury can disrupt visual processing at the primary levels of oculomotor control and visual acuity.

Because of the unity of the hierarchy, a disruption of skill function at one level will affect the entire structure. If an eye or brain injury disturbs a lower level skill, the skills above it will also be compromised. Evaluation and treatment of visual deficits require an understanding of the integration of vision at each skill level; thus this is the responsibility of the registered occupational therapist (OTR). The following background information is provided to prepare the certified occupational therapy assistant (COTA) to assist in treatment, as directed by the OTR.

## DEFICITS IN PRIMARY VISUAL SKILLS

### Oculomotor Control

Oculomotor control deficits result in decreased speed, control, and coordination of eye movements. The eye is unable to move in the direction of the paretic (weakened) muscles and may drift toward one side of the eye socket (i.e., drift either in or out). To maintain a single visual image, the eyes must always move together and line up evenly. When the movement of one eye does not match that of the other, the person sees a double image. This condition is known as *diplopia,* or double vision.[20] To eliminate the double image, the patient often holds the head in a position that reduces the need to use the paretic muscle. The patient may have difficulty using the eyes together in a coordinated manner. *Dysmetric* eye movement, in which the eye undershoots or overshoots a target, may also be observed.[3,17]

These disturbances in control of the eye muscles can create a variety of functional deficits. The patient may be slower to scan the environment and take in visual information because of reduced speed and range of eye movement; this causes delays in responding. The patient may have difficulty maintaining a clear image and may experience doubling and blurring of visual images. The patient also may have difficulty focusing at different distances from the body, and depth perception may be diminished. All these conditions create significant visual stress for the patient, reducing concentration and endurance for activities. The patient may respond to this increased stress by becoming agitated and uncooperative in therapy sessions or complaining of headaches, eye strain, or neck strain. Treatment for this type of dysfunction should be coordinated by the OTR with the guidance of an optometrist or ophthalmologist who specializes in visual impairment caused by neurological conditions.[12,21]

### Visual Acuity

Visual acuity is more than just the ability to read a line on the letter chart. It represents a complex interaction between the optical system, which focuses light on the retina, and the CNS processing, which transforms that light into the visual images seen.

The first stage of CNS processing begins at the retina, where photoreceptors respond to discrete visual stimuli in the environment and activate only when that stimulus occurs. It is estimated that the retinal field contains almost 1 million discretely coded photoreceptors sending detailed information on the spatial components of objects to the CNS for visual processing. This neural specificity enables the CNS to detect minute differences between patterns. Thus, for example, a person is able to tell a "b" from a "d" and a tangerine from an orange.[6]

In order for the retina to resolve spatial information, visual images must be focused precisely. A defect in the optical system can cause the images to be poorly focused on the retina.[6] The optical system consists of the cornea, lens, and optic media.

The four most common optical defects reducing acuity are myopia (nearsightedness), hyperopia (farsightedness), presbyopia (farsightedness associated with aging), and astigmatism. In **myopia** the image of an object is focused at a point in front of the retina and is blurred when it reaches the retina. Myopia is corrected by placing a concave lens in front of the eye. In **hyperopia** the image comes into focus behind the retina, causing the image to remain out of focus on the retina.[6] **Presbyopia** is caused by reduced elasticity of the lens of the eye. Hyperopia and presbyopia are corrected by placing a convex lens in front of the eye.

In **astigmatism,** light cannot be focused clearly because the cornea is not totally spherical (more spoon shaped). It results in a blurring of the image and is corrected by placing a cylindrical lens in front of the eye.[6]

**Cataracts** are a clouding of the lens. Cataracts and corneal opacities, cloudy media, and other conditions can also reduce the quality of the image projected onto the retina.

**Glaucoma** is caused by increased pressure within the eye, pinching the optic nerve. Poor peripheral or side vision results.

The health and integrity of the retina also influence the image quality sent on to the CNS. The **macular area** of the retina is particularly critical for identification of visual detail. Unfortunately, this structure is also vulnerable to several diseases that destroy its function, including age-related diseases (e.g., macular degeneration) and systemic diseases (e.g., diabetic retinopathy, hypertension).

Damage to the macular area of the retina does not result in blindness but causes poor central vision and significantly reduces the patient's ability to distinguish visual details such as variations in colors, pattern frequency, and contrast.[10] Accurate identification of patterns and objects becomes difficult because the CNS does not receive sufficient information to identify salient features. For example, human faces contain little differentiation in contrast between the facial features; that is, the nose is the same color as the forehead, cheeks, and chin, and eye and hair color are designed to blend with skin tones. Because of the reduced contrast between facial features, patients with macular loss almost universally have difficulty identifying faces of even close friends and family members. They must rely on other characteristics of the person, such as height, weight, hair color, clothing preferences, and voice, to make identification. Approximately one in four persons over age 80 years has a visual impairment affecting the retina that is so significant that the individual is unable to read standard print.[10] This is an important statistic because many older patients experiencing cerebrovascular accident (CVA) or other neurological insults may also have a retinal pathology that adds to their other impairments.

### *Treatment Strategies*

Myopia, hyperopia, presbyopia, cataracts, and other refractive errors can generally be corrected with the use of lenses or surgery. Glaucoma is treated with medication. A vision specialist such as an ophthalmologist or an optometrist can correct these deficiencies.

Reduced ability to see contrast or color and the loss of central or peripheral vision cannot be resolved by prescribing a pair of lenses. Instead, the environment must be adapted and the patient taught compensatory strategies. Three factors can be manipulated to make the environment more "user friendly" to the patient with reduced acuity: background contrast, illumination, and background pattern.[9]

Increasing *background contrast* is as simple as using a black cup for milk and a white cup for coffee. The key to using contrast effectively is first to identify the critical items needed for orientation or identification in the environment and then to increase their contrast with surrounding features. For example, if the patient has difficulty walking down stairs because of the reduced contrast between the risers, a line of bright fluorescent tape or paint can be applied to the end of each step to distinguish between them. A carrot on a white cutting board is easier to see and safer to chop up than one placed on a wood cutting board.

Increasing the intensity of available light for better *illumination* enables objects and environmental features to be seen more readily and reduces the need for high contrast between objects. For example, facial features can be more easily identified if the person's face is fully illuminated. The challenge in providing light is to increase illumination without increasing glare. Halogen and fluorescent lighting provide the best sources of high illumination with minimal glare and are recommended over standard incandescent lighting for both room and reading illumination.

In addition to reducing glare, it is also important to minimize shadows. The use of single bulb or recessed "can" lighting in hallways and rooms should be avoided; instead, long panels of fluorescent lights should be used. When fluorescent lighting cannot be used, 300- to 500-watt torchiere halogen lamps provide excellent illumination with minimal shadow. These lamps are relatively inexpensive and can be strategically placed in each room to provide the broadest amount of illumination. For reading, 50-watt halogen desk lamps provide the best illumination. Halogen bulbs generate intense heat and must be firmly anchored (so that they will not fall over) and not placed near flammable materials such as curtains.

*Patterned backgrounds* have the effect of camouflaging objects lying on them; a person who has searched for a sewing needle dropped on a patterned rug can attest to this fact. Solid colors should be used for background surfaces such as bedspreads, place mats, dishes, counter tops, rugs, towels, and furniture coverings.

Clutter in an environment causes the same problems as a pattern. A patient who has difficulty identifying objects will perform better when asked to scan a kitchen shelf with a few orderly items than one with dozens of items. The same is true of closets, drawers, sewing baskets, desks, bookshelves, counter tops, and clinic areas.

## Visual Fields

**Homonymous hemianopsia** (or hemanopia), the loss of visual field in the corresponding right or left half in each eye, is the most common visual impairment observed after a CVA.[37] Although often considered to be a mild impairment compared with the dramatic loss of limb use, a visual field deficit can limit the patient's ability to adapt to the environment and remain independent.

Patients with visual field deficits experience changes in several areas of performance that affect their ability to complete ADLs accurately and safely. The most significant change occurs in the area of **scanning** to compensate for the blind portion of the visual field. Instead of spontaneously adopting a wider scanning strategy, turning the head farther to see around the blind field, patients tend to narrow their scope of scanning.[36] They adopt a more protective strategy, turning their heads very little, limiting their scanning to areas immediately adjacent to the body, and concentrating more on sensory input from the tactile, proprioceptive, and vestibular senses. This may seem like an odd strategy to adopt after a vision loss but occurs because the brain fills in (perceptually completes) any portion of the visual field that is missing, thus providing the viewer with the illusion of seeing a complete visual scene.[27] The person experiencing visual field loss is not immediately aware of the absence of vision and experiences it only through interaction with the environment.[18] The person may run into walls or other obstacles when navigating in the environment or may not be able to find items placed within the blind field.

Patients with field loss do not notice a boundary between the seeing and nonseeing field. Instead, they (incorrectly) perceive a complete visual scene in which objects always seem to be appearing, disappearing, and reappearing without warning. Uncertainty regarding the accuracy of visual input on the affected side causes the person to adopt a protective strategy that is more midline and body centered.[22] This midline fixation creates problems in activities such as driving a car and moving about in a busy environment, which require scanning and awareness of a wider environment.

If the central and particularly the macular portion of the visual field is affected, the patient tends to miss or misidentify detail when viewing objects. Reading presents the greatest challenge and frustration for the patient in this regard.[37] For example, a patient with a left visual field deficit may read the number "8" as a "3" or the word "radish" may be seen as "dish." Words can often be guessed from context. Inaccurate reading of numbers is the more functionally limiting problem because numbers appear without context. The person is often unaware of a mistake in reading a number until presenting a store clerk with $30 for an item that costs $80. Patients experiencing these types of errors quickly lose confidence in their ability to pay bills and manage their checkbook and turn over these important ADLs to someone else.

Depending on the size of the visual field loss and the side on which the loss occurs, the patient may experience difficulty guiding the hand in writing and other near-vision tasks such as cutting. The top envelope in Figure 24-2 illustrates the handwriting of a patient with right visual field loss. In attempting to address the envelope, the patient would lose sight of the hand in the hemianopic field on the right side and subsequently begin to drift downward on that side. The bottom envelope in Figure 24-2 illustrates the patient's performance after training.

Evaluation of visual field integrity is performed by the OTR or other qualified professional.[33] In observing the patient, the COTA may note signs of the presence of a visual field deficit, including (1) changing head position when asked to view objects placed in a certain plane, (2) consistently bumping into objects on one side, (3) misplacing objects in one field, and (4) making consistent errors in reading.

### Treatment Strategies

In providing treatment for patients with visual field deficits, a combination of strategies is used. Remedial strategies focus on increasing the speed and scope of the scanning pattern. The patient must learn to turn the head to compensate for the limitation in field and to do so as quickly as possible. Activities may include ball games in which balls are passed quickly from player to player and balloon batting.

Visual field deficits affect three specific activities: driving, reading, and writing. Driving is a complex skill that involves the interaction of physical, cognitive, emotional, and visual abilities.[30] A patient's ability to resume driving safely requires a specialized evaluation completed by qualified personnel. Patients with field deficits experience difficulty primarily in three aspects of driving: (1) changing lanes, (2) merging on and off roadways, and (3) monitoring traffic in multilane situations. The extent to which the patient has difficulty with these maneuvers depends on the size of the field deficit and the patient's awareness of and ability to compensate for the deficit. Speed and scope of scanning are required for compensation. Training focuses on increasing scanning speed and scope and teaching the patient specific strategies to handle the three traffic situations.

The patient's primary complaints in reading center on difficulty locating and maintaining the correct line of print and accurately identifying words and numbers.[37] Patients with left visual field deficit experience difficulty returning to the left-hand margin of the reading material to begin a new line of text. Drawing a bold red line down the side of the left-hand margin provides the patient with an "anchor" to find the left margin.[34] The same technique used on the right-hand margin assists patients with right visual field loss, who are often uncertain whether they have reached the end of a line of print.

If the patient has difficulty staying on line or moving down to the correct line, a ruler or card can be held under the line of print to keep the patient's place. These techniques can be employed when the patient is required to read a bill or financial statement or a recipe or instructions during cooking.

Difficulty staying on line when writing is addressed by teaching the patient to monitor the pen tip and maintain visual fixation as the hand moves across the page and into the blind side. Activities that require the patient to trace lines toward the side of the field loss are effective in reestablishing the eye-hand lock. Devices that offer feedback such as a talking pen* also work well to train the patient to monitor the pen tip during handwriting.

*Wayne Engineering, Northfield, Ill.

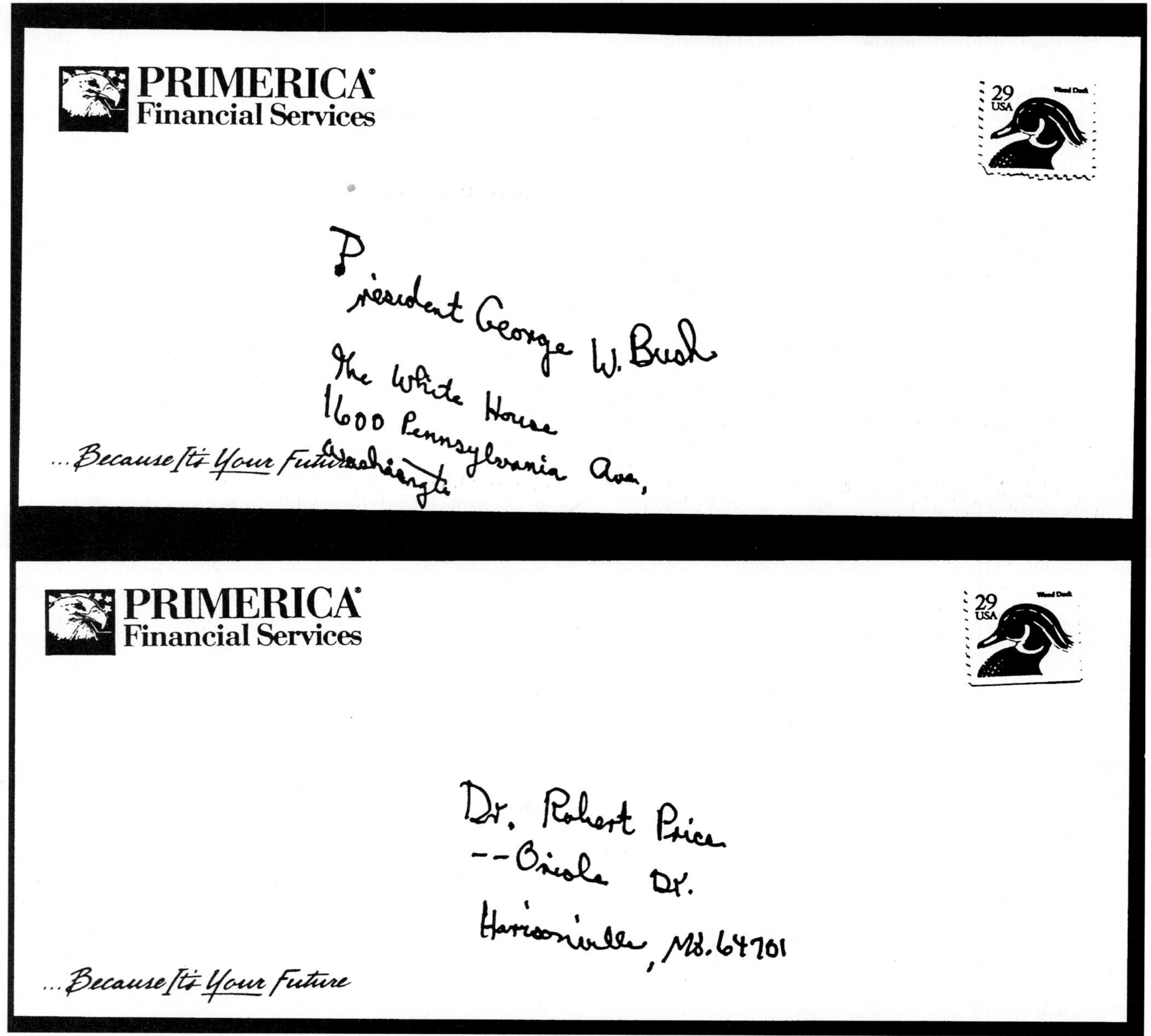


*Figure 24-2* Handwriting completed by a patient with right-sided hemianopsia (hemanopia). Upper drawing depicts typical slant as pen moves into hemianopic field. Lower drawing shows improvement after training. (From Warren M: Visuospatial skills: assessment and intervention strategies. In Royeen CB, editor: *AOTA self-study series: cognitive rehabilitation,* Rockville, Md, 1994, American Occupational Therapy Association.)

Reading and writing and ADL performance can be enhanced by modifying the patient's visual environment. Adding color and contrast to the key structures in the environment needed for orientation (door frames, furniture, etc.) assist the patient in locating these structures. Contrast in writing materials can be heightened by using black felt-tip pens and boldly lined paper to help the patient in monitoring handwriting. The simple addition of more light often increases reading speed and reduces errors. Reduction of pattern in the environment by eliminating clutter and using solid-colored objects enhance the patient's ability to locate items.

## DEFICITS IN CENTRAL NERVOUS SYSTEM VISUAL SKILLS

### Visual Attention and Scanning

Visual attention can be divided into two categories: (1) focal or selective visual attention and (2) ambient or peripheral visual attention.[16] *Focal or selective attention* is used for object recognition and identification and enables persons to distinguish visual details accurately, such as differences between letters and numbers. It contributes greatly to academic achievement. *Ambient or peripheral attention* is used to detect and locate items in the environment. It relies on input from the peripheral visual field. To have a fully operational and efficient visual system, the two modes of visual attention must work together.

Research has shown that in normal adults, scanning is consistently completed in an organized, systematic, and efficient pattern.[5,11,23,31] The type of scanning pattern used depends on the demands of the task. In reading, a left-to-right and top-to-bottom rectilinear strategy is used. In scanning an open array (e.g., a room), a circular, left-to-right strategy is generally employed, with the eye following either a clockwise or a counterclockwise pattern.

Studies have shown that disruption in the normal scanning strategy can occur after brain injury. The characteristics of the disruption vary depending on which hemisphere was damaged. Visual scanning deficits associated with right-sided brain injury are characterized by an avoidance in shifting the eye toward the left half of the visual space.[4,8,14] This creates an asymmetrical scanning pattern. Instead of starting the scanning pattern on the left side of a visual array, where most adults do, individuals with right-sided brain injuries tend to begin on the right side of the array and stay on the right side. The person misses both detail and configuration in viewing objects on the left side and may fail to note some visual information needed to make accurate identification and decisions.

The visual inattention associated with right-sided brain injuries is often referred to as *visual neglect, unilateral spatial neglect,* or *hemi-inattention.*[11] Although neglect is often used to describe inattention to visual space occurring after left or right hemisphere lesions, research indicates that the condition only occurs with right-sided brain injuries.[14,28] The condition of neglect is often confused with the presence of a visual field deficit in the patient. Although both conditions may cause the patient to miss visual information on one side, they are distinctly different conditions and do not have the same effect on the patient's performance. When a visual field deficit occurs, the patient attempts to compensate for the loss by engaging visual attention.[15] The patient directs eye movements toward the side of the vision loss in an attempt to gather visual information from that side. Because of the field deficit, however, the patient may not move the eye far enough to see the needed visual information and thus misses visual input on that side. This may create a false impression of hemi-inattention or neglect.

In contrast, the patient with true hemi-inattention or neglect has lost the attentional CNS mechanisms that drive the search for visual information. The inattentive patient makes no attempt to search for information on the left side of the visual space; no eye movements or head turning are observed toward the left side.[15]

The greatest challenge to the clinical staff is when the two conditions occur together in the patient. In this case the patient is missing visual information on the left side because of the field deficit and has no means to compensate for it by directing attention toward the left side. The presence of a visual field deficit exaggerates the inattentive behavior observed in the patient with neglect.[13,35]

### Pattern Recognition

When a patient does not thoroughly and efficiently scan objects, the result is decreased pattern recognition. Patients with right-sided brain injury may not tune into the presence of objects and may fail to recognize an object or pattern because they do not notice or "see" it. Patients with left-sided brain injuries may be aware of objects but have difficulty with identification.[7,26] For example, these patients may realize that they are seeing a letter but may not be able to distinguish that letter from the one next to it.

### Visual Memory

Visual memory depends on accurate pattern recognition. When a critical aspect of an object is overlooked, the result is an inaccurate representation in the brain. If the representation is not accurate, the CNS may not recognize it or may misidentify it. When this occurs, the CNS has difficulty establishing a visual memory of the object. For example, a patient with a dense left-central visual field deficit often misses the first letters of words and thus may read a word such as "delicious" as "licious." Whereas "delicious" elicits pleasant associations, the word "licious" has no counterpart in memory and so is discarded by the CNS as a nonsense word and not stored in memory.

Fortunately from a treatment standpoint, persons do not store information or learn everything exclusively through the visual channel. The models stored in memory can be retrieved through more than one sensory channel. For example, if I want you to go into the kitchen to get a cup for me, I can tell you to get me a "cup" (verbal); I can show you a cup and ask you to get me one like it (visual); or I could put a cup in a bag, ask you to feel its features, and get me one like it (physical). Any one of these three methods would be successful.

In real-life daily situations, information about objects is available through several sensory channels. If a person does not recognize an object by looking at it, the person can pick it up and feel it or can ask someone to explain what it is. Because of this, a patient with a visual deficit that results in inaccurate pattern recognition can still function reasonably well in ADLs in which a variety of sensory information is available. However, as discussed earlier, three daily living skills rely almost exclusively on vision for completion: reading, writing, and driving. Without accurate visual input, these skills cannot be performed, and thus the patient may experience limitations in activities that require these skills, such as shopping, completing a check or a form, cooking with recipes, or administering medications.

### Visual Cognition

Visual cognition is the end product of the integration of foundation skills, visual attention, visual scanning, pattern recognition, and memory. Any deficit in these lower level skills diminishes the person's ability to apply these skills cognitively to adapt.

Deficits in visual cognition result in difficulties in identifying the spatial properties of objects and mentally manipulating these properties in thought. Many terms are used to describe the deficits that occur in visual cognition, such as spatial agnosia; alexia; and disorders of spatial analysis, visual closure, and figure-ground perception. These terms, however, do little more than label the deficit; they do not explain why it has occurred. To treat a deficit, it is necessary to identify what is causing it.

Patients with brain injuries demonstrate changes in three areas of selective attention: (1) an inability to attend to the critical features and variables among objects, (2) a tendency to restrict scanning to objects on the ipsilateral (sound) side, and (3) an inability to superimpose a structure in scanning and unstructured array.[23,25] These changes cause the patient to commit errors in viewing and manipulating complex visual input. For example, when trying to find a specific puzzle piece in a difficult 500-piece puzzle, a person looks for certain salient features, such as a certain color or shape. The person also must superimpose some sort of organizational structure on the task, such as putting together the border first. Deficits in the ability to attend selectively to such aspects significantly affect the ability to complete the puzzle.

Evaluation of visual perceptual deficits is performed by the OTR.[33]

### Treatment Strategies

Treatment of CNS visual perceptual skills must ensure that the patient learns to take in visual information in a consistent, systematic, and organized manner. Treatment approaches are designed by the OTR, who may direct the COTA to carry out certain aspects. The following information may assist the COTA in understanding the context and reasons for specific treatment methods.

Patients with inattention caused by right-sided brain injuries are taught to reorganize their scanning pattern by beginning scanning in the impaired space (or left side) first.[34] Two scanning strategies are taught: a left-to-right rectilinear pattern for reading and a left-to-right circular pattern for scanning an unstructured array. The COTA can use activities such as solitaire, double solitaire, dominoes, and checkers to help establish the correct scanning strategy.

Patients with left-sided brain injuries are given activities that emphasize conscious attention to detail and careful inspection and comparison of objects. These include any type of matching or sorting activity, such as form boards and puzzles and such games as dominoes.

To help the patient orient to a broad visual space, as is needed in many ADLs, the scanning activities should also require the patient to scan as broad a visual space as possible. The working field should be large enough to require the patient either to turn the head or to change body positions to accomplish the task. Many activities and games can be enlarged to require head turning for scanning. For example, form boards can be enlarged to $3 \times 2$ feet or a tic-tac-toe game can be expanded.

Any therapeutic activity chosen to reestablish an organized scanning pattern will be more effective if the patient is required to manipulate physically the objects scanned. Research has shown that a stronger mental representation of a visual image is formed if what is seen is verified by tactile exploration.[2] Whenever possible the treatment should be designed to be interactive. Games such as solitaire or dominoes, ball games, or activities such as putting together large puzzles are examples of treatment activities with interactive qualities.

To improve selective attention, patients may be taught to study objects consciously, emphasizing those placed in the impaired space. Matching activities that require discrimination of subtle details are especially effective. Many games have these qualities, such as solitaire, double solitaire, Concentration, Connect Four, checkers, Scrabble, and dominoes. Large 300- to 500-piece puzzles, word or number search workbooks, crossword puzzles, and needlecrafts such as latch-hooking also require these skills. Throughout their performance of these tasks, patients should be encouraged to double-check their work to make sure that critical details are not missed. Success in regaining selective attention depends on the patient's ability to learn and employ a conscious strategy to compensate for the deficits created by inattention.

According to Toglia,[29] patients with brain injury may overestimate their abilities, believing these are unaffected by the injury. Without a true understanding of their limitations, patients will not see the purpose of compensatory strategies. To increase insight, Abreu and Toglia[1] advocate teaching a patient how to monitor and control performance by learning to recognize and correct for errors in performance. The clinician gives the patient immediate feedback about performance and points out deficiencies. The patient is taught self-monitoring techniques such as *activity prediction,* in which the patient predicts how successfully an activity will be performed and identifies aspects of the activity where errors are likely to occur. The patient then compares actual performance with predicted performance. Use of this technique helps the patient become aware and anticipate how the deficit will affect functional capabilities.

A final treatment guideline is to practice the skill within context to ensure carry-over of application to ADLs. Research has shown that brain-injured patients generally do not spontaneously transfer skills from one learning situation to the next. The OT practitioner should have the patient apply the learned strategy to different ADL contexts. For example, the patient can be required to use the strategy of initiating the scanning pattern in the impaired space when selecting clothes from a closet, searching for items in a refrigerator or on a shelf, shopping for groceries, reading, and driving. Repetition under varied circumstances assists in generalizing the skill and transferring it to new situations. No substitute exists in therapy for the practice of real-life situations in helping the patient develop insight into abilities and compensation for limitations. This may require some creative scheduling to take the patient out of the clinic. Cafeterias, gift shops, and office areas within the facility and streets, fast-food restaurants, and shops near the facility can be used to expose the patient to more realistic and demanding visual environments. Independent-living apartments, simulated work areas, and kitchens within the clinic should also be used regularly in treatment.

## VISION LOSS: COMPENSATORY TECHNIQUES FOR ACTIVITIES OF DAILY LIVING*

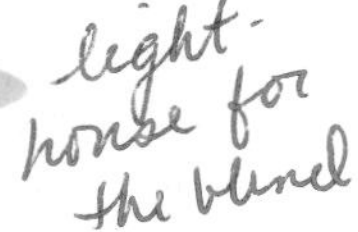


Performing ADLs may be an overwhelming task for the person with a new vision loss. Patients should be encouraged to use the remaining senses (hearing, taste, touch, smell) to gather and filter information. The OTR or COTA must teach safety techniques first, break each activity into small parts, and organize all materials before beginning each activity.

### Eating

The newly impaired individual is concerned about whether eating behaviors will be socially acceptable. Lack of confidence may lead the person to avoid social situations that involve eating and to restrict feeding to foods that can be finger-fed.

#### *General Suggestions*

The person should be taught to do the following:

1. Establish a point of reference with an object at the table, such as a dinner plate. From this object, the placement of other objects can be determined.
2. Always maintain contact with the table.
3. Bend forward while eating so that any food falling from the fork will land on the plate.
4. Estimate the weight, temperature, and texture of the food from the way it feels on the fork or spoon.
5. Use a "pusher" (e.g., piece of bread or roll) to stabilize food that will be picked up by the fork.
6. When necessary, be assertive and ask what is on the plate and where food on the plate is located. Ask to have meat cut and liquids poured as needed.

#### *Exploring Contents of a Plate*

1. Hold fork with the tines turned downward.
2. Insert fork into food starting with the 12-o'clock position and working around the plate clockwise.
3. Identify food by texture and smell.
4. If meat is on the plate, turn the meat to the 6-o'clock position, where cutting will be easier.

#### *Cutting Food With a Knife and Fork*

1. Locate knife and turn cutting edge downward toward the table. Hold knife in the right hand.
2. Hold knife in the right hand with index finger firmly along the handle and thumb by the side of the handle.
3. Hold fork in the left hand with the tines turned downward to the table and the index finger along the top surface of the handle.
4. Use knife to locate food to be cut (preferably placed at the 6-o'clock position).
5. Place fork about 1 inch (2.5 cm) from the outer edge of the food to be cut, and cut bite-sized pieces by placing knife against the back of fork's tines and sawing back and forth firmly and slowly.

### Simple Food Preparation

A large tray should be used to prepare foods. This keeps all items together, minimizes the area to be cleaned up, and makes it easy to carry items to the sink.

#### *Pouring Cold Liquids*

1. Use a tall glass and center the container of liquid over the glass.
2. Before pouring, place the glass in the sink or a bowl to catch spills.
3. To estimate the level of the liquid as the glass fills, place the index finger (up to the first joint) over the lip of the glass.
4. Note changes in weight, temperature, and sound as glass is being filled.

#### *Opening a Container of Milk*

1. Locate the seam of the milk carton. The side that should be opened is directly opposite this seam.
2. Alternately, locate the two indented lines on the top of the milk carton. These lines indicate that this is the side to be opened.

#### *Buttering a Piece of Bread*

1. Soften a stick of butter or margarine by taking it out of the refrigerator for a few minutes to make it easier to spread.
2. Use a knife warmed in hot water to make the butter spread easier.
3. Use fingers or the feel of the knife's weight to determine the amount of butter on the knife.

*Information in this section is modified from Powell S: *A handbook for the homemaker–home health aide working with adults who are visually impaired or hearing impaired,* New York, 1982, LaGuardia Community College.

4. Place butter either in the palm of the hand or on a plate. Spread the butter from the top right-hand corner to the lower right-hand corner. Then turn the bread 90° counterclockwise and repeat the procedure.

#### *Making a Sandwich*

1. Apply sandwich spreads in same manner as for butter.
2. Use presliced cold cuts.
3. Cut a sandwich safely by first placing the thumb and index finger on either side of the bread so that an arch is formed. Then place the knife under the fingers in the center of the arch and cut the bread.

### Mobility and Safe Travel

In a large city, it is not unusual to encounter someone with vision loss crossing the street. How do these persons know when it is safe to cross? How do they remember where they are and how to reach their destination? Most visually impaired persons receive training in techniques of orientation and mobility (O&M). This is a specialized regimen, and COTAs who are interested might pursue training in these techniques. However all OT practitioners should understand the basics of **hand trailing** and **sighted guiding,** techniques that can be used with the patient in the home and when traveling together outdoors.

#### *Hand Trailing*

This technique uses the hands to trail along a smooth, stationery object in a straight line, such as a wall or table edge.

1. Use the arm closest to the smooth trailing surface.
2. Patient should hold the arm straight but not rigid, extending down in a diagonal.
3. The hand should lightly touch the trailing surface.

#### *Sighted Guiding*

The following is the recommended technique for guiding a vision-impaired person when traveling together in the community.

1. Patient grasps guide's arm lightly but firmly above the elbow, with thumb outside and fingers wrapped to inside of arm.
2. Guide holds arm relaxed, with elbow bent.
3. Patient stands at side of guide. Guide walks in front with patient following a half step behind to ensure safety.
4. Always allow visually impaired patient to take your arm. Never push or shove patient ahead of you. Try and set a comfortable pace. If patient's grip tightens or if patient pulls back, slow down.

### Protective Techniques for Safe Mobility

These techniques are used to warn the visually impaired person of unexpected and potentially harmful objects in the environment. They are used most often in unfamiliar areas or areas that may have been changed because of activities of other people (e.g., repositioning of furniture). The two techniques given may be used separately or together.

#### *Upper Body Protection (Upper Chest, Head)*

For upper body protection the vision-impaired person is instructed to do the following:

1. Bend forearm across the chest and touch the opposite shoulder.
2. Move hand forward so that it is about 12 inches (30 cm) from the shoulder, with the palm facing outward and the fingers held loosely.

#### *Lower Body Protection*

For lower body protection the vision-impaired person is instructed to do the following:

1. Extend one arm forward and downward, placing it about 12 inches (30 cm) in front of the opposite thigh.
2. Turn palm to face the body, with fingers pointing toward the feet.

### Telling Time

Low-vision aids such as magnifying glasses and telescopes may be used. Special timepieces with Braille or large print are also available, but practice may be needed to use these well. Adapted large **punt watches** and **punt clocks,** which have large numbers with contrasting background colors, and talking watches and clocks can be obtained from the American Foundation for the Blind.

### Money Identification

The ability to manage money independently is very important. The OTR or COTA may use the following suggestions.

#### *Bills*

Dollar bills cannot be identified without assistance. The person must be told the denominations and then can use a system of folding, as follows:

1. Singles should remain flat in the wallet.
2. Fives can be folded in half horizontally.
3. Tens can be folded in half vertically.
4. Twenties can be folded in half twice.

#### *Coins*

Coins can be identified through stereognosis, as follows:

1. Quarters are large with rough edges.
2. Dimes are small and thin with rough edges.
3. Nickels are thicker and wider than dimes and have smooth edges.
4. Pennies are smaller and thinner than nickels and have smooth edges.

### Clothing Identification

Various methods may be used to mark clothing to assist in color matching, such as the following:

1. Safety pins (e.g., one for red, two for green) may be attached to the label. Alternatively, French knots or iron-on patches may be used. Braille labels from the American Foundation for the Blind are also available.
2. Texture or identifying marks (e.g., fasteners, trimmings) may be used to identify certain garments.
3. A strip of sandpaper may be attached in front of the heel of the shoe to identify the color.

## SUMMARY

Many different structures in the eye and the brain are responsible for the processing of visual information. Whether or not a deficit in visual perceptual processing will require therapy intervention depends on the patient's lifestyle and whether the visual deficit prevents successful completion of ADLs.

The framework for evaluation and treatment rests on the concept of a hierarchy of visual perceptual skill levels that interact with and subserve one another. Because of the unity of the hierarchy, a skill function cannot be disrupted at one level without an adverse effect on all perceptual processing. Treatment focuses on increasing the accuracy and organization of the sensory input into the system by manipulating the environment and providing the patient with strategies to compensate for or minimize the effect of the deficit in ADLs.

The COTA may teach compensatory techniques to persons with vision loss to enable ADL performance.

## *Selected Reading Guide Questions*

1. Compare and contrast the roles of the OTR and the COTA in the treatment of patients with deficits in performance components.
2. Contrast remedial and compensatory treatment.
3. Give four examples of compensatory strategies used to prevent injury in the patient with sensory loss from a central nervous system (CNS) lesion.
4. Describe some remedial treatments used for patients with sensory loss.
5. List some safety precautions used for patients with sensory loss in the hand.
6. Describe some of the activities used to remediate astereognosis.
7. Give examples of activities and strategies used for the patient with unilateral neglect.
8. List some activities used to treat patients with body scheme disorders.
9. Describe in detail how you would teach a patient with ideational and ideomotor apraxia to comb the hair.
10. List some activities used to treat the patient with constructional apraxia.
11. Describe how you would lay out clothing for a patient with dressing apraxia.
12. Explain what is meant by "providing structure" for the patient with cognitive deficits.
13. Describe the role of environmental cues in the treatment of patients with cognitive deficits, and give two examples of such cues.
14. List some activities and strategies used for patients with problems in orientation.
15. Contrast vision and visual perception.
16. Describe what happens to the eye that lacks oculomotor control, and describe what happens to vision as a consequence.
17. List three environmental factors that can be changed to help the patient with a deficit in visual acuity.
18. Describe the typical strategy of a patient with a visual field loss, and explain what you would direct the patient to do instead.
19. Contrast the effects of a visual field loss with the effects of true hemi-inattention.
20. Name the three areas of selective attention that typically are changed in the patient with brain injury.
21. Describe the scanning pattern used to train patients with right-sided brain injuries to compensate for inattention.
22. Describe compensatory strategies for the patient with visual loss in the areas of eating, food preparation, mobility, telling time, and identifying money and clothing.

## *REFERENCES*

**Section I**

1. Barber LM: Desensitization of the traumatized hand. In Hunter JM, Mackin EJ, Callahan AD, editors: *Rehabilitation of the hand,* ed 4, St Louis, 1995, Mosby.
2. Callahan AD: Methods of compensation and reeducation for sensory dysfunction. In Hunter JM, Mackin EJ, Callahan AD, editors: *Rehabilitation of the hand,* ed 4, St Louis, 1995, Mosby.
3. Chusid JG: *Correlative neuroanatomy and functional neurology,* ed 19, Los Altos, Calif, 1985, Lange.
4. Dellon AL: *Evaluation of sensibility and re-education of sensation in the hand,* Baltimore, 1981, Williams & Wilkins.
5. Eggers O: *Occupational therapy in the treatment of adult hemiplegia,* Rockville, Md, 1984, Aspen.
6. La Croix E, Helman J: Upper extremity orthopedics. In Logigian MK, editor: *Adult rehabilitation: a team approach for therapists,* Boston, 1982, Little, Brown.
7. Ruskin A: Understanding stroke and its treatment. In Ruskin A, editor: *Current therapy in physiatry,* Philadelphia, 1984, Saunders.
8. Schutt AH, Opitz JL: Hand rehabilitation. In Goodgold J: *Rehabilitation medicine,* St Louis, 1988, Mosby.
9. Turner A: *The practice of occupational therapy,* ed 2, New York, 1987, Churchill Livingstone.
10. Wynn Parry CB: *Rehabilitation of the hand,* London, 1981, Butterworth.

**Section II**

1. Ayres AJ: *Sensory integration and learning disorders,* Los Angeles, 1972, Western Psychological Services.

2. Baum B, Hall K: Relationship between constructional praxis and dressing in the head injured adult, *Am J Occup Ther* 35:438, 1981.
3. Eggers O: *Occupational therapy in the treatment of adult hemiplegia,* Rockville, Md, 1984, Aspen.
4. Fall CC: Comparing ways of measuring constructional praxis in the well elderly, *Am J Occup Ther* 41:500, 1987.
5. Farber SD: *Neurorehabilitation: a multisensory approach,* Philadelphia, 1982, Saunders.
6. Ferreri JA: Intensive stereognostic training, *Am J Occup Ther* 16:141, 1962.
7. Hécaen H, Albert ML: *Human neuropsychology,* New York, 1978, Wiley and Sons.
8. Miller N: *Dyspraxia and its management,* Rockville, Md, 1986, Aspen.
9. Neistadt ME: Normal adult performance on constructional praxis training tasks, *Am J Occup Ther* 43:448, 1989.
10. Neistadt ME: A critical analysis of occupational therapy approaches for perceptual deficits in adults with brain injury, *Am J Occup Ther* 44:299, 1990.
11. Vinograd A, Taylor E, Grossman S: Sensory retraining of the hemiplegic hand, *Am J Occup Ther* 16:246, 1962.
12. Zoltan B: Remediation of visual, perceptual and perceptual motor deficits. In Rosenthal M, editor: *Rehabilitation of the adult and child with traumatic brain injury,* ed 2, Philadelphia, 1989, Davis.
13. Zoltan B, Siev E, Freishtat B: *Perceptual and cognitive dysfunction in the adult stroke patient,* ed 2, Thorofare, NJ, 1986, Slack.
14. Zoltan B et al: *Perceptual motor evaluation for head injured and other neurologically impaired adults,* rev ed, San Jose, Calif, 1987, Santa Clara Valley Medical Center.

**Section III**

1. Abreu BC, Hinojosa J: The process approach for cognitive perceptual and postural control dysfunction for adults with brain injuries. In Katz N: *Cognitive rehabilitation: models for intervention in occupational therapy,* Boston, 1992, Andover.
2. Abreu BC, Toglia JP: Cognitive rehabilitation: an occupational therapy model, *Am J Occup Ther* 41:439, 1987.
3. Allen CK: Cognitive disabilities. In Katz N: *Cognitive rehabilitation: models for intervention in occupational therapy,* Boston, 1992, Andover.
4. Allen CK, Earhart CA, Blue T: *Occupational therapy treatment goals for the physically and cognitively disabled,* Rockville, Md, 1992, American Occupational Therapy Association.
5. Arenberg D, Robertson-Tchabo E: Learning and aging. In Birren J, Schaie K, editors: *Handbook of the psychology of aging,* New York, 1977, Van Nostrand Reinhold.
6. Ayres AJ: *Sensory integration and learning disorders,* Los Angeles, 1980, Western Psychological Services.
7. Ball K, Sekuler R: Improving visual perception in older observers, *J Gerontol* 41:176, 1986.
8. Ben-Yishay Y, Piasetsky EB, Rattock J: A systematic method for ameliorating disorders in basic attention. In Meier MJ, Benton AL, Diller L, editors: *Neuropsychological rehabilitation,* New York, 1980, Guilford.
9. Beyer BK: *Practical strategies for the teaching of thinking,* Boston, 1987, Allyn & Bacon.
10. Craine JF, Gudeman HE: *The rehabilitation of brain functions: principles, procedures and techniques of neurotraining,* Springfield, Ill, 1981, Thomas.
11. DLM Teaching Resources: *Apple computer resources in special education and rehabilitation,* Allen, Tex, 1988, DLM.
12. Doughtery PM, Radomski MV: *The cognitive rehabilitation workbook,* Rockville, Md, 1987, Aspen.
13. Giles GM: A neurofunctional approach to rehabilitation following severe brain injury. In Katz N: *Cognitive rehabilitation: models for intervention in occupational therapy,* Boston, 1992, Andover.
14. Harrell M et al: *Cognitive rehabilitation of memory: a practical guide,* Gaithersburg, Md, 1992, Aspen.
15. IBM National Support Center for Persons with Disabilities, Atlanta, Ga.
16. Levin W: Computer applications in cognitive rehabilitation. In Kreutzer JS, Wehman PH: *Cognitive rehabilitation for persons with traumatic brain injury,* Baltimore, 1991, Brookes.
17. Lezak MD: *Neuropsychological assessment,* New York, 1983, Oxford University Press.
18. Lundgren CC, Persechino EL: Cognitive group: a treatment program for head injured adults, *Am J Occup Ther* 40:397, 1986.
19. Lynch WJ: Ecological validity of cognitive rehabilitation software, *J Head Trauma Rehabil* 7:36, 1992.
20. Matthews CG, Harley JP, Malec JF: Guidelines for computer-assisted neuropsychological rehabilitation and cognitive remediation, *Clin Neuropsychol* 5:3, 1991.
21. Neistadt ME: Occupational therapy for adults with perceptual deficits, *Am J Occup Ther* 42:434, 1988.
22. Neistadt ME: A critical analysis of occupational therapy approaches for perceptual deficits in adults with brain injury, *Am J Occup Ther* 44:299, 1990.
23. Parente R, Anderson-Parente J: *Retraining memory: techniques and applications,* Houston, 1991, CSY.
24. Parente R, Stapleton M: An empowerment model of memory training, *Appl Cogn Psychol* 7:585, 1993.
25. Parente R, Stapleton MC, Wheatley CJ: Practical strategies for vocational reentry after traumatic brain injury, *J Head Trauma Rehabil* 6:35, 1991.
26. Riege WH et al: Decision speed and bias after unilateral stroke, *Cortex* 18:345, 1982.
27. Schacter DL, Glisky EL: Memory remediation: restoration, alleviation, and the acquisition of domain-specific knowledge. In Uzzell BP, Gross Y, editors: *Clinical neuropsychology of intervention,* Boston, 1986, Martinus Nijihoff.
28. Sohlberg MM, Mateer CA: *Attention process training,* Puyallup, Wash, 1986, Association for Neuropsychological Research and Development.
29. Toglia JP: Visual perception of objects: an approach to assessment and treatment, *Am J Occup Ther* 43:587, 1989.
30. Toglia JP: Generalization of treatment: a multicontext approach to cognitive perceptual impairment in adults with brain injury, *Am J Occup Ther* 45:505, 1991.
31. Toglia JP: A dynamic interactional approach to cognitive rehabilitation. In Katz N: *Cognitive rehabilitation: models for intervention in occupational therapy,* Boston, 1992, Andover.
32. Toglia JP, Golisz K: *Cognitive rehabilitation: group games and activities,* Tucson, Ariz, 1990, Therapy Skill Builders.
33. Wehman PH: Cognitive rehabilitation in the workplace. In Kreutzer JS, Wehman PH: *Cognitive rehabilitation for persons with traumatic brain injury: a functional approach,* Baltimore, 1991, Brookes.
34. Wheatley CJ, Rein JJ: Intervention in traumatic head injury: learning style assessment. In Hertfelder S, Gwin C, editors: *Work in progress: occupational therapy in work programs,* Rockville, Md, 1989, American Occupational Therapy Association.
35. Wilson BA: *Rehabilitation of memory,* New York, 1987, Guilford.
36. Wilson BA, Moffat N, editors: *Clinical management of memory problems,* Rockville, Md, 1984, Aspen.
37. Ylvisaker M et al: Topics in cognitive rehabilitation therapy. In Ylvisaker M, Gobble EM: *Community re-entry for head injured adults,* Boston, 1987, Little, Brown.
38. Zoltan B, Siev E, Frieshtat B: *The adult stroke patient: a manual for evaluation and treatment of perceptual and cognitive dysfunction,* rev ed 2, Thorofare, NJ, 1986, Slack.

**Section IV**

1. Abreu BC, Toglia JP: Cognitive rehabilitation: a model for occupational therapy, *Am J Occup Ther* 41:439-448, 1987.
2. Ayres AJ: *Sensory integration and learning disorders,* Los Angeles, 1972, Western Psychological Services.
3. Baker RS, Epstein AD: Ocular motor abnormalities from head trauma, *Surv Ophthalmol* 36:245-267, 1991.
4. Belleza T et al: Visual scanning and matching dysfunction in brain damaged patients with drawing impairment, *Cortex* 15:19-36, 1979.

5. Chedru F, Leblanc M, Lhermitte F: Visual searching in normal and brain damaged subjects, *Cortex* 9:94-111, 1973.
6. Cotman CW, McGaugh JL: *Behavioral neuroscience: an introduction,* New York, 1980, Academic.
7. Delis DC, Robertson LC, Balliet R: The breakdown and rehabilitation of visuospatial dysfunction in brain injured patients, *Int Rehabil Med* 5:132-138, 1983.
8. DeRenzi E: *Disorders of space exploration and cognition,* New York, 1982, Wiley and Sons.
9. Dickman IR: *Making life more livable,* New York, 1985, American Foundation for the Blind.
10. Fletcher D et al: Low vision rehabilitation: finding capable people behind damaged eyeballs, *West J Med* 154:554-556, 1991.
11. Gianutsos R, Matheson P: The rehabilitation of visual perceptual disorders attributable to brain injury. In Meier MJ, Benton AL, Diller L, editors: *Neuropsychological rehabilitation,* New York, 1987, Guilford.
12. Gianutsos R, Ramsey G, Perlin RR: Rehabilitative optometric services for survivors of acquired brain injury, *Arch Phys Med Rehabil* 69:573-578, 1988.
13. Halligan PW, Marshall JC, Wade DT: Do visual field deficits exacerbate visuo-spatial neglect? *J Neurol Neurosurg Psychiatry* 53:487-491, 1990.
14. Heilman K, Van Den Abel T: Right hemisphere dominance for attention: the mechanism underlying hemispheric asymmetries of inattention (neglect), *Neurology* 30:327-330, 1980.
15. Ishial S, Furukawa T, Tsukagoshi H: Eye fixation patterns in homonymous hemianopia and unilateral spatial neglect, *Neuropsychologia* 25:675-679, 1987.
16. Julesz B: Preconscious and conscious processing in vision. In Chagas C, Gattass R, editors: Pattern recognition mechanisms, *Exp Brain Res* III (suppl), 1985.
17. Leigh RJ, Zee DS: *Neurology of eye movements,* Philadelphia, 1983, Davis.
18. Levine DH: Unawareness of visual and sensorimotor deficits: a hypothesis, *Brain Cogn* 13:233-281, 1990.
19. Moore JC: *The visual system: in relation to rehabilitation,* Cincinatti, June 18-20, 1993, Franciscan Health System of Cincinnati (workshop).
20. Neger RE: The evaluation of diplopia in head trauma, *J Head Trauma Rehabil* 4:27-34, 1989.
21. Padula WV: *A behavioral vision approach for persons with physical disabilities,* Santa Anna, Calif, 1988, Optometric Extension Program Foundation.
22. Pommerenke K, Markowitsch HJ: Rehabilitation training of homonymous visual field defects in patients with postgeniculate damage of the visual system, *Restor Neurol Neurosci* 1:47-63, 1989.
23. Posner MI, Rafal RD: Cognitive theories of attention and the rehabilitation of attentional deficits. In Meier MJ, Benton AL, Diller L, editors: *Neuropsychological rehabilitation,* New York, 1987, Guilford.
24. Powell S: *A handbook for the homemaker–home health aide working with adults who are visually impaired or hearing impaired,* New York, 1982, LaGuardia Community College.
25. Rapesak SZ et al: Selective attention in hemispatial neglect, *Arch Neurol* 46:178-182, 1989.
26. Sergent J: Inferences from unilateral brain damage about normal hemispheric functions in visual pattern recognition, *Psychol Bull* 96:99-115, 1984.
27. Sergent J: An investigation into perceptual completion in blind areas of the visual field, *Brain* 111:347-373, 1988.
28. Spier PA et al: Visual neglect during intracarotid amobarbital testing, *Neurology* 40:1600-1606, 1990.
29. Toglia J: Generalization of treatment: a multicontext approach to cognitive perceptual impairment in adults with brain injury, *Am J Occup Ther* 45:505-516, 1991.
30. van Zomeren AH et al: Fitness to drive a car after recovery from severe head injury, *Arch Phys Med Rehabil* 69:90-96, 1988.
31. Warren M: Identification of visual scanning deficits in adults after cerebrovascular accident, *Am J Occup Ther* 44:391-399, 1990.
32. Warren M: A hierarchical model for evaluation and treatment of visual perceptual dysfunction in adult acquired brain injury. Parts 1 and 2, *Am J Occup Ther* 47:42-66, 1993.
33. Warren M: Evaluation and treatment of visual deficits. In Pedretti LW, editor: *Occupational therapy: practice skills for physical dysfunction,* ed 4, St Louis, 1995, Mosby.
34. Weinberg J et al: Visual scanning training effect on reading-related tasks in acquired right brain damage, *Arch Phys Med Rehabil* 60:479-486, 1979.
35. Weintraub S, Mesulam MM: Visual hemispatial inattention: stimulus parameters and exploratory strategies, *J Neurol Neurosurg Psychiatry* 51:1481-1488, 1988.
36. Zangemeister WH et al: Eye head coordination in homonymous hemianopsia, *J Neurol* 226:243-254, 1982.
37. Zihl J: Rehabilitation of visual impairments in patients with brain damage, 1993 (unpublished).

# Part VI

# Treatment Applications

# Chapter 25

# Cerebrovascular Accident

*Lori M. Shiffman*

## Chapter Objectives

*After studying this chapter, the student or practitioner will be able to:*

1. Define CVA and list potential causes of CVA.
2. List specific risk factors for CVA.
3. List and describe common problems found in a patient after CVA.
4. Explain the role of the occupational therapy practitioner in preventing common complications after CVA.
5. Understand the effects of sensory deficits of stroke on function.
6. Understand the common visual perceptual, cognitive, and behavioral impairments after stroke, and identify occupational therapy treatment strategies.
7. Describe the role of the occupational therapy practitioner and patient in the treatment of dysphagia after CVA, and list feeding precautions.
8. Explain how aphasia may affect communication skills, and describe interaction guidelines for stroke patients with aphasia.
9. Understand the role of the occupational therapy practitioner in providing emotional support and education to stroke patients and members of their social support system.
10. Describe the effects of deficits commonly experienced after left-sided CVA and right-sided CVA in performance of familiar and new tasks.
11. Identify occupational therapy treatment strategies for stroke patients in the following occupational therapy performance areas: activities of daily living, work, and leisure.
12. Understand occupational therapy treatment strategies and selection of adapted equipment in treatment of performance area deficits after CVA.
13. Appreciate the emphasis of occupational therapy treatment planning on promoting a balance among work, rest, and play with patients after CVA.

## Key Terms

cerebrovascular accident (CVA, stroke)
hemiplegia/hemiparesis
flaccid paralysis/hypotonicity
deep venous thrombosis (DVT)
shoulder subluxation
synergy
spasticity/hypertonicity
hemianopsia
apraxia (dyspraxia)
perserveration
emotional lability
dysphagia
aphasia

**Cerebrovascular accident (CVA, stroke)** is the most common disabling medical condition of adulthood,[34] accounting for at least half of patients hospitalized with neurological disease. There are about three million stroke survivors in the United States.[2] Of the estimated 500,000 new strokes every year,[7] 33% to 40% cause death. At least half of the survivors have permanent disability. Adult stroke survivors are the single largest diagnostic group seen by occupational therapy practitioners in physical dysfunction.[68]

## DEFINITION

CVA, or stroke, occurs when the blood supply is compromised in the brain. Catastrophic reduction of nutrients carried by the blood causes damage to brain tissue, resulting in various neurological deficits. Stroke results in **hemiplegia** (one-sided paralysis) or **hemiparesis** (partial motor loss on one side of the body). These effects are experienced in the side of the body opposite to the hemisphere of the brain that suffered the lack of blood supply. A lesion on the left side of the brain produces right-sided hemiplegia and a right-sided CVA produces left-sided hemiplegia. The term CVA is used to describe a completed stroke.[34]

Incomplete strokes or transient ischemic attacks (TIAs) are temporary. The symptoms of TIA are usually mild, develop suddenly, and last from a few minutes up to 24 hours. There are no remaining symptoms. Approximately one third of persons with TIAs will have a stroke, another third will continue to have more TIAs without stroke, and one third will have no further problems.[55]

## ETIOLOGY

TIAs occur when the blood supply to the brain is temporarily reduced.[34] CVA occurs when the blood supply to the brain is interrupted. This may be caused by a thrombus (blood clot that causes blockage), an embolus (traveling blood clot), or a hemorrhage (rupturing of a blood vessel). Brain tissue dies as a result of the lack of blood supply. Most strokes are caused by clots, but hemorrhagic strokes result in a significantly higher death rate, especially for the elderly.[60]

### Risk Factors

Risk factors that contribute to stroke are classified as uncontrollable or controllable. Uncontrollable risk factors include age, gender, heredity, and race.[57] The most significant risk factor for stroke is age. Risk increases with age, especially into late adulthood when most strokes occur.[57] Men have a slightly higher risk of stroke than women.[57] Blacks tend to have a much higher frequency of stroke than other ethnic groups because of the increased incidence of predisposing diseases such as hypertension and diabetes.[34,60] Controllable factors for CVA are hypertension, cerebrovascular disease, coronary artery disease, diabetes, TIAs, previous CVA, high cholesterol, diet, cigarette smoking, alcohol abuse, obesity, cardiac disease, and use of birth control pills.[34,38,57,60] Measures that reduce the risk and help to prevent CVA include control of blood pressure and diabetes, elimination of smoking and obesity, regular exercise, proper diet, and reduction of high cholesterol levels.

## EFFECTS

Stroke can cause severe loss of function of many bodily systems.

### Warning Signs

Before stroke, many adults experience warning symptoms[15] that may be ignored. Generally, individuals may experience headache, nausea, vomiting, seizures, loss of consciousness,[15] or fatigue. Common specific symptoms include one-sided weakness, facial palsy, slurred speech, swallowing problems, and sensory losses.[15] Sensory changes include numbness, burning, or tingling on one side. Blurred vision or blind spots may occur. Cognitive symptoms such as lethargy, disorientation, confusion, or impaired memory may be experienced.

### Dysfunction

Immediately after stroke, there is **flaccid paralysis** (absence of muscle tone), or **hypotonicity** of the affected side with reduced or absent reflexes.[15] Other losses may include impaired postural control, sensory deficits, visual impairments, perceptual dysfunction, cognitive dysfunction, behavioral and personality changes, and impaired speech and language skills.[34]

### Outcome

The outcome and severity of CVA depend on the type, size, location, and density of the brain damage,[7] the timing and success of medical care, other medical or neurological problems, and the patient's current state of health. The area of the brain affected by stroke is determined by the cerebral blood supply involved.[15] Spontaneous recovery of motor function occurs mostly in the first 3 months after CVA,[41] but can continue for up to 1 year. Improvement in functional abilities may continue years after stroke. Factors associated with a poor prognosis are advanced age, coma, poor perceptual or cognitive functions, lack of motor return, absent sensation, prior history of CVA, and chronic diseases.[34,50]

## MEDICAL MANAGEMENT

Emergency medical treatment of CVA includes maintenance of an open airway, establishment of fluid balance, and treatment of medical problems. Drugs are often used to prevent or reduce damage to cerebral tissues.[49] Surgery may be indicated to repair damaged blood vessels to reduce bleeding and to prevent additional damage to intact cerebral tissues.

### Medical Complications

Stroke survivors are prone to complications, and extended bedrest increases the risk. The most common complication after CVA is **deep venous thrombosis (DVT)**,[34] which usually develops in the veins of the legs. Blood clots called *pulmonary emboli*, released from deep veins and lodged in the lungs, are the most common cause of death within the first month after CVA.[11] After a DVT is diagnosed, the affected limb must be elevated and non–weight bearing until the clot is resolved. DVT may be prevented by early exercise, medication, or use of elastic stockings.[53]

Scarred brain tissues can cause seizures in about 10% of stroke survivors.[60] Medical care stresses prevention or control of seizure activity with anticonvulsant drugs. Side effects cause drowsiness and may impair thinking skills.[34]

**Subluxation** commonly occurs in the glenohumeral (GH) joint of the affected upper extremity. The GH joint is between the glenoid fossa of the scapula and the head of the humerus. Subluxation is a dislocation or separation of the joint as a result of paralysis or weakness of the rotator cuff muscles and spasticity of the scapular muscles. Shoulder subluxation may cause the joint to be painful and, if not treated, can lead to deformity and adhesive capsulitis. Shoulder subluxation may be diagnosed medically with x-ray and may be palpated (felt) by the OT practitioner.

For patients with cardiac problems and stroke, treatment should be individualized with precautions taken to avoid straining the heart (see Chapter 30). Immobility, poor inhalation because of weakness of respiratory muscles from hemiparesis, and impaired swallowing after CVA increase risk for lung infections such as pneumonia.[8,60]

After stroke, bowel and bladder incontinence is common. Retention of urine can lead to urinary tract infection. Medical care involves regular toileting, diet and fluid control, and drug treatment.

There are several risk factors for the development of decubitus ulcers (pressure areas that tend to develop over bony prominences). These factors affect individual stroke survivors and include bedrest, sensory loss, impaired movement, loss of range of motion (ROM), visual losses, and perceptual-cognitive impairments. Regular weight shifting, turning, early exercise, daily skin checks, proper nutrition, and monitoring of all positioning devices can significantly reduce the risk of developing pressure areas.[34]

## OCCUPATIONAL THERAPY INTERVENTION

### Role of Occupational Therapy

Occupational therapy in the treatment of CVA focuses on improving motor function of the affected side; integrating sensory, visual perceptual, and cognitive functions; facilitating maximal level of functional independence; and encouraging return to life roles as possible. When the patient is identified as medically stable by the physician, the OT practitioner may begin treatment. At the acute care level, occupational therapy stresses early exercise, prevention of complications, basic self-care, and gathering of information to determine the patient's rehabilitation potential. Inpatient rehabilitation OT focuses on activities of daily living (ADL), work, and leisure skills. Outpatient services and home health care continue rehabilitation goals until maximum functional performance is achieved. This may involve special programming such as job reentry or driver's training.

### Goals of Occupational Therapy

Occupational therapy services with the stroke patient focus on preventive and rehabilitative goals in occupational performance. Overall goals are the following:

1. Prevention of deformity
2. Prevention of injury
3. Encouragement of normal postural and movement patterns
4. Achievement of maximal active and passive ROM, strength, and coordination
5. Achievement of maximal functional use of the affected side
6. Remediation of visual perceptual and cognitive dysfunction
7. Achievement of maximal level of independence in self-care
8. Achievement of maximal mobility skills
9. Achievement of functional communication skills and social interactive skills
10. Facilitation of realistic adjustment to remaining problems
11. Facilitation of reentry into meaningful roles in family and community
12. Facilitation of a balance between work, rest, and play[35,63,69]

### Occupational Therapy Programming Considerations

The occupational therapy treatment program is based on the evaluation results in performance components (sensory motor components, cognitive integration, and psychosocial skills) and performance areas (activities of daily work, leisure skills).[3] Stroke patients are receiving OT treatment earlier than in the past, as a result of more aggressive, immediate medical care characteristic of current health care trends.

#### *Confounding Factors*

More stroke patients are surviving, and many have a higher level of medical acuity or illness. Medical status can change daily. The physician usually determines whether the patient is well enough to receive OT on any particular day. Therefore treating OT practitioners must know signs and symptoms of all diagnoses as well as current emergency procedures. Careful attention must be given in treatment planning to avoid activities that may worsen symptoms.

The majority of stroke patients are older persons who statistically have high rates of additional disabilities[35] because of chronic medical problems. Older patients do benefit from rehabilitation[35] but often experience more severe symptoms or disability that may require more time for recovery.

### *Gradation of Treatment*

Treatment is graded by increasing the length and complexity of the activity. The starting level of difficulty is based on the evaluation results. Time for completion, amount of set-up, number of steps, amount of physical assistance, number and frequency of verbal cues, and use of adaptive equipment are adjusted as needed. Age, medical status, and symptoms of disease or complications may change the gradation of treatment. Stroke survivors may experience setbacks and require readjustment of the treatment program, restarting at a lower level of skill demand. As improvements in endurance and skills increase, task complexity increases until maximum benefit has been achieved.

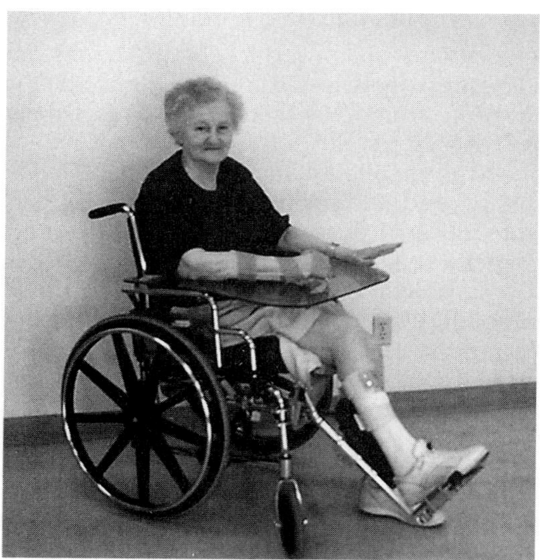

*Figure 25-1* Patient using a lapboard to support hemiplegic arm while sitting in wheelchair. A lapboard promotes proper wheelchair positioning and symmetrical trunk alignment.

## OCCUPATIONAL PERFORMANCE DOMAIN OF CONCERN FOR TREATMENT

Occupational therapy treatment for the stroke patient is based on the domain of concern of occupational performance (see Chapter 2 and the *Uniform Terminology for Occupational Therapy—Third Edition*).[3] Treatment begins with activities to prepare the patient for purposeful, functional tasks, and leads to practicing previous roles and community reintegration as possible.

## DYSFUNCTION CHARACTERISTICS AND OCCUPATIONAL THERAPY INTERVENTIONS

### Abnormal Reflexes and Postural Mechanisms

Postural mechanisms are often changed by CVA. Normal righting, equilibrium, and protective responses can be delayed or absent on the hemiplegic side. Without the ability to maintain and recover balance, body alignment and mobility skills can be significantly impaired.

### Positioning Techniques

Proper positioning after CVA is important to minimize the effects of abnormal muscle tone on the involved side. Positioning of the spastic extremities can reduce the risks of developing contractures or skin ulcers. Positioning of the hypotonic extremities can reduce the risk of overstretching muscles. In bed, alternating between supine, sidelying on the affected side, and sidelying on the unaffected side at 2 to 4 hour intervals is recommended. Symmetry of trunk alignment is desirable in all positions. The affected arm should be supported in supine and in sidelying while on the unaffected side to reduce edema and prevent injury. The affected leg should be positioned to encourage hip and knee flexion in all positions. During positioning changes, excessive effort should be avoided to prevent the influence of abnormal muscle tone on the affected side. Patients may require adaptive devices such as wedges, bolsters, extra pillows, towel rolls, or splints to maintain proper alignment and positioning.

In upright sitting, the trunk should be symmetrical and erect. The affected arm should be supported with pillows, a bedside table, or laptray. The affected leg should be positioned in flexion at the hip and knee joints. A properly fitting wheelchair significantly improves a patient's sitting posture. A lumbar support, a hard seat and back, or a custom cushion can maximize comfortable sitting. The feet should be supported on foot rests at all times while the patient is sitting. Wheelchair lapboards or an arm trough may be required (Figure 25-1).

The resting hand splint is the most commonly used splint for protection of the affected forearm, wrist, and hand, and for prevention of contractures or deformities (Figure 25-2). Whether prefabricated or custom made, the resting hand splint supports the distal arm in a functional position of wrist extension, slight metacarpophalangeal (MP) flexion, proximal interphalangeal (PIP) and distal interphalangeal (DIP) extension, and thumb opposition with flexion.

### *Abnormal Muscle Tone*

After CVA, flaccid paralysis is often replaced by spastic paralysis or paresis, resulting in a nonfunctional extremity. Patients move the affected extremities in flexion or extension patterns called **synergies.** Flexor spasticity of the arm musculature is more dominant

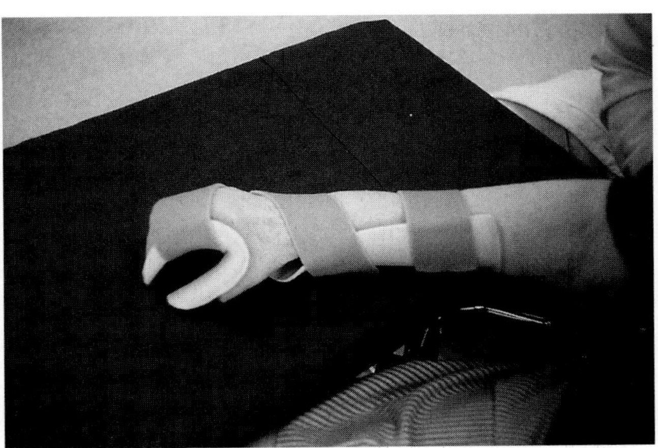

*Figure 25-2* A resting hand splint properly supports hemiplegic forearm, wrist, and hand in a functional position.

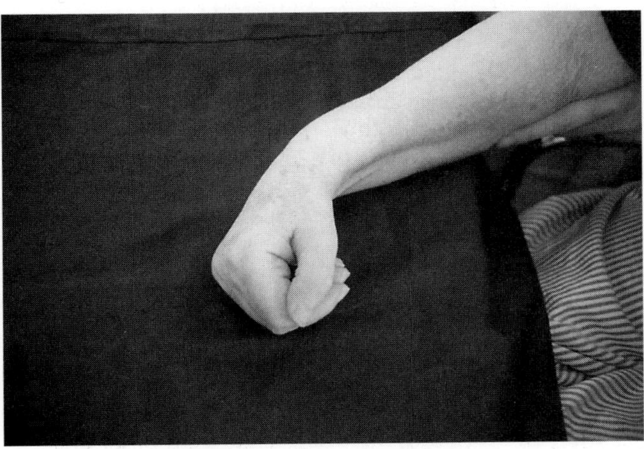

*Figure 25-3* Typical upper extremity flexion synergy.

and can result in a strong involuntary adducted and flexed positioning of the upper extremity (UE) (Figure 25-3).

Functionally, synergy influence or overlay is more obvious in movements against gravity, especially those requiring more effort and reach. Extension synergy is more dominant in the lower extremity (LE). In walking, as the patient attempts to flex the hip, knee, and ankle to step, the unintended response is hip extension and adduction, knee extension, and plantar flexion of the ankle. Without intervention, synergy patterning may progress to contractures and deformities in the affected extremities as well as asymmetries in the trunk.

**Spasticity** can be described as minimal, moderate, or severe and may fluctuate between levels daily. **Hypertonicity** (high muscle tone) tends to increase with stressful bodily changes such as fatigue, infections, injury, ulcers, bowel dysfunction, or in response to some medications. A significant increase in tone may indicate the presence of a urinary tract infection, a developing decubitus pressure sore, or bowel impaction. Spasticity usually reduces to previous levels after successful medical treatment of the underlying problem. Tone may also decrease during rest.

### *Motor Skills Deficits*

Immediately after stroke, voluntary control of the affected UE is usually absent. Motor function returns in stages and may stop at any stage. Typically as motor function returns, it develops from the trunk, into the shoulder and hip, and down into the extremities (proximally to distally). Motor recovery begins with partial active movements and may progress to stronger more coordinated movements against gravity. Most patients experience some return in scapular retraction, shoulder horizontal adduction, and shoulder elevation. Although complete recovery is rare, some patients regain full functional UE use, especially when sensation is intact and awareness of the hemiplegic side is normal.[9]

### *Balance Impairment*

After a stroke, the patient may have problems sitting or standing erect. Because of poor automatic and postural adjustments against gravity,[8] patients tend to compensate by a reluctance or decreased ability to bear weight on the hemiplegic side, often leaning away from that side. Balance is poorer if sensation is impaired. Patients unaware of their poor vertical sense may assume they are upright despite leaning and may need to use vision to correct positioning. Balance training incorporating the affected UE will encourage more automatic use of motor and cognitive perceptual skills.[1] Supportive devices such as lateral trunk supports, chest belts, or lapboards can increase stability while sitting and may be required until balance improves. Balance impairments significantly increase risk for falls, especially for patients with multiple problems.

### *Common Motor Problems*

The person with hemiplegia lacks the ability to perform a wide variety of normal movement combinations.[10] As motor function returns, gross and fine motor coordination problems or incoordination, such as ataxia, may occur. Chapters 10 and 23 delineate the types of coordination problems that can occur in a person with hemiplegia. The quality of movement is also affected by muscle weakness, fatigue, infection, and certain drugs. Quicker, finer movements are the last to recover.

### *Occupational Therapy Treatment Techniques*

Treatment of the motor dysfunction focuses on improving balance and voluntary control of the hemiplegic side for maximum function.

*Passive and active range of motion* Maintenance of full joint ROM and prevention of deformity are important early goals in occupational therapy. Passive ROM (PROM) exercises should be performed twice daily and continued indefinitely if sufficient active movement does not return. ROM can be limited by fluctuating tone, subluxation, pain, edema, fractures, joint diseases, and reduced scapular and clavicular mobility. Full mobility of the scapula, clavicle, and humerus is required for pain-free shoulder motion. If the scapula does not protract (abduct) and rotate upward and outward with shoulder movements, then ROM exercises past 90 degrees of shoulder flexion are contraindicated because of the risk for injury.

PROM exercises of the affected UE are performed by the patient (using the unaffected arm) or by another person. PROM or self-ROM (SROM) exercises are required when active movement is weak or absent. During SROM exercises the unaffected UE fully supports the affected UE through all exercises. When there is minimal active movement, active assisted ROM (AAROM) exercises are performed. This involves partial assist from the unaffected UE or from another person. Active ROM (AROM) is performed by the patient only and requires voluntary movement of the hemiplegic UE. ROM exercises generally include 10 repetitions of all movements, beginning at the shoulder and proceeding to elbow, forearm, wrist, and hand.

*Treatment of shoulder subluxation and pain* As discussed previously, when the hemiplegic shoulder moves and normal scapular motion does not occur, the GH joint can become subluxed. Factors that contribute to subluxation include severe sensory loss, poor UE support, poor alignment of GH joint during ROM exercises, arthritic shoulder joint, and incorrect handling of the involved UE by staff or untrained family members.[21,52]

The presence of pain of a subluxed GH joint depends on the type of sensory loss and severity of the subluxation. Shoulder pain can be present during movement and/or at rest and may range from minimal to severe. The patient with shoulder pain may reduce or refuse participation in therapy. Shoulder pain can be prevented through proper positioning; passive PROM exercises; and education of patient, staff, and family on proper handling techniques. The affected UE should be fully supported at all times on pillows in bed and on a lapboard or arm trough while sitting. Use of arm slings is controversial because they tend to increase the flexed adducted posture while reducing sensory feedback without reducing subluxation.[7,10] Patients who have severe edema, have a heavy flaccid upper extremity, or are at high risk for injury may require a sling temporarily for mobility activities.

*Motor retraining* Motor retraining programs encourage normal postural mechanisms, normal movement, and use of the affected side in functional activities. Retraining is accomplished with sensorimotor (see Chapter 23) or functionally based approaches.[16,24,72]

*Influencing muscle tone* OT treatment techniques can influence muscle tone. Active movement of hypotonic muscles can be facilitated through stimulation of various sensations. Inhibition (reduction) of hypertonic muscles can be accomplished through positioning and handling. Tactile and proprioceptive input can help to decrease high tone. Specialized training is required to perform these techniques.

*Bilateral integration* Bilateral integration of the upper extremities can be an early goal in stroke rehabilitation, even if the affected arm is nonfunctional. Increased tactile and visual input will encourage development of movement sense. The affected UE should be properly positioned and kept within the patient's view during one-handed activities.[10] UE activities with hands clasped, such as pushing a ball on a tabletop[10] or using a hemiskate incorporate the affected arm passively (or with active assistance). As motor functions return, the affected arm initially serves as a stabilizer and progresses to being a gross assist, then a partial assist, and may eventually become functional in all tasks.

*Strengthening and endurance* Therapeutic goals for patients with normal tone after stroke emphasize strengthening both arms. If spasticity is present in the affected UE, resistive activities will increase tone and are contraindicated. Strengthening of the unaffected side is appropriate if increased resistance does not cause spasticity of the hemiplegic side. Stroke survivors often experience loss of strength on the unaffected side and a significant reduction of endurance as a result of disuse. Endurance training is basic to every stroke program. It is most effective when graded according to the patient's medical, physical, and cognitive abilities and designed to address postdischarge lifestyle needs. Programming that ignores these factors may contribute to anger, frustration, and noncompliance. Rest periods are a very important part of the stroke rehabilitation schedule.

*Elevation and retrograde massage* Edema or fluid accumulation in extremities due to immobility, poor circulation, and dependent positioning is a common preventable complication after a stroke. Swelling causes an increase in diameter of the skin, which becomes soft and puffy. Prolonged edema results in shiny hard skin, stiff joints, and ROM loss. Sensory loss, poor positioning, obesity, and conditions that increase fluid retention are the chief risk factors for the development of edema. Edema can be prevented by elevation of extremities. In bed, the affected UE and LE should be propped up on pillows. While the patient is sitting, the UE should be supported on an elevated lapboard and the LE on an extended legrest. AROM tasks, especially those involving upward reach, are most effective in preventing or reducing edema. Retrograde manual massage of the elevated hand, beginning at the fingertips and moving toward the elbow with a smooth and even touch, can be performed by the patient, the family, or a clinician. Elastic stockings or sleeves and pneumatic compression devices such as airsplints reduce edema through constant pressure. Splints and positioning devices should be closely monitored to prevent edema.

*Compensatory techniques* For some stroke survivors, the dominant side is also the hemiplegic side. Such patients may require training in one-handed performance and possibly dominance retraining because they may have to rely on one hand permanently.[10] The nondominant UE may have poorer fine motor control, especially in right-handed persons. Strategies for one-handedness include learning methods of stabilizing objects and compensating with adapted equipment.

### Sensory System Dysfunction

Stroke can cause absent or impaired sensation. If sensation returns, it usually does so in a proximal to distal pattern. Pain usually returns first.

#### *Visual Deficits*

OT practitioners should be aware of many factors that affect visual performance. Because 95% of the elderly either wear or need corrective lenses,[32] usually to improve visual acuity (clarity of vision), many patients who suffer stroke already wear glasses. To maximize vision, all corrective lenses should be current prescriptions, well-fitting, and clean. Environmental factors such as lighting and contrast should be considered. Older adults require more light to see and are more affected by glare. Adding light sources behind them tends to reduce glare. Increasing contrast can improve visual discrimination.

Stroke affects many aspects of vision. Complete visual evaluation should be performed by vision care specialists such as ophthalmologists or optometrists. The registered occupational therapist (OTR) may often be the first rehabilitation team member to screen vision after stroke. Weakness of the eye muscles controlling the upward, downward, and side movements of the eyeballs may cause diplopia (double vision) or decreased accommodation (ability to use eyes together to focus on images at any distance). Double vision may be present in some directions of gaze but not others. Patching of either eye as prescribed by the vision specialist will eliminate double vision immediately, and patients often follow a graded program with the use of patches. Accurate judgment of distance and the speed of moving objects in the environment may be difficult after CVA.

The ability to see objects in the center of vision is usually not affected by CVA, but peripheral vision losses are common. These visual field cuts or **hemianopsia** are permanent areas of absent vision, and size and quantity may vary. Homonymous hemianopsia is a loss of the visual field of the lateral (temporal) aspect of the hemiplegic side and the medial (nasal) aspect of the unaffected side, resulting in a loss of one half (R or L) of the visual field. Headaches are a common complaint of the elderly who have peripheral field losses.[46] Patients may not see objects in the affected area of vision, often ignoring or hitting them accidentally, and visual losses after CVA usually reduce safety. Visual deficits related to perception are discussed later in this chapter.

#### *Auditory Deficits*

Generally, stroke does not seem to affect hearing, even in patients with aphasia (language disorders).[25] If hearing deficits exist in patients after stroke, they are usually a result of normal aging, especially in men.[25] Previous hearing loss may be exaggerated by the stroke and may lead to communication problems.

#### *Tactile Deficits*

Changes in the senses of touch, pain, pressure, temperature, vibration, and proprioception (position sense) are common after CVA.[41] Without sensory feedback, patients experience difficulty using affected extremities, even when motor recovery is good. Risk for injury increases with increased sensory loss.

#### *Olfactory and Gustatory Deficits*

After stroke, the senses of smell and taste may become dulled as a result of brain damage.[26] OT practitioners can instruct patients about changes in taste or smell that could contribute to poor appetite, hygiene problems, safety problems, (e.g., inability to smell dangerous odors), or a reduced ability to enjoy pleasurable odors and tastes.

#### *Occupational Therapy Treatment Considerations*

*Sensory retraining and compensatory techniques* The occupational therapy program for the stroke patient may include sensory reeducation and compensatory techniques as described in Chapter 24.

### Perceptual Dysfunction

Perception is the complex process of interpreting sensory information from the environment. Stroke may affect a variety of visual perceptual and perceptual motor skills. Changes in visual perception seen after CVA are a result of the stroke and not normal aging.[66]

#### *Visual Perceptual Impairments*

Normal human visual behavior involves visual attention and search. Visual attention is a purposeful visual response to the environment and in normal adults can be sustained as desired. Visual search, or tracking, is the process of selecting objects on which to focus attention by scanning the environment. A common visual perceptual problem after CVA is hemi-inattention. Patients with a visual attention deficit have difficulty shifting their gaze or attending to objects.[59] Their eye movements tend to be slower. When patients cannot attend, search, and scan, the ability to identify objects or people is reduced.

### *Spatial Relations Deficits*

The ability to identify shapes and recognize the relationship between objects and between object and self is affected by CVA. Patients may have trouble judging the distance between objects or following a familiar route.[67] Deficits in understanding concepts such as over, under, through, and behind can cause dressing problems.[69]

Visual figure-ground perception is the recognition of forms hidden within a complicated background.[28] Patients with impairments have difficulty selecting the correct visual information.[6] They may appear distractible but could be responding to irrelevant visual information.[22,74]

Difficulty with vertical or horizontal orientation (directionality) may be present, especially in patients with left-sided hemiplegia who tend to see vertical objects as tilted left of center.[9,63] Because visual orientation is important to the righting reactions for upright posture, directional disturbances interfere with balance and ambulation.[9]

### *Color Discrimination Deficits*

Problems discriminating color after CVA are less common. However, because the majority of stroke survivors are elderly, age-related changes in color vision may be present. After age 60, the older adult experiences difficulty with red-green and blue-green discrimination.[58] Blues seem darker and duller[43] and are often perceived as red.[37] The yellowing of the lens makes distinguishing white objects from yellow objects difficult, but yellow and red colors are still easily seen.[43]

## Perceptual Motor Impairments

Perceptual motor skills rely on the processing of sensation to develop adaptive motor responses. A person who has suffered a CVA may have perceptual motor deficits that interfere with functional independence.

### *Unilateral Neglect*

Unilateral neglect is the inability to interpret perceptual messages from the hemiplegic side of the body or space. Unilateral neglect is more frequent in persons with left-sided hemiplegia and can occur with or without visual inattention and hemianopia. Patients show a gaze preference, keeping their head turned away from the affected side and ignoring the affected half of the body and of space.

### *Apraxia (Dyspraxia)*

**Apraxia** is an impairment in the ability to plan motor acts. Patients can have difficulty performing purposeful movement on command, understanding the concept of a task, or drawing or constructing two- or three-dimensional designs. Apraxia occurring with body scheme problems can cause dressing apraxia and problems with ADL.[71,74]

### *Body Awareness Deficits*

Body scheme disorders affect knowledge of body construction, spatial relationships, awareness of bodily parts in relation to one another, and right and left discrimination.[4] Because bodily awareness is basic to all motor function, poor body scheme causes many functional deficits, particularly evident in basic self-care.[42]

### *Agnosia*

Agnosia refers to the inability to recognize objects by vision, hearing, touch, or proprioception (position sense) despite intact senses. Symptoms are worsened when the patient has an impaired body scheme and unilateral neglect. One of the more common problems is tactile agnosia or astereognosis, the inability to recognize familiar objects by touch without vision. (Additional information on these and other sensory and perceptual problems can be found in Chapters 11 and 24.)

### *Occupational Therapy Treatment Considerations*

*Remediation of visual perceptual deficits* Perceptual difficulties are often not well understood by patients and their families or friends. Remediation of deficits focuses on the goal of restoration of skills; OT practitioners also educate families and others about these problems.

*Compensatory strategies for visual perceptual and perceptual motor impairments* Treatment of perceptual problems can be lengthy and complex. Compensatory strategies use intact skills to substitute for deficits. Selection of treatment activities should be based on the patient's previous lifestyle, remaining strengths and deficits, living situation, and goals.

Patients or family members may mistakenly assume that field cuts can be "fixed with better glasses." New eye glasses cannot alter the permanent absence of vision. Some patients can compensate automatically and may require minimal or no intervention. Others with gaze preference can learn to turn their heads toward the affected side and use auditory and tactile cues and remaining vision. Patients with apraxia can learn tasks with tactile cues from others to assist them through familiar basic functional tasks until they become more automatic. Persons with mild neglect can learn strategies such as verbally cuing themselves to attend to the affected side or wearing a watch on that side. Persons with persistent neglect require continual supervision for safety. For patients with unilateral neglect, use of functional activities and feedback from videotaping such activities can improve awareness.[56,62]

Use of a mirror and clothing labels to identify parts (e.g., right sleeve) can compensate for body awareness deficits. Patients with spatial relations problems may learn routes in their environments using the same route each time and taking notice of signs to mark the way. Patients with agnosia can learn to use other senses to compensate for problems. For example, patients who do not recognize their family members by sight may identify them by their voices. Labelling family pictures can be useful.

Garments can be labelled to avoid mismatching clothing for individuals with impaired color discrimination. Customizing treatment materials and the environment to address color contrasts needs of the older adult is recommended.[19]

## Cognitive Dysfunction

Cognition requires the integration of numerous abilities, many of which may be impaired by CVA.

### *Initiation and Motivation Deficits*

Impaired initiation is characterized by difficulty starting and finishing tasks. Patients require physical assistance or verbal cues to begin and are often unable to restart after stopping. These behaviors may be mistaken for noncompliance or poor motivation. Step-by-step assistance to complete even familiar basic self-care tasks may improve skills. Many patients show a decrease in intrinsic motivation, or the inner drive to act spontaneously. Such patients should not be labelled "unmotivated" or "resistant," because their lack of drive is a result of brain damage.

### *Attention and Concentration Deficits*

Deficits in the abilities to attend to information and to maintain that focus affect every aspect of performance. Distractibility is common, especially in a stimulating environment. Attention problems are worsened by fatigue, depression, illness, disinterest, and certain medications.

### *Disorientation and Confusion*

Orientation involves awareness of person, place, time, and situation. Awareness of person includes being aware of information such as full name, birthdate, age, marital status, telephone number, number of children, and education. Place concepts involve knowing current location, (e.g., hospital), address, city, state, and country. Time orientation includes day, date, time, month, year, season, and next holiday. Situational information includes identifying reason for hospitalization or verifying employment or general knowledge, such as naming the president. Orientation is often documented as the abbreviation "0" times the number of oriented areas (e.g., 0 × 2). Patients tend to retain personal information longest and forget situational information first.

### *Memory Deficits*

CVA can affect reception, integration, and retrieval of information for short- or long-term memory skills. Patients may have difficulty recalling persons, objects, and procedures learned.

### *Sequencing and Organization Deficits*

Sequencing involves planning, organizing, and completing the steps of a task in correct order. It includes temporal concepts such as first, second, and third, and spatial ordering such as top, bottom, left to right, and around.[5] Sequencing errors can occur in any task, even familiar ones. The more complex the activity, the greater the number of errors.

Effective organization requires higher levels of attention, concentration, orientation, memory, and correct sequencing. Patients who are disorganized have severe difficulty in activities such as maintaining schedules, fulfilling responsibilities, and completing projects. Categorization involves the organizational ability to group similar objects or concepts. Deficits in this area can affect higher level skills such as shopping or budgeting.

### *Abstract Reasoning and Problem-Solving Deficits*

When abstract thinking is impaired, patients show concrete literal thinking. They may propose extremely ineffective, unrealistic, or unsafe answers to questions or solutions to problems.

### *Thought Inflexibility*

Thinking involves the flow of thoughts or ideas and may be affected by stroke. Thought inflexibility or rigidity is the inability to adapt thinking patterns or behavior in response to change. The patient may be labelled as "difficult" as a result of problems accepting new concepts. Changing from one activity to another, changing environments, or following more complex conversation is also impaired.

### *Insight Deficits*

After stroke, insight into lifestyle changes and limitations may be reduced. Dysfunction may be denied despite obvious disability. Continued denial can prolong or prevent the patient's progress toward adjustment to disability.

### *Judgment and Safety Awareness Deficits*

Poor judgment and decreased safety awareness impair the ability to understand consequences of behavior. Patients may be unreceptive to feedback and become argumentative or noncompliant. Family education is very important for patient safety.

### *Generalization and Learning Deficits*

One of the main focuses of stroke rehabilitation is generalization for use after discharge of all skills learned in the hospital. If learning ability is also impaired, carry-over of new techniques may be reduced. To effectively plan treatment to maximize learning, the clinician must understand previous and current learning styles.

### *Cognitive Fatigue*

Performance errors due to cognitive fatigue are common after CVA. Occupational therapy practitioners should be familiar with signs of fatigue and make adjustments in programming accordingly. Signs may include decreased attention and concentration, increased lethargy, increased distractibility, increased performance errors, decreased quality control, decreased performance speed, decreased frustration tolerance, and complaints of fatigue.

### *Occupational Therapy Treatment Considerations*

Occupational therapy intervention for cognitive deficits focuses on maximizing long-term generalization of learned skills and safety procedures.

*Cognitive retraining* Different aspects of cognitive rehabilitation are provided by neuropsychologists, speech-language pathologists, and OT practitioners. Treatment methods for cognitive dysfunction are described in Chapter 24.

*Compensatory strategies for cognitive deficits* Verbal and tactile cues may stimulate patients with decreased initiation to begin an activity. Cues are reduced as skills improve. Establishing realistic, meaningful, achievable treatment goals and giving frequent positive feedback improve motivation. The patient and therapist should plan and modify treatment goals together.

Patients with impaired attention can benefit from brief, frequent sessions in activities of high interest in a nondistracting environment. Time and difficulty are increased as the patient's capacity increases. These activities can be provided in a group format or individually. Orientation methods include reality orientation, reminiscence therapy, use of family pictures, labelling patient's belongings, using calendars and watches, or using props for holidays. Family members and friends can help to individualize the treatment program.

Memory strategies often involve devices. Some of the many commercially available products include notebooks, daily calendars, watches, posted schedules, labels, and pocket memory mates. Occupational therapy intervention for organizational deficits focuses on gradual increase of task complexity. Treatment for sequencing and categorization errors involves building skill level from one step to multiple step tasks. Problem-solving also involves a graded approach with the use of simulations. Patient who are concrete problem-solvers benefit more from a functional approach.

Easing transitions from one activity to another and increasing patient control can reduce anxiety for patients with rigid thinking. Patients with thought inflexibility perform better when breaks between activities are longer to allow time for adaptation. Intervention for insight deficits involves gradual introduction to performance problems, beginning with nonthreatening information and progressing as the patient tolerates. A matter-of-fact approach addressing safety issues is useful. Training should take place in the real-life situations.

Increasing instruction time, repeating instructions, and using written instructions are helpful in addressing learning problems. Understanding the cause of functional problems will suggest treatment strategies. For example, patients may experience difficulty in UE dressing primarily as a result of perceptual and cognitive problems, and deficits in LE dressing may be more related to motor recovery deficits.[70]

## Behavioral Manifestations

After CVA, cognitive deficits may lead to behavioral problems that impair interaction skills. Patients have a limited understanding of the motives and consequences of their behavior. Inappropriate behavior reduces the ability to participate in rehabilitation.

### *Impulsivity and Perseveration*

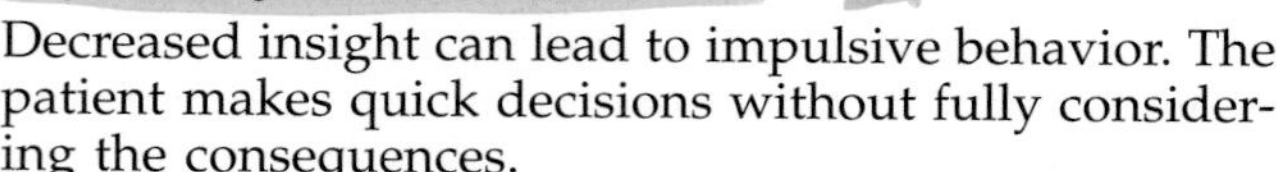

Decreased insight can lead to impulsive behavior. The patient makes quick decisions without fully considering the consequences.

Motor **perseveration** is the meaningless, nonpurposeful repetition of an act.[18,51] The patient usually continues until someone or something intervenes. Perseveration is more obvious during activities that are repetitive in nature, such as writing or combing hair.

### *Mood Impairments*

Many stroke survivors show **emotional lability**,[47] or diminished ability to control the expression of emotions. Inappropriate, uncontrolled outbursts of laughing (euphoria) or weeping are common. Emotionally charged situations, whether pleasant or unpleasant, can cause such responses. Some patients may become agitated, often as a result of confusion. Behaviors may include random movements, yelling, verbal abuse, hitting, biting, spitting, kicking, pulling out medical appliances, removing restraints, or trying to escape. Medications can reduce these behaviors, but some patients may need to be restrained for safety. Brief treatment sessions can be scheduled when medication effects peak and should focus on improving one aspect of function at a time. Frequent treatment sessions throughout the day or cotreatment with other team members is recommended.

Depression after stroke is one of the most underidentified and undertreated conditions. Depression can be reactive, an appropriate grieving response to losses, but it is more often the result of cerebral damage.[27] Strokes of the left hemisphere are much more likely to cause major depression.[33] Poststroke depression affects approximately 20% to 60% of patients annually.[27] Without intervention, severity peaks between 6 months and 2 years after stroke.[27] Early identification and drug treatment can be very effective. Symptoms of depression include lethargy, apathy, extreme fatigue, excessive sadness, forgetfulness, disorganization, loss of appetite, and sleep disturbance.

### *Frustration Tolerance Deficits*

Recovery after CVA can be stressful and frustrating. Some patients with reduced frustration tolerance may act out their negative feelings. Treatment must be individualized to suit the patient's frustration tolerance, which may vary from day to day.

### *Quality Control Errors*

CVA also affects the ability to judge the quality of performance. Patients may show decreased ability to identify errors and may ignore poor performance. They tend to show errors of omission (leaving out details). Inattention, poor memory, lowered frustration tolerance, or depression can increase errors.

### *Behavioral Implications*

Behavioral problems that result from CVA may reduce a patient's ability or willingness to participate in therapy. A history of previous behavior and usual coping methods during crisis helps the OT practitioner understand the current behavior of the patient with cognitive deficits. Shifts in behavior may be viewed as losses by patient and family. The most effective strategy is for health care providers and family members to use the same approaches in responding to behavioral problems of the stroke survivor.

### *Psychosocial Adjustment*

An important role of the OT practitioner is to aid in the patient's adjustment to disability. Treatment approaches and performance expectations should match the patient's level of adjustment. Patients and families may take months to cope with the many personal and social changes. Much repetition may be needed to clarify questions and reduce concerns. Throughout the rehabilitative process, there can be a wide range of reactions such as denial, anger, noncompliance, psychosomatic illness, extreme sadness, complaints of pain or acting out.

Equally important are the patient's social and family circumstances. Caregivers have stated that receiving stroke information and counseling regarding care issues is important to them.[45] Coping with extreme reversals in functional abilities after the CVA is challenging for all involved. Caregivers are at risk for stress-related conditions and burnout. Options such as taking turns in the family, hiring professional help in the home, or using respite care can reduce stress. Some stroke survivors and families choose to participate in community stroke support groups, often after discharge. Engaging family and friends early in the rehabilitative process can reduce stress levels and help to improve generalization of skills to the home environment.

### *Occupational Therapy Treatment Considerations*

Occupational therapy programming for behavioral problems of adult stroke patients focuses on the development of appropriate behaviors and generalization to daily life.

*Behavioral intervention strategies* Strategies for impulsivity include giving directions slowly, verbally, or in written form one step at a time and using a calm approach in a nondistracting environment. Verbal and tactile cues and avoidance of repetitive tasks can reduce perseveration. Some patients with reduced frustration tolerance perform better with new activities in which they have no preconceived ideas about expected performance. The OT practitioner should provide activities that involve choice, using a matter-of-fact approach and immediate positive reinforcement. To improve attention to detail, a graded approach would initially focus on recognition of errors, progressing to correcting errors, and then to checking quality of performance. Checklists provide an ongoing written record of responses that gives the patient feedback on progress.

When treating combative patients, OT practitioners should obtain information regarding their current behavioral state before every session and decide whether treatment is possible at that time. It is recommended that OT practitioners work with one unrestrained extremity at a time in a calm, nondistracting environment. Cotreatment can reduce risk of injury. Soothing music and reduced lighting that begin several minutes before and continue throughout treatment may improve relaxation. If agitation increases, treatment should be immediately discontinued and reattempted only when the patient is calmer.

Many patients and families are unfamiliar with OT services. They may question the value of therapy or express reluctance to participate in activities that seem simple or tedious. OT practitioners must provide ongoing education with respect to these issues. Many patients focus on the possibility of full recovery despite the fact that it is very likely problems may remain. The therapist may approach this matter by discussing it openly and honestly in objective terms but without eliminating hope. Repeated reviews may be needed before the patient begins to apply the information to personal recovery.

*Social skills training* The multiple deficits of stroke can have a major impact on social skills. Common behaviors include acting out, emotional outbursts, interrupting others, seeking constant immediate reinforcement, flirting, or other attention-seeking behaviors. These behaviors can be minimized with consistent limit setting. Social skills training individually or in a group setting can be very effective in improving appropriate behavior.

## Oral-Motor Dysfunction

Oral-motor control is the coordination of movement for speech, facial expression, sucking, chewing, and swallowing. This involves the muscles and other structures of the face, throat, and tongue.

### *Dysarthria*

Normally, the coordination of facial muscles, lips, tongue, and jaw produces articulated speech that can be understood by listeners. After stroke, oral-motor weakness on the affected side causes facial palsy or drooping, especially of the corner of the mouth. Reduced sensation often accompanies muscle weakness. Patients with dysarthria have difficulty pronouncing many sounds or combinations of sounds, causing slurred speech. These patients may be difficult to understand.

### *Dysphagia*

**Dysphagia** is caused by sensory loss and muscle weakness in the structures of the mouth and throat that control swallowing.[12] Patients with dysphagia are at high risk for aspiration (breathing into lungs) of saliva or food,[40] which often leads to aspiration pneumonia. To protect the airway, some patients receive a temporary or permanent tracheostomy ("trach") tube—a tube surgically placed through the skin of the neck and into the trachea. The primary physician determines whether the patient can eat orally or must be tube fed. Many stroke patients with dysphagia are given nutrient liquids and medications by a nasogastric (NG) tube, which passes through the nose into the stomach. NG tubes can cause increased gagging and irritation of the nasal and upper gastrointestinal tract.[23] Confused patients often remove their NG tubes repeatedly unless restrained. Gastrostomy tubes (G-tubes) placed surgically through the abdominal wall into the lower stomach are used by dysphagic patients who cannot eat anything by mouth (NPO).

### *Occupational Therapy Treatment Considerations*

Dysphagia often occurs in association with dysarthria and cognitive impairments.[44] These problems contribute to poorer oral control, increased communication difficulties, and decreased safety while eating.

*Oral-motor control* Patients who have difficulty keeping their lips closed tend to drool saliva and leak food from the affected corner of the mouth. This problem can be minimal to severe and is worsened by impaired sensation. Many patients, especially those with unilateral neglect, may be unaware of the problem. Treatment for dysphagia involves a feeding program and ongoing instruction of patient, family, and staff to promote carryover of feeding techniques. OT practitioners should be aware of the roles of the therapist, patient, and family in the treatment of dysphagia (Table 25-1) (see also Section 1 of Chapter 19).

Safe eating is also related to diet and food choices. Items such as dry foods (bread, crackers, chips), chewy foods (meat, candy), thin liquids (water, soda), and foods with mixed consistencies (casseroles, soups) are problematic. Softer foods such as Cream of Wheat, gelatin, mashed potatoes, applesauce, custards, puddings, popsicles, or ice cream are easier to chew and swallow. Sensory loss may reduce ability to detect hot and cold foods. A variety of diet types and diet modifications can be offered to patients based on individual needs, as determined by the physician, the dysphagia therapist, and the dietitian (see Chapter 19).

*Safety issues* All patients with dysphagia should be supervised by staff at all times to prevent complications and maximize safety. Some patients may be self-conscious about their appearance while eating and may prefer a more private dining setting. Patients with visual perceptual and cognitive problems may show impaired safety, increased spillage (especially with hotter foods or liquids), and noncompliance with dietary changes. OT practitioners should be familiar with all patient precautions, dietary restrictions, symptoms of dysphagia, and emergency procedures in case of choking. Facilities that treat dysphagic patients should have the proper emergency equipment, such as a suction machine, readily available.

## Speech and Language Dysfunction

CVA causes several types of language disorders, varying from mild to severe, often in combination with speech problems. Language dysfunction occurs most frequently in left-sided CVA, but can occur with damage to the right hemisphere. The speech-language pathologist recommends the best communication techniques. The role of the OT practitioner is to reinforce these techniques and adapt communication devices.

### *Aphasia*

**Aphasia** is a language disorder that may result in deficits in verbal comprehension, reading comprehension (alexia), oral expression, written expression (agraphia), ability to interpret gestures, or mathematical skills (acalculia). There are several different types of aphasia. Anomia, or word-finding difficulty, occurs in all types. Patients with expressive aphasia have difficulty speaking, and those with receptive aphasia have problems understanding language. Global aphasia is characterized by a loss of both language skills. The ability to speak is often absent. Patients with global aphasia may *seem* to respond to gestures, voice tone changes, and facial expression. They may appear to understand more than they actually do.[30]

### *Occupational Therapy Treatment Considerations*

Recovery from aphasia is variable. Family education to improve understanding of aphasia by spouses seems to improve adjustment and marital satisfaction.

*Communication guidelines for patients with aphasia* Most patients with aphasia use a variety of communication methods, including alphabet boards, lap typewriters, picture boards, gestures, and writing. Some are able to speak single words or phrases. Patient responses may be less than 100% accurate and become

Table 25-1

## Clinical Considerations for Safe Feeding for Patients with Dysphagia

| OT practitioner | Patient and family roles |
|---|---|
| Determine proper and necessary equipment to promote the best position for eating/feeding. | Patient should be sitting upright with trunk supported and head and neck aligned and slightly flexed to aid swallowing (chin tuck). |
| Know emergency procedures for choking and aspiration. | Understand the causes of choking (one of the signs of difficulty with swallowing) and the potential for aspiration. |
| Know feeding precautions and discuss with patient, family, and team. | Understand feeding problems and need for supervision at all times while eating. |
| Understand food and liquid consistencies of diet. | Comply with prescribed diet to prevent complications. |
| Determine sitting endurance. | Patient should show ability to sit up while eating, and for 30 to 45 minutes afterward. |
| Determine eating/feeding endurance. | Patient should show ability to eat all food and drink items without fatigue, and gradually increase food intake. |
| Determine order of food and drink intake. | Understand why order of food intake improves eating and prevents choking. |
| Determine whether patient should be fed or should begin self-feeding. | Understand that being fed leads to self-feeding with progress. |
| Determine whether training will be individual or in a group setting. | Understand that feeding training is chosen based on individual needs. |
| Select environment in which feeding training will occur. | Understand the dining setting can reduce stress and improve performance. |
| Determine type of eating utensil(s), cup, or devices needed for patient, and train patient, family, and staff with that equipment. | Understand that adaptive equipment can improve eating skills, increase eating safety, and may be needed temporarily. |

less accurate with fatigue. The OT practitioner can engage in meaningful interaction with aphasic patients (Table 25-2).

## HEMISPHERIC LATERALIZATION

### Left-Sided CVA

The left cerebral hemisphere of most right-handed persons is primarily responsible for language, time concepts, and analytical thinking.[17] Patients with right-sided hemiplegia (left brain damage) often achieve self-care independence earlier than patients with left-sided hemiplegia (right brain damage) but are more likely to experience depression.

### Right-Sided CVA

The right cerebral hemisphere primarily controls visual perceptual skills and perception of the whole.[17] Damage to this hemisphere results in difficulties in tasks requiring spatial analysis and orientation and dressing praxis.[69,74] Patients with left-sided hemiplegia may retain good verbal skills, which may tend to hide perceptual dysfunction, and may show poorer functional performance.

### Comparison of Left- and Right-Sided CVA

Although the left and right cerebral hemispheres show specialization, both control several of the same abilities. This may explain how patients who apparently have permanently lost brain function for certain skills are able to regain function. Left-hand dominant adults tend to exhibit less specialization than right-handed adults.[48] (Table 25-3 presents similarities and differences between left and right CVA.)*

### Bilateral CVA

Some patients experience multiple strokes affecting both hemispheres. Patients with significant left- and right-sided hemiplegia and numerous deficits may have functional losses that are more like those of patients with traumatic brain injuries than of patients who have had left- or right-sided CVAs. Treatment interventions for patients with head injury may be used after bilateral CVA (see Chapter 37).

*References 3, 14, 29, 31, 39, 61, 64, 65, 73, 74.

### Recurrent CVA

Despite decreases in the occurrence of new stroke, recurrence rates have not changed.[20] Approximately one third of stroke survivors will have a second stroke.[60] Incidence of death and recurrence are highest for 30 days after the new stroke.[37] Risk of recurrence increases with more strokes.[57] The elderly have the highest recurrence rate, and this rate increases with age.[36] Because of decreased death rates and the increasing elderly population, the numbers of stroke survivors may continue to grow in the next three decades.

*Table 25-2*

**General Communication and Interaction Guidelines for Patients with Aphasia**

| *Clinical approach* | *Therapeutic purpose* |
|---|---|
| Use a calm approach in a nondistracting environment. | Reduces environmental distractions and increases comfort level |
| Use face-to-face interaction at eye level. | Establishes visual attention with visual cues |
| Establish eye contact before conversation. | Maintains visual attention with visual cues |
| Use communication techniques and devices per speech-language pathologist recommendation. | Carries over communication goals |
| Keep messages short and simple. | Improves understanding |
| Encourage patient response and allow time to respond. | Allows sufficient time for patient response |
| Use gestures if simpler than verbal message. | Facilitates communication |
| If message is unclear to patient, rephrase with different words. | Clarifies message with other wording |
| If patient's message is unclear or inaccurate, clarify with the use of other means of communication. | Clarifies patient's message with the use of other senses |
| Give instructions one step at a time. | Prevents memory overload |
| Incorporate family or friends as much as possible. | Establishes better rapport, improves patient's motivation, and increases communication accuracy |

*Table 25-3*

**Differences and Similarities Between Left- and Right-Sided CVA**

| *Left-sided CVA and right-sided hemiplegia* | *Skills* | *Right-sided CVA and left-sided hemiplegia* |
|---|---|---|
| Right-sided paralysis/paresis, decreased motor control of repetitive movements (dysphagia*) | Motor | Left-sided paralysis/paresis, more severe motor problems, decreased motor response time, (dysphagia) |
| Right-sided sensory losses | Sensory | Left-sided sensory loss |
| Right visual field cuts (visual neglect) | Visual | Left field cuts, visual neglect |
| Impaired right/left discrimination, verbal apraxia, (hemi-inattention, motor apraxia) | Perceptual | Unilateral neglect, hemi-inattention, motor apraxia, constructional apraxia, dressing apraxia, agnosia, disorientation for directionality, difficulty crossing midline |
| Decreased analytical thinking, impaired logic, impaired time concepts, impaired memory associated with language | Cognitive | Impaired attention span, impaired understanding of whole, decreased creativity, impaired memory for performance, poor insight, poor safety awareness, poor judgment |
| Slow performance, cautious behavior, depression | Behavioral | Impulsivity, emotional lability |
| Aphasia, agraphia, dyscalculia, decreased understanding of gestures, impaired reading, decreased ability to learn new information, singing without words | Speech and language | Decreased ability to differentiate between gestures, decreased learning for familiar (old) information, singing with words |

*Conditions in parentheses play a lesser role.

## FUNCTIONAL PERFORMANCE AREAS AND OCCUPATIONAL THERAPY TREATMENT TECHNIQUES

Treatment of the stroke patient focuses primarily on occupational performance areas, ADL, work, and leisure.[3] Functional skills are often severely impaired.

### Activities of Daily Living

Occupational therapy intervention often begins with basic self-care, progressing to higher level skills. Many ADL tasks require use of a mirror. The OT practitioner may be the first to introduce new stroke patients to their appearance, which may be considerably changed. Sensitivity to the patient's readiness is needed.

Treatment strategies for stroke patients should be adapted for use of the unaffected dominant UE (one-handedness), use of the unaffected nondominant UE (dominance retraining), and use of both UEs (bilateral integration). The affected limbs should be incorporated into treatment as much as possible and tasks adapted as needed. Functional tasks can be used as treatment for a range of deficits (Table 25-4).

### Work and Productive Activities

Home evaluation early in rehabilitation can assist treatment planning because it allows the OT practitioner to gain a clearer understanding of the discharge environment setting. (See Table 25-4 for treatment strategies in work skills related to stroke.)

### Leisure Activities

Leisure is freely chosen and provides a method of coping with problems.[13] After stroke, disability may prevent participation in previously enjoyed leisure activities. The therapist can provide the patient with information, skills training, and adapted equipment.

*Table 25-4*

**Functional Performance Areas and Treatment Techniques**

| *Performance areas* | *Treatment considerations and activities* | *Adapted equipment and strategies* |
|---|---|---|
| **ADL** | | |
| Grooming: shaving, putting on cosmetics, brushing hair, polishing nails, caring for skin, putting on deodorant | Use mirror for all tabletop and bathroom activities. | Small, adjustable double-sided mirror with magnifying and regular sides; angled wall mirror |
| | Shave face or trim beard and moustache using small scissors. | Electric safety razor, razor holder with strap (for higher-level patients using a manual razor); aerosol can dispenser handles for can such as shaving cream, small scissors or electric nose trimmer |
| | Use patient's own make-up when possible. Practice removing make-up first and progress to applying it; make changes for facial palsy. | Lighted mirror with magnifying side |
| | Comb or brush hair, and practice putting on and taking off hair clips, bobby pins, headbands. | Large-handled comb/brush, extended-handled comb/brush, comb/brush with velco strap |
| | Scrub nails with stationary brush, file nails with stationary nail file, cut nails with stationary nail clipper, and paint nails with stationary nail polish brush. | Suction nail brush, suction nail file, suction nail clipper, small C-clamp |
| | Open and close deodorant, adjust deodorant level, and apply deodorant. | Stick or cream deodorant or baby powder stabilized with suction cup or velcro while applying to uninvolved side |
| Performing oral hygiene: rinsing mouth, caring for teeth or dentures | Open and close mouthwash containers and rinse mouth; open and close toothpaste and brush teeth; and remove, reinsert, and clean dentures. | Built-up handle on toothbrush, diluted mouthwash with water if too strong, pump-style toothpaste dispenser, denture brush, denture tablets (reduced need for brushing), suction denture brush, glycerine swabs |

*Continued.*

Table 25-4

## Functional Performance Areas and Treatment Techniques—cont'd

| *Performance areas* | *Treatment considerations and activities* | *Adapted equipment and strategies* |
|---|---|---|
| Bathing and showering | Wash face, hands (can soak unaffected one), upper body, trunk, and lower body. | Wash mitt, soap-on-a-rope, octopus soap holder, pump-style soap dispenser, long-handled sponge, bath bench, handheld shower, grab rails, suction pillow for back support |
| Performing toileting hygiene: using bedpan, catheters, commode; participating in bladder and bowel program | Roll side to side, bridging and lifting hips to use bedpan. | Bedrails, fracture pan |
| | Empty legbag, change soiled clothing, and receive bladder and bowel program training.<br>Practice clothing management while standing, cleaning after toileting, and toilet transfers. | Legbag straps, catheter clamps, bedside commode, suppository inserter, digital stimulator, Depends panty liners, loose-fitting clothes without fasteners for easier use, raised toilet seat, toilet rails, wall grab bars, handheld toilet paper holder |
| Caring for personal devices: maintaining personal items | Practice cleaning, caring for, and learning sources for repair or replacement of eyeglasses, splints, braces, slings, edema gloves, communication devices, and durable medical equipment, such as wheelchairs or bath seats. | Wash mitt, magnifying lens, notebook with written directions, address book with phone numbers and contact persons |
| Dressing: dressing and undressing, using fasteners, donning and doffing devices | Avoid tight clothing. Take off items first (easier) using hemiplegic methods and progress to putting on—begin with eyeglasses, hats, jewelry, upper body dressing with loose button shirt or sweater, or T-shirt. Use full-length mirror while sitting supported, progressing to unsupported (i.e., edge of bed, fastener boards, shoes [one-handed shoe tie] and socks, lower body dressing while supine or sidelying progressing to edge of bed with feet supported on floor). | Hemiplegic dressing techniques; buttonhook, zipper pull, velcro shoes or loafers; adapted shoelaces; shoe zippers; sock aid; dressing stick; reachers; shoe horn<br>Adapted straps on splints to improve one-handed use<br>Clothes adapted with velcro |
| Feeding and eating: setting up food, using utensils, eating and drinking | Follow dietary guidelines. Eating with spoon may be safer. Cut softer food items and progress to tougher, open seasoning packets and all containers, prepare liquids (i.e., coffee, soups), wipe face as needed, check mouth regularly for trapped food in affected cheek during and after meal, eat small bites and take small sips leaving time to swallow completely, *stop* eating or drinking if choking occurs and take appropriate action, and brush teeth after meal to rid mouth of residual food particles. | Plateguard or scoop dish, adapted cups with lids or easy grip handles, cup holders, extended straws, adapted fork or spoon, rocker knife, dycem matt, thickened liquids, proper positioning, oral motor intervention |

*Table 25-4*

## Functional Performance Areas and Treatment Techniques—cont'd

| *Performance areas* | *Treatment considerations and activities* | *Adapted equipment and strategies* |
|---|---|---|
| Managing medication: obtaining medication, managing containers, taking as scheduled | Understand drug uses and precautions; understand how to adhere to schedule; practice opening and closing containers (removing appropriate dosage); practice simulated administration; carryover skills with nursing; and use consumer skills to learn to ask questions about medications, report side effects, and obtain refills. | Segmented pillboxes with daily and weekly dosage, timers, wristwatch alarms, calendars |
| Maintaining health maintenance and preventing illness | Identify patient's risk factors for stroke and strategies to reduce controllable ones; improve knowledge of nutrition and understanding of prescribed diet; plan and prepare meal, applying information learned; and develop a home-exercise program incorporating SROM and resistive activities and endurance training as indicated. | Cookbooks with low-salt, low-fat, and low-sugar recipes, Theraband, hand exerciser, cuff weights |
| Using functional communication skills: writing; using telephones, typewriters, emergency systems, computers | Establish pen/marker grip; use graded writing beginning with printing, script exercises, writing games, mazes, tracing; copying signature, writing from memory, and handwriting short passages; fold letters and put into envelopes, address, seal and reopen envelopes; complete forms; use pencil and eraser; dial phone number and use telephone book and directory assistance; perform one-handed typing; practice emergency system use; and receive computer training as appropriate to lifestyle. | Enlarged-grip writing utensils, writing aids, clipboard, enlarged telephone dial, phone holders, speaker phone, portable telephone, adaptive hardware (expanded keyboard, touch window), specialized software |
| Performing functional mobility tasks: transferring, functionally ambulating, transporting objects | Participate in progressive mobility training from bed to functional activities while ambulating; roll while supine to sidelying toward unaffected side; roll toward affected side; bridge hips while supine; sit from supine; perform sitting balance activities with back and feet supported using bilateral UEs (hemi-skate, counterbalance slings); sit in balance without back support; sit and then stand, transferring weight between LEs; per form stand-pivot transfer to/from chair toward unaffected side; perform stand-pivot transfer to/from chair toward affected side; and propel wheelchair indoors short distances on flat surface using unaffected UE to push and unaffected LE to steer, progress to longer distances, uneven surfaces, and steeper grades. | Bedrails, overhead trapeze bars, pull straps for LE management, hemi-wheelchair that is 2 inches lower to floor for easier propulsion, wheelchair seat cushion, seatbelt, transfer belt, removable wheelchair brake extension on the affected side, wheelchair accessories, possibly ramp for home<br>Requirements for some patients: recliner, one-arm drive, or electric wheelchair; transfer board; lapboard |

*Continued.*

*Table 25-4*

## Functional Performance Areas and Treatment Techniques—cont'd

| *Performance areas* | *Treatment considerations and activities* | *Adapted equipment and strategies* |
|---|---|---|
| | Perform safe, functional indoor ambulation with assistive device (per physical therapy) while doing ADL or safely carrying items such as toiletries, laundry, and cooking supplies. | Backpack, apron, cup with lid, cart, walker bag or tray |
| Performing community mobility tasks: using public and private transportation | In wheelchair or while ambulating, practice going in/out all types of doors; using the elevator; performing car transfers; ambulating outdoors; calling for a taxi ride or getting information regarding the bus schedule; and riding city bus, taxi, or train (if appropriate). | Grade aids and treated wheelchair tires, shoes with good tread, transfer board, reachers, notebook for information, wheelchair carrier for car, portable or electric ramp for van |
| | Obtain a wheelchair sticker for car or license plate for disabled from state Department of Motor Vehicles if approved by doctor. | Driving evaluation by MD, referral and possibly driver's training by OTR, possibly special controls for driving car or van |
| Responding to emergencies: recognizing sudden hazards, acting to reduce threat to safety | Discuss circumstances regarding admission for stroke and what actions were taken; brainstorm safeguards at home and in community that can improve personal safety, such as inviting local police to visit home and make suggestions to improve security; recommend patient carry valuables on body rather than in backpack on back of wheelchair to prevent theft; recommend patient take self-defense course for disabled patients (often offered by local karate schools or YMCA); and assist patients who are unsafe alone in planning for home supervision. | Personal defense items if desired, home security items, waistpack purse, telephone with patient at all times, touch lamps, door alarms, nightlights, railings on stairs on both sides |
| **Work activities** | | |
| Managing home and caring for clothing | Fold towels, clothes, sheets, blankets; put clothes on hangers; handwash small items; measure laundry detergent and softener; wash and dry clothes; and put clothes in drawers and closet. | Reachers, pull-down ironing board, lightweight iron; work station for laundry |
| Cleaning | Use hand-held vacuum, and vacuum with full-size model; sweep, dust, mop from wheelchair or while ambulating; straighten up room; remove linens from beds, put pillow into pillowcase, and replace linens; and bag trash and throw out. | Lightweight upright vacuum cleaner, long-handled dust pan, wonder-mop (for use with one hand), long-handled cleaning sponge, extra-large pillow cases, fitted bedsheet, trash bags with built-in tie |
| Preparing and cleaning up meal | Cooking involves a graded program beginning with planning and preparing a cold snack, progressing to a light hot snack, a cold meal, a hot meal, and clean-up; full training involves use of all appliances patient would use at home and kitchen mobility and may involve adapting patient's kitchen for easier accessability. | Paring board, jar openers, pot handle holder, rolling cart, one-handed electric can opener, one-handed mixer, angled wall mirror, paring rocker knife, one-handed paring board, built-up handle utensils, oven mitt, labelled drawers and refrigerator, rearrangement of items used most frequently to most accessible place in refrigerator or cabinets |

Table 25-4

Functional Performance Areas and Treatment Techniques—cont'd

| *Performance areas* | *Treatment considerations and activities* | *Adapted equipment and strategies* |
|---|---|---|
| Shopping: selecting and purchasing items, performing money transactions | Perform simulated catalog or telephone shopping, list items to be purchased, count various amounts of money, make change, and shop in hospital store if feasible. | List and money in accessible purse or wallet such as hip pouch, shopping cart |
| Managing money: budgeting, paying bills | Perform commercially available budgeting exercises, write checks, and balance accounts. | Calculator with large numbers and bright number display, flow chart of monthly bills |
| Maintaining household: maintaining home, yard, garden, appliances, and household items | Practice lighter responsibilities such as changing a lightbulb, replacing batteries, watering plants, and cleaning refrigerator—progress as possible; and determine capabilities for certain jobs and assistance options for the remaining jobs. | Ergonomic garden tools (in adapted equipment catalog), electric shears and other tools, riding lawnmower |
| Performing safety: performing prevention and emergency procedures | Develop an emergency plan for medical, fire, and police for home; eliminate fire hazards in the home; practice fire/rescue procedures; post emergency numbers by all telephones on speed dial if possible with code printed on phone; post name, address, and home telephone number by each telephone; and use family or neighbors to check daily on patient living alone. | Fire extinguisher, smoke alarms, rope ladders, generator or battery back-up for medical equipment, call bell to alert others in home for help, emergency alert system membership |
| Caring for others: caring for children, spouse, parent, or others | Care of other adults is probably not possible. Improve care of infant, child, pet, or others. | Baby doll with added cuff weights, adapted games and stories to use with children, adapted animal care products such as larger handled brushes and leashes with solid grips |
| Performing vocational activities: working, planning retirement | Perform simulated work tasks and work hardening.<br>Prepare for retirement. | Adapted work setting to accommodate wheelchair; adapted writing devices; telephone aids; adapted hand tools; wrist supports; UE supports, padding, or wrist glides for computer keyboard use; electric pencil sharpener; calculator with large numbers |
| **Leisure activities** | | |
| Participation in leisure activities | Practice previous leisure tasks adapted by technique or equipment as needed, and develop new leisure skills as indicated. | Bookholders; cardholders, magnifying lenses, adapted games and equipment such as bowling ramps, leather-lacing T-frames, one-handed embroidery hoop, large print playing cards |

Table 25-5

Occupational Performance Domain of Concern—Partial Treatment Plan

| *Stages* | *Occupational therapy emphasis* | *Example of occupational therapy treatment* | *Example of patient goals* |
|---|---|---|---|
| Stage 1—adjunctive methods | Rehabilitation of performance components | Practice bilateral antigravity UE reaching activities in all directions and bilateral fine-motor tasks requiring tip and lateral pinch. | Patient will increase overhead reach of UEs to full and pick up and place 1-inch diameter objects using tip and lateral pinch bilaterally. |
| Stage 2—enabling activities | Rehabilitation of performance components and introducing performance skills (i.e., simulations) | Practice putting on and taking off hospital gown, fastening and unfastening buttonboard on table, and using buttonboard on lap in midline. | Patient will put on and take off hospital gown independently and fasten and unfasten buttonboard independently. |
| Stage 3—purposeful activity | Rehabilitation of performance skills using relevant functional tasks | Practice putting on and taking off a button-down shirt and other UE clothing. | Patient will put on and take off buttondown shirt and put on sweater independently. |
| Stage 4—occupational performance and community reintegration | Renewal of premorbid occupational roles to maximum potential using performance skills | Generalize UE dressing skills to residence at discharge. | Patient will show independent carryover of UE dressing training skills at discharge. |

Continuation of participation in enjoyable activities can reduce stress, improve coping skills, and maximize quality of life after CVA.

### Occupational Therapy Treatment Plan

An example of a partial sample of occupational therapy treatment using the occupational performance domain of concern is shown in Table 25-5.

## SUMMARY

CVA results in a complex set of dysfunctions. The achievement of treatment goals depends on multiple factors including patient recovery and application of appropriate treatment by health professionals.

Within the last decade, inpatient hospital stays have been reduced, with continuation of any further treatment on an outpatient basis. In stroke rehabilitation, much emphasis is placed on maximizing mobility and self-care skills to accelerate the discharge process through intensive physical rehabilitation. Occupational therapy practitioners may be pressured toover-emphasize these physical gains, neglecting other areas, such as cognitive skills, that affect the quality of life after discharge.[54] Motor and functional goal achievement is dependent on integration of perceptual, cognitive, and psychosocial skills.

Rehabilitation goals should not be based on motor improvements only. Rather, the total scope of the disability must be considered, including sensory, perceptual, cognitive, psychological, emotional, and intellectual capabilities. Therapists can adjust programming to accommodate changes in service delivery while still providing professional expertise in maximizing functional performance and facilitating resumption of meaningful occupational roles.*

## *Selected Reading Guide Questions*

1. Explain the difference between a complete CVA and an incomplete CVA or TIA.
2. Name three common warning signs of CVA.
3. Explain why stroke survivors are at higher risk for developing medical complications.
4. Describe how occupational therapy treatment would change for a patient who develops a DVT of the unaffected lower extremity.
5. Describe the effects of long-standing edema of the hemiplegic forearm and hand.
6. How are the occupational therapy goals of prevention of deformity and injury important to the achievement of rehabilitation goals for the stroke patient?
7. Discuss the differences in roles of the OT practitioner treating the stroke survivor in acute care and home health settings.

*We thank Jean Solomon, OTR, for her review and suggestions in writing this chapter.

8. What are the effects of abnormal reflexes and impaired postural mechanisms on the sitting balance of the CVA patient?
9. State and discuss the important considerations for positioning the stroke patient in bed and in the wheelchair.
10. What are the purposes of the lapboard and resting hand splint for the patient with hemiplegia?
11. Explain why PROM is recommended for the patient with a flaccid UE.
12. Why is scapular mobility required for pain-free ROM activities for the shoulder?
13. What can the OT practitioner do to prevent subluxation of the shoulder?
14. What causes a reduction in strength and endurance after CVA?
15. Describe some methods of positioning the affected arm and leg to reduce edema.
16. Why is it important to know the results of visual screening when treating the stroke patient?
17. How does stroke affect vision?
18. Describe how to educate family members about hemianopsia.
19. How would apraxia affect the ability of a patient to learn exercises from a videotape?
20. What treatment strategies could be used to help patients with poor sequencing to brush their teeth?
21. Explain how to increase the attention of a patient who is easily agitated.
22. Explain why consistency in behavioral intervention is important.
23. What could the OT practitioner do to assist a working family to provide a safe home environment for a patient who requires 24 hour supervision and ambulates independently?
24. What factors would prevent a patient from using adaptive equipment for dressing?

## REFERENCES


1. Abreu B: The effect of environmental regulations on postural control after stroke, *Am J Occup Ther* 49(6):517-525, 1995.
2. American Heart Association: *1991 Heart and stroke facts*, Dallas, 1990, The Association.
3. American Occupational Therapy Association: *Uniform* terminology for occupational therapy—third edition, *Am J Occup Ther* 41(11):1047-1059, 1994.
4. Ayres AJ: Perceptual motor training for children. In *Approaches to the treatment of patients with neuromuscular dysfunction.* Proceedings of study course IV, Third International Congress, World Federation of Occupational Therapists, Dubuque, Ia, 1962, William C Brown.
5. Banus BS, editor: The developmental therapist, Thorofare, NJ, 1971, Charles B Slack.
6. Bardach JL: Psychological factors in hemiplegia, *J Am Phys Ther Assoc* 43:792, 1963.
7. Basmajian JV: The winter of our discontent: Breaking intolerable time locks for stroke survivors, *Arch Phys Med Rehabil* 70:92-94, 1989.
8. Bierman SN: Cerebrovascular accident. In Hansen RA, Atchison B, editors: *Conditions in occupational therapy: effect on occupational performance,* Baltimore, 1993, Williams & Wilkins.
9. Birch GH et al: Perception in hemiplegia. 1. Judgment of the vertical and horizontal by hemiplegic patients, *Arch Phys Med Rehabil* 41:19, 1960.
10. Bobath B: *Adult hemiplegia: Evaluation and treatment,* ed 3, Oxford, 1990, Butterworth-Heinemann Ltd.
11. Bornstein NM, Norris JW: Deep vein thrombosis after ischemic stroke: Rationale for a therapeutic trial, *Arch Phys Med Rehabil* 68:955, 1988.
12. Buchholz DW: Dysphagia associated with neurological disorders, *Acta Otorhinolaryngol Belg* 48(2):143-155, 1994.
13. Bundy AC: Assessment of play and leisure: Delineation of the problem, *Am J Occup Ther* 47(3):217-222, 1993.
14. Cadalbert A et al: Singing with and without words: Hemispheric asymmetries in motor control, *J Clin Neurophysiol* 16(5):664-670, 1994.
15. Carpenter MB: Upper and lower motor neurons. In Downey JA et al, editors: *Physiological basis of rehabilitation medicine,* Boston, 1994, Butterworth-Heinemann.
16. Carr JH, Shepherd RB: *A motor relearning programme for stroke,* Rockville, Md, 1987, Aspen.
17. Charness A: *Stroke/head injury.* Rehabilitation Institute of Chicago Procedure Manual, Rockville, Md, 1986, Aspen.
18. Chusid J: *Correlative neuroanatomy and functional neurology,* ed 19, Los Altos, Calif, 1985, Lange Medical Publications.
19. Cooper BA: A model for implementing color contrast in the environment of the elderly, *Am J Occup Ther* 39(4):253-258, 1985.
20. Davidoff GN et al: Acute stroke patients: Long-term effects of rehabilitation and maintenance of gains, *Arch Phys Med Rehabil* 72:869-873, 1991.
21. Daview PM: *Steps to follow: a guide to the treatment of adult hemiplegia,* New York, 1985, Springer-Verlag.
22. Delacato C, Doman G: Hemiplegia and concomitant psychological phenomena, *Am J Occup Ther* 11(186):196, 1957.
23. Dorsher PT, McMichan JC: Pulmonary considerations in rehabilitation. In Sinaki M, editor: *Basic clinical rehabilitation medicine,* St Louis, 1993, Mosby.
24. Flinn N: A task-oriented approach to the treatment of a client with hemiplegia, *Am J Occup Ther* 49(6):560-569, 1995.
25. Formby C, Phillips DE, Thomas RG: Hearing loss among stroke patients, *Ear Hear* 8(6):326-332, 1987.
26. Foulkes MA: Design issues in chemosensory trials, *Arch Otolaryngol Head Neck Surg* 116(1):65-68, 1990.
27. Francisco GS: An overview of poststroke depression, *N J Med* 90(9):686-689, 1993.
28. Gilfoyle E, Grade A: Cognitive-perceptual-motor behavior. In Willard H, Spackman C, editors: *Occupational therapy,* ed 4, Philadelphia, 1971, JB Lippincott.
29. Goldberg E: Associative agnosias and the functions of the left hemisphere, *J Clin Exp Neuropsychol* 12(4):467-484, 1990.
30. Halper AS, Mogil SI: Communication disorders: diagnosis and treatment. In Kaplan PE, Cerullo LJ, editors: *Stroke rehabilitation,* Boston, 1986, Butterworth.
31. Harrington DL, Haaland KY: Hemispheric specialization for motor sequencing: Abnormalities in levels of programming, *Neurophysiologica* 29(2):147-163, 1991.
32. Health JM: Vision. In Ham RJ, Sloane PD, editors: *Primary care geriatrics: A case-based approach,* ed 2, St Louis, 1991, Mosby.
33. Herrmann M et al: Poststroke depression: Is there a pathoanatomic correlate for depression in the post acute stage of stroke? *Stroke* 26(5):850-856, 1995.
34. Jann BB, Rusin MJ, Kovan BS: Rehabilitation and the stroke patient. In Fletcher GF et al, editors: *Rehabilitation medicine: Contemporary clinical perspectives,* Philadelphia, 1992, Lea & Febiger.
35. Kalra L: Does age affect benefits of stroke unit rehabilitation?, *Stroke* 25:347-351, 1994.
36. Kalra L: The influence of stroke unit rehabilitation on functional recovery from stroke, *Stroke* 25:821-825, 1994.
37. Keeney VT, Keeney AH: Emotional aspects of visual impairment in the population over sixty years of age. In Kwitko ML, Weinstock FJ, editors: *Geriatric ophthalmology,* Orlando, 1985, Grune & Stratton.

38. Kent TH, Hart MN: *Introduction to human disease,* ed 3, East Norwalk, Conn, 1993, Appleton-Century-Crofts.
39. Khader MS, Tomlin GS: Change in wheelchair transfer performance during rehabilitation of men with cerebrovascular accident, *Amer J Occup Ther* 48(10):899-905, 1994.
40. Kidd D et al: Aspiration in acute stroke: a clinical study with videofluoroscopy, *Q J Med* 86(12):825-829, 1993.
41. Lieberman JS: Hemiplegia: rehabilitation of upper extremity. In Kaplan PE, Cerullo LG, editors: *Stroke rehabilitation,* Boston, 1986, Butterworth.
42. MacDonald JC: An investigation of body scheme in adults with cerebral vascular accidents, *Am J Occup Ther* 15:75, 1960.
43. Marmor MF: Visual changes with age. In Caird FI, Williamson J, editors: *The eye and its disorders in the elderly,* Bristol, Great Britain, 1986, John Wright & Sons.
44. Martin BJ, Corlew MM: The incidence of communication disorders in dysphagic patients, *J Speech Hear Disord* 55(1):28-32, 1990.
45. McLean J et al: Service needs of stroke survivors and their informal careers: A pilot study, *J Adv Nurs* 16(5):559-564, 1991.
46. Michaels DD: Ocular disease of the aged. In Rosenbloom AA, Morgan MW, editors: *Vision and aging: general and clinical perspectives,* New York, 1986, Fairfield Publications.
47. Morris PL, Robinson RG, Raphael B: Emotional lability after stroke, *Aust N Z J Psychiatry* 27(4):601-605, 1993.
48. Naugle RI, Raymond MJ: Neuropsychological sequelae [sig] of stroke as a function of handedness, *Percept Mot Skills* 73(2):555-562, 1991.
49. Nozer M, Materson RS, Caplan LR: Nature of the problem. In Nozer M, Materson RS, Caplan LR, editors: *Management of persons with stroke,* St Louis, 1994, Mosby.
50. Olsen TS: Arm and leg paresis as outcome predictors in stroke rehabilitation, *Stroke* 21(3):247-251, 1990.
51. Olson DA: Management of non-language behavior in the stroke patient. In Kaplan PE, Cerullo LJ, editors: *Stroke rehabilitation,* Boston, 1986, Butterworth.
52. Pelland MJ: Occupational therapy and stroke rehabilitation. In Kaplan PE, Cerullo LJ, editors: *Stroke rehabilitation,* Boston, 1986, Butterworth.
53. Piambianco G, Orchard T, Landau P: Deep vein thrombosis: prevention in stroke patients during rehabilitation, *Arch Phys Med Rehabil* 76(4):324-330, 1995.
54. Radomski MV: There is more to life than putting on your pants, *Am J Occup Ther* 49(6):487-490, 1995.
55. Rubenstein E, Federman D, editors: *Scientific American: Neurocerebrovascular diseases,* New York, 1994, Scientific American.
56. Rubio KB, Van Dueson J: Relation of perceptual and body image dysfunction to activities of daily living of persons after stroke, *Am J Occup Ther* 49(6):551-559, 1995.
57. Sacco RL: Ischemic stroke. In Gorelick PB, Alter M: *Handbook of neuroepidemiology,* New York, 1994, Marcel Dekker.
58. Sadun AA, Miao M, Johnson BM: The effects of age on parallel processing in the human optic nerve. In Armstrong D, Marmor MF, Ordy JM, editors: *The effects of aging and environment on vision,* New York, 1991, Plenum Press.
59. Schlesinger B: *Higher cerebral functions and their clinical disorders,* New York, 1962, Grune & Stratton.
60. Sinaki M, Dorsher PT: Rehabilitation after stroke. In Sinaki M, editor: *Basic clinical rehabilitation medicine,* St Louis, 1993, Mosby.
61. Sine RD: Disability syndrome of hemiplegia. In Sine RD et al, editors: *Basic rehabilitation techniques: a self instructional guide,* ed 3, Rockville, Md, 1988, Aspen.
62. Soderback I et al: Video feedback in occupational therapy: its effects in patients with neglect syndrome, *Arch Phys Med Rehabil* 73(12):1140-1146, 1992.
63. Spencer EA: Functional restoration. In Hopkins HL, Smith HD, editors: *Willard and Spackman's occupational therapy,* ed 8, Philadelphia, 1993, JB Lippincott.
64. Sterzi R et al: Hemianopsia, hemianasethesia, and hemiplegia after right and left hemisphere damage: a hemispheric difference, *J Neurol Neurosurg Psychiatry,* 56(3):308-310, 1993.
65. Stone SP, Halligan PW, Green RJ: The incidence of neglect phenomena and related disorders in patients with acute right or left hemisphere stroke, *Age Ageing* 22(1):46-52, 1993.
66. Su C-Y et al: Performance of older adults with and without cerebrovascular accident on the test of visual-perceptual skills, *Am J Occup Ther* 49(6):491-499, 1995.
67. Sutin JA: Clinical presentation of stroke syndromes. In Kaplan PE and Cerullo LJ: *Stroke rehabilitation,* Boston, 1986, Butterworth.
68. Trombly CA: *Occupational therapy for physical dysfunction,* ed 3, Baltimore, 1989, Williams & Wilkins.
69. Turner A: *The practice of occupational therapy,* ed 2, New York, 1987, Churchill Livingstone.
70. Walker MF, Lincoln: Factors influencing dressing performance after stroke, *J Neurol Neurosurg Psychiatry* 54(8):699-701, 1991.
71. Williams SE: The impact of aphasia on marital satisfaction, *Arch Phys Med Rehabil* 74(4):361-367, 1993.
72. Yongblood L, Stacey S, Brighton C: Stroke rehabilitation: sensorimotor inegrative treatment versus functional treatment, *Am J Occup Ther* 43(6):391-397, 1989.
73. York CD, Cermak SA: Visual preception and praxis in adults after stroke, *Am J Occup Ther* 49(6):543-550, 1995.
74. Zoltan B, Siev E, Freishtat B: *The adult stroke patient: a manual for evaluation and treatment of perceptual and cognitive dysfunction,* ed 2 rev, Thorofare, NJ, 1986, Slack.


## *RECOMMENDED READING*


Anderson R: *The aftermath of stroke: the experience of patients and their families,* New York, 1992, Cambridge University Press.

Carr JH, Shepherd RB: *Early care of the stroke patient: a positive approach,* London, 1983, Heinemann.

Eggers O: *Occupational therapy in the treatment of adult hemiplegia,* Rockville, Md, 1984, Aspen.

Gordon NF: *Stroke: your complete exercise guide,* Champaign, Ill, 1993, Human Kinetics Publishers.

Okkema K: *Cognition and perception in the stroke patient: a guide to functional outcomes in occupational therapy,* Gaithersburg, Md, 1993, Aspen.

Ozer M, Masterson RS, Caplan LR, editors: *Management of persons with stroke,* St Louis, 1994, Mosby.

Van Deusen J: *Body image and perceptual dysfunction in adults,* Philadelphia, 1993, WB Saunders.

Zoltan B: *Vision, perception, and cognition—a manual for the evaluation and treatment of the neurologically impaired adult,* ed 3, Thorofare, NJ, 1996, SLACK.

Chapter 26

# Arthritic Diseases

Wendy Buckner

## Chapter Objectives

*After studying this chapter, the student or practitioner will be able to:*

1. Identify common symptoms and differences between arthritis, osteoarthritis, and gout.
2. Identify common joint and hand deformities seen in arthritis.
3. Recognize medications commonly used in the treatment of arthritis and their side effects.
4. Recognize surgical interventions commonly performed on persons with arthritis.
5. Identify psychological impact of arthritis.
6. Identify important areas to evaluate in patients with arthritis.
7. Identify treatment objectives of occupational therapy intervention for persons with arthritis.
8. Identify appropriate treatment methods for persons with arthritis, on the basis of diagnosis, stage of disease, functional limitations, type of deformity(ies), and lifestyle.
9. Identify resources helpful to persons with arthritis.
10. Identify treatment precautions.

## Key Terms

connective tissue
inflammation
chronic
systemic
autoimmune
synovitis
tophi
crepitation
osteophytes
joint laxity

Although arthritis literally means *joint inflammation,* it is used to describe many different conditions that cause aching and pain in joints and **connective tissues** throughout the body. Many of these diseases, such as osteoarthritis, do not involve **inflammation.** Three of the more common forms of arthritis are rheumatoid arthritis, osteoarthritis, and gout.[3,20]

## DESCRIPTION OF MAJOR ARTHRITIC DISEASES

### Rheumatoid Arthritis

Rheumatoid arthritis (RA) is a **chronic, systemic, autoimmune** disorder. It is long lasting, involving multiple body systems. In RA, the immune system of the body attacks itself. The course of the disease is different for each person. Some may have a single episode of joint inflammation and a long-lasting remission. The majority of persons with RA will experience inflammation of the joints over long periods of time. The disease process may continuously progress or may follow a series of flare ups or exacerbations and complete or incomplete remissions. Remissions provide a period of pain relief, but this does not mean the condition has been cured. It may flare up again. In addition, any damage done during an active stage remains. The patient's functional skills may vary depending on the course of the disease and the severity of the symptoms.[2,7,20]

The systemic symptoms characteristic of RA include fatigue, loss of appetite, fever, overall achiness or stiffness, and weight loss. Morning stiffness, an overall stiffness that occurs on awakening, is another indicator of systemic involvement. The severity of the systemic symptoms usually matches the severity of joint involvement. As in many chronic diseases, there may also be a resulting depression or lack of motivation. In a small percentage of persons, the blood vessels, heart, lungs, or eyes may be involved.[2,7,20]

The cause of RA is unknown. It occurs most frequently between the ages of 30 and 40, and women are three times more commonly affected than men.[2,7,18] Its outstanding clinical feature is **synovitis,** or inflammation of the synovial tissue surrounding the joints. The function of the synovial tissue is to produce fluid to lubricate the joint. Joint swelling results from an abundance of synovial fluid, enlargement of the synovium, and thickening of the joint capsule. This weakens the joint capsule, tendons, and ligaments. Inflamed joints will be warm, swollen, tender, often red, and difficult or painful to move. There is usually a loss of range of motion (ROM), strength, and endurance. As the inflammation continues it invades the cartilage, bone, and tendons and secretes enzymes that damage them. If the inflammation is not stopped, the cartilage, bone, tendons, and ligaments surrounding the involved joint(s) can be destroyed. Scar tissue can form between the bone ends, and the joint can become fused, permanently rigid, and immovable.[2,5,7,20]

Joint involvement is frequently bilateral.[5] If one hand is involved, the other one is also. However, the disease progression is often different on the two sides. One side may be more involved than the other and have different deformities. The joints most affected by RA are the wrist, thumb, and hand. RA is frequently seen in the proximal interphalangeal (PIP) and metacarpophalangeal (MCP) joints, whereas the distal interphalangeal (DIP) joints are usually spared severe damage. The elbows, shoulders, neck, jaw, hips, knees, ankles, and feet also may be involved. The spine is usually not directly affected.[2,5,20]

### Osteoarthritis (Degenerative Joint Disease)

Osteoarthritis (OA) is a disease that causes the breakdown of cartilage in joints, leading to joint pain and stiffness. Unlike RA, OA is not inflammatory or systemic, but limits its attack to individual joints. It is often referred to as the *wear and tear* disease because the involved joints wear down with age or overuse. Up to the age of 45 years, OA is more common in men; beyond age 54, it is more common in women.[2]

In OA the breakdown of joint tissue occurs in several stages. First, the smooth cartilage softens and loses its elasticity. This allows it to be more easily damaged. Eventually, large sections of the cartilage wear away completely and permit the bones to rub together, causing pain. The joint may lose its normal shape. As the ends of the bone hypertrophy (thicken), spurs (bony growths) are formed where the ligaments and capsule attach to the bone (Figure 26-1). These spurs are also referred to as *osteophytes.* Fluid-filled cysts may form in the bone near the joint. Bits of bone or cartilage may float loosely in the joint space. The joint becomes stiff or unstable. Joint motion becomes restricted and painful. Occasionally, the process of osteoarthritis causes irritation of the joint, and local inflammation may occur.[1,20]

OA can affect any joint and is most frequently seen in the weight-bearing joints of the hips, knees, spine, and the metatarsal phalangeal joint of the big toe, producing bunions.[1,5] In the hand, the DIP joints, PIP joints, and the carpometacarpal joint at the base of the thumb are most likely to be affected. Hip and knee involvement cause the most severe disability and may require surgery for joint replacement.

The symptoms of OA usually begin slowly and may appear as a minor ache or soreness with movement. Pain is most frequently felt in the affected joint(s) after overuse or long periods of inactivity. The joint becomes stiff, although movement is possible. If the joint is not moved, surrounding musculature becomes weak. Coordination and posture may also be impaired.[1,5]

Degenerative joint disease (DJD) occurs in some degree among many people over the age of 60. Although it is most common in the elderly, other factors such as obesity, heredity, injury, and overuse of joints can aggravate the disease process.[1,5,20]

### Gout

Gout is a metabolic disease marked by urate (a by-product of the kidneys) deposits that cause recurrent acute episodes of arthritis. It occurs most frequently in middle-aged men (40 to 50 years old). It rarely occurs in women until after menopause.[4,5,20]

The exact cause of gout is unknown. It appears to be the result of a genetic defect in body chemistry that causes uric acid, a normal body substance, to be either overproduced or produced faster than the kidneys can dispose of it. The increased concentration of uric acid leads to the formation of **tophi** (needlelike crystals of sodium urate) in joints or tissues. This causes severe inflammation.[4,5,20]

Gout follows an intermittent course and often leaves patients free of symptoms for years between attacks. The acute onset is very rapid. The inflamed joint displays extreme heat, pain, redness, and swelling within

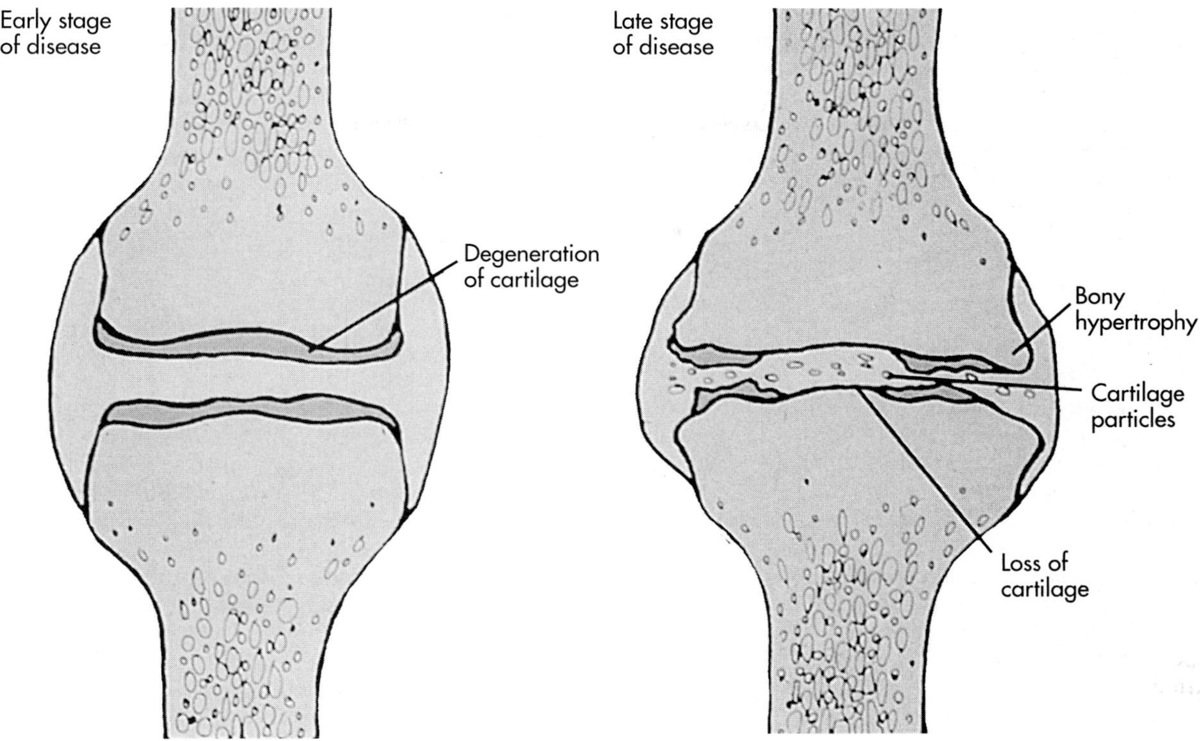


*Figure 26-1* Joint involvement in osteoarthritis. (From the ARHP Arthritis Teaching Slide Collection, American College of Rheumatology.)

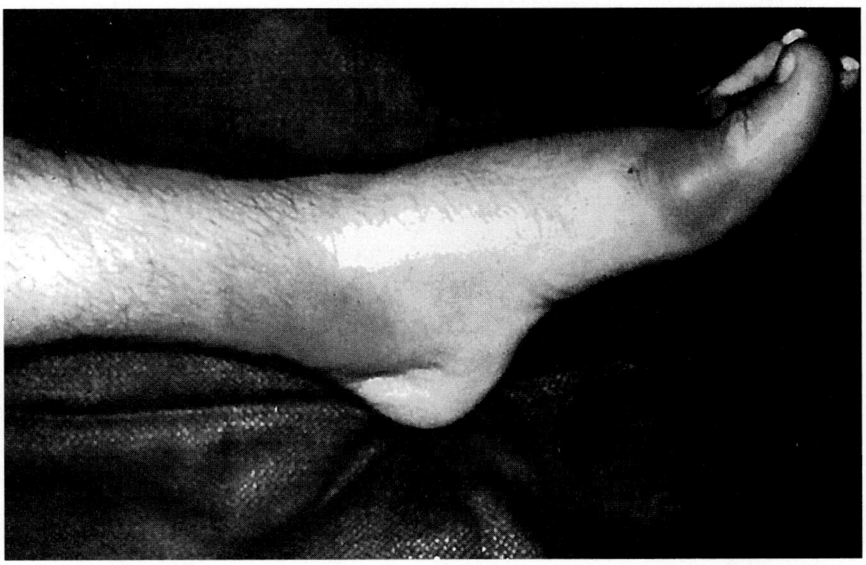

*Figure 26-2* Podagra—gout. (From the ARHP Arthritis Teaching Slide Collection, American College of Rheumatology.)

several hours. The attack of gout is an extremely painful arthritis; it usually affects one joint. The most common site of involvement is in the big toe. The metatarsophalangeal joint of the big toe becomes inflamed first (podagra), then the instep, ankle, heel, knee, or wrist joints (Figure 26-2). With treatment, the prognosis is good. Appropriate medication can limit the initial attack to a few days and prevent further attacks.[4,5,20]

Without proper medication, recurrent episodes may affect more than one joint. Severe attacks may persist for days or weeks. The accumulation of urate crystals can erode into the joints, cartilage, synovial membranes, tendons, and soft tissue, with resulting joint deformity. This can lead to chronic disability, severe hypertension, and progressive renal failure.[4,5,20] Occupational therapy is seldom needed for an acute attack of gout, unless resting splints are required. Referral to occupational therapy may be for decreased hand function as a result of tophi. Adapted equipment and assistive techniques may be beneficial for the patient's functioning.[4,5,20]

## Description of Common Upper Extremity Joint and Hand Deformities

The destructive processes seen in arthritis can result in tendon, muscle, and nerve dysfunction and many joint deformities. A brief explanation of some of the most common deformities follows.

**Crepitation** is seen in both RA and OA and occurs as the joints degenerate. It is characterized by a grating, crunching, or popping sensation (and/or sound) that occurs during joint or tendon motion. When documenting the presence of crepitus, the location and/or motion that caused the sensation should be noted.[1,20]

### *Osteoarthritis*

In osteoarthritis, **osteophytes** or bone spurs may form in the fingers or at the base of the thumb.[1,5,20] This indicates there has been cartilage damage. Osteophytes are hard to the touch and generally are not painful. They are most commonly seen at the DIP joint and are called *Heberden's nodes* (Figure 26-3). If seen at the PIP joint they are called *Bouchard's nodes* (Figure 26-3).

Osteoarthritis may also involve the carpometacarpal (CMC) joint at the base of the thumb. This joint is highly mobile and is subject to a large amount of stress during pinch activities. The most common symptom is pain with motion. Patients may be limited in many activities, because the thumb accounts for 45% of hand function.[20] As the disease progresses, osteophytes may form and the joint can sublux, giving a squared appearance (Figure 26-4).[6]

### *Rheumatoid Arthritis*

The hands are the most severely affected sites of RA.[2,5,20] A typical sign of RA is the fusiform (spindle-shaped) swelling in the PIP joints (Figure 26-5). Swan neck and boutonniere deformities may also result from muscle and tendon contractures. The swan-neck deformity involves a flexion contracture of the MCP joint, hyperextension of PIP joint, and flexion of the DIP joint (Figure 26-6). Patients who have a swan-neck deformity will be unable to make a fist or to flex the PIP joint to hold small objects. The boutonniere deformity may look worse than a swan-neck deformity, but it does not impair function as much. It is a combination of PIP flexion and DIP hyperextension (Figure 26-7). Its cause is the detachment of the central slip of the extensor tendon, so the patient is unable to extend the PIP joint.[2,5,20]

Trigger finger is caused by a nodule or thickening of the tendon at the entrance of the tendon sheath. The tendon's gliding motion through its sheath is hindered, and this results in a snapping or catching of the finger during active flexion or extension (Figure 26-8). If persistent triggering occurs, it may result in lost ROM or tendon rupture.[5,20]

The MCP and CMC joints are the most common sites

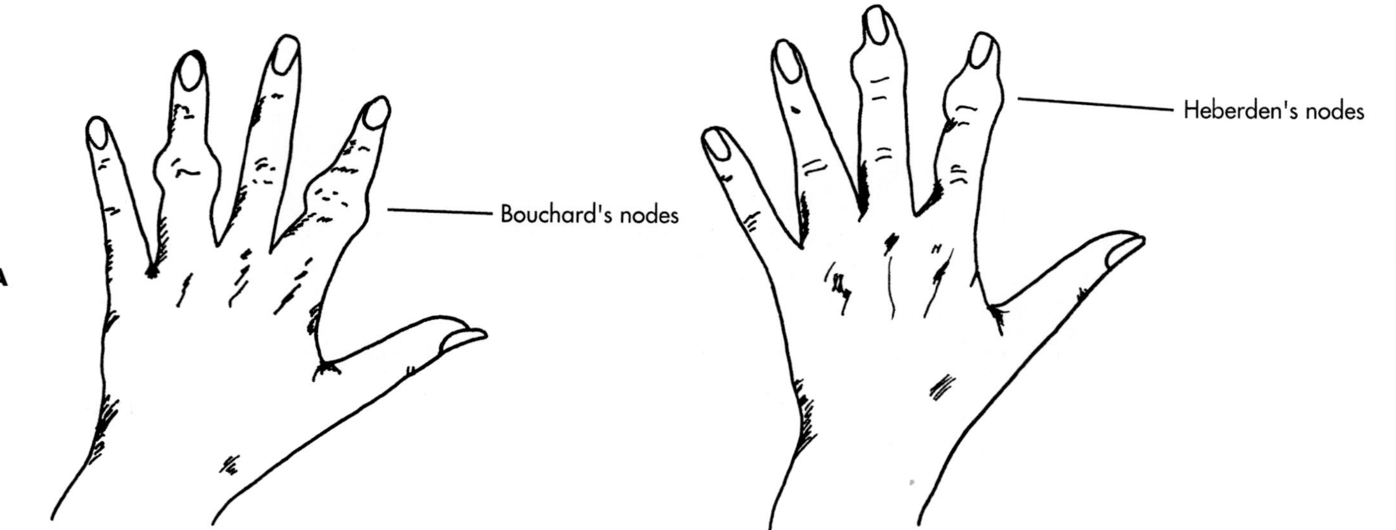


*Figure 26-3* Osteophyte formation in the **(A)** proximal interphalangeal joints (Bouchard's nodes) and **(B)** distal interphalangeal joints (Heberden's nodes) are characteristic of osteoarthritis.

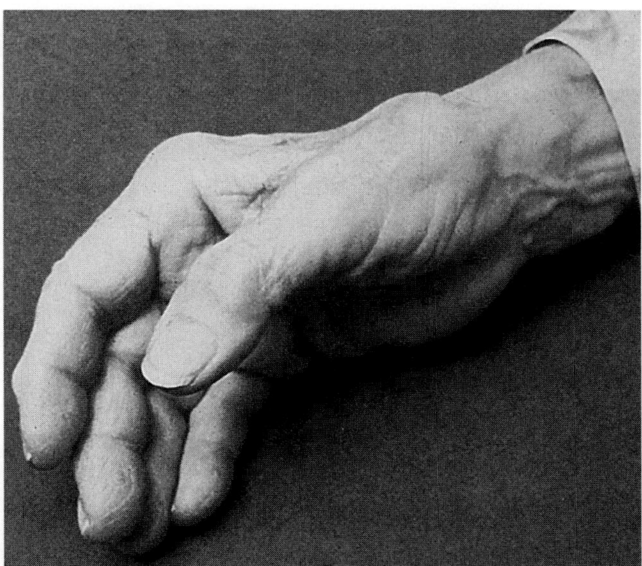

*Figure 26-4* Arthritic changes in the carpometacarpal joint of thumb result in a squared appearance. (From the ARHP Arthritis Teaching Slide Collection, American College of Rheumatology.)

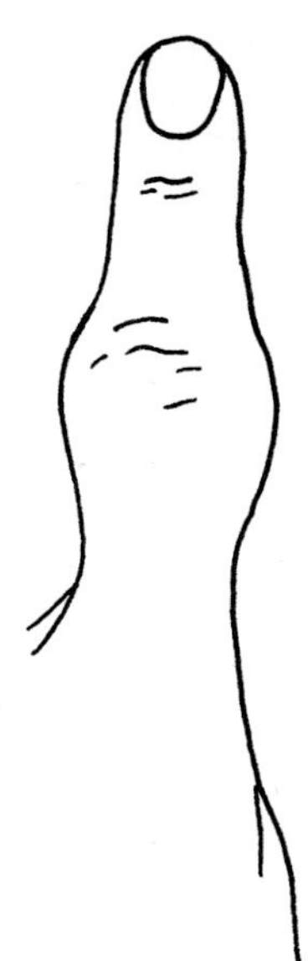

*Figure 26-5* Fusiform swelling.

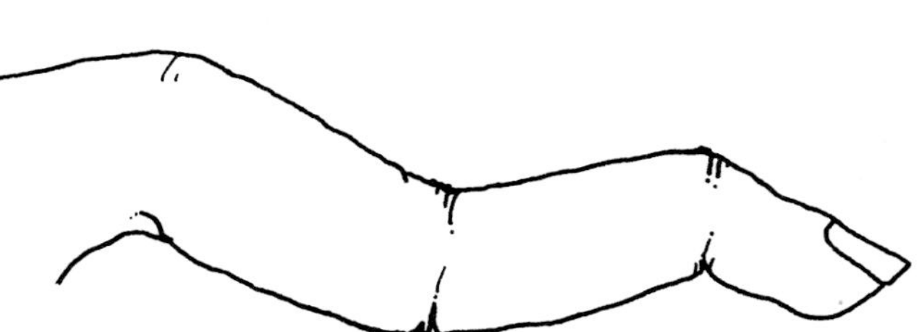

*Figure 26-6* Swan-neck deformity results in PIP hyperextension and DIP flexion.

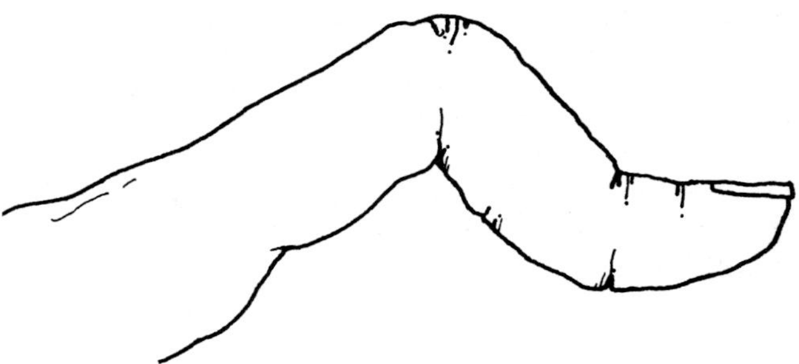

*Figure 26-7* Boutonnière deformity results in DIP hyperextension and PIP flexion.

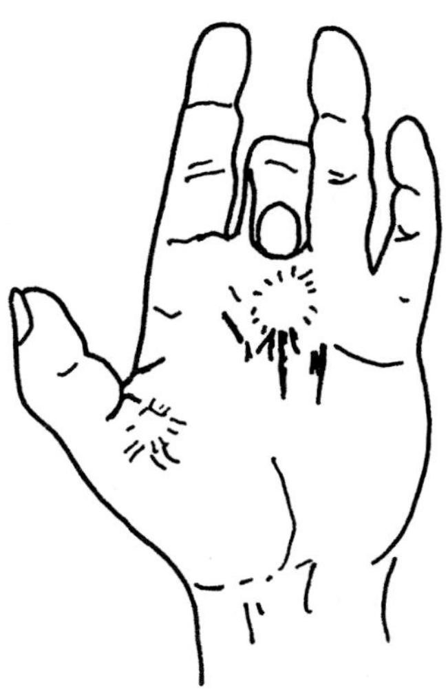

*Figure 26-8* Trigger finger. (From Melvin JL: *Rheumatic disease in the adult and child: occupational therapy and rehabilitation,* ed 3, Philadelphia, 1989, FA Davis.)

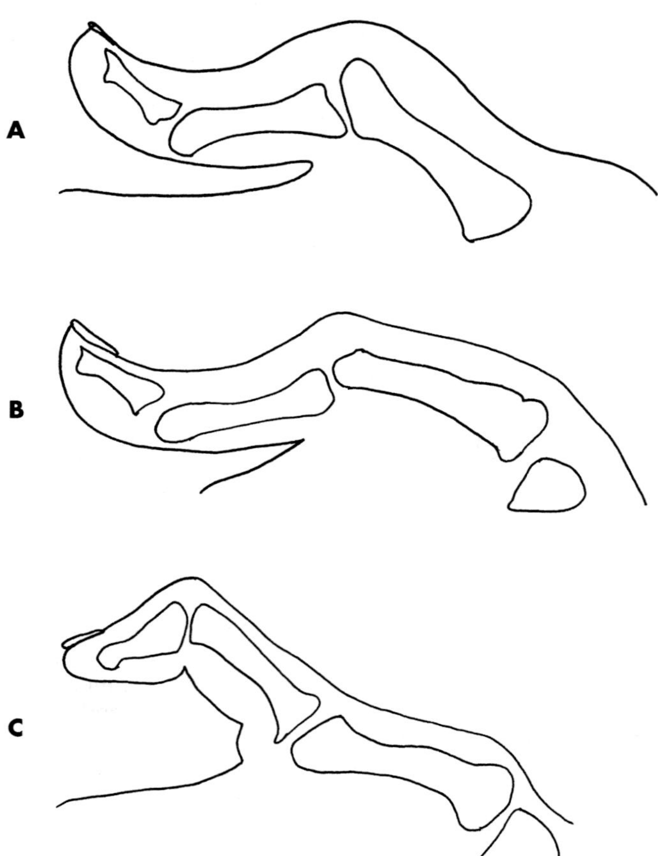


*Figure 26-9* Common rheumatoid thumb deformities. **A,** Type I—IP Hyperextension, MP Flexion. **B,** Type II—IP Hyperextension, MP Flexion, Carpometacarpal Subluxation. **C,** Type III—IP flexion, MP hyperextension, Carpometacarpal Subluxation. Type I is the most common deformity seen in RA, followed by Type III. Although Type II is seen infrequently in RA, it is a common sequela of OA of the CMC joint. (From Melvin JL: *Rheumatic disease in the adult and child: occupational therapy and rehabilitation,* ed 3, 1989, Philadelphia, FA Davis.)

of inflammation in the thumb.[2,5,20] Thumb deformities are referred to by several names. Many clinicians use the same terms that are used with the fingers. The Nalebuff classification uses three categories (Figure 26-9). Type I is the most commonly seen deformity in RA. It begins with chronic synovitis of the MCP joint, leading to stretching of the joint capsule and flexion of MP joint with hyperextension of the interphalangeal (IP) joint. The type II deformity is rarely seen. It involves subluxation of the CMC joint that lead to a fixed adduction contracture with hyperextension of the distal phalanx.[20] The type III deformity is seen in both RA and OA. It is characterized by MCP flexion and hyperextension of the DIP joint.[7,20,22]

**Joint laxity** is a term that describes ligamentous instability and is a major cause for loss of hand function. In the fingers and thumb, the collateral ligaments support the joint capsule on either side. Chronic synovitis can result in stretching or lengthening of the ligaments and abnormal lateral movement. When the thumb IP joint becomes unstable, the thumb tip can easily be wiggled by the therapist, but the patient loses the ability to oppose the thumb and manipulate small objects (Figure 26-10). Joints may also become subluxed or dislocated (Figure 26-11) due

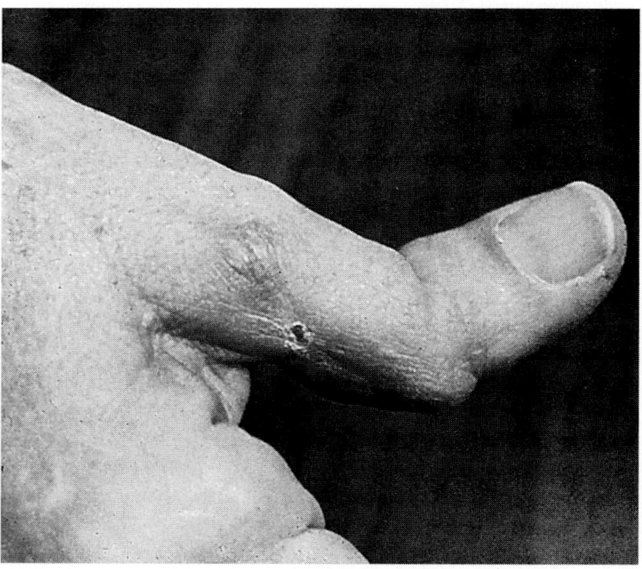

*Figure 26-10* Joint laxity (instability). (From the ARHP Arthritis Teaching Slide Collection, American College of Rheumatology.)

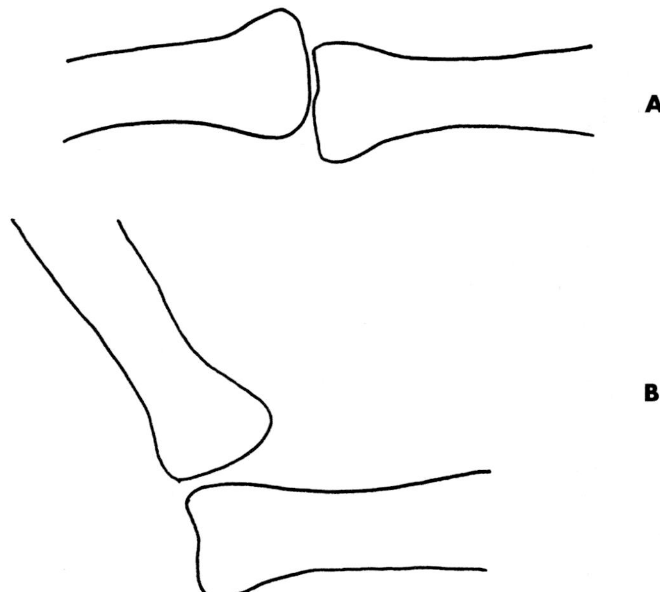


*Figure 26-11* **A,** Subluxation. **B,** Dislocation. (From Melvin JL: *Rheumatic disease in the adult and child: occupational therapy and rehabilitation,* ed 3, 1989, FA Davis.)

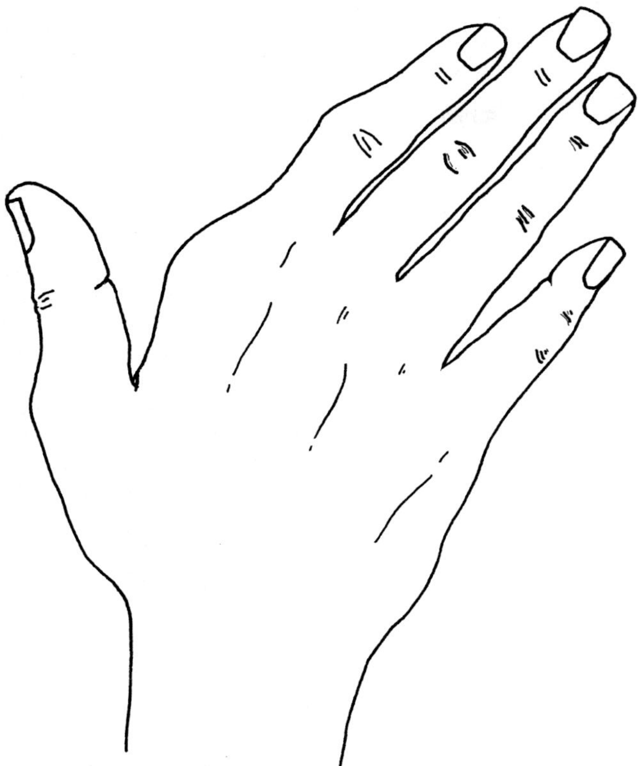

*Figure 26-12* MP joint ulnar drift.

to weakened ligaments. The most common sites of subluxation are in the wrist and MCP joints.[5,7,20]

A characteristic sign of RA is ulnar drift or deviation of the MCP joint (Figure 26-12). Synovitis of the MP joints leads to weakness or destruction of the ligaments. Normal muscle forces acting on these unstable joints can pull the joint toward the little finger. Forced contractions and especially forceful hand grip increase this tendency.[5,20,30]

Loss of elbow and shoulder motion because of weakness, pain, and contractures are also common occurrences in RA. Secondary conditions such as tendonitis and bursitis are frequent causes of pain. Frozen shoulder is a complication of shoulder synovitis. This is characterized by very restricted ROM.[20] In addition, most patients with RA develop muscle weakness as a result of disuse, bed rest, and drug effects.[16]

## MEDICAL MANAGEMENT

There is no known cure for arthritis. Treatment is geared toward reducing inflammation, pain, and joint damage. Treatment methods include medication, exercise, use of heat and cold, joint protection techniques, weight control, surgery (when necessary), and coping strategies.[2,4,5,20] When making treatment decisions, both the benefits and risks (or costs) of one form of treatment over another must be considered.

### Drug Therapy

Many drugs are used in treating arthritis. Drug therapy is constantly changing, and no single method is recommended over all other methods.[20] Patients' needs and reactions change and each physician develops his or her own philosophy and regimen. Allied health professionals need to be aware of the medical protocols used in their facilities and of the specific medications (and their side effects) taken by their patients.

In large doses, aspirin is one of the most frequently prescribed medications because it reduces pain and inflammation with tolerable side effects. Inflammation can also be reduced with the newer nonsteroidal antiinflammatory drugs (NSAIDs) that are used individually or in conjunction. Some side effects include stomach pain, diarrhea, dizziness, headache, nausea, ringing in the ears, and dark stools (bleeding).[2,7,20]

Steroids are effective as antiinflammatory and pain reducing agents but have serious side effects such as bone erosion, diabetes, weight gain, emotional problems, and hypertension. Steroids are used most frequently on a temporary basis if the disease is not adequately controlled by other medications alone.[2,20] Gold salts and antimalarials are slow-acting medications that suppress inflammation and can alter the course of the disease.[20] Two to three months of drug therapy may be required before their full benefit is seen. These drugs are toxic and must be given in carefully regulated doses. Side effects include diarrhea, skin rashes, mouth ulcers, bone marrow suppression, and possible blindness. Any of these symptoms should be promptly reported to the physician.

### Surgical Intervention

Treatment of the patient with long-term RA will often include operative procedures to repair soft tissue or replace joints destroyed by the rheumatoid process.[3,20] Several surgical procedures may be of benefit to patients with RA. Synovectomy (removal of the diseased synovium) and tenosynovectomy (removal of diseased tendon sheath) are performed to prevent further complications. These surgeries relieve symptoms and slow down the process of joint destruction or tendon rupture and help preserve vascular supply to the joint. The removal of the excessive tissue does not prevent the progression of the disease. A synovectomy may be performed on the ankle, knee, hip, MCP, wrist, elbow, or shoulder.[3,20]

Tendon surgery (including tendon relocation, tendon repair, tendon transfer, and tendon release) is considered a corrective strategy for specific hand impairments. Tendon surgery is most frequently performed on the extensor tendons of the hand and wrist.[3,20] Arthroplasty (joint reconstruction) and arthrodesis (joint fusion) may be done when joint restoration is not possible. Both types of surgery may be performed to relieve pain, provide stability, correct deformity, and improve function. Common sites for these types of surgery are the ankle, knee, hip, first MCP, PIP, and wrist.[3,20]

## PSYCHOLOGICAL FACTORS

The "rheumatoid personality" was once characterized as rigid and hostile. This description is no longer considered valid as those same personality characteristics are found in many other persons, both with and without a chronic illness.[17] Any person with a chronic illness must develop coping strategies to deal with the disability. The effects of arthritis on a patient's function and lifestyle can cause an adjustment process similar to the grief process after a death. Because the disease is both painful and unpredictable, reactions such as depression, denial, and anxiety are common. Psychological stressors may also contribute to an exacerbation of the disease.[26]

Family relationships and culture will influence the patient's response to the disability.[17] Occupational therapy practitioners need to understand their patients' responses and work to facilitate their adjustment to the disease. (See Chapter 13 for information on psychosocial adjustment to physical disability.) It is important for the patients and their families to learn all they can about the disease and to have opportunities to share their concerns.[5,20] The arthritis support groups available through the Arthritis Foundation will be helpful for many (see Resources list at the end of chapter).

## OCCUPATIONAL THERAPY INTERVENTION

### Evaluation of Functional Abilities and ADL

The functional abilities of the patient with arthritis must be the first consideration in evaluation. Deformity and decreased function do not necessarily go hand in hand. For example, impaired ROM and joint deformities may be seen in the patient who functions well independently. Such a patient may use substitute motions to complete tasks. In contrast, the patient with no apparent deformities may be severely disabled for routine tasks because of pain, edema, or joint laxity.[5,20] It is also important to consider the effect of medication on performance.[20]

The initial interview should consider such factors as the medical history, joints involved, presence of pain, medication, functional abilities, and the current symptoms the patient is experiencing.[20] It is also important to find out how much the patient already knows about arthritis, and if any exercise or splinting program is being followed. If the patient reports pain, it is important to ask "Where is it?" "When does it occur?" and "How does it limit your abilities?" The patient may also be asked to complete a pain rating on a scale of 0 (no pain) to 10 (greatest pain) at different times of the day or with different activities. The patient should be asked if morning stiffness is experienced. Morning stiffness that lasts less than an hour would be more characteristic of OA. With RA, the stiffness would last for longer than an hour. The interview should address present abilities and the potential for independence in self-care. The patient's tolerance for activity should be noted. This type of interview may be conducted by either the registered occupational therapist (OTR) or the certified occupational therapy assistant (COTA) with a structured format such as the Arthritis Evaluation Checklist (Figure 26-13).

The patient should be observed for signs of acute inflammation. These include pain, heat, swelling, and redness.[2,20] When observing the patient's movements, look for signs of pain, loss of ROM, decreased muscle strength, and the presence of joint deformities. Strength of the lower extremities can be observed in the patient's gait pattern and when the patient rises from a chair. If the patient must use arms and hands to push off, this indicates weakness. The patient's use of joint protection techniques can be observed during functional activities.[5,20]

The OTR determines whether objective measurements of ROM, strength, gross and fine coordination, sensation, and cognition should be taken (see Chapters 8, 9, 10, and 11). The actual testing may be done by the OTR or by a COTA who has met service competencies in the specific areas. When completing these measurements, the occupational therapy practitioner should be careful not to stress the joints. For this reason, grip and pinch strength may be tested with an adapted blood pressure cuff and measured in mm Hg.[5,20] Manual muscle testing may not be possible because of joint instability and alterations in the line of muscle pull. Touch, pain, temperature, and proprioceptive sensations may be impaired as a result of nerve damage. Depression may cause deficits in attention span, short-term memory, and problem-solving skills.[7]

The evaluation of activities of daily living (ADL) for patients with arthritis is similar to ADL evaluations for other physical disabilities (see Chapter 17). However, the evaluation should consider such factors as morning stiffness, medication schedule, activity tolerance, and proper positioning.[17,20] Patients with arthritis may report both "good days" and "bad days." It is important to find out the relative percentage of each and how the patient's functional abilities differ on good and bad days. Such information may help the patient learn how to prevent pain and stress to the joints and to increase functional independence.[17,20]

Evaluations for ADL, work, and leisure activities should consider both psychological and social factors. What is the patient's attitude toward the disability? What specific goals does the patient have? What strategies are used to deal with pain and fear? The patient's abilities may be determined in part by interview. The actual performance should be observed at the normal time each activity is performed because the patient's abilities may change at different times of the day. Ideally, a home evaluation should be done in the patient's home. On site or simulated experiences may be used to assess job performance. In all areas of ADL, it is essential to determine whether the patient is using energy conservation and joint protection techniques.[5,17,20]

## ARTHRITIS EVALUATION CHECKLIST

Name: ______________________ Diagnosis: ______________________

Referral: ______________________

**Initial Interview:**

Which joints bother you the most? ______________________

Pain: at rest _____ on movement _____ constant _____ Description ______________________

Do you experience morning stiffness? _____ Duration? ______________________

Which medications are you presently taking? ______________________

Since taking the medication, have you noticed any of the following? (circle)

headaches nausea itching rash ringing in ears other __________

Surgeries? ______________________

Exercise program? ______________________

Splints? ______________________

What do you know about arthritis? ______________________

What are your goals? ______________________

**UPPER EXTREMITY ROM:**

| | | RIGHT | | LEFT | | COMMENTS |
|---|---|---|---|---|---|---|
| | | Active | Passive | Active | Passive | |
| **Shoulder** | Extension/flexion | | | | | |
| | Adduction/abduction | | | | | |
| | Internal rotation | | | | | |
| | External rotation | | | | | |
| **Elbow** | Extension/flexion | | | | | |
| **Forearm** | Supination | | | | | |
| | Pronation | | | | | |
| **Wrist** | Flexion | | | | | |
| | Extension | | | | | |
| | Ulnar/radial deviation | | | | | |

**Limitations:**

**HAND PLACEMENT EVALUATION:**

Key: 0—Easily
1—With minimal difficulty
2—With moderate difficulty
3—Unable

| | RIGHT | LEFT | COMMENTS |
|---|---|---|---|
| Reach overhead | | | |
| Touch top of head | | | |
| Touch mouth | | | |
| Touch back of neck | | | |
| Touch behind back | | | |

*Figure 26-13* Arthritis evaluation checklist.

*Continued.*

**HAND**

| | RIGHT | LEFT |
|---|---|---|
| 9 hole peg (seconds) | | |
| Grip strength | | |
| Pinch: lateral, 3-jaw | | |
| Opposition | | |

COMMENTS

**Sensation:**

Soft tissue and hand deformities noted: (including flexion contractures, swan neck, boutonniere, ulnar deviation, subluxation, edema, redness, warmth)

________________________________________

________________________________________

FUNCTIONAL ABILITIES: Key: 0—Easily 1—With minimal difficulty 2—With moderate difficulty 3—Unable

| | |
|---|---|
| Grasp spoon or fork | |
| Carry to mouth | |
| Cut meat | |
| Drink from glass/cup | |
| **Bilateral activities** | |
| Button | |
| Manipulate coins | |
| Turn key in lock | |
| Write name | |
| Turn pages | |
| Use telephone | |
| Open doors | |
| Open jars | |

COMMENTS

Endurance: ____________________

Marital status: ______ Family members/supportive persons at home: ____________

Household responsibilities: ____________________

Do you have difficulty in ADL? ____________________

Architecture: ____________________

Vocational responsibilities: ____________________

RECOMMENDATIONS: Adaptive equipment (circle): key extension feeding device writing device telephone device car door opener dressing stick buttonhook other ____________

Splints: ____________________

Joint protection: ____________________

Home program: ____________________

Evaluation completed by: ____________________ Date: __________

*Figure 26-13, cont'd* Arthritis evaluation checklist.

### Treatment Objectives

Treatment of the patient with arthritis must take into account the chronic and progressive nature of the disease.[17] An overall goal of treatment is to decrease pain and inflammation. According to Hittle et al,[17] the general objectives of treatment in occupational therapy are to (1) maintain or increase joint mobility and strength; (2) increase physical endurance; (3) prevent, correct, or minimize the effect of deformities; (4) maintain or increase ability to perform activities of daily living; (5) increase knowledge about the disease and the best methods of dealing with the physical, psychological, and functional effects; and (6) assist with stress management and adjustment to physical disability.

The treatment plan should be designed for the individual patient and be based on the severity of the symptoms as well as the general health status, lifestyle, and personal goals of the patient. The patient should be an active participant in the treatment process. Both the patient and significant others need to understand the disease process and treatment methods. Rehabilitation intervention will most likely be intermittent so that the patient's ability to follow through with the treatment methods between visits will greatly influence the success of the treatment.[5,20]

### Treatment Methods

A number of treatment strategies are used in occupational therapy for the management of arthritis. Traditional methods include rest, positioning, physical agent modalities, exercise, therapeutic activity, splinting, and ADL training. The choice of methods will depend on the patient's condition and reaction to the various procedures.

#### *Rest*

Rest is an important part of treatment and should be considered a very effective way of reducing inflammation. Rest can take several forms. The required amount of systemic rest varies with individuals—from complete bed rest to a short nap during the day. Localized rest to individual joints might include wearing a splint to support the involved joint during activity or lying in non–weight-bearing positions to prevent joint stress. Psychological rest may be experienced with a short diversion from routine activities or a refocusing of attention on enjoyable instead of stressful events.[7,9,16]

#### *Positioning*

Positioning against the patterns of deformity is recommended to prevent contractures. To prevent flexion contractures, persons with arthritis should *not* sleep with a pillow under the knees and should use only a small pillow under the neck. Prone lying is recommended for both the hip and knee joints. Maintaining good postural alignment when standing and sitting will discourage the development of deformities and prevent undue stress to the muscles and joints. Patients may benefit from using chairs with high seats and armrests as these will make it easier for them to stand up.[17,20]

#### *Physical Agent Modalities*

Physical agent modalities (PAMs) such as heat, transcutaneous electrical nerve stimulation (TENS), and biofeedback, are helpful in relieving pain.[7,20] Local applications of heat, including paraffin wax treatments and moist or dry heat packs, help to reduce stiffness and increase mobility. At home, patients may enjoy the benefits of heat by taking a warm bath or shower. The application of heat should be limited to 20 minutes, as longer periods of warmth can cause an increase in inflammation and edema.[7,20,21] Ice packs are used both for pain relief and to decrease edema. OTRs and COTAs must be aware of their state licensure requirements and be trained in the use of PAMs if they plan to use them with their patients.

#### *Therapeutic Activity and Exercise*

Therapeutic activity and exercise are used to promote joint function, muscle strength, and endurance. Any functional program needs to be coordinated with the physical therapy program to avoid overworking any group of muscles. The specific types of activity that might be prescribed will depend primarily on the stage of disease the patient is experiencing. The stages of the inflammatory process have been described as acute, subacute, chronic active, and chronic inactive.[10,20]

Clinical symptoms seen in the acute stage include limited movement, pain and tenderness at rest that increases with movement, overall stiffness, weakness, tingling or numbness, and hot, red joints. In the subacute stage, limited movement and the tingling remains. A decrease in pain and tenderness indicates that inflammation is subsiding. Stiffness is limited to morning stiffness, and the joints appear pink and warm. The chronic-active stage is characterized by reduced tingling, pain, and tenderness, and increased activity tolerance, although endurance remains low. No signs of inflammation are present in the chronic-inactive stage. The patient's low endurance, pain, and stiffness at this stage are due to disuse. Overall functioning may be decreased because of fear of pain and limited ROM, muscle atrophy, and contractures.[17,20,29,31]

Any treatment program should begin slowly, and gradually increase in intensity, duration, and frequency of the various activities.[5] Splints, braces, and positioning devices may be used throughout the stages to provide joint rest and stability. The patients may perform self-care activities as tolerated. During the acute stage, active assistive exercises and exercises with gravity eliminated may be performed within the limits of pain tolerance. As the patient's abilities improve, the activities will progress to include active and resistive exercises. The exercises should be done at the best time of the day for the patient, that is, when the patient feels more limber and has the least pain, such as after a warm shower or a short time after receiving pain medication).[5,20]

In the acute stage, gentle passive and active ROM exercises to the point of pain (without stretch) should be done twice a day. As few as one to two repetitions of complete joint range are needed to prevent loss of ROM.[17,20] However, several attempts at movement may be needed before full range is achieved. The patient may complete self-ranging exercises of the neck, elbows, and hands, but the therapist should passively range the shoulder to promote muscle relaxation.[20] Some believe that isometric exercises without resistance may be attempted to preserve strength. One to three contractions per muscle group per day are recommended.[17,20] Resistive exercises and stretching at the end range should be avoided.[17,20]

Active and passive ROM exercises that include a gentle passive stretch may be started in the subacute stage. Isotonic exercises and graded isometric exercises may be done provided there is minimal stress to the joints.[17,20]

In the chronic-active and chronic-inactive stages, stretch at the end of the range may be included during ROM. Resistive isotonic and isometric exercises may be done as long as they do not overstress the joints.[5,17,20]

There is some controversy over the use of isotonic resistive exercise for patients with arthritis.[17,20] The occupational therapist must determine whether stable inactive joints will benefit from a strengthening program, without jeopardizing other joints. If pain resulting from exercise lasts longer than 1 hour, the vigor of the exercise should be reduced.[17,20]

Whether choosing therapeutic activities or exercise, the OTR and COTA should apply the same principles to treatment.[20] Activities should not overstress the joints but should offer enough repetition of movement to help improve ROM and strength. The activities should be nonresistive and avoid patterns of deformity. In general, resistive squeezing of the hand should be avoided as it can promote ulnar deviation, MP subluxation, and extensor tendon displacement.[11,20] When choosing an activity, it is important to consider how it will affect all joints. Although sanding a board on an inclined board may be helpful in increasing shoulder and elbow range, it could be harmful for the hand to grip a piece of sandpaper. This could be remedied with the use of a sanding block.

It is recommended that patients with arthritis avoid activities that require the use of the hand in prolonged static contractions. However, sometimes the psychological benefits of doing activities one enjoys may outweigh the risks involved, especially if the risks can be minimized. According to Melvin,[20] activities such as knitting and crocheting are only contraindicated if there is active MP synovitis, developing swan-neck deformity, or thumb CMC joint involvement. Problems may be avoided by having the patient wear a hand or thumb splint while performing the activity. In addition, frequent rest breaks and stretching exercises for the intrinsic muscles will help to prevent complications.[7,20]

Other leisure activities may be introduced to patients as a means of helping them to cope with their disabilities. An interest survey completed by the patient can be analyzed to determine appropriate activities. The patient may need help modifying or substituting similar activities.

### *Splinting*

The goals of splinting are to support the joint in an optimal position for function and to reduce inflammation by providing rest or support to the joint.[17,20] Dynamic splints are also used to correct deformity. Splints can be useful for the wrist, fingers, neck, elbows, knees, and ankles. The OTR should determine the need for splinting on the basis of a thorough evaluation and consultation with the patient's physician. The inappropriate use of splints can be harmful.[13,27] The splinting of one joint may put added stress to the surrounding joints (for example, increased stress to the MP joints when splinting the wrist).[20]

Some of the more commonly used splints in the treatment of the arthritic hand include the resting splint, wrist immobilization splint, wrist cock-up splint with MCP support, and ulnar drift positioning splint. Specific directions for these and other splints may be found in several sources.[20,33] In addition, several splints designed for the arthritic hand are available commercially.

The resting hand splint (see Chapter 22) is useful for the treatment of acute synovitis of the wrist, fingers, and thumb as it helps to prevent ulnar drift and maintains the thumb web space. Its primary use is to provide rest for the involved joints but may also help to prevent the development of multiple joint contractures. Because it restricts movement, it is usually worn during sleep. If the patient requires resting splints for each hand, each splint should be worn on alternate nights so that the patient has one free hand.[20,33]

A wrist immobilization splint (Figure 26-14) is used to immobilize a painful wrist while allowing the hand to remain functional. It supports the wrist in extension and relieves compression of the carpal tunnel.[20,33] If the MPs are also involved a wrist cock-up splint with MCP support may be necessary (Figure 26-15). It places the MCP joints in normal alignment, allowing them 0 to 25 degrees of MP flexion.

During pinch and grasp activities, an ulnar drift positioning splint (Figure 26-16) may be used to prevent ulnar drift. To prevent stiffness from occurring, it is important to remove splints and other orthoses on a regular basis to carry out ROM exercises to the involved joints.[20,33] Table 26-1 describes specific splinting and treatment strategies for upper extremity deformities previously described.[17]

### *Occupational Performance*

An effective method of minimizing the effects of disuse and bedrest is to have patients perform ADL through-

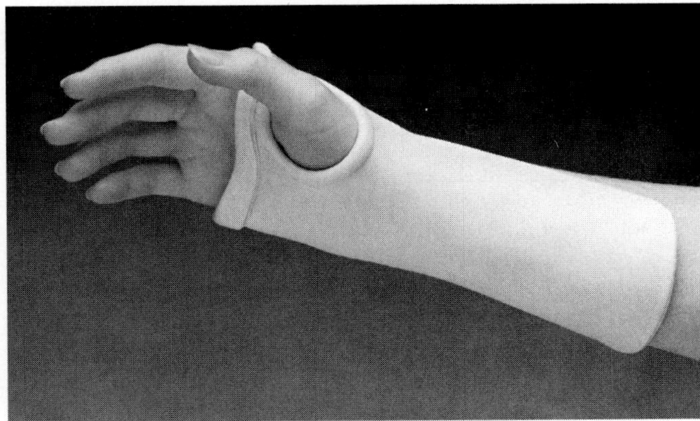

*Figure 26-14* Wrist immobilization splint. (From North Coast Medical, Inc., San Jose, Calif.)

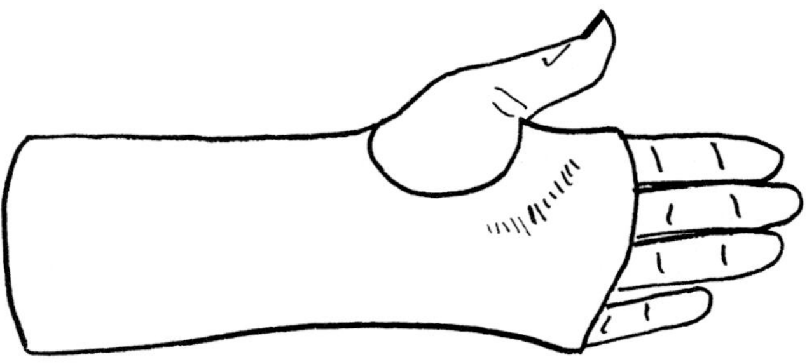

*Figure 26-15* Wrist cock-up splint with MCP support. (From Melvin JL: *Rheumatic disease in the adult and child: occupational therapy and rehabilitation,* ed 3, 1989, FA Davis.)

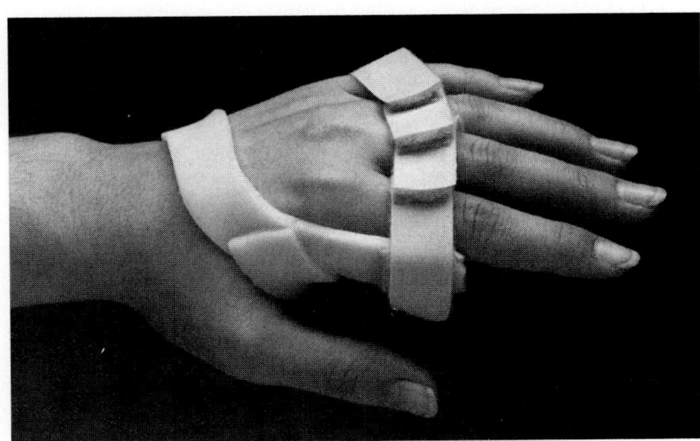

*Figure 26-16* Ulnar drift positioning splint. (From North Coast Medical, Inc., San Jose, Calif.)

*Table 26-1*

### Treatment for Specific Deformities

| *Deformity* | *Possible medical care* | *Treatment methods* | *Splinting* | *Methods to avoid* |
|---|---|---|---|---|
| Swan neck | Synovectomy in early stages | Daily PROM and gentle stretching for the DIPs<br>Daily AROM to each finger joint<br>Active muscle contraction with stretch for flexion contractures | Small, short, dynamic splint for the PIPs during daily activity to prevent hyperextension<br>Three-point finger splint to maintain range of PIP flexion | Isotonic, isometric, and resistive exercise<br>Passive or device stretch to flexion contractures |
| Boutonnière deformity | Synovectomy for the second and third fingers | Daily PROM to all joints of the involved finger(s) | Dynamic extension splints for second and third fingers may improve function and opposition | Isotonic, isometric, and resistive exercise |
| Trigger finger | Steroid injections | Tendon protection techniques—heat/ice for immobility/ inflammation | Trigger finger splint | — |
| MP ulnar drift | Synovectomy<br>Tendon replacement<br>Joint replacement | Daily PROM to MP joints if AROM lacks full flexion and extension<br>Joint protection | Dynamic ulnar deviation splints during the day<br>Static splints with the MPs in neutral deviation and 45 degree of flexion at night | Isotonic, isometric, and resistive exercise<br>Positions of deformity |
| MP palmar subluxation-dislocation | Joint replacement or repair | PROM and AROM of the MPs<br>Joint protection | — | — |
| Wrist subluxation | — | — | Flexible splint during the day and rigid splint at night | — |
| Elbow synovitis | Steroid injections<br>Synovectomy and resection of the radial head<br>Arthroplasty | Rest for acute synovitis<br>Use of cold<br>Daily AROM and PROM exercises<br>Isotonic or isometric exercise | Splint to provide joint rest or prevent instability | Overuse |
| Shoulder synovitis | Steroid injections<br>Applicable surgery | AROM and isotonic exercises preceded by hot packs<br>Joint protection | — | Slings |

out their hospitalization.[5,7,17,20] When the patient's condition is acute, activities may be limited to feeding and facial hygiene. As the patient's condition improves, ADL should be resumed to help maintain muscular tone and improve endurance. Adaptive equipment and methods may be used with bathing, dressing, feeding, work/home management, and leisure activities to promote independence and to prevent pain and further injury to the joints. Both occupational therapists and occupational therapy assistants working with the arthritic population should be familiar with adaptive equipment and joint protection and work simplification techniques described in this chapter. Two additional resources are the *Guide to Independent Living for People with Arthritis* available from the Arthritis Foundation and *A Workbook for Persons with Rheumatoid Arthritis* available from the United States Government Printing Office. Both books are reasonable in cost and are excellent teaching tools for patients with arthritis (see Resources at end of chapter).

An important but often neglected aspect of self-care training is sexual counseling (see Chapter 14). Patients may approach any member of the health care team with questions related to sexual concerns. In addition to open discussion of sexual problems, patients and their partners are often helped by illustrations of more comfortable positions for intercourse. Several excellent treatments of this subject are available.[8,25,28]

*Energy conservation* Because patients with arthritis have a decreased energy supply and may require more energy to do things,they can benefit from using energy conservation techniques (Figure 26-17).[16,17,20] Occupational therapy practitioners can teach the techniques to their patients and help the patients to apply the principles to daily activities. Patients may have difficulty fitting the principles into their lifestyle as they often require a change in lifelong habits. Practice in using the techniques during hospitalization will help with carryover after discharge.

*Assistive devices* Assistive devices should be used only when necessary and must be selected with the patient's needs in mind.[5,17,19,20] Patients are less likely to use equipment that is expensive or cumbersome. Patients will need to be taught to use some of the assistive devices, (such as those that compensate for loss of ROM) when they are experiencing a flare-up. When the inflammation has subsided, patients should be encouraged to stop using the devices and to begin using their own ROM and muscle power in order to maintain their strength and mobility. Table 26-2 describes the principles used in selecting devices and examples for each.[5,17,20]

*Joint protection* Joints affected by arthritis have an increased potential for developing further damage. Joint protection (or joint saver) techniques are taught to patients to minimize their risk of injury during daily activities. These techniques are especially helpful for patients with rheumatoid arthritis or with osteoarthritis involving the hands.[7,9,17,30]

1. *Respect pain.*
   Pain is one way that the body signals there is something wrong. Many patients with arthritis may feel that they can "tough it out," but ignoring pain will often lead to more pain. As a rule of thumb, pain that lasts for more than 1 or 2 hours

*Table 26-2*

## Assistive Devices

| *Problem* | *Principle* | *Examples* |
|---|---|---|
| Decreased ROM | Lengthen the handle on objects. | Reachers, long-handled shoe horn, extended mop handle |
| | Organize objects within easy reach. | Revolving space saver, pegboards |
| Impaired grasp | Enlarge the circumference of handles. | Built-up soft handles, large pens, universal cuffs, stocking aids |
| Instability | Stabilize objects and provide support for safety. | Nonskid mats, suction brushes, handrails, grab bars |
| Decreased energy | Facilitate ease of performance. | Lightweight tools, electrical tools, Zim jar opener |
| Potential for joint deformities | Increase leverage. | Extended faucet handles, adapted key holder, vegetable peeler held at MPs |
| | Prevent static or prolonged holding. | Book stand, bowl holder |
| Decreased strength | Modify work heights. | Raised toilet seats |
| | Raise the height of beds and chairs to make standing easier. | |

**Attitudes and Emotions**
- Remove yourself from stressful situations.
- Avoid concentrating on things that make you tense.
- Close your eyes and visualize pleasant places and thoughts.

**Body Mechanics**
- When lifting something that is close to the floor, bend your knees and lift by straightening your legs. Try to keep your back straight.
- Avoid reaching (or use reachers). Avoid stretching, bending, carrying, and climbing. If you have to bend, keep your back straight.
- Incorporate good posture into your activities.
- Sit while working whenever possible.
- To get up from a chair, slide forward to the edge of the chair. With your feet flat on the floor, lean forward and push with your *palms* on the arms or seat of the chair. Stand by straightening your legs.
- *Before* you get tired, stop and rest.

**Work Pace**
- Plan on getting 10 to 12 hours of rest daily (through naps and sleeping at night).
- Work at your own pace.
- Spread tedious tasks throughout the week.
- Do the tasks that require the most energy at the times you have the most energy.
- Alternate easy and difficult activities, and take a 10 to 15 minute rest break each hour.

**Leisure Time**
- Devote a portion of your day to an activity that you enjoy and find relaxing.
- Check out what activities are available in the community.

**Work Methods**
- Keep items within easy reach.
- Provide good light, proper ventilation, and a comfortable room temperature.
- Use joint protection techniques.
- Make sure work surfaces are at the correct height.

**Organization**
- Plan ahead—do not rush or push yourself.
- Decide which jobs are absolutely necessary.
- Share your work load with family and friends.

*Figure 26-17* Principles of energy conservation.

**How to Begin**

- Plan ahead by charting your daily routine.
- Make a list of tasks and spread them out in your schedule.
- Include daily rest periods and rest breaks during energy-consuming times.

**Weekly Schedule**

| TIME | Sunday | Monday | Tuesday | Wednesday | Thursday | Friday | Saturday |
|---|---|---|---|---|---|---|---|
| 7:00 AM | | | | | | | |
| 8:00 | | | | | | | |
| 9:00 | | | | | | | |
| 10:00 | | | | | | | |
| 11:00 | | | | | | | |
| 12:00 PM | | | | | | | |
| 1:00 | | | | | | | |
| 2:00 | | | | | | | |
| 3:00 | | | | | | | |
| 4:00 | | | | | | | |
| 5:00 | | | | | | | |
| 6:00 | | | | | | | |
| 7:00 | | | | | | | |
| 8:00 | | | | | | | |
| 9:00 | | | | | | | |
| 10:00 | | | | | | | |

Check your schedule for the following:

- Is one day longer than another?
- Are heavier tasks distributed through the week?
- Is there a long task that could be done in several steps?
- Will your plan allow flexibility?
- Have you devoted part of your day to a relaxing activity?
- Does your plan use the principles of energy conservation?

*Figure 26-17, cont'd* For legend see opposite page.

after completing a task indicates that the activity was too stressful and that it should be changed. This might include breaking the task into steps or using less effort to complete the task. Activities that put strain on an already painful joint should be avoided.[7,9,17,30]

2. *Maintain muscle strength and joint ROM.*

   This may be accomplished by using each joint to its maximal available ROM and strength during daily activities. When ironing, sweeping, or mopping, the patient should use long, flowing strokes, straightening and bending the arms as

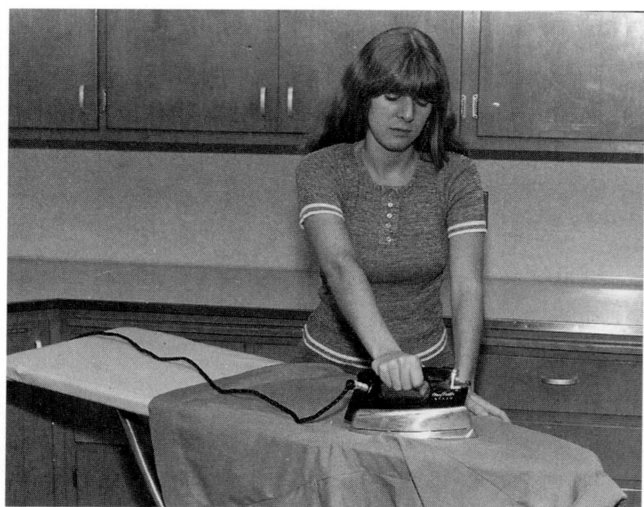

*Figure 26-18* During ironing, full extension at elbow can be practiced.

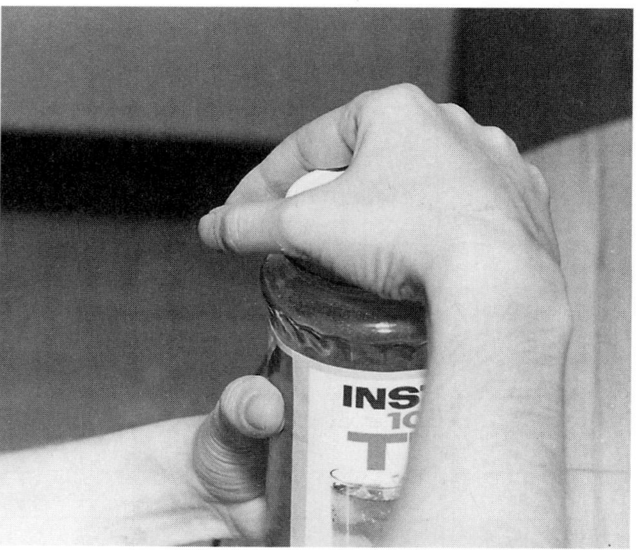


*Figure 26-19* Jar cap is twisted off with palm of hand and opened with right hand to prevent ulnar drift.

much as possible (Figure 26-18). Light items, such as cereal or noodles, can be stored in high cabinets so that full shoulder ROM will be used when reaching.[7,9,17,30]

3. *Avoid positions that put stress on involved joints.* The "normal way" of doing things may need to be changed so that joints are used in their most stable position. Activities involving a tight grip can be avoided by using items with enlarged handles.[7,9,17,30]

Holding a knife in the traditional manner puts too much direct pressure on the fingers. Instead the patient should use the knife as if it were a dagger, or use a pizza cutter. A vegetable peeler should be held parallel to MP joints and not diagonally across the palm. A butter knife can be used to open milk cartons. The palm of the hand (not just the fingers) should be used when pushing from a chair to stand up.[7,9,17,30]

Other hand positions to avoid are those that involve tight pinching, squeezing, or twisting motions. A dusting mitt will help to keep the fingers extended while dusting. Sponges or rags may be wrung out by spreading the hand flat over them or by squeezing them between the palms. Several methods may be used to open a screw-top jar. The person can lean on the jar with the palm of the hand and turn the lid with shoulder motion (Figure 26-19), or hold the jar in a drawer as the cap is twisted.[7,9,17,30]

To discourage the development of ulnar drift deformities, patients are taught to turn their hands toward the thumb when turning doorknobs. When opening jars, the right hand is used to open the jar and the left hand to close it. When stirring, the spoon is moved counter clockwise (right hand) or clockwise (left hand) (Figure 26-20). Patients should be discouraged from leaning their chins on the hands or fingers and from using their fingers to pick up a mug because pressure on the thumb side of the fingers may promote ulnar deviation.[7,9,17,30]

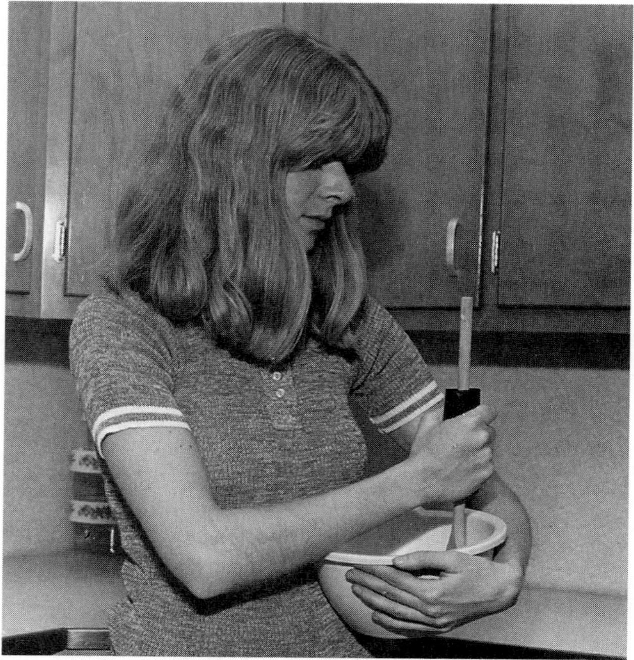

*Figure 26-20* Mixing bowl is stabilized with forearm. Spoon with soft, built-up handle is held so that pressure is toward radial side of the hand.

4. *Avoid staying in one position for a long time.*
   Staying in one position can cause excess fatigue and stiffness. Instead, use a book stand to hold a book, or when stirring, place the bowl in a partially opened drawer or on a rubber mat to eliminate holding. Never begin an activity that cannot be stopped immediately if pain or fatigue sets in.[7,9,17,30]
5. *Use the strongest joints and muscles available.*
   The use of the larger joints reduces the stress on the smaller joints. One example is carrying a purse on the shoulder instead of in the hands. (Backpacks and fanny packs are also helpful.) The weight should be either balanced between both shoulders or frequently alternated between the two sides. Other examples include pushing doors open with the side of the arm instead of the hand, adding cloth loops to drawer pulls so they can be opened with the forearm, using palms instead of fingers to pick up a coffee mug, and using the stronger leg first to go up the stairs and last to go down the stairs. It is also important to keep weight under control to avoid stress on the weight-bearing joints.[7,9,17,30]
6. *Distribute the work load over several joints.*
   For example, use the palms of both hands to lift and hold cups, plates, pots, and pans instead of grasping them with the fingers. Use oven mitts to carry hot dishes. Carry heavy loads close to the body in the arms instead of holding them with your hands. Slide objects along the counter instead of carrying them. If necessary, lift objects by scooping them up with both palms turned upward. Stress may also be reduced by wearing a wrist splint.[7,9,17,30]

### *Discharge Planning*

Discharge planning begins as soon as the patient is referred to occupational therapy. Patients who are encouraged to be active participants throughout their treatment program are more likely to follow through with treatment once discharged.[7,28] Patient education will help patients to use the many appropriate resources available to them.

Education of the patient and family should provide information about the disease process including signs of inflammation, potential disability, and realistic treatment options.[7] It is important for families to understand the patient's abilities and when they should help (or not help) the patient do things.[23,24] They must be cautioned against medical quackery that promotes worthless arthritis remedies. Because over 30 million Americans suffer from arthritis, health fraud in this area is a very lucrative business.[1]

When providing patient education, particular attention should be paid to questions the patient may ask. Information should be reviewed even if the patient may have heard it before.[5] Repetition and reinforcement are the keys to education. Approach the topics in a variety of ways. Use examples that relate directly to the patient's interest and experiences.[5]

Group treatment, such as movement or exercise classes, home management classes, or arthritis education classes, can use group processes for mutual support and problem solving. Seeing others with similar problems may serve as a powerful motivational tool.[5,14,17,20] Occupational therapy practitioners may lead or participate with other members of the rehabilitation team in such activity groups.

One group program, designed by an occupational therapist, is the ROM Dance Program.[15] Based on the principles of T'ai-Chi Ch'uan, it promotes involvement in daily exercise and rest. Components include the ROM dance itself, relaxation techniques, group sharing, and health education. Information on the ROM Dance Program can be obtained from the address listed at the end of the chapter.

Both the OTR and the COTA should develop a home program and train the patient in its use. A variety of topics including energy conservation, joint protection, and appropriate activities and exercises might be included. An example of a home exercise program can be found in Figure 26-21. Verbal and written directions should be geared to the patient's level of understanding. The patient should be made aware of the resources available from the local or national chapter of the Arthritis Foundation. The Foundation supports research and offers literature and classes designed to improve the quality of life for patients with arthritis. (See address at end of chapter.)

#### Treatment Precautions

The following is a list of treatment precautions to be followed when working with patients with arthritis.[17] More specific information on each can be found in the appropriate sections in this chapter.

1. Avoid fatigue.
2. Respect pain.
3. Avoid static, stressful, or resistive activities.
4. Limit the application of heat to 20 minutes.
5. Use resistive exercises with caution and never with unstable joints.[32]
6. Be aware of sensory impairments.

## SUMMARY

Three of the more common forms of arthritis are rheumatoid arthritis, osteoarthritis, and gout. Although their causes and symptoms differ, methods for treating the joint involvement are similar. Potential for further injury can be reduced by proper medication, a balance between rest and activity, exercise, and surgery. In occupational therapy, patients learn how to protect their joints while performing day-to-day tasks at work and at home. Successful treatment depends on early intervention and ongoing care and reassessment.

ARTHRITIS RANGE OF MOTION EXERCISES

The following exercises will help you to maintain your mobility. Do only those checked by the therapist.

**INSTRUCTIONS**

1. Start doing five of each exercise two times per day.
2. Progress to ten of each, two times per day.
3. Do all exercises *slowly* while sitting.
4. If having an active flare-up, cut down or eliminate exercises. After symptoms subside, start at the beginning to build up tolerance.

**Shoulder**

___ Hold your hands on your shoulders and make small to large circles with your elbows. Go clockwise and then counterclockwise.

___ With your hands on your shoulders, bring your elbows together in front of you and then spread your elbows apart to the side and as far back as you can reach.

___ Roll up a newspaper and hold onto the ends of it with each hand facing down. Rest the paper on your knees. Bend your elbows to bring the paper to your right shoulder and back to your knees. Bend your elbows to your left shoulder and back to your knees.

**Elbow**

___ Hold your hands on your shoulders. Bring them out straight in front of you with your palms up.

___ With your elbows bent at your side, turn your palms up and down.

**Wrist**

___ Hold your hand facing down. Make a fist as you bend your wrist up. Open your fingers as you bend your wrist down.

___ Hold your hands together in a praying position. Keeping your hands together and moving only your wrist, point your fingertips away from and toward you.

**Hands**

___ Touch your thumb to each finger.

___ Make a fist and stretch your fingers open and out.

Please call if you have any questions.

*Figure 26-21* Arthritis range of motion exercises.

## Sample Treatment Plan

The following treatment plan[17] is not comprehensive as it deals with only four of the eight problems identified and two stages of the disease process. The reader is encouraged to add objectives and methods to the plan to make it more complete.

### Case study

Mrs. J. is a 36-year-old woman with a diagnosis of RA. The onset was 3 years ago. She is a wife and the mother of an 8-year-old girl. She lives with her husband and daughter in a three-bedroom, single-level tract home. Mrs. J.'s primary role is that of homemaker. However, she has held a part-time job at a florist shop designing and constructing wreaths and arranging flowers. She both enjoys this work and sees her salary as a necessary adjunct to the family income.

Mrs. J. experiences intermittent acute disease episodes that have primarily involved the elbows, wrists, MP, and PIP joints bilaterally. There are slight losses of ROM and strength in all involved joints.

To date there is no permanent deformity, but ulnar deviation, MP subluxation, boutonnière deformity, wrist subluxation, and further limitation of ROM at all involved joints are possible deformities.

Medical management has been through rest and medication. Medical precautions include no strenuous activity, no resistive exercise or activity, and prevention of fatigue.

Mrs. J. was referred to occupational therapy during the acute phase of her most recent episode for prevention of deformity and loss of ROM and maintenance of maximal function. She continued with occupational therapy services during the subacute period with the same goals.

#### *Personal data*

Name: Mrs. J.
Age: 36
Diagnosis: Rheumatoid arthritis
Disability: Limited ROM, decreased strength, potential deformity of elbows, wrists, MP and PIP joints bilaterally
Treatment aims stated in the referral: Prevent deformity, prevent loss of ROM, maintain maximal function.

### Other services

Physician: Supervise medical management and rehabilitation therapies.
Physical therapy: Used if needed for specific exercise program.
Social services: Provide patient and family counseling if needed, and explore financial arrangements if appropriate.
Vocational counseling: Explore feasibility of return to same or modified occupation in floral work.

#### *Treatment approach*

Biomechanical and rehabilitation approaches

### OT evaluation

#### *Performance components*

Sensorimotor Components
- Active and passive ROM: test
- Muscle strength: observe, test
- Hand deformities: observe, test MP stability
- Ulnar drift (measure if present): wrist subluxation, MP subluxation, boutonnière deformity, swan-neck deformity, thumb deformities
- Hand function: test
- Endurance: observe, interview
- Sensation: test

Cognitive Functioning
- Memory: observe, interview
- Functional language skills: observe, interview comprehension of written/spoken language

Psychosocial Functioning
- Role performance: observe, interview
- Adjustment to disability: observe, interview
- Coping and time management skills: observe
- Family and community support: interview

#### *Performance areas*

ADL: observe, interview
Home management: observe, interview
Work performance: observe, interview
Play/leisure: observe, interview

### Evaluation summary

Weakness is noted particularly in wrist and finger extensors (F+) and to a lesser degree in flexor groups (G). Mild ROM limitations are present in elbows, wrists, and fingers with some MP instability noted (10 degree ulnar drift). No subluxation or other deformities were noted. Hand function testing revealed difficulty with fingertip prehension, and pinch and grip are good but not normal in strength. Forceful use of the thumb in opposition enhances ulnar drift and produces MP discomfort.

Sensation is intact. Cognitive state is within normal limits. The patient's family has noted that the patient demonstrates withdrawal from social situations during flares and has limited patience when fatigued and in pain. Her family appears to be supportive, and her daughter helps with household tasks. During inactive disease periods the patient is independent for light housekeeping, self-care, and work. She fatigues after 2 hours of light to moderate activity and requires a 20-minute rest period. During flares she is severely limited in ADL, leaves home management tasks to her family, and is unable to work. She manages to do only light self-care activities independently.

*Continued.*

## Sample Treatment Plan—cont'd

Observation of the job by another worker and Mrs. J. in simulated tasks revealed that some aspects of her job would contribute to development of deformity. Cutting and twisting floral wire, forcing stems and stem supports into floral foam, and binding wreaths were thought to be likely to enhance ulnar drift and MP subluxation because of the resistance and direction of joint forces. However, wreath design and layout and fresh flower arrangement are possible alternatives. Mrs. J.'s employer is willing to retain her on a part-time basis to perform these duties.

**Assets**

No lower extremity involvement
Good preservation of function
Supportive and intact family unit
Potential job skills, flexible employer
Intelligence, motivation

**Problem list**

1. Muscle weakness
2. Limited ROM
3. Potential deformity
4. Fluctuating vocational role
5. Limited ADL independence
6. Fluctuating role as wife and mother
7. Tendency to social withdrawal
8. Limited endurance

**Acute stage—problem 1**

Muscle weakness

***Objective***

Maintenance muscle strength

***Method***

Isometric exercise without added resistance to elbow and wrist flexors and extensors, one to three repetitions once a day; active ROM exercise to elbows and wrists, two to three repetitions once a day; self-care to tolerance

***Gradation***

Increased number of exercise sessions or repetitions as synovitis and pain subside

**Acute stage—problem 2**

Limited ROM

***Objective***

Maintenance ROM of affected joints

***Method***

Active or active-assisted ROM exercises to elbow, MP and PIP flexion and extension, wrist flexion, extension, radial and ulnar deviation; may carry out active ROM exercises in a warm bath or shower or immediately after bathing

***Gradation***

Graded to active exercises and addition of gentle active and passive stretching during subacute stage

**Acute stage—problems 3 and 5**

Potential deformity
Limited ADL independence

***Objective***

With adaptive equipment and use of joint protection techniques, performance of self-care activities independently and without causing stress to involved joints

***Method***

Instruction from occupational therapy practitioner in joint protection and specific recommendations for modifications to existing equipment (building up handles on toothbrush, hairbrush, eating utensils, etc); provision of necessary self-care adaptive equipment (button hook, washing mitt, etc.) and instruction in their use; treatment sessions within the clinic that include dressing and grooming tasks to facilitate problem solving and permit patient to demonstrate competence in the use of adaptive equipment and joint protection techniques

***Gradation***

As synovitis subsides, gradual tapering off from the use of adaptive equipment and increase in activity level

**Subacute stage—problem 1**

Muscle weakness

***Objective***

Increase in strength of weakened muscles by a half grade as compared with the initial evaluation

***Method***

Light housekeeping activities (ironing, dust mopping, dish washing) to increase home activity level; isometric exercise with resistance to elbow and wrist flexor and extensors, MP and PIP extensors, 3 to 10 repetitions 3 times daily

**Subacute stage—problem 2**

Limited ROM

***Objective***

Increase in or maintenance of ROM of affected joints

***Method***

Active ROM exercise to elbow, wrist, MP and PIP joints; gentle passive stretching to elbow flexion; and extension and PIP extension; instructions to use full ROM for light resistance ADL such as dust mopping, folding linen, and ironing

***Gradation***

Increased resistance for stretching exercise as tolerated

## Selected Reading Guide Questions

1. What is the outstanding clinical feature that causes joint damage in rheumatoid arthritis?
2. What are the major differences between osteoarthritis and rheumatoid arthritis?
3. When is occupational therapy indicated for the treatment of patients with gout?
4. What are three systemic signs of rheumatoid arthritis?
5. What are the clinical signs of joint inflammation?
6. When is resistive exercise appropriate for persons with rheumatoid arthritis?
7. Why are activities such as crocheting and knitting controversial for patients with rheumatoid arthritis?
8. What adaptive equipment would be useful for patients with arthritis?
9. Why is it important to know the type and schedule of medication the patient is taking?
10. Why should patients with rheumatoid arthritis avoid opening doors in the usual method?
11. What are important areas to evaluate in patients with arthritis?
12. Why is grip strength measured with an adapted blood pressure cuff for patients with rheumatoid arthritis?
13. Why is rest an important part of treatment for patients with arthritis?
14. Identify five principles of joint protection.
15. Describe how energy conservation techniques can be applied to daily activities.
16. Identify five assistive devices and describe why they are useful for patients with arthritis.

## REFERENCES


1. *Arthritis information: osteoarthritis,* Atlanta, 1994, The Arthritis Foundation.
2. *Arthritis information: rheumatoid arthritis,* 1993, The Arthritis Foundation.
3. *Arthritis surgery information: information to consider,* Atlanta, 1981, The Arthritis Foundation.
4. *Arthritis: the basic facts,* Atlanta, 1974, The Arthritis Foundation.
5. Arthritis Health Professions Selection Task Force: *Arthritis teaching slide collection for teachers of allied health professionals,* New York, 1980, The Arthritis Foundation.
6. Banwell B: Physical therapy in arthritis management. In Ehrlich G, editor: *Rehabilitation management of rheumatic conditions,* ed 2, Baltimore, 1986, Williams & Wilkins.
7. Batts C: Rheumatoid arthritis. In Hansen RA, Atchison B, editors: *Conditions in occupational therapy: effect on occupational performance,* Baltimore, 1993, Williams & Wilkins.
8. Comfort A: *Sexual consequences of disability,* Philadelphia, 1978, George F. Stickley.
9. Cordery JC: Joint protection: a responsibility of the occupational therapist, *Am J Occup Ther* 19:285, 1965.
10. Engleman E, Shearn M: Arthritis and allied rheumatic disorders. In Krupp M, Chatton M, editors: *Current medical diagnosis and treatment,* Los Altos, Calif, 1980, Lange Medical Publications.
11. Fries JF: *Arthritis: a comprehensive guide to understanding your arthritis,* Reading, MA, 1986, Addison-Wesley.
12. Reference deleted in proofs.
13. Hanten DW: The splinting controversy in rheumatoid arthritis. *Physical Disabilities Special Interest Newsletter* 5:4, 1982.
14. Harcom TM, et al: Therapeutic value of graded aerobic exercise training in rheumatoid arthritis, *Arthritis Rheum* 28:32, 1985.
15. Harlowe D: The ROM dance program, *Physical Disabilities Special Interest Newsletter* 5:4, 1982.
16. Harris E: *Rheumatic arthritis: the clinical spectrum.* In Kelly WH, editor: *Textbook of rheumatology,* Philadelphia, 1981, WB Saunders.
17. Hittle JM, Pedretti LW, Katch MC: Rheumatoid arthritis. In Pedretti LW, Zoltan B: *Occupational therapy practice skills for physical dysfunction,* St Louis, 1995, Mosby.
18. Lipsky P: Rheumatoid arthritis. In Harrison TR, Braunwald, editors: *Principles of internal medicine,* ed 11, New York, 1987, McGraw-Hill.
19. Mann WC, Hurren D, Tomita M: Assistive devices used by home-based elderly persons with arthritis, *Am J Occup Ther* 49(8):810, 1995.
20. Melvin JL: *Rheumatic disease in the adult and child: occupational therapy and rehabilitation,* ed 2, Philadelphia, 1989, FA Davis.
21. Michlovitz SL: *Thermal agents in rehabilitation,* ed 2, Philadelphia, 1990, FA Davis.
22. Nalebuff EA: Diagnosis, classification and management of rheumatoid thumb deformities, *Bull Hosp Joint Dis* 24:119, 1968.
23. Navarro A: *Rheumatic conditions causing hip pain.* In Rigg G, Galle E, editors: *Rheumatic diseases: rehabilitation and management,* Boston, 1984, Butterworth.
24. Potts MG: *Psychosocial aspects of rheumatic diseases: rehabilitation and management,* Boston, 1984, Butterworth.
25. Richards JS: Sex and arthritis, *Sexuality Dis* 3:97, 1980.
26. Rudolph M: The psychosocial affects of rheumatoid arthritis, *OT Forum* 2:24, 1987.
27. Seeger M: Splints, braces and casts. In Riggs G, Gall E, editors: *Rheumatic diseases: rehabilitation and management,* Boston, 1984, Butterworth.
28. Sidman JM: Sexual functioning and the physically disabled adult, *Am J Occup Ther* 31:81, 1977.
29. Sliwa J: Occupational therapy assessment and management. In Ehrlich G, editor: *Rehabilitation management of rheumatic conditions,* ed 2, Baltimore, 1986, Williams & Wilkins.
30. Slonaker D: *Arthritis information: using your joints wisely,* Atlanta, 1992, The Arthritis Foundation.
31. Talbott JH: *Clinical rheumatology,* ed 2, New York, 1981, Elsevier.
32. Wickersham B: The exercise program. In Riggs G, Gall E, editors: *Rheumatic diseases: rehabilitation and management,* Boston, 1984, Butterworth Publishers.
33. Ziegler EM: *Current concepts in orthotics: a diagnosis-related approach to splinting,* Chicago, 1984, Rolyan Medical Products.


## RECOMMENDED READING


Lorig K, Fries J: *The arthritis help book,* Reading, Mass, 1990, Addison Wesley Publishing Co.

Marx H: *Arthritis: Best use of the hands,* Phoenix, 1988, Video Education Specialist (videotape).

Melvin JL: *Rheumatic disease in the adult and child: occupational therapy and rehabilitation,* ed 3, Philadelphia, 1989, FA Davis.


## RESOURCES

Arthritis Foundation
P.O. Box 7669
Atlanta, GA 30357-0669
(1-800-283-7800)

The ROM Dance Program
ROM Institute
New Ventures of Wisconsin, Inc.
3601 Memorial Drive
Madison, WI 53704
(608) 249-6670

*A Workbook for Persons with Arthritis*
Superintendent of Documents
US Government Printing Office
Washington, DC 20402

Chapter 27

# Amputation and Prosthetics

Patricia Ann Morris
Laurie Muhn

## Chapter Objectives

*After studying this chapter, the student or practitioner will be able to:*

1. Appreciate the role of occupational therapy within the context of the rehabilitation team.
2. Understand the relationship between levels of amputation and the function of the amputee.
3. Appreciate the importance of maximizing the amputee's skill with prosthetics.
4. Understand why recovery can be slow and physically draining for the patient and family.
5. Teach new methods for basic and advanced activities of daily living with prosthetics.

## Key Terms

phantom pain
cosmesis
mechanical prosthesis
terminal devices (TDs)
socket
myoelectrical prosthesis
electrode
early postoperative prosthesis
above-knee amputations (AKAs)
below-knee amputations (BKAs)
Symes amputation
rigid removal dressing
SACH foot
ischial weight-bearing prosthesis
pylon

The vast majority of people who undergo amputations do not know what to expect when they come to the medical center. This traumatic crisis will affect not only the patient but also the family. A successful rehabilitation program requires the coordinated effort of the rehabilitation team. This chapter addresses teamwork, surgical management, psychological adjustment, levels of losses in upper and lower extremities, mechanical versus myoelectric prostheses, and treatment planning.

We will also consider the ongoing collaboration between the registered occupational therapist (OTR) and certified occupational therapy assistant (COTA) in amputation and prosthetics programs.

## THE TEAM MEMBERS

The rehabilitation of the individual with limb loss requires the skills of many health care professionals: general or vascular surgeon, orthopedic surgeon, physiatrist, prosthetist, OTR and COTA, physical therapist, social worker, psychologist, pastoral counselor (spiritual guidance), and vocational counselor. Ideally these health care specialists function together as an integrated team.

Successful amputee rehabilitation programs focus on individual needs, development of new surgical techniques, improvements in technology, and a better understanding of the psychosocial implications of limb loss.

## CONGENITAL AND ACQUIRED AMPUTATIONS

### Incidence and Cause

The cause of limb loss and associated medical conditions varies. Loss of a limb is generally divided into two broad categories: congenital and acquired.[16]

Congenital amputation is the absence of a limb or part at birth, usually the result of a defect in development.[20] The loss of part or all of an extremity as the direct result of trauma or by surgery is known as an acquired amputation.[16] This chapter will discuss and focus only on acquired amputations sustained in adulthood and will consider both upper and lower extremities. Acquired amputations result from surgery and trauma.[33] Surgical amputations of both upper and lower extremities are performed in cases of severe infections or gangrene, to remove cancerous tumors, and in cases of severe injury to extremities that have no hope of salvage.

In 1990, national hospital discharge data reported 54,000 amputations in diabetic patients. This data did not include Veterans Administration medical centers that average 8,997 amputations per year in patients with diabetes. Furthermore, accidents and disease result in more than 156,000 amputations each year. Various estimates place the amputee population at over 2 million within the United States.[22] The incidence of lower extremity amputations is expected to increase with individuals living into their 80s and 90s.[22]

Traumatic amputations are often results of motor vehicle accidents (MVAs), work-related injuries, recreational injuries, tumors, burns, and electrical injuries. In the lower extremity, approximately 75% of all acquired amputations are related to diabetes or peripheral vascular disease, especially in the age 60 and over population.[12]

Surgical amputation is a last resort after all conventional treatments have been tried. Conventional treatments include testing, medication adjustment, and therapy. When these treatments have not improved the medical situation, the physician will reassess the individual for surgical intervention. If amputation is required, the physician will consult with the internist, neurologist, and orthopedic surgeon. The orthopedic surgeon will determine the level of the amputation on the basis of the potential for wound healing and optimal prosthetic fit and function. During the surgery, attention will be directed to the management of the various tissues involved, with an eye toward rehabilitation and prosthetic restoration. This includes beveling the ends of bones, sharp transection of the nerves (which are allowed to retract into proximal soft tissues so they do not adhere to the scar or remain in a location where they might be traumatized by a prosthesis), appropriate myofascial closure of muscle or myodesis to provide good control of the remaining bone in the residual limb, and appropriate placement of skin incision line(s) to avoid bony prominences and prevent adherence of skin to the underlying bone.[7] Such attention to detail results in a well-shaped residual limb that can be fitted with a prosthesis permitting maximum prosthetic function. During and after medical and surgical interventions, the team members try to facilitate the psychosocial adjustment of the patient and family members.

## PSYCHOLOGICAL ADJUSTMENT

Responses to upper and lower extremity amputations have often been compared to the grieving process. The amputee experiences identifiable stages of denial, anger, depression, coping, and acceptance.[6] Some individuals will progress through these stages and ultimately adapt to the loss. The cause of the amputation may contribute significantly to the individual's response. The psychosocial adjustment of an individual depends on various factors: the individual's character and inner strength, the quality of the social support systems available, and the comprehensive care provided by the team.

## POSTOPERATIVE COMPLICATIONS

The following conditions may occur in upper and lower limbs following amputation.

### Neuromas

A swelling or tumor along the course of a nerve or at the end of a divided nerve.

### Phantom Sensation

One of the biggest surprises after an amputation can be discovering that sensations still seem to come from the missing limb and that it feels as though its movement can be controlled. Just after amputation, the phantom can feel so real that fresh (recent/new) leg amputees may try to stand up and walk again. Occasionally, the missing limb feels as though it is in a very uncomfortable position. Nearly all amputees report that they can sense the shape of the amputated limb for at least a few months after amputation. Many continue to sense it all their lives.

### Phantom Pain

Pain seems to come from the amputated portion of the limb. The patient may experience burning, stinging, cramping, shooting, twisting, or other unpleasant sensations.

### Weakness

Prolonged muscle inactivity leads to weakness. The individual is encouraged to get out of bed and move around as soon as possible. Generally the amputee will be up the day after surgery. The longer the amputee stays in bed, the longer it will take to recover and more debilitated the person will be. It is vital that the amputee get up and start moving around as soon as possible.

### Skin Breakdown

This condition is mainly caused by excess pressure. Poor blood supply from lack of mobility might also cause breakdown, and decreased sensation leading to poor awareness is another cause.

## UPPER EXTREMITY AMPUTATIONS

### The Role of the COTA

Upper extremity amputee training is a specialized area of treatment. A program is usually directed by a skilled and experienced senior clinician. Under guidelines established by the American Occupational Therapy Association (AOTA) the OTR would complete the evaluation and prosthetic checkout and establish the goals and treatment plan. Under close supervision the COTA may implement a program for the patient with an amputation. Close supervision is essential because of the complex problems and degree of change frequently seen that may require a modified treatment approach or re-evaluation by the OTR. It is the responsibility of the COTA to keep the supervising therapist informed of all changes in patient performance and any other pertinent facts. As treatment progresses and changes are noted the assistant may contribute suggestions for program modifications or additions that will help the patient reach the established goals. Communication and feedback between OTR and COTA are the keys to a successful program.

### Levels of Amputation

The amputations of the upper extremity may be at one of several levels (Figure 27-1). The higher the level of amputation the greater the functional loss and the more the amputee must depend on the prosthesis for function and **cosmesis** (appearance). The higher level amputations require more complex and extensive prostheses and prosthetic training. The more complex prostheses can be more difficult to operate and use effectively.[28]

The shoulder forequarter and shoulder disarticulation (SD) amputations will result in the loss of all arm and hand functions. The short above-elbow (AE) amputation will result in the loss of all hand, wrist, and elbow functions and rotation of the shoulder. The long AE and elbow disarticulation amputations will result in the loss of hand, wrist, and elbow functions, but good shoulder function will remain.

The short below-elbow (BE) amputation will result in loss of hand and wrist function, forearm pronation and supination, and reduction in the force of elbow flexion. Shoulder function will be intact and good. The long BE amputation will result in loss of hand and wrist function and most forearm pronation and supination. Elbow function and force of elbow flexion will be good. The wrist disarticulation will result in incomplete loss of hand and wrist function and about 50% loss of pronation and supination.

Amputations below the wrist, across the metacarpal bones, are called transmetacarpal or partial hand amputations. Functions of all the joints of the arm are intact, and there may be some hand function available depending on whether the thumb was amputated or left intact. Many types of prostheses are available for each level of amputation. Each prosthesis is individually prescribed according to the client's needs and lifestyle and is individually fitted and custom-made.[28]

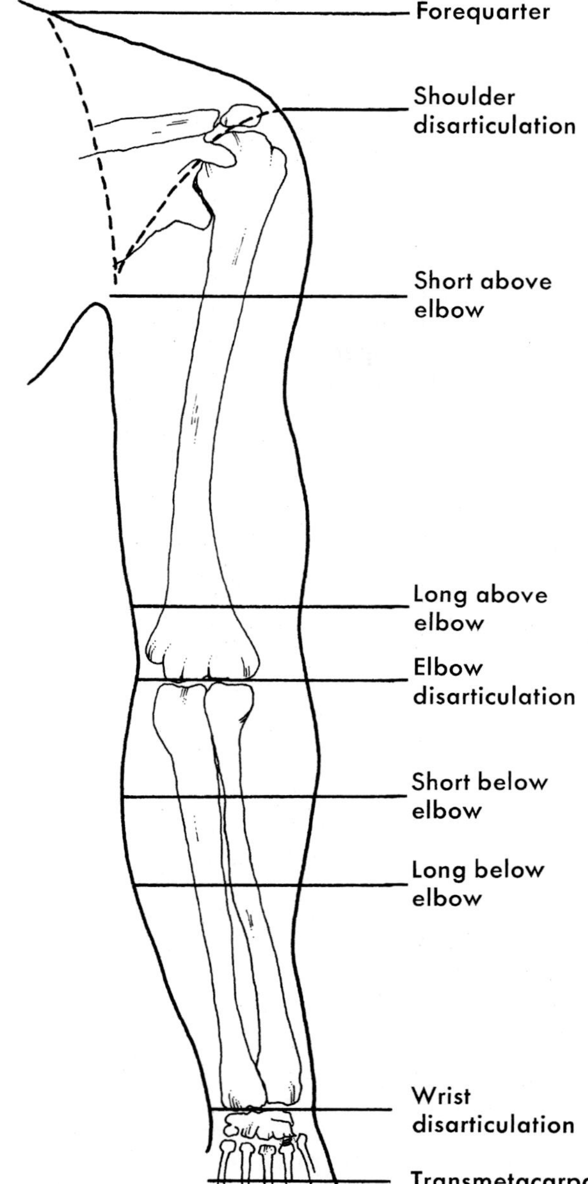


*Figure 27-1* Levels of upper extremity amputation.

### Rehabilitation Philosophy

There is a "golden period" of fitting for upper-limb prosthetic devices that appears to be within the first 30 days after amputations.[19] Until recently, the standard approach for providing a prosthetic device was to wait for complete wound healing and stump maturation, which might take 3 to 6 months. Waiting often resulted in late fitting of amputees and poor rehabilitation results. By the time amputees were fitted with a prosthetic device, they had become one-handed individuals who could see very little use for an assistive prosthetic device. The current philosophy is that the patient should be fitted as soon as possible (within 30 days) with a postoperative prosthetic device. There are multiple advantages to early prosthetic fit and they include the following:

- Decreased edema
- Decreased postoperative and phantom pain
- Accelerated wound healing
- Maintenance of two-handed function
- Decreased length of hospital stay
- Increased prosthetic use and acceptance
- Increased proprioceptive input through the residual limb
- Improved psychological adjustment
- Improved patient rehabilitation

Prosthetic fitting within the first 30 days of amputation appears to be the most important element in achieving successful upper-limb amputation rehabilitation.[19]

## Component Parts of a Mechanical Prosthesis

### *Terminal Devices*

Two types of **terminal devices (TDs)** available are the hook and the cosmetic hand (Figure 27-2).

The hook TD may be made of aluminum or steel. It may have canted or lyre-shaped fingers and usually has a neoprene lining to protect grasped objects and prevent slippage. The hook is the most functional and most frequently prescribed and used TD. Several types of hooks are available to meet individual needs. The farmer's and carpenter's hooks make handling tools easier, and narrow-opening hooks may be used for handling fine objects.

On the hook TD, the number of rubber bands controls the amount of grasp pressure. Training usually begins with one rubber band, and the number increases to three to four rubber bands as training progresses.

A cosmetic TD, designed to duplicate the amputee's hand as nearly as possible, is also available. The mechanical hand is a functional hand that may be attached to the wrist unit and is activated by the same control cable that operates the hook. The fingers are controlled at the metacarpophalangeal (MP) joints by the prosthesis control cable. The hand TD sacrifices grip force (2 lbs maximum) for improved cosmesis. A natural-looking plastic glove fits over the mechanical hand.[28]

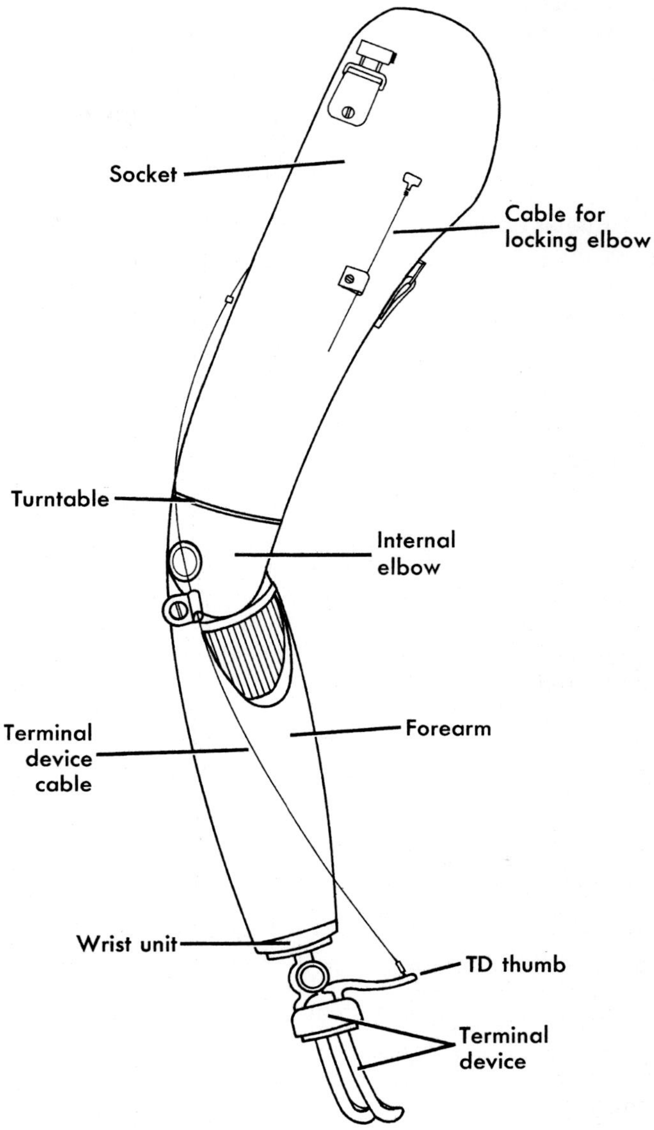


*Figure 27-2* Component parts of standard above-elbow prosthesis. (Modified from Santschi W, editor: *Manual for upper extremity prosthetics*, ed 2, Los Angeles, 1958, University of California Press.)

### *Wrist Unit*

The wrist unit joins the TD to the forearm socket. There are three basic types of wrist units: friction, locking, and oval types. The wrist unit allows prepositioning of the TD to accommodate the task to be performed. It serves as a disconnecting unit so that TDs may be interchanged.

The wrist unit is usually selected for its ability to meet the use needs of the amputee in daily living and vocational activities.[28]

### *Elbow Unit*

The elbow unit on the AE prosthesis allows the maximal range of motion (ROM) possible, locking of the elbow in various degrees of motion, and prepositioning of the prosthesis for arm rotation by a manual control friction turntable unit.

### *Socket*

The forearm **socket** for the BE amputee is made of plastic resins and may have a single or double wall. The socket must be anchored stably on the stump to allow the wearer full power and control of the prosthesis. The BE stump socket may be constructed to allow any remaining pronation and supination to be used. The single wall socket is used when the outside diameter of the distal end of the stump is sufficient to permit tapering to the wrist unit. The double wall socket is used when the stump is too short or slender to achieve the desired contour or tapering. The inner wall conforms to the stump, and the outer wall gives the required length and contour for the forearm replacement. The socket must fit snugly and firmly but allow full ROM at the first available joint.

### *Cable and Components*

The cable is made of stainless steel and is contained in a flexible stainless steel housing. It is fastened to the prosthesis by a retainer unit made of a base plate and a retainer butterfly or a housing crossbar and a leather loop. A ball or ball swivel fitting at one end of the cable attaches it to the TD while a T-bar or hanger fittings at the other end attach it to the harness.[25,34]

### *Harness*

The purposes of the harness are to suspend the prosthesis and provide the anchor point of the control cables. The figure eight Dacron harness is a commonly used design, although others are available. Extra straps may be added to the figure eight as needed. The higher the level of amputation is, the more complex the harnessing system. Variations in available muscle power and ROM may necessitate variations in the harness design. A properly fitted harness is important for both comfort and function.

### *Stump Sock*

A stump sock of knit wool, cotton, or Orlon-Lycra is usually worn by the amputee. It absorbs perspiration and protects from discomfort or irritation that could result from direct contact of the skin with the socket of the prosthesis. It accommodates volume change in the stump and aids with fit and comfort of the stump in the socket.[28,35]

## Component Parts of a Myoelectrical Prosthesis

A **myoelectrical prosthesis** is controlled by electrical signals from muscles. The first practical myoelectrically controlled prosthesis was demonstrated in 1948.[10] In the next several decades a considerable research effort followed and, as a result, myoelectric prostheses have been improved so much that their clinical value is no longer in doubt.[10] The concept of myoelectric control is very simple: an electric signal from a muscle is used to control the flow of energy from a battery to a motor. The muscles in the residual limb produce the control signal by contracting through voluntary control. The motor is activated by the signal and a prosthetic hand, wrist, or elbow is directed to move into action.

### *Terminal Devices*

Most myoelectric prostheses use an electric hand as a terminal device (Figure 27-3). They are available in various sizes to fit small children to adults. A latex glove covers the mechanism and is made to look as similar to the sound hand as possible, with skin tone choices and male or female features. The hand offers a simple open/close function. No individual finger movements are available, and there is no gradation of grip force. The hand does open at varying widths to provide for grasp of small objects such as a piece of paper or large objects such as a can of soda. The grip is strong (25 lb of force). For adults who are active and perform heavy upper body activities, a Greiffer is recommended. It can be used for heavy work in industry or farming and provides quick handling and precise manipulation of small objects. Features of the Greiffer include a 38-lb grasp, parallel gripping surfaces, and a flexion joint for dorsal and volar wrist flexion.[24] There are also endless accessories available for specific activities such as sports, unusual work tasks, and leisure activities. The prosthetist is a good resource for these specialized TDs.

### *Wrist Unit*

Several wrist unit options are available: (1) passive friction wrist, (2) quick disconnect wrist, (3) flexion wrist, (4) electric wrist rotator.

The quick disconnect wrist is the most frequently used wrist component in a myoelectric prosthesis. Several reasons for this are that (1) it is quicker to manually position the wrist than wait for a myoelectric signal to activate a motor to turn a component, (2) it eliminates an additional movement that would have to be incorporated into the amputees repertoire for prosthetic movement, and (3) it provides for easy exchange of TDs.

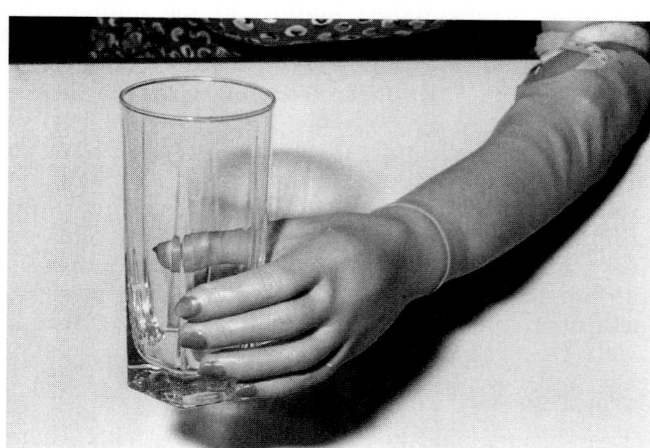

*Figure 27-3* Myoelectrical hand.

### *Elbow Unit*

Myoelectrically controlled elbow units are available for AE amputees. The amputee with a high-level amputation requires an electric elbow because of insufficient residual limb length to operate a mechanical prosthetic elbow. In other words, the force required to pull the mechanical prosthetic cable to operate a TD or mechanical elbow is too great for a short residual limb. Previously, prosthetic choices for these individuals were greatly limited. The development of the electric elbow has made it possible to restore upper limb function to even the highest level amputee.

The motions of elbow flexion and extension are controlled by electrical signals from the muscle surface. When a muscle contracts, the muscle membrane generates an electric potential. This is sensed, amplified, and processed by the control unit. The same muscle sites used for hand control are used for elbow movement. Therefore no retraining of new muscle sites is needed. No large shoulder movements are required, only the natural contraction of the triceps and biceps. The elimination of awkward gross body movements allows more natural, smooth, body movements. The elbow has 21 available stopping positions within the range of 15 to 150 degrees of elbow flexion.[10] Currently the elbow unit is capable of performing only flexion and extension movement patterns through myoelectrical control. A passive humeral rotation joint provides side to side positioning of the forearm. The elbow, when locked, has the capacity to sustain a maximum load of 50 pounds and a live-lift of 2 pounds.[10] A common complaint about the electric elbow is its weight. The elbow unit itself adds 2 pounds of weight to the prosthesis, with an additional 1 pound for the electric hand. The finished product usually weighs a total of 3 to 4½ pounds. However, the amputee who develops competence in operating the unit usually finds its functional worth more than compensates for the initial discomfort.

### *Shoulder Unit*

When a patient has a shoulder disarticulation or a forequarter amputation, a shoulder unit is used. It provides cosmesis for a symmetrical body appearance. There are passive and friction components permitting manual positioning of the shoulder but no active function.

### *Electrodes*

Surface electrodes (Figure 27-4) are mounted inside the socket at predetermined muscle sites that display strong myoelectric signals. Good electrical contact is the key to achieving a usable myoelectric prosthesis. The **electrode** reads the muscle activity and sends a message to the controller that moves the motor at the terminal device. For instance, for a BE amputee, electrodes are placed on the wrist extensors and flexors. With normal movement, the flexors when activated would close the hand and the extensors would open the hand. In other words, when the electrodes read a signal from the flexors, the message would be sent to the motor and the hand would respond by closing. In the case of AE amputation the electrodes are placed on the triceps to open the hand and the biceps to close the hand. These sites are also used to send the signal to the elbow device triggering elbow flexion from the biceps and elbow extension from the triceps.

### *Battery*

The battery (Figure 27-5) provides the energy from which the motor runs to operate the component parts of the prosthesis. A removable rechargeable 6-V battery is used. The battery operates the prosthesis during the day and is recharged at night. The amputee may have several batteries to interchange as needed. The normal charge life of a battery is 6 hours of active use. The capacity of these batteries to hold a charge will decrease in time, eventually requiring complete re-

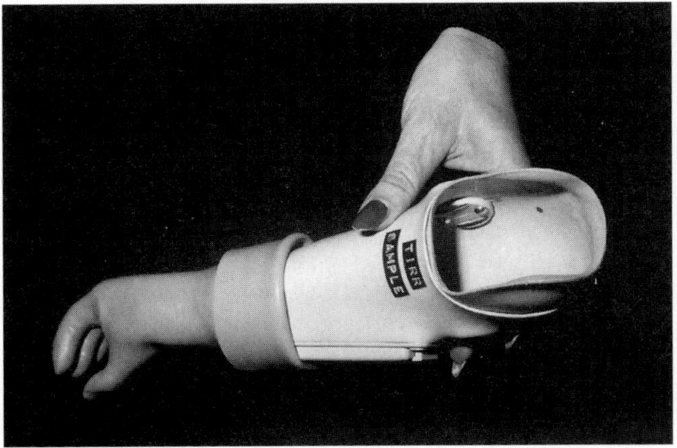


*Figure 27-4* Surface electrodes recessed within the wall of a myoelectric socket detect muscle contractions.

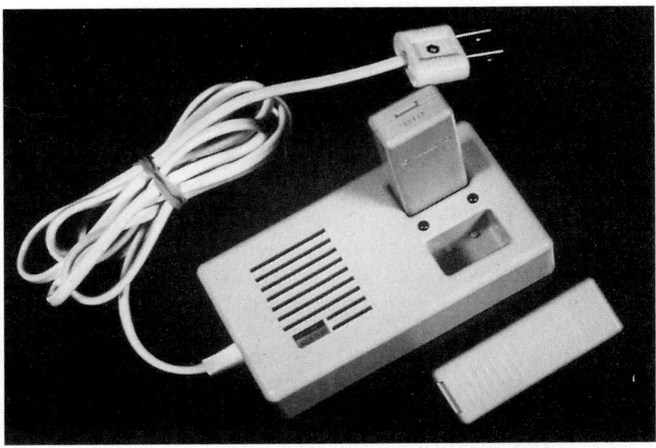

*Figure 27-5* Battery of a myoelectrical arm is inserted in a battery charger and charged overnight.

placement of the battery approximately every 2 years, depending on the patient's use and care patterns of the battery itself.[10] The battery is normally positioned at the surface of the prosthesis to allow for easy removal for charging. On the below elbow prosthesis, the battery is located on the forearm; on the above elbow prosthesis, the battery is fitted at the elbow joint or is internal. The goal of the prosthetist in positioning the battery is two-fold—easy removal and good cosmetic appearance.

#### *Socket/Suspension*

Socket design is very important to the functional use of the myoelectric prosthesis. When the prosthetist is designing the socket for the patient, the following areas must be considered: (1) residual limb comfort, (2) overall cosmesis, (3) electrode contact, (4) suspension style.

Residual limb comfort within the socket will often determine the wear and use pattern of the prosthesis. The socket must not compromise skin integrity by causing pressure points or pressing on sensitive areas of the residual limb. The amputee will not wear or use the device if it is not comfortable.

The same principle applies to the overall appearance of the prosthesis. The prosthetic socket should be pleasing in skin tone, size, length, and muscle bulk so as to encourage the person to accept the prosthesis.

It is most essential that the socket design provide constant contact between the skin and the electrodes with very little movement of the arm within the socket. Without careful design and fit of electrode to muscle site contact, the operation of the prosthesis will be difficult (if not impossible), setting the patient up for failure.

Finally, the socket design determines the type of suspension to be used. For BE amputees, self-suspension is always an option. This means the total elimination of a harness and its restriction of movement. In most cases the AE amputee still requires a harness in addition to self-suspension to distribute the weight of the prosthesis. The type of suspension used should be determined by the length of the residual limb, the patient's preference based on comfort and ease of prosthetic application and removal, and the prosthetic use pattern. There are three types of suspension: sleeve suspension, supracondylar suspension, and suprastyloid suspensions.[3]

The prosthetist is the expert on the various socket suspensions available. However, the therapy practitioner must know the suspension options to assist the patient and the prosthetist in choosing one that will best meet the functional demands of the patient.

### Mechanical vs. Myoelectrical Prostheses

There are many positive and negative aspects of both the mechanical and myoelectrical prostheses (Box 27-1). The best solution for an amputee is to have both prosthetic devices available to meet the changing demands of specific activities. An amputee may use the mechanical prosthesis when he is working on a car but later that day might wear the myoelectric prosthesis to go out with his friends to play pool. Different tools are used for different applications—both have value.

*Box 27-1*

**Advantages and Disadvantages of Myoelectrical Prostheses**

**Advantages**

- Improved cosmesis
- Increased grip force (approximately 25 lb in an adult myoelectrical hand)
- Minimal or no harnessing
- Ability to use overhead
- Minimal effort needed to control device
- Closely corresponds to human physiological control

**Disadvantages**

- Cost of prosthesis
- Frequency of maintenance and repair
- Fragile nature of glove and need for frequent replacements
- Absence of sensory feedback (some sense of proprioceptive feedback provided in a *body-powered* prosthesis)
- Slow response of electric hand
- Increased weight

### Progression of the Prosthesis

Many factors interfere with the preferred prosthetic progression. Assuming an amputee enters the prosthetic rehabilitation process at the time of surgery and has no complications, has good funding sources, has an optimal length of the residual limb, and is motivated for treatment, the progression would proceed as follows: (1) immediate/early postoperative (postop) prosthesis, (2) preparatory mechanical prosthesis, (3) preparatory myoelectrical prosthesis, (4) definitive mechanical prosthesis, (5) definitive myoelectrical prosthesis. In many cases this progression is not practical or realistic. The progression differs from patient to patient depending on variables such as stump length, funding sources, patient motivation, and time of entry into the rehabilitation process. A patient can start or stop at various points in the progression as a result of these factors.

#### *Immediate/Early Postoperative Prosthesis*

An immediate prosthesis and an **early postoperative prosthesis** are identical in fabrication. The name given varies with the time of fabrication. The immediate prosthesis is applied in surgery at the time of final closure. The early postoperative prosthesis is applied sometime after surgery but before suture removal. In both cases the socket is made out of fiberglass casting tape wrapped around the residual limb. A thermoplastic frame is attached to the socket, and the terminal device and elbow unit are stabilized onto this frame.[3] If an elbow unit is needed, a lightweight manual hinge elbow is placed on this prosthesis with eight set-locking points to position the elbow. A figure-eight harness with a simple cable to control the TD is used. Only one rubber band is provided for grip force at this stage. The prosthesis is used mainly as a gross stabilizer. The immediate/postoperative prosthesis serves to introduce the patient to prosthetic use and wear and to provide a rigid dressing for edema control and proprioceptive input.[3]

### *Preparatory Mechanical Prosthesis*

The preparatory mechanical prosthesis is applied when full healing is complete and the sutures are removed, usually 10 to 14 days after surgery. The socket is fabricated from a plaster mold of the residual limb for a customized fit. The socket is made out of clear plastic to allow for monitoring of stump changes in volume and socket fit. The preparatory prosthesis is made out of more durable materials than the postop prosthesis and can be used like a definitive (final) prosthesis. Its construction permits easy interchangeability of parts and components to evaluate which works best for this patient. The purposes of the preparatory mechanical prosthesis are the following:

- To continue edema control
- To condition tissues to accept forces exerted by the prosthetic socket
- To help the patient and clinic team determine which parts will functionally be the best
- To demonstrate the patient's level of motivation and compliance
- To give the patient a chance to see the value and limitations of a mechanical prosthesis[3]

The preparatory prosthesis allows the patient to develop skill and strength while determining which specifications work best. It is more cost effective to make changes to this (temporary) prosthesis. Thus patients are free to evaluate his or her prosthetic needs.

### *Preparatory Myoelectrical Prosthesis*

Once the patient has demonstrated good muscle site control and funding is ensured for a myoelectrical prosthesis, a preparatory myoelectrical prosthesis is fabricated. A preparatory myoelectrical prosthesis is a cost-effective way to analyze the patient's ability to use the prosthesis and to evaluate the components best suited to the patient's needs. The preparatory myoelectrical prosthesis is fitted similarly to the definitive prosthesis, except it has a transparent test socket to monitor electrode contact and evaluate socket stability. A fitting frame is attached to the socket to provide a surface for the electronic components to be attached. A standard protective outer glove is placed over the electronic hand for cosmesis and protection of the inner shell of the hand. Suspension, socket design, and electrode placement are all easily changeable to allow the patient to explore options. The purposes of the preparatory myoelectric prosthesis are the following:

- To determine patient's motivation and commitment to get the maximum use out of the prosthesis
- To evaluate in a cost-effective way appropriate components and suspension systems
- To condition the tissues in a self-contained socket
- To determine the patient's use, skill, and wear patterns with myoelectrical control[3]

### *Definitive Mechanical Prosthesis*

Once the patient has determined the components needed, has established a full wear pattern with good prosthetic skill, and had reached full residual limb maturation, a definitive mechanical prosthesis is considered. The definitive prosthesis is designed on the basis of choices the patient made during the preparatory stage. The definitive prosthesis is fabricated with durable parts and provides a good cosmetic appearance.

### *Definitive Myoelectrical Prosthesis*

The cost of a definitive myoelectrical prosthesis in 1996 was approximately $40,000 for an AE prosthesis and $20,000 for a BE prosthesis. The preparatory myoelectrical prosthesis is an essential step in determining whether myoelectrical control is functional enough for the patient to incur this cost. The decision is based on the patient's wear, use, and skill patterns during the preparatory stage. The design incorporates the components that best suited the patient during the use of the preparatory myoelectrical prosthetic.

## The Upper Extremity Prosthetic Training Program

### *Preoperative Care*

Seventy-five percent of amputations result from trauma, and an opportunity to treat a patient before amputation is unusual. However, some amputations are the result of elective or needed surgery (after cancer or unsuccessful upper extremity (UE) reattachment). Intervention before surgery emphasizes psychological support, education on prosthetic options available, training for the postoperative exercise program, and introduction to one-handed survival techniques for activities of daily living (ADLs).

### *Postoperative Care*

The usual patient length of stay in the hospital after an amputation is 3 to 4 days if there are no complications. Within these several days, patients are fitted with a prosthesis, and the therapist or assistant makes the initial contact with them. The initial contact should focus on emotional and psychological support. Patients usually are overwhelmed with feelings of uncertainty and anxiety about the future. Answers to unspoken questions will begin to put them at ease about starting a rehabilitative process. During the postoperative period, patients may be counselled about the acceptance of the amputation and about the prosthesis and its benefits. It is important for the clinician to be aware of what the amputation and the prosthesis may mean to the client.

A preprosthetic evaluation is completed by the occupational therapist, and the training program is introduced at this time. Based on this evaluation and with the patient's input, a treatment program is established that is designed to promote stump shrinkage, desensitize the stump, maintain ROM of proximal joints, and begin building prosthetic skill. Adjusting to the loss and achieving independence in self-care are other important aspects of the training program.[23] The following areas should be addressed in the postoperative training stage before the patient is discharged from the acute care hospital.

*Stump care/skin hygiene* The client is encouraged to move and use the stump as much as possible during the healing period. This movement will help give normal proprioceptive input to the brain and prevent muscle atrophy and contractures that result from guarding the residual limb at the side of the body. Instruction in proper residual limb hygiene is provided.

*Stump wrapping* Shrinking and shaping the residual limb is necessary to form a tapered-shaped limb that will tolerate a prosthesis. Compression aids in the shrinking and shaping process, with either an elastic ace bandage, tubular bandage, or a shrinker sock applied to the residual limb. A figure-eight method is used when an elastic bandage is applied to the limb. Care must be taken to apply the bandage smoothly, evenly, and not too tightly from the distal to the proximal end of the residual limb. The elastic bandage should be rewrapped several times a day to keep the correct tension. The patient is instructed to wrap the stump when not wearing the postoperative prosthesis.

*ROM exercise* With medical approval, stump exercises may begin. These are designed to encourage use of the stump, maintain ROM of joints proximal to the amputation site, and strengthen muscles of the arm and shoulder. Many of these muscles will ultimately be used to operate the prosthesis, so strength and endurance are the desired results of training.[23] A simple AROM routine without resistance is recommended, involving all the nonaffected muscles and available movements.

*Desensitization* A program is established to normalize sensation in the residual limb, which often is hypersensitive after surgery with extreme discomfort in response to normal tactile stimulation. Treatment aims to decrease hypersensitivity. Graded stimuli are introduced; materials are graded from soft to hard and force of application is graded from light touch to rubbing to tapping to prolonged pressure. A desensitization program is best carried out by the patient so that tolerance is increased without pain.

*Wear schedule and use schedule* The patient is instructed to wear the postoperative prosthesis three times a day beginning with 15 minute periods with 5 minutes of active use. The wear schedule is increased to 30 minutes of wear three times a day with 10 minutes of active use by the third day. Wear and active use progressively increase on an individual basis. The patient is instructed to check the residual limb after wear periods to identify pressure spots and any problems with healing. An activity list is provided giving suggestions for skill building. Examples of appropriate activities are picking up small objects such as paper clips, wrapping a present, and playing cards. The early use of a temporary prosthesis aids in psychological adjustment and will increase the likelihood of acceptance and use of the prosthesis by the amputee.

*Prosthetic skill training* The patient will need instruction in the use of the early postoperative prosthesis. The mechanical training section in this chapter provides specifics of prosthetic use training. The postoperative prosthesis is basic in design, with a lightweight working hook TD that requires very little excursion to operate. The TD has only 1 lb of grip force and therefore has limited practical use. The patient must be made aware of this limitation to prevent undue frustration. The patient should also be reassured that the next prosthetic device will be more functional. The patient is encouraged to incorporate the prosthesis in two-handed patterns and use it actively as much as possible. Most of the prosthetic skill training will occur on an outpatient basis and only simple instructions are provided at first to avoid overwhelming the patient and to encourage prosthetic use.

### Components of Mechanical Prosthetic Training

A preparatory mechanical prosthesis is fabricated at the time the sutures have been removed. Once the patient has this device, training can begin full force with emphasis on prosthetic wear, skill, use, acceptance, grip-strength tolerance, a two-handed pattern, and a return to independence in ADL, work, and leisure activities. Other goals include retraining dominance if necessary, normalizing sensation in the residual limb, and strengthening the residual limb.

*Training the unilateral BE amputee*

- *Introduction to prosthetic parts:* The amputee should learn the names and functions of the parts of the prosthesis so that communication can occur with the therapist, physician, or prosthetist, using terminology understood by all. This is especially important if the amputee is having difficulties with the prosthesis or if it is in need of repairs.

- *Donning and removing the prosthesis:* The amputee dons the stump sock with the sound arm. To apply the prosthesis the amputee places it on table or bed and pushes the stump between the control cable and Y strap from the medial side into the socket (Figure 27-6, *top*). The sound arm is then slipped into the axilla loop. The amputee grasps the harness and lifts it over the head so it is positioned properly in back (Figure 27-6, *bottom*). The shoulders are shrugged to shift the harness forward and into the correct position. To remove the prosthesis the amputee slips the axilla shoulder strap off on the sound side with the TD and then slips the shoulder strap off on the amputated side. The harness is slipped off like a coat.
- *TD control training*: Bi-scapular abduction and humeral flexion on the amputated side are the motions necessary to operate the TD. The clinician moves the patient through the motions passively (Figure 27-7). During this procedure the amputee watches the TD operate and gains a sense of the tension on the prosthesis control cable. The amputee then repeats the motions without assistance and verbalizes the actions that occurred during operation. The clinician instructs the amputee to repeat all of the motions in one continuous sequence in both sitting and standing positions until they are smooth and natural.[34] The amputee will then be instructed to open and close the TD in a variety of ranges of elbow and shoulder motion. TD opening and closing should be accomplished easily with the elbow extended, at 30 degrees, 45 degrees, 90 degrees, and with full elbow flexion, as well as with the arm overhead, down at the side, out to the side, and leaning over to floor level.[35]

*Training the unilateral AE amputee*

- *Elbow control training:* Learning to flex the mechanical elbow is the first step in the training process. Once again humeral flexion and scapular abduction are the control motions. The clinician passively flexes the prosthesis into full elbow flexion, noting that the control is slackened by this maneuver (Figure 27-8). The clinician then flexes the amputee's shoulder forward and asks the amputee to hold this position while the clinician lets go (Figure 27-9). The amputee gains a sense of the control cable tension across the scapula from

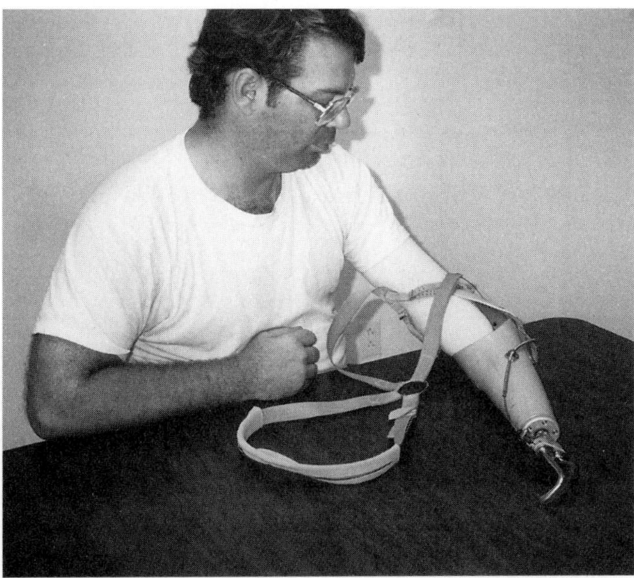

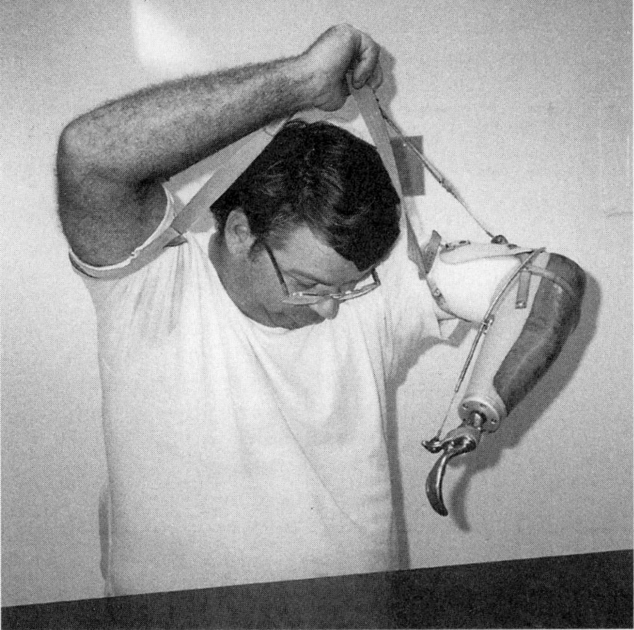

*Figure 27-6* Donning a mechanical prosthesis.

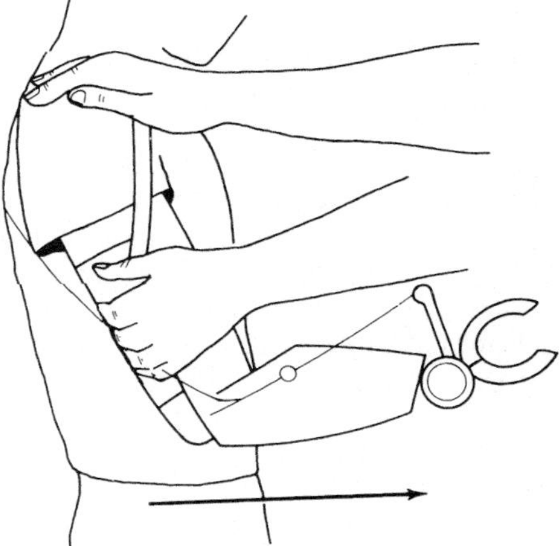

*Figure 27-7* Therapist moves stump forward to attain cable tension and TD opening.

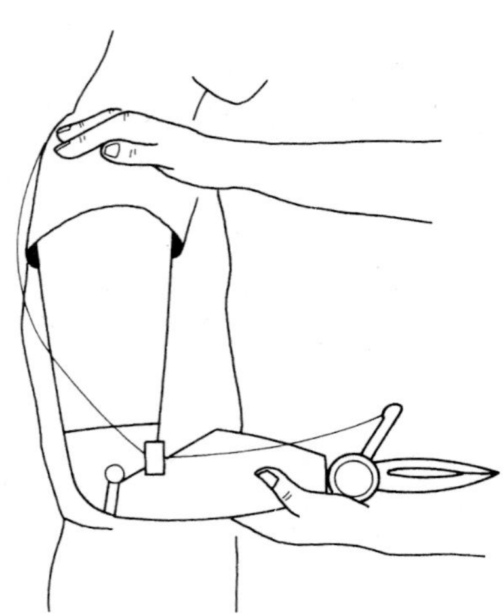

*Figure 27-8* Therapist passively flexes elbow to cause slackening of control cable.

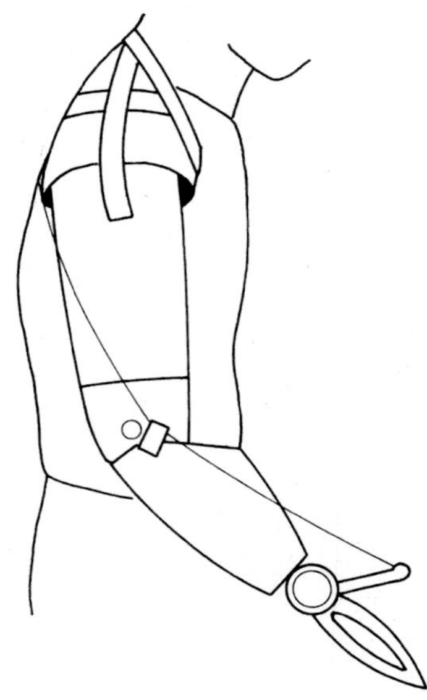

*Figure 27-10* Amputee relaxes stump to allow controlled extension of forearm.

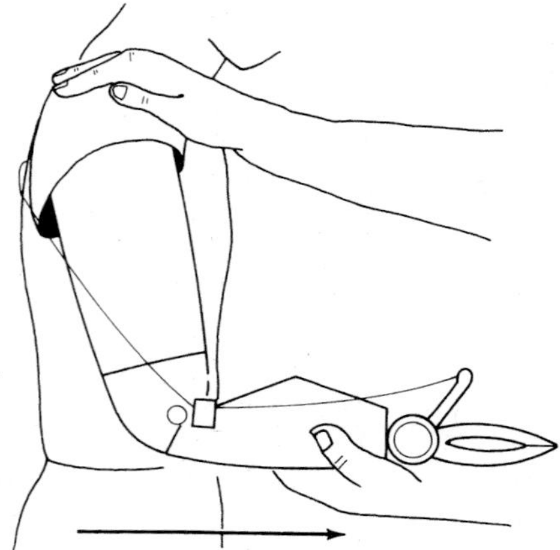

*Figure 27-9* Forearm is moved forward to maintain elbow flexion; this causes tension on control cable.

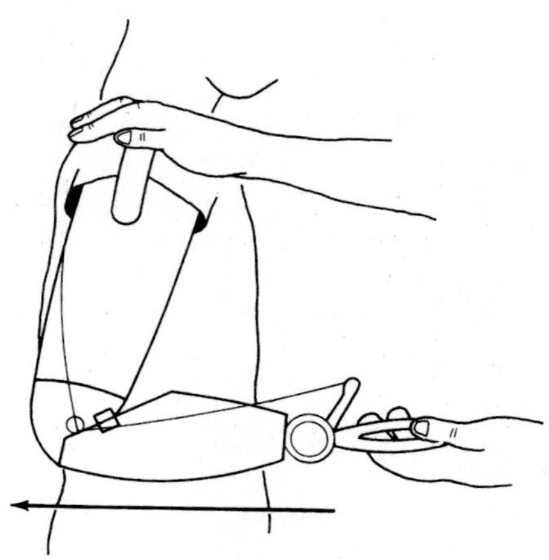

*Figure 27-11* Therapist pushes humerus into hyperextension to lock elbow.

this maneuver. The amputee is asked to relax the stump to the side of the body once again, slowly allowing the forearm to extend (Figure 27-10). The amputee is then asked to again flex the humerus and abduct the scapula to accomplish elbow flexion and relax the stump back slowly into shoulder extension to achieve elbow extension. This is repeated until the amputee gains enough control of cable tension to accomplish elbow flexion and extension smoothly and with ease.[35] The clinician then teaches elbow locking by passively pushing the humerus into hyperextension with the elbow flexed thus locking the elbow (Figure 27-11).

The clinician brings the arm back to the neutral position and then lets go, demonstrating that the elbow mechanism is locked. The clinician repeats this maneuver, demonstrating that the elbow is now unlocked. The amputee is then asked to lock the elbow by moving the humerus into hyperextension and rolling the shoulder forward, using scapular depression and abduction at the same time to lock the elbow. The amputee is then asked to practice locking and unlocking the elbow in various ranges of elbow flexion and extension until full flexion and extension are obtained (Figure 27-12).[35]

- *Use training:* Once the controls are mastered, use training begins. The first stage is prepositioning the TD. This involves rotating the TD to the best

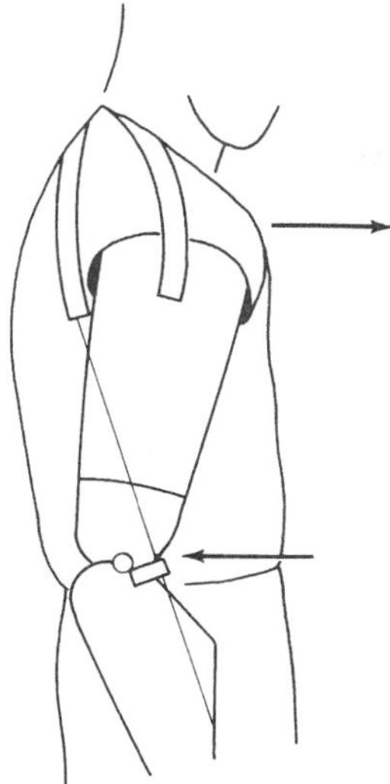

*Figure 27-12* Shoulder is rolled forward, scapula abducted, and humerus hyperextended to lock or unlock elbow at various points in ROM.

position to grasp an object or perform a given activity. The goal of prepositioning the TD should be to allow amputees to approach an object or activity as they would with a normal hand and to avoid awkward body movements that might be used to compensate for poor prepositioning. Along with prepositioning, prehension training should begin with large, hard objects such as blocks, cans, and jars and progress to soft, then to crushable objects such as rubber balls, sponges, paper boxes, cones, and paper cups. These objects should be placed at various heights and positions that demand prepositioning and TD opening and closing, elbow flexion, and locking and unlocking, at various heights.

The amputee should be encouraged to use a problem-solving approach to these and other tasks to determine the best position for the TD as well as appropriate use of the sound arm and the prosthesis in activities. Use training should progress to performance of necessary ADL. The amputee is encouraged to analyze and perform activities of personal hygiene and grooming, dressing, feeding, home management, communication and environmental hardware use, avocation, and vocation as independently as possible. The COTA may help the amputee achieve success by training with a special method or gadget or repetitious practice.[34]

### *Components of Myoelectrical Prosthetic Training*

Myoelectrical prosthetic training takes place simultaneously with mechanical prosthetic training. Once the patient has developed good skill and use with the mechanical prosthesis and can tolerate learning another skill, muscle site testing and weight training is introduced. A typical treatment session at this point might focus on mechanical prosthetic functional use training for 15 minutes, muscle site training for 15 minutes, and weight training for the remaining 30 minutes. It is important that the therapist have a complete understanding of the myoelectrical prosthesis and an ability to differentiate patient errors from possible equipment malfunctions. The ability to pinpoint the source of the problem (whether it be equipment or operator error) is the key to successfully teaching and training the amputee about myoelectrical control.

The goals of the myoelectrical training program are the following:

1. To operate the prosthesis automatically with minimal effort
2. To care for the prosthesis
3. To use the prosthesis smoothly and efficiently for frequently encountered tasks
4. To analyze the best methods for unusual or new tasks[27]

*Signal training* Signal training is the process of learning to produce the muscle signals necessary to operate the myoelectrical prosthesis.[27] Electrodes placed on the residual limb are connected to a feedback system that lets the patient know when the control muscles are contracting and at what level of intensity. Signal training helps the patient develop the ability to produce clear, strong contractions without wasting energy and to relax the control muscles even when the rest of the arm is actively moving.[27] Once the muscle sites are located by the OTR, the COTA uses the same biofeedback device for training. It is essential that individuals with an amputation receive adequate training and practice in initiating the desired muscle contractions before receiving the myoelectrical prosthesis. The patients' success and effectiveness in using the prosthesis is closely related to the quality of the muscle site training process.

*Weight training* The OTR designs a strengthening program to be carried out at home to strengthen the shoulder so that the added weight of a myoelectrical prosthesis can be managed. The COTA may implement the weight training program, providing instruction to ensure follow-through. Theraband, free weights, or weight training equipment all work equally well to accomplish this goal. The prosthetist often provides a socket with weights equalling the myoelectrical prosthesis attached to it for patients to wear several weeks before receiving the prosthesis to accustom them to the additional weight.

*Care of prosthesis* When patients are given the myoelectrical preparatory prosthesis, they are instructed in the basic care of the prosthesis, including how to charge the batteries, clean the prosthesis, and take care of the glove.

*Donning/doffing* The method of application is determined by the type of suspension and socket design that the patient uses. Therefore no one method can be discussed. Regardless, donning the prosthesis should be done with the electronics in the "off" position.

*Use training* Training focuses on a combination of skill-building activities to learn prosthetic control and functional activities to encourage carryover of skills in daily tasks. Training must begin with learning to use the myoelectrical hand in simple approach, grasp, and release activities. Classic therapeutic activities for hand control can be used, such as the pegboard or Velcro checkers. The patient should be able to judge the amount of hand opening or closing required to pick up an item. For instance, if the patient is trying to pick up a cotton swab, full hand opening would not be necessary and would demonstrate a lack of control. The clinician emphasizes good problem-solving skills for the patient to preposition the TD in the optimum position for the specific activity. It is a common error for the amputee to "adjust" the body with compensatory large body motions rather than adjusting or prepositioning the hand first.

Another important aspect in training is mastery of the gripping force of the terminal device. This involves close visual attention to grade the muscle contraction to get a specific result in the myoelectric hand. Too strong a grasp will result in crushing an object that is being held (Figure 27-13). Training with foam cups, sponges, and cotton balls will help develop the control needed to handle paper cups, eggs, potato chips, sandwiches, and even to hold someone's hand. Eventually the movements will take less cognitive effort and become automatic. Each session should focus on both functional training and skill-building activities. Functional two-handed tasks are selected according to the patients' interests or the activities that they are finding difficult. The therapist should observe the patient closely when performing a functional task and ask the following questions: (1) Is the patient using the prosthesis spontaneously in the activity? (2) Is it being used as a gross stabilizer or in a nonactive pattern of use? (3) Does the patient use large compensatory body movements instead of prepositioning the components to the optimal position? (4) Is the patient overshooting the target? (5) Is the patient using the proper grip force? On the basis of the answers to these questions, appropriate activities can be selected to focus on deficit areas.

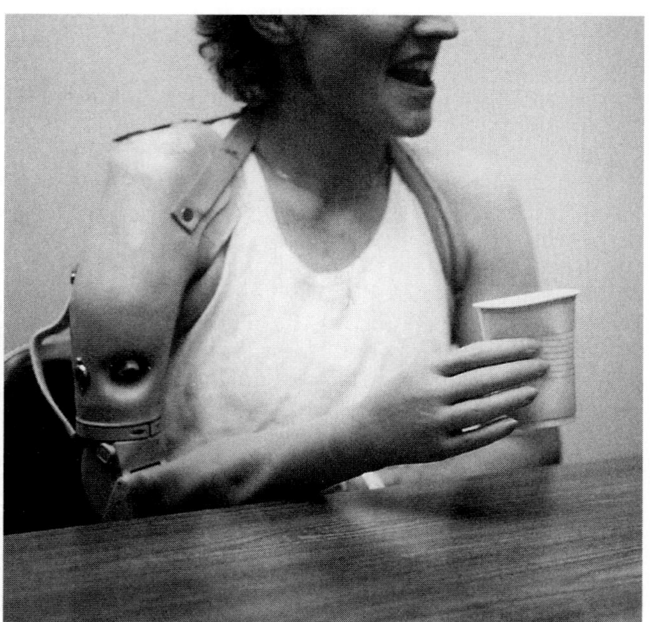

*Figure 27-13* Above elbow amputee demonstrates how too strong a grasp will crush the object being held.

*Vocational and leisure activities* As training proceeds and the patient develops a sense of self-acceptance and comfort with the amputation, the clinician should broach the subject of return to work. If possible, job requirements can be discussed and then practiced in a simulated step-by-step process. Ideally, an on-site visit could be made by the clinician, and several requirements of the job could be practiced. If changes and adjustments to the work environment are necessary, the clinician could advise in these modifications.

Recreational activities are also critically important because they contribute to significant physical and psychological well-being. The terminal devices for recreational activities are not myoelectrical but can be placed on the socket of a myoelectrical prosthesis. Therapeutic Recreation Systems (TRS) has some excellent adaptation components.[23]

**Expected Outcomes**

At the completion of a training program, patients should be proficient in the use and care of both the mechanical and myoelectrical prostheses and should demonstrate a full-day wear pattern. Patients should incorporate the use of a prosthesis in all areas of their premorbid lifestyle. They should demonstrate good spontaneous prosthetic use with skilled precision of movement. They should also have resolved psychological issues related to limb loss and have a realistic outlook on the usefulness of the prosthesis as a replacement arm.

## LOWER EXTREMITY AMPUTATIONS

The management of a lower-extremity (LE) amputee will be addressed by occupational therapy differently from the UE amputee. Occupational therapy will focus primarily on positioning, basic activities of daily living (BADL), dynamic balance (with and without a prosthesis), strengthening the UE for the amputee to perform advanced ADL (with and without a prosthesis), driving, prevocational and vocational activities, leisure education, facilitating reintegration into the community, family education, home program, durable medical equipment (DME) for the home, and a home visit. The COTA may assist the OTR or assume responsibility for many of these areas once service competency with this population is achieved.

Physical therapy assumes major responsibility for the preprosthetic preparation and prosthetic training of the LE amputee. Physical therapy manages the wound care and application of any physical modalities to minimize the pain and promote healing. Understanding the levels of an LE amputation is important in the management of an LE amputee in occupational therapy.

### Levels of Amputation and Functional Losses in the Lower Extremity

The higher the level of amputation is (Figure 27-14) the greater the functional loss of the part and the more the amputee will depend on the prosthesis for function and cosmesis. The higher level amputation requires more complex and extensive prostheses and prosthetic training. Hemipelvectomy and hip disarticulation amputation results in loss of the entire LE, thus hip, knee, ankle, and foot functions are lost.[20,21] **Above-knee amputations (AKAs)** and knee disarticulation amputations result in loss of knee, ankle, and foot motion.

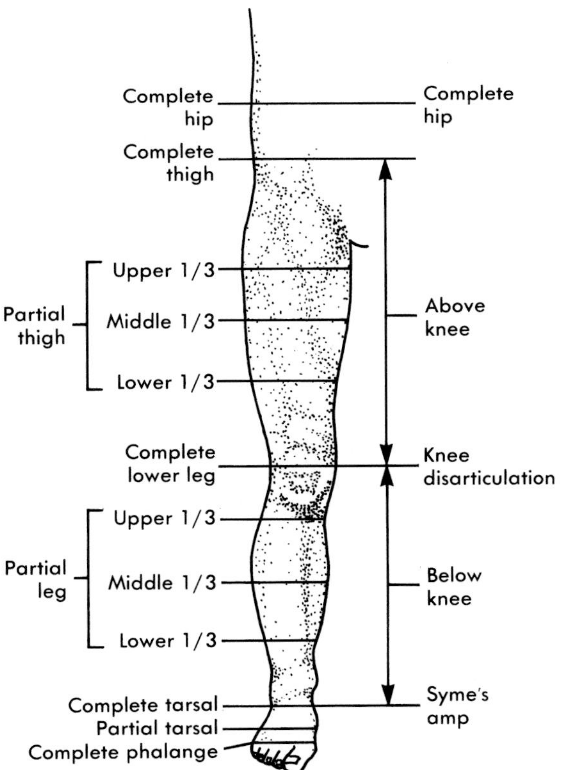


*Figure 27-14* Levels of amputation and functional losses in lower extremity. (From O'Sullivan SB, Cullen K, Schmitz T: *Physical rehabilitation: evaluation and treatment procedures,* Philadelphia, 1981, FA Davis.)

The stump of the AKA can vary in length from 10 to 12 inches (5.4 to 30.5 cm) below the greater trochanter.[20,21]

**Below-knee amputations (BKAs)** result in a stump that is approximately 4 to 6 inches (10.1 to 15.2 cm) in length from the tibial plateau.[20,21] Other classification systems further delineate the amputations into thirds. Upper, middle, and lower ⅓ indicate the distance below the ischium for AKAs. For the BKAs, these divisions indicate the distance below the tibial plateau.[20] The **Symes amputation** is equivalent to an ankle disarticulation.[2] These individuals lose ankle and foot function. In a transmetatarsal amputation, the foot is severed through the metatarsal bones and the ankle function remains intact.[2] Loss of the small toes does not result in functional impairment. Loss of the great toe, however, prevents toe-off during ambulation.[29]

### Component Parts of the Lower Extremity Prosthesis

#### *Rigid Removal Dressing*

The major component parts in the immediate postoperative prosthesis for lower extremity amputee can include the **rigid removal dressing** (i.e., cast or a stiff solid dressing of plaster of paris or other material) that is applied just after surgery to assure control of swelling, to apply firm pressure, and to contour the stump in preparation for the permanent prosthesis. The cast is changed approximately every 10 days or earlier if the cast becomes loose until the stump is healed and ready for a permanent artificial leg (Figure 27-15). The cast is held in position with a canvas band and secured with a Velcro strap. Another method to overcome the weight of the cast is using suspension straps.

#### *Suspension Straps*

The suspension straps can go to the waist or shoulder belt to keep the cast in position. The end of the cast can be made to take a simple training prosthesis (usually

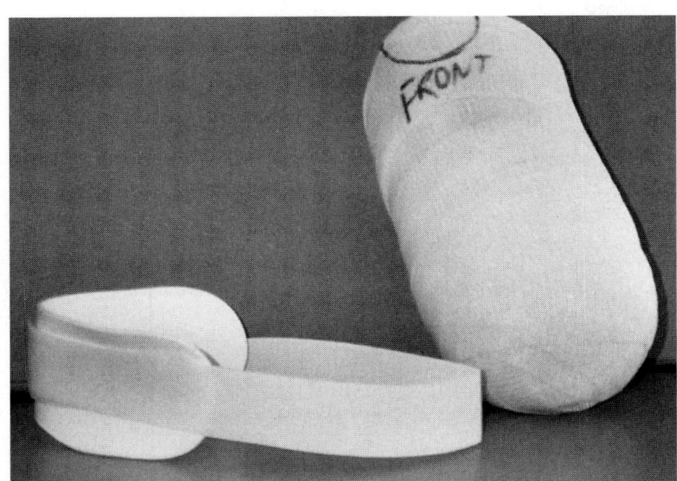


*Figure 27-15* Rigid removal dressing with velcro strap.

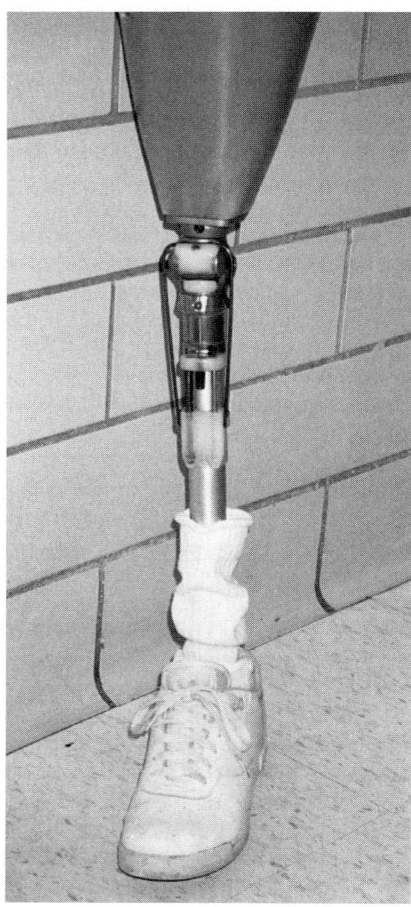

*Figure 27-16* A typical pylon.

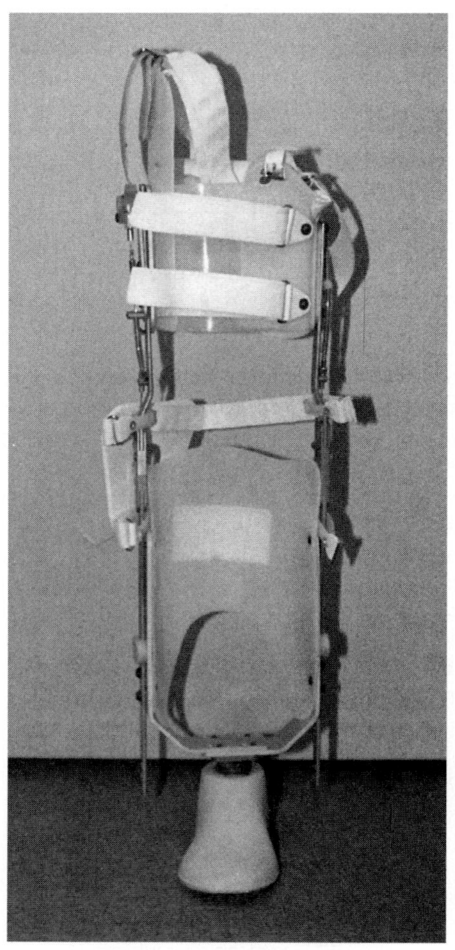

*Figure 27-17* Immediate postoperative ischial weight-bearing prosthesis.

called a pylon) so that training in standing and walking can be started immediately. A typical pylon is shown in Figure 27-16.

The casts are normally designed to take only 30 to 45 lb of the body weight. Too much weight on the cast may result in slow healing or even cause the wound to open. An adjustment quadrilateral socket attached to the upright of a bail suspension and a solid ankle cushion heel **(SACH foot)** are used for the foot.[21] An immediate postoperative prosthesis for the lower extremity amputee allows greater independence early on in the rehabilitation program.

### Types of Prostheses

The immediate postoperative **ischial weight-bearing prosthesis** (IWBP)[30] (Figure 27-17), designed by Dr. Madan Telikicherla, is an early fitting prosthesis that is prefabricated and totally adjustable to an individual's height and build. It can be fit to below-knee, above-knee, and knee disarticulation amputees as early as the first postoperative day. Previous methods of early weight bearing and ambulation have been associated with such complications as wound dehiscence (the separation of the layers of a surgical wound). The unique design of the IWBP bypasses weight bearing through the stump, thus protecting the surgical wound and preventing the pain usually associated with early weight bearing through the residual limb. Use of the IWBP under the supervision of a physician, an occupational therapist, a physical therapist, and a prosthetist enables the amputee to achieve functional ambulation and independent mobility. Within 1 week of surgery, stairs and uneven terrain can be negotiated, almost a full month before the amputee could even be fitted for a conventional prosthesis. This early independence results in increased self-esteem and dignity and enhances the quality of life for the recent amputee. Furthermore, early mobility with the prosthesis can potentially reduce the rehabilitation stay as well as the risk of medical complications associated with immobility.[30]

The **pylon** is a temporary artificial leg. The pylon will serve as a working prosthesis to allow the amputee to use the stump and proximal musculature, maintain

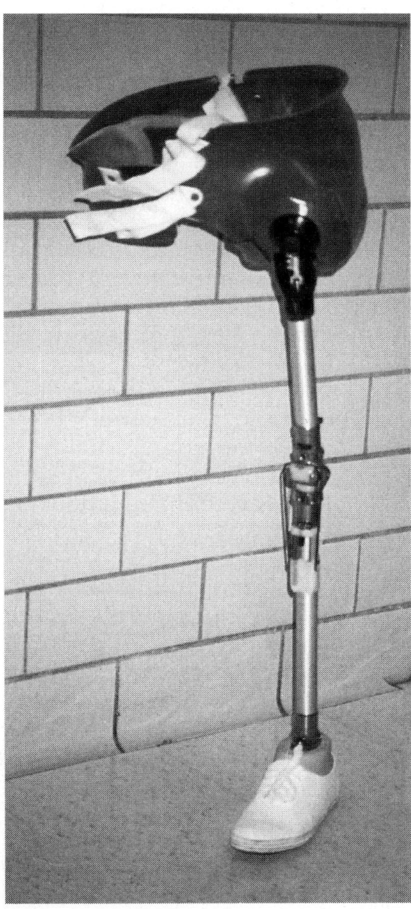

*Figure 27-18* The Canadian prosthesis meets the needs of the hemipelvectomy and hip disarticulation amputee.

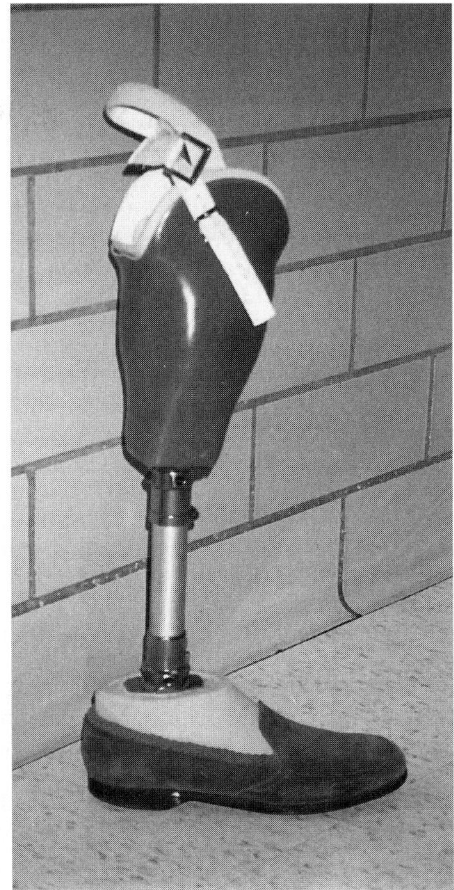

*Figure 27-19* Plastic Syme.

joint ROM, and provide a sense of pressure, motion, and weight that may be similar to that of the actual prosthesis.[29]

The Canadian-type disarticulation prosthesis meets the needs of the hemipelvectomy and hip disarticulation amputee (Figure 27-18). This prosthesis is suspended from the pelvis and equipped with hip and knee joints and a SACH foot. Pelvic movements provide energy for the limb use.[29]

The Syme's amputee uses the Canadian-type Syme prosthesis or a plastic Syme (Figure 27-19). This prosthesis consists of a total contact plastic socket and SACH foot; there is no ankle joint.[29]

Transmetatarsal and toe amputation do not require prostheses. These amputees need a shoe-toe-filler.[29] In the complete tarsal, the amputation is the same as in the Syme. In the partial tarsal the instep is intact. In the complete phalanage all the toes are amputated.

### Lower Extremity Preoperative Training

Preoperative care includes psychological support; keep in mind that individuals' cultural background and lifestyle will influence their ability to cope with the loss of a limb. If amputations are viewed with aversion in individuals' culture or lifestyle, they are likely to have the same feelings.[6] Support groups can help them express feelings. Group members are generally sensitive to others' needs and encourage constructive and creative thinking, which helps to motivate initiative and self-assurance. Visits by other amputees who have adjusted to the loss of a limb can also offer support.

Postoperatively, the therapy practitioner trains the individual in edema management, exercise, balance, and pain management. For AK and BK with swelling (edema) at the stump site, the practitioner instructs the amputee on how to apply the elastic wrap(s) in a figure-eight pattern to prevent a tourniquet effect. The elastic wrap(s) should be placed around the stump site with firm pressure distally that decreases as the wrapping continues proximally. Reapply bandages three or four times a day.[22] If the amputee cannot wrap properly, a stump shrinker (an elastic stocking to control edema) is worn when the prosthesis is not on. Postoperatively, maintaining ROM in the involved extremity is necessary to maintain joint integrity and prevent contractures. Because balance can be affected by the loss of the LE, additional training will be required for ADLs. Pain management is important and should decrease pain whenever possible. Evaluation will be the next step in the occupational therapy program.

### Occupational Therapy Evaluation

The OTR and COTA will work in close partnership with *all* the rehabilitation team members to obtain information on the new amputee in the rehabilitation unit. The OTR and COTA have important and distinct roles in the practice setting. The COTA's responsibilities in the initial evaluation process may include data collection from chart review, interviews with patient and family members, general observations, behavioral checklists, and administering standardized tests once competency is demonstrated (in accordance to the COTA's experience and the facility's regulations). The COTA and OTR should both have the following knowledge of the patient's medical condition: (1) date and level of amputation, (2) reasons for amputations, (3) exact site and level of amputation, (4) periods of dependent positioning allowed by physician, and (5) other medical conditions that might influence treatment (e.g., fractures, vascular involvement, medication, edema, infection).[18] The occupational therapy evaluation will cover the following areas: physical components, BADL, assessment of vocational interests/pursuits, home safety and accessibility, and architectural barriers within the community.

The assessment of the ROM, muscle strength, sensation, vision, pain, and endurance of the amputee will be performed by the OTR. The OTR will prepare the treatment plan for any complex problem involving performance components. The treatment plan will be reviewed and implemented by the COTA with supervision from OTR. The COTA will observe for any changes from the initial assessment and collaborate with the OTR. The COTA will perform the routine/structured techniques for the basic ADL, bed mobility, wheelchair mobility, transfers, hygiene, and dressing, with supervision from the OTR.

Balance and pain management are assessed by the OTR. Advanced ADL assessment including avocational interests and pursuits can be conducted by an experienced COTA. The COTA can lead groups on home safety and accessibility and document the participant's participation.

Home assessment for architectural barriers within the individual's home and community and while driving is performed by the OTR or experienced COTA if permissible by law. When indicated the OTR assesses cognition, psychological adjustment to amputation and its limitations, and visual/perceptual components.

The OTR and COTA will formulate the occupational therapy discharge and follow-up plan and report factual data at time of discharge orally and in writing.[5] A partnership between the OTR and COTA will accelerate the amputee's rehabilitation. The OTR and COTA can also work effectively in another area of importance—sexual counseling—at the individual's request.[9]

#### *Basic ADL*

*Positioning* Prevention of muscle contracture is an immediate postoperative concern.[18] Joint contracture is a common preprosthetic problem among LE amputees.[21] The AKA typically develops a flexion, external rotation, and abduction contracture of the affected hip. The BKA develops an external rotation deformity of the hip and flexion of the knee.[21] Daily ROM exercise is encouraged. One should avoid placing pillows beneath the knee in a BK amputee and under the stump in an AK amputee. Proper positioning reduces excessive edema in a limb when the individual is up in a wheelchair (Figure 27-20).[21]

*Stump hygiene* Once the wound is healed and sutures are removed, the stump should be washed with warm water and dried with a towel. The use of lotions or alcohol is not recommended. Evening care is recommended so that the stump is not softened before prosthetic use.[16]

*Dressing training* Most LE amputees are independent in UE dressing but require assistance for LE dressing. Grade LE dressing from performing in bed, to sitting, to standing.[21] Socks and shoes should be donned while sitting. A sock aid and elastic shoelaces may ease donning for the individual with loss of flexibility, poor sitting balance, or impaired vision. A footstool may also be useful.

*Bed mobility* Individuals are taught bed mobility activities to promote independence without the use of rails or an overhead trapeze bar. They are encouraged to roll from side to side, perform bridging activities

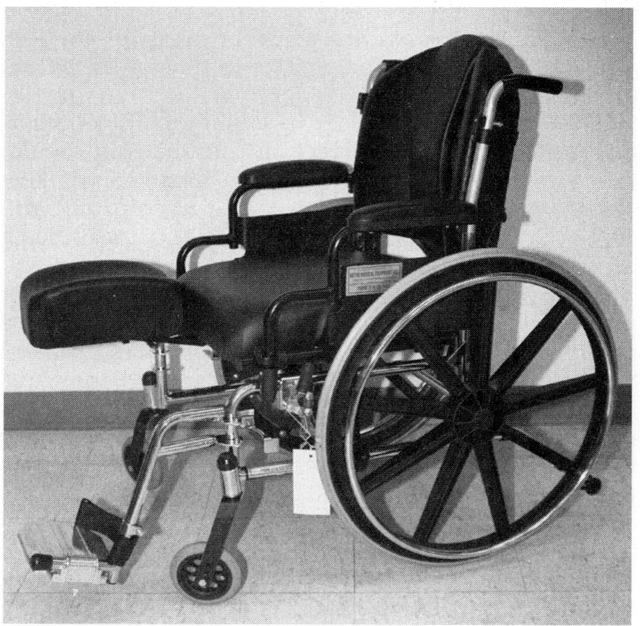

*Figure 27-20* Proper positioning reduces excessive edema in a limb when individual is in a wheelchair.

with knee and hip flexion, and push the foot of the existing limb so that they can push up in bed and don LE clothing over the hips (Figure 27-21).[21]

*Wheelchair mobility and parts management* Postoperatively the wheelchair will be the main source of mobility. (See Chapter 18 for information on wheelchair training.)

*Transfer training* The unilateral LE amputee generally uses a standing pivot transfer (90-degree pivot), transferring toward the existing limb when possible. Having the individual practice transfers toward the amputated side or 180-degree pivots increases independence when transferring in more restrictive environments (e.g., a bathroom or bedroom).[21] Sliding board transfers may be taught to the individual whose existing limb is very weak and to bilateral amputees. Bilateral amputees may consider purchasing a wheelchair with a zippered or removable back to allow transfer by sliding backward to a surface and by sliding forward to return to the wheelchair (anterior/posterior).[18]

*Bathing* Bathing is a self-care activity that includes dressing and undressing, transferring to and from shower chair or tub transfer bench, and balancing while managing the water controls (faucets) and body parts. Adaptive devices (i.e., long-handled bath brush, flexible shower hose, and a tub transfer bench) can be beneficial for independence and safety.[21]

*Balance activities* The prerequisite to performing basic and advanced ADL is balance. The amputee must have good dynamic balance while performing LE dressing activities and while bathing, transferring, reaching for objects in cupboards overhead, and retrieving objects from the floor. These tasks may be done from the wheelchair and while wearing an immediate postoperative prosthesis. It is imperative that the OT practitioner provide graded functional activities to facilitate postural adjustment in all planes.[21]

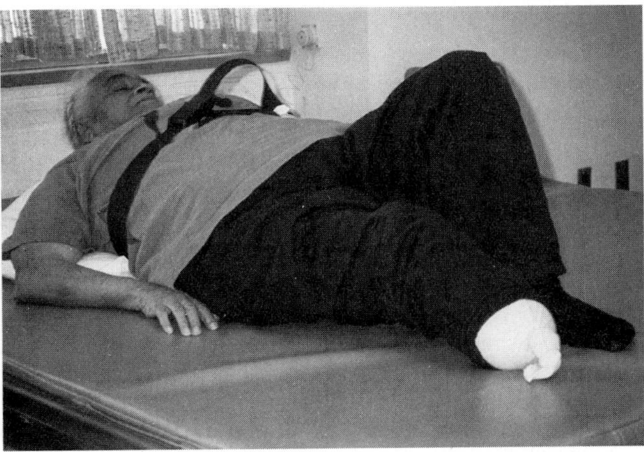

*Figure 27-21* Bed mobility skill called bridging to perform pushing up in bed and to don lower extremity.

*Pain management* There is no specific protocol for the treatment of phantom sensation and pain. Medication, biofeedback, and other compensatory techniques are used to decrease the pain and sensation. In treatment the OTR can instruct the amputee on techniques such as applying pressure (to tolerance), rubbing, tapping, and other modalities such as heat or cold applications on the stump for relief.[18] An experienced COTA will monitor the amputee's performance and collaborate with the OTR when problems arise.

*Energy conservation and work simplification* The amputee will expend more energy during ADL than a person of the same sex, age, and stature who has no amputations.[2] Energy expenditure increases with age and obesity.[21] The COTA should incorporate pacing in all activities to prevent fatigue and injury.

*Home management* Living alone will require the individual to be independent and safe while performing homemaking tasks. Home management should be addressed near discharge and may involve a combination of individual and group sessions. Areas discussed and practiced are preparing simple and full meals, purchasing food, cooking, serving, cleaning, doing laundry (light and heavy), cleaning house, stripping and making beds (a hospital and double bed), and working at various levels (e.g., with a wheelchair, walker, cane, and axillary crutches with or without prosthesis).[21]

*Driving* State laws vary regarding driving after LE amputation. The OTR practitioner should know the law before recommending that the individual resume driving. When appropriate, the individual should be referred to a driver safety specialist for a driving assessment (see Chapter 19).

*Prevocational and vocational activities* The evaluation will determine whether the amputees can return to their previous job. The basic elements are psychological testing including interest and achievement; establishment of an initial vocational plan; vocational counseling; work evaluation including definition of functional skills and assessment of architectural barriers in the work environment; driver education and vehicle modification as needed; communication with state vocational rehabilitation agencies, insurance companies, and other sponsors; job analysis and modifications; and follow-up.

*Recreation/leisure activities* Recreation and the constructive use of leisure time enhance quality of life. Many individuals may view mobility limitations as obstacles to returning to premorbid leisure activities. Thus the overall program should include using community recreational resources, learning new leisure skills, making adaptations for previous leisure skills and interst, and refining of functional abilities related to specific leisure activities. Community skills groups feature both discussion and reentry trips to develop the skills necessary to take an active role in recreational opportunities.[14] Recreational LE prostheses are available for golf, swimming, and skiing.[21]

*Reintegration into community* Ultimately, the individual must gain independence in and accessibility to the community. Here the amputee attempts to manage curbs, inclines, uneven surfaces, and elevators. The individual should be encouraged to problem solve specific architectural barriers.

*Discharge planning* Discharge planning includes educating the family, providing home exercise programs, and securing necessary DME. A home visit may be completed in anticipation of discharge.[21]

*Family education* During family education, the therapist (OTR or COTA) demonstrates transfers and encourages the family to practice using recommended DME with the individual. The therapist observes closely how the family and individual perform the activities and corrects any unsafe practices. If the therapist feels the family will benefit from additional family education it should be discussed at that time. Exercise programs are reviewed with the family in clear and understandable language, and a written copy is provided. DME is discussed in great detail with the family as are locations to purchase equipment in the community. To ensure accessibility in and out of the home and in tight spaces a home visit is essential.

## Case Study

The OTR and COTA work collaboratively as the following case study situation illustrates.

Mrs. M. is a 76-year-old African American woman. She had a surgical right BKA because of poor circulation. The stump is well healed and there is good stump shrinkage. There are no significant medical issues.

Mrs. M. is a retired postal worker. She reported having completed 1 year of college. She enjoys the following leisure activities: playing cards and visiting friends, bowling, and traveling with her husband (Mr. M.) to Georgia visiting family members. Mrs. M. will need to be moderately independent with self-care skills and transfers with the IWBP and a standard walker.

A referral was sent to occupational therapy to increase function in basic ADL, mobility, transfers, and advanced ADL with a prosthesis and walker. The estimated length of stay was 5 to 10 days.

Mrs. M. was assigned to the amputee unit. The OTR assigned a COTA to review Mrs. M.'s medical chart to obtain data sent from the acute facility.

Mrs. M. lives with her husband in a single-family home. The husband is in poor health and in a wheelchair. He was unable to assist her physically. Mrs. M. needed to be moderately independent with her basic self-care to return home. Mrs. M.'s niece was able to perform the heavier home management activities, marketing, and other personal business in the community.

The COTA's admissions interview included an introduction to the OT program. Mrs. M. was aware of her deficits and appeared motivated. The assessment began with the upper extremities passive ROM and active ROM, manual muscle test, sensory, coordination, visual, and cognition performance by the OTR. The BADL were assessed by the COTA. A treatment plan was developed after completion of all the assessments. Areas of deficits were identified. Short-term and long-term goals were identified with Mrs. M. She played an active part in setting her goals.

Mrs. M. was treated in daily, 45- to 60-minute OT sessions. The COTA collaborated with the OTR daily on her progress.

Adaptive devices (i.e., long-handled bath brush, dressing stick, stocking aid, reacher) were issued to improve Mrs. M.'s self-care skills at bed or wheelchair levels. Transfers were initially performed with a sliding board to compensate for Mrs. M.'s decreased endurance. At discharge, Mrs. M.'s mobility and transfers were moderately independent at walker level with prosthesis. Dressing the lower extremity posed some problems initially, but Mrs. M. was moderately independent at discharge. Mrs. M. was reassessed daily for areas that required more improvement. Family instruction was completed with her husband and niece present. DME was ordered for the home (i.e., stationary commode chair, tub transfer bench). Mrs. M. made significant progress in the rehabilitation program. She returned home with good family support. Outpatient OT was recommended for further prosthetic training in light home management at walker level three times a week. The team members were aware that transportation might be a problem and requested orders to be written for home therapy.

Three weeks after discharge, Mr. M. informed the staff that his wife had passed away. Mrs. M. will be remembered for her determination to regain her skills and return to the community.

## SUMMARY

Rehabilitation and prosthetic training of the UE amputee is a complex speciality practice area and is managed by an experienced OTR in collaboration with the prosthetist and other rehabilitation team members. The COTA may assist, particularly in use training, donning and doffing, and transfer of skills to ADL and work and leisure activities.

The rehabilitation of an individual with LE loss requires the skills of many health care specialists including occupational therapy practitioners. Occupational therapy evaluation and training for the LE should focus on positioning, ADL training, and maintaining and improving the ROM and strength in the UE for training with the prosthesis in purposeful activities. The occupational therapy practitioner also assesses the feasibility of the amputee returning to work and resuming or exploring leisure skills.

Facilitating psychological adjustment is another major role of the clinician working with the UE and LE amputees and their family members. It is essential that OTR and COTA collaborate to maximize the amputee's skills for reentry into work force and community.

## Selected Reading Guide Questions

1. What do the following abbreviations mean: AE, TD, BE?
2. Which arm functions are lost and which functions are retained in a long BE amputation?
3. List the advantages and disadvantages of a myoelectrical prosthesis.
4. Which motions accomplish TD opening with a mechanical prosthesis?
5. Which five questions should be asked when observing an amputee in an activity?
6. What is the recommended initial wearing period for the postoperative prosthesis?
7. What does "prepositioning the TD" mean?
8. Why is it important to wrap the stump?
9. What are the responsibilities of the COTA in initial evaluation of the LE amputee?
10. Which method can be used postoperatively to ensure control of stump swelling and to contour the stump for the permanent prosthesis?
11. Why is the LE amputee patient instructed *not* to place pillows under the hip and knee?
12. Amputees sometimes feel as if their missing limb is moving. What is this phenomenon called?
13. Which adaptive devices can ease donning of an LE prosthesis for an individual with loss of flexibility?
14. Which method can be used to teach the LE amputee to don pants in bed?
15. Which transfer approach is generally used by the LE amputee?
16. For which activities must the LE amputee have good dynamic balance?
17. For the LE amputee, which areas are assessed, discussed, and practiced in home management?
18. What will be reviewed by the OTR or COTA during family education?
19. Describe what is included in discharge planning for the LE amputee.

### REFERENCES


1. American Occupational Therapy Association: *The roles and function of occupational therapy personnel,* Rockville, Md, 1973, The Association.
2. Banerjee SJ: *Rehabilitation management of amputees,* Baltimore, 1982, Williams and Wilkins.
3. Brenner CD: *Atlas of limb prosthetics,* ed 2, St Louis, 1992, Mosby.
4. Davies EJ, Friz BR, Clippinger FW: Amputees and their prostheses, *Artif Limb* 14:19-48, 1980.
5. DiDomenico R, editor: Lower limb amputation in the elderly: meeting the rehabilitation challenge, *Focus Geriatr Care Rehabil,* 4:1-8, 1989.
6. Friedman LW: *The surgical rehabilitation of the amputee,* Springfield, Ill, 1978, Charles C. Thomas.
7. Friedman LW: *The psychological rehabilitation of the amputee,* Springfield, Ill, 1978, Charles C. Thomas.
8. Glanttly HW: Statistical study of 12,00 new amputees, *South Med J* 57:1373-1378, 1964.
9. Gurgold GD, Harden DH: Assessing the driving potential of the handicapped, *Am J Occup Ther* 32:41-46, 1978.
10. Jacobsen S et al: Development of Utah Artificial Arm, *IEEE Trans Biomed Eng* 29(4):5, 1982.
11. Jones MS: *An approach to occupational therapy,* ed 2, London, 1964, Butterworth.
12. Kay HW, Newman JD: Relative incidences of new amputations: statistics comparison of 6000 new amputees, *Orthot Prosthet* 59:109, 1978.
13. Kegel B, Carpenter ML, Burgress EM: Functional capabilities of lower extremity amputees, *Arch Phys Med Rehabil* 59:109, 1978.
14. Kegel B, Webster J, Burgress EM: Recreational activities of lower extremity amputees: survey, *Arch Phys Med Rehabil* 61:258, 1980.
15. Kostuik JP, editor: *Amputation surgery and rehabilitation,* New York, 1981, Churchill Livingstone.
16. Larson CB, Gould M: *Orthopedic nursing,* ed 8, St Louis, 1974, Mosby.
17. Leonard JA, Meier RH III: *Rehabilitation medicine: Principles and practice,* New York, 1988, JB Lippincott. Amputees: survey, *Arch Phys Med Rehabil* 61:258, 1980.
18. Lyons BG: The issue is: purposeful versus human activity, *Am J Occup Ther* 37:493, 1983.
19. Malone J et al: Immediate, early and late postsurgical management of upper limb amputation, *J Rehab Res Dev* vol 21, 1984.
20. O'Sullivan S, Cullen K, Schmitz T: *Physical rehabilitation: evaluation and treatment procedures,* Philadelphia, 1981, FA Davis.
21. Pedretti L, Pasquinelli S: Amputations and prosthetics. In Pedretti L, Zoltan B, editors: *Occupational therapy: Practice skills for physical dysfunction,* ed 3, St Louis: 1990, Mosby.
22. *Project to delineate the roles and functions of occupational therapy personnel,* 1972, Rockville, Md, American Occupational Therapy Association.
23. Rock L, Atkins A: Upper extremity amputations and prosthetics. In Pedretti L, Zoltan B, editors: *Occupational therapy: practice skills for physical dysfunction,* ed 4, St Louis, 1995, Mosby.
24. Rusk H, Taylor E: *Rehabilitation medicine: a textbook of physical medicine and rehabilitation,* ed 2, St Louis, 1964, Mosby.
25. Santschi WR, editor: *Manual of upper extremity prosthetics,* ed 2, Los Angeles, 1958, University of California Press.
26. Scott R: An introduction to myoelectric prosthesis, *UNB Monogr Myoelectric Prostheses,* 1984.
27. Scott R et al: Understanding and using your myoelectric prosthesis, *UNB Monogr Myoelectric Prostheses,* 1985.
28. Spencer E: Amputations. In Hopkins HL, Smith HD, editors: *Willard and Spackman's occupational therapy,* ed 5, New York, 1978, JB Lippincott.
29. Stoner EK: Management of the lower extremity amputee. In Kottke FJ, Stillwell GK, Lehmann JF: *Krusen's handbook of physical medicine and rehabilitation,* ed 3, Philadelphia, 1982, WB Saunders.
30. Telikicherla M: *Immediate postoperative prosthesis for lower extremity amputation,* Detroit, 1993, Rehabilitation Institute of Michigan.
31. The American Academy of Orthotists and Prosthetists, Duke University Medical Center, Durham, NC, 1991.
32. United States Department of Health and Human Services: *Vital and health statistics: prevalence of selected chronic conditions, United States,* 1979-1981, Series 10, 155-29, 1986.
33. United States Department of Health and Human Services: *Vital and health statistics: prevalence of selected impairments,* United States, 1977, Series 10, 155-29, 1993.

34. Wellerson TL: *A manual for occupational therapists on the rehabilitation of upper extremity amputees,* Dubuque, Ia, 1958, Brown.
35. Wright G: *Controls training for the upper extremity amputee,* San Jose, Calif, Instructional Resource Center, San Jose State University (film).

## RECOMMENDED READING

Atkins DJ, Meier RH, editors: *Comprehensive management of the upper-limb amputee,* New York, 1989, Springer-Verlag.

Pedretti LW: *Occupational therapy: Practice skills for physical dysfunction,* ed 4, St Louis, 1996, Mosby.

Pedretti LW, Zoltan B: *Occupational therapy: practice skills for physical dysfunction,* ed 3, St Louis, 1990, Mosby.

Reed KL: *Quick reference to occupational therapy,* Gaithersburg, Md, 1991, Aspen.

Willard HS, Spackman CS, editors: *Occupational therapy,* ed 4, Philadelphia, 1971, JB Lippincott.

Chapter 28

# Degenerative Diseases of the Central Nervous System

Phyllis Ber

## Chapter Objectives

*After studying this chapter, the student or practitioner will be able to:*

1. Name and describe four degenerative diseases.
2. List the signs and symptoms of these diseases.
3. List the goals of occupational therapy in the treatment of degenerative diseases.
4. Be aware of the precautions that must be observed in the treatment of these diseases.
5. Be familiar with the occupational therapy modalities used to treat patients with degenerative diseases.
6. Understand the role of long-term care in the treatment of degenerative diseases.
7. Identify potential safety problems in the homes of patients with degenerative diseases.

## Key Terms

degenerative neurological disease
multiple sclerosis (MS)
progressive disease
demyelination
exacerbation
remission
Parkinson's disease (PD)
bradykinesia
cog-wheel rigidity
micrographia
dementia
amyotrophic lateral sclerosis (ALS)
Lou Gehrig's disease
dementia
Alzheimer's disease (AD)
catastrophic reactions
sundowning
dysphagia
task segmentation

**Degenerative neurological disease** causes progressive pathological changes in the central nervous system. These changes result in loss of functioning in one or more of the following areas: sensation, motor functioning, and cognition. The diseases addressed in this chapter are multiple sclerosis, Parkinson's disease, amyotrophic lateral sclerosis, and Alzheimer's disease. Although no cures exist for these diseases, their debilitating effects can be partially ameliorated with effective medical and rehabilitative management. The role of occupational therapy in the treatment of degenerative neurological diseases is to assist in managing symptoms, maintain function, and help the patient to compensate for lost abilities.

## MULTIPLE SCLEROSIS

**Multiple sclerosis (MS)** is a chronic, **progressive disease** of the central nervous system resulting from inflammation and destruction of the fatty protein tissue called *myelin* that surrounds the nerve fibers.[2,8,10,38] This process, which is called **demyelination,** occurs in random and disseminated (scattered) areas throughout the central nervous system. When the body attempts to repair the damaged myelin sheath with glial cells, sclerotic lesions or plaques are formed. The two processes of demyelination and plaque formation impede the transmission of nerve impulses to and from the brain.[10,38]

### Incidence

MS most commonly affects young people in the prime of their life. It is the third largest cause of major disability in adults of working age.[33,37] The estimates of the number of Americans with this disease vary from 300,000 to 500,000.[8,28,38] Statistical evidence indicates that women are more likely to develop the disease than men, whites are at greater risk than African-Americans or Asian-Americans, and those that live above the thirty-seventh parallel are more than twice to three times as likely to get MS as those that live below that latitude.[28,31,33]

### Cause

The cause of MS is unknown. Current research has been unable to isolate a specific cause for this disease although several theories have emerged. These include a hereditary factor, a possible viral cause, and a disturbance of the immune system. Research has not been able to link any virus with MS, but studies continue on the HTLV-1 virus that is known to trigger autoimmune reactions. At the present time, some researchers believe that the cause of MS is multifactorial.[8,33,37]

### Signs and Symptoms

The signs and symptoms of MS vary depending on the areas of the central nervous system that have been affected by demyelination. Each patient will present with a unique set of clinical manifestations depending on the locations of the lesions and the stage of the disease process.[10,33,37] Symptoms can be divided into primary, secondary, and tertiary symptoms. Primary symptoms are those that are directly caused by demyelination. These include transient fatigue, double vision, paresthesia, weakness, ataxia, unsteady gait, bowel and bladder dysfunction, pain, and decreased cognition. Other primary symptoms are spasticity, fatigue, trigeminal neuralgia, and speech and swallowing disorders. Some of the early symptoms may occur years before the disease is diagnosed. Patients in the early stage of the disease often have these symptoms attributed to psychological or hysterical factors by their families and physicians.[8,10,33,37]

Secondary symptoms result as complications of the primary symptoms. Secondary symptoms include contractures, urinary tract infections, decubitus ulcers, pain, and cognitive impairments. Tertiary symptoms encompass the emotional, social, and vocational impact of the disease on the patient, family, and community.[33,38]

The course of the disease varies widely. Approximately 20% of patients have the benign type of MS with a brief occurrence of symptoms of the disease, followed by recovery and no recurrence. Thirty percent of patients with MS have a relapsing-remitting form of the disease with periods of exacerbations of symptoms followed by remissions. Forty percent have a chronic relapsing form that is characterized by a slow and steady deterioration over many years. Ten percent of the MS population have a rapid decline in functioning related to the chronic progressive type of MS. The type of MS and the symptoms present govern the course of the patient's medical treatment.[8,20,28,31,33]

### Medical Management

The treatment of MS is primarily focused on the alleviation of the patient's symptoms. For many years **exacerbation** has been treated with corticosteroids to diminish the duration and severity of relapses.[10,20,37] Experimental studies with immunosuppressants, such as Betaseron, have demonstrated reduced frequency of acute exacerbation.[16,36] Other medications are prescribed for treatment of muscle spasticity, depression, pain, constipation, and urinary incontinence. Pharmacological treatment of MS symptoms requires careful monitoring. The certified occupational therapy assistant (COTA) can assist the physician by reporting changes in the patient's behavior and physical status.

Medical management of the MS patient also includes patient education. Patients are encouraged to observe good health habits. The proper mix of exercise, rest, stress management, and good nutrition is important.[31] There is no proof, however, that specific diets or vitamins affect the frequency or severity of exacerbation.[8,38]

During the chronic stages of MS, medical management of the disease may include catheterization for urinary dysfunction, tube feeding for swallowing disorders, and nerve blocks or surgical release of tendons for treatment of severe contractures.

### Long-Term Care

The increasing loss of function that results from the chronic progressive and chronic relapsing forms of MS places a severe strain on the patients' families. Chronic patients "often exhaust all of their financial, supportive, and psychological resources. . . . In desperation, early nursing home placement often follows."[33] Long-term care facilities are equipped to provide for the skilled care needs of patients in advanced stages of the disease. The patient in a long-term care center will receive the medical, nursing, psychosocial, and rehabilitative care required to treat complications of the disease. Those receiving restorative rehabilitation may show improvement in their ability to dress, bathe, eat, toilet, and transfer themselves.[33] Maintenance rehabilitation is provided to residents in long-term care centers to prevent decreased function.[33,42]

### Occupational Therapy Intervention

The patient with MS offers a challenge to the occupational therapy practitioner. The disease follows a variable and unpredictable course that causes changes in the patient's functional ability from morning to night, from day to day and of course, over a lifetime. These changes demand frequent adjustments to the patient's therapy program.[29,42]

#### *Precautions*

The functional status of a MS patient may be affected by stress, heat, pain, fatigue, and exacerbations.[31] The occupational therapy program must be tailored to the patient's capabilities at the present moment. Flexibility in both goals and treatment modalities is essential to prevent both injury to the patient and frustration for patient and clinician.[33] The COTA must rely on good observational skills to determine if the patient is able to proceed with the planned therapeutic modalities. A patient who is able to transfer one day may have serious difficulties with transfers the next. The occupational therapy schedule must be adjusted to allow MS patients to receive therapy in the morning when they are most rested. Excessive use of progressive exercises is unwise, because this can also lead to fatigue, increased weakness, and potential injury.

The COTA must also guard against injury related to the patient's possible loss of sensation. Patients with sensory loss (e.g., from cerebrovascular accident [CVA] or peripheral nerve injury) are generally taught to use their vision to compensate for their tactile losses. But many MS patients also have deficits in visual function, and this approach may be ineffective. Care must be taken to avoid injury from sharp objects. Patients with pain, temperature, and tactile sensation deficits should not receive physical agent modalities that use heat. The patient who has problems in coordination, balance, and gait requires careful monitoring during transfers, bathroom, and kitchen activities.

#### *Evaluation*

The initial evaluation process for the MS patient sets the tone and prepares both the patient and the occupational therapy (OT) practitioner for the treatment sessions to follow. It is important that the evaluation determine areas that may be remediable and those for which compensatory techniques should be taught. The evaluation should be done when the patient's endurance is highest, preferably in the morning. Because the patient may have cognitive deficits or may be experiencing anxiety or stress, the practitioner must be careful to explain the reason for the evaluation and to describe what is going to be done during the evaluation. Rest periods may be required if the patient becomes fatigued or agitated. If necessary, the evaluation may be broken up into two or more sessions. At the conclusion of the evaluation process, the therapist and the patient should agree on the goals for the occupational therapy program. The practitioner should emphasize that the occupational therapy program is going to help the patient fight the disease through exercise and the learning of compensatory techniques. The continuous changing status of the MS patient makes periodic reevaluations necessary.[27,29,33,42]

The evaluation includes assessment of physical abilities, sensory functioning, cognitive functions, and occupational performance levels. Physical abilities include strength, muscle tone, coordination, joint range of motion, endurance, and balance. Because persons with MS have decreased endurance, manual muscle testing is not an effective measurement of strength. The measurement of grasp strength with a dynamometer requires the averaging of three trials.[33]

Sensory functions to be evaluated include visual and perceptual skills, tactile sensation, pain and temperature sensation, and proprioception. Cognitive functions to be assessed are memory, behavior, communication skills, attention span, and intellectual functioning.

Proficiency in the occupational performance areas of activities of daily living, vocational tasks, and leisure skills must also be determined during the evaluation.[29,33] The occupational performance and sensory parts of the evaluation may be performed by an experienced COTA who has demonstrated competency in these evaluation techniques. The coordination and interpretation of the evaluation results is the role of the registered occupational therapist (OTR).

#### *Treatment Goals*

After the evaluation is completed, the OTR should have a thorough understanding of the MS patient's strengths and weaknesses. In collaboration with the patient, the therapist establishes realistic goals with the overall purpose of increasing or maintaining the patient's present functional status. Both long- and short-term goals are addressed. Treatment goals are to increase or maintain strength, endurance, coordination, ADL status, range of motion (ROM), and mobility; to increase or maintain the ability to work and participate in leisure pursuits; to prevent contractures, deformities, and decubiti; and to assist the patient and family in their emotional adjustment to changes in their roles over the course of the disease.[17,29] The success of the OT program depends somewhat on the patient's perceived sense of accomplishment and a positive attitude. The progressive nature of MS requires that treatment goals be established in small enough increments so that the patient is assured of some measure of progress.

#### *Treatment Methods and Modalities*

The treatment methods and modalities selected for MS patients are determined by individual goals for the patient. The patient's cognitive level and emotional state obviously have a major influence on the choice of treatment activities.

*Cognition* Decreased cognitive functioning significantly impedes the rehabilitation process because the patient is less able to store and receive new information.[33] Short- and long-term memory deficits contribute to confusion and agitation. Specific memory-enhancing techniques may be successful in improving memory, but the most effective approach is to encourage the patient to compensate for memory loss with paper and pen. New information should be presented to the patient simply and repetitively. Consistency in the therapy program as to day, time, and modalities helps to orient the patient and minimize frustration.[29,33,42]

*Sensory perception* The patient with MS may have a variety of sensory and perceptual disorders. In most cases, therapists aim to make the patient and family aware of the problem and to teach the patient to use compensatory techniques. Loss of tactile sensation, especially stereognosis, interferes with performing fine motor tasks such as buttoning. If there is no visual loss the patient may be able to compensate visually, but using a button aid, changing the style of shirt worn, or replacing the buttons with Velcro fasteners may be easier to manage. Patients with loss of pain and temperature sensation need to be cautioned to avoid situations that could cause burns or other injuries. Those who experience poor sensation or numbness and tingling of the extremities may benefit from activities that increase sensation to these areas.

Visual deficits such as double vision, blurring, decreased acuity, and nystagmus may make even simple activities of daily living (ADL) difficult. Patients can be taught compensatory techniques such as closing or covering one eye to minimize double vision or using devices for the blind such as magnifying glasses, large print books, and talking books.

*Coordination* Decreased coordination may be due to a number of factors. The quality of movement and the speed of fine motor tasks are influenced by the patient's visual function, tactile and proprioceptive sensation, and the degree of upper extremity weakness, spasticity, and tremors. The COTA might give the patient graded coordination exercises. Weighted wrist cuffs are used to enhance the quality of movement for patients with minor tremors. Weighted utensils may be helpful in self-feeding.[33] Patients with severe ataxia, however, generally do not find weights helpful in improving coordination. In some cases, the patient may be taught to perform fine motor tasks with the nondominant upper extremity or to compensate in other ways. Patients who find it difficult to write can use adaptive writing devices, substitute a keyboard for a pen, or use a recording device. The COTA will help guide the patient in choosing the most appropriate compensatory techniques. Coordination deficits related to MS are not limited to the upper extremities. Tremors of the head may be minimized through the use of a cervical collar.

*Strength and endurance* Patients with MS are taught by the COTA to plan their day and pace themselves accordingly. Planning and energy conservation help the patient budget strength and endurance to meet daily needs. Important activities, including exercises, are done in the morning or after a scheduled nap or rest period. Graded resistive exercises increase the strength of upper extremity and trunk muscles. To increase endurance, emphasis should be placed on increasing repetitions rather than increasing weights.[33]

Patients with severe loss of muscle strength are sometimes able to perform functional activities with the help of devices that substitute for weak muscles. The COTA may encourage the patient to use an overhead suspension sling or mobile arm support to increase independence.

*Contracture prevention and treatment* Patients with decreased active ROM and spasticity will inevitably develop contractures unless preventive measures are taken. Whenever possible, the patient should perform self-ranging techniques. Passive ROM (PROM) of each joint through the full range must be done daily.[33,37] The OT or physical therapy (PT) department may be responsible for teaching the family or a nursing assistant techniques of ROM. The OTR may administer inhibition techniques (such as icing or positioning to decrease tone before PROM) to patients with severe spasticity. Splints to maintain range or provide sustained stretch may be indicated to treat or prevent contractures of the elbow, wrist, or hand.[33]

*Activities of daily living* Independence in ADL promotes self-esteem and quality of life. Occupational therapy may provide assistive devices and adaptive techniques to enable MS patients to be more independent in transfers, dressing, grooming, and toileting. Cups with lids, scoop dishes, and adapted utensils facilitate eating. Long-handled shoe horns, reachers, sock aids, and elastic shoe laces are just some of the devices that can increase independence in dressing. The COTA needs to work with the patient to evaluate the effectiveness of equipment and provide training on an individual basis. As the disease progresses, modifications in equipment and techniques will be needed. A severely disabled patient may require an environmental control unit (ECU) to operate lights, television, or radio with a simple switch. The OT practitioner may be asked to determine which body part should activate the switch and what type of switch should be used (see Chapter 21).

*Home evaluation* The purpose of the home evaluation is to help the MS patient continue to reside at home safely and to facilitate independence. The use of a wheelchair in the home frequently requires modifications to doorways or the removal of the bathroom vanity cabinet or the cabinet under the kitchen sink. In the bathroom, grab bars may be needed to assist in toilet and bathtub transfers. Toilet safety frames, a transfer tub bench, and a raised toilet seat provide additional safety in the bathroom.[29,33] The COTA who has had training and experience in home evaluations may be involved in this aspect of the patient's treatment.

*Communication* In MS, both written and verbal communication skills may be affected. The OT frequently works closely with the speech therapist to devise a method of improving the patient's communication skills. Patients with dysarthria may be given communication boards or computers that speak for them. The COTA may provide equipment that enables the patient to use these devices, such as splints for upper extremity stabilization or head or mouth pointers. Adaptive writing devices (built-up and weighted pens, pen holders, and magnetized wrist stabilizers) compensate for decreased coordination and weakness. Special computer keyboards and large-button and speech-activated telephones facilitate independent communication for patients with motor deficits.

*Mobility and positioning* Many patients with MS will require the use of a wheelchair for mobility as their disease progresses. The primary considerations in recommending a wheelchair for a MS patient are the patient's upper extremity status and the medical prognosis. Patients with sufficient upper extremity strength should have a lightweight manual wheelchair if they are to propel their own wheelchair. Patients with a rapidly progressive type of the disease may require a wheelchair with a reclining back to compensate for diminished trunk strength. In some cases an electric wheelchair may be indicated. Modifications to the wheelchair that are helpful with the MS population include oblique rim projections, lateral supports, solid back inserts, head positioners, and brake extensions. Training in wheelchair mobility and transfer techniques may be taught as part of the patient's OT program. In a long-term care setting, MS patients with poor alignment and no wheelchair mobility skills may be positioned in gerirecliners for proper alignment and comfort.

Proper positioning of the patient both in and out of the wheelchair is under the scope of the OT department in many facilities. MS patients are at high risk for decubitus ulcers because of their diminished sensation, incontinence, and poor ability to reposition themselves. Pressure-relieving cushions and mattresses should be provided to all MS patients. Patients with sufficient strength should be taught and encouraged to do periodic wheelchair push-ups as part of their OT training. Use of bed positioners for sidelying further assists in decubitus prevention.

*Leisure skills* Leisure skills provide mental and social stimulation and substitute avocational interests for vocational skills. The COTA can assist the patient by stressing the importance of activity and by recommending adaptive devices such as card holders and shufflers and adapted board games. The patient should be encouraged to manage time effectively, planning for social events with naps and limited exercise on days when evening activities are scheduled.[33]

*Work skills* MS patients may be able to maintain their ability to work during the early stages of the disease or during **remission,** with changes to their schedule and adaptive devices for communication. Worksite modifications for wheelchair accessibility may be required. The COTA may assist the OTR in conducting the vocational evaluation, which may be used to determine a worker's ability to continue the job and make recommendations for adaptive equipment.

*Psychosocial issues* Initially, a diagnosis of MS will be received by the patient and his family with shock, denial, and anger.[37] However, in some cases the patient may feel some relief in finally knowing that the symptoms were not psychosomatic. As the disease progresses, the patient frequently becomes resentful of the caregiver, may be embarrassed by the condition, and frequently becomes depressed. The COTA can offer emotional support to both the patient and family. The patient should be encouraged to maintain a daily schedule of activity. Referral to MS support groups sponsored by the local MS society may be helpful in dealing with the daily stress of having a chronic progressive disease. Additional support and information are available on the internet in the reference and health sections and with chat groups.

The members of the rehabilitation team, including the COTA, have an obligation to help the family and the patient adjust to the disease and to provide encouragement, emotional support, training, and exercise programs. Occupational therapy can help the MS patient function as productively as possible within the limits of the disease.

## PARKINSON'S DISEASE

**Parkinson's disease (PD)** is a slow, progressive disease of the nervous system that was first described by James Parkinson in 1817.[6] The disease is caused by the degeneration of neurons in the part of the brain called the *substantia nigra,* resulting in damage to the basal ganglia. These neurons produce the chemical called *dopamine* that transmits messages in the brain.[5,18,41]

### Incidence

Approximately 1.5 million Americans have PD. One of every 1000 Americans will have the form of PD that has no known cause, with the ratio rising to 1 of 100 over the age of 60 years. Three quarters of all the patients with PD develop it between the ages of 50 and 70 years.[7,24] Diagnosis may be made as early as age 20 and as late as 80. Whites have a higher incidence of this disease than African-Americans or Asian-Americans.[7,24] Persons of Jewish and Spanish backgrounds also have increased risk.[7,24]

### Cause

A small percentage of PD cases are known to be caused by intoxication with poisons such as herbicides, inflammation of the brain from encephalitis, and drug-induced reactions that are sometimes reversible.[30,40] The cause of the majority of the cases of PD remains a mystery. A viral link has been suggested, but research has been unable to prove this theory. Heredity does not seem important. Environmental factors continue to be studied, but no common agent has been identified.[40]

### Signs and Symptoms

There are three major symptoms of Parkinsonism: **bradykinesia** (slowness of movement), muscle rigidity, and resting tremor.[40] Early symptoms of the disease include hand tremor, difficulty performing fine motor skills, a "heavy feeling" or stiffness in the legs, and increasing rigidity especially in the neck area. The patient develops a stooped posture and does not swing the arms when walking. There are episodes of freezing—sudden difficulty in walking through doorways or making turns. Postural dysfunction and rigidity result in typical gait patterns that are characterized by a slow, shuffling gait or a festinating gait that includes small, fast steps, which propel the patient forward with ever-increasing speed. The patient has difficulty in stopping the forward motion short of falling or hitting a wall.[5-7,24,40]

Other characteristic signs of PD include a mask-like face (a lack of facial expression), pill-rolling motion of the thumb and fingers, **cog-wheel rigidity** (a rhythmic jerking quality of movement exhibited during passive ranging), and an inability to perform rapid, repetitive movements. Patients frequently demonstrate **micrographia**—small, crowded writing. As the disease progresses, the patient experiences problems with oral musculature, resulting in drooling, dysphagia, and monotone speech with low volume. The patient may demonstrate disorders in bowel and bladder control.[5-7,24] Approximately 50% of PD patients also experience depression. Dementia is evident in 20% of the patients, and up to 30% have memory deficits. Disturbances in the autonomic system may result in excessive sweating, oily skin, and hot and cold flashes.[5,7,24,40]

### Medical Management

There is no cure for PD. Medical management concentrates on relieving the symptoms of the disease primarily through medication, although there have been recent advancements in surgical interventions.[6,10,24,30,41] Pharmacological treatments for Parkinson's disease were first introduced in the late 1960s. Levodopa (l-dopa, Sinemet), designed to augment the decreased amount of dopamine in the brain, revolutionized the treatment of parkinsonism.[24] It is still widely used today, but clinical observations and studies indicate that it tends to lose its effectiveness after 5 years and increasing the dosage at that time causes adverse reactions such as confusion and hallucinations.[24,41] Other dopaminergic drugs such as bromocriptine (Parlodel) may be prescribed to give the patient a "drug holiday" from the l-dopa. In 1989, deprenyl (Eldepryl) was introduced with some success in slowing the progression of the disease and easing the symptoms. Some physicians are prescribing this drug as a preliminary treatment, hoping to hold off the use of l-dopa for the latter stages of the disease.[5] During the early stages of the disease, the physician may prescribe anticholinergic drugs, which reduce rigidity and tremors but are not effective in treating bradykinesia.[5,10,24,41] In addition to antiparkinsonian drugs, medication for treatment of depression, nutritional supplements, and pain medication may be prescribed.[5,10]

Two different types of experimental surgery have demonstrated some potential in the treatment of PD. The transplant of fetal cells into the brain has resulted in the growth of dopamine producing neurons.[24] There are legal and ethical concerns with this approach. A second form of surgery, called pallidotomy, involves inserting an electric probe in the brain. Both types of surgery are used as a last resort for patients with severe, debilitating forms of the disease. Because of their experimental designation, these surgical procedures may not be covered by medical insurance. The procedures are risky, and some physicians believe further quantitative studies are needed.[21,24,26]

### Long-Term Care

Persons in the latter stages of Parkinson's disease may have frequent falls and resulting fractures, incontinence, sleep disturbances, skin integrity problems, **dementia,** depression, visual problems, and dysphagia. Placement in a long-term care facility is indicated when the patient and family can no longer cope with these symptoms in the home. Nursing homes offer speech, physical, and occupational therapy, daily PROM, decubitus ulcer prevention and treatment, tube feedings, counseling programs, and the 24 hour supervision necessary for patient safety.

### Occupational Therapy Intervention

Inactivity is a serious problem for the PD patient. The patient withdraws in response to the increased difficulty of initiating movement, fear of falling, psychological affects of the changes in appearance, and the difficulty communicating.[12] Even in the early stages of the disease, parkinsonian patients find safety in the house, watching television for the majority of the day.

Occupational therapy can help to improve the PD patient's quality of life by retraining in ADL and encouraging daily exercises to maintain muscle tone, strength, coordination, and ROM, and helping to provide a safe environment in the home.[1,6,12]

### *Precautions*

The parkinsonian patient has diminished proprioception and balance. Ten to fifteen percent of parkinsonian patients have orthostatic hypotension, usually from the Levodopa. There is a significant risk for falls.[6,9,18,27] Care must be taken during ambulation and transfers. Doorways and elevators may trigger freezing behavior.[7] The patient may have dysphagia and should not be offered food or drink unless the clinician is sure of the patient's ability to swallow. The patient's tendency toward immobility (coupled with incontinence) increases the risk of pressure ulcers. Patients need to be encouraged to stand or reposition themselves at least hourly.

### *Evaluation*

The registered occupational therapist will perform the OT evaluation, which should include measurement of active ROM (AROM) and PROM and assessment of tremors and rigidity, standing and sitting balance and righting reactions, cognitive skills, fine motor coordination, and functional performance level in work-related and ADL.[1,29] The COTA may participate in the evaluation of occupational performance areas.

### *Treatment Goals*

The goals of occupational therapy with the parkinsonian patient are to maintain or increase strength and ROM, prevent contractures and deformities, improve coordination skills, increase level of productivity in ADL, maintain maximum level of mobility, improve ability to participate in leisure activities, and provide education and support to the patient and family.[27,29]

### *Treatment Methods and Modalities*

*Motor skills/prevention of deformities* The increased rigidity and tendency toward immobility puts the parkinsonian patient at great risk for contracture development and general deconditioning. This patient requires a daily home exercise program for AROM and stretching as well as clinic appointments in which the exercise program can be closely supervised by the COTA or OTR.[24,29] The frequency of the therapy is determined by the physician in consultation with the OTR. AROM exercises may be done in an individual or a group setting. Passive stretching of the upper extremities and the neck and trunk muscles may be required if the patient is unable to achieve full active range. In the later stages of the disease, splinting may be indicated to maintain joint ranges and skin integrity. Verbal prompting and use of visual cues (sitting patient in front of mirror) can be used to promote improvement in posture. Encourage the patient to take deep breaths, and offer breathing exercises if indicated.[10,12,27]

Clinicians can use visual, tactile, and auditory cues to help patients initiate movement. Auditory cues should be short, firmly spoken commands such as "Stop," "Step up," etc. Rhythmic music and counting can also help to initiate movement. Auditory commands coupled with counting are especially helpful in teaching the patient transfer techniques. Graded, resistive exercises and gross motor activities, particularly sports activities, are used to develop strength and general mobility. Functional fine motor tasks, such as stringing beads, removing nuts from bolts, and picking up coins assist in developing and maintaining hand strength and coordination.[12,24] These tasks can be graded by changing the size of the objects. The clinician should monitor and record the time it takes for the patient to complete the task assigned. Other hand-strengthening modalities include hand grippers and therapeutic putty exercises. Handwriting exercises may help to control or reduce the patient's micrographia. Patients should stop writing and stretch the hand muscles when the letters become small and cramped. There is some evidence that exercises such as whistling, raising the eyebrows, and opening the mouth wide help to maintain ability to make facial expressions.[12] The OTR may use facilitation techniques on the oral musculature to improve swallowing and minimize drooling.

*Activities of daily living* Parkinsonian patients may increase self-feeding skills with adaptive feeding devices such as weighted utensils, scoop dishes, and cups with lids. Wrist weights (1 lb) can also be used to minimize tremors. Clothing with easy-to-use fasteners (Velcro closures, elastic shoe laces) increases independence. Because of balance deficits, patients should be discouraged from bending down to don shoes and socks. Patients should instead be taught to use long-handled shoe horns, reachers, sock aids, and dressing sticks and to always be seated when dressing. Patients with a shuffling gait should not wear rubber- or crepe-soled shoes because they may cause tripping. Grooming tasks are simplified with electric toothbrushes and electric razors. Long-handled brushes, "soap on a rope," and terry cloth mitts are recommended for the shower.[5,7,29]

*Communication* Parkinsonian patients frequently develop a monotone, low-volume speech. OT practitioners can increase the benefits of speech therapy by providing breathing and postural exercises. Diminished blinking responses and disturbances of the ocular muscles impair the patient's ability to read. Large-print and audio books are useful with these patients. Computers and word processors offer an alternative for patients who have difficulty writing. Felt tip markers are easier to use than regular pens. A signature stamp is helpful in the workplace. Cordless and automatic dialing telephones simplify communication.[5]

*Home evaluation* The home evaluation must help to eliminate any hazardous conditions that could trigger a fall.[10] Patients with a shuffling gait have difficulty with uneven floor surfaces. Special care should be taken to remove all throw or scatter rugs. Bathroom mats should be replaced with wall-to-wall carpeting. Doorway thresholds should be even with the floors. On the outside of the home, gravel or cobblestone walkways represent a safety hazard. In the bathroom, grab bars, a raised toilet seat with a safety frame, and a shower chair or tub transfer bench are recommended. In the bedroom, a sturdy chair with armrests should be used while dressing. For patients who have difficulty getting out of bed, satin sheets coupled with silk or satin nightwear help to reduce friction and make it easier to slide out of bed. A firm mattress and a trapeze over the bed also help with bed mobility. A bedside commode or urinal should be considered when the patient makes frequent nighttime trips to the bathroom. In the living room, the patient should be advised not to sit in deep, low chairs. The preferred chair has firm cushions, a straight back, and padded arm rests. The height and depth of the chair should allow the patient to maintain feet on the floor with knees flexed at ninety degrees. For those patients who are unable to get out of the chair independently, automatic lift chairs are available. In the kitchen, frequently used items should be placed so that excessive bending and reaching are not required. Patients with severe tremors should not be handling sharp or hot objects. The patient's walker can be fitted with a bicycle basket to make it easier to carry objects.[5,7,12,24,29]

*Mobility* The patient should attend physical therapy for gait training.[6,24] OT can supplement this training by using verbal cues to remind the patient to stand erect, lift the feet, etc. Bed mobility skills, transfer training, and wheelchair mobility skills should be taught by the COTA if indicated. As the patient's ambulation status declines, the PT may decide that a wheelchair is required. The patient should be advised to purchase a lightweight wheelchair. Oblique rim projections, a pressure-relieving cushion, elevating swing-away leg rests, and reclining backs are options that should be considered.

*Leisure skills* PD frequently makes it difficult for patients to pursue their hobbies and interests. Adaptive devices for card playing, gardening, board games, and crafts are available through various vendors. The COTA may have to encourage the patient and family to develop new interests.

*Psychosocial issues* The parkinsonian patient has a tendency to withdraw from society because of embarrassment, difficulty in mobility, and depression. The patient and family need a daily schedule that encourages exercise, outside activity, and social contacts. Information and support groups for patients with PD and their families are available through local chapters of Parkinson's Disease Foundation. The National Parkinson Foundation and the online computer network for PD also offer advice and education.[24] Group counseling and day treatment programs provide emotional and social outlets.

*Advanced parkinsonism* In the latter stages of the disease, patients have severe deficits in communication, mobility, swallowing, and cognition. Social isolation becomes a serious problem. Secondary complications, such as decubitus ulcers, aspiration pneumonia, fractures from falls, and contractures may arise.[5,6,24] The COTA may help to prevent some of these problems. Use of a pressure-relieving mattress and cushion for the wheelchair, proper head alignment, and use of a flow control cup at meals, daily PROM, and splinting are interventions that should be explored with this population. Group activities at the patient's cognitive level help minimize the social isolation frequently experienced by patients with advanced parkinsonism.

## AMYOTROPHIC LATERAL SCLEROSIS

**Amyotrophic lateral sclerosis (ALS)** is a progressive disease characterized by the degeneration of the motor neurons in the anterior horn cells of the spinal cord, brain stem and corticospinal tracts.[9,23,34] ALS is also called **Lou Gehrig's disease,** named after the famous baseball player who had the disorder. Patients with this disease have progressive muscle weakness and paralysis. Half will die within 3 to 5 years of onset.[34]

### Incidence

ALS is the most common form of motor neuron disease. Men are 1½ times more likely to have the disease than women. The average age of onset is 56 years, with most victims between the ages of 40 and 70 years. The incidence of the disease is 7 of 100,000 people.[10,23,34]

### Cause

Approximately 10% of ALS victims have an inherited form of the disease, transmitted on a dominant gene.[10,32] The cause of the remaining forms of the disease is unknown. Researchers have proposed many theories including a slow-acting virus, an autoimmune reaction, toxic exposure to heavy metals, and enzyme or hormone deficiencies.[34,39]

### Signs and Symptoms

Early symptoms of the disease include difficulty walking, picking up objects, and performing fine motor tasks. The patient complains of weakness and stiffness. There is atrophy of the intrinsic muscles of the hands. The patient exhibits hyperactive reflexes and fasciculations (twitching). The weakness spreads to the other muscle groups relatively quickly, involving all the limbs and the neck and trunk muscles. With bulbar involvement, there is difficulty in swallowing, speaking, coughing, and breathing. Eventually the patient's muscles become flaccid. Bowel and bladder functions remain intact, as do mental status and sensory functions. ALS patients may consider themselves prisoners of their bodies. Death generally results from respiratory complications.[34]

### Medical Management

There is no cure for ALS. Treatment is primarily palliative. The Federal Drug Administration has recently allowed two new drugs, riluzole and myotrophin, to be marketed to ALS patients to slow the disease progression.[14,15] Medication is also prescribed to control muscle spasms and pain, minimize drooling, and treat depression.[23,34] Respiratory and swallowing problems may require tracheostomy and gastrostomy procedures. Frequent suctioning to clear the airway may be needed. Because of the patient's compromised respiratory system, care should be taken to avoid exposure to respiratory infections.[34]

### Long-Term Care

In the latter stages of the disease, the patient becomes increasingly dependent on caregivers, eventually becoming quadriplegic and requiring 24-hour care.[10,23] Many families are unable to meet the complex needs of the ALS patient in the home. Placement in a long-term care facility may become the only way to deal with the patient's needs for frequent positioning and suctioning, transfers with mechanical lifters, tube feedings, and ADL assistance.

### Occupational Therapy Intervention

The role of occupational therapy with the ALS patient is to enable the patient to adapt and to maintain the maximal level of functioning throughout the course of the disease.[1,29]

#### *Evaluation*

The initial occupational therapy evaluation establishes a baseline of active and passive ROM, muscle strength and tone, ADL skills, and chewing and swallowing abilities.[1,29] Frequent reevaluation of the patient's status is required as the disease progresses. The COTA may assist in the evaluation of occupational performance areas.

#### *Treatment Goals*

Treatment goals for the ALS patient are to maintain ROM and prevent contractures, maintain strength, preserve independence in activities with the use of adaptive equipment, provide emotional support to the patient and family, and facilitate the patient's comfort through proper positioning both in and out of bed.[1,29]

#### *Treatment Methods and Modalities*

*Motor skills and prevention of deformities* In the early stages of the disease, emphasis is placed on strengthening unaffected muscle groups through a graded exercise program. Care should be taken to avoid fatigue. Orthotic devices provide stabilization and support for weakened muscles. Cock-up splints and short opponens splints may be needed for weak intrinsic hand muscles and wrist extensors. General conditioning and mild aerobic exercises are recommended. PROM is provided when the patient is unable to actively move the joint to the end of the range. Relaxation and deep breathing exercises should be taught. Use of suspension slings or mobile arm supports is indicated as the disease progresses. Exercises should be done over several, short periods throughout the day, rather than in one long session, to avoid fatigue. In the latter stages of the diseases more intensive passive stretching and ranging and splinting are required to prevent contracture development.[1,23,29,34]

*Feeding issues* In the early stages of the disease the patient will require adaptive feeding devices and orthotics to feed themselves independently. Lightweight, angled, built-up handles, or long-handled utensils may be required. A universal cuff is helpful when gross grasp is impaired. A scoop dish or plate guard may also be useful. As the disease progresses, the patient will develop chewing and swallowing deficits, requiring changes in food texture (first chopped and then pureed foods). Swallowing facilitation techniques should precede the meal. Tube feeding is generally inevitable in the final stages of the disease.

*Communication* The trauma associated with the loss of verbal communication skills is compounded by the fact that the patient retains full mental capacity.[9] The OT and speech therapy departments need to work jointly on establishing an alternative method to help the patient communicate thoughts and needs. Initially the patient may be able to write. A communication board, electronic communication aid, or a computer with a voice module offer other alternatives. The COTA may be involved in positioning the patient and fabricating the upper extremity equipment and switches that enable the patient to use these devices. It is important that the patient be able to call for help. Call bells that can be controlled with any part of the body with a minimal amount of pressure are available and become necessary when the patient can no longer speak.

*Assistive technology* Computers enable the ALS patient to perform a variety of tasks from speech to turning on lights and appliances. Computers can be activated by a variety of different types of keyboards and switches. The COTA can assist in determining the patient's functional capacity to operate these devices and may be called on to make recommendations as to the type of device to purchase. ECUs decrease dependency on the caregiver.[29]

*Mobility and positioning* In the early stages of the disease, the patient will continue to ambulate with the help of a cane or walker. Eventually the patient will require a wheelchair. Although initially the patient may have sufficient strength to sit and propel a standard wheelchair, the progressive nature of the disease will inevitably necessitate the use of a reclining or motorized wheelchair. For financial reasons, it may be wise to plan ahead when consulting on a wheelchair purchase. Proper positioning of the head may require a cervical collar and head support. Lateral supports to the wheelchair may have to be supplied in the latter stages of the disease. Pressure relieving cushions are indicated.

*Psychosocial issues* Reactive depression is common among victims of terminal diseases such as ALS. Medication and counseling may help ameliorate depression. The rehabilitation team needs to provide psychological support to help in coping with the devastating effects of the disease. Independence in ADL may increase the patient's self-esteem in addition to improving functional status.

## ALZHEIMER'S DISEASE

Medical science has revealed approximately 70 causes of **dementia,** the loss or impairment of mental powers.[2,25] The most common known cause of irreversible dementia in adults is **Alzheimer's disease (AD).** Also known as *senile dementia of the Alzheimer type* (SDAT), this disease was first described by Dr. Alors Alzheimer in 1907.[2,4,41] Alzheimer's disease is a progressive, slow deterioration of brain tissue resulting in decreased cognitive abilities including language and memory deficits, disturbances in the sense of time and place, personality changes, and emotional instability.[2,25]

### Incidence

The Alzheimer's Association estimates that there are presently 4 million Americans afflicted with Alzheimer's disease.[2] One of every 10 persons over the age of 65 years has been diagnosed with the disease.[2,25] The incidence increases with age, with 50% of all persons over the age of 85 having Alzheimer's.[2] Youth, however, is not a defense against this disease. Persons as young as 30 years old have been diagnosed with Alzheimer's.[2,41] It is anticipated that by the middle of the next century, 14 million Americans will have this disease. The Alzheimer's Association indicates that men and women are equally affected by this disease, but other sources suggest that women are more likely to be diagnosed with Alzheimer's disease. This may be attributed to women having longer lifespans. The incidence of this disease is unaffected by racial or ethnic heritage.[2]

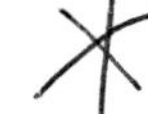

### Cause

The cause of Alzheimer's disease continues to elude scientists. It is possible that Alzheimer's may be a family of diseases with different causal factors triggering the symptoms. Recent genetic studies have identified chromosomal defects in persons with the familial type of Alzheimer's.[2,22,25] Approximately 5% to 10% of all Alzheimer's patients appear to have hereditary factors.[2] The odds of developing Alzheimer's increase fourfold if a close relative has been diagnosed with the disease. Early onset of the disease in some families has been identified with defects of chromosomes 14, 19, and 21.[22] Chromosome 21 is associated with the production of a protein called *amyloid.* Abnormal deposits of this protein have been found in the brains of patients with Alzheimer's disease.[2,22,25]

Scientists have theorized that other causal factors of the disease include a deficiency in neurotransmitters (particularly acetylcholine), head trauma, viral infection, exposure to toxins such as aluminum, and immunological defects.[25,41] None of these theories has been proven.

### Signs and Symptoms

Over a period of from 3 to 20 years, the victims of Alzheimer's disease experience a loss of memory, inability to perform routine tasks, disorientation, a loss of language skills, personality changes, and decreased strength and coordination. In the early stages of the disease, the patient commonly develops short-term memory loss and may exhibit difficulty learning new tasks or dealing with abstract concepts. Depression or other mood changes may occur. Patients may be aware that they are having cognitive problems and are frequently embarrassed by their limitations.[25]

As the disease progresses the patient demonstrates more behavioral changes, with bouts of anger, restlessness, antisocial behavior, anxiety, depression, and paranoia. The patient may have hallucinations and frequently overreacts to minor events, becoming severely agitated and violent. These types of behavior are known as **catastrophic reactions.**[4,25] The patient may wander, especially at night. Increased agitation and pacing that may accompany the onset of the evening is referred to as **sundowning.** Language skills continue to decline. Antisocial behavior is common. The patient may develop problems with walking and balance. There is a marked deterioration in the patient's ability to perform ADL, and the forgetfulness and disorientation associated with the disease now mandate close supervision to prevent injury.[2,4,25]

In the final stages of the disease the patient becomes severely impaired, unable to ambulate, to recognize loved ones, and to make needs known. Additional neurological changes at this stage lead to incontinence, dysphagia, and decreased motor function. The patient no longer interacts with the environment and is generally bed or chair bound. He or she requires total assistance in ADLs and may require tube feeding. The patient lacks sufficient language skills to comprehend speech or make needs known. The average patient with Alzheimer's disease dies within 7 to 10 years, although victims of the early onset type generally have a more rapidly fatal course.[25,41]

### Medical Management

Treatment of the patient with Alzheimer's disease is primarily symptomatic. There is no cure or any treatment that will slow the progression of the disease.[2,25] Pharmacological management of the disease focuses on minimizing depression, delusions, hallucinations, and violent behavior with antidepressants and major and minor tranquilizers. Drugs that reduce acetylcholine in the brain have been shown to have some beneficial effect on memory for brief periods. One such drug, THA (tacrine), has recently been touted as a treatment for Alzheimer's disease.[13] The physician must also treat symptoms associated with the disease, such as **dysphagia** and decubitus ulcers, and should be available to assist the family and the patient in best coping with the disease.

### Long-Term Care

The 24 hour supervision and skilled nursing care required for patients with Alzheimer's disease frequently leads the family to seek long-term care placement in a nursing home.[4,19,25] Many nursing homes have specialized dementia units and typically provide programs and diversional activities that help to keep the patient involved in the environment. They provide toileting, diapering, and positioning schedules to deal with patients who are incontinent and prone to developing decubitus ulcers. The staff of long-term care facilities helps to ensure the safety and dignity of patients with Alzheimer's disease and to minimize suffering as the disease progresses.

### Occupational Therapy Intervention

The role of occupational therapy in the treatment of patients with Alzheimer's disease varies according to the stage of the disease but aims to maximize independence and to provide guidance and support to the family.

#### *Occupational Therapy Evaluation*

The occupational therapy evaluation of the patient with Alzheimer's disease establishes a baseline of cognitive, motor, self-care, and sensory skills. This evaluation is not only used to establish treatment guidelines and goals but also may help to determine the level of care and supervision necessary for the patient. The information in the evaluation may assist the family in making the difficult decision of whether to maintain the patient in the home or to seek placement in an assisted living or a long-term care facility.[29]

Evaluation of cognition may be done through formalized assessment tools such as the Mini-Mental Status Examination or the Allen Cognitive Level Test or through informal testing, which includes assessing the patient's orientation to person, place, and time, determining the patient's ability to follow one, two, or multi-stepped commands, and evaluating task focus. Motor functioning should be evaluated by assessing active and passive ROM, coordination, balance, transfer skills, and praxis.[1,29] The speech-language pathologist and the physical therapist may have additional information to supplement the OT evaluation. Self-care evaluation includes observation of the patient's ability to feed, dress, groom, and toilet. In the early stages of the disease the OT evaluation may also include the patient's ability to perform housekeeping and work-related tasks.

Leisure skills, including the patient's ability to continue to participate in previously enjoyed hobbies, should also be assessed. A thorough history should be obtained from the patient's family before evaluation.[1,25,29]

The occupational therapy evaluation is performed by the OTR. The COTA may be asked to complete the occupational performance part of the evaluation or to assist in determining the patient's perceptual and sensory skills. The OTR coordinates the findings of the evaluation and determines the recommendations and treatment goals for the patient.

#### *Treatment Goals*

Occupational therapy goals for the patient with Alzheimer's disease are to improve or maintain ADL skills; increase or maintain muscle strength, coordination, and ROM; foster socialization skills; assist in the maintenance of leisure skills; and provide education and support to the family. The progressive nature of the disease requires periodic reassessments and frequent revision of each patient's specific goals.[1,25,29]

#### *Treatment Methods and Modalities*

*Activities of daily living* In the middle stages of Alzheimer's disease the patient begins to demonstrate difficulty performing simple ADL. Frequent reminders to initiate a task may be required, such as "Wash your face" or "Put on your shirt." As the disease progresses, the patient has problems sequencing multistepped tasks and needs help breaking the tasks down into one step segments. This process, known as **task segmentation,** helps the patient complete ADL tasks with the verbal prompting of the therapist and also helps to train and refocus on the task at hand. Instead of saying, "Wash your face," the patient is instructed, "Pick up the wash cloth. Put the wash cloth in the water. Now put some soap on the wash cloth. Wash around your mouth." These instructions are offered in a calm, reassuring manner. Positive feedback in the form of praise is provided after each step. Physical prompts (hand-over-hand assistance) may also be given if the patient permits it. The OT should instruct patients' caregivers in these task segmentation methods and may need to remind them of the importance of allowing patients to perform as much of their own daily care as possible.

Typically, a patient with Alzheimer's disease demonstrates poor frustration tolerance. It is important to avoid situations that may trigger catastrophic reactions. Activities should be analyzed and graded to ensure that the patient has sufficient physical and cognitive skills to perform the task requested.

The patient's physical deterioration may contribute to safety problems in the home. Bathroom safety devices should be prescribed if indicated. The family should be advised of hazards in the home or patient's environment that need to be removed or safeguarded. Scatter rugs, power tools, electric appliances, medications, stairways, windows, balconies, household cleansers, smoking materials, and the kitchen stove are just some of the items that represent a serious potential hazard to the patient.[25]

Mealtimes can be difficult for both the patient and the caregiver. Confused patients are frequently messy, fussy eaters. The provision of adaptive eating devices such as scoop dishes, spill-proof cups, and built-up utensils may be helpful. If the patient no longer uses utensils it may be easier to have the caretaker provide finger foods than to try to force use of a fork.[25] The patient may demonstrate swallowing difficulties. The OTR can instruct the caregiver in feeding techniques for the dysphagic patient. These may include changing the food consistency, maintaining the head in neutral position, putting small amounts of food on the spoon, ensuring that the previous mouthful of food has been swallowed before offering the next spoonful, encouraging swallowing with verbal prompting and facilitation techniques, using a thickening agent in liquids, and using a flow control cup. Dysphagia is discussed further in Chapter 19.

*Environmental design* The COTA can help the caregiver structure the environment to help maximize the patient's functioning. Eliminating clutter in the environment helps to minimize confusion. Contrasting colors make it easier for the patient to differentiate an object from the background. Simple changes such as eliminating the condiments from the kitchen table and ensuring contrast of color between the plate and table (and the plate and the food) simplify mealtime. Contrasting the color of the toilet seat and bowl with the bathroom floor helps to aid in toileting. Minimizing the amount of furniture and maintaining traffic areas free of obstacles decreases the risk of falls in the home. Gates and locks on stairways and doors may need to be installed for safety. Signs identifying the patient's room and bathroom may be helpful.[4,11,25] The OT clinic should also incorporate some of these design features.

*Day care and group activities* Adult day care facilities offer the caregiver a respite from the daily pressure and stress of taking care of a loved one with Alzheimer's disease.[25] These programs offer a variety of group activities within a structured environment, striving to provide the patient with positive social opportunities. Group activities, whether offered in a day care setting or as part of the activity program in a long-term care facility, may be administered by occupational therapy clinicians. The patients frequently enjoy music-based activities, simple and familiar games, and crafts. Teaching new activities is not recommended. Also enjoyed are sensory stimulation, reminiscing games, and pet therapy visits. Childish activities that may be demeaning to the patient should be avoided. The OT working in this area should consult the numerous books on activity programs for the dementia patient for further suggestions.[1,43]

*Reality orientation* Patients with Alzheimer's disease become less oriented as the disease progresses. Formal daily orientation programs to review the patient's name, the date, the weather, and the location may be helpful. In addition, the patient should always be addressed by name, and all staff should introduce themselves and tell the patient their function regularly as if they have just met. Frequently review the names of the patients' close family members and show them their room, the dining room, etc. Clocks and calendars should be clearly displayed.

*Exercise programs* Exercise, whether offered as a group or individual activity, is important to maintain strength, coordination, and ROM. Simple group calisthenics can be done in a standing or sitting position. The addition of rhythmic music helps to keep the patient involved in the activity. Parachute activities and ball, scarf, or balloon tosses are good group exercise activities. Dancing and walking are activities that the caretaker can easily do with the patient. There is evidence that the patient who engages in physical activity during the day sleeps better at night and has fewer periods of restlessness.[25] If the patient is unable to participate in group exercise programs or if there are joint contractures, the patient should be involved in a daily PROM program. It is recommended that exercise programs be offered at the same time each day to help establish a routine.[1,25,29,43]

*Psychosocial issues* Patients with Alzheimer's disease may demonstrate a variety of behavior problems including agitation, physical aggression, depression, inappropriate sexual behaviors, "stealing," paranoia, and hallucinations. The patient may receive some form of medication for these problems but behavioral interventions are frequently preferable to chemical interventions that may have serious side effects.[25] Always approach the patient using a calm, reassuring voice. Do not become angry or argue with the patient. Redirect and refocus the patient to a different topic. Clear instructions on how to behave or what is acceptable should be offered. Using the name of the patient's spouse in your request frequently helps to achieve the desired behavior (e.g., "Mary wants you to take a bath now."). Reducing the amount of stimulation, noise, or unstructured time sometimes helps to decrease agitation and antisocial behavior. The patient should be seen in OT when the clinic is relatively quiet and distractions are minimal.[29]

*End-stage Alzheimer's disease* In the final stages of the disease, the patient most often requires long-term and skilled nursing care. The patient may receive occupational therapy services in the form of nursing rehabilitation programs for ROM, positioning recommendations, splinting to prevent contractures or maintain ROM and skin integrity, and sensory stimulation.[19,25]

Throughout the course of the disease, the family will need guidance and support to help cope with the effect of the Alzheimer's disease on the patient and the family structure. The nature of the disease demands changes and role reversals in the family. The COTA and other team members should be prepared to provide this support. Families may also seek advice from the Alzheimer's Organization and online chat groups and informational services.[2,3]

## SUMMARY

Treating patients with degenerative diseases can take an emotional toll on health care providers. At all times the practitioner must maintain a positive attitude while acknowledging the feelings of the patients and their families. This is not always an easy thing to do. However, the occupational therapy practitioner can gain great satisfaction from working with this population, knowing that such a significant improvement can be made in the quality of life of these patients and their families.

This chapter has focused on four degenerative diseases: multiple sclerosis, Parkinson's disease, amyotrophic lateral sclerosis, and Alzheimer's disease. Although there are other neurological diseases that result in progressive loss of function, the occupational therapy practitioner will find that the treatment goals and interventions for the diseases outlined in this chapter will be helpful in treating all patients with degenerative disorders.

## Case Study

The patient, Ms. S., is a 36-year-old woman who has been admitted to the nursing home from a hospital after an exacerbation of MS that has left her with an inability to ambulate. Ms. S. is married and has two children. Her first symptoms of MS began 8 years ago, but the disease was not accurately diagnosed until 2 years later when symptoms reappeared and she began to have visual disturbances. She had to leave her job as a high school math teacher at that time. Ms. S. appears fearful and depressed since her admission to the nursing home. She is worried about her children and anxious to go home.

The occupational therapy evaluation reveals that Ms. S. has severe ataxia in both upper extremities with her dominant right upper extremity more involved. Tactile sensation is impaired bilaterally, with deficits in temperature, pain, and stereognosis abilities. She has difficulty maintaining proper body alignment when seated because of weakness in her trunk muscles. She has difficulty in all ADL but is most concerned with the problems she has trying to feed herself. At the present time, the nursing assistants are using a mechanical lifter to transfer Ms. S from bed to wheelchair. She has periods of incontinence related to a neurogenic bladder. She fatigues easily and requests to take a nap in the afternoon. Cognitive testing reveals some short-term memory loss.

Discharge plans for Ms. S. are uncertain at this time. The family has indicated that she needs to be more independent before they can consider taking her home. Mr. S. is caring for his two children alone and has indicated to the discharge planner that he believes his wife will have to stay in the nursing home indefinitely.

**Assets**

Good intelligence and educational background
Family support
Good family relationships
Good motivation to return home

**Problems**

1. Ataxia
2. Tactile sensation deficits
3. Poor alignment/weak trunk musculature
4. Dependence in all ADL
5. Unable to feed self
6. Dependence in transfers
7. Incontinence
8. Fatigues easily
9. Mild short-term memory loss
10. Expectation to return home probably not realistic

**Treatment planning and interventions**

1. Star (*) the problems of most concern to the patient.
2. Place problems in order of priority and select the first three. State a short-term goal for each. Describe one or more treatment methods the COTA could use to address this goal.
3. Describe the type of wheelchair and the wheelchair features that would be appropriate for Ms. S. at this time.
4. Describe how you would respond to the patient when she expresses her wish to return home.

## Selected Reading Guide Questions

1. List the precautions that need to be observed when treating a patient with multiple sclerosis.
2. Briefly describe the three clinical signs associated with Parkinson's disease and explain how these impact on the treatment process.

3. Discuss the psychosocial aspects of treating patients with degenerative diseases.
4. Describe how assistive technology can be used to increase the functional level of the patient with amyotrophic lateral sclerosis.
5. Explain *catastrophic reactions* and *sundowning* in relationship to Alzheimer's disease.
6. Describe the treatment goals associated with each of the diseases discussed in this chapter: MS, PD, ALS, and Alzheimer's disease.
7. Describe the ways the COTA can help the MS patient cope with fatigue.
8. Explain how the COTA can use adaptive devices to promote independence in feeding skills for patients with degenerative diseases.
9. Describe the techniques used by the OT practitioner to promote proper positioning and the prevention of decubitus ulcers in patients with degenerative diseases.
10. Describe the role of the COTA in the treatment and prevention of contractures with patients with MS, PD, ALS, and Alzheimer's disease.
11. List some of the environmental changes that the COTA may recommend in the home of a patient with Alzheimer's disease.

## *REFERENCES*

1. Allen CK: *Occupational therapy treatment goals for the physically and cognitively disabled,* Rockville, Md, 1992, American Occupational Therapy Association.
2. Alzheimer Organization: *Alzheimer disease fact sheet,* Case Western Reserve University—Alzheimer Disease Resource. E-mail address: cwru.edu/orgs/adsc/intro.html
3. Alzheimer Association e-mail address: http:/www.alz.org/
4. Aronson MK: *Understanding Alzheimer's disease: what it is, how to treat it, how to cope with it,* New York, 1988, Scribners.
5. Atwood GW: *Living well with Parkinson's,* New York, 1991, John Wiley and Sons.
6. Burrows A, et al: Treating Parkinson's disease and its side effects: complicated but worth it, *Brown University Long-Term Care Quality Letter* vol 6, July 1994.
7. Carrol DL: *Living with Parkinson's,* New York, 1992, Harper Collins.
8. Carrol DL, Dorman J: *Living well with MS, a guide for patient, caregiver and family,* New York, 1993, Harper Collins.
9. Chipps EM, et al: *Neurological disorders,* St Louis, 1992, Mosby.
10. Cochran JW, Kessler ES: *Five scenarios to manage patient care* 28:32, 1994.
11. Cohen U: *Holding on to home: designing environments for people with dementia,* Baltimore, 1991, Johns Hopkins University Press (pamphlet).
12. Cote L, Reidel G: *Exercises for the Parkinson patient,* New York, The Parkinson Disease Foundation.
13. Davis KL: Tacrine, *Lancet* vol 345, March 1995.
14. Investigational drugs available, *FDA Consumer* vol 29, September 1995.
15. Fisher LM: Maker says biotech drug slows Lou Gehrig's disease, *The New York Times,* p.D2, June 13, 1995.
16. Goodkin DE: Role of steroids and immunosuppression and effects of the interferon beta-1b in multiple sclerosis, *West J Med,* vol 161, September 1994.
17. Harmon JE: Multiple sclerosis—laying a foundation for occupational therapy, *Occupational Therapy Forum,* October 4, 1991.
18. Hutton JT, Dippel RL: *Caring for the Parkinson patient,* Buffalo, NY, 1989, Prometheus Books.
19. Jackson E, et al: *Alzheimer's disease: Long term care,* San Diego, 1991, San Diego University Press.
20. Kalb R, Scheiner LC: *Multiple sclerosis and the family,* New York, 1992, Demos Publications.
21. Kolata G: Parkinson's suffers gamble on surgery with great risks, *New York Times,* p. A1, March 16, 1995.
22. Levy L, et al: *Science,* August 1995.
23. Livingstone D: ALS a patient's guide. E-mail address: http:/httpl.brunel/.ac.uk:8080/~hssrsdn/alsig/guidel.html.
24. National Parkinson Foundation: *The Parkinson handbook,* Miami, Fla, (pamphlet).
25. Mace NL, Rabins P: *The thirty six hour day,* New York, 1991, Warner Books.
26. Meyer H: Boom in surgery raises concerns, *Am Med News,* vol 38, April 1995.
27. McDowell FH: Neurorehabilitation, *West J Med,* 161, September 1994.
28. MS Society: *Multiple sclerosis: A guide for patients and their families,* ed 2, New York, The Society, (pamphlet).
29. Pedretti LW: *Practice skills for physical dysfunction,* ed 4, St Louis, 1996, Mosby.
30. Quinn N: Parkinsonism—recognition and differential diagnosis, *Br Med J,* 310, February 1995.
31. Richert J: *Multiple sclerosis, 1990,* US Department of Health and Human Services.
32. Rosen DR, et al: Genetic linkage analysis of familial ALS using human chromosome 21 microsatellite DNA markers, *Am J Med Genet* vol 51, May 1994.
33. Schapiro R: *Multiple sclerosis—a rehabilitation approach to management,* New York, 1991, Demos Publications.
34. Schellenberger T, Stover J: ALS demands diligent nursing care, *RN,* vol 58, March 1995.
35. Reference deleted in proofs.
36. Segal M: Multiple sclerosis: New treatment reduces relapses, *FDA Consumer* vol 28, June 1994.
37. Shuman R, Schwartz J: *Understanding MS—a new handbook for families,* New York, 1988, Charles Scribner's Sons, MacMillan Publishing.
38. Soll R, Grenoble P: *MS—something can be done and you can do it,* Chicago, 1984, Contemporary Books.
39. Takahashi H: Evidence for a dopaminergic deficit in sporadic amyotrophic lateral sclerosis, *Lancet* vol 342, October 1993.
40. Stern G, Lees A: *Parkinson's disease—the facts,* Oxford, England, 1990, Oxford University Press.
41. Van der Cammen TJM, et al: *Manual of geriatric medicine,* New York, 1991, Churchill Livingstone.
42. Wolf B: Occupational therapy for patients with multiple sclerosis. In Maloney FP et al: *Interdisciplinary rehabilitation of multiple sclerosis and neuromuscular disorders,* Philadelphia, 1985, JB Lippincott Co.
43. Zgola J: *Doing things, a guide to programming activities for person's with Alzheimer's disease and related disorders,* Baltimore, 1991, The Johns Hopkins Press.

Chapter 29

# Hip Fractures and Lower Extremity Joint Replacement

*Sonia Coleman*
*Deborah Morawski*
*Karen Pitbladdo*
*Elizabeth Maria Bianchi*
*Sheri L. Lieberman*
*Jan Polon Novic*
*Helen Bobrove*

## Chapter Objectives

*After studying this chapter, the student or practitioner will be able to:*

1. Outline the cause of hip fractures and joint replacements.
2. Outline the medical management for these disabilities.
3. Describe occupational therapy treatment goals.
4. Understand the medical precautions associated with hip fractures and joint replacements.
5. Describe appropriate activities of daily living (ADL) techniques for these conditions.
6. Identify areas of intervention for the occupational therapist and the occupational therapy assistant.

## Key Terms

open reduction and internal fixation (ORIF)
weight-bearing restrictions
articular capsule
osteoarthritis
ankylosing spondylytis
arthroplasty
knee immobilizer
hip precautions
leg lifter
commode chair
abduction wedge

Hip fractures and lower extremity (LE) joint replacements occur with more frequency now than in years past because of an increasing elderly population and medical advances. In all of these types of injuries or surgeries, a large weight-bearing joint is unstable for a period of time, which limits an individual's mobility and ability to complete ADLs.

The elderly population is at greatest risk for hip fractures, because of already impaired mobility and the presence of osteoporosis. Osteoporosis is reduced bone density that causes the bones to be more brittle and susceptible to fracture. Elderly women are more likely to develop osteoporosis than men and thus tend to have more hip fractures when they fall.

Adults with a history of arthritis or other joint disease are primary candidates for LE joint replacement. These individuals have lived with increasing pain in their joints for many years and are already limited in their ability to perform daily tasks. They hope that having the painful joint replaced will return them to a more active and satisfying lifestyle.

The occupational therapist and occupational therapy assistant play key roles in defining and remediating functional problems and returning the patient to optimal performance of safe and independent ADLs.

This chapter discusses hip fractures and LE joint replacement, medical and surgical management, the psychological implications of hospitalization and disability, and the health care team approach in acute hospital and rehabilitation settings.

## FRACTURES

It is important for the occupational therapy assistant working with orthopedic patients to have a good understanding of the site, type, and cause of the fracture before starting treatment. A basic understanding of fracture healing and medical management is also necessary to appreciate risks, precautions, and complications involved. The occupational therapy assistant is advised to consult an orthopedic manual for specific information with respect to the fracture healing process. In general, a fracture occurs when the bone's ability to absorb tension, compression, or shearing forces is exceeded. Osteoblasts are cells that form bone and begin the healing process. A good blood supply is necessary for proper healing. The fracture site is protected during the healing process by a cast and/or pins and wires. Several months may be required for a bone fracture to completely heal. The time required varies with the age of the patient, site and configuration of the fracture, initial displacement of the bone, and the blood supply to the fragments.[7,11]

### Cause

Trauma is the major cause of fractures. Osteoporosis, a type of metabolic bony atrophy and another cause of fractures, is a common bone disease of people over 65 years of age. It involves mostly the vertebral bodies and cancellous metaphyses of the neck of the femur, humerus, and distal end of the radius. Because the bone becomes porous and thereby fragile, the affected bones are prone to fracture. A pathological fracture can occur in a bone weakened by disease or tumor, such as osteomyelitis and lytic tumors of bone caused by deposition of metastatic carcinoma.[7]

### Medical Management

The aims of fracture treatment are to relieve pain, maintain good position of the fracture, allow for bony union, and restore optimal function to the patient.[17]

Reduction of a fracture refers to restoring the fragments to normal alignment.[7] This can be done by a closed procedure (manipulation) or by an open procedure (surgery). A closed reduction is performed by applying a force to the displaced bone opposite to the force that produced the fracture. Depending on the nature of the fracture, the reduction is maintained in a cast, brace, traction, or skeletal fixation.

With open reduction, the fracture site is exposed surgically so that the fragments can be aligned. The fragments are held in place with internal fixation by pins, screws, a plate, nails, or a rod. Further immobilization by a cast or a brace may be necessary. Usually an **open reduction and internal fixation (ORIF)** must be protected from excessive forces, so weight bearing is restricted.[10]

There are several levels of **weight-bearing restrictions.** The physician will indicate the level and will reduce the restrictions as the fracture site heals and becomes stronger. The levels of weight-bearing restrictions are listed in Box 29-1.

### Hip Fractures

In a hip fracture the articular surfaces of the hip may need to be removed and replaced by a prosthesis called an *endoprosthesis.* This is necessary when there are complications of avascular necrosis, nonunion, or degenerative joint disease. Avascular necrosis occurs when cells die as a result of poor blood supply. Often after the fracture, soft tissue trauma, edema, and ecchymosis (bruising) develop around the fracture site and can result in increased pain.[15]

#### *Types of Hip Fractures*

A knowledge of hip anatomy is necessary to understand medical management of hip fractures. The hip is an endothrodial or ball-and-socket joint formed by the head of the femur and the acetabulum.[9] The **articular capsule** of the hip joint refers to the dense connective tissue enclosing the joint. It provides stability and

*Box 29-1*

**Weight-Bearing Restrictions**

**NWB** (non–weight bearing) indicates that no weight at all can be placed on the extremity involved.

**TTWB** (toe touch weight bearing) indicates that only the toe can be placed on the ground to provide some balance while standing—90% of the weight is still on the unaffected leg. In toe touch weight bearing, patients are instructed to imagine that an egg is under their foot.

**PWB** (partial weight bearing) indicates that only 50% of the person's body weight can be placed on the affected leg.

**WBAT** (weight bearing at tolerance) indicates that patients are allowed to judge how much weight they are able to put on the affected leg without causing too much pain.

**FWB** (full weight bearing) indicates that patients should be able to put 100% of their weight on the affected leg without causing damage to the fracture site.

assists with hip motion. The capsule extends from the margins of the acetabulum downward anteriorly to the intertrochanteric ridge and posteriorly to the middle of the neck. The hip abductors; gluteus medius and gluteus minimus; and the external rotators, piriformis, gemellus, and obturators attach to the greater trochanter. The hip flexors, psoas major, and iliacus (iliopsoas) attach to the lesser trochanter. Blood is supplied to the femoral head by the ligamentum teres, capsular vessels, and femoral shaft vessels (Figure 29-1).

The levels of fracture lines are shown in Figure 29-2. The names of the fractures generally reflect site and severity of injury and may signal which medical treatment will be used.[5] For example, a femoral neck fracture will be treated with femoral neck stabilization.

*Femoral neck fractures* Femoral neck fractures (subcapital, transcervical, and basilar fractures) are common in adults over 60 years of age and occur more frequently in women. Even slight trauma or rotational force causes fracture in osteoporotic bone.[3] Treatment of a displaced fracture in this area is complicated by poor blood supply. The osteoporotic bone is not suited to hold metallic fixation, and the thin periosteum limits fracture healing. The type of surgical treatment used is based on the amount of displacement and the circulation in the femoral head.

The age and health of the patient are considered in deciding on the surgical procedure. Generally, hip pinning or application of a compression screw and plate is used when displacement is minimal to mod-

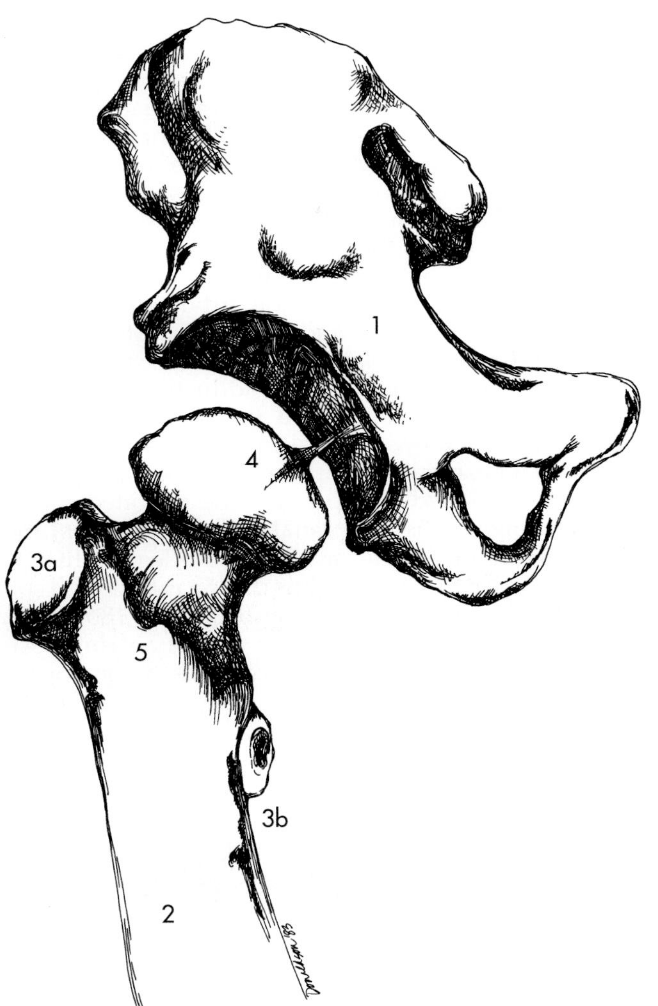


*Figure 29-1* Normal hip anatomy. *1,* Acetabulum; *2,* femur; *3a,* greater trochanter; *3b,* lesser trochanter; *4,* ligamentum teres; *5,* intertrochanteric crest. (Modified from Crouch JE: *Functional human anatomy,* ed 3, Philadelphia, 1978, Lea & Febiger; and Grant LC: *Grant's atlas of anatomy,* ed 6, Baltimore, 1972, Williams & Wilkins.)

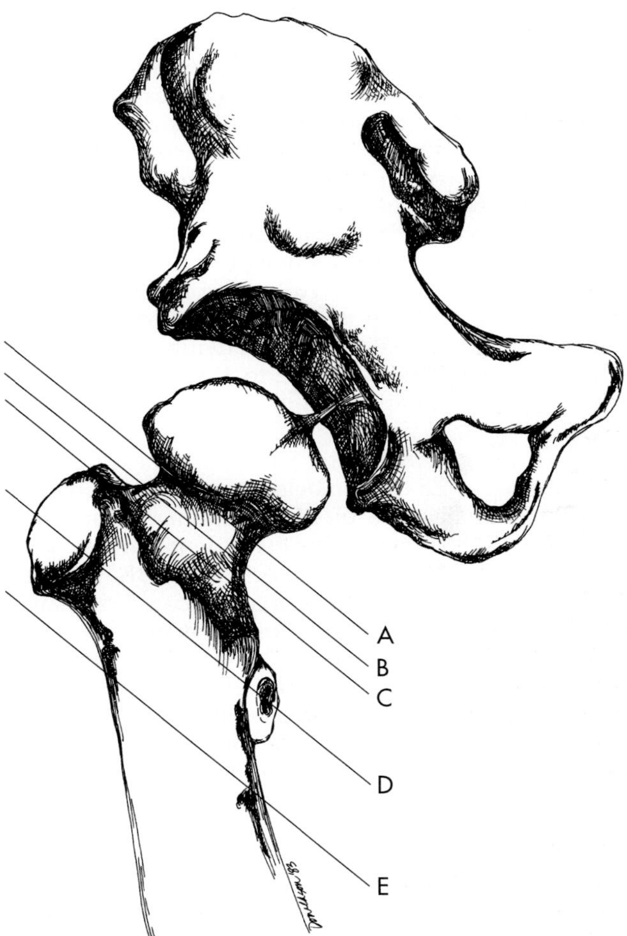


*Figure 29-2* Levels of femoral fracture. *A,* Subcapital; *B,* transcervical; *C,* basilar; *D,* intertrochanteric; *E,* subtrochanteric. (Modified from Crow I: Fracture of the hip: a self study, *ONA J* 5:12, 1978.)

erate and blood supply is intact. With physician approval the patient is usually able to begin out-of-bed activities 2 to 4 days after surgery. Per physician orders, weight-bearing restrictions may need to be observed with the aid of crutches or a walker for at least 6 to 8 weeks while the fracture is healing. Weight-bearing restrictions may extend beyond this time if precautions are not observed or a delayed union occurs.[10]

With severe displacement or poor blood supply the femoral head is surgically removed and replaced by an endoprosthesis. This is referred to as a *bipolar arthroplasty*.[15] Several types of metal prostheses can be used; each has its own shape and advantages. Weight-bearing restrictions are sometimes indicated. Because of the surgical procedure, precautions for positioning the hip must be observed to avoid dislocation. The precautions will vary according to the surgical approach. Patients who have had a prosthesis implanted can usually begin out-of-bed activity, with a physician approval, about 2 to 4 days after surgery.[10]

*Intertrochanteric fractures* Intertrochanteric fractures between the greater and lesser trochanter are extracapsular (or outside the articular capsule of the hip joint), and the blood supply is not affected. Like femoral neck fractures, intertrochanteric fractures occur mostly in women who are in a slightly older age group. The fracture usually is caused by direct trauma or force over the trochanter as can occur in a fall. ORIF is the preferred treatment. A nail or compression screw with a sideplate is used. Weight-bearing restrictions must be observed, sometimes for as long as 4 to 6 months, when a patient is ambulating. Again, the patient is allowed out of bed 2 to 4 days after surgery pending physician approval.[10]

*Subtrochanteric fractures* Subtrochanteric fractures (1 to 2 inches or 2.5 to 5 cm below the lesser trochanter) usually occur because of direct trauma, which may result from falls, motor vehicle accidents, or any other situation in which there is a direct blow to the hip area. These fractures occur most often in persons less than 60 years old. Skeletal traction followed by an ORIF is the usual treatment. A nail with a long sideplate or an intramedullary rod is used. The rod is inserted through the central shaft of the bone to help maintain proper alignment for bone healing. This condition may require further immobilization after surgery.

### *Hip Joint Replacement*

*Cause* Restoration of joint motion and treatment of pain by total hip replacement or arthroplasty is sometimes indicated in patients with osteoarthritis, rheumatoid arthritis, and ankylosing spondylitis.[6] **Osteoarthritis** or degenerative joint disease may develop spontaneously in middle age and progress as the normal aging process of joints is exaggerated. It may also develop as the result of trauma, a congenital deformity, or a disease that damages articular cartilage. Weight-bearing joints, such as the hip, knee, and lumbar spine, are usually affected. In the hip, cartilage is lost centrally on the joint surface and osteophytes (bone spurs) form on the periphery of the acetabulum. Pain arises from the bone, synovial membrane, fibrous capsule, and muscle spasm. When movement of the hip causes pain, movement is restricted and muscles shorten from disuse. The osteoarthritic hip may assume a flexed, adducted, and internally rotated position that also causes a painful limp.[11]

**Ankylosing spondylitis,** a chronic progressive polyarthritis, primarily involves the sacroiliac and spinal joints. The soft tissues eventually ossify and produce a bony ankylosis. The proximal joints of the extremities, particularly the hips, may also be affected.[17]

Rheumatoid arthritis (see Chapter 26) may also involve the hip joint. Surgery is often performed early in the disease process to limit fibrotic damage to joint and tendon structures.[6,17]

*Medical management* Total joint replacement or **arthroplasty** may be necessary in various types of arthritis. This surgery is designed to alleviate pain and restore joint motion. There are two components to a "total hip." A high-density polyethylene socket is fitted into the acetabulum and a metallic prosthesis replaces the femoral head and neck. Methylmethacrylate or acrylic cement fixes the components to the bone. Various surgical approaches are used according to the surgical skill or technique of the orthopedist, severity of the joint involvement, and history of past surgery to the hip. With an anterolateral approach the patient will be unstable in external rotation, adduction, and extension of the operated hip and usually must observe precautions to prevent these movements for 6 to 12 weeks. If a posterolateral approach is used, the patient must be cautioned not to move the operated hip in specific ranges of flexion (usually 60 to 90 degrees) and not to internally rotate or adduct the leg. Failure to maintain these **hip precautions** during muscle and soft tissue healing may result in hip dislocation (Box 29-2).

Most surgeons do not restrict weight bearing postoperatively when cement fixation is used. One of the major problems with total joint replacement is the loss

*Box 29-2*

**Hip Precautions**

**Posterolateral approach**

- No hip flexion greater than 90 degrees
- No internal rotation
- No adduction (crossing legs or feet)

**Anterolateral approach**

- No external rotation
- No adduction (crossing legs or feet)
- No extension

of fixation at the prosthesis interface (the "glue" breaks down). The most recent development is the use of biological fixation. Bony ingrowth instead of cement secures the prosthesis. New bone grows into openings in the prosthesis and thus attaches the prosthesis to the bone. The precautions after the surgery are those of the anterior or posterior hip replacements with an additional restriction on weight bearing for 6 to 8 weeks. The restrictions on weight bearing will vary. A walking aid, usually a walker or crutches, is necessary for at least the first month while the hip is healing and muscles are becoming stronger. Patients with total joint replacements usually begin out-of-bed activity 1 to 3 days after surgery.[11]

It is important for therapy practitioners to be aware of complications or special surgical procedures and to inquire about additional precautions and risks. For example, if a trochanteric osteotomy is necessary and the greater trochanter is removed and rewired down, active abduction is prohibited.[11] Another special procedure involves using a spica cast to immobilize the hip joint for individuals who are at high risk for a dislocation.

Total joint surface replacements, which are rarely used, are a variation of the total hip replacement.[7] The surface of the femur is capped by a metallic shell, and the acetabular cavity receives a plastic cup. Both are held in place by methylmethacrylate. This technique preserves the femoral head and neck. This technique has no weight-bearing restrictions.

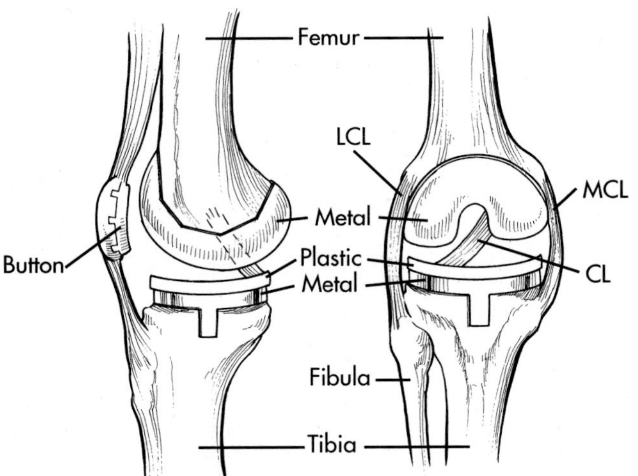


*Figure 29-3* Total knee replacement prosthesis. The metal aspects of the prosthesis cover the distal portion of the femur and the end of the tibia. There is a polyethylene plastic-bearing surface *(plastic)* between the metalic aspects of the two surfaces. The patella is replaced by a polyethylene button. The medial collateral ligament *(MCL)*, lateral collateral ligament *(LCL)*, and cruciate ligaments *(CL)* are retained. (Modified from Calliet R: *Knee pain and disability*, ed 3, Philadelphia, 1992, FA Davis.)

### *Total Knee Replacement*

*Medical management* The cause for a total knee replacement is similar to that for the total hip replacement except that the degenerative changes occur in the knee joint. Total knee replacement or arthroplasty (TKA) is designed to alleviate pain, regain motion, and maintain alignment and stability of the knee joint. The process involves cutting away the damaged bone (as little bone as possible) and attaching a prosthesis for the new joint. There are various types of prostheses. The type used depends on the severity of joint damage. (Figure 29-3). The prosthesis can be cemented to the bone or not cemented. In a cemented prosthesis, patients are usually able to bear weight at tolerance on the operated leg. In a noncemented prosthesis, non–weight bearing is usually the restriction initially.[4]

Emphasis in rehabilitation is on maintaining or regaining joint motion, slowly increasing the strength of surrounding musculature, decreasing swelling, and increasing independence in ADL. Occupational therapy's role in this process is primarily in educating the knee replacement patient of adaptive techniques for ADL as a result of limited knee flexion. Patients may use a **knee immobilizer** (Figure 29-4) when moving in and out of the bed and ambulating to provide support to the knee. The patient should avoid any rotation at the knee up to 12 weeks after surgery.[16]

Individuals with joint changes that result in increasing pain may have multiple joint involvement (i.e., both knees or hips). Some individuals opt to have both joints replaced during the same hospitalization, and procedures are usually 1 week apart. This can complicate the rehabilitation process because the patient will not have a stronger leg to rely on for ambulation and performing ADL.

## PSYCHOLOGICAL FACTORS

Psychological issues affect the overall treatment of the orthopedic patient. A large number of such patients are faced with either a chronic disability (e.g., rheumatoid arthritis), a life-threatening disease (e.g., cancer), or the aging process. Loss or potential loss of mobility and physical ability is a major concern. Adjusting to loss is stressful and requires an enormous amount of physical and emotional energy.[13] An awareness of and a sensitivity toward the orthopedic patient is critical to the delivery of optimal patient care.

The occupational therapy practitioner must realize that each patient's experience of loss varies with intrinsic makeup (personality, physical diseases, specific changes, and body image). Environmental factors such as personal losses or gains, family dynamics, and the home environment affect the patient also.[13]

Patients with a chronic orthopedic disability often experience one or all of the following: a disease of a body part, fear, anxiety, change in body image, decreased functional ability, deformity, and pain. These may occur at a relatively young age and often in rapid succession. Orthopedic patients often consider them-

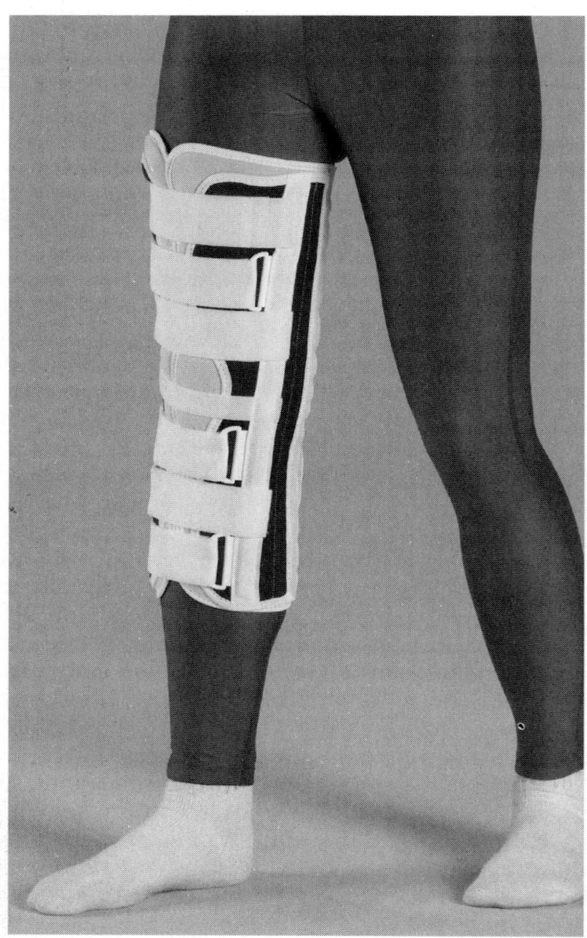

*Figure 29-4* A knee immobilizer is used to support and stabilize the knee joint during mobility. (Courtesy DeRoyal, Powell, Tenn.)

selves prisoners of their own bodies and are left with accumulated layers of unresolved grief, fatigue, and a sense of emptiness.[3] When treating a patient with a chronic orthopedic disability, it is important to address these issues and to provide the support needed for the mourning and grieving process to take place. Without an opportunity to confront these issues, the patient is likely to become depressed, filled with guilt and anxiety, and paralyzed with fear. These emotions inhibit the patient's progress and further damage self-image. Clinicians can help patients acknowledge and experience some of these feelings and ultimately enhance the treatment process.

The same holds true when working with the disabled elderly patient, but the following additional issues are specific to the aging process: life review, fear of dependency, and relocation trauma.

The elderly patient often experiences the need to reflect on and review past life experiences.[2] This activity is central to the resolution of Erikson's stage of ego integrity versus despair.

A second important issue experienced by the elderly disabled individual is dependency. With the onset of a disability late in life, the patient may be forced to let go of years of independence and self-sufficiency.[13] For some, this can be a devastating experience, requiring prolonged grieving before adjustment. Others may use dependency for secondary gain, remaining in the hospital for extra attention or manipulating their support systems to avoid taking responsibility for themselves and others.

A third psychosocial phenomenon experienced by the aged when hospitalized is relocation trauma. Older people, when removed from their familiar environment, will often decompensate cognitively and may experience confusion, emotional lability, and disorientation. Therefore it is important that their new environment be made as familiar as possible. Decorating it with familiar objects from their home and providing a calendar and current newspapers and magazines are often helpful in reducing this traumatic effect.

Learning to cope and adjust to the changes resulting from chronic disability or the aging process is a critical aspect of recovery. Practitioners must realize that a great deal of a patient's functional independence has been relinquished as a result of disease or disability. The psychosocial issues resulting from this loss must be addressed while focusing on increasing the patient's functional level of independence.

## REHABILITATION MEASURES

Good communication and clear role delineation among members of the health care team are essential for an efficient and smooth therapy program. The health care team usually consists of a primary physician, nursing staff, a physical therapist, and possibly a physical therapy assistant, an occupational therapist or assistant, a nutritionist, a pharmacist, a discharge planner, and possibly a social worker. Regular team meetings to discuss each patient's ongoing treatment, progress, and discharge plans are necessary to coordinate individual treatment programs. Members from each service usually attend to provide information and consultation.

The role of the physician is to inform the team of the patient's medical status. This includes information regarding a medical history, diagnosis of the present problem, and a complete account of the surgical procedure performed. This would include the type of appliance inserted, the anatomical approach, and any movement or weight-bearing precautions that could endanger the patient. The physician is also responsible for ordering specific medications and therapies. Any change or progression in therapy or changes in the patient's medication regimen should be approved by the physician.

The nursing staff is responsible for the actual physical care of the patient during hospitalization. Responsibilities of the nurse include administering medications, assisting the patient with bathing and hygiene, and constantly monitoring vital signs and physical status. Each patient's blood pressure, pulse, and respiratory status are checked every 1 to 2 hours immediately after surgery.[11] During the rehabilitation phase, vital signs are usually checked once every 8 hours unless otherwise ordered by the physician.[11] Wound and skin care, such as the changing of dressings or the sterilization of wounds, are performed by the nurse. The orthopedic nurse must have a thorough understanding of the surgical procedures and movement precautions for each patient. Proper positioning with pillows and wedges is carried out by the nurse, especially in the first few days after surgery. As the therapy program progresses, the patient can start to take more responsibility for proper positioning and physical care. The nurse works closely with the physical and occupational therapists and occupational therapy assistants to carry through self-care skills that the patient has already learned in therapy.[11]

The physical therapist is responsible for evaluation and treatment in the areas of musculoskeletal status, sensation, pain, skin integrity, and mobility (especially gait). In many cases involving total joint replacements and surgical repair of hip fractures, physical therapy is initiated on the first day after surgery. The physical therapist obtains baseline information including range of motion (ROM), strength of all the extremities, muscle tone, mental status, and mobility, and adheres to the prescribed precautions of protocol. A treatment program that includes therapeutic exercises, ROM activities, transfer training, and progressive gait activities is established. The physical therapist is responsible for recommending the appropriate assistive device to be used during ambulation. As the patient's ambulation status advances, instruction in stair climbing, managing curbs, and outside ambulation is given.[8,11,15]

The nutritionist consults with each patient to ensure that adequate and appropriate nutrition is received to aid the healing process. The pharmacist monitors the patient's drug therapy and provides information and assistance with pain management.[11]

The role of the discharge planner is to ensure that each patient is being discharged to the appropriate living situation or facility. Usually the discharge planner is a registered nurse or social worker with a thorough knowledge of community resources and nursing care facilities available. With input from the health care team, the discharge planner makes the arrangements for ongoing therapy after hospitalization, admission to a rehabilitation facility for further intensive therapy, or nursing home care if necessary. The discharge planner works closely with the health care team and is instrumental in coordinating the program after the patient's discharge from the hospital.[11,15]

### The Role of Occupational Therapy

After a total joint replacement or surgical repair of a fractured hip, occupational therapy usually begins when the patient is ready to start getting out of bed, about 2 to 4 days after surgery. The actual time varies depending on age, general health, and surgical events or medical complications. Before any physical assessment, it is important for the occupational therapy practitioner to introduce and explain the role of occupational therapy, establish rapport, and then gather by interview any information pertinent to the patient's prior functional status, home environment, and living situation. The goal of occupational therapy is for the patient to return home independently performing ADLs and observing all movement precautions during activities. It is the role of the occupational therapist and assistant to teach the patient ways and means of performing ADL safely.[11,14,15]

The role of the occupational therapist and certified occupational therapy assistant (COTA) can be clearly defined in the cases of total joint replacement and hip fractures. The occupational therapist is responsible for performing any evaluations that are needed. A baseline physical evaluation is necessary to determine whether any physical limitations not related to surgery might prevent functional independence. UE ROM, muscle strength, sensation, coordination, and mental status are assessed before a functional evaluation is made. The COTA participates in the ADL evaluation. During evaluation, it is also important to observe any signs of pain and fear at rest and/or during movement.[8]

Occupational therapy treatment involves a progression of functional activities that simulate a normal daily regimen, applying all the movement precautions.[11,14,15] The COTA plays a major role, introducing and training patients in the use of assistive devices, proper transfer techniques, and ADL techniques, while maintaining hip precautions. Both the occupational therapist and the occupational therapy assistant are involved in treatment planning, documentation, and discharge planning (including recommending equipment and home exercise programs).

Total joint replacements are usually preplanned and scheduled to be performed on a specific date. The COTA can play a role along with the occupational therapist in providing education classes. Persons who may be at risk for falling may attend a class on fall prevention. The COTA can coordinate and facilitate this type of group. Topics can include home modifications (such as removing throw rugs, telephone cords, clutter), safe transfer techniques, use of public transportation, and community mobility tips. The person who is having an elective total joint replacement can benefit from a class offered before surgery that explains the procedures, introduces assistive devices, and describes therapy procedures.

### Guidelines for ADL Training

Some common assistive devices are useful for many people with hip fractures or joint replacements (Figure 29-5). The occupational therapy clinic should have samples of these and should be able to issue them to patients for use during the training process. Helpful assistive devices or adaptive aids include a dress-

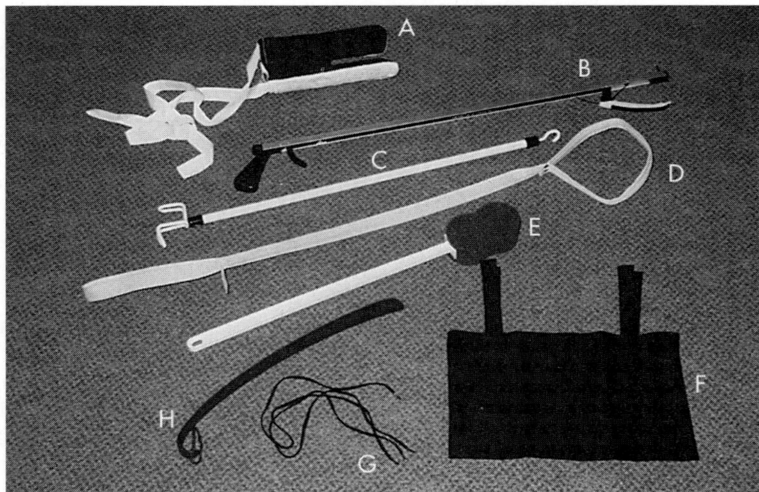


*Figure 29-5* Assistive devices for ADL. *A,* Sock aid; *B,* reacher; *C,* dressing stick; *D,* leg lifter; *E,* long-handled sponge; *F,* walker bag; *G,* elastic shoe laces; *H,* long-handled shoe horn.

ing stick, a sock aid, a long-handled sponge, a long-handled shoe horn, a reacher, elastic shoe laces, an elevated toilet or commode seat, a **leg lifter,** and a shower chair or bench. Walker bags are helpful for people who are using walkers and need to carry small items from one place to another.[11,15]

### *Hip Joint Replacement Procedure*

Procedures for training outlined below apply to both types of hip joint replacement (posterolateral and anterolateral) unless otherwise noted. It is important to remember the positions of hip instability for both types of surgical procedures. For the posterolateral approach, positions of instability include adduction, internal rotation, and flexion greater than precautions. For the anterolateral approach, positions of instability include adduction, external rotation, and excessive hyperextension.

*Bed mobility* The supine position with the appropriate wedge or pillow in place is recommended. If patients sleep on their side, sleeping on the operated side is recommended if tolerable. When sleeping on the nonoperated side, the legs must be abducted with the wedge or larger pillows and the operated leg supported to prevent rotation. The patient is instructed on getting out of bed on both sides, although initially it may be easier to observe precautions by moving toward the nonoperated leg. Careful instruction is given to avoid adduction past midline. It is important to determine the type and height of the patient's bed at home. When getting in and out of bed initially, the patient may use a leg lifter to assist the operated leg in moving from one surface to another.

*Transfers* It is always helpful for the patient to first observe the proper technique for transfers before attempting the movement.

- *Chair:* A firmly based chair with armrests is recommended. The patient is instructed to extend the operated leg forward, reach back for the armrests, and sit slowly. For the person with a posterolateral approach, care should be taken to not lean forward when sitting down (Figure 29-6). To stand, the patient extends the operated leg and pushes off from the armrests. Because of the hip flexion precaution for the posterolateral approach, the patient should sit on the front part of the chair and lean back (see Figure 29-6, C). Firm cushions or blankets can be used to increase the height of chairs and may be especially needed if the patient is tall. Low, soft, reclining, and rocking chairs should be avoided.
- *Commode chair:* Over-the-toilet **commode chairs** with armrests are to be used in the hospital and at home (see Figure 17-4). For the person with a posterolateral approach, the height and angle can be adjusted so that the front legs are one notch lower than the back legs; thus with the patient seated hip flexion will not exceed 90 degrees. A person with an anterolateral approach may have enough hip mobility to safely use a standard toilet seat at the time of discharge. All patients should wipe between the legs in a sitting position or from behind in a standing position with caution to avoid rotation of the hip. The patient is to stand up and step to turn to face the toilet to flush.
- *Shower stall:* Nonskid strips or stickers are recommended in all shower stalls and tubs. When enter-

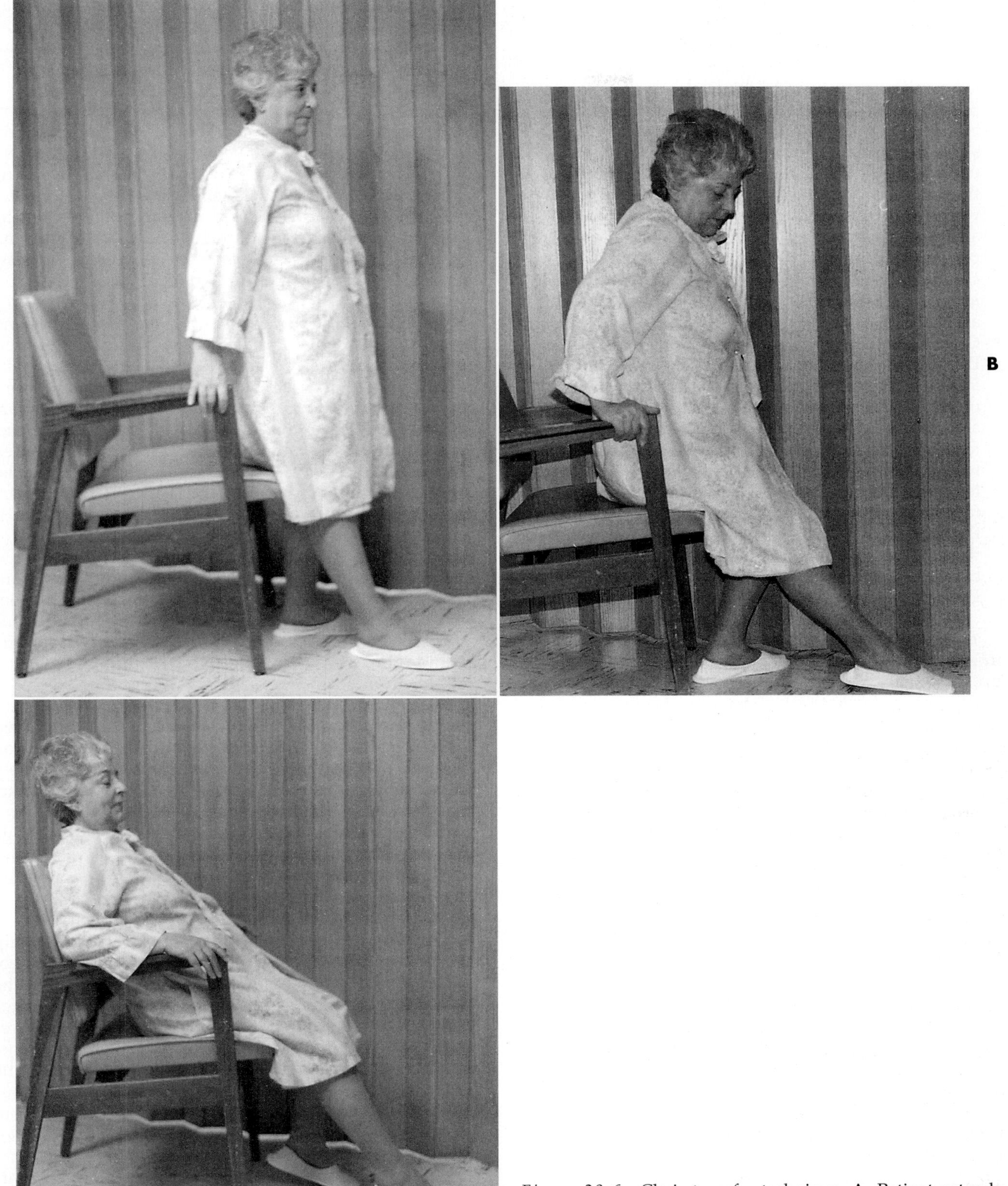


*Figure 29-6* Chair transfer technique. **A,** Patient extends operated leg and reaches for arm rests. **B** and **C,** Bearing some weight on arms, patient sits down slowly while maintaining some extension of operated leg.

ing, the walker or crutches go first, then the operated leg followed by the nonoperated leg. A shower chair with adjustable legs or a stool and grab bars should be installed if balance is a problem or if weight-bearing precautions are necessary.

- *Shower-over-tub (without shower doors):* The patient is instructed to stand parallel to the tub facing the shower fixtures. Using the walker or crutches, the patient is to transfer in sideways by bending at the knees, not at the hips. For patients with weight-bearing precautions or poor balance, use of a tub bench may be considered, which allows the patient to sit on the edge of the bench and then swing the legs over the tub while observing flexion precautions. Sponge bathing at the sink is an alternate activity.
- *Car:* Bucket seats in small cars should be avoided. Bench-type seats are recommended. The patient is instructed to back up to the passenger seat, hold onto a stable part of the car, extend the operated leg, and slowly sit in the car. Remembering to lean back, the patient then slides the buttocks toward the driver's seat. The upper body and lower extremities then move as one unit to turn to face the forward direction. It is helpful to have the seat pushed back and reclined to accomodate the hip flexion precaution. Pillows in the seat may be necessary to increase the height of the seat. Prolonged sitting in the car should be avoided.

*Lower body dressing* The patient is instructed to sit in a chair with arms or on the edge of the bed for dressing activities. The patient is instructed to avoid adduction and rotation or crossing the legs to dress. Crossing the operated extremity over the nonoperated extremity at either the ankles or knees is to be avoided. Assistive devices may be necessary to observe precautions (see Figure 29-5). To follow hip precautions, a reacher or dressing stick is used to aid in donning and removing pants and shoes. When putting on pants, the operated leg is dressed first by using the reacher or dressing stick to bring the pants over the foot and up to the knee. A sock aid is used to don socks or kneehigh nylons, and a reacher or dressing stick is used to doff. A reacher, elastic laces, and a long-handled shoe horn can also be provided.

*Lower body bathing* Refer to transfer section for method to get in/out of shower or tub. Sponge bathing at the sink is indicated until approved by the physician to shower. A long-handled bath sponge or back brush is used to reach the lower legs and feet safely; soap-on-a-rope is used to prevent the soap from dropping; and a towel is wrapped on a reacher to dry the lower legs.

*Hair shampoo* Until patients are able to shower, they are instructed to obtain assistance for shampooing hair. If unable to have any assistance, the patient may shampoo hair while standing or sitting on a stool at the kitchen or bathroom sink, while observing hip precautions at all times.

*Homemaking* Heavy housework, such as vacuuming, lifting, and bed making, should be avoided. Commonly used items for kitchen activities should be kept at counter top level. Items can be moved by using aprons with large pockets, sliding along the counter top, using utility cart, attaching a small basket or bag to a walker, or wearing a pouch ("fanny pack") around the waist. Reachers are used to grasp items in low cabinets or to pick them up from the floor.

*Family orientation* A family member or friend should be present for at least one occupational therapy treatment session so that any questions may be answered. Appropriate supervision recommendations and instruction regarding activity precautions are given at this time. Instructional booklets on hip fractures and total hip and knee surgery can be purchased from the American Occupational Therapy Association[1] and Krames Communications[12] to supplement training.

### *Total Knee Replacement Procedures*

Following are procedures for ADL training for persons with total knee replacement. Many of the techniques used with a hip replacement can be used for someone with a knee replacement. Positions of knee instability include internal and external rotation and flexion greater than ROM permits.

*Bed mobility* Supine position is recommended with leg slightly elevated via balanced suspension with or without a knee immobilizer. This will help to reduce edema and prevent knee flexion contractures. Sleeping on the operated side is not recommended. As in hip replacement, a pillow or wedge can be placed in between the legs if this is necessary for sidelying and the person lies on the nonoperated side.

*Transfers* In general, patients can bend at the hip during transfers as much as they are able. Because of decreased knee flexion, the patient may need to use the same techniques as described for hip replacements for commode and car transfers. Grab bars and a shower chair or bench are recommended especially for transferring to the shower over the tub as well as for the individual with decreased standing endurance or inability to bend the knee enough to sit on the bottom of the tub.

*Lower body dressing* Lower body dressing presents a problem only if patients are unable to reach their toes. In such a case, techniques described for the hip replacement can be used. The patient should practice donning and doffing the knee immobilizer.

The techniques for homemaking and family training are the same as those used for hip replacement.

### *Special Equipment*

The occupational therapy practitioner should be familiar with the following equipment that is commonly used in the treatment of hip fracture and total hip replacement.

*Nelson bed* An adjustable bed that allows for chair or 90 degree vertical tilt positions may be used in some programs in the initial postoperative days to facilitate a change in the patient's position and allow a progressive tilting program before ambulation.

*Hemovac* During surgery a plastic drainage tube is inserted at the surgical site to assist with drainage of blood postoperatively. It has an area for collection of drainage and may be connected to a portable suction machine. The unit should *not* be disconnected for any activity because this may create a blockage in the system. The Hemovac is usually left in place for 2 days after surgery.

*Abduction wedge* Large and small triangular **abduction wedges** are used when the patient is supine to maintain the LEs in the abducted position.

*Balanced suspension* Balanced suspension is fabricated and set up by the physical therapist or cast-room technician and physician and is often used for about 3 days after surgery. Its purpose is to support the affected LE in the first few postoperative days. The patient's leg should *not* be taken out of the device for exercise until the device's use has been discontinued by the physician.

*Reclining wheelchair* A wheelchair with an adjustable backrest that allows a reclining position is used for patients who have hip flexion precautions while sitting.

*Commode chairs* The use of a commode chair instead of the regular toilet aids in safe transfers and allows the patient to observe necessary hip flexion precautions. The two front legs of the commode chair may be adjusted slightly lower than the back legs to increase the patient's ability to observe hip flexion limitations and decrease the risk of dislocation.

*Sequential compression devices (SCDs)* SCDs are used postoperatively to reduce the risk of deep vein thrombosis. They are inflatable, external leggings that provide intermittent pneumatic compression of the legs.[11]

*Antiembolus hose* Antiembolus hosiery is thigh-high hosiery that is worn 24 hours a day and removed only during bathing. Its purpose is to assist circulation, prevent edema, and thus reduce the risk of deep vein thrombosis.[11]

*Patient-controlled administration (PCA) IV* The amount of medication is predetermined and programmed by the physician and nursing to allow the patient to self-administer pain medication by pushing a button.

*Incentive spirometer* An incentive spirometer is a portable breathing apparatus used to encourage deep breathing and prevent the development of postoperative pneumonia.

## SUMMARY

The protocol for occupational therapy is determined by the surgical procedure performed and the precautions prescribed by the physician. Patients who have weight-bearing precautions must be trained to observe these during all ADL. A simulation of the home environment or a home assessment is helpful to prepare the patient for potential problems that may arise after discharge. Areas to assess include the entry, stairs, bathroom, bedroom, sitting surfaces, and the kitchen. It is recommended to remove throw rugs, other slippery floor coverings, and obstacles because the patient will most likely be going home with an ambulatory assistive device. A kitchen stool or utility cart may be indicated. It is important to assess and instruct the patient and caregiver in ADL with adaptive equipment while observing any movement precautions.

Sexuality is an area that is often overlooked. Diagrams of positions that observe hip precautions can be provided, with additional instruction regarding the method to get in and out of the recommended positions. Psychosocial reactions to hip fracture and total hip surgery can impact the success of therapy and must be considered in treatment planning. Home therapy may be indicated after a hospital stay to ensure safety and independence in ADL if these goals were not met during hospitalization.

Preoperative teaching programs are invaluable in aiding patient adjustment. The group class orients and familiarizes the patient to the hospital, nursing, physical therapy, occupational therapy, respiratory therapy, and discharge planning. Procedures and equipment, concerns regarding the hospitalization and discharge, and therapy are addressed. Participation in this type of class has been shown to relieve anxiety and fear, empower the patient during the hospitalization, and decrease the hospital length of stay.

## Sample Treatment Plan

This sample treatment plan is not comprehensive. It deals with four of eight problems identified. The reader is encouraged to add objectives and methods to the plan that deal with these and the other problems.

**Case study**

Mr. B. is an 82-year-old man who has noticed increased right hip pain over the past year. A week ago he fell on ice just outside of his home. He was unable to bear weight on his right leg. He was admitted to the emergency room. A hip x-ray examination showed degenerative arthritis and a right femoral neck fracture. He was admitted to the orthopedic unit of the hospital for elective right total joint replacement using the posterolateral approach.

Mr. B. is a widower from Kentucky whose wife died shortly after they moved to California 6 months ago. Mr. B. lives in his own cottage behind his son's home. Mr. B. has been independent in meal preparation, self-care, and homemaking. He enjoys gardening, walking in the neighborhood, and visiting with his two grandchildren. His increased hip pain has limited his daily activity. He must take frequent rests during the day and use a cane.

*Personal data*

Name: Mr. B.
Age: 82
Diagnosis: Right femoral neck fracture and degenerative arthritis affecting right hip, right total hip replacement
Disability: Limited LE ROM and ambulation
Precautions: Avoidance of right hip internal rotation, flexion greater than 90 degrees, and adduction for 6 to 8 weeks after surgery; weight bearing as tolerated
Treatment aims as stated in referral: orient patient to rehabilitation program, evaluate patient's function, instruct patient in maintaining hip precautions for ADL postoperatively.

**Other services**

Medical: Perform right total hip replacement surgery; prescribe rehabilitation therapies and medication.
Nursing: Provide nursing care, positioning, and supervision in activities and exercises after therapist instructs patient.
Physical therapy: Provide LE ROM and strengthening exercises and transfer and gait training.
Discharge planner: Arrange for home care follow-up.
Family: Provide emotional support and physical assistance after discharge from hospital; encourage patient to observe precautions for hip movements at home.

**Treatment approach**

Occupational performance/rehabilitative approach

**OT evaluation**

*Occupational therapist and assistant*

Role of occupational therapy and rehabilitation program: Orient patient.
Patient's goals from this surgery: Interview.
General appearance: Observe ease of movement, personal hygiene, hospital equipment in use, and patient's position and expression

*Occupational therapist*

Mental and behavioral state: Observe.
Communication, vision, and hearing: Observe.
Sensation and pain: Test and observe.
Strength of UEs and trunk: Test.
Muscle tone: Test.
Posture: Observe.
Bulbar function: Screen.
Perceptual and cognitive function: Test and observe.

*Occupational therapist and/or assistant*

Avocational and vocational activities and endurance: Interview.
Home layout and accessibility: Interview.
Bed mobility: Demonstrate and interview.
Transfers (bed, chair, toilet, shower, and car): Demonstrate or interview.
Dressing: Interview.
Personal hygiene: Interview.

**Evaluation summary**

UE active ROM after surgery was limited to 160 degrees of shoulder flexion bilaterally, and strength was grades 4 to 5 (G to N).

Mr. B. was very cooperative during treatment. He was tearful at times when discussing the loss of his wife. Mr. B. currently requires assistive equipment for independence in self-care. Endurance is improved for homemaking, but assistance is still required for heavy household tasks because of hip precautions. After 8 weeks of recovery, he is expected to be independent in most household tasks and in all self-care without equipment. For the first 8 weeks of recovery, Mr. B. will be cautioned against activities such as gardening and heavy lifting that may violate hip precautions. After 8 weeks, he will be allowed to resume all of his leisure activities with less pain, and increased endurance is expected.

## Sample Treatment Plan—cont'd

**Assets**

Strives for independence
Has a good understanding of rehabilitation program
Has a supportive family
Has good safety awareness and judgment

**Problem list**

1. Pain
2. Limited independence because of pain
3. Anxiety about surgery and dependence
4. Unable to ambulate without aids
5. ADL dependence
6. Limited leisure activities
7. Mild memory deficit
8. Limited endurance
9. Impaired standing balance
10. Grief over loss of spouse

**Problem 3**

Anxiety about surgery and dependence

*Objective*

Patient will be independent in stating and explaining hip precautions as related to functional activity.

*Method*

Surgery and hip precautions are described to the patient. The occupational therapy program and progression of functional activities both in the hospital and at home are explained; a sound-slide module or written material may be used to help clarify explanations. Post signs in patient's room to help with mild memory deficit.

**Problems 4 and 5**

Unable to ambulate without aids, ADL dependence

*Objective*

Patient will not require any verbal cueing for safety during dressing, bathing, transfers, and ambulating with aids. Patient will be independent in using assistive aids for self-care while observing hip precautions.

*Method*

Correct use of assistive aids and transfer methods are demonstrated to the patient. Patient practices under supervision, with the assistive aids and transfer methods. Patient ambulates safely with assistive aid during ADL with verbal cueing as needed. Encourage patient to problem solve on his own.

**Problems 4 and 6**

Unable to ambulate without aids, limited leisure activities

*Objective*

The patient will state two ways he may modify gardening, visiting with grandchildren, and walking in the neighborhood to ensure observance of hip precautions and safety.

*Method*

Patient participates in simulated gardening by bending, reaching, and carrying items in clinic. Safety skills for ambulating with a walker or crutches around children are discussed and demonstrated; patient practices maneuvering in clinic obstacle course. Therapist discusses the methods for pacing and awareness of safe surfaces for ambulating in neighborhood with patient; patient practices pacing and maneuvering on various surfaces in hospital.

*Gradation*

Patient solves problems through discussion, then in simulated situations.

## *Selected Reading Guide Questions*

1. Why is it critical for the occupational therapy assistant to understand hip anatomy and treatment of hip fractures?
2. When reviewing the patient's medical history, what information should be obtained?
3. Identify four factors that will influence fracture healing.
4. What is a pathological fracture, and in which diseases can it occur?
5. Describe the differences in approach and maintenance of closed and open reductions.
6. Define the levels of weight-bearing restrictions.
7. Why are weight-bearing restrictions observed with ORIF hip pinnings?
8. List areas of occupational therapy in intervention for hip fractures and joint replacements.
9. Why must hip position precautions be observed during activity by patients with total hip replacements?
10. In which diagnostic groups other than fractures will there be frequent indication for total joint replacement? What are the goals for this surgical approach in these diagnostic conditions?
11. Briefly describe the positions of instability in both the anterolateral and posterolateral approaches to hip replacement orthoplasty.
12. Briefly describe a total joint surface replacement and indications for its application.
13. Briefly describe a wedge and the indications for its use and application.
14. After initial postoperative assessment, which functional activities are generally assessed in planning the initial treatment program?
15. Briefly describe the transfer method to a chair after total hip replacement with a posterolateral approach. What is the rationale applied here? What types of chair should be avoided? Why?
16. Briefly describe a car transfer recommended for the patient with hip replacement orthoplasty with an anterolateral approach.
17. Which pieces of adaptive equipment might help a patient who has had a posterolateral total hip replacement achieve independence in LE dressing?
18. What suggestions could be made for carrying items when ambulation aids are necessary?
19. Describe techniques for completing home management tasks for someone with a total hip replacement.
20. Outline the psychosocial issues faced by the elderly person with a hip fracture or joint replacement.

### *REFERENCES*


1. American Occupational Therapy Association: *Daily activities after your hip surgery,* ed rev, Rockville, Md, 1990, The Association.
2. Butler RN: *The life review: an interpretation of reminiscence in the aged.* In Kastenbaum R, editor: *New thoughts on old age,* New York, 1964, Springer.
3. Butler RN: *Aging and mental health,* ed 3, St Louis, 1982, Mosby.
4. Calliet R: *Knee pain and disability,* ed 3, Philadelphia, 1992, FA Davis.
5. Crow I: Fractures of the hip: a self study, *ONA J* 5:12, 1978.
6. Ehrlich G: *Rehabilitation of rheumatic conditions,* ed 2, Baltimore, 1986, Williams & Wilkins.
7. Garland JJ: *Fundamentals of orthopedics,* Philadelphia, 1979, WB Saunders.
8. Goodgold J: *Rehabilitation medicine,* St Louis, 1988, Mosby.
9. Gray H: *Gray's anatomy,* Philadelphia, 1974, Running Press.
10. Hogshead HP: *Orthopaedics for the therapist,* Unpublished manuscript, 1973.
11. Jones M, et al.: *The total hip replacement protocol,* Stanford, Calif, 1982, 1986, Stanford University Hospital (unpublished material).
12. Krames Communications: *After total hip replacement and after hip fracture,* Daly City, Calif, 1989, Krames Communications.
13. Lewis SC: *The mature years: a geriatric occupational therapy text,* Thorofare, NJ, 1979, Charles B Slack.
14. Melvin J: *Rheumatic disease: OT and rehabilitation,* ed 2, Philadelphia, 1982, FA Davis.
15. Morawski D: *The total hip replacement protocol and hip fracture protocol,* Unpublished manuscript, 1990.
16. Richardson J, Iglarsh Z: *Clinical orthopaedic physical therapy,* Philadelphia, 1994, WB Saunders.
17. Salter RB: *Textbook of disorders and injuries of the musculoskeletal system,* Baltimore, 1970, Williams & Wilkins.


### *RECOMMENDED READING*


American Occupational Therapy Association: *Daily activities after your knee surgery,* Rockville, Md, 1990, The Association.

Chapter 30

# Cardiac Dysfunction and Chronic Obstructive Pulmonary Disease

*Maureen Michele Matthews*

## Chapter Objectives

*After studying this chapter, the student or practitioner will be able to:*

1. Briefly describe the cardiovascular system and its function.
2. Identify the significance of ischemic heart disease and valvular diseases of the heart.
3. Differentiate between modifiable and nonmodifiable risk factors.
4. Identify signs and symptoms of cardiac distress.
5. Describe the course of action to take if signs and symptoms of cardiac distress are present.
6. List the psychosocial considerations for persons with cardiovascular or pulmonary disease.
7. Describe methods for taking heart rate and blood pressure.
8. Determine rate pressure product, given heart rate and blood pressure.
9. Give a brief overview of the respiratory system and identify its primary function.
10. Define chronic obstructive pulmonary disease.
11. Identify pulmonary risk factors and psychosocial considerations.
12. Describe dyspnea control postures, pursed-lip breathing, and diaphragmatic breathing.
13. Describe a relaxation technique and its purpose.
14. List interview questions that will help the clinician know what the patient understands about treatment.
15. List the principles of energy conservation.
16. Explain the significance of a basal metabolic equivalent chart in the progression of activity and describe how to use it.

## Key Terms

myocardium
ischemia
myocardial infarction (MI)
cardiac rehabilitation
congestive heart failure (CHF)
cardiac risk factors
signs of cardiopulmonary distress
heart rate
blood pressure
rate pressure product (RPP)
rate of perceived exertion (RPE)
chronic obstructive pulmonary disease (COPD)
pulmonary rehabilitation
dyspnea control postures
pursed-lip breathing (PLB)
diaphragmatic breathing
cardiovascular responses to activity
basal metabolic equivalent (MET)
energy conservation

Individuals with disorders of the cardiovascular or pulmonary system can be severely limited in endurance and performance of activities of daily living (ADL). Occupational therapy services can benefit such individuals. An understanding of the normal function of the cardiopulmonary system, the pathology of cardiopulmonary disease, common risk factors, clinical terminology, medical interventions, precautions, and standard treatment techniques will guide the certified occupational therapy assistant (COTA) in providing effective care and promoting recovery of function in persons with compromised cardiovascular or pulmonary systems.

Every cell of the body has three major requirements for life: (1) a constant supply of nutrients and oxygen, (2) continual removal of carbon dioxide and other waste products, and (3) a relatively constant temperature. The cardiovascular and pulmonary systems play key roles in these processes.

## THE CARDIOVASCULAR SYSTEM

### Anatomy and Circulation

The heart and blood vessels work together to maintain a constant flow of blood throughout the body. The heart, located between the lungs, is pear shaped and about the size of a fist. It functions as a two-sided pump. The right side pumps blood from the body to the lungs; simultaneously the left side pumps blood from the lungs to the body. Each side of the heart has two chambers, an upper atrium and a lower ventricle.

Blood flows to the heart from the venous system. It enters the right atrium, which contracts and squeezes the blood into the right ventricle. Next, the right ventricle contracts and ejects the blood into the lungs where carbon dioxide is exchanged for oxygen. Oxygen-rich blood flows from the lungs to the left atrium. As the left atrium contracts, it forces blood into the left ventricle, which then contracts and ejects its contents into the aorta for systemic circulation (Figure 30-1). Blood travels from the aorta to the arteries and through progressively smaller blood vessels to networks of very tiny capillaries. In the capillaries, blood cells exchange their oxygen for carbon dioxide.

Each of the ventricles has two valves, an input valve and an output valve. The valves open and close as the heart muscle **(myocardium)** contracts and relaxes. These valves control the direction and flow of blood.

The heart is living tissue and requires a blood supply (arterial and venous system) of its own or it will die. Coronary arteries cross over the heart muscle to supply the myocardium with oxygen-rich blood. The coronary arteries are named for their location on the myocardium (Figure 30-2). Cardiologists tend to call these arteries by abbreviations, such as LAD for left anterior descending. A blockage of the LAD will interrupt the blood supply to the left ventricle. Because the left ventricle supplies the body and brain with blood, a heart attack caused by LAD blockage can have serious consequences.[3,13,17]

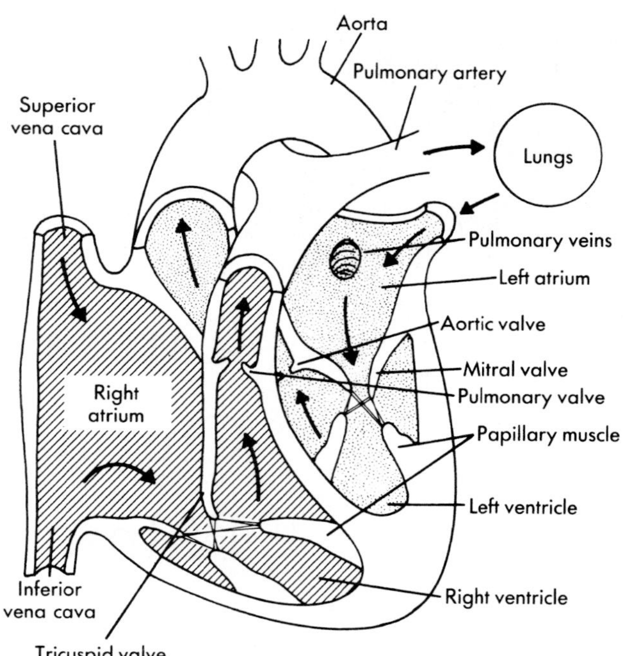


*Figure 30-1* Anatomy of the heart. (Modified from Guyton AC: *Textbook of medical physiology,* ed 8, 1991, Saunders.)

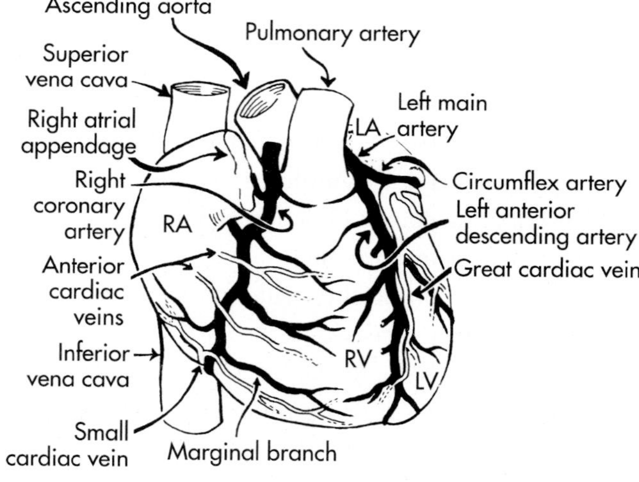


*Figure 30-2* Coronary circulation (From Underhill SL et al, editors: *Cardiac nursing,* Philadelphia, 1982, JB Lippincott.)

### Mechanism of Heart Contraction

The heart has an electrical conduction system that causes it to contract and relax (Figure 30-3). Electrical impulses usually originate in the right atrium at the sinoatrial (SA) node, travel along internodal pathways to the atrioventricular (AV) node, through the bundle of His, to the left and right bundle branches, and finally to the Purkinje fibers. Nerve impulses normally travel this pathway 60 to 100 times every minute, causing

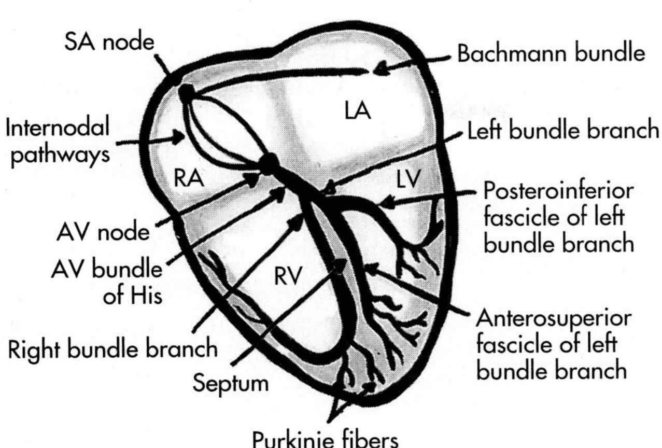


*Figure 30-3* Cardiac conduction. (Modified from Andreoli KG et al: *Comprehensive cardiac care: a text for nurses, physicians, and other health practitioners,* St Louis, 1983, Mosby.)

both atria to contract and then both ventricles. The SA node responds to vagal and sympathetic nervous system input.[3] Heart rate increases in response to exercise and anxiety and decreases in response to relaxation techniques, such as deep breathing and meditation.

Electrical impulses generated below the SA node cause the heart to contract abnormally. Some conduction irregularities can be life threatening. Impulses generated by the heart's conduction system can be studied by electrocardiography (ECG). ECG is used to assist in diagnosing cardiac disease.[3,13,17]

## PATHOLOGY OF CARDIAC DISEASE

### Ischemic Heart Disease

Coronary artery disease (CAD) develops over a period of many years. The internal wall of an artery can become injured by years of cigarette smoking or high blood pressure. Once the wall is damaged, it becomes irregular in shape and prone to collecting plaque (fatty deposits, like cholesterol). Platelets also gather along the arterial wall and clog the artery (which is called a *lesion*). The artery narrows and allows less blood to pass through it. This disease process is called *atherosclerosis.*

If a coronary artery is partially or completely blocked, the heart may not get enough oxygen (a condition called **ischemia**). Persons with CAD may be free of symptoms at rest but develop angina, a type of chest pain, while eating or during exercise, exertion, or exposure to cold. Angina varies from individual to individual. Rest, medication, or both may relieve angina, usually without permanent heart damage. However, angina is a warning sign and should not be ignored.

Chest pain that is not relieved by rest or medication is indicative of a **myocardial infarction (MI),** or heart attack. The patient should be evaluated promptly by a physician. During an MI, part of the heart muscle dies. If a substantial section of the heart is damaged, the heart will stop (cardiac arrest) and the person may die.

For about 6 weeks after an MI, tissue damage is easily extended if the heart works too hard. A delicate balance of rest and activity must be maintained for **cardiac rehabilitation** so that the heart can heal without the patient becoming deconditioned.

In about 6 weeks, scar tissue forms and the risk of extending the MI decreases. Scar tissue does not contract with each heart beat, so the heart will not pump as well. Graded exercise can strengthen the healthy part of the myocardium and improve cardiac output.

**Congestive heart failure (CHF)** results when the heart is unable to pump effectively and fluid backs up into the lungs or the body. Fluid overload is serious because it puts a greater workload on the heart. Straining causes further congestion. Usually, CHF can be controlled with diet, medications, and rest. Patients who experience difficulty resuming their former level of activity after acute CHF may limit their own recovery. Persons with acute CHF can attain optimal function through graded activity.

### Valvular Disease

Heart valves may become damaged with disease or infection. Two complications result from valvular disease: volume overload and pressure overload.

Volume overload results when fluid accumulates in the lungs and causes shortness of breath. Volume overload increases the potential for irregular and ineffective contractions in both atria (atrial fibrillation). Consequently, blood flow through the heart slows, and blood clots (emboli) may develop in the ventricles. Many cerebrovascular accidents are caused by emboli ejected from the heart into the circulatory system of the brain.

If the aortic valve fails to close properly (aortic insufficiency), CHF or ischemia may result. In another disorder of the aortic valve, aortic stenosis (calcification) pressure overload occurs. The left ventricle, which is working harder to open the sticky valve, enlarges and cardiac output decreases. Ventricular arrhythmia, cerebral insufficiency, confusion, syncope (fainting), and sudden death may result. Surgery to correct valve problems may be recommended.

### Cardiac Risk Factors

The Framingham study[8] identified many factors that put people at risk for developing atherosclerosis. **Cardiac risk factors** fall into three major categories: (1) unchangeable factors—heredity, male gender, and age; (2) changeable factors—cholesterol levels, cigarette smoking, high blood pressure, and an inactive lifestyle; and (3) contributing factors—diabetes, stress, and obesity. The more risk factors people have, the greater their risk of developing CAD.

The team should support patients' attempts to reduce risk factors. Prevention of cardiac disease is ultimately in the hands of the individual. Health care professionals, aware of the changes that persons with heart disease must make to reduce risk factors, can facilitate these changes via education, dialogue, and affirmation of the individual's responsibility.

### Medical Management

Persons who experience a heart attack are initially managed in a coronary care unit where they are closely observed for complications. Ninety percent of all persons who have had an MI will develop arrhythmia.[5] Close medical management is imperative.

Various surgical options can correct circulatory problems associated with CAD. Balloon angioplasty (pericutaneous transluminal coronary angioplasty—PTCA) and coronary artery bypass grafts (CABGs) are most common. In a PTCA, a balloon catheter is guided through the circulatory system into the coronary arteries. The site of the lesion is pinpointed and the balloon inflated, pushing plaque against the arterial wall. When the balloon is deflated, improved circulation to the myocardium usually results.

In a CABG, the surgeon opens the patient's chest by sawing through the sternum and spreading the ribs to expose the heart. Diseased sections of the coronary arteries are bypassed with healthy blood vessels from the saphenous veins or the internal mammary arteries. Improved coronary circulation results.

When the heart's pumping ability is severely reduced, a heart or heart lung transplantation may be performed. If successful, the patient may be rehabilitated to a level of function that is significantly higher than in the months before surgery.

### Cardiac Medications

Knowledge of the purpose and side effects of cardiac medication provides a framework for understanding the patient's response to activity. Table 30-1 lists common cardiac medications. Cardiac medications are frequently adjusted until an optimal therapeutic response has been attained. Adverse signs and symptoms should be reported to the physician or nurse promptly. In most settings, the nurse is responsible for contacting the physician.

### Psychosocial Considerations

Persons who have experienced an MI pass through a number of phases of adjustment to disability. Fear and anxiety present initially as patients confront their mortality. Education and supportive communication will do much to reduce anxiety.[12]

As patients begin to resume more normal activities, feelings of helplessness may begin to subside. Patients feel more secure when familiar coping mechanisms

*Table 30-1*

**Common Cardiac Medications**

| *Category* | *Common names* | *Purpose/uses* | *Side effects* |
|---|---|---|---|
| Diuretics | Furosemide (Lasix)<br>Dyazide and hydrochlorothiazide (HCTZ) | Lowers BP, decreases edema | Orthostatic hypotension, muscle spasms, dehydration |
| Vasodilators | Hydralazine<br>Captopril | Lowers BP, controls CHF | Palpitations, tachycardia, orthostatic hypotension |
| Cardiac glycosides | Digoxin<br>Lanoxin | Lowers heart rate, controls ventricular heart rate | Anorexia, nausea, arrhythmia, heart block |
| Anticoagulants | Coumadin<br>Heparin<br>Aspirin<br>Persantine | Prevents blood clots | Hemorrhage, nausea/vomiting, abdominal cramps |
| Antiarrhythmic | Procainamide<br>Quinidine<br>Propanolol (Inderal)<br>Lidocaine | Controls heart rhythm | Can aggravate ventricular arrhythmias, bradycardia |
| β-blockers | Atenolol (Tenormin)<br>Propanolol (Inderal) | Manages angina, hypertension, arrhythmia | Worsening of peripheral vascular disease, dyspnea, CHF |
| Calcium channel blockers | Verapamil<br>Diltiazem<br>Nifedipine | Manages angina, coronary artery spasms, arrhythmia | Orthostatic hypotension, bradycardia |
| Nitrates | Nitroglycerin (NTG) sublingual<br>Nitropaste<br>Isordil | Manages angina and CHF | Orthostatic hypotension, headache |

allow them to respond to the stress; but some former coping mechanisms (smoking, drinking, or consuming fatty foods) are harmful. These patients must learn new strategies.

Denial is common in patients with cardiac disease. Persons in denial must be closely monitored during the acute phase of recovery as they may not believe precautions are necessary and could further damage their cardiovascular system by not complying with them.

Depression is not uncommon in the third to sixth day after an MI and can last many months.[4] Forced inactivity during the recovery phase can frustrate a person who previously used exercising to exhaustion as a way to deal with stress. Including the patient's family in the education will correct misconceptions and decrease anxieties.

## CARDIAC REHABILITATION

Acute, inpatient rehabilitation consists of monitored ADLs and instruction in cardiac and postsurgical precautions, energy conservation, graded activity, and risk factor management. The patient is also instructed in guidelines for discharge activities. The ill effects of prolonged inactivity can be averted by means of monitored activity, while medical problems, poor responses to medications, and atypical chest pain can be rooted out. Cardiac rehabilitation may continue in the home, community, or outpatient setting.

Prompt, accurate identification of the signs and symptoms of cardiac distress and modification of treatment are imperative. If any **signs of cardiac distress** (Table 30-2) are observed during treatment, the proper response is to stop the activity, have the patient rest, seek emergency medical help if the symptoms do not resolve, report the symptoms to the team, and modify future activity to decrease the workload on the heart.

The Borg Rate of Perceived Exertion (RPE) scale measures perception of workload. Patients are shown the scale (which ranges from 6 to 20) and instructed that a rating of 6 means no exertion at all and a 19 equals the most strenuous activity they have ever performed. After the activity, they are asked to appraise their feelings of exertion and rate the task.

### Tools for Measuring the Patient's Response to Activity

Heart rate, blood pressure, rate pressure product, and ECG readings are other measures for evaluating the cardiovascular system's response to work.

#### *Heart Rate*

**Heart rate** (beats per minute) can be monitored by palpating the radial, brachial, or carotid pulse. The radial pulse is located on the volar surface of the wrist, just lateral to the radial head. The brachial pulse is slightly medial to the antecubital fossa. The carotid pulse, located lateral to the Adam's apple, should be palpated gently because overstimulation can cause the heart rate to fall. The COTA must establish service competency in palpating the carotid pulse.

Heart rates can be regular (even) or irregular. Although an irregular heart rate is not normal, many persons function quite well with one. To determine the heart rate, apply the second and third fingers flat (not

*Table 30-2*

**Signs and Symptoms of Cardiac Distress**

| *Sign/symptom* | *What to look for* |
|---|---|
| Angina | Chest pain may be squeezing, tight, aching, burning, and choking in nature. Pain is generally substernal and may radiate to the arms, jaw, neck, or back. More intense or long-lasting pain forewarns of greater ischemia. |
| Dyspnea | Patient will have shortness of breath with activity or at rest. If the resting respiratory rate is >30 breaths per minute, seek emergency medical help. |
| Orthopnea | Dyspnea will result by lying supine. The severity is graded by the number of pillows the patient sleeps on to breathe comfortably. |
| Nausea/emesis | Patient will feel sick to the stomach or be vomiting. |
| Diaphoresis | Patient will experience cold, clammy sweat. |
| Fatigue | Patient will have a generalized feeling of exhaustion. |
| Cerebral signs | Patient will experience ataxia, dizziness, confusion, and fainting (syncope), which indicate that the brain needs more oxygen. |
| Orthostatic hypotension | The systolic blood pressure will fall more than 10 mm Hg with change of position (i.e., sit to stand). |

tips) to the pulse site. If the pulse is even (regular) count the beats for 10 seconds and multiply the finding by 6. When the heart rate is irregular, the number of beats should be counted for a full minute.

A sudden change in heart rate from regular to irregular should be reported to the physician. In addition, patients can be taught to take their own pulse and monitor their heart rate's response to activity. As a general rule of thumb, the heart rate should rise in response to activity.

#### *Blood Pressure*

**Blood pressure** is the pressure that the blood exerts against the artery walls as the heart beats. A stethoscope and blood pressure cuff (sphygmomanometer) are used to determine blood pressure indirectly. Place the cuff snugly around the patient's upper arm just above the elbow, centering the bladder of the cuff above the brachial artery. Inflate the cuff while palpating the brachial artery to 20 mm Hg above the point at which a pulse is last felt. With the ear pieces of the stethoscope angled forward in your ears, place the dome of the stethoscope over the patient's brachial artery. Support the patient's arm in extension with the brachial artery and the stethoscope gauge at the patient's heart level. Deflate the cuff at a rate of approximately 2 mm Hg per second. Listen carefully. The first two sounds heard correspond to the systolic blood pressure. Listen until the pulse fades (diastolic blood pressure). This procedure should be practiced under immediate supervision until competency is established.

#### *Rate Pressure Product*

Heart rate and blood pressure will fluctuate in response to activity. Cardiac output is affected by both. **Rate pressure product (RPP)** measurement gives a more accurate indication of how well the heart is pumping. RPP is the product of heart rate and systolic blood pressure (RPP = HR × SBP). It is usually a five-digit number but is reported in three digits by dropping the last two digits (for example HR 100 × SBP 120 = 12000 = RPP 120). During any activity RPP should rise at peak and return to baseline in recovery.

It takes hours of learning and practice to become proficient in EKG reading and interpretation. See Dubin's *Rapid Interpretation of EKG*[9] as a resource on the subject.

There are many similarities in the evaluation and treatment of persons with cardiac disease and those with pulmonary dysfunction. A review of the pulmonary system and chronic obstructive pulmonary disease follows.

## THE ANATOMY AND PHYSIOLOGY OF RESPIRATION

While the heart provides oxygen-rich blood to the body and transports carbon dioxide and other waste products to the lungs, the respiratory system exchanges oxygen for carbon dioxide. The cardiac and pulmonary system are interdependent. If no oxygen were delivered to the blood stream, the heart would soon stop functioning for lack of oxygen; conversely, if the heart were to stop pumping, the lungs would cease functioning for lack of a blood supply.

The respiratory system supplies oxygen to the blood and removes waste products, primarily carbon dioxide, from the blood. Air enters the body through the nose and mouth and travels through the larynx to the pharynx or voice box. From there it continues downward into the lungs by way of the trachea or windpipe. If the trachea or pharynx becomes blocked, a small incision may be made into the trachea to allow air to freely pass into the lungs. This procedure is called a *tracheotomy.*

Two main bronchi branch off from the trachea, carrying air into the left and right lungs. The bronchi continue to branch off into smaller tubes called *bronchioles.* Bronchioles segment into smaller passages called the *alveolar ducts.* Each alveolar duct divides and leads into three or more alveolar sacs. The entire respiratory passageway from bronchi to alveolar ducts is often referred to as the *pulmonary tree.*

Each alveolar sac contains more than 10 alveoli. A very fine, semipermeable membrane separates the alveolus from the capillary network. Across this membrane, oxygen is transported and exchanged for carbon dioxide. Carbon dioxide is exhaled by traveling upward through the pulmonary tree.

The muscle power for breathing air into the lungs, or inspiration, is primarily provided by the diaphragm. Originating from the sternum, ribs and lumbar vertebrae, and the lumbocostal arches, it forms the inferior border of the thorax. The muscle fibers of the diaphragm insert into a central tendon. Innervated by the left and right phrenic nerves, the diaphragm domes downward as it contracts, enlarging the volume of the thorax and causing a drop in pressure in the lungs. Air then enters the lungs, equalizing lung and outside air pressures. Accessory muscles, the intercostals and scalene, are also active during inspiration. They maintain the alignment of the ribs and help elevate the rib cage, respectively.

At rest, expiration is primarily a passive relaxation of the inspiratory musculature. Forced expiration requires active contraction of the abdominal muscles to compress the viscera and squeeze the diaphragm upward in the thorax. Expiration can be further forced by flexing the torso forward and pressing with the arms on the chest or abdomen. As the volume of the thorax decreases, air is forced out of the lungs. Figure 30-4 shows the structure of the respiratory system.[5,17]

### Innervation of the Respiratory System

Breathing is mostly involuntary. A person does not have to think to take a breath. The autonomic nervous system has control over breathing. With anxiety and

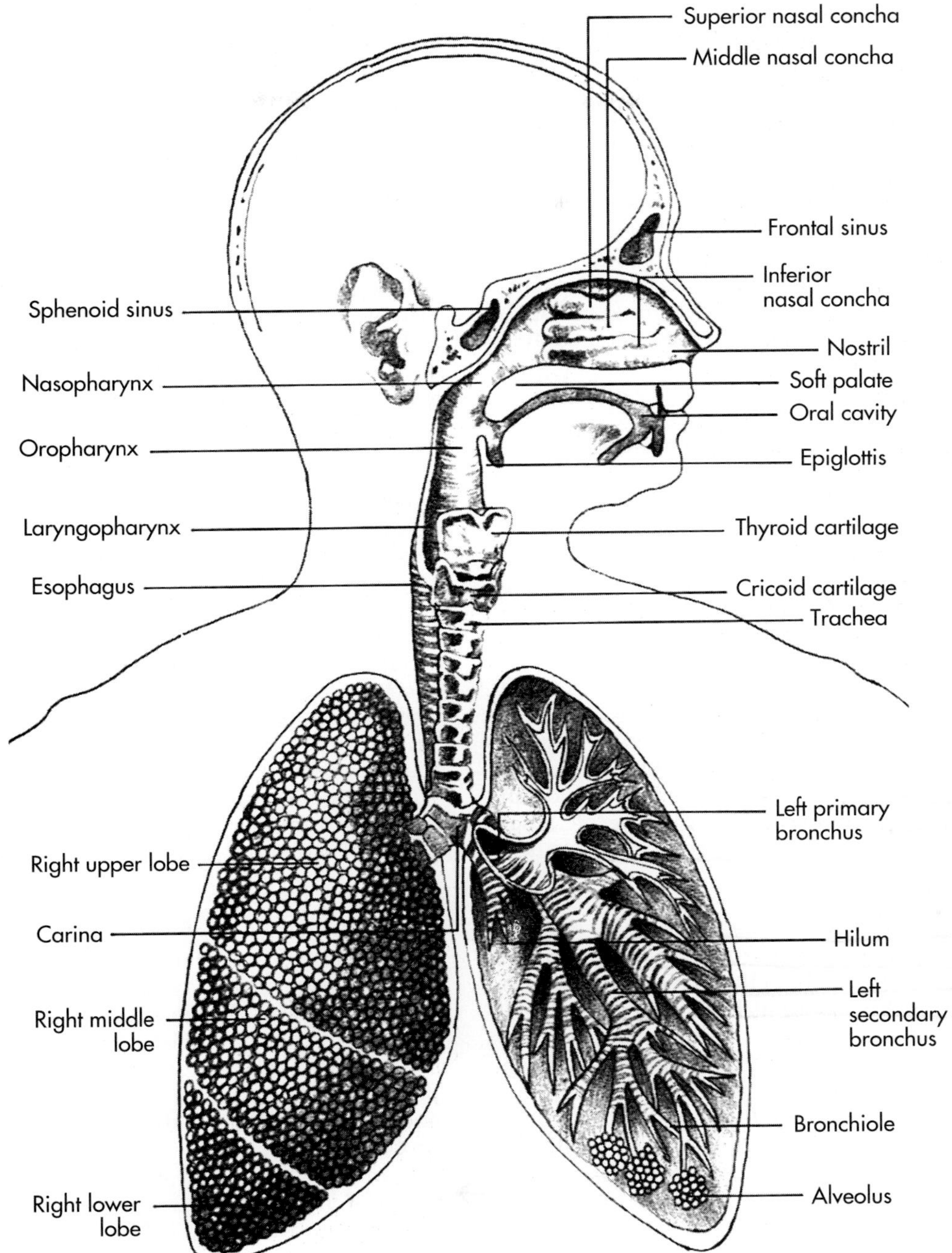


*Figure 30-4* Major structures of the respiratory system. (From *Respiratory support*, 1991, Springhouse.)

increased activity, the sympathetic nervous system will automatically increase the depth and rate of inspiration. Parts of the brain provide the central control for breathing; they adjust their response to input from receptors in the lungs, the aorta, and the carotid body.

Although the act of breathing is primarily involuntary, there is also a volitional component. This allows us to control the outflow of breath during activities requiring controlled breathing, such as swimming or playing the harmonica.[5,17]

## CHRONIC OBSTRUCTIVE PULMONARY DISEASE

Common chronic disorders of the lungs for which pulmonary rehabilitation is ordered include: **chronic obstructive pulmonary disease (COPD)** and asthma.[5] COPD is characterized by "damage to the alveolar wall and inflammation of the conducting airways"[2] and includes emphysema, peripheral airway disease, and chronic bronchitis. More than 15 million Americans have been diagnosed with COPD.

In COPD the onset of physical disability is typically gradual, with dyspnea on exertion representing the initial phases of disability and evolving to shortness of breath at rest.

Asthma is characterized by irritability of the bronchotracheal tree and is typically episodic in its onset. Individuals with asthma may be free of symptoms for periods of time between the episodes of wheezing and dyspnea.[11] There appears to be a genetic predisposition of some individuals to develop asthma. Allergic causes of asthma may include pollens and respiratory irritants such as perfume, dust, pollen, and cleaning agents. If left untreated a severe asthmatic episode may result in death.[2,5]

### Pulmonary Risk Factors

Cigarette smoking is the number one cause of COPD, and smoking cessation will slow the progression of disability in persons with COPD.[18] Because cigarette smoke is a pulmonary irritant, it may also be a causative agent in asthmatic episodes. Other environmental irritants such as air pollution and chemical exposure are contributory risk factors in the development of COPD and asthma.[2,5]

### Medical Management

COPD is a progressive, chronic disease process. The onset of the disease process is gradual. Medications prescribed for persons with pulmonary disease include antiinflammatory agents (steroids, cromolyn sodium etc.), bronchodilators (albuterol, theophylline etc.) that help to open the air ways, and expectorants (iodides, guaifenesin, etc.) that help loosen and clear mucus. Oxygen therapy, at a specific liter flow, may also be prescribed. Some persons on oxygen therapy may be tempted to increase the liter per minute flow, erroneously thinking that more is better. This can result in $CO_2$ retention and lead to right heart failure.

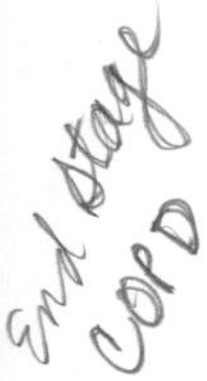


Persons with acute respiratory distress may initially be managed on a ventilator before being weaned to oxygen. Ventilators provide the mechanical assist to the process of inspiration and do not increase the number of healthy alveolar sacs. Ventilators will not slow down the end stage disease process of COPD.

When a patient's endurance decreases enough to impair ADL performance, the physician may refer the patient to occupational therapy.[2,5]

### Signs and Symptoms of Respiratory Distress

Dyspnea is the most obvious sign that an individual is having difficulty breathing. In its most severe form, the patient is short of breath at rest. Persons with this level of dyspnea will be unable to utter a short phrase without gasping for air. When reporting that a patient has dyspnea, note the precipitating factors (e.g., "Mr. S. becomes short of breath when washing his face while seated in front of the sink.")

Other signs that the body is not getting enough oxygen include extreme fatigue, a nonproductive cough, confusion, impaired judgment, and cyanosis (a blue tinge to the skin).[2,5]

### Psychosocial Considerations

COPD is a progressive and debilitating physical illness, and the psychosocial effects of the disease are considerable. Depression and anxiety are not uncommon; 96% of patients with COPD have reported disabling anxiety.[1] Others complain of faintness or difficulty concentrating.[10] Progressive muscle relaxation has been shown to be successful for controlling dyspnea and anxiety and for lowering heart rate.[20]

Most persons with end stage COPD realize that they will die of their disease. Individuals with $CO_2$ retention usually die peacefully in their sleep[14] rather than from suffocation.[2,5]

## PULMONARY REHABILITATION

The goal of **pulmonary rehabilitation** is to stabilize or reverse the disease process and return the patient's function to its highest capacity. A multidisciplinary rehabilitation team working with the patient can design an individualized treatment program to meet this end. An accurate diagnosis, medical management, therapy, education, and emotional support are components of a pulmonary rehabilitation program. Occupational therapy personnel are frequently part of the team that also includes the physician, the nurse, and the patient. Respiratory therapists, dietitians, physical therapists, social workers, and psychologists may also be team members. Their roles will vary slightly from facility to facility. Knowledge of specialized pulmonary treatment techniques is imperative when treating persons with pulmonary disease.

### Treatment Techniques

#### *Dyspnea Control Postures*

Breathlessness can be reduced in patients with COPD by adopting certain postures such as the **dyspnea control postures**. When sitting, the patient bends forward slightly at the waist while supporting the upper body by leaning the forearms on the table or thighs. When standing, leaning forward and propping the body on a counter or shopping cart may relieve the problem.

#### *Pursed-Lip Breathing*

**Pursed-lip breathing (PLB)** is thought to prevent tightness in the airway by providing resistance to expiration. This technique increases use of the diaphragm and decreases accessory muscle recruitment.[6] PLB is sometimes instinctively adapted by persons with COPD, whereas others may need to be instructed in the technique. Instructions for PLB are as follows: (1) Purse your lips as if you are going to whistle. (2) Slowly exhale through pursed lips; you should feel some resistance. (3) Inhale deeply through your nose. (4) It should take you twice as long to exhale as it does to inhale.

#### *Diaphragmatic Breathing*

Another breathing pattern that calls for increased use of the diaphragm to improve chest volume is **dia-**

**phragmatic breathing.** Many persons learn this technique by placing a small paperback novel on the abdomen just below the thorax. The patient lies supine and is instructed to inhale slowly and make the book rise. Exhalation through pursed lips should cause the book to fall.

#### *Relaxation*

Progressive muscle relaxation in conjunction with breathing exercises can be effective in decreasing anxiety and in controlling shortness of breath. One technique involves tensing muscle groups while slowly inhaling, followed by relaxation of the muscle groups when exhaling twice as slowly through pursed lips. It is helpful to teach the patient a sequence of muscle groups to tense and relax. One common sequence involves tensing and relaxing the face; followed by the face and the neck; next the face, neck, and shoulders and so on down the body to the toes. A calm, quiet, and comfortable environment is important for learning.

#### *Other Treatments and Considerations*

Physical therapists may teach chest expansion exercises, a series of exercises intended to increase the flexibility of the chest. Percussion, postural drainage, and vibration are other techniques used to loosen secretions and assist with draining them from the lungs. These techniques are usually taught by other team members.

Humidity, pollution, extremes of temperature, and lack of air movement have been reported to have a deleterious effect on persons with respiratory ailments. These factors should be taken into consideration when planning activities.

## OCCUPATIONAL THERAPY EVALUATION AND TREATMENT OF PERSONS WITH CARDIOPULMONARY DYSFUNCTION

Occupational therapy intervention can promote improvements in performance of ADL for persons with limitations caused by chronic respiratory or cardiovascular limitations.

### Evaluation

#### *Review of the Medical Record*

A review of the medical record will identify the patient's medical history (diagnosis, severity, associated conditions, and secondary diagnoses), social history, test results, and precautions. Although the COTA may not perform the initial evaluation of the patient, being familiar with changes in the patient's condition as documented in the medical record should be standard practice.

#### *Patient Interview*

It is common courtesy and good medical practice to begin every patient encounter with an introduction and an explanation of the purpose of treatment. Good interview skills include asking the right questions, listening to the patient's response, and observing patients as they respond. Look for signs of anxiety, shortness of breath, confusion, difficulty comprehending, fatigue, posture, endurance, ability to move, and family dynamics. Interview questions should not only seek clarification of information that was not clear in the medical record, but should also clarify the patient's understanding of their condition and treatment.

Patients with a history of angina should be asked to describe their angina. If they have also had an MI, they should be asked if they can differentiate between their angina and their MI chest pain. Clarification of symptoms before treatment can prove invaluable should symptoms arise.

Asking patients to describe a typical day, identify activities that bring on shortness of breath or angina, and tell how their physical limitations interfere with the things they enjoy doing most in life will reveal problems that are relevant to the patient.

#### *Clinical Assessment*

The purpose of the clinical assessment is to establish the patient's present functional ability and limitations. The content of a registered occupational therapist's (OTR) clinical assessment will vary from patient to patient and setting to setting. Persons with impairments of the cardiovascular system will be monitored for heart rate, blood pressure, and signs and symptoms of cardiac distress during an evaluation of tolerance to postural changes, and a functional task. Table 30-3 summarizes appropriate and inappropriate **cardiovascular responses to activity.** Individuals with disorders of the respiratory system must be monitored for signs and symptoms of respiratory distress. Range of motion, strength, and sensation may be grossly assessed within the context of the ADL evaluation. The patient's cognitive and psychosocial status will become apparent to the skilled clinician through interview and observation.

On completion of the evaluation, the occupational therapist has sufficient information to formulate a treatment plan. By consulting the patient about the treatment plan, the clinician informs the patient of the expected outcome of treatment and verifies that goals will be meaningful and relevant to the patient.

### Treatment

Progression of treatment for persons with cardiovascular impairment or respiratory impairment is guided by present clinical status, recent functional history, response to current activity, and prognosis. Persons with significant cardiac or pulmonary impairment, limited recent functional ability, inappropriate responses to activity or orthostats (changes in position, e.g., sit to stand) and a poor prognosis will progress very slowly when compared with individuals with little impairment of the heart or lungs, a recent history of normal functional ability, appropriate responses to orthostats and activity, and a good prognosis. The COTA should keep these factors in mind when treating persons with cardiopulmonary deficits.

*Table 30-3*

### Cardiovascular Responses to Activity

| *Category* | *Appropriate* | *Inappropriate* |
|---|---|---|
| Heart rate | Increases with activity to no more than 20 beats above resting rate | Rises >20 beats above resting rate with activity, resting heart rate >120, drop in pulse or failure of pulse to rise with activity |
| Blood pressure | Rises (systolic) with activity | Systolic blood pressure >220 mm Hg, diastolic blood pressure >110 mm Hg, orthostatic hypotension (>10-20 mm Hg drop in systolic blood pressure), any decrease in systolic blood pressure with activity |
| Signs and symptoms | Absence of adverse symptoms | Excessive shortness of breath, angina, excessive sweating, nausea/vomiting, extreme fatigue, RPE >15, cerebral symptoms |

*Table 30-4*

### MET Table of Self-Care and Homemaking Tasks

| *MET level* | *Self-care* | *MET level* | *Ambulation and household tasks* |
|---|---|---|---|
| 1.2 | Eating, seated[16] | 1.2 | Hand sewing[7] |
| 1.6 | Transferring from bed to chair[15] | 1.5 | Machine sewing or sweeping floors[7] |
| 2 | Washing face and hands, brushing hair[16] | 2.5 | Dusting[16] |
| 2 | Seated sponge bath[21] | 2.5 | Kneading dough[7] |
| 2.5 | Standing sponge bath[21] | 2.5 | Hand washing, small items[7] |
| 2.5 | Dressing/undressing[15] | 2.6 | Vacuuming (electric)[16] |
| 3 | Seated warm shower[21] | 3 | Preparing a meal[15] |
| 3.5 | Standing warm shower[15] | 3.5 | Climbing stairs (24 feet/min)[7] |
| 3.6 | Bowel movement on toilet[7] | 3.9 | Making a bed[15] |
| 4.2 | Hot shower[15] | 4.4 | Changing bed linens[16] |
| 4.7 | Bowel movement (bedpan)[15] | 5 | Walking up stairs (30 feet/min)[21] |
| 5 | Sexual intercourse[21] | | |

Energy costs of an activity and the factors that influence them can further guide the COTA in the safe progression of activity. Oxygen consumption suggests how hard the heart and lungs are working, providing an indication of the amount of energy required to complete a task. Resting quietly in bed requires the least amount of oxygen per kilogram of body weight, 1 **basal metabolic equivalent (MET),** roughly 3.5 ml $O_2$ per kilogram of body weight. As activity increases more oxygen is required to meet the demands of the task. For instance, dressing requires 2 METs or roughly twice the amount of energy that lying in bed takes. Guided by a MET table (Table 30-4) and the patient's response to activity, prognosis, and goals, the COTA will be able to determine a logical treatment progression. As a general rule, once patients tolerate an activity (i.e., seated sponge bathing) with appropriate responses, they can progress to the next higher MET level activity (i.e., standing sponge bath).

The duration of any physical activity must also be taken into account when determining activity guidelines. Obviously, persons who have difficulty performing a 2 MET activity must still use a commode (3.5 METs) or bedpan (5 METs) for their bowel management. A person can perform at a higher than usual MET level for brief periods without adverse effects.

Sexual activity at 5 METs is frequently a grave concern to persons with impaired cardiovascular function and their partners. Sexual intercourse is intermittent in its peak demands for energy. Patients are frequently able to return to sexual intercourse once they can climb up and down two flights of steps in 1 minute with appropriate cardiovascular responses.[22] Providing the patient with information as to when it is safe to resume sexual activity can reduce anxiety surrounding the resumption of sexual intercourse. Discussing sexual activity guidelines with the patient and partner may further decrease anxiety. The patient should be instructed to monitor heart rate and symptoms of cardiac distress before and after intercourse. In addition, the patient and partner should be informed that cardiac medications can effect the patient's libido. The patient should be encouraged to inform the physician of problems related to sexual activity. Medications can frequently be adjusted to alleviate these problems.

### Energy Conservation

When patients learn to conserve their energy resources, they can perform at a higher functional level without expending more energy. The principles of **energy conservation** and work simplification are based on knowledge of how specific factors increase the body's workload. Ogden[19] has identified the following six variables that increase oxygen demand: increased work rate or activity pace, increased resistance, increased use of large muscles, increased involvement of trunk musculature, raising the arms, and isometric work (straining). Arm activity has also been shown to require a greater cardiovascular output than lower extremity activity, and standing activity requires more energy than seated activity. Extremes of temperature, high humidity, and pollution make the heart work harder. By applying this information, a skilled COTA can make suggestions for modifying activity that will decrease the amount of energy required for the task.

Energy conservation should be personalized for each patient. Time management involves preplanning activities so that tasks with high energy expenditure are intermingled with lighter tasks, and rest breaks are plotted throughout the day, especially after meals. Patient involvement in planning the day grounds the program toward realistic goal attainment.

Written material may augment energy conservation instruction. However, until the patient has successfully applied energy conservation principles to activity, expect little follow-through with recommendations. Practice and practical application of skills are critical to changing behavior.

Exhaling with exertion is another breathing principle for persons with cardiac or pulmonary compromise. This technique is more energy efficient and helps control the rate of increase of systolic blood pressure with activity. It is important for the patient to practice these skills during treatment. Therapeutic support is critical in learning.

### Patient and Family Education

Occupational therapy personnel, as members of the health care team, share the responsibility for patient and family education. Cardiac or pulmonary anatomy, disease process, symptom management, risk factors, diet, exercise, and energy conservation must be taught and reinforced to patient and family members by the team. Including family members in an education program provides support indirectly to the patient through the family unit. Such support is critical when a patient is dependent on the help of a family member to accomplish everyday tasks.

## SUMMARY

Healthy individuals are able to meet the varying demands of their bodies for oxygen because their heart and respiratory rates adjust to meet oxygen demand. When the cardiovascular or pulmonary system is compromised, the ability to perform normal activity declines. This chapter is designed to guide the COTA in the treatment of persons with impairments of the heart or lungs.

## Sample Treatment Plan

**Case study (cardiovascular disease)**

An occupational therapist has evaluated Mr. F., a 48-year-old auto mechanic who experienced 10/10 substernal chest pain, nausea, and shortness of breath while working under an automobile 1 week ago. He was diagnosed with an acute anteriolateral MI complicated by subsequent CHF.

He is married and the father of three children, ages 9, 5, and 4. His wife works full-time and was unable to manage his care at home, so he was placed temporarily in a skilled nursing facility. He was referred to occupational therapy for ADL evaluation and progression of activity.

**Treatment approach**

Rehabilitative

**Evaluation summary**

*Medical history:* Unremarkable. *Risk factors:* Age, sex, family history, and a sedentary lifestyle. *Current clinical status:* Normal sinus rhythm, enlarged left ventricle, and diffuse coronary artery disease. He performed a 2 MET seated sponge bath with minimal assistance. Vital signs were appropriate during the evaluation, except systolic blood pressure fell 20 mm Hg in recovery (3 minutes after completion of bathing), and patient became symptomatic (nausea and shortness of breath). Symptoms and vital signs stabilized after 5 minutes of rest.

Mr. F. is anxious. He eats his meals in bed. He transfers independently and per physical therapy can safely walk to the bathroom. He expressed concern that he will die "before I'm 50, just like Dad." Before his MI, Mr. F. enjoyed playing catch with the kids and occasional walks with his wife. He describes himself as a weekend warrior.

**Problem list**

1. Decreased functional capacity and endurance for self-care
2. Lack of ability to pace activity and monitor own signs and symptoms
3. Potential for alteration in sexual function
4. Positive risk factor of sedentary lifestyle
5. Anxiety amplified by family history of cardiac death

**Problem 1**

Decreased functional capacity for self-care

***Objective***

Mr. F. will shower standing (3.5 METs) and tolerate being out of bed for most of the day.

***Method***

Daily practice and instruction in graded self-care activity with monitoring of heart rate, blood pressure, and sign and symptoms. Mr. F. will receive instruction in energy conservation with emphasis on slowing the pace of the activity

***Gradation***

Progressive activity to standing shower: Mr. F. will take all meals out of bed. Self-care tasks will be graded by MET level, initially repeating 2 MET level seated sponge bath (awaiting an appropriate response) and progressing through standing sponge bathing to standing shower. Emphasis will be placed on decreasing pace (rate) of work performed.

**Problem 2**

Lack of ability to pace activity and monitor own signs and symptoms.

***Objective***

Mr. F. will independently pace activity and respond appropriately to symptoms of cardiac distress.

***Method***

Instruction and dialogue regarding symptoms of cardiac distress and purpose of pace activity: COTA will review symptoms of cardiac distress with Mr. F. and instruct him to stop and rest if he experiences any symptoms. Should he fail to stop when he experiences symptoms during treatment, activity will be interrupted. Mr. F. will be asked if he can identify why treatment was stopped. COTA will guide Mr. F. to perform activity more slowly. He will be asked to contrast his symptoms at the slower pace with his symptoms when he rushes.

## Sample Treatment Plan

**Case study (COPD)**

Mrs. P. is a 64-year-old woman with a 3 year history of COPD. She was released from the acute hospital 3 days ago, having been stabilized after an acute exacerbation of COPD. She is widowed and lives alone in a small one-bedroom apartment. She has one daughter who is married, works full-time, and has one child. Mrs. P. was referred to occupational therapy for pulmonary rehabilitation. An occupational therapist evaluated her and established a treatment plan for the COTA to follow.

**Evaluation summary**

Mrs. P. has been smoking cigarettes since age 20 and currently smokes one pack per day. She has had three prior exacerbations of COPD. She states that she is unable to quit smoking because all of her friends smoke. Her apartment is on the first floor and is across the street from a grocery store. There is a first floor laundry room in her building. Mrs. P.'s daughter lives three blocks away and checks on her daily. She empties the bedside commode and provides groceries and dinner. Mrs. P. wants to empty the commode herself. The home health aide provides total assistance with a bed bath. Mrs. P. experiences dyspnea on exertion and is unable to apply breathing techniques to activity. She gets herself a light breakfast and snack with a complaint of severe dyspnea on exertion. Mrs. P. does not use her prescribed oxygen during activity because it is too heavy to carry around. According to physical therapy, she was a limited community ambulator before her recent hospitalization.

**Assets**

1. Potential for improved endurance and function in ADL
2. Good living situation
3. Adequate family support

**Problem list**

1. Inability to empty bedside commode
2. Inability to coordinate breathing techniques with self-care
3. Decreased endurance for self-care
4. Positive risk factors of smoking

**Problem 1**

Inability to empty bedside commode

*Objective*

Mrs. P. will be able to independently empty the commode.

*Method*

Graded practice in emptying the bedside commode

*Gradation*

Instruction in removing a clean, empty commode bucket from the commode: Have Mrs. P. practice cleaning commode bucket. Help Mrs. P. identify logical rest breaks during task (e.g., removing bucket from commode, placing it on floor, and resting seated on commode; carrying commode bucket to bathroom and resting seated on toilet). Mrs. P. empties and cleans commode independently with a decreasing number of rest breaks needed as endurance improves.

**Problem 2**

Inability to coordinate breathing with self-care

*Objective*

To spontaneously use breathing techniques during self-care

*Method*

Demonstration, return demonstration, verbal cueing, and discussion; 50-foot $O_2$ line

*Gradation*

Review and practice of breathing techniques: COTA will first review appropriate breathing techniques without activity. Mrs. P. will practice breathing techniques initially during low MET activity (e.g., brushing hair), with emphasis on exhaling on exertion, and gradually progressing to using PLB during dressing, bathing, and meal preparation. Patient will be verbally cued to use dyspnea control positions as need arises. Verbal cues will be decreased as patient's responses become more spontaneous.

## Selected Reading Guide Questions

1. Describe the heart's size and explain the function of its right and left sides.
2. What do the heart valves control?
3. Explain the significance of the coronary arteries in heart disease and heart attacks.
4. Identify the symptoms of cardiac distress. Explain why it is important to modify activity in response to them.
5. Explain the significance of left ventricular dysfunction.
6. Using the MET chart, determine what would be a safe self-care task to perform on a person who can function at 2.5 METs.
7. If the patient was able to perform a seated sponge bath but was unable to stand because of a secondary disability, which activity would you choose to help them progress in rehabilitation and why?
8. Describe the appropriate therapeutic response when a patient develops chest pain during activity.
9. What is COPD?
10. Name the breathing techniques used in pulmonary rehabilitation and their purposes.
11. Describe dyspnea control postures.
12. List at least three energy conservation principles.
13. Using the cardiac medications chart, explain how cardiac medications might affect heart rate or blood pressure.
14. What are some cerebral signs and why are they significant?

## Exercises

1. Demonstrate dyspnea control postures in sitting and standing.
2. Teach your partner pursed-lip and diaphragmatic breathing.
3. Choose a cooking task. Explain how to modify the activity by using three energy conservation principles.
4. Determine your partner's heart rate and respiratory rate.
5. Have your partner run in place for 3 minutes. Immediately take your partner's blood pressure and heart rate. Calculate the rate pressure product for before and immediately after activity. Was your partner's response appropriate?
6. Pretend that your partner is Mr. F. from the Sample Treatment Plan and that he has questions about when it will be safe for him and his wife to resume sexual activity. How will you respond?
7. Pretend your partner is Mrs. P. from the Sample Treatment Plan and she has a resting respiratory rate of 33. While panting, she tells you to "Leave" (pant) "me" (pant) "alone" (pant). Demonstrate an appropriate response.

## REFERENCES


1. Agle DP, Baum GL: Psychological aspects of chronic obstructive pulmonary disease, *Med Clin North Am* 1977; 61:749.
2. American Thoracic Society: Definitions and classifications of chronic bronchitis, asthma, and pulmonary emphysema, *Am Rev Respir Dis* 85:762-68, 1962.
3. Andreoli KG, et al: *Comprehensive cardiac care: a text for nurses, physicians and other health practitioners,* St Louis, 1983, Mosby.

3a. Borg et al: *Med Sci Sports Exerc* 14:376, 1982.

4. Bragg TL: Psychological response to myocardial infarction, *Nurs Forum* 14(4):383-395, 1975.
5. Brannon FJ et al: *Cardiopulmonary rehabilitation: basic theory and application,* ed 2, Philadelphia, 1992, FA Davis Company.
6. Breslin EH: The pattern of respiratory muscle recruitment during pursed-lip breathing, *Chest* 101(1):75-8, 1992.
7. Colorado Heart Association: *Exercise equivalent 1970 cardiac reconditioning & work evaluation unit,* Spaulding Rehabilitation Center.
8. Dawber R: *The Framingham study: the epidemiology of atherosclerotic disease,* Cambridge, Mass, 1980, Harvard University Press.
9. Dubin D: *Rapid Interpretation of EKGs,* ed 4, Tampa, Fla, 1989.
10. Dudley DL et al: Psychosocial concomittants to rehabilitation in chronic obstructive pulmonary disease—part 2: psychosocial treatment, *Chest* 77:544, 1980.
11. Farzan S: *A concise handbook of respiratory diseases,* ed 2, Teston, Va, 1985, Reston.
12. Gentry WE, Haney T: Emotional and behavioral reaction to acute myocardial infarction, *Heart Lung* 4:738, 1975.
13. Goldberger E: *Essentials of clinical cardiology,* Philadelphia, 1990, JB Lippincott.
14. Hodgkin JE et al: *Pulmonary rehabilitation guidelines to success,* ed 2, Philadelphia, 1993, JB Lippincott.
15. Kottke FJ: *Common cardiovascular problems in rehabilitation.* In Krusen FH, Kottke FJ, Elwood PM, editors: *Handbook of physical medicine and rehabilitation,* Philadelphia, 1971, WB Saunders.
16. Maloney FP, Moss K: *Energy requirements for selected activities,* Unpublished manuscript, 1974.
17. Mythos for SoftKey: *BodyWorks 4.0: human anatomy leaps to life,* Cambridge, Mass, 1993-95, SoftKey International.
18. Nemeny B, et al: Changes in lung function after smoking cessation: an assessment from a cross sectional survey, *Am Rev Respir Dis* 125:122-124, 1982.
19. Ogden LD: *Guidelines for analysis and testing of activities of daily living with cardiac patients,* Downey, Calif, 1981, Cardiac Rehabilitation Resources.
20. Renfroe KL: Effect of progressive relaxation on dyspnea and state anxiety in patients with chronic obstructive pulmonary disease, *Heart Lung* 17:408, 1988.
21. Santa Clara Valley Medical Center: *Graded activity sheets,* San Jose, Calif, 1994.
22. Scalzi C, Burke L: *Myocardial infarction: behavioral responses of patient and spouses.* In Underhill SL et al, editors: *Cardiac nursing,* Philadelphia, 1982, JB Lippincott.

Chapter 31

# Oncology

*Ann Burkhardt*

## Chapter Objectives

*After studying this chapter, student or practitioner will be able to:*

1. Describe cancer and its diagnosis and medical-surgical treatments.
2. Identify strategies for helping patients cope with side effects of chemotherapy and radiation.
3. Describe the role of occupational therapy in the treatment of cancer patients.
4. Identify techniques to be used in addressing a variety of occupational therapy goals with cancer patients.

## Key Terms

neoplasm
cancer
carcinoma
sarcoma
lymphoma
leukemia
paraneoplastic syndrome
chemotherapy
blood levels
radiation therapy
palliative care
mastectomy
radical neck dissection
stomas
colostomy
urostomy

Cancer is a broad category of conditions found when a tumor, or **neoplasm** (new abnormal growth of cells) is present in the body. A **cancer (carcinoma)** is an abnormal tissue that grows and spreads or that may metastasize (move and start in new sites) throughout the body. They may be "low grade," with a natural history of slow development and spread, or they may be "high grade," with a tendency to grow very quickly and spread rapidly. The cancer type is diagnosed by the tissue from which it first develops. For example, if a person has breast cancer that metastasizes to the lung, the biopsy of the lung lesion will contain breast cancer cells, not lung cancer cells. This condition would be labeled "breast cancer metastatic to the lung."

The type of cancer is further defined by the tissue in which it arises. For example, a carcinoma arises from epithelial tissue, a **sarcoma** arises from connective tissue, a **lymphoma** arises from the cellular components of lymph nodes, and **leukemia** arises from the blood-forming organs such as the bone marrow. Many cancers are solid tumors or masses in the tissue of origin. Cancers arising in the bone marrow are often characterized by abnormal blood cell counts, such as those associated with anemia. When cancers arise in endocrine tissues (glands), the cancer may produce a pseudohormone that mimics a hormone that normally present in the bloodstream. In these instances, the free-circulating hormone level will be abnormally elevated in the blood. Occasionally people will have neurological signs (e.g., seizures, cognitive changes) caused by the free circulation of the pseudohormones. This creates a **paraneoplastic syndrome,** a group of symptoms caused by the presence of the cancer cells in the bloodstream. Occasionally, the paraneoplastic syndrome is the first clinical sign of cancer and may be difficult to diagnose because there is no solid tumor present.

## MEDICAL BACKGROUND INFORMATION

A variety of x-rays and scans are used to assist in the diagnosis of cancer. A lung cancer, for instance, may initially be detected by chest x-ray. The x-ray is the initial screening test. It is crude and not clear in its definition but still sensitive enough to be used for cancer screening, and much less expensive than a computerized axial tomography (CAT or CT) scan or magnetic resonance imaging (MRI) procedure. Mammograms—x-rays of the breast tissue—are a form of x-rays used to detect breast tumors.

CAT or CT scans may be done with or without the use of contrast dye. Contrast dye is a radioactive dye that circulates in the blood stream and outlines all vascular (blood vessel) structures. Tumors have a higher rate of metabolism than normal tissues. To receive the nutrients tumors need to grow, they usually develop vascular networks that are highlighted by dye during this test. CT with contrast dye is a fairly good tool to diagnose the presence of a solid tumor.

MRIs are helpful in the diagnosis of soft tissue lesions. No radiation is used in an MRI. In contrast, this scan uses magnetic properties of biological tissues to form the basis of an image. Abnormal tissues respond to magnetic radio frequencies differently than do normal tissues and produce a different image in an MRI. The scan cannot differentiate, however, between blood clots, cancers, or demyelinating plaques (like those found in patients with multiple sclerosis). Gadolinium is a magnetically active material used with the MRI as a contrast dye. It enhances the image of the vascular system with magnetic properties of the dye. MRIs are particularly helpful in diagnosing spinal disorders.[16]

Bone scans are tomographic scans (serial x-rays that, when viewed in composite, produce a three-dimensional representation of the segment of the body scanned) of the skeletal system. Contrast dye is injected 2 hours before the scan is taken. Bone scans are helpful in diagnosing metastatic lesions to bone and some primary bone tumors. They are used to stage cancers that metastasize to bone, such as breast cancer and prostate cancer. They are also used for regular, routine follow-up for persons with an initial diagnosis of these cancers to check for recurrence of the cancer.

Biopsies are surgical procedures in which a section or segment of tumor is removed so that a pathologist may examine it to determine a diagnosis. There are a number of ways in which biopsies may be done (e.g., scrape, smear, or needle biopsy).

Regional lymph nodes may be suspected of involvement, either from a primary cancer such as lymphoma, or a sign of regional spread of disease, as in breast cancer. Lymph nodes are dissected at the time of a surgery to detect regional spread of the cancer and to stage the cancer. In the future, imaging with ultrasound may be used instead of biopsy of lymph nodes for staging a cancer.

### Staging the Disease

There are a few systems in use for staging cancers but most are based on the same underlying principles. At diagnosis, the cancer may be localized to one region. This is usually an early stage and may be classified as stage I disease. When there is spread of the cancer to an adjacent local region of the body, such as from the right breast to the right axilla, then stage II disease is present (a tumor and one metastasis). If the disease spreads to another organ, such as from the breast to the lung, then stage III disease is evident. When multiple systems/organs are involved, and the disease is widespread, stage IV is present.[9]

Another staging system commonly used is the tumor, metastasis, and node system (TMN). Tumor (T) represents the number of actual tumor sites, primary and metastatic. Metastasis (M) may be regional or widespread. Nodes (N) refers to the number of positive or involved lymph nodes that have cancer present in a surgical pathology sample.

Staging of the disease is helpful, along with other information concerning the specific cancer, in determining a treatment course and prognosis for the cancer.

### Treatment

After a diagnosis and staging of cancer, choices concerning treatment are made. Most tumors with a solid mass are treated by surgery. The mass may be resected and a margin of normal tissue taken from the surrounding area to remove the risk of local spread to normal tissues. When a tumor is encapsulated, tightly localized in its own capsule, sometimes a limited resection or lumpectomy is sufficient. If a tumor has invaded some of the local region or structures, a resection of the tumor and the involved structures as a whole mass may be done. If the surgery removes bone, sometimes reconstructive or joint replacement surgeries may be needed to improve cosmetic appearance or function. When a tumor is aggressive but interferes with a normal body function, a surgical bypass procedure may be performed to prolong function or alleviate pain. If a tumor has invaded surrounding tissues and structures and the neurovascular bundle (nerves and their blood supply), sometimes an amputation is the surgery of choice.

#### *Medical Oncology and Chemotherapy*

Tumors are composed of different types of tissue, so the same treatment will not work for all tumors. Some tumor cells are sensitive to chemotherapy agents.

**Chemotherapy** is a means of affecting change with chemicals. Most chemotherapeutic agents are toxic to normal tissues as well as cancer cells, so there are inevitable side effects. The chemotherapy drug can interfere with the tumor cells' genetic material, so the tumor cells stop dividing, multiplying, and surviving. The tumor cells often have a higher metabolic rate than normal cells, so they take up the chemicals and die first before the normal tissue shows signs of destruction.

Other chemotherapies work by bonding with the surface of the cancer cells and blocking their interaction with other cells. Because many cells rely on interactions with other cells to travel through membranes and become biologically active, this mechanical blocking mechanism stops their ability to act. Monoclonal antibodies, hormones, and some antitumor antibiotics act in this manner.[12]

Patients who accept the concept of chemotherapy will typically dread the side effects. The drugs are poisonous to normal tissues and can affect almost any body organ. For instance, many chemotherapies deplete the bloodstream of platelets, cells that help to clot blood. A person whose platelet count is low bleeds easily.[1] Simple activities, such as brushing teeth, may result in abnormal bleeding. Overuse of a joint can cause bleeding into a joint space or a muscle compartment. This can abnormally raise the pressure in the enclosed area and cause the normal tissues to die. In extreme cases, a compartment syndrome may result. If this goes undetected and the tissues become necrotic, an amputation may be necessary to save the person's life. Therapy personnel need to stay informed about the person's blood cell counts, monitor the sensory and motor function, and inform the doctor of any changes involving a limb. It is helpful to use **blood levels,** such as white blood cell and platelet counts and hematocrit, to guide treatment choices in therapy (Table 31-1). The crisis with platelets may last only a few days, when the chemotherapy is at the maximum level in the blood stream. Once the platelets begin to recover, more normal and increasingly stressful activities may be graded to adjust to the change and restore normal function.

*Neutropenia* is a severe impairment of the immune response with decreased resistance to infection. A cold can cause severe illness in someone who is immunosuppressed. Often neutropenic patients are kept on protective isolation to limit the risk of cross infection.[15]

*Anemia* reduces an individual's tolerance for treatment. The oxygen level in the system is depleted because of reduced hemoglobin. Fatigue should be respected, and activities paced and prioritized to encourage a sense of self-direction and to maximize functional ability. With overactivity, the person may require oxygen to recover from shortness of breath.

*Peripheral neuropathy* is a frequent side effect of neurotoxic chemotherapeutic agents. The person may have both motor and sensory involvement of the peripheral nerves, experiencing diminished (hypoesthesia) or heightened (hyperesthesia) sensory awareness, particularly in the hands and feet.[6] Diminished awareness can lead to a loss of protective sensation, and the person may be at risk for cutting, burning, or entrapping a limb, depending on which neurological components are involved. Patients with heightened sensation often complain of pain and burning sensations so much that it interferes with tolerance for even basic activities of daily living (ADL). Mild compression garments (toning gloves or tubular support bandages) may muffle the sensation that is causing the pain and provide comfort and protection of the limb. In addition, sensory stimulation may decrease pain; examples include massage and exposure to graded textures (very soft to somewhat rough).

Another difficult side effect of some chemotherapies is *alopecia*—hair loss—which may also affect eyebrows, pubic hair, and extremity hair. Alopecia is one of the most obvious outward signs that identifies a person who has a serious illness and may signal the social stigma of cancer. Hair is also a significant element of individual identification. Hair usually grows back after completion of chemotherapy treatment, but the person may experience premature graying, other color changes, and changes in texture and distribution of hair. Some people respond well to the suggestion to use wigs or hairpieces; others prefer to wear hats, scarves, or turbans; some prefer to go bald. It is a very personal choice. Identifying the choices and providing community resources, names of stores, and access to catalogs, is often helpful.

*Table 31-1*

Blood Values Reference Chart

| *Complication* | *Normal range* | *Precaution* |
|---|---|---|
| Neutropenia (WBC count) | 47.6%-76.8% | Avoid exposure to infection. |
| Platelets (thrombocytopenia) | <130,000 | Avoid resistive activities.<br>Avoid skin breakage. |
| Hematocrit (anemia) | Men: 40%-54%<br>Women: 37%-47% | Monitor vitals and respiratory rate. |

Some chemotherapies and radiation can cause detrimental changes to reproductive organs. Patients should be informed of the effects of the cancer treatment on the ability to reproduce (have children by natural means). Men can have sperm frozen in a sperm bank for future use. Embryos can also be frozen for later use. Even adolescents who do not currently have a sexual partner may chose this option to keep future choices open. For those who do not save eggs or sperm, parenting is still possible through donors or adoption.

### *Radiation Therapy*

**Radiation therapy** is the use of radioactive materials to kill or control the growth of cancer cells. Only some cancers are sensitive to radiation, so this is not always the treatment of choice. However, when a tumor is sensitive to its beams, radiation can be curative on its own or in combination with a chemotherapeutic agent.

The radioactive isotope may be placed in a machine that pinpoints the location of the tumor. A lead plate protects tissues from exposure until the person is correctly positioned and ready for treatment. External beam radiation directs the radiation over a set field, exposing the tumor and surrounding tissues to treatment. The beam can also be directed to a specific spot by placing a cone over the lens of the linear accelerator (radiation machine), thus concentrating the beam in one specific region. Exposure is given over a period of days, weeks, or months to deliver a total dose of radiation that cannot all be done at once (because the radiation burns the tissues). Near the completion of treatment, the person may experience radiation burning. The radiologist will ask the patient to avoid using lotions, creams, perfumes, and soaps on the treatment zone because these products could increase the probability of a burn by changing the surface composition of the skin.[4]

Radiation can also be administered through implantation of radioactive seeds into the tumor bed or affected gland *(brachytherapy)*. The seeds are removed when treatment is completed. The treatment course for brachytherapy is usually a few days to a week. The radioactive seed is either implanted directly into the tissues or is inserted through a flexible straw. Brachytherapy is used in the treatment of thyroid cancer, prostate cancer, some cancers of the genitourinary tract in women, and in soft tissue carcinomas. While a patient is radioactive with the seed implanted, special precautions must be taken by personnel. Lead aprons are often available for short-term direct contact with the patient. The chart usually states the maximum time allowed for exposure to health care providers, thus limiting the rads delivered to the caregiver. Lead chariots (shields) are often provided at the doorway of the patient's room. The caregiver is protected behind the chariot but can speak with the patient inside the room.

In addition to its curative effect, radiation can also be used to treat cancer pain. Radiation may reduce pain in two ways: (1) by decreasing the size of a mass that is pressing on structures or nerves, or (2) or by deadening the perception of the nerve. This is particularly helpful with spinal tumors and bony metastases.[6]

The side effects of radiation may be seen immediately (as in the case of radiation burns), over time, or in conjunction with the healing process. Fibrosis is a form of scarring that may result from radiation. Some of the modalities used to treat burns have been found helpful in treating radiation fibrosis in its early stages. Silicone gel pads, for instance, keep the tissues soft, hydrated, and pliable.

Normal activity during the scar management phase may help to reverse the soft tissue contracture effect.[5] Soft tissues are, in part, soft because of their elastic properties and their relationship to fascia, the tissue layer beneath the skin. Fascia covers the muscle compartments and reduces the effect of friction that occurs with normal movement and work. When the soft tissues are irradiated, they are burned. On healing, the tissues stiffen and harden. Beneath the skin, the fascia may also loose its elasticity and resilience. The person who receives radiation therapy may report pulling, tightening, or stiffness associated with the fibrotic change. The patient may describe the body as feeling hard, even like wood.

Radiation to the region of the head and neck may contribute to the development of dysphagia, or swallowing disorders (see Chapter 19). Initially, the irradiated tissues are inflamed and swollen. Open sores can result in the oral cavity and oropharyngeal cavity. This can slow down the swallowing reflex and diminish the function of the musculature supporting the swallowing mechanism. Food can spill into the airway and be aspirated (breathed into the lungs).[11]

Head and neck irradiation can also cause stiffening of the muscles of the jaw, mouth, neck, and shoulder. Scar management, range of motion, and movement activities are helpful in restoring normal function and preventing pain and discomfort.

Radiation may also cause neutropenia, so care should be taken to protect the neutropenic patient from cross infection. If the caregiver has an infection, good handwashing technique and the use of masks is expected. If the patient participates in a group activity, avoiding proximity with a patient who has an infection is important.

*Myelopathy* (pathological loss of the myelin surrounding a nerve) and *neuropathy* (weakness or sensory loss) can also result in the short-term or long-term after radiation therapy. Permanent nerve damage usually results, so restoration of function is unrealistic. A patient with a *brachial plexopathy* (sensory or motor dysfunction of nerves arising at the proximal level of division of the peripheral nerves of the arm), can benefit from positioning and comfort measures as well as adapted equipment to compensate for lost function. The nerves will not regenerate, therefore the goals will be (1) to support the remaining function, (2) to prevent subluxation and pain, and (3) to compensate for loss of arm function. Chronic pain syndromes may accom-

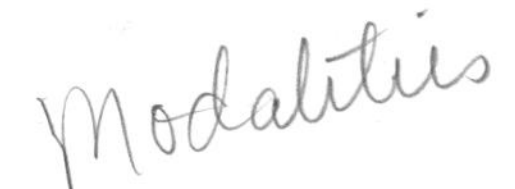



pany this condition. Restoration of function is often the primary goal, rather than total relief of pain. Treatments administered by the registered occupational therapist (OTR) or physical therapist (PT) such as transcutaneous electrical nerve stimulation (TENS) can help to alleviate pain. The certified occupational therapist (COTA) may provide stress reduction techniques such as relaxation breathing or guided imagery.

Cancer treatment and survival with a diagnosis of cancer often interrupts and alters normal activities. The patient may experience change in expectations concerning future roles and may need to define new roles. The therapy practitioner can help by determining the activities that are most important to the individual and enabling participation in those that are realistic. Counseling patients may empower them to recognize their ability to strive for new goals and accept their inability to resume some activities.

Patients who receive radiation may experience alopecia. The response and management is the same in this instance as in the management of alopecia after chemotherapy.

## REASONS FOR REFERRAL TO OCCUPATIONAL THERAPY

The reasons for referral to occupational therapy may be described along a continuum of expected functional gain and prognosis of disease—prevention, restoration, support, and palliation.[8] Reference to this continuum is helpful in guiding treatment choices and determining realistic goals for the individual undergoing treatment (Box 31-1).

Prevention is an optimal goal in treatment because it supports normal living and avoids the development of conditions or complications that could otherwise arise from high-risk behaviors. An example of prevention in terms of cancer is a smoking cessation program to prevent lung cancer.[18] Occupational therapy practitioners might work with healthy adolescents in a smoking-prevention program. An occupational therapist in a community-based practice could run a women's health group and train women to do breast self-examination.

Restoration focuses on a return to normal functioning without the need for adaptive equipment or techniques. This is appropriate for individuals who may have mild sequelae after medical treatment, but who are expected to recover completely. For example, women who are diagnosed with breast cancer in the early stages, receive medical treatment, and are declared in remission often are physically deconditioned. They may not have had good exercise habits before treatment. Now they are invested in health-promoting behaviors and wellness.

Supportive goals become the focus of treatment when individuals cannot resume doing things normally without adaptations because of medical, surgical, or disease-specific sequelae. For example, a patient who has lost intrinsic hand function after surgical resection and radiation therapy for a soft tissue sarcoma in the forearm may become independent in ADL again. Function may be supported by a wrist support or tenodesis splint and adaptive devices to substitute for fine mobility loss in the affected hand.

Palliation is emphasized when the disease has widely metastasized, and the patient may have only a limited time to live. Occupational therapy intervention may provide the patient with control over the environment or may reduce pain to allow increased activity for part of the day. **Palliative care** focuses on empowering the patient to determine which activity is personally important. Palliative care can sustain realistic hope and interest, and ward off overwhelming depression and accompanying feelings of helplessness and hopelessness.

*Box 31-1*

### Key Concepts for Treatment Planning with Cancer Patients

**Prevention**

Treatment that can decrease a risk behavior for development of a disease

**Restoration**

Treatment that can restore function with little or no evidence that the dysfunction existed

**Support**

Treatment that uses substitution actions or equipment to optimize function

**Palliation**

Treatment that provides physical comfort or peace of mind by empowering patients to focus on goals of their choosing

## SPECIFIC DIAGNOSES OF CANCER AND THE ROLE OF THE COTA

### Breast Cancer

During the early postoperative phase after breast cancer surgery, the arm on the side of surgery is at risk for loss of range of motion because the surgical incision may extend under the arm and thus limit chest wall and myofascial (soft tissue) gliding. Within the first 2 to 3 weeks after surgery, the patient should move gently to protect the incision and promote healing. In the next phase, the patient should stretch to regain normal movement in the arm. Because inpatient hospitalization is short (2 days for a **mastectomy** [removal of a breast]; a 1-day surgical procedure for a lumpectomy), outpatient and community group programs to encourage movement are appropriate and needed. In addition, education is needed about sensory

Table 31-2

## Peripheral Neuropathy and ADL Precautions

| Clinical sign | Functional problem | Solution |
|---|---|---|
| Numbness | Loss of sharp and dull perception, at risk for cutting and burning limb | Use vision, cueing, and adapted equipment. |
| Burning pain | Cannot tolerate anything touching hand or foot | Wear toning gloves, cloth gloves, soft padding, and socks. Use relaxation techniques. |
| Proprioceptive loss | Unaware of where arm and leg are in space | Teach cueing and position for safety. |

changes perceived as discomfort or pain that occur normally after breast surgery. Education helps to encourage movement and allay fear as to the meaning of the pain.

Education concerning lymphedema (swelling of the arm on the side of surgery that can occur because lymph nodes were removed or damaged) is also crucial. Patients with lymphedema should follow arm and hand precautions, avoiding trauma (cuts, insect bites, burns, and repetitive strain injuries) to the arm on the surgical side.[3] Community agencies may provide support groups and exercise programs. Putting patients in touch with these programs can be very beneficial. Examples of programs include the Reach to Recovery or Look Good Feel Better program of the American Cancer Society, SHARE, or ENCORE. Patients will appreciate information about resources available for breast prostheses (e.g., corsettiers), wigs, salons, and other camouflage (hats or turbans). Occupational therapy practitioners may initiate, coordinate, and lead groups for a Look Good Feel Better program if one does not currently exist.[17]

During chemotherapy and radiation therapy treatment, patients can benefit from movement programs to restore normal motion to the arm on the side of treatment. Radiation therapy can result in adhesive capsulitis (a stiffening and hardening of the glenohumeral joint capsule resulting in a loss of rotation and mobility of the shoulder joint) and lead to frozen shoulder in the irradiated shoulder as radiation fibrosis develops. Continuing stretching exercises is important, especially overhead and shoulder rotation movements. Otherwise, patients may develop reflex muscle spasm and pain syndromes.

Chemotherapy can cause peripheral neuropathy, resulting in lost or diminished sensation or motor function of the arms or legs. Patients may complain of nerve-related pain, such as burning, tingling, or numbness. In some instances, this pain can be intense enough to limit participation in ADL. Providing the patient with isotonic gloves or tubular support bandages can sometimes soothe this pain enough to allow resumption of more normal activity. Sensory reeducation with textures can be soothing (see Chapter 24). Adapting assistive devices with large handles and soft grips may be helpful in supporting function until the person completes chemotherapy and the peripheral nerve function improves or returns to normal.

If protective sensation (perception of hot, cold, sharp, dull, and position sense) is lost, participation in activities that rely on these sensations may put the person at risk for injury. For example, cooking activities rely on the patient's ability to use sharps. Patients are taught to use vision to avoid cutting themselves and oven mitts to prevent burns. Tables 31-2 and 31-3 provide summaries of side effects, precautions, and techniques.

The psychosocial adjustment aspect of care is too often overlooked with cancer patients. Most are in the process of role adjustment and redefining themselves during the treatment phase of their disease. Encouraging group interaction and discussion as well as providing opportunities to develop new hobbies or interests may be beneficial. Research has shown that women with breast cancer who attend support groups tend to have a better quality of life and extended longevity even if they are in the advanced stage of disease. From a research perspective, very little is known about the healing power of prayer and spiritual development.

Improved perception of the value of complementary medicine is promoting research in several allopathic medical centers on the value of techniques such as stress reduction, massage, and energy therapies (e.g., therapeutic touch, Reiki). This is another potential area of development and participation for occupational therapy practitioners who use groups in treatment settings. Functionally based standardized tests can be used to demonstrate improved functional outcomes with the use of complementary techniques.

In addition, some patients may have defined psychiatric diagnoses and may require occupational therapy intervention based on that diagnosis. For instance, adjustment disorder occurs in many patients who are emotionally reacting to their diagnosis or to a change in their condition. This is frequently seen in patients who develop acute lymphedema and experience anxiety with a tendency to overfocus on details.

*Table 31-3*

**Functional Impact and Management of Side Effects from Cancer Treatment**

| *Treatment* | *Side effect* | *Functional impact* | *Rehabilitation management* |
|---|---|---|---|
| Radiation stretching | Burn (acute) | Avoid touch | Active range of motion |
| | Burn (subacute) | Soft tissue contracture | Scar management, stretching |
| | Myelopathy | Plexopathy | Positioning, ADL compensatory strategies |
| Chemotherapy | Neutropenia | Immunocompromise fatigue | Protective isolation, paced activity |
| | Thrombocytopenia (low platelet count) | Decreased activity tolerance | Avoidance of skin breaks, paced activity |
| | Anemia | Shortness of breath; decreased activity tolerance | Frequent rest periods |
| | Peripheral neuropathy | Decreased sensation | Safety education and activity modification |
| Surgery | Incision | Movement limitation | Time for incision to heal (approximately 10 days), stretching after healing |
| | Referred pain | Reluctance to move | Coordination of pain medications with treatment, education regarding actual risk |
| | Phantom pain | Sleep disturbance, decreased activity tolerance | Application of light pressure to the area, education regarding meaning and actual risk |

These patients may require some counseling and limit-setting in addition to drug therapy to overcome their anxiety. Depression is another diagnosis that is often encountered. It may be reactional and appropriate to the situation, or it may be organically based.[14] Using activities with successful outcomes can be helpful to foster the development of self-esteem. In addition, structured activity is also sometimes helpful because it can limit distractions and redirect the focus of the individual from a feeling of being overwhelmed to an ability to tolerate life in the present—to cope. Successful completion of a structured activity may also provide hope because concrete evidence of a positive change results.

Family and caregiver training is also important for breast cancer patients who will be responsible for participating in a home exercise program. The caregiver who is educated about the home program can better appreciate its value and assist the patient with specific recall of exercises or activities. Compliance with self-treatment may improve if a caregiver reminds the person about the importance of the home program.

### Lung Cancer

In the early postoperative phase, patients who have undergone surgery to remove a portion of the lung may be dependent on oxygen because of shortness of breath.[3] ADL should focus on energy conservation and work simplification. It is advisable to monitor the patient's vital signs including respiratory rate (the number of breaths per minute), pulse, and blood pressure. In inpatient rehabilitation settings, it may be possible to monitor their activity tolerance with a pulse oximeter (a digital machine with a finger electrode that measures the percentage of oxygen consumed). The goal is for the patient to do as much activity as physical tolerance allows.

The surgery for lung cancer, a thoracotomy, involves a wide excision from the center of the chest to under the arm that terminates laterally at the spine. After the initial healing of the incision, the patient may benefit from scar management. Patients may complain of burning paresthesias and stabbing sensations in the scar. Silicone gel pads worn on the scar 22 hours a day for 4 to 6 weeks may prevent adhesion and soften and flatten the scar tissues while the collagen beneath the scar remodels. The silicone may also provide neutral warmth, a relaxing or comforting sensation that occurs from absorption and reflection of body heat. Sensory reeducation with textures may also help to reduce scar-related discomfort.

Gentle general conditioning exercises (GCEs) may assist the patient with increasing activity and respiratory tolerance. A program of GCEs may be taught to the patient or caregiver for a self-treatment regimen to support the occupational therapy program. The caregiver and patient can also be instructed in a range of motion and positioning program for the shoulder on the side of surgery.

### Head and Neck Cancer

Cancers of the head and neck region require surgical resection, usually augmented by radiation therapy and in some cases chemotherapy. The procedures most commonly done with oropharyngeal cancer patients require removal of cervical and submaxillary lymph nodes. The procedures for which occupational therapy is consulted most often are neck dissections (radical or modified radical) and resections involving the oral-pharyngus and tongue.

**Radical neck dissection** involves removing the lymph nodes and vessels from the border of the jaw, the strap muscles of the neck, and the trapezius muscle. The spinal accessory nerve is usually impaired after a radical dissection. When this nerve does not work, the scapula wings. Winging of the scapula results in instability of the arm in overhead planes of motion because the scapula is unsupported. Therefore patients who have this surgery can develop painful shoulders and loose shoulder movement above 90 degrees of flexion and abduction. After surgery, it is necessary to allow some scar tissue to develop in the neck to substitute for the lost function of the sternocleidomastoid muscle, which aligns the head at midline. Some neck stiffness tends to result and is necessary. However, what is not necessary is hardening of the tissues that are radiated. Scar management through the use of silicone gel pads, gentle active range of motion, and positioning with cervical support pillows is helpful for restoring more normal skin quality and preventing pain and deformity of the neck.[4]

Head and neck cancer patients also are at risk for developing oral-motor dysphagia. The swallowing team may find the patient can eat only if the diet is limited in consistency or food will be aspirated. Some of these patients not be able to eat orally and may need to be tube fed for some time. If the patient's diet is limited, liquids may have to be thickened with a thickening agent to guarantee the consistencies of the bolus. In addition, the patients may require special positioning or timed sitting after eating so that they do not aspirate after meals. The swallowing specialist, usually the speech or occupational therapist, provides the instructions. The COTA may be responsible for following through on the feeding program based on these instructions. (See Chapter 19 for more information on dysphagia).

Again, training of the caregiver and patient is very important for follow-through on exercise and activity programs. This is essential with dysphagia because the ability to swallow and protect one's airway is a vital (life-supporting) function.

### Bone Tumors and Soft Tissue Sarcomas

Bone tumors and soft tissue sarcomas are usually first seen in the extremities. The surgical management depends on numerous factors including the type of tumor, the aggressiveness of the tumor, the status of the circulatory supply to the limb, the age and general health of the patient, and the functional prognosis. Some of the bone tumors are primary in bone, but most are metastases from other cancers. Soft tissue tumors are usually primary in nature. Some develop from prenatal influences and are called *embryonic in origin*. Some of these tumors are highly malignant and difficult to treat effectively.

If a tumor is aggressive and the blood or nerve supply to the limb is impaired, the patient may require an amputation. If the tumor is present, but the blood and nerve supply are intact, it may be possible to salvage the limb. In this instance, the distal portion of the limb is preserved, the portion of bone is removed with some healthy tissue (a margin), and a prosthesis is implanted and cemented into place.[13] Amputees from cancer are rehabilitated similarly to amputees from other causes. However, some cancer amputations remove the total hindquarter or forequarter.

Occupational therapy focuses on positioning and ADL. The patient will require training in positioning with the fracture brace and the sling, as well as self range of motion (with precautions as prescribed by the surgeon) and activities to restore hand strength and function. Cosmetic shoulder pads are also helpful in restoring the illusion of bulk to the arm because there will be loss of muscle and soft tissue with surgery.[4]

Because many of these patients are children or adolescents, parent training is important. Compliance with the use of the fracture brace and sling is crucial to prevent fracture of the limb and dislocation of the indwelling prosthesis.

### Colon and Bladder Cancers

Patients with colon or bladder cancer have **stomas**—openings from the surgically resected site to the outside of the body, after surgery. **Colostomy** stomas (which have an opening between the colon and body surface) and **urostomy** stomas (which have an opening between the body surface and the organs that produce and collect urine) are common. Patients may also undergo chemotherapy as part of their treatment. They may develop peripheral neuropathy and lose fine motor sensibility and function—the very type of feeling and movement they must rely on to independently remove and clean their colostomy and urostomy bags and sites.

The occupational therapy practitioner may be asked to work collaboratively with the enterostomal nurse and the patient to develop strategies to restore independent function in stoma care and hygiene. Changing a clamp or using a built-up tool and practicing this adapted technique is often the single skill needed for discharge of these patients to the community.

This group can also benefit from peer support group activities because the presence of the stomas and the side effects of the disease and treatment affect body image, self-perception, sexual functioning, and life roles. A summary of cancer conditions frequently seen in occupational therapy settings appears in Table 31-4.

Table 31-4

**Cancer Conditions Commonly Treated in Rehabilitation Settings**

| *Type of cancer* | *Side effect causing physical disability** | *Possible rehabilitation diagnoses* |
|---|---|---|
| Brain | Mass effect of the tumor displacing brain tissue | Hemiparesis, quadriparesis, cognitive impairment |
| | Postradiation necrosis | Visual impairment, sensory impairment, ADL impairment, dysphagia |
| Head and neck | Facial disfigurement, sensory and motor loss (surgery) | Decreased movement of face or neck, shoulder pain and instability |
| | Oropharyngeal loss | Facial/regional disfigurement, dysphagia, ADL impairment |
| Spinal | Sensory and motor loss below the level of the tumor | Paraparesis, quadriparesis, bowel and bladder dysfunction, pain, ADL impairment |
| Leukemia and lymphoma | Blood cell count changes, neurological signs | Weakness, fatigue, deconditioning, neuropathy, dysphagia, ADL impairment |
| Bone | Amputation, limb-sparing postsurgical complications | Mobility impairment, ADL impairment, wounds and scars, pain |
| Soft tissue | Amputation, scar adhesions, radiation fibrosis | Mobility impairment, ADL impairment, wounds and scars, pain |
| Colon and bladder | Colostomy, urostomy | Peripheral neuropathy, impaired mobility, ADL changes—toileting, bathing, and dressing |
| Lung | Postsurgical oxygen dependence and thoracic surgical movement limitations | Shortness of breath, ADL impairment, decreased mobility |
| Breast | Myofascial and joint changes in chest wall and shoulder | Decreased mobility in arm, pain, myofascial scarring |
| | Sensorimotor compromise in arm (brachial plexopathy) | Muscle imbalance, sensory changes |
| | Uncontrolled lymphedema in arm, ADL impairment | |
| Metastatic | Multiple organ and system involvement | Pain, fatigue, deconditioning, pain, impaired mobility, sensorimotor changes<br>Cognitive changes |

*There may be accompanying psychological sequelae: depression (situationally or organically based), anxiety (including adjustment disorders), and hallucinations (medication-related or organic/disease process-related). In addition, people with diagnoses of cancer frequently have issues concerning role adjustment and adaptation.

## ISSUES CONCERNING DEATH AND DYING

People who confront life-threatening illnesses are forced to face their own mortality. Grief is a common reaction and a necessary part of the adjustment process and is preceded by a dynamic interplay of behaviors or stages described by Kübler-Ross[10] as denial, bargaining, anger, depression, hope, and acceptance. At any given point the patient may exhibit one or several of these behaviors. Usually one stage prevails at a given time over the others. Denial is characterized by thoughts like, "A mistake has been made. This cannot be happening to me." Bargaining is manifested by thoughts such as, "If I do this one thing then it will be all right." Anger may be volatile at times and may also be outwardly directed at a number of objects, including at times the therapist. When people are predominantly angry, they may not be tolerant of therapy.

Depression is manifested by feelings of helplessness and hopelessness. When people are depressed, motivation generally wanes. Hope implies that some change for the good is possible. This restores motivation and participation in therapeutic goals. Acceptance is rarely achieved.[2,4] Great faith or self-actualization must be possessed for a person to accept the inevitable. Once acceptance is reached, therapy may no longer be a goal, unless the person has personal goals or requires the intervention of the therapist for comfort measures.

It may be hard for the therapy staff to react normally around the dying patient. It is difficult for most people to feel comfortable around death because it forces each of us to face our own individual issues, beliefs, and fears. Knowing the right thing to do or say is part of the art of practice. For some people, it is enough for a caregiver to be accountable and present; the physical act of following up indicates caring and support.

Some patients may seek existential (religious and spiritual) meaning.[2] The response of the caregiver is individualized and depends on the individual caregiver's comfort and willingness to engage in the therapeutic use of self. If the caregiver is uncomfortable, the patient could be assisted in contacting a spiritual or religious advisor and the clinician should just say, "I am not comfortable discussing this with you" or "I don't feel comfortable speaking about this topic."

Providing or facilitating activities that help the person deal with issues concerning death can be helpful. Some examples are creating memory books for significant others who will be left behind and writing personal diaries with humorous or special events—the stories that define the dying individual's life roles and experiences. Patients may also wish to write letters to family members or friends to resolve issues or say goodbye.

Palliative care also has its physical aspects. Techniques of comfort care that could be used are positioning, massage, complementary medicine (e.g., guided imagery, stress management, aromatherapy, therapeutic touch), adaptive devices, and rearrangement of the physical environment to allow maximum access for the patient with limited mobility. The practitioner can help maintain the patient's dignity by helping with toileting activities and strategies.

## SUMMARY

Cancer is a cluster of diseases with unique and identifiable problems for the occupational therapy practitioner to evaluate and treat. Although at one time many people did not survive cancer, with advances in medical care, diagnoses are being made earlier, and patients are being successfully treated for many cancer conditions.

The role of occupational therapy for the person with cancer is ever changing. The occupational therapy practitioner must be a good detective and to search out the clues in each instance that may guide treatment. Elements of physical disability and mental health practice are inextricably woven together.

The partnership of the OTR and COTA is imperative in cancer treatment, perhaps even more than in other areas of practice, because the case management for these conditions is highly technical. The certified occupational therapy assistant may perform many of the evaluations and treatments used with the general physically disabled and mental health populations.

## *Selected Reading Guide Questions*

1. List three tests commonly used to diagnose cancer.
2. What is the purpose of dissecting lymph nodes during cancer surgeries?
3. Which blood values are important to monitor in a cancer patient who is actively undergoing chemotherapy treatment?
4. What safety concerns would you have with a patient who has a chemotherapy-induced neuropathy?
5. List and describe the common effects of chemotherapy.
6. List and describe the common effects of radiation therapy.
7. What skin precaution should you follow when helping a cancer patient who is undergoing radiation therapy treatment perform basic self-care tasks?
8. A patient who has head and neck cancer is referred to your feeding group. What feeding problems might you expect this person to have? Do you need to follow any precautions?
9. Should your cancer patient who has neutropenia participate in the leisure group with patients of mixed diagnostic categories? Explain.
10. Are the goals for a patient with brachial plexopathy as a complication of breast cancer restorative, preventative, or palliative? Explain.
11. Give an example of a complementary treatment technique that can be used to reduce stress.
12. What approach could be used in counseling a cancer patient who cannot return to previous life roles?
13. What is alopecia, and is it a permanent condition in cancer patients?
14. List one restorative goal for a cancer patient (any diagnosis).
15. List a palliative goal for a patient who is confined to bed and has a progressive disease.
16. What education could you provide to a breast cancer patient to prevent lymphedema?
17. Which concern regarding ability to move should you have for a breast cancer patient who is receiving radiation to her breast and shoulder?
18. Which strategies might you use to manage anxiety in a cancer patient who is diagnosed with an adjustment disorder?
19. Which ADL problems might be observed in a person with a diagnosis of lung cancer who has had a thoracotomy to remove the tumor?
20. List three ADL that are difficult for the head and neck cancer patient to perform after a radical neck resection and spinal accessory nerve dysfunction.
21. A head and neck cancer patient has winging of the scapula on the side of the surgery. What movement will be difficult for this patient?
22. Describe an activity that could be helpful for a patient who is coping with issues of death and dying.
23. From an occupational therapy perspective, what are the common functional problems of patients with cancer?

## REFERENCES


1. Bierenger A: Cancer and impaired independence. In Abreu BC, editor: *Physical disabilities manual,* New York, 1981, Raven.
2. Buckman R: *I don't know what to say: how to help and support someone who is dying,* New York, 1989, Random House.
3. Burkhardt A: *Lymphedema: self care and treatment: a patient education booklet.* Memorial Sloan-Kettering Cancer Center, New York, 1992.
4. Burkhardt A, Joachim L: *A therapist's guide to oncology: medical issues affecting management,* San Antonio, 1996, Harcourt Brace.
5. Burkhardt A, Weitz J: Oncological applications for the use of silicone gel-sheets in soft-tissue contractures, *Am J Occup Ther* 45(5):460-2, 1991.
6. Carr JA et al: *Management of cancer pain: adults; quick reference guide no 9, ACHP & R 94-0593,* Rockville, Md, United States Department of Health and Human Services, 1994.
7. Cook A, Burkhardt A: The effect of cancer diagnosis and treatment on hand function, *Am J Occup Ther* 48(9):836-9, 1994.
8. Dietz JH: Rehabilitation of the cancer patient: its role in the scheme of comprehensive care, *Clin Bull* 4:104-7, 1974.
9. Grunberg SM, Groshen S: *Concepts of cancer staging.* In Calabrese P, Schein PS, eds: *Medical oncology,* ed 2, New York, 1993, McGraw Hill.
10. Kübler-Ross K: *On death and dying,* New York, 1969, McMillan.
11. Logemann JA et al: Impact of the diagnostic procedure on outcome measures of swallowing rehabilitation in head and neck cancer patients, *Dysphagia* 7:179-186, 1992.
12. Lowitz B, Casciato D: Cancer chemotherapeutics. In Casciato D, Lowitz B: *Manual of clinical oncology,* Boston, 1991, Little Brown.
13. Marcove R: En bloc upper humeral intrascapular resection: the Tikoff-Limberg Procedure, *Clin Orthop* 124:219-28, 1977.
14. Margary CJ: Aspects of psychiatric management of breast cancer, *Med J Australia* 148:239-42, 1988.
15. Mehls J: Occupational therapy in the rehabilitation of cancer patients. In American Occupational Therapy Association: *Cancer information packet,* Rockville, Md, 1987, The Association.
16. Miller GM, Forbes GS, Onofrio BM: Magnetic resonance imaging of the spine, *Mayo Clin Proc* 64:986-1004, 1989.
17. Shea B, Kleban R, Knauer C: Breast cancer rehabilitation, *Sem Surg Onc* 7:326-30, 1994.
18. Williams V, Burkhardt A, Royce J: Helping you call it quits, *OT Week,* p. 18, 1995.

Chapter 32

# HIV Infection and AIDS

Michael Pizzi

## Chapter Objectives

*After studying this chapter, the student or practitioner will be able to:*

1. Discuss the physical, psychosocial, and environmental factors associated with HIV disease that impede occupational performance.
2. Understand the occupational therapy process for adults with HIV disease.
3. Understand the stages of HIV disease and the corresponding occupational therapy response to enhance occupational performance.
4. Develop wellness strategies (in collaboration with the OTR) for adults with HIV disease.

## Key Terms

human immunodeficiency virus (HIV)
acquired immunodeficiency syndrome (AIDS)
occupational role
control
occupational choices
functional activity
wellness
adaptation

In 1982, five gay men from New York and California were diagnosed with a rare form of cancer and pneumocystis pneumonia (PCP), diagnoses not commonly seen in younger men. Soon thereafter, people with hemophilia, intravenous (IV) drug users, and children were becoming infected at dramatic rates with the same disease that did not have a name. This mysterious illness claimed the lives of hundreds before it was discovered to be fast and insidious and transmitted sexually or through blood products, essentially always transmitted from blood to blood and highly infectious. The disease came to be known as the **human immunodeficiency virus,** or **HIV,** from which the **acquired immunodeficiency syndrome,** or **AIDS,** arises.

HIV attacks a person's immune system, the body's system that wards off infections and calls on T cells and B cells to help out when it recognizes a foreign substance. The virus often goes unrecognized and when it is finally recognized, it has already attacked the system that helps a person get well. The virus can lie dormant in the body for up to 15 years with the person showing no symptoms but always being a carrier of the virus. Consequently, in the 1990s, the emphasis has shifted to "living well with your disease" and to the view that HIV disease is a chronic and *not* a terminal illness. Occupational therapy was founded on the belief that it can help people with chronic diseases lead productive and active lives, and thus we have an important role to play with people with HIV disease.

Although HIV was first noted in the gay population, that population was quick to identify prevention and health promotion strategies that have decreased the number of new cases of HIV in their population. However, recent infection in women, minorities, and heterosexual males has increased dramatically. The virus does not discriminate. The "worried well" fear they may be infected because of a past or current history of high-risk behavior (behavior that puts them at higher risk for being infected with HIV). The prominent high-risk behavior is unprotected sex, the cause of increased numbers of cases in adolescents and young adults. Another high-risk behavior is sharing needles and injectables with others (including sharing a steroid needle with workout partners).

A person who is HIV infected does not necessarily have AIDS. HIV disease has several stages; AIDS is the latter stage. The stages can be rapidly experienced or can be drawn out over time. The first is a mononucleosis-like syndrome with fatigue, high fever, and some lymphadenopathy (swollen lymph glands). This usually occurs within a few weeks of being infected. Then a person may be asymptomatic for years, later developing persistent generalized lymphadenopathy (PGL). Finally, the last stage is characterized by clinical medical symptoms leading to the diagnosis of full blown AIDS. These medical problems can include opportunistic infections like Kaposi's sarcoma or PCP. The person can also have medical complications like high fevers, chronic diarrhea, painful neuropathies (that can affect sensation), and severe weight loss.

The assistant may work with individuals at any one of these stages, helping the person attain the highest level of occupational functioning possible. An emphasis on holism and mind-body-spirit is essential to help people attain that level of functioning. The occupational therapy goals of mastery and independence celebrate wellness, life, and living (and not illness, death, and dying). It is vital that practitioners value individuals for their unique worth and contribution to the world and examine each person within the context of their environment and culture.

## CONSIDERATIONS FOR PERSONS WITH HIV DISEASE AND AIDS

The following are the physical, psychosocial, and environmental factors that the assistant might note in working with people with HIV disease.

### Physical Considerations

There are many physical impairments that a person with HIV may experience over time. Given that each person is uniquely affected by disease, not all individual factors may be noted. They include the following:

- Fatigue
- Peripheral and central nervous system disorders
- Visual impairments
- Cardiac problems
- Pain
- Weakness (neuromuscular)
- Changes in posture, gait, range of motion, strength, coordination, balance
- Changes in cognition (particularly affecting safety in carrying out tasks)

These physical problems lead to changes in occupational routines, such as self-care, leisure, and work performance, often increasing the time needed to complete activities of daily living (ADL).

### Psychosocial Considerations

Physical changes may impair psychosocial functioning because there is continuous interplay between mind and body. A person can become immobilized from carrying out daily routines or activities while "waiting for the next shoe to drop" (i.e., waiting for the next diagnosis, symptom, or blood test to come back). Persons with HIV often feel overwhelmed with the numbers of medical appointments and tests and can easily fall into the "sick role" of not being able to see the positive in anything. Their identity becomes wrapped up in their T-cell count or how many red and white blood cells there are instead of how they can function on a day-to-day basis. Occupational therapy assists people with managing their daily lives while helping them cope with the many new challenges of living with HIV. Other psychosocial considerations can include the following:

- Anxiety (which is often manifested in physical symptoms)
- Depression
- Guilt over being infected or the possibility of having infected others
- Preoccupation with illness or death
- Lack of treatments, limited access to health care, lack of insurance
- Anger (at the disease, lack of treatment, lack of social support, etc.)
- Neuropsychiatric problems (forgetfulness, apathy, withdrawal, memory loss)
- Altered self-image because of cancer or severe weight loss
- Lack of control over environment
- Hopelessness and helplessness
- Lack of meaning in daily activity and sense that "life is meaningless"
- Altered goals, plans, dreams for the future
- Grief and bereavement issues

It seems that people who have high standards of performance (the perfectionists) or those who have a very rigid schedule or routine of activity do not fare very well in coping with illness. They are less able to adapt to the many changes that occur, sometimes on a daily basis. Occupational therapy can help them identify how to adapt more easily.

### Environmental Considerations

The environment is not just the physical setting in which a person lives but the social and cultural environment as well. People with HIV can function much better when the assistant incorporates environmental observations and awareness into treatment.

#### *Physical Environment*

People with symptomatic HIV (and associated physical impairments) might have difficulty negotiating steps, going around corners, going shopping, and traveling into the community. Mobility could be decreased because of impaired vision, reduced strength, or fatigue. Sensory problems like neuropathies can alter balance, and taking a few steps can be painful.

### *Social Environment*

Stigma and discrimination often cause people with HIV to be seen as social pariahs or outcasts. Many people with HIV have already been victims of discrimination—gay men, persons of color, women, and IV drug users. This is important for the assistant to note in treatment. Relationships with significant others, family members, and work associates may change because of an HIV diagnosis. Health care providers may discriminate, consciously or unconsciously, which can make going to the hospital a fearful prospect instead of one that is welcomed for care and relief. The occupational therapy assistant may be one of the first people to physically touch a person with HIV—through ADL, ROM, or some creative treatments. Tactile contact that is accepting and caring can be as important to the person with HIV as any medication.

### *Cultural Environment*

A person with HIV may be gay or bisexual as well as a minority. Developing culturally specific and uniquely defined treatments and interventions enhances health and promotes a sense of well being. Such interventions symbolically demonstrate that the assistant cares and is attentive to the particular needs of that one individual and helps to establish rapport.

## THEMES IN OCCUPATIONAL THERAPY

When Adolph Meyer, one of the founders of occupational therapy, created the paradigm of occupation, he recognized several aspects of human behavior that today can be applied to work with people with HIV disease. These include the following:

1. An individual's health is measured by involvement in life tasks in the social and physical environments.
2. The focus must be on a person's *lifestyle.*
3. A healthy balance between work, rest, sleep, and play is necessary to fully function.
4. Occupation can restore function, maintain functioning, and prevent dysfunction.
5. Occupation helps people make better use of time and reorganize time.

These aspects of behavior, along with the following occupational themes that guide treatment, help to create a healthier lifestyle for people with HIV disease.

### Environment

The physical, social, and cultural environments are essential to consider in treatment. Occupations provide the most meaning when they are developed within the context of a familiar environment. For example, facilitating a homemaker in a wheelchair to make a home-cooked meal for a family gathering can include all aspects of the environment with the task holding meaning for the individual.

### Occupational Roles

Role functioning (mastery and progress toward developing an **occupational role**) should be incorporated in treatment goals and activities. For example, if a patient is a worker, treatments designed to restore work habits, routines, and task performance would be appropriate. If a patient has no occupational role, role development might be important if that patient has no habits, routines, or meaningful activity during the day.

### Wellness

Occupation that holds meaning and in which the person can successfully engage promotes wellness. The immune system can be supported and thus wellness created when a person engages in productive occupations and functions in tasks adapted by the assistant and registered occupational therapist (OTR). For example, stacking cones in a clinic is not a wellness-oriented, meaningful occupation for a weight lifter with HIV (unless cones were stacked for a living), but a strengthening program (in collaboration with the physical therapist) and balancing that with rest and periods of leisure and good nutrition is a more appropriate wellness-oriented treatment.

### Temporal Rhythms

Time is often organized through activity, and activity is often organized through time. A person with HIV might perceive that there is a dearth of time and time cannot be wasted. The assistant can help the person to organize routines, prioritize goals, and make the best use of time by using different techniques, such as a time log or activity log that corresponds to how time is used by the person. This can give the person with HIV an insight into how time can best be used and not wasted on a day-to-day basis. It is also important to recognize that many persons with HIV have an immediate need to get on with life and living, so practitioners need to offer practical, functional, and meaningful occupations to people with HIV throughout the therapy process.

### Control

HIV disease often takes **control** away from a person, by the sheer magnitude of the disease process. The health care system also takes control away, especially in most hospitals, because it dictates how a person will spend waking moments. From the start of occupational therapy treatment, control must be shared with the patient through **occupational choices** every session. For example, the COTA can have a list of five to ten tasks that the person can engage in to increase physical or psychosocial well being and can ask the person to choose three for that session.

## OCCUPATIONAL THERAPY ASSESSMENT AND EVALUATION

The OTR can assess all of the aforementioned areas with a variety of tools, from physical assessment tools like goniometry, balance, strength, and ADL evaluations through psychosocial assessment, including a neuropsychiatric battery and coping assessments. It is also important to examine assessments done by other disciplines. The Pizzi Assessment of Productive Living (PAPL) for adults with HIV disease (Figure 32-1) gives the assistant an overview of other areas that need to be assessed for people with HIV and suggests how those areas can be addressed in treatment. Pizzi has also developed the Occupational Loss Assessment, the Wellness Spiral, and the HIV Stress Assessment (Pizzi, 1994), which are often used in HIV care. The assistant can contribute to the assessment process by doing an occupational history, an observational and written ADL evaluation, and a caregiver interview to determine level of social support and type of home environment (if possible) to which the person with HIV may be discharged.

The assistant then works with the assessment information and the plan of care and goals set up by the OTR to develop the treatment sessions in collaboration with the person with HIV. It can also be appropriate for the OTR and assistant to coassess although it is not necessary. It is always important to collaborate with persons with HIV on their goals, plans, and desired functional outcomes from treatment.

Before assessment, it is vital that the assistant be aware of precautions for infection control. Masks are needed if the person with HIV has tuberculosis or other airborne infectious disease or when the assistant has a cough, cold, or other symptom that might infect the person with HIV. Gloves are needed to wipe up blood or other body fluid spills but are not normally worn for traditional treatment or written assessments or treatments. Gloves should always be readily available. Always check with your department and facility policy on universal precautions (see Chapter 12).

## TREATMENT

Goal and treatment planning and implementation must take on a positive and supportive spirit; this is the responsibility of the individual therapist. Assistants help to create environments and approaches toward health, wellness, and positive living for people with HIV disease. "Persons with HIV are often devastated physically, psychologically, and spiritually and most likely have encountered prejudice and discrimination before and after diagnosis. We have an opportunity to support people with HIV through nonjudgmental, positive approaches to life and living and to use our power as a catalyst for transformation. We can provide hope and meaning to patients through adaptation and a positive spirit without providing false hope for a cure."[1] Restoring and maintaining function and preventing dysfunction in self-chosen occupations related to the person's life and lifestyle are the focus of clinical interventions. Generally, traditional clinical interventions used with other diagnoses are implemented, with the use of the guidelines thus far set forth in this chapter. Other considerations must also be noted during treatment. These include the following:

1. Incorporating nutritional education in treatment. Good nutrition maintains the body in good emotional and physical shape and is important to the immune system. This education can be incorporated into adaptive homemaking skills and ADL.
2. Use of alternative medicine therapies to complement traditional care. These can include visualization, imagery, massage, meditation, herbs, therapeutic touch, and several manual therapies. The assistant can ask people with HIV if they currently use any alternative or complementary techniques and if so learn from that person as well as introduce other techniques. The assistant should acquire service competency before administering any techniques and should discuss these with the OTR.
3. Providing control and choices at each session conveys a healthy respect for the person with HIV and helps to establish rapport. It also symbolizes caring at its very best.
4. Helping the person to adapt a routine or habit of daily living can promote healthier living. Illness of any kind disrupts a routine of activity. A progressive and chronic disease constantly interrupts routine. The COTA should work with the person with HIV to determine the best and worst times of day for activity and energy output. Is the person a morning or evening person? What is the normal routine of the person's day? How can you as a health care provider help to adapt the routine to make it as comfortable as possible? This is an often overlooked but vital part of treatment and overall caring that the assistant can implement.
5. Generalized weakness and fatigue disrupt routines and activity performance. Incorporating energy conservation, work simplification, and other strategies and adaptive devices can help maintain task performance.
6. Positioning for the bedbound or frail patient can prevent decubitus ulcers and promote healthier sleep and rest patterns. Positioning for tasks will optimize comfort and engagement in functional activity.
7. Learning the use of adaptive equipment is vital for any person with functional limitations. Reachers for wheelchair-bound persons; lap trays, feeding equipment, and writing implements for people with hand neuropathies; and dressing sticks and sock aids for lower extremity dressing are just some examples of commonly used equipment. The COTA must make sure that the person accepts the equipment and knows how to use it.

**Demographics**
Name: Age: Sex:
Lives with (relationship)
Identified caregiver:
Race: Culture: Religion: —practicing?
Primary occupational roles:
Primary diagnosis:
Secondary diagnosis:
Stage of HIV:
Past medical history:
Medications:

**Activities of Daily Living** (using ADL performance assessment)
Are you doing these now?
Do you perform homemaking tasks?
For areas of difficulty: Would you like to be able to do these again like you did before? Which ones?

**Work**
Job: When last worked:
Type of activity at job:
Work environment:
If not working, would you like to be able to?
Do you miss being productive?

**Play/Leisure**
Types of leisure activities engaged in:

Are you doing these now?
If not, would you like to? Which ones?
Would you like to try other things as well?

Is it important to be independent in daily living activities?

**Physical Function**
Active and passive range of motion:
Strength:
Sensation:
Coordination (gross and fine motor/dexterity):
Visual/perceptual:
Hearing:
Balance (sit and stand):
Ambulation/transfers/mobility:
Activity tolerance and endurance:
Physical pain:
Location:
Does pain interfere with doing important activities?
Sexual function:

**Cognition** (attention span, problem solving, memory, orientation, judgment, reasoning, decision-making, safety awareness)

**Time Organization**
Former daily routine (prior to diagnosis):
Has this changed since diagnosis? If so, how?

Are there certain times of day that are better for you to carry out daily living tasks?

Do you consider yourself regimented in organizing time and activity or pretty flexible?

What would you change if anything in how your day is set up?

*Figure 32-1* Pizzi Assessment of Productive Living (PAPL) for adults with HIV infection and AIDS. (Courtesy Michael Pizzi.)

*Continued.*

**Body Image and Self-Image**
In the last six months, has there been a recent change in your physical body and how it looks? How do you feel about this?

**Social Environment** (Describe support available and utilized by patient.)

**Physical Environment** (Describe environments in which patient performs daily tasks and level of support or impediment for function)

**Stressors**
What are some things, people, and situations that are or were stressful?
What are some current ways you manage stress?

**Situational Coping**
How do you feel you are dealing with:
a. Your diagnosis
b. Changes in the ability to do things important to you
c. Other psychosocial observations

**Occupational Questions**
What do you consider to be important to you right now?

Do you feel you can do things important to you now? In the future?

Do you deal well with change?

What are some of your hopes, dreams, aspirations? What are some of your goals?

Have these changed since you were diagnosed? How?

Do you feel in control of your life at this time?

What do you wish to accomplish with the rest of your life?

Plan:

Short-term goals:

Long-term goals:

Frequency:

Duration:

Therapist:

*Figure 32-1, cont'd* For legend see opposite page.

8. Unique psychosocial factors must be considered. These can include (1) the fact that there is no known cure for the disease, (2) routines are interrupted by treatment regimens that may include 30 pills three times a day, (3) constant doctor and clinical appointments, (4) real and perceived discrimination, (5) work roles and relationships that are lost because of the diagnosis. These are all very real factors for people living with HIV disease—factors that are not commonly seen with other diagnoses. Perhaps the most important is that the person may have lost many, many friends and perhaps significant relationships to the same disease. Unresolved grief and bereavement issues and anger may exacerbate anxiety and other psychosocial factors related to HIV. The assistant must always note this possibility in clinical care.

The following case study will illustrate the integration of the concepts and clinical considerations discussed in this chapter.

## Case Study*

Mr. P., a 38-year-old white male, was admitted to the hospital 6 months after an initial diagnosis of AIDS and after his first incident of PCP. He was referred to OT

*From Pizzi M: The model of human occupation and adults with HIV infection and AIDS, *Am J Occup Ther* 44(3):42-49, 1990.

because of neuropathy in both feet. Mr. P. is a well-educated and well-traveled bank executive of French descent who speaks five languages. He was Catholic but left formal religion years ago because of the conflict between his gay lifestyle and the church's position on homosexuality. He rarely communicates with members of his nuclear family, who live outside the United States, and he lives with his supportive partner of 5 years. Mr. P. was referred to OT on the day of his hospital discharge. Because of this acute care situation (i.e., referred to OT in the morning and discharged that afternoon), assessment consisted only of interview and role, ADL, and biomedical assessments.

Assessment revealed Mr. P. to be independent in all self-care, home maintenance, and mobility activities except for minor standing balance deficits. No cognitive or sensory deficits were noted other than mild lower extremity neuropathy. Strength, active range of motion, and coordination were all functional for task performance. Mr. P. complained of diminished endurance, which affected his occupational habits and pursuits of interests including exercise, history, collecting, photography, movies, concerts, classical music, and swimming. He had narrowed leisure activities to listening to classical music when he "felt up to it." He felt out of control and believed that HIV had taken over. He openly discussed his prognosis and his religious beliefs, examining his unresolved relationship with God and the possibilities of an afterlife. The occupational therapist referred him to Dignity (a gay Catholic organization), the unit social workers, and the hospital chaplain.

OT recommendations included adaptive equipment for safety during bathing. Physical activity was tailored to his interests, values, and occupational choices. A new routine of daily living included a balance of activity and rest to maintain productivity. Adaptations of the worker role from office to home were also suggested because Mr. P. highly valued the work role.

Mr. P. was admitted to the hospital 6 weeks later with his third episode of PCP and severe neuropathy in both feet. This caused considerable pain even at rest. Physical limitations resulted in increased dependence.

This time the OT assessment was performed with the primary nurse and Mr. P.'s partner, Mr. J., in attendance. This gave a more comprehensive perspective and helped meet the needs and goals of both Mr. P. and his caregiver.

#### Assessment

Mr. P. had poor endurance and severe pain in both feet, which limited standing tolerance to less than 2 minutes. His active range of motion, strength, coordination, vision, and cognition were within functional limits. No neuropathy was noted in his hands, but he had a flexion contracture as a result of a painful tubercular nodule that caused difficulties with writing and holding utensils.

Mr. P.'s daily living routine was severely altered, and his occupational roles of worker, home maintainer, and hobbyist were affected. His partner related he did nothing with his day except lie in bed and watch television or listen to music. He would not come to the dining room table for meals but demanded that Mr. J. bring them to the bedroom. Mr. J. related that he felt obligated to help Mr. P. but guilty about supporting Mr. P.'s dependent state.

Mr. J. reported that Mr. P. seemed to have much unresolved anger and depression related to helplessness and hopelessness but refused to acknowledge this or see a mental health professional. He participated in no leisure activity, was apathetic, and felt hopeless regarding current and future occupational functioning. He was manipulating people into supporting his maladaptive style of dependency. He would often perform tasks for the occupational therapist yet tell nurses he could not perform these tasks, creating a division among staff regarding his functional abilities. Discussion among team members led to development of a structured and consistent approach that focused on sharing control of timing and choice of activities with Mr. P. The program of care was adapted to his preferences and promoted wellness by making treatment more meaningful to Mr. P.

The physical environment of the hospital was adapted and items from Mr. P.'s home were brought in to create a more familiar, physical space. Throughout the rehabilitation process, the OT worked with Mr. P.'s partner in his caretaker role. Attention was given to restructuring Mr. J.'s other roles, routines, time management, and activities to diminish his stress level, validate his own caregiving abilities, and work through impending loss of a partner. Mr. J. found these interventions helpful. He also stated that he felt like withdrawing from Mr. P. because of guilty feelings and impending loss. OT helped him focus on positive aspects of life and living.

One month before Mr. P.'s death, his mother, father, and sister visited him. The OT discussed the rehabilitation program with them; treatment was expanded to meet their needs to assist Mr. P. with his personal care, passive range of motion, and work and leisure tasks and to incorporate their support for Mr. P.

Despite Mr. P.'s ability and choice to eat independently, his mother was observed feeding him. In acknowledging her overwhelming need to resume the role of caregiver, a role soon to be relinquished, the treatment team continued to learn the lesson of asking, "Whose need is it? Whose need is greater?"

#### Treatment

Mr. P.'s treatment focused on OT and PT, including a balance among self-care, mobility, work, and leisure tasks. The program incorporated rest and his medical regimen including vital signs and IV medications. As much as possible, he was given the opportunity to organize his schedule, which helped him to normalize his routine and incorporate new activities. Mr. P. chose to follow a program of holistic activities that included massage and back rubs, imagery and visualization, therapeutic touch, exercise, balance and gait training, and personal and instrumental ADL. Important leisure and social activities such as listening to classical music, attending plays at the hospital, praying and meditating, reading, working, spending time with loved ones, resting, and sleeping were included. The treatment team included OT and PT, a nurse, a chaplain, a physician, a social worker, a recreation therapist, and Mr. P.'s significant others.

In addition, the OT program included the following:

1. Provision of and teaching in use of adaptive equipment (tub bench, hand-held shower, built-up handles for utensils, writing adaptations)
2. Joint self-ranging, exercise and upper extremity strengthening occupations
3. Energy conservation
4. Development of new leisure tasks and engagement in those formerly enjoyed
5. Discussion and activities centered around role changes and adaptation of favored roles (e.g., setting up tasks at bedside to continue his work in banking)
6. Family and partner education to develop competence and confidence and to reduce fear in caring for Mr. P.

At the beginning of Mr. P.'s second hospitalization, a home program was designed to give direction, focus, and purpose and to establish goals for his hospitalization. (This is realistic and does not provide false hope to people with HIV because HIV is a process with great variability). Although Mr. P. hoped he would be discharged home, he came to accept that this was not possible as his medical condition rapidly worsened. His OT program was adapted accordingly.

At his highest level of function during his 6 weeks of hospitalization, Mr. P. participated in daily exercise, walked to and from therapy, engaged in work-related tasks, and was independent in personal care. At his lowest level of functioning, Mr. P. was positioned for comfort, had classical music at his bedside, and participated in as much personal care as he chose, which occasionally consisted of finger feeding while in bed.

As the nuclear family slowly became involved in Mr. P.'s care, the benefits of an occupation-centered approach were evident. The family was able to restore their own forsaken occupational roles (particularly that of caregiver), and participation in occupations once enjoyed by the entire family assisted in healing old wounds. Open communication and self-expression were facilitated by the restoration of these roles and occupations. Mutual love, forgiveness, and support were shared among all family members, which assisted Mr. P. in envisioning his life as complete. The nuclear family first met Mr. P.'s partner at the bedside, and they immediately supported each other, which eased the loss felt by everyone when Mr. P. died.

## SUMMARY

As highlighted by the case study, assistants have an important role in treatment sessions and may develop sessions to promote health and well-being for people with HIV. Assistants must primarily remember the guidelines set forth in this chapter and implement them without judgment, stigma, or discrimination. Communication with the OTR on a consistent basis, including asking questions or voicing concerns about protection from HIV and how to protect the person with HIV, should be continuous. Maintaining an occupation-centered approach to care will enhance health and well-being and promote a positive way of coping with HIV.

## *Selected Reading Guide Questions*

1. Describe the stages of HIV disease.
2. Describe the physical, psychosocial, and environmental factors to consider when working with adults with HIV.
3. Discuss the three types of environment that need to be considered when implementing treatment.
4. Describe and discuss several themes related to occupational therapy intervention when working with people with HIV.
5. Describe and explain various treatments used in occupational therapy when working with adults with HIV.
6. Discuss and explain how wellness approaches in occupational therapy guide clinical interventions for adults with HIV.

### *REFERENCES*

1. Pizzi M: Nationally speaking: the transformation of HIV infection and AIDS in occupational therapy: beginning the conversation, *AJOT* 44(3):1-5, 1990.
2. Pizzi M: The model of human occupation and adults with HIV infection and AIDS, *AJOT* 44(3):42-49, 1990.

### *RECOMMENDED READING*

DeVita VT et al: *AIDS: etiology, diagnosis, treatment and prevention,* ed 2, Philadelphia, 1988, JB Lippincott.

Galantino ML, Levy J: HIV infection: neurological implications for rehabilitation, *Clin Manage Phys Ther* 8(1):6-13, 1988.

Galantino ML, Pizzi M: Occupational and physical therapy for persons with HIV disease and their caregivers, *J Home Health Care Practice* 3(3):46-57, 1991.

Gutterman L: A day treatment program for persons with AIDS, *AJOT* 44(3):234-237, 1990.

Miller HG et al: *AIDS: The second decade,* Washington, DC, 1990, National Academy Press.

Pizzi M: *HIV infection and AIDS: a professional's guide to wellness, health and productive living,* Silver Spring, Md, 1996. Positive Images and Wellness.

Pizzi M: Women and AIDS, *AJOT* 46(11):1021-1026, 1992.

Pizzi M: Occupational therapy: creating possibilities for adults with HIV infection, ARC, and AIDS, *AIDS Patient Care* 3:18-23, 1989.

Pizzi M: Adaptive human performance and HIV infection: considerations for therapists. In Galantino ML, editor: *Clinical assessment and treatment in HIV: rehabilitation of a chronic illness,* Thorofare, NJ, 1991, Slack.

Pizzi M, Hinds-Harris M: Infants and children with HIV infection: perspectives in occupational and physical therapy. In Pizzi M, Johnson J, editors: *Productive living strategies for people with AIDS,* New York, 1990, Haworth Press.

Pizzi M et al: HIV infection and occupational therapy. In Mukand J, editor: *Rehabilitation for patients with HIV disease,* New York, 1991, McGraw-Hill.

Schindler V: Psychosocial occupational therapy intervention with AIDS patients, *AJOT* 42:507-512, 1988.

Spence DW et al: Progressive resistance exercise: effect on muscle function and arthropometry of a select AIDS population, *Arch Phys Med Rehabil* 71:644-648, 1990.

Solomon GF, et al: An intensive psychoimmunologic study of long surviving persons with AIDS, *Annals of the New York Academy of Science,* 496, 647-655, 1987.

Villarino ME et al: AIDS, infection control and employee health: considerations in rehabilitation medicine. In Munkand J, editor: *Rehabilitation for patients with HIV disease,* New York, 1991, McGraw-Hill.

# Chapter 33

# Older Adults and Multidiagnosis Patients

*Angela M. Peralta*

## *Chapter Objectives*

*After studying this chapter the student or practitioner will be able to:*

1. Explain the developmental psychology theories regarding the aged.
2. Describe various stages of old age.
3. Understand the biological changes related to aging.
4. Understand the sensorimotor changes related to aging.
5. Describe occupational therapy interventions with the aged.
6. Discuss the variety of settings that provide services to the aged.
7. Describe the methods used in a fall prevention program.
8. Explain the federal regulation concerning restraint-free environments.
9. Describe various interventions for the reduction of restraint use.
10. Use communication strategies with family, client, supervisor, and other staff members in long-term care.
11. Discuss the purpose and makeup of the minimum data set.

## *Key Terms*

aging
adult day care
home and community care
assisted living
subacute care
minimum data set
resident assessment protocols
physical restraints
restorative programs
maintenance programs
enhanced environments

Old age is generally a period of reorganization of life styles. Not all persons will age in exactly the same way. Health factors greatly influence how a person will experience old age. **Aging** is an obvious and complex process that begins as soon as an individual is conceived. Health and disease, however, determine the quality of life individuals will have as they reach maturity. Aging by itself does not necessarily precipitate an increase in disease. Rather, age-associated changes in various organs and age-associated diseases contribute to the belief that old age means illness, dependency, and dementia.

It is important to view illness separately from reduced abilities. Although some diseases are more common in the elderly (e.g., stroke, hypertension, diabetes mellitus, osteoporosis), they should not be confused with normal aging. Generally, changes from normal aging cause a slow down in normal functioning, whereas changes from illness and disease may cause temporary or permanent inability to function.

Many of us know people who are extremely healthy and productive through their 80s and 90s and others who are totally dependent at age 65 or younger. Despite this range in ability to participate in life roles, normal aging is associated with many physiological changes as well as a decline in function in many organs. Understanding that old age does not mean illness is important because it clarifies the importance of a healthy lifestyle. Nutrition, exercise, good relationships with others, and meaningful involvement in activities that are personally important are the foundation of a healthy old age.

Lewis[18] described four stages of old age. Stage I, from 50 to 65 years, is the preretirement age in which a person begins to plan for the use of leisure time and may begin to assume new roles such as grandparent or caretaker of elderly parents. In stage II, from 65 to 74 years, the individual may begin to encounter increased health problems and may experience grief as spouse, friends, or siblings die. Stage III, from 75 to 84 years, may be when independent living is jeopardized. The person may begin to require assistance in life tasks. Stage IV, 85 years and older, may be when the individual becomes increasingly dependent on others. Institutional living arrangements may need to be made or the individual may need to live with a family member.

## DEVELOPMENTAL FACTORS

For certified occupational therapy assistants (COTAs), an understanding of developmental psychology theories can help in anticipating some of the needs of the elderly.

Human development is widely described in the literature and is often presented with a model that goes from birth to childhood to adolescence to early adulthood to adulthood and to old age. Many theories postulate that a person must first master the tasks required of each stage before progressing to the next. Tasks may be mastered in isolation and may be carried over to another developmental stage.

Havighurst defines a developmental task as one "which arises at or about a certain period in the life of the individual, successful achievement of which leads to his happiness and to success with later tasks, while failure leads to unhappiness in the individual, disapproval by the society, and difficulty with later tasks."[23] Havighurst identified the following six tasks related to "later maturity": (1) adjustment to decreased physical strength and health, (2) adjustment to retirement and reduced income, (3) adjustment to the death of a spouse, (4) establishment of affiliation with own age group, (5) flexible adaptation to social role in a flexible way, and (6) establishment of satisfactory physical living arrangements.[23]

Havighurst feels that development is a cognitive learning process. Tasks develop out of a combination of pressures arising from physical development, cultural expectations, and individual values and goals. He postulates that the occurrences of "teachable moments" of a special sensitivity or readiness to learn a task arise from the unique combination of physical, social, and psychic readiness.[23]

Roger Gould developed a model comprising six stages of adulthood in which individuals progressively abandon one childhood myth after another, manage to confront reality to a greater degree than before, and eventually succeed in raising their levels of consciousness.[19]

Erik Erikson formulated a theory of human development with a model of eight stages of life. "The three adult stages of the model are viewed as struggles devoted to the accomplishment of a primary task; young adulthood, a struggle between intimacy and isolation; middle age, a struggle between generativity and stagnation; and old age, a struggle to achieve a sense of ego integrity"[23] against despair. He identifies the basic virtue of old age as renunciation and wisdom.

Carl Jung postulates three stages of life: youth, middle age, and old age. Jung views youth as a period of expanding consciousness, middle age as a period of questioning long-held convictions, and old age as a period of increased introspection and preoccupation with self-evaluation.[19]

Biological and sociological theories also seek to explain the aging process. Biological theories are generally concerned with how the cells age and how the aging process affects the various organs. Sociological theories are concerned with the types of activities the elderly engage in and how the elderly disengage from familiar roles.

Expected biological changes are well documented in the literature. As age increases, various body functions decrease. The type and rate of change, however, vary with the individual. Many of these changes do not necessarily affect an individual's ability to function except when illness or disease occurs.

Occupational therapy practitioners must be aware of how normal aging and pathological conditions affect the individual client to develop an occupational therapy treatment program that (1) does not aggravate the condition, and (2) compensates for any functional deficit that may have developed as a result of the disease process.

## NORMAL AGE-RELATED CHANGES

Normal age-related changes are not pathological and should not be seen as illness. These changes, however, form the base on which specific pathological conditions are superimposed; thus the signs and symptoms and clinical course of the disease may be modified to a significant extent by physiological aging. Pneumonia can be used to illustrate how the aging person's body reacts to disease compared to a younger person's body. In a younger person, pneumonia may resolve in a few weeks, whereas in an older person it may be fatal.

Normal age-related changes in various systems include decreased functioning of the heart in times of stress and exercise. The strength of the heart muscle is reduced; the heart needs a longer time to relax between contractions. Normal aging also reduces the elasticity of the cardiovascular system.[4]

Decalcification causes the bones to become more porous, resulting in a decrease in the normal quantity and quality of bone structure.[10] As the demineralization of bone proceeds, bones become brittle and fractures may be common.[10]

Decreased hormone levels, decreased basal metabolic rate, decreased overall use of glucose, and decreased adrenal activity under stress are some of the endocrine changes seen in the elderly.

With advancing age, there are changes at all levels of the nervous system. There is a gradual decrease in bulk of individual muscles. (The changes in muscle seen with aging do not produce clinically symptomatic muscle weakness.) There is a slowing of nerve conduction velocity and oxygen consumption.[7]

In the elderly, the body appears to become less efficient in receiving, processing, and responding to stimuli. The elderly person experiences neurological changes related to temperature regulation and ability to perceive pain. The older person feels cold more easily; it is common to see an older person wrapped in blankets and keeping the room temperature quite warm. Pain perception and reaction to painful stimuli are decreased with age. The number and sensitivity of sensory receptors are reduced in the aging process. The sense of balance and the ability to use fine movements are affected by the aging process. The aged person may reach for doorways, chairs, and hand railings to maintain balance and ensure stability.[10]

Elderly persons may experience a decrease in function of various senses. Visual acuity usually decreases with age. The incidence of cataracts increases with age. The lenses of the eye also become somewhat rigid; therefore the eye accommodates less efficiently. (See Table 33-1 for suggestions regarding environmental adaptations for vision impairment.)

Overlaid on these normal changes are a number of pathological conditions that can affect the elderly person's health status.

## PATHOLOGICAL CONDITIONS

### Cardiovascular Conditions

The cardiovascular system undergoes several physiological alterations with advancing age. Cardiovascular disease accounts for 50% of all adult deaths in the

*Table 33-1*

**Environmental Adaptations for Visual Impairments**

| *Condition* | *Problem* | *Intervention* |
| --- | --- | --- |
| Glare | May distract older people, especially those who have difficulty concentrating | Reducing glare will make it easier to recognize faces, which may improve communication. |
| Dark/light adaptation | Delayed for the older person when moving from a light to a darker area or vice versa | Freeing the entrance of furniture or other objects will make it easier to move from light to dark areas. |
| Color perception | Decreased for the aged | If colors are being used to enhance orientation, contrasting colors should highlight only those areas that are important to the person. For example, the utility room door may be painted the same color as the wall and the bathroom door may be painted in a contrasting color.<br>Color contrast is helpful not only in public areas, but also in activities of daily living such as dressing. Other tasks can also be made easier by creating a contrast between objects such as a toothbrush and a sink, a handrail and a wall, and a plate and a tablecloth. |
| Depth perception | Decreases with age and is more dependent on brightness and contrast | With age, more attention must be given to floor surfaces and steps. Figure-ground illusions are created when patterns are used. For example, when a floor surface is patterned, it may appear to be an object or several objects. Older people who have a cognitive impairment may perceive patterns as objects but not be able to ask questions or otherwise determine which objects are truly present in an environment. |

Modified from Christenson MA: Adaptations for vision changes in older persons, *OT Practice* 1:1, 1996.

United States, with atherosclerosis accounting for 80% of those deaths.[9]

Cardiovascular conditions in the elderly include hypertension, congestive heart failure (CHF), arteriosclerotic heart disease (ASHD), valvular problems that may lead to the client using a pacemaker, peripheral vascular disease (PVD), and cardiac arrest.

### Pulmonary Conditions

The development of pulmonary disease in the elderly is determined by the maximum level of pulmonary function developed during early adulthood.[25] In other words, a young adult who exercises and does not smoke has a greater chance of maintaining healthy lungs through old age.

The most common pulmonary condition associated with old age is chronic obstructive pulmonary disease (COPD). COPD results in airflow obstruction and often hyperreactive airways, usually with bronchitis or emphysema.[24] COPD is a functional diagnosis that includes a variety of disease processes that affect the upper and lower respiratory tracts and are characterized by cough, expectoration, wheezing, and dyspnea, first on exercise and later at rest. These conditions may severely limit the person's stamina and endurance, thus impairing the ability to participate in self-care, work, and leisure activities.

### Musculoskeletal Conditions

Pathological changes that may develop as a person ages include osteoarthritis and osteoporosis. These conditions affect the joints. Decreased mobility, joint stiffness, and deformities contribute to difficulty participating in physical daily living activities.

### Endocrine System Conditions

The most prevalent disorder of the endocrine system in the aged is diabetes mellitus (DM). Diabetic neuropathy commonly results in segmental injury to nerves and may cause decreased sensation.

### Nervous System Conditions

Nervous system disorders include cerebrovascular accidents (CVAs), multiple sclerosis, Parkinson's disease, and reflex sympathetic dystrophy syndrome. These conditions severely affect the person's ability to perform activities of daily living (ADL).

### Sensory Changes

Sensory changes may include a decrease in visual acuity, hearing loss, changes in taste and smell, decreased proprioception, decreased sensory awareness, sensory processing and difficulties with perception, as well as deficits in the vestibular system.

#### *Vision*

Changes in vision may include glaucoma and cataracts. The older person may have difficulty adjusting to changes in light and may experience impaired depth perception. These conditions can severely limit the person's ability to engage in activities outside the home. See Table 33-1 for suggestions on how to modify the environment.

#### *Hearing*

Changes in hearing often affect a person socially as well as physically. Even a slight hearing loss can be emotionally upsetting, particularly if it interferes with understanding family, friends, or television. Hearing loss can lead to isolation, depression, and anxiety. People with impaired hearing may withdraw from group situations because listening is a chore.[16]

#### *Taste and Smell*

Declining ability to taste and smell food is compounded by disease or use of medications, both of which can adversely affect these senses. Changes in the taste mechanism include difficulty in perceiving and identifying odor. Smelling food is a large part of enjoying it. Because of these decrements, many older people do not eat enough food to meet their nutritional needs. In addition, changes in the sense of taste and smell may cause the person to eat spoiled food. This in turn can lead to poor health.

#### *Sensorimotor*

Sensorimotor changes may include a decrease in sensory awareness, sensory processing, and perceptual skills (see Chapters 11 and 24).

### Cognitive Changes

Some pathological conditions that occur more frequently in the elderly are dementias such as Alzheimer's (see Chapter 28), memory disorders, and delirium.

#### *Dementia*

Dementia is described as a structurally caused permanent or progressive decline in several dimensions of intellectual function that interferes substantially with the individual's normal social or economic activity. Conditions such as drug intoxication, hyperthyroidism, and insulin shock also result in symptoms of dementia. When these conditions are treated, the symptoms of dementia are usually resolved. There are several types of dementia frequently seen in the elderly, the most common being Alzheimer's type dementia. Memory loss is the most prominent early symptom. Multi-infarct dementia is more common in men and begins most frequently in the seventh decade. It tends to progress in a steplike manner, each step accompanied by intellectual worsening and perhaps the development or aggravation of neurological signs. In the early stages of the illness, personality and insight tend to be better preserved than in dementia of the Alzheimer's type. Depressive symptoms are common and suicide is possible. As the condition advances, neurological features may develop, especially hemiplegia, pseudobulbar palsy, pathological laughing and crying, or other signs of extrapyramidal dysfunction.[21]

### *Delirium*

Delirium is characterized by extreme disturbances of arousal, attention, orientation, perception, intellectual function, and affect; most are commonly accompanied by fear and agitation. It is occasionally seen with large right hemispheric parietal occipital infarcts in the elderly.[21]

### *Memory*

Memory disorders (see Chapters 11 and 24) are defined as partial or total inability to encode (process), store, or retrieve (recall) information. Encoding determines which stimuli are noticed or attended to and which ones are selected for storage. Storage concerns the saving of information. Retrieval concerns the recall of information from a memory store. Memory can be divided into the following three major psychological components: immediate—the past few seconds; intermediate—the period from a few seconds past to a few days before; and remote or long-term—extending further back in time.[21]

## COMMUNICATION TECHNIQUES

Because of the number and severity of conditions that affect the elderly, communication is especially important. Elderly patients may be of a different culture than the practitioner and often have strongly held values and beliefs derived from a lifetime of experiences. Occupational therapy practitioners constantly communicate with patients and others both verbally and nonverbally. Verbal communication is used to provide directions, explain a treatment method, or express an idea. Nonverbal communication such as smiles, frowns, and posture is used to reinforce or discourage a behavior or provide information regarding pleasure or displeasure.

How we communicate can enhance the occupational therapy process by providing the patient, the family, and other caregivers with information regarding what they should expect from the occupational therapy intervention and by allowing them to express their questions or fears in a nonthreatening environment. By explaining methods, suggesting alternatives, and giving the older person the opportunity to communicate with us, we empower them to participate in their treatment process (Box 33-1).

*Box 33-1*

**Six Techniques for Communicating**

In 1996, Cheryl Joiner and Mary Hansel described the following six techniques that can be used to enhance the communication process between therapist and patients.

1. *Use active listening techniques.* Let people know you are interested in what they have to say and that you want to fully understand them. Free the area of distractions. Positioning yourself at their level and making eye contact tells them that you are attentive. Once patients know that you are interested in them as people and care about their needs, they are often more willing to engage in therapy.
2. *Make a written or verbal contract.* The contract should specify the number of treatment sessions and the modalities involved. Contracting with patients helps them feel as though they are active participants in deciding how their treatment will be provided.
3. *Give choices.* No matter how trivial they may seem, choices are important. If possible, offer selections among predetermined modalities. This helps patients have more control over what happens to them.
4. *Problem solve to encourage involvement in the therapy process.* Encourage patients to brainstorm to reinforce their worth and primary importance in the treatment effort.
5. *Be consistent whenever possible.* Having the same practitioners and schedules helps patients feel secure. If a decision must be made to change therapists or treatment times, the patients must be informed before the change occurs.
6. *Educate.* Education helps patients feel more comfortable in the long-term care setting. Providing them with as much information as possible helps them to understand their illness and know what to expect from treatment. Some clients are not familiar with nursing homes and need instruction in routine policies and in their own rights.

Modified from Joiner C, Hansel M: Empowering the Geriatric Client, *OT Practice* 1:2, 1996.

### Communicating With Family

Family members are perhaps the most trusted individuals for many elderly persons. This trust is based on a common history. Occupational therapy practitioners can make use of these individuals when encouraging a patient to participate in the treatment process, when explaining a method for treatment, and when follow-through needs to be monitored by someone close to the patient.

In addition, new health care regulations require that both the nursing-home resident and family members be informed with respect to the type of intervention the resident receives. It is important for the COTA to develop skill in conveying information to the family.

When communicating with families, COTAs must be aware of the impact the patient's disability may have had on the family unit. Explanations should be given in lay terms. Jargon and medical terminology should be kept to a minimum and clearly explained. It is especially important that explanations be given respectfully. Remember, the purpose of communicating with the family is to enhance the treatment process.

## DEVELOPING APPROPRIATE OCCUPATIONAL THERAPY GOALS

Treatment planning can be a relatively easy process if a systematic approach is followed. This approach includes (1) the evaluation of performance areas, performance components, and performance context; (2) development of a plan of care that includes identified problems, long-term goals, short-term goals, and intervention strategies; (3) intervention according to the plan, and; (4) reassessment of progress or lack of progress and termination of services.

In occupational therapy, it is the responsibility of the registered occupational therapist (OTR) to determine when an evaluation is indicated. The OTR is also responsible for verifying the competency of the COTA in performing specific procedures. The OTR can assign the COTA specific performance areas or performance components to assess following a structured format. Although the OTR maintains the responsibility for the treatment plan, it can be a collaborative effort between both practitioners. OT practitioners have the responsibility to ensure that the treatment plan is clear and that the COTA has the knowledge and expertise to carry out the intervention program.

One of the challenges of working with the elderly is developing a treatment plan that addresses normal aging as overlaid with (often) several pathological conditions.

When developing treatment plans for patients with multiple diagnoses, the practitioner must be aware of how one diagnosis will affect another and of how one medication may affect or cause symptoms that interfere with functional abilities. For example, someone who is recovering from a CVA may also have a diagnosis of ASHD, CHF, and DM. If part of the treatment plan is to have the person perform light cooking or meal preparation, there may be a need for education on proper diet to deal with DM. It must be ensured that the patient takes rest periods as necessary to prevent shortness of breath and that the patient is able to recognize symptoms of CHF such as swelling of the feet. In addition, safety precautions with the use of kitchen knives is essential; a simple cut may take a longer period to heal because of the diabetes, thereby increasing the risk of infection.

The following case studies may help the reader integrate the information on practice models given in Chapter 3.

### *Case Study*

**Biomechanical model**

Mrs. S. is an 81-year-old woman with a diagnosis of DM, ASHD, and hypertension. She was recently hospitalized for CHF and has been discharged to a nursing home for rehabilitation. She now requires assistance with self-care activities as a result of generalized weakness. Mrs. S. is expected to return to the community.

The occupational therapy treatment plan includes the following goals:

1. Mrs. S. will be independent in dressing, grooming, and bathing.
   - She will be able to select, don, and doff her dress independently.
   - She will be able to brush her hair independently.
   - She will be able to reach for her clothing in the closet and grooming supplies in the cabinet independently.

The intervention plan includes the following:

1. Therapeutic activities to increase range of motion (ROM) of all joints
2. Progressive resistive exercises to increase muscle strength of bilateral upper extremities
3. Practice sessions in dressing, grooming, and bathing

### *Case Study*

**Rehabilitation model**

Mrs. C. is a 65-year-old woman with a diagnosis of COPD, arthritis, and hypertension. She lives at home with her three children, and her mother lives in the second floor apartment. Her mother is homebound and receives full-time home care. Mrs. C. stopped working as a bookkeeper 8 years ago and retired this year. Mrs. C. presents with +2 edema in both ankles, ROM within functional limits for all joints, and F–F+ muscle strength in both upper extremities. At this time, she exhibits a significant decrease in ADL participation. She does not go outside the house. She no longer visits her mother because of the difficulty going up the stairs. She is no longer participating in housekeeping activities.

The occupational therapy goals are the following:

1. Mrs. C. will engage in grooming, dressing, and bathing activities independently on a daily basis.
   - She will be able to retrieve clothing from the closet.
   - She will be able to wash her hair independently.
   - She will be able to enter the bathtub and shower independently.
2. Mrs. C. will engage in light housekeeping on a daily basis.
   - She will be out of bed for at least 3 hours in the morning and 3 hours in the afternoon.
   - She will make the bed in the morning on a daily basis.
   - She will dust at least one room per day.
   - She will wash and put away dishes at least one time per day.

- She will actively supervise the housekeeper on a daily basis.

3. Mrs. C. will engage in an exercise routine at least four times per week.
   - She will walk to the front stoop (approximately 100 feet) and pick up the mail daily.
   - She will visit with her mother at least once per day by going up one flight of stairs.
   - She will walk to the grocery store at least three times per week with another person (approximately 500 feet).
   - She will engage in isometric exercises three times per week.

The intervention plan includes the following:

1. Practice sessions in self-care skills
2. Provision of adaptive equipment to assist with housekeeping, bathing, and grocery shopping
3. Training in energy conservation and work simplification activities
4. Instruction in health maintenance and safety

## TREATMENT SETTINGS

### Occupational Therapy Assistant Role in Long-Term Care

According to the Bureau of the Census,[6] in 1990 there were 31,241,831 people aged 65 years and over in the United States. This segment of the population is currently growing faster than any other and will continue to grow through the year 2030 when the baby boom cohort will be aged 65 or over. The number of elderly will have doubled to over 65 million people.[11]

Occupational therapy practitioners have responded not only by increasing the numbers of practitioners working with the elderly (Table 33-2) but also by developing a variety of programs to deal with their changing needs. The elderly patient may be seen in a continuum of environments including the home, extended care facilities, day care centers, senior centers, and nursing homes. These programs are considered to be part of long-term care services. Long-term care refers to services provided over a long period of time to persons with chronic illnesses who need assistance with regular everyday activities such as eating, bathing, and getting dressed. Long-term care can be provided in the home (for example, by a visiting nurse), in the community (e.g., as adult day care), or an institution (e.g., nursing home).

*Table 33-2*

**Number of OT Practitioners Working in Long-Term Care Settings***

| Year | OTR | COTA |
|---|---|---|
| 1986 | 5.8% | 20.1% |
| 1996 | 18.2% | 42.2% |

Modified from Americal Occupational Therapy Association: *Member survey*, Bethesda, Md, 1996, The Association.
*Skilled nursing facility/intermediate care facility.

Long-term services and support encompass a wide spectrum, including assistance with basic activities and routines of daily living, such as bathing, dressing, meal preparation, and housekeeping as well as facilitating full functioning in family, work, school, and leisure. Long-term services may also include skilled and therapeutic care for the treatment and management of chronic conditions.[3]

The COTA or OTR might also coordinate services or provide case management to assist clients in using long-term services and supports. OT practitioners are qualified to provide specialized services such as training and consultation on the use of assistive technology and modification of homes and other environments.[3]

The COTA, under the supervision of the OTR, can provide services to the patients in any of the settings described below after an OTR has conducted an evaluation and established a treatment plan. The COTA may treat residents on site without the physical presence of the occupational therapist (assuming state or other local jurisdictions permit this). The COTA provides treatment activities to improve abilities in identified performance areas and components with the final goal of returning the patient to the optimal level of independent functioning within the home. The COTA may administer standardized tests in a noninterpretive manner with the OTR's supervision once service competence has been established. Other aspects of the COTA's role include assisting in ADL evaluation, ordering equipment, providing adaptations to equipment and the environment, and training caregivers.[2]

### Day Care Centers

**Adult day care** is a program of care during the day for the impaired adult in a group setting away from home. Although in many ways these adults will be like the aged who attend senior centers, they are more handicapped by physical, mental, or social problems and sometimes require rehabilitation services not offered in senior centers.[20]

### Home Health Care

**Home and community care** for functionally disabled elderly individuals generally is defined as care provided to financially eligible people 65 years of age or over who require substantial human assistance in performing two of three specified ADL. Individuals with Alzheimer's disease may qualify for the program under somewhat more liberal eligibility criteria (requiring assistance in two of five specified ADL or being sufficiently cognitively impaired as to require substantial supervision because of inappropriate behaviors that pose serious health or safety hazards to themselves or others). Home and community care includes homemaker, home health aide, chore, and personal care services; nursing care services provided by or under the supervision of a registered nurse; respite care; training for family members in managing the individual; adult day care; and for the chronically mentally ill, day treatment partial hospitalization, psychosocial rehabilitation services, and clinic services.[12]

### Assisted Living

**Assisted living** is an innovative approach to meeting the housing and care needs of frail older persons and individuals with disabilities in a residential rather than an institutional environment, while maximizing independence, choice, and privacy.

Assisted living is defined as a group residential program that is not licensed as a nursing home, that provides personal care to persons with needs for assistance in ADL (bathing, dressing, feeding, transferring, toileting, continence), and that can respond to unscheduled needs for assistance. For many individuals with modest to substantial care needs, assisted living offers an alternative to nursing homes and board and care homes.

### Subacute Care

**Subacute care** is defined as a comprehensive inpatient program designed for the individual who has had an acute event as a result of an illness, injury, or exacerbation of a disease process, has a determined course of treatment, and does not require intensive diagnostic and invasive procedures. The severity of the individual's condition requires an outcome-focused interdisciplinary approach using a professional team to deliver complex clinical interventions (medical and rehabilitation).

The majority of residents in subacute care settings will have conditions with diagnoses generally associated with rehabilitation, such as stroke, orthopedic procedures (including joint replacements), general and degenerative neurological disorders (including multiple sclerosis, muscular dystrophy, Parkinson's disease), amputations, severe arthritis, neuromuscular disorders, and general debilitation.

### Nursing Homes

Nursing homes are residential facilities that provide skilled nursing care, rehabilitative services, or health-related care on a daily basis to individuals who are injured, disabled, or sick. Services include those that are given to an individual who needs daily basic nursing care or other rehabilitative services that can be provided practically only in a nursing facility on an inpatient basis. These include nursing and related services; specialized rehabilitative services; medically related social services; and activities to attain or maintain to the fullest extent possible the physical, mental, and psychosocial well-being of each resident.[12]

## MEDICARE, MEDICAID, AND THE RESIDENT ASSESSMENT INSTRUMENT

### Medicare

The Medicare program helps pay medical costs for people 65 years and older and about 3 million disabled people. Medicare Part A covers inpatient hospital services, home health services, and other institution-based services. Part B covers physician, outpatient hospital, and various other health services such as diagnostic tests. Practitioners should check with individual state Medicare providers because guidelines are frequently changed.

### Medicaid

Medicaid is a federally aided, state-administered medical assistance program intended, among other things, to provide the poor with access to health care. The services provided by the Medicaid program include inpatient and outpatient hospital, home health, physician, and skilled nursing facility services.

### Resident Assessment Instrument

At this time, Medicare is in the process of developing a joint assessment form and reimbursement strategy with Medicaid. With this program, long-term care reimbursement rates will be based on patient grouping called *Case Mix.* The Case-Mix classification system is called the *Resource-Utilization Groups (RUGs III).* Both Medicaid and Medicare patients will be grouped on the basis of the level of care needed when a patient enters a long-term care program.[14]

Patients entering long-term care will be assessed using the Resident Assessment Instrument (RAI) (Box 33-2), which is a congressionally mandated resident assessment tool used to conduct a comprehensive assessment of all residents in federally certified nursing homes. It includes the **minimum data set** (MDS) and the **resident assessment protocols** (RAPs). The MDS provides data for classifying residents into RUG III groups. The RAPs provide guidelines for the clinician to assess the patient, concentrating on conditions that affect physical, cognitive, and psychosocial functioning. The RAPs selected for inclusion in the RAI are clinical entities (such as falls) frequently encountered by caregivers in nursing home settings.

## COMMUNICATING WITH SUPERVISORS

Nursing home practice in the United States has seen a rapid change in the way occupational therapy services are provided. Before 1990, when the Omnibus Budget Reconciliation Act of 1987 (OBRA 87) became law, many occupational therapy programs in nursing homes were staffed by COTAs with OTR consultants.

Box 33-2

**How the Resident Assessment Instrument is Used in Clinical Practice**

A. Perform initial assessment with RAI.
   1. Perform a comprehensive assessment encompassing completion of the MDS and problem identification RAPs.
   2. Develop a care plan.
B. Begin to deliver care.
   1. Implement a care plan.
   2. Evaluate care provided; reassess based on time frames for each goal/approach to care established in the care plan.
   3. Modify plan of care as necessary.
C. Review resident status.
   1. Review resident status at least every 3 months (quarterly review) to ensure that assessment remains accurate, revising plan of care as necessary.
D. Perform reassessment with RAI.
   1. Reassessments (including MDS and RAPs) are conducted according to the utilization guidelines.
   2. Identify problems using RAPs.
   3. Evaluate whether care plan addresses current needs of resident.
   4. Review and revise the care plan as needed.

From Lee S, Dichter B: The multistate nursing home case mix and quality demonstration, 1996, Eliot Press.

This model required that the COTA coordinate the occupational therapy service with the OTR providing overall supervision. The recent requirement that restorative occupational therapy services be provided only while the OTR is on the premises has changed this model, because the COTA now has more frequent access to OTR supervision. This change, however, has not necessarily increased the amount of time the COTA has to discuss issues with the OTR or the frequency of supervisory meetings. The current health care trend to reimburse for direct services only minimizes the time available for supervisory meetings.

All of these changes, coupled with the increased expectation that occupational therapy programs be outcome oriented, challenge occupational therapy practitioners to maintain communication. Clarity is important. The COTA must have a clear job description and must develop clear and effective communication strategies in collaboration with the OTR.

One effective strategy for communicating with supervisors is using a "communication book." In this book, both practitioners jot down concerns, questions, or information important to the other. Both practitioners review the book daily and are able to respond to concerns either in writing or in person. This method reduces the risk of forgetting something.

## COMMUNICATING WITH OTHER PROFESSIONALS

COTAs are expected to communicate with other professionals within the facility, including nurses, social workers, physical therapists, speech pathologists, and others.

Communication often involves the COTA demonstrating or teaching specific methods for working with the patient to nursing assistants. It may mean teaching passive ROM, splint application, or the use of an assistive device. Communication with others may also include gathering information about how a resident is able to manage a specific activity, finding out the funding source for the resident, or participating in treatment planning meetings.

## ENVIRONMENTAL SAFETY/FALL PREVENTION AND THE RESTRAINT-FREE ENVIRONMENT

### Fall Prevention

Falling is the most common cause of fatal injury in the elderly according to the National Safety Council. Moreover, thousands are left permanently disabled from falls, most often by hip fractures. About 300,000 Americans—most of them elderly—fracture their hips each year. About 20% of those individuals die within 1 year of the fracture, according to government statistics. This type of injury can transform an active person into a bedridden one. The National Osteoporosis Foundation reports that half of all people with hip fractures who could walk without assistance before the accident cannot walk independently afterward. Of those injured, 41% need nursing home care during their rehabilitation.[22]

Elderly people are highly susceptible to falls because of health problems such as arthritis, poor eyesight and hearing, frailty, poor balance and coordination, senility, dementia, and weakness or dizziness caused by medications.[22]

In 1994, Brungardt[5] described the following as increasing the risk factor for falls in the elderly: mental status factors including disorientation, depression, and dementia; medical factors including more than one disease, acute illness, or orthostatic hypotension; sensory factors including a change in vision, vestibular or proprioceptive dysfunction; musculoskeletal factors including increased activity, decreased mobility, foot disorders, and cervical disk disease; neurological factors including changes in gait and peripheral neuropathy; environmental factors including stairs, undifferentiated steps, slippery surfaces, poor lighting, and unexpected obstacles; and other factors including confinement, history of falls, and ill-fitting shoes.

Occupational therapy practitioners participate in the fall prevention program by assessing and developing a plan of care for residents who are at high risk for falls.

The occupational therapy assessment includes information on the sensorimotor, cognitive, and psychological performance components.

The COTA, in conjunction with the OTR, assists in developing a plan of care geared toward the remediation of deficits or compensation for any loss of function.

Occupational therapy practitioners provide intervention in environmental safety and fall prevention by assessing residents in the context of their environment. Intervention includes the remediation of deficits, instruction in compensatory techniques, and the provision of adaptive equipment such as reachers, stocking aids, or carts for carrying heavy loads.

OT practitioners also assess and plan intervention in home design and modification. Modifications may include the removal of obstacles such as throw rugs, the rearrangement of cabinets to place heavier things on the bottom rather than on top shelves, and bathroom aids such as a call bell, bathtub seat, grab bars, and raised toilet seats (Figure 33-1).

## *Case Study*

**Fall prevention**

Mrs. G. is an 86-year-old woman who sustained a hip fracture 2 weeks ago and was admitted to the nursing home for rehabilitative care. Mrs. G.'s family hopes to be able to take her home as soon as she is able to walk again. It is Mrs. G.'s and her family's hope that she will be able to continue to participate in social activities such as going to the senior center, and to perform physical ADL such as dressing, grooming, bathing, and light meal preparation. Mrs. G. lives alone in a barrier-free (i.e., no steps) senior citizen building. Before the fall she was independent in all self-care activities and traveled frequently by bus.

During her hospitalization, Mrs. G. underwent a right total hip replacement. Because of her diabetes, healing was slow and despite her being able to bear weight on the right leg she had to be confined to bed during the first week to promote healing of the surgical scar. During her hospitalization, Mrs. G. spent the days alone and was visited by family and friends in the late afternoon and evening.

On admission to the nursing home, Mrs. G. was assessed as being disoriented, unable to participate in any self-care activity except eating, and unable to transfer from the bed independently. She had decreased ROM on the right hip and exhibited poor endurance and impaired postural control. She was incontinent and nonambulatory. Because of her disorientation, Mrs. G. made several attempts to climb out of bed, and there was fear that she might fall and reinjure herself.

Each discipline assessed Mrs. G. and a plan of care was instituted. The recreational staff formulated and implemented an activity plan that included arts and crafts and social activities. The occupational therapy staff was able to suggest activities that included both mental and physical stimulation. The nursing and social service staff provided reality orientation and encouragement for continued participation in therapy and activities.

The occupational therapy evaluation included an assessment of Mrs. G.'s physical and daily living skills including dressing, grooming, and bathing. The sensorimotor evaluation included assessment of ROM, muscle strength, endurance, transfer skills, and mobility. The cognitive evaluation included assessment of orientation, ability to follow directions, and ability to conceptualize safety issues.

The occupational therapy plan included increasing ROM, muscle strength and endurance, topographical orientation, and mobility while at the same time providing practice sessions in self-care activities such as dressing, bathing, grooming, and transfer training.

As Mrs. G.'s mental and physical status improved, she was increasingly able to make her own decisions and was able to work with the OT staff to develop an activity schedule to be followed at home. She was able to describe her apartment and where her furniture was located and was able to make decisions about what could and could not be moved. She participated in the rearrangement of her home to eliminate obstacles and increase safety. Mrs. G. was discharged from the nursing home and was referred to a home health service that provided occupational therapy. The home-care occupational therapist was able to assist Mrs. G. in readjusting to community life by assessing her ability to perform self-care activities and use public transportation and by offering suggestions for modifying the home.

### Restraint Use

OBRA 87 made restraint use the exception rather than the rule. The law requires nursing homes to provide quality care and quality of life for each resident. This includes maintaining the well-being of each resident and ensuring (to the greatest practical extent) a good quality of life by providing services and activities.

**Physical restraints** were defined as any manual method or physical or mechanical device, material, or equipment attached or adjacent to the resident's body that the individual cannot remove easily; they restrict freedom of movement or normal access to the body.

Physical restraints are devices that restrict independent movement, including vests, belts, wheelchair seat belts, wheelchairs, hand mitts, wheelchair safety bars, bed rails, and other devices used to position a resident.

#### *Risks of Restraint Use*

Haddad[13] in 1994 described several risks of restraint use. The resident may become agitated and more

**Patient** ______________________ **Age** ______ **Room** ______________________

**Triggered Problems** ______________________

Assessment goals are (1) to ensure that a treatment plan is in place for patients with history of falls, and (2) to identify patients who are at risk for falls and are not currently enrolled in a fall prevention program.

1. Is there a previous history of falls? Yes _____ No _____
2. Was the fall an isolated event? Yes _____ No _____

**Internal Risk Factors**

| **Does patient have?** | **YES** | **NO** |
|---|---|---|
| Cardiovascular abnormalities | | |
| Cardiac dysrhythmia | | |
| Hypotension | | |
| Syncope | | |
| Neuromuscular | | |
| Cerebrovascular accident | | |
| Hemiplegia | | |
| Unsteady gait | | |
| Incontinence | | |
| Seizure disorder | | |
| Parkinson's disease | | |
| Chronic/acute condition causing instability | | |
| Loss of leg or arm movement | | |
| Decline in functional status | | |
| Orthopedic impairments | | |
| Arthritis | | |
| Osteoporosis | | |
| Joint pain | | |
| Hip fracture | | |
| Perceptual abnormalities | | |
| Impaired hearing | | |
| Dizziness or vertigo | | |
| Psychiatric or cognitive impairments | | |
| Alzheimer's | | |
| Decline in cognitive skills | | |
| Delirium | | |
| Manic depression | | |
| Other dementia | | |

*Figure 33-1* Sample of a falls protocol worksheet.

*Continued.*

**External Factors**

| | YES | NO |
|---|---|---|
| Medications | | |
| Psychotropic medications | | |
| Cardiovascular medications | | |
| Diuretics | | |
| Where medication administered before fall | | |
| Where medication administered after the fall | | |

If medications were administered before the fall, how much time before the fall were they first administered? ______________

List all medications and note possible side effects ______________________________________________

______________________________________________

______________________________________________

______________________________________________

**Appliance and Devices**

| | YES | NO |
|---|---|---|
| Pacemaker | | |
| Walker or cane | | |
| Physical restraints | | |
| Other | | |
| Restraints before fall | | |

Observe patient's use of the device for possible problems and describe performance ______________________________

______________________________________________

______________________________________________

**Environmental and Situational Hazards**

| | YES | NO |
|---|---|---|
| Glare | | |
| Poor illumination | | |
| Slippery floors | | |
| Uneven floors | | |
| Patterned carpets | | |
| Objects in walkway | | |
| Recent move | | |
| New arrangement of objects | | |
| Proximity of aggressive residents | | |
| Type of activity | | |
| Standing still/walking | | |
| In a crowded area | | |
| Responding to bladder/bowel urgency | | |
| Reaching/not reaching | | |

*Figure 33-1, cont'd* Sample of a falls protocol worksheet.

Is there a pattern of falls in any of the above circumstances (environmental and situational hazards)?

If you know what the resident was doing during the fall, have resident repeat the activity and observe

**Vital Signs**

Measure patient's blood pressure and heart rate:

Supine

1 minute after standing

3 minutes after standing

**Resident Interaction with the Environment**

Observe resident and check "able or not able" and "safe or unsafe."

| Activity | Able | Not able | Safe | Unsafe |
|---|---|---|---|---|
| Moving in and out of bed | | | | |
| Walking | | | | |
| Turning | | | | |
| Transferring | | | | |
| Toileting | | | | |

**IDENTIFIED PROBLEMS**

**Suggested Multidisciplinary Treatment Interventions**

**Nursing**

**OT/PT**

*Figure 33-1, cont'd* For legend see opposite page.

*Continued.*

**Activities** ______________________________________________

______________________________________________

______________________________________________

**Medical** ______________________________________________

______________________________________________

______________________________________________

______________________________________________

**Social Services** ______________________________________________

______________________________________________

______________________________________________

______________________________________________

*Figure 33-1, cont'd* Sample of a falls protocol worksheet.

disoriented. The resident might be embarrassed, which would diminish self-esteem. Restrained residents may experience increased injuries while attempting to break free from the restraints. The resident may suffer the effects of immobility, including skin breakdown, decreased circulation, and incontinence. The nursing staff may end up with more work, not less, if the resident becomes injured while trying to remove the restraints, or develops skin and other problems from restraint use.

### *Occupational Therapy Role*

Many facilities require that an occupational therapy evaluation be completed before using or removing a physical restraint. The evaluation will determine the resident's positioning needs and transfer skills, as well as other needs associated with the resident's ability to safely negotiate the environment. There are many instances in which residents are restrained because they slide out of the wheelchair. The clinician will need to assess whether this is caused by an inappropriate seating system, inappropriate wheelchair, or whether there are other physiological, neurological, or orthopedic reasons that cause the resident to slide forward.

In evaluating and reconsidering the use of restraints for a resident, the practitioner must consider the needs of the resident, as well as any problems, conditions, and risk factors. The clinician must be able to explain why the restraint is being used; the type of restraint being used; when, where, for how long, and under what circumstances the restraint is being used; and who suggested the restraint. It may be possible to eliminate the restraint if the underlying problem is identified and resolved. If the restraint is being used to control a behavior, the clinician must bear in mind that many behaviors are caused by unmet needs and can often be eliminated by having those needs met. The MDS restraint protocol guidelines include a review of the resident's record and the condition associated with restraint use, which includes problem behaviors, risk of falls, and treatment regimens. The MDS protocol also includes conditions under which a restraint may be used, and these include enhancement of independent ADL performance.

### *Alternatives to Restraints*

Alternatives to restraints include restorative and maintenance programs, supportive devices, enhanced environment, and a variety of staff approaches.

*Restorative programs* **Restorative programs** are individualized programs that address and remediate underlying conditions such as proprioceptive deficits, balance problems, mobility problems, positioning problems, and ADL problems.[17]

*Maintenance programs* **Maintenance programs** are designed to maintain the resident at the highest possible level by providing exercise and cognitive programs as well as activity programs.[17]

*Enhanced environments* **Enhanced environments** may include changes in the resident's room and immediate environment such as color coding walls, arranging furniture to reduce obstacles, decreasing glare in corridors, labeling doors, reducing noise, providing conversational seating, and allowing furnishings to be brought from the home.[17]

*Staff approaches* All staff should be trained to support each resident. Staff should learn what residents want and how to meet their needs. Some staff will be better at interacting with residents or a particular resident than others.[17]

## SUMMARY

Aging is a complex process that begins as soon as the individual is conceived. Health and disease, however, determine the quality of life individuals will have as they reach maturity.

It is important to view illness separately from reduced abilities. Although some diseases are more common in the elderly, this should not be confused with normal aging.

Occupational therapy practitioners must have an understanding of the developmental needs of the elderly person. In addition, practitioners must be aware of what constitutes normal aging and how superimposed pathological conditions affect the elderly person. The practitioner must be cognizant of cultural differences and be able to communicate information clearly.

COTAs collaborate with the OTR in developing treatment plans for the elderly resident. Under the supervision of the OTR COTAs may perform a variety of assessments following a structured format. When developing treatment plans for elderly clients with multiple diagnoses, the clinician must be aware of how one diagnosis will affect another and of how one medication may affect or cause symptoms that interfere with functional abilities.

Occupational therapy practitioners may work in a variety of settings within the long-term care continuum. These settings may include day care centers, the home, assisted living centers, subacute care units, and nursing homes.

Occupational therapy services may be funded under a variety of programs including Medicare and Medicaid. Elderly clients residing at federally or state-funded nursing facilities receive a comprehensive, multidisciplinary assessment—the RAI. This assessment process includes the completion of the MDS form and the development of a multidisciplinary treatment plan. Occupational therapy practitioners are involved in facility-wide, federally mandated programs such as fall prevention and the promotion and assessment of and environmental adaptations that promote a restraint-free environment.

## *Case Study*

**Multidiagnosis**

The resident is a 70-year-old woman admitted with a diagnosis of right CVA, CHF, ASHD. At this time, the resident is residing in a nursing home with no plans for discharge home.

Before hospitalization, she was living with a niece in the community. She was able to participate in light housekeeping, attended a senior citizen center four times each week, participated in frequent family get-togethers, attended church on Sundays, and socialized with neighbors. The patient reports that she always liked to dress nicely and often shopped through catalogs. At this time, she is able to make some of her needs known. She requires minimal assistance for a stand pivot transfer. She is able to groom herself after set up. She is able to feed herself with adaptive equipment and after tray preparation by staff. She requires moderate assistance with dressing.

*Performance area deficits: ADL*

1. Requires assistance to transfer from wheelchair to bed and toilet and back
2. Unable to reach toothbrush and toothpaste on sink
3. Unable to cut meats and to open sugar and milk container during meals
4. Unable to reach clothing in closet
5. Unable to fasten shoes
6. Unable to don stockings
7. Unable to dress without assistance

*Performance component deficits: sensorimotor*

1. Limited ROM in left shoulder
2. Flaccid left upper extremity
3. Decreased endurance
4. Decreased postural control

*Performance context*

1. Change of living environment
2. Decreased opportunity to socialize with friends and relatives

*Occupational therapy treatment plan: long-term goals (for resident)*

1. Will be independent with transfer from wheelchair to bed and toilet and back, grooming, feeding, and dressing
2. Will exhibit ROM within functional limits of left shoulder
3. Will be able to bear weight on left upper extremity
4. Will demonstrate segmentation when transitioning from one position to another
5. Will be able to maintain upright sitting on wheelchair for at least 4 hours at a time
6. Will develop new leisure-time skills

*Occupational therapy intervention plan*

1. Passive and then active ROM of left upper extremity
2. Weight-bearing activities for left upper and lower extremities
3. Rotational exercises for trunk
4. Practice sessions on one-handed self-care including dressing, grooming, and feeding
5. Practice sessions on wheelchair mobility
6. Leisure skills exploration
7. Provision of adaptive equipment as needed

## REFERENCES


1. American Occupational Therapy Association: *Member survey,* Bethesda, Md, 1996, The Association.
2. American Occupational Therapy Association: Teamwork, personnel issues, and supervision in the home setting. In *Guidelines for occupational therapy practice in home health,* Rockville, Md, 1995, The Association.
3. American Occupational Therapy Association: Position paper: Occupational therapy and long-term services and supports, *Am J Occup Ther* 48:1035, 1994.

4. Berger KS: *The developing person through the life span,* ed 3, New York, 1994, Worth.
5. Brungardt GS: Patient restraints: new guidelines for a less restrictive approach, *Geriatrics,* 49:44, 1994.
6. Bureau of the Census: *Age by sex for all persons in the U.S. in 1990,* Summary tape file, 1991, America Online.
7. Caplan LR: Neurology. In Rowe JW, Besdine RW, editors: *Health and disease in old age,* 1982, Little, Brown.
8. Christenson MA: Adaptations for vision changes in older persons, *OT Practice* 1:30-31, 1996.
9. Damjanov I: *Pathology for the health related professions,* Philadelphia, 1996, WB Saunders.
10. Flynn JE, Mabry ER: Biophysical development of later adulthood. In Schuster CS, Asbum, SS: *The process of human development,* ed 2, Canada, 1986, Little, Brown.
11. Fulks JS: *Putting a definition to aging,* Document Number: 285072485, Department of Family and Human Development, Utah State University, 1993, America Online.
12. Gurny P, Hirsch MB, Gondek KE: A description of medicaid covered services, *Health Care Financing Rev* 1:1, 1992.
13. Haddad A: Acute care decisions—ethics in action, *RN* 57:19, 1994.
14. Health Care Financing Administrations: *Nursing home case—mix and quality demonstration medicare skilled nursing facility (SNF) supplementary provider manual,* 1995, The Administrations.
15. Joiner C, Hansel M: Empowering the geriatric client, *OT Practice* 1:2, 1996.
16. Kessel G: Visual problems can become social problems, Document Number: 800111501, West Virginia University Extension Service, 1995, AOL.
17. Lee S, Dichter B: *The multistate nursing home case mix and quality demonstration manual,* 1992, Eliot Press.
18. Lewis SC: *Elder care in occupational therapy,* Thorofare, NJ, 1989, Slack.
19. Naylor M: *Changing views on adult development: an ERIC digest publication,* Document Number: 285072634, 1993.
20. Padula H: Developing day care for older people, *Tech Assist Monogr,* 1972.
21. *The Merck Manual,* ed 15, Rahway, NJ, 1987, Merck, Sharp, & Dohme.
22. Roan S: A serious slip for the elderly, *Los Angeles Times,* Tuesday May 10, 1994, Home Edition, Life & Style.
23. Schuster CS, Ashburn SS: *The process of human development—a holistic life-span approach,* ed 2, 1986, Little Brown.
24. Snyder GL: Defining chronic obstructive pulmonary disease. In Caverley P, Pride N, eds: *Chronic obstructive pulmonary disease,* London, 1996, Chapman & Hall.
25. Weiss ST: Pulmonary system. In Rowe JW, Besdine RW, editors: *Health and disease in old age,* 1982, Little Brown.

## RECOMMENDED READING

American Occupational Therapy Association: Occupational therapy services for persons with Alzheimer's disease and other dementias, *Am J Occup Ther* 48:1029-31, 1994.

American Occupational Therapy Association: Uniform terminology for occupational therapy—third edition, *Am J Occup Ther* 48:1043-59, 1994.

Barney KF: From Ellis Island to assisted living: meeting the needs of older adults from diverse cultures. *Am J Occup Ther* 45(7):594-606, 1991.

Cook EA, Luschen L, Sikes S: Dressing training for an elderly woman with cognitive and perceptual impairments. *Am J Occup Ther* 45(7):652-654, 1991.

Reed KL: *Quick reference to occupational therapy,* Gaithersburg, Md, 1991, Aspen.

Trace S, Howell T: Occupational therapy in geriatric mental health, *Am J Occup Ther* 45(9):933-837, 1991.

## Selected Reading Guide Questions

1. List three theories that address the developmental needs of the elderly.
2. Describe four conditions that affect the aged.
3. List four sensory changes commonly seen in the aged.
4. Define cognition.
5. Define dementia.
6. Describe three practice models used when working with multidiagnosis patients.
7. Describe four treatment settings in which the COTA may provide services to the aged.
8. Describe one method that may be used to prevent falls in the elderly.
9. Define restraints.
10. List the risks of restraint use.
11. Describe three types of programs that may be used to prevent restraint use.
12. Describe the importance of communicating with the family.
13. Describe one method of communicating with a supervisor.
14. Name and discuss six techniques that can be used to communicate with patients.
15. What is the Resident Assessment Instrument?
16. What is the Minimum Data Set?
17. Define RAPs.
18. Who is responsible for completing the MDS?
19. Name the components of the comprehensive care plan.

# Chapter 34

# Motor Unit Dysfunction

Guy L. McCormack
Lorraine Williams Pedretti
Regina M. Lehman

## Chapter Objectives

*After studying this chapter, the student or practitioner will be able to:*

1. Describe the causes of lesions that result in motor unit dysfunction.
2. Name the clinical conditions that are characterized as motor unit dysfunction.
3. Identify the clinical manifestations of motor unit dysfunction conditions.
4. Contrast the goals and methods of occupational therapy treatment programs for the various motor unit conditions.

## Key Terms

motor unit
neurogenic
myopathic
lower motor neuron dysfunction
poliomyelitis
contracture
postpolio syndrome
Guillian-Barré syndrome
peripheral nerve injury
atrophy
regeneration
pain syndrome
myasthenia gravis
muscular dystrophies

The **motor unit** is the elementary functional unit in the motor system.[34] Its components are the motor neurons and the muscle fibers that it innervates.[28] Diseases of the motor unit generally cause muscle weakness and atrophy of skeletal muscle and may be **neurogenic** (originating in the nerves) or **myopathic** (originating in the muscle). Neurogenic disorders affect the nerve cell bodies or the peripheral nerves. Myopathic diseases affect the neuromuscular junction or the muscle itself.[34] These conditions are commonly seen in clinical practice and the certified occupational therapy assistant (COTA) should be familiar with their symptoms, course, and treatment.

## NEUROGENIC DISORDERS: LOWER MOTOR NEURON DYSFUNCTION

A lesion to any of the neurological structures of the lower motor neuron system will result in **lower motor neuron dysfunction.**[9,34] Lesions can result from (1) nerve root compression; (2) trauma—bone fractures and dislocations, lacerations, traction, penetrating wounds, and friction; (3) toxins—lead, phosphorus, alcohol, benzene, and sulfonamides; (4) infections—poliomyelitis, Guillain-Barré syndrome; (5) neoplasms—neuromas and multiple neurofibromatosis; (6) vascular disorders—arteriosclerosis, diabetes mellitus, peripheral vascular anomalies, and polyarteritis nodosa; (7) degenerative diseases of the central nervous systems—amyotrophic lateral sclerosis; and (8) congenital malformations.[10,18,45,50]

### Poliomyelitis

The active immunization program (using the Salk and Sabin vaccines) in the United States since the mid-1950s has essentially eradicated poliomyelitis in the western hemisphere; new cases are rare.[45,53] However, some new cases have been identified among those who have not been immunized. Adults who had poliomyelitis in early life in the United States and those from countries that lacked the benefits of immunization and rehabilitation, are referred to occupational therapy for vocational evaluation or improvement of quality of life.[41,50]

**Poliomyelitis** is a contagious viral disease that affects the anterior horn cells of the gray matter of the spinal cord and the motor nuclei of the brainstem. The cervical and lumbar enlargements of the cord are primarily affected. It results in a flaccid paralysis that may be local or widespread. The lower extremities, accessory muscles of respiration, and muscles that promote swallowing are primarily affected, but there may be upper extremity involvement as well. Marked atrophy may be seen in the involved extremities, and deep tendon reflexes may be absent. Because poliomyelitis destroys the anterior horn cells, sensory roots are spared and sensation is intact. **Contractures** (permanent shortening of the muscles, tendons, ligaments) can occur very early in the course of the disease. In cases of local paralysis, the asymmetry of muscles pulling on various joints may promote deformities, such as subluxation, scoliosis, and contractures. In severe cases, osteoporosis (bone atrophy) may weaken the long weight-bearing bones (tibia and femur) and pathological fractures can occur.[26]

The medical treatment for poliomyelitis during the acute phase includes bed rest, positioning, and applications of warm packs to reduce pain and promote relaxation. Because there is no known cure for poliomyelitis, the disease must run its course. There is an incubation period of 1 to 3 weeks; the recovery is dependent on the number of nerve cells remaining intact. Paralysis may begin in 1 to 7 days after the initial symptoms. The medical aspects of rehabilitation may include reconstructive surgery such as tendon transfer, arthrodesis, and surgical release of fascia, muscles, and tendons. Other rehabilitation measures may include therapeutic stretching, casts, muscle reeducation, orthoses, and bracing for standing or stability.[20]

#### *Occupational Therapy Intervention*

The poliomyelitis virus is infectious during the acute stage of the disease. It is therefore essential that isolation procedures be carefully followed by all medical and therapy personnel who have contact with the patient. During this phase, the patient is confined to bed and treated symptomatically. Hot packs and bed positioning are used to relieve muscle spasms and to prevent contractures and deformity. Bed positioning needs are assessed by the physical or occupational therapist with consultation from nursing. The main goals of bed positioning are to prevent contractures and protect weakened muscles. The therapist or assistant should provide gentle passive range of motion (PROM) to the extremities at the patient's physical tolerance level. Care should be taken not to grasp the involved muscle bellies because they will be extremely tender and painful. The muscles may also be prone to spasm when painfully stimulated.[41]

Muscle fatigue, which can result in further weakness, should be avoided. If the patient has bulbar poliomyelitis, which affects the muscles of respiration, a respirator may be used or a tracheostomy performed to provide an airway. If the muscles necessary for swallowing are impaired, tube feeding may also be prescribed. The registered occupational therapist (OTR) or COTA should collaborate with the nursing staff when carrying out treatment to ensure proper functioning of the equipment necessary for the life support.[8,20,23,41]

Psychological support for both the patient and family should be a part of the treatment program. The patient's fears and anxieties about the disabling effects of the disease should not be underestimated. The patient may need encouragement and positive experiences to promote an optimistic outlook during the rehabilitation process. The family may also need assistance in adjusting to the patient's disability. The OTR or COTA should address these psychosocial issues with both the patient and the family during treatment. Additional support may be secured through a referral to the psychology service in the rehabilitation facility.

As the rehabilitation process progresses, the precautions against physical and body fatigue continue. Assistive devices, splints, and mobile arm supports may be used to gain independence in the activities of daily living (ADL). After the acute medical problems have subsided, the recovery stage may last as long as 2 years.[8] Because the damage to the anterior horn cells is permanent, the clinician should assist the patient in making the best possible use of whatever muscular function remains. Before treatment is started, an evaluation of the existing disability must be made. A thorough manual muscle test, performed by the occupational therapist, provides a baseline for measuring gains in muscle strength and detects joint deformities caused by contractures. Manual muscle tests should be repeated monthly for the first 4 months and bimonthly for the next 4 months. After 8 months of therapeutic exercises the average patient has probably responded maximally.[6,18]

Movement for the patient who is recovering from acute poliomyelitis proceeds from PROM to active ROM (AROM), depending on the patient's level of voluntary control. Muscle reeducation should be preceded by gentle stretching exercises. All active motions should be performed under careful supervision of the therapist or assistant. Compensatory movement should be avoided. A limited but correct movement is preferred to a larger but incorrect movement. Active movements should be done in front of a mirror so that the patient may observe and correct motions accordingly.[20,23,42]

Muscle reeducation is accomplished in a graded fashion. At first the patient should learn "muscle-setting" exercises—alternating contraction and relaxation of muscles without moving the joints. Isometric exercises and electromyographic (EMG) biofeedback may be beneficial. As the patient progresses, light resistance can be applied manually by the clinician before the use of resistance equipment. This allows the clinician to directly estimate the patient's physical strengths and weaknesses. Weakened muscles must be protected at all times. Muscles that cannot resist the force of gravity are supported during exercise and rest periods. As a rule, resistive exercises are not attempted until the muscle is able to carry out a complete ROM against gravity. Weakened or flaccid muscles can be splinted at night to counteract the force of gravity or the pull of the stronger antagonist muscles. During resistive exercises the clinician should stress correct body positioning, joint alignment, and energy conservation. Periods of rest should be included in the exercise program. Activities that incorporate the same movements and musculature as the exercises are encouraged.[14]

The goals for resistive exercises in the rehabilitation of the patient who has poliomyelitis are (1) to strengthen undamaged muscles and (2) to reinforce the slightest contraction by integrating it into a larger movement that permits the performance of a given activity. After eight months, if the muscle is unable to contract completely against gravity, it is doubtful that additional muscle strength will return. At this point the emphasis should be placed on maintenance of existing muscles and functional ADLs.

A self-care evaluation should be administered by the OTR or COTA to achieve a baseline of function. Dressing activities may include donning and removing orthoses. Assistive devices should be tailored to the needs of the patient.[32] It may also be advantageous to begin activities for prevocational and vocational exploration. Patients' quality of life can be improved if they are employed and productive. The prognosis for successful rehabilitation depends on the personality of the patient and the perseverance of the clinician.

### Postpolio Syndrome

Occupational therapy practitioners are seeing more patients with postpolio syndrome in rehabilitation centers. Patients who had polio earlier in life are experiencing additional weakness and other disabling symptoms years after the initial disease.[45,53] The numbers of such persons has increased, in part because of the influx of immigrants from Southeast Asia and Latin America who suffered the original infection in their native lands.[15] It is estimated that there are more than 250,000 polio survivors in the United States. Of those, some 75,000 persons are experiencing symptoms of postpolio syndrome. Postpolio syndrome causes health and functional problems, and patients who are affected are likely to be referred for occupational therapy services.[53]

The primary symptom of **postpolio** syndrome is progressive weakness.[15] There may be slowly progressive muscular weakness in muscles that were thought to be spared in the original illness as well as in those previously affected. Pain, fatigue, cold intolerance, and new breathing difficulties may accompany the muscle weakness. Other symptoms include musculoskeletal problems such as joint, limb, or trunk deformities that can cause pain, decreased endurance, nerve entrapment, degenerative arthritis, falls, and unsteady gait.[53]

Fatigue is the most debilitating symptom because it limits activity yet is not apparent to others. The fatigue may be severe and out of proportion to the apparent physical demands of the activity and can be overwhelming.[15,53] An increase in difficulties with ADL accompanies the symptoms. Problems with ambulation, transfers, using stairs, home management, driving, dressing, eating and swallowing, and bladder and bowel control may occur.[53]

The cause of postpolio syndrome is not fully understood. Unless there is severe pulmonary or swallowing involvement, postpolio syndrome is not life threatening. The symptoms can range from a very mild weakness that is only slightly annoying to profound weakness that is severely incapacitating, with risks of additional disabling problems such as fractures, osteoporosis, contractures, and depression. Effective remedies aim to prevent muscle fatigue, improve body mechanics, and conserve energy. In general, it has been observed that patients who adjust their life styles experience improvement of symptoms and stabilization of function.[15]

#### *Occupational Therapy Intervention*

When a diagnosis of postpolio syndrome has been made, the affected person may be referred for rehabilitation services. The physical and occupational therapists are called on to assess strength, ROM, endurance, activities of daily living (ADL), occupational performance, and psychosocial status. Gait and orthotic needs should be evaluated as well.[15] The COTA may participate in this assessment process in specific areas where proficiency and competence have been demonstrated.

The occupational therapy practitioner should begin by interviewing the patient to ascertain valued occupational roles and obtain an activity profile of daily life. The clinician should ask the patient which activities cause pain or fatigue, which activities have been curtailed or eliminated because of symptoms, when symptoms are most likely to occur (time, circumstances), and what kinds of aids, equipment, and human assistance are presently used. Manual muscle testing of the upper extremities may be indicated if there is weakness. It should be noted that postpolio muscles may actually function at levels of strength lower than estimated from scores on the manual muscle test and that upper extremity strength varies markedly throughout the ROM.[53] Joint ROM measurements are important if there are contractures and muscle imbalances.

An assessment of psychosocial status is necessary to select the best approach for the patient to facilitate rehabilitation efforts and to adjust to new limitations. Changes in physical capacities and curtailment of valued life skills confront the individual with psychological issues of coping, adjustment, and adaptation. These may be as traumatic as they were at the time of the original illness. Feelings of denial, anger, frustration, and hopelessness must be recognized, worked through, and processed.

As a group, persons who originally had polio assumed that the disease was over, that disability was in the past, and that any residual weakness would not worsen. They worked hard to overcome the effects of the initial paralysis and often performed well, achieved high levels of personal fulfillment, became well integrated into society, and so "disappeared" as a disabled group. The onset of new symptoms disrupts the performance and lifestyle achieved through years of hard work. Old remedies do not work to ameliorate these new limitations. It is often difficult for the patient to confront the reality of the circumstances. As a result, the clinician should introduce change gradually. Small changes may be more easily accepted than major ones, even if the latter are obviously necessary.[15]

The patient is confronted, for a second time, years after the disability was thought to be stabilized, with the notion of being "disabled" and limiting function and valued life activities. A supportive and realistic approach and patient education are key to lifestyle modification.[53]

The benefits of exercise are controversial. Exercise may aggravate pain. Overwork of muscles that have a decreased number of motor units may be damaging. However, muscles weakened by disuse may benefit from a nonfatiguing trial of gentle exercises for strengthening purposes. Strength may be maintained by performance of ADL. Muscles used for ADL should not be stressed further.[53] Patients should be encouraged to be active within limits of comfort and safety. A regular routine of activity or nonfatiguing exercise is important and affords the patient the feeling of doing something positive. Exercise programs must be carefully supervised. Long-term strengthening or maintenance exercises are recommended only in muscles that show no EMG evidence of prior polio involvement. Further weakness, discomfort, pain, muscle spasm, or chronic fatigue resulting from exercise are signs of excessive activity.[15,53]

Pain can be managed or alleviated by improving body mechanics, supporting weakened muscles, and promoting lifestyle modification. The COTA can teach correct body mechanics in daily living tasks such as work and home management, ambulation, and transfers. Orthoses may be used to support weakened muscles. Activities and lifestyle should be modified to reduce fatigue, stress, and overuse of muscles. Weight reduction is necessary for some patients.[15]

Perhaps the most important contribution of the occupational therapy practitioner is guiding and facilitating lifestyle modifications. Patients must avoid overuse of muscles. Evaluation and retraining in all aspects of ADL is important. Assistive devices for self-care and home management may be indicated. Home and workplace modifications can help prevent muscle overuse and decrease fatigue and potential deformity. Energy conservation and work simplification techniques should be taught. The patient and clinician should set priorities for occupational role performance. Energy conservation for the most valued activities may mean sacrificing less valued ones to be done by others or to be done with the assistance of equipment such as orthoses, assistive devices, or ambulation aids.[53]

### Guillain-Barré Syndrome

**Guillain-Barré syndrome** (also known as *acute ideopathic neuropathy, infectious polyneuritis,* and *Landry's syndrome*) is an acute inflammatory condition involving the spinal nerve roots, peripheral nerves, and, in some cases, selected cranial nerves. Guillain-Barré syndrome often follows a viral illness, immunization, or surgery, and may affect both sexes at any age.*

Guillain-Barré syndrome has a rapid onset. Initially there is no fever, but pain and tenderness of muscles, weakness, and a decrease in deep tendon reflexes occur. As the disease progresses, it produces motor weakness or paralysis of the limbs, sensory loss, and muscle atrophy. The prognosis is varied. In severe cases, cranial nerves 7, 9, and 10 may be involved, and the patient may have difficulty speaking, swallowing, and breathing. If vital centers in the medulla are affected, the patient may experience respiratory failure and require tracheostomy or assisted ventilation. In the majority of the cases, the patient completely recovers within a few weeks to a few months with relatively few residual effects.[18,45]

#### *Occupational Therapy Intervention*

Once the patient is medically stabilized, rehabilitation can be initiated. Comprehensive rehabilitation goals should be coordinated with the nurse, physical therapist, and other members of the team. The patient may be referred to occupational therapy while still totally paralyzed. This initial phase of treatment focuses on PROM, positioning, and splinting to prevent contracture and deformity and to protect weak muscles. Passive activities such as watching television, and light social activities such as visits from friends are encouraged. As improvement occurs and more active motion

*References 6, 8, 18, 36, 41, 42, 45, 50.

is possible, occupational therapy interventions include gentle, nonresistive activities, and light ADL to alleviate joint stiffness and muscle atrophy and to prevent contractures. The occupational therapist or assistant should grade the activity program to the patient's physical tolerance level. Fatigue should be avoided and psychological support provided.[41]

The occupational therapy evaluation should include a test of strength, ROM measurement, and sensory tests. During the early stages of recovery the evaluation process itself may be fatiguing. It is often best to spread the evaluation over a few days. Sensory testing should also be conducted because the sensory pathways are often affected. In most cases this formal testing is performed by the OTR.

PROM should begin with gentle movement of the proximal joints and should proceed only to the point of pain. As the patient's tolerance increases, AROM and light exercises may be introduced. The program should stress joint protection, and the clinician should look for muscle imbalance and substitution patterns. Progressive resistive exercises should be used conservatively. Throughout the course of recovery the clinician should guard against fatigue and irritation of the inflamed nerves.

As the patient's strength and tolerance increase, resistance can be gradually and moderately increased. The clinician may also introduce sedentary or tabletop activities during the early stages of recovery. As the patient's strength increases, activities promoting more resistance, such as leather work, textiles, and ceramics, can be added. Grooming, self-care, and other ADL should be included as soon as the patient is capable of some independence and graded to include more activities as strength and endurance improve. Slings and mobile arm supports may be used to alleviate muscle fatigue and promote independence. Activities should be varied between gross and fine and resistive and nonresistive to prevent undue fatigue. Ongoing assessment of ADL status is important to determine which activities the patient is capable of performing, where assistive or adaptive equipment is needed, and in which cases independence can be maximized.

Psychological support is important throughout the treatment program. The clinician should try to facilitate the feeling of self-worth, a positive attitude, and encouragement throughout the therapeutic process. Because the prognosis for recovery is good, the activities should be mentally stimulating and purposeful to the patient. The clinician should also respect the patient's level of pain tolerance during stretching and ROM exercises.[48]

## Peripheral Nerve Injuries

### *General Characteristics*

Regardless of the origin of the injury, peripheral nerve lesions produce similar clinical manifestations. The most obvious manifestation of **peripheral nerve injury** is muscle weakness or flaccid paralysis, depending on the extent of the nerve damage. Because of the loss of muscle innervation, **atrophy** will follow and deep tendon reflexes will be absent or depressed. Sensation along the cutaneous distribution of the nerve will also be lost. Trophic changes, such as dry skin, hair loss, cyanosis, brittle fingernails, painless skin ulcerations, and slow wound healing in the area of involvement may also be present. Occasionally, minute muscle contractions called *fasciculations* may be seen on the surface of the skin overlying the denervated muscle belly. As a result of disturbances of sympathetic fibers of the autonomic nervous system, there will be a loss of the ability to sweat above the denervated skin surfaces.

The patient may experience paresthesias, that is, sensations such as tingling, numbness, and burning or pain (causalgia), particularly at night. In addition, if the nerve damage was caused by trauma, edema will be a prominent clinical manifestation. EMG examinations may reveal extremely small muscle contractions called fibrillations.*

Extensive peripheral nerve damage may produce deformity if contractures, joint stiffness, and poor positioning are allowed to occur. Disfigurement of the hands is particularly noticeable and may produce some psychological complications. Other complications may include osteoporosis of bone and epidermal fibrosis of the joints.

The medical-surgical management of peripheral nerve lesions depends on the type of injury that has occurred and may include microsurgery, nerve grafts or transplants, and injections of alcohol, vitamin $B_{12}$, and phenol.

Peripheral nerve **regeneration** begins about 1 month after the injury has occurred. The rate of regeneration depends on the nature of the nerve lesion. If the nerve root has been cleanly severed and surgically repaired, the rate of regeneration will vary from ½ inch (1.3 cm) to 1 inch (2.6 cm) per month. Peripheral nerve injuries caused by burns, sepsis, or crushing will present other complications to the healing process. Age is another factor; children usually have a faster rate of regeneration than adults.[29] In addition, proximal lesions regenerate faster than distal lesions, and injuries to mixed nerves are slower to recover than single nerves.[5,27] Early medical treatment may require suturing the nerve and immobilizing the involved extremity to ensure good apposition of the severed nerves. In the past, full recovery of muscles was not probable because regenerated fibers lose about 20% of their original diameter and conduct impulses at a slower rate.[9,28] Microsurgery has improved the regenerative process in recent years.

Because peripheral nerves have the capacity to regenerate, the course of recovery can be somewhat predictable. The clinical signs of regeneration do not always follow a specific sequence. The following clinical signs of nerve regeneration can be expected:

*References 3, 4, 8, 9, 13, 21.

- *Skin appearance:* As the edema subsides and collateral blood vessels develop, the circulatory system should become more normalized. The skin should improve in its color and texture.
- *Primitive protective sensations:* The first signs of cutaneous sensation will usually be the gross recognition of crude pain, temperature, pressure, and touch.
- *Paresthesias:* Tingling or paresthesias ("pins and needles") distal to the presumed site of lesion may indicate regeneration is occurring.
- *Scattered points of sweating:* As the parasympathetic fibers of the autonomic nervous system regenerate, the sweat glands will recover their functions.
- *Discriminative sensations:* The more refined sensations, such as the ability to identify and localize touch, joint position (proprioception), recognition of objects in the three-dimensional form (stereognosis), movement (kinesthesia), and two-point discrimination, should be returning at this point.
- *Muscle tone:* Flaccidity will decrease and muscle tone will increase. An important principle is that paralyzed muscles must first sense pressure before tone and movement can be realized.
- *Voluntary muscle function:* The patient will be able to move the extremity first with gravity eliminated, and then proceed to full ROM as strength increases. At this point graded exercises can begin.

### *Specific Peripheral Nerve Injuries*

*Brachial plexus injury* The nerve roots that innervate the upper extremity originate in the anterior rami between the C4 and T1 vertebrae. This network of lower anterior cervical and upper dorsal spinal nerves is collectively called the *brachial plexus.* This very important nerve complex can be palpated just behind the posterior border of the sternocleidomastoid as the head and neck are tilted to the opposite side.[6,8,20,40]

Lesions to the brachial plexus usually result from a variety of traumatic injuries. Most brachial plexus injuries in children are caused by birth trauma. Such injuries are called *Erb's palsy* and *Klumpke's paralysis.* Erb's palsy is indicative of lesions to the fifth and sixth brachial plexus roots. Paralysis and atrophy occur in the deltoid, brachialis, biceps, and brachioradialis muscles. Clinically the arm hangs limp, the hand rotates inward, and functional movement is extremely limited.

Klumpke's paralysis affects the more distal aspect of the upper extremity. The disorder results from injury to the eighth cervical and first thoracic brachial plexus roots. Consequently, there will be paralysis to the distal musculature of the wrist flexors and the intrinsic muscles of the hand.[6,8]

*Long thoracic nerve injury* The long thoracic nerve (C5 to C7) innervates the serratus anterior muscle, which anchors the apex of the scapula to the posterior of the rib cage. Although injury to this nerve is not common, it can be injured by carrying heavy weights on the shoulder, neck blows, and axillary wounds. The resulting clinical picture is winging of the scapula, difficulty flexing the outstretched arm above shoulder level, and difficulty protracting the shoulder or performing scapular abduction and adduction.

Injuries involving the long thoracic nerve are usually treated by stabilizing the shoulder girdle to limit scapula motion. The clinician must avoid activities that promote shoulder movements. If nerve regeneration is not complete, surgery may be indicated to relieve the excessive mobility of the scapula. After medical treatment the occupational therapist or assistant encourages maximal functional independence and teaches the patient to use long-handle devices to compensate for shoulder limitations.

*Axillary nerve injury* The axillary nerve is composed of the C5 and C6 spinal nerves and derived from the posterior region of the brachial plexus. The motor branches of the axillary nerve innervate the superior aspect of the deltoid muscle and the teres minor muscle. Although the axillary nerve is rarely damaged by itself, it is often damaged along with traumatic lesions to the brachial plexus. As a result, the patient will experience weakness or paralysis of the deltoid muscle, which causes limitations in horizontal abduction and hyperesthesia on the lateral aspect of the shoulder. In addition to the loss of muscle power, atrophy of the deltoid muscle produces asymmetry of the shoulders. If the nerve damage is permanent, a muscle transplantation may be required to provide some abduction of the arm.[6,8,36]

The occupational therapy practitioner should maintain ROM to prevent deformity and improve circulation. Passive abduction of the shoulder should be done daily. The teres minor and deltoid muscles should be protected from stretch during the manual ROM activities. The patient may be taught to use long-handled assistive devices to compensate for the abduction deficit. If a surgical transplant is performed, the clinician should be familiar with the surgical procedure to assist in muscle reeducation. An EMG biofeedback machine can be beneficial in providing the patient with visual and auditory incentives during muscle reeducation sessions. The clinician may also assist the patient in dressing activities. If the asymmetry of the shoulders presents a cosmetic problem when wearing shirts or jackets, a foam rubber or thermoplastic pad can be fabricated to fill in the space that was once occupied by the deltoid muscle. The patient should be encouraged to learn self-ranging techniques and implement an exercise program to maintain the integrity of the unimpaired muscles of the involved extremity.

Lesions of the radial, median, and ulnar nerves and cumulative trauma disorders affecting the hand are discussed in Chapter 35.

*Volkmann's contracture* A fracture of the lower end of the humerus (in the supracondylar region) may result in a diminished supply of well-oxygenated blood to the muscles of the forearm. This phenomenon can occur when the fracture has been tightly cast and bandaged. Edema sets in near the site of the injury and shuts down the blood supply to the muscle bellies because the cast will not allow the tissue to swell outward. Ischemia deprives tissues of oxygen and nourishment. The muscle can become necrotic, causing atrophy and contractures of the wrist, fingers, and forearm. The flexor digitorum profundus and flexor pollicis longus muscles are severely affected. The median nerve is often more impaired than the ulnar nerve.[8,20]

Shortly after a fracture of the humerus has been immobilized, the patient may have a cold, distal extremity with a smooth, glossy, or dusky appearance of the skin. If the clinician observes these symptoms and cannot detect a radial pulse, the physician should be informed immediately, and the cast should be removed. Early detection and prevention of this problem can prevent or minimize what would otherwise become a very severe deformity. If, for example, the ischemia lasts 6 hours, some contracture will follow. Ischemia lasting 48 hours or more will result in a permanent deformity of the forearm. If mild ischemia has occurred, the physician may prescribe vigorous, active exercises to increase circulation, activate musculature, and prevent joint stiffness.[6]

### *Occupational Therapy Intervention for Peripheral Nerve Injuries*

Peripheral nerves convey sensory information from the environment to the central nervous system and then control the motor response of the muscles and glands to this sensory input.[28] Peripheral nerve injury occurs most commonly as the result of trauma to the shoulder complex, upper extremity, or hand. Management of peripheral nerve injury may involve surgery, orthopedic stabilization or immobilization, and occupational and physical therapy.

The aim of treatment for peripheral nerve injuries is to assist the patient in regaining the maximum level of motor function and independence in performance areas. Treatment is directed to the stage of recovery and focuses on remediation and compensation for sensory, motor, and performance deficits. The rate of return and the residual impairments depend largely on the severity of the lesion and the quality of care during the rehabilitation process. Table 34-1 is a useful summary of the major nerve roots and clinical manifestation of their lesions.

The occupational therapy practitioner may be involved during the acute and rehabilitation phases of treatment. During the acute phase (immediately after surgery), treatment is aimed at preventing deformity. Initially, static splints are used to immobilize the extremity and protect the site of injury.[42,46] See Chapter 35 for more information on postoperative management of peripheral nerve repair.

Reduction of edema is important and is achieved by elevating the extremity above the level of the heart. This will decrease the hydrostatic pressure in the blood vessels and promote venous and lymphatic drainage. Manual massage while the extremity is elevated may also reduce edema. The massage should entail centripetal (small, circular) strokes to gently force the excess fluids toward the proximal aspects of the body. Care must be taken not to disturb the healing process of the site of injury. External elastic support can also be used to alleviate the edema. PROM will assist in the prevention of edema by promoting venous return.[49]

As the patient's muscle function returns, an appropriate exercise program can be established. Resistive activities, such as woodworking, ceramics, leather work, and copper tooling may be used in conjunction with isometric and isotonic exercises when muscle function is adequate. The clinician should not overtax the musculature where nerve regeneration and motor return is apparent and should protect the weaker muscle groups from stretch and fatigue. The clinician may fabricate splints or slings to protect weakened musculature from overstretching and to maintain functional position.

ADL assessment is necessary to identify difficulties with essential performance tasks. One-handed methods of dressing, eating, and hygiene activities may be necessary temporarily or permanently. Assistive devices, such as long-handled reaching aids and one-handed kitchen tools, can be beneficial to increase independence.

Sensory reeducation is used to assist the patient in establishing appropriate responses to sensory stimuli. Sensory reeducation for peripheral nerve injuries is discussed in Chapters 24 and 35.

### Peripheral Nerve Pain Syndromes

Pain is a common complication in peripheral nerve injuries.[7,52] For some patients the pain itself becomes an overwhelming disability. The types of **pain syndromes** that have been associated with peripheral nerve injuries are causalgia and neuroma pain.[37,43,52] Causalgia is pain of great intensity that commonly results from injury to the brachial plexus, median, and ulnar nerves.[5]

In the upper extremity, causalgia is described as an intense burning sensation so excruciating that the patient holds the affected limb immobile for fear of stimulating the pain. The affected limb becomes extremely sensitive to temperature change, wind, and even noise.[12,27] Causalgia is also exacerbated by emotional stress.

Neuromas are incompletely regenerated nerve endings and fibers at the site where the peripheral nerve was damaged. Neuromas are particularly problematic in nerve endings serving the fingers and in amputated limbs. Phantom limb pain is often the result of neuroma formation.

### *Occupational Therapy Intervention*

Research on pain management has revealed that certain activities and noninvasive techniques can

*Table 34-1*

## Clinical Manifestations of Peripheral Nerve Lesions

| *Spinal nerves* | *Nerve roots* | *Motor distribution* | *Clinical manifestations* |
|---|---|---|---|
| **Brachial plexus** | | | |
| C5-C7 | Long thoracic | Shoulder girdle, serratus anterior | Winged scapula |
| C5, C6 | Dorsal scapular | Rhomboid major and minor, levator scapulae | Loss of scapular adduction and elevation |
| C7, C8 | Thoracodorsal | Latissimus dorsi | Loss of arm adduction and extension |
| C5, C6 | Suprascapular | Supraspinatus, infraspinatus | Weakened lateral rotation of humerus |
| C5, C6 | Subscapular | Subscapularis, teres major | Weakened medial rotation of humerus |
| C6-C8, T1 | Radial | All extensors of forearm, triceps | Wrist drop, extensor paralysis |
| C5, C6 | Axillary | Deltoid, teres minor | Loss of arm abduction, weakened lateral rotation of humerus |
| C5, C6 | Musculocutaneous | Biceps brachii, brachialis, coracobrachialis | Loss of forearm flexion and supination |
| C6-C8, T1 | Median | Flexors of hand and digits, opponens pollicis | Ape-hand deformity, weakened grip, thenar atrophy, unopposed thumb |
| C8, T1 | Ulnar | Flexor of hand and digits, opponens pollicis | Claw-hand deformity, interosseus atrophy, loss of thumb adduction |
| ***Lumbosacral plexus*** | | | |
| L2-L4 | Femoral | Iliopsoas, quadriceps femoris | Loss of thigh flexion, leg extension |
| L2-L4 | Obturator | Adductors of thigh | Weakened or loss of thigh adduction |
| L4, L5, S1-S3 | Sciatic | Hamstrings, all musculature below the knee | Loss of leg flexion, paralysis of all muscles of leg and foot |
| L4, L5, S1, S2 | Common peroneal | Dorsiflexors of foot | Foot drop, steppage gait, loss of eversion |
| L4, L5, S1-S3 | Tibial | Gastrocnemius, soleus, deep plantar flexors of foot | Loss of plantar flexion and inversion of foot |

modulate pain perception.[22,43,44] A better understanding of pain control mechanisms has provided therapists with new techniques for patients with peripheral nerve pain.[1,7,22,30,39]

The occupational therapy practitioner can modulate pain perception in several ways. An evaluation, by the OTR of the intensity, quality, and location of pain is done during an interview. The patient is asked to mark the point of pain on an anatomical drawing and then estimate pain intensity on a numerical scale. The patient is told to describe the personal experience of the pain with terms such as sharp, dull, aching, throbbing, sore, or burning. Factors that seem to contribute to pain should also be explored during the interview. These might be things such as specific foods and drinks, positions, and activities.[22]

Several intervention techniques can alter pain messages. Peripheral pain emitting from neuromas is managed with intervention from both the OTR and the COTA. The OTR may provide graded sensory input such as tapping or vibration over the neuroma, transcutaneous electrical nerve stimulation (TENS), or localized stimulation to acupoints and trigger points.* The COTA may instruct the patient to obtain pain relief by protecting the tender regions of the body during daily activities and by using protective devices fabricated from splinting materials.

Involving the patient in successful and purposeful activities may help manage pain by providing cognitive diversion from the pain experience. Engagement

*References 1, 19, 24, 25, 38, 39, 43.

in purposeful activities can influence moods and emotions, an effect that in turn will alter the perception of pain intensity in causalgia and ultimately modify the pain threshold.[16,22,27,43] The clinician can also use background music or music with earphones as a therapeutic modality. While the patient is engaged in activities, the volume of the music can be increased or decreased as a diversion to accommodate the pain intensity.[22]

Causalgia is related to tension and stress. To decrease these factors, the clinician can also instruct the patient in relaxation techniques[7,12] such as deep breathing, progressive relaxation, and visualization.[22,27,43] When the relaxation response is elicited, the patient's muscles relax, the heart rate and respiration rate slow, and the patient experiences a sense of well-being. By learning relaxation techniques, the patient can control emotional tension and depression, both contributors to causalgia and the perception of pain.[22]

## DISEASE OF THE NEUROMUSCULAR JUNCTION

Some motor unit disorders originate in diseases of the junction between the motor nerve and the muscle it innervates.

### Myasthenia Gravis

**Myasthenia gravis** is a disease of chemical transmission at the nerve-muscle synapse or neuromuscular junction. It results in weakness of skeletal muscle.[33] It occurs at all ages but primarily affects younger women and older men.[18,45] Medical management of these patients varies and may include removal of the thymus gland (thymectomy), treatment with pharmacological agents, or plasmapheresis (blood filtering).*

Myasthenia gravis is characterized by abnormal fatigue of voluntary muscle.[14] The disease can affect any of the striated skeletal muscles of the body but in particular targets the muscles of the eyelids and eyes and oropharyngeal muscles. Therefore the muscles most often affected are those that move the eyes, eyelids, tongue, jaw, and throat. The limb muscles may also be affected. The muscles that are used most often fatigue sooner.[14,33,51] Therefore the patient may have double vision, drooping of the eyelids, and difficulty with speech or swallowing as muscles fatigue. Patients with myasthenia gravis may experience life-threatening respiratory crises that require hospitalization and the use of a ventilator. The incidence of these crises has declined significantly in recent years, probably because of increased use of thymectomy.[33,51] The intensity of the disease fluctuates and its course is unpredictable.[51] Spontaneous remissions occur frequently but relapse is usual.[8] Remissions or decrease in symptoms and improvement in strength and function can last for years. However, there may be exacerbations of unpredictable severity induced by exertion, infection, or childbirth.[41] The prognosis for myasthenia gravis varies with each individual, but for most it is a progressively disabling disease; the patient may ultimately become bedridden with severe permanent paralysis. Death usually occurs as a result of respiratory complications.[8,41,45]

*References 2, 17, 18, 33, 45, 51.

#### *Occupational Therapy Intervention*

The primary role of the occupational therapy practitioner is to help the patient regain muscle power and build endurance. It is important that the therapeutic program not cause fatigue. The clinician should monitor the patient's muscle strength on a regular basis, taking into account factors that would contribute to fatigue and the effects of medications. A running record noting any significant changes in muscle strength should be kept. The clinician should report any changes in the patient's physical appearance (such as ptosis of the eyelids, drooping facial muscles, or alterations of breathing or swallowing) to the physician.

The clinician should provide gentle, nonresistive activities that are intellectually and psychologically stimulating. The activities should be graded so that they do not fatigue the patient. Overexertion must be avoided and respiratory problems prevented. The treatment plan should include energy conservation, work simplification, and necessary adaptive and assistive devices to reduce effort during daily activities. If appropriate, electronic communication devices can be installed in the patient's home so that contact with community agencies can be maintained. In addition, the clinician may assist with home planning to determine architectural barriers, bathroom adaptations, and furniture rearrangements. Mobile arm supports and splints may be used to protect weakened musculature from overstretching and to aid in positioning for function.[41]

The clinician should assist in educating the patient about the disease. The patient should avoid emotional stress, overexertion, fatigue, and excessive heat or cold because they may exacerbate the symptoms of the disease. All clinicians should follow infection control procedures because minor infections can also exacerbate the symptoms.

## MYOPATHIC DISORDERS

Another group of motor unit disorders is caused by disease of the muscles.

### Muscular Dystrophies

The **muscular dystrophies** are a group of uncommon inherited conditions. The four major types of muscular dystrophy (MD)[34,51] have in common the progressive degeneration of muscle fibers while the neuronal innervation to muscle and sensation remain intact. As the number of muscle fibers declines, each axon innervates fewer and fewer of them, resulting in progressive weakness.[31]

### *Duchenne's Muscular Dystrophy*

This type of MD affects males only; it is inherited as an X-linked recessive trait. The disease begins at birth and is usually diagnosed between the ages of 18 to 36 months. It begins in the muscles of the pelvic girdle and legs and then spreads to the shoulder girdle. The child has difficulty walking, has a waddling gait, and usually must use a wheelchair by age 12. Ultimately the child becomes bedridden, and death usually occurs by the age of 30.[34,41,51]

### *Facioscapulohumeral Muscular Dystrophy*

This form of MD has its onset in adolescence and primarily affects the muscles of the face and shoulder girdle, hence its descriptive name. It progresses slowly, and there is a normal life expectancy for its victims.[51] It is inherited through an autosomal dominant gene and affects both males and females equally.[34]

### *Myotonic Muscular Dystrophy*

This type of MD not only causes weakness but has another component, myotonia (tonic spasm of muscles), that makes relaxation of muscle contraction difficult. It is inherited through an autosomal dominant gene and affects males and females. Its unique features, besides the myotonia, are that it involves the cranial muscles and shows a pattern of limb weakness that is distal rather than proximal. Associated symptoms are cataracts, found in almost all patients, and testicular atrophy and baldness found in men. The disease may be mild or severe and can occur at any age.[34,51]

### *Limb-Girdle Dystrophy*

This type of MD is probably a group of disorders that do not fit readily in the other types described. Affected persons differ in age of onset, extent of weakness, and familial inheritance patterns. It is inherited by an autosomal recessive gene.[34,51]

### Occupational Therapy Intervention

Because this group of diseases is degenerative, decline of muscle function cannot be prevented. Medical management is largely supportive, and rehabilitation measures are vital in delaying deformity and achieving maximal function within the limits of the disease and its debilitating effects. The primary goal of occupational therapy is assisting the patient to attain maximal independence in ADL for as long as possible. Self-care activities, assistive devices for independence, and leisure activities are key elements of the treatment program. Wheelchair prescription and mobility training may be included; power wheelchairs are necessary in some instances. The wheelchair may require a special seating system or supports to minimize scoliosis and to prevent or reduce hip and knee flexion contractures and ankle plantar flexion deformity. A wheelchair lap board, suspension slings, or mobile arm supports are indicated to facilitate self-feeding, writing, reading, use of a computer, and table top leisure activities when there is significant shoulder girdle and upper limb weakness. Built-up utensils may be helpful when grip strength declines.[41] Home and workplace modification may be necessary for some patients.[11]

Active exercises may be helpful, but overexertion and fatigue must be avoided. For patients with respiratory involvement, exercise for breathing control may be administered by the physical therapist.[47]

Psychosocial problems and educational and vocational requirements also need attention by the occupational therapy practitioner. Deficits in cognitive function and verbal intelligence have been reported in some types of MD. Depression and personality disorders may be concomitant problems.[11] Patient and family education is an important part of the occupational therapy program. A supportive approach to the patient and family is helpful as function changes and new mobility aids, assistive devices, and community resources become necessary.[41]

## SUMMARY

The motor unit consists of the lower motor neuron, neuromuscular junction, and muscle. Some motor unit disease conditions are reversible and others are degenerative. The OTR and the COTA both play vital roles in the management of patients with motor unit dysfunction. Formal assessment of functional capabilities in all performance areas is coordinated by the OTR. Specific interventions may be implemented by either the OTR or COTA as stated. Provision of positioning, exercise, pain management techniques, and orthoses are a necessary part of the treatment of these patients. ADL skills including self-care, home management, mobility, and work-related tasks are central to recovery of function. Compensatory measures such as energy conservation, work simplification, and joint protection techniques are important elements of the occupational therapy intervention program. Assistive devices, communication aids, and mobility equipment as well as training in their use may be necessary. Psychosocial considerations and patient and family education are important aspects of the occupational therapy program.

## *Selected Reading Guide Questions*

1. Name three causes of lesion that will result in motor unit dysfunction.
2. Describe the differences in the occupational therapy treatment programs for patients with poliomyelitis and postpolio syndrome.
3. Describe the symptoms of postpolio syndrome.
4. What are the elements of the occupational therapy program for the patient with postpolio syndrome?
5. Describe the occupational therapy intervention for Guillain-Barré syndrome.

6. List at least six clinical manifestations of peripheral nerve injury.
7. Describe the sequential signs of recovery after peripheral nerve injury.
8. Describe some treatment strategies for peripheral nerve injuries.
9. Describe four noninvasive methods of modulating pain perception.
10. Discuss the clinical signs of myasthenia gravis.
11. Describe the role of occupational therapy for patients who have myasthenia gravis.
12. What is the primary treatment precaution in myasthenia gravis?
13. Name and differentiate four types of muscular dystrophy. Which one primarily affects children?
14. What are the occupational therapy treatment goals for muscular dystrophy?

## REFERENCES


1. Adler M: Endorphins, enkephalins and neurotransmitters, *Med Times* 110:32, 1982.
2. Barone D: Steroid treatment for experimental autoimmune myasthenia gravis, *Arch Neurol* 37:663, 1980.
3. Barr ML: *The human nervous system,* ed 2, New York, 1974, Harper & Row.
4. Bateman J: *Trauma to nerves in limbs,* Philadelphia, 1962, WB Saunders.
5. Birch R, Grant C: Peripheral nerve injuries—clinical. In Downie P, editor: *Cash's textbook of neurology for physiotherapists,* ed 4, Philadelphia, 1986, JB Lippincott.
6. Brashear RH, Raney RB: *Shand's handbook of orthopaedic surgery,* ed 9, St Louis, 1978, Mosby.
7. Brena SF, editor: *Chronic pain: America's hidden epidemic,* New York, 1978, Atheneum.
8. Chusid JG: *Correlative neuroanatomy and functional neurology,* ed 19, Los Altos, Calif, 1985, Lange.
9. Clark RG: *Clinical neuroanatomy and neurophysiology,* ed 5, Philadelphia, 1975, FA Davis.
10. deGroot J: *Correlative neuroanatomy,* ed 21, Norwalk, Conn, 1991, Appleton & Lange.
11. Fowler WF, Goodgold J: Rehabilitation management of neuromuscular diseases. In Goodgold J, editor: *Rehabilitation medicine,* St Louis, 1988, Mosby.
12. Gandhavadi B: Autonomic pain: features and methods of assessments, *Postgrad Med* 71:85, 1982.
13. Gardner E: *Fundamentals of neurology,* ed 6, Philadelphia, 1975, WB Saunders.
14. Gilroy J, Meyer J: *Medical neurology,* ed 3, New York, 1979, Macmillan.
15. Halstead LS: Late complications of poliomyelitis. In Goodgold J, editor: *Rehabilitation medicine,* St Louis, 1988, Mosby.
16. Heck SA: The effect of purposeful activity on pain tolerance, *Am J Occup Ther* 42(9):577-581, 1988.
17. Kornfeld P: Plasmapheresis in refractory generalized myasthenia gravis, *Arch Neurol* 38:478, 1981.
18. Krupp MA, Chatton MJ: *Current medical diagnosis and treatment* 1984, Los Altos, Calif, 1984, Lange.
19. Lampe G: Introduction to the use of transcutaneous electrical nerve stimulation devices, *Phys Ther* 1:357, 1975.
20. Larson CB, Gould M: *Orthopedic nursing,* ed 9, St Louis, 1978, Mosby.
21. Laurence TN, Pugel AV: Peripheral nerve involvement in spinal cord injury: an electromyographic study, *Arch Phys Med Rehabil* 59:209, 1978.
22. McCormack GL: Pain management by occupational therapists, *Am J Occup Ther* 42(9):582-590, 1988.
23. Melville ID: Clinical problems in motor neurone disease. In Obeham P, Rose FC, editors: *Progress in neurological research,* London, 1979, Pitman.
24. Melzack R: Prolonged relief from pain by brief, intense transcutaneous somatic stimulation, *Pain* 1:357, 1975.
25. Melzack R, Wall PD: Psychophysiology of pain, *Int Anesthesiol Clin* 8:3, 1970.
26. Morrison D, Pathier P, Horr K: *Sensory motor dysfunction and therapy in infancy and early childhood,* Springfield, Ill, 1955, Charles C Thomas.
27. Newberger P, Sallan S: Chronic pain: principles of management, *J Pediatr* 98:180, 1981.
28. Noback CR, Demares RJ: *The nervous system: introduction and review,* ed 2, New York, 1977, McGraw-Hill.
29. Phelps PE, Walker C: Comparison of the finger wrinkling test results to establish sensory tests in peripheral nerve injury, *Am J Occup Ther* 31:465, 1977.
30. Piercey MF, Folkers K: Sensory and motor functions of spinal cord substance P, *Science* 214:1361, 1981.
31. Portney L: Electromyography and nerve conduction velocity tests. In O'Sullivan SB, Shmitz TJ: *Physical rehabilitation: assessment and treatment,* ed 2, Philadelphia, 1988, FA Davis.
32. Robinault I: *Functional aids for the multiply handicapped,* New York, 1973, Harper & Row.
33. Rowland LP: Diseases of chemical transmission at the nerve-muscle synapse: myasthenia gravis. In Kandel ER, Schwartx JH, Jessell TM: *Principles of neural science,* New York, 1991, Elsevier.
34. Rowland LP: Diseases of the motor unit. In Kandel ER, Schwartz JH, Jessell TM: *Principles of neural science,* New York, 1991, Elsevier.
35. Schmidt RF: *Fundamentals of neurophysiology,* ed 2, New York, 1978, Springer-Verlag.
36. Schumacher B, Allen HA: *Medical aspects of disabilities,* Chicago, 1976, Rehabilitation Institute.
37. Seddon HJ: *Surgical disorders of the peripheral nerves,* ed 2, Edinburgh, 1975, Churchill Livingstone.
38. Shealy C: Transcutaneous electrical nerve stimulation for control of pain, *Surg Neurol* 2:45, 1974.
39. Sjolund B, Erikson M: Electroacupuncture and endogenous morphines, *Lancet* 2:1985, 1976.
40. Smith B: *Differential diagnosis in neurology,* New York, 1979, Arco Publishing.
41. Spencer EA: Functional restoration, section 2. In Hopkins HL, Smith HD: *Willard and Spackman's occupational therapy,* ed 8, Philadelphia, 1993, JB Lippincott.
42. Spencer EA: Functional restoration, specific diagnoses. In Hopkins HL, Smith HD: *Willard and Spackman's occupational therapy,* ed 6, Philadelphia, 1983, JB Lippincott.
43. Swerdlow M: *The therapy of pain,* Philadelphia, 1981, JB Lippincott.
44. Tappan FM: *Healing massage techniques: a study of eastern and western methods,* Reston, Va, 1978, Reston.
45. Tierney LM, McPhee SJ, Papadakis MA: *Current medical diagnosis and treatment,* ed 33, Norwalk, Conn, 1994, Appleton & Lange.
46. Trombly CA, Scott AD: *Occupational therapy for physical dysfunction,* Baltimore, Md, 1977, Williams & Wilkins.
47. Turner A: *The practice of occupational therapy,* ed 2, New York, 1987, Churchill Livingstone.
48. Van Dam A: Guillain-Barré syndrome: a unique perspective, *Occup Ther Forum* 2:6, 1987.
49. Vasudevan S, Melvin JL: Upper extremity edema control: rationale of the techniques, *Am J Occup Ther* 33:520, 1979.
50. Walter JB: *An introduction to the principles of disease,* Philadelphia, 1977, WB Saunders.
51. Walter JB: *An introduction to the principles of disease,* ed 3, Philadelphia, 1992, WB Saunders.
52. Wynn-Parry CB, Withrington R: Painful disorders of peripheral nerves, *Postgrad Med J* 60:869, 1984.
53. Young G: Occupational therapy and the postpolio syndrome, *Am J Occ Ther,* 43(2):97-103, 1989.

# Chapter 35

# Acute Hand Injuries

*Mary C. Kasch*
*Sally E. Poole*
*Marianne Hedl*

## Chapter Objectives

*After studying this chapter, the student or practitioner will be able to:*

1. Differentiate the roles of the registered occupational therapist and the certified occupational therapy assistant in the evaluation and treatment of the patient with an injured hand.
2. Explain the general principles for conducting assessments of range of motion, strength, sensibility, edema, soft tissue, and function.
3. Explain the treatment principles for selected acute hand injuries.
4. Practice conducting specific assessments and treatment techniques under supervision.
5. Explain the impact of a hand injury on overall function.

## Key Terms

observation
range of motion
total active ROM (TAM)
total passive ROM (TPM)
edema
grip strength
pinch strength
joint assessment
sensibility
sympathetic function
evaluation of hand function
Coban
sensory desensitization
Baltimore Therapeutic Equipment (BTE)
weight well
theraband
flexor tendons
extensor tendons
peripheral nerve injuries
contracture
fracture
reflex sympathetic dystrophy (RSD)
cumulative trauma disorders (CTDs)

Three days before he is to be married, a 32-year-old police officer falls down a short flight of stairs at home while taking out the garbage. In an attempt to break his fall, he extends both arms. His right arm goes through the window pane of the back door at the bottom of the steps, resulting in a deep laceration at the level of the wrist that cuts all the flexor tendons to the wrist and hand and the median nerve. He is referred to occupational therapy for splinting and treatment 2 days after the accident, 24 hours after the surgical repair of all damaged structures. What are the therapists to do? Will this patient make it to his wedding? Will he ever return to work?

The case illustrated is not at all unusual for a registered occupational therapist (OTR) and certified occupational therapy assistant (COTA) working in a facility where people with acute hand injuries are treated. Treatment of the upper extremity is important to all occupational therapists who work with physically disabled persons. Upper extremity injuries account for about one third of all injuries. The nearly 16 million upper extremity injuries that occur annually in the United States result in 90 million days of restricted activity and 12 million visits to physicians. The upper extremities are involved in about one third of work-related farm injuries and one third of disabling industrial injuries. Other causes of upper extremity dysfunction include disease and congenital anomalies. Estimates suggest that only 15% of those with severe cerebrovascular accidents recover hand function.[36]

The hand is vital to human function and appearance. It flexes, extends, opposes, and grasps thousands of times daily, allowing the performance of necessary daily activities. The hand's sensibility allows feeling without looking and provides protection from injury. The hand touches, gives comfort, and expresses emotions. Loss of hand function through injury or disease thus affects more than the mechanical tasks that the hand performs. Hand injury may jeopardize a family's livelihood and at the least affects every daily activity. The occupational therapist with training in physical and psychological assessment, prosthetic evaluation, fabrication of orthoses, and assessment and training in activities of daily living (ADL) and functional restoration is uniquely qualified to treat upper extremity disorders.

Hand rehabilitation, or hand therapy, has grown as a specialty area of both physical therapy and occupational therapy. Many of the treatment techniques evolved from both disciplines. Although hand therapists may use physical agent modalities, the purpose of this chapter is to provide fundamental knowledge about treating hand-injured patients. It is assumed that these treatment techniques will be provided by the therapist best trained to provide them. Hand rehabilitation requires advanced and specialized training by either physical therapist assistants (PTAs) or occupational therapy assistants (OTAs). The OTA or PTA, with close supervision of the therapist, may assist in providing care for these patients. The American Occupational Therapy Association's (AOTA's) position is that physical agent modalities may be used in preparation for or an adjunct to purposeful activity.[1] It is within this context that physical agent modalities will be discussed in this chapter.

Successful treatment of the injured hand requires timing and judgment. After trauma or surgery, the body must repair the wound. This is called the *healing phase.* Once the tissues are healed at a cellular level, the wound enters its restorative phase. It is in this phase that hand therapy is most beneficial. Early treatment in the restorative phase is ideal and in some cases essential for optimal results. Although sample timetables are often available, the therapist should always coordinate the application of any treatment with the referring physician. Surgical techniques may vary, and inappropriate treatment of the hand patient can result in failure of a surgical procedure. Communication between a surgeon, therapist, and patient is critical. Without the patient's cooperation, gains will be limited. The psychological loss suffered by the patient with a hand injury must be recognized and addressed. A comfortable environment in which group interaction is possible may increase patient motivation and cooperation.

Hand therapy is provided in treatment settings ranging from private therapy offices to outpatient rehabilitation clinics and hospitals. Reimbursement for services may come directly from the patient, through private medical insurance, worker's compensation insurance, or a variety of managed care programs. The number of authorized visits may be limited. Therapists will be asked to provide outcome data that support the need for services. Continuous quality improvement may be a condition for participation in managed care programs. With fewer authorized visits, the therapist must be more adept at instructing the patient in self-management of the condition being treated. Occupational therapy practitioners should anticipate a greater need to justify treatment in the future as part of the national challenge to control medical costs. Certified assistants, aides, and other support personnel will be used increasingly, but the quality of service must continue to meet all professional and ethical standards.

## INFORMATION GATHERING AND OBSERVATION

### Information Gathering

The COTA must clarify the diagnosis either by reading the medical chart or operative report or by communicating with other health professionals—that is, the physician or registered therapist. Only then can the COTA accurately understand and carry out the treatment. Looking at the x-rays or other test results may help the COTA to more fully understand the patient's condition. The COTA should also make note of any further surgery or conservative treatment that is planned.

The COTA may be asked to gather demographic information about the patient, such as age, hand dominance, general medical conditions, occupation, living situation, and avocational interests. This will assist the therapist in setting appropriate goals, as well as in selecting appropriate treatment activities with the patient. When working with a hand-injured patient, it is important to understand not only the medical condition but also the patient's concerns.

### Observation

**Observation** of the patient by the clinician takes two forms. First, if possible, the patient is observed entering the clinic or office. Is the patient alone and able to negotiate the contact with the office personnel? Or does the patient enter the office with an entourage of family and friends who negotiate the system for the patient? How does the patient hold the injured hand? Is it carefully guarded and over protected or ignored? Is the hand wrapped in a silk scarf? Or is the patient attempting to use the hand within the confines of the injury? The position of the hand and arm at rest as well as the carrying posture can yield valuable information about the dysfunction and the patient's response to it.

Second, the hand must be carefully observed. The skin condition of the hand and arm should be noted. Are there lacerations, sutures, or evidence of recent surgery? Is the skin dry or moist? Are there scales or crusts? Does the hand appear swollen? Does the hand have an odor? Palmar skin is normally less mobile than dorsal skin. The degree of mobility, elasticity, and adherence of scars is determined. Trophic changes in the skin should be observed. The vascular system is assessed by observing the skin color and temperature of the hand and evaluating for presence of edema. Are there contractures of the web spaces? The therapist should observe the relationship between the hand and arm function as the patient moves about and performs test items or tasks.

The therapist should ask the patient to perform some simple bilateral ADL such as buttoning a button, putting on a shirt, opening a jar, and threading a needle, and observe the amount of spontaneous movement and use of the affected hand and arm.

## PHYSICAL EVALUATIONS

The effect of trauma or dysfunction on anatomical structures is the first consideration in evaluating hand function. To administer a thorough evaluation of the hand-injured patient, each of the following areas must be investigated: joints, ligaments, tendons, and muscles. Usually, the OTR would perform the formal initial evaluation and subsequent interim evaluations.

The joints must be assessed for active and passive mobility, fixed deformities, and any tendency to assume a position of deformity. The ligaments must be evaluated for laxity or contracture and their ability to maintain joint stability. Tendons must be examined for integrity, contracture, or overstretching; muscles are tested for strength and function.

The results of these individual assessments will be crucial in determining the patient's overall function in the areas of work, play, and leisure.

### Range of Motion Assessment

When indicated, goniometric measurements are part of an initial assessment. There may be times clinically when it is impossible to use the goniometer because of the patient's position, pins in place, or edema. It is generally accepted to measure **range of motion** (ROM) with a goniometer in the field of hand therapy. In the hand, goniometric measurements give information about the joint and also about the soft tissue surrounding the joint, as well as the long finger flexors and extensors.

Unless it is medically contraindicated, active ROM is usually measured first, to assess the ROM available at the joints when they are moved volitionally.[16] Passive ROM need not be measured when full active ROM is present. There is also a specific method of recording finger ROM known as **total active ROM (TAM)** and **total passive ROM (TPM).** This method, which requires additional clinical training, considers the dynamics of tendon excursion, as well as joint mobility (Figure 35-1). In addition to goniometric measures, a gross measurement of finger flexion would be to measure in centimeters the distance between the finger pulp and the distal palmar crease (Figure 35-2).

### Edema Assessment

One consequence of an acute hand injury is **edema,** which Brand defines as "the collection of water and electrolytes in the tissues."[58] Hand volume is measured to assess the presence of edema and may also be used to determine the effect of treatment and activities. By measuring the volume at different times of the day, the effects of rest versus activity may be determined, as well as the effects of splinting or treatment designed to reduce edema.

A commercially available volumeter[20] may be used to assess hand edema (Figure 35-3). The volumeter has been shown to be accurate to 10 ml [9] when used in the prescribed manner. Variables that have been shown to decrease the accuracy of the volumeter include (1) the use of a faucet or hose that introduces air into the tank during filling, (2) movement of the arm within the tank, (3) inconsistent pressure on the stop rod, and (4) the use of a volumeter in a variety of places. The same level surface should *always* be used.[29] The evaluation is performed as follows:

1. A plastic volumeter is filled and allowed to empty into a large beaker until the water reaches spout level. The beaker is then emptied and dried thoroughly.
2. The patient is instructed to immerse the hand in the plastic volumeter, being careful to keep the hand in the midposition.
3. The hand is lowered until it rests gently between the middle and ring fingers on the dowel rod. It is important that the hand does not press onto the rod.
4. The hand remains still until no more water drips into the beaker.
5. The water from the beaker is poured into a graduated cylinder. The cylinder is placed on a level surface, and a reading is made.

Not all patients are candidates for the volumeter. Patients who have open wounds, sutures, staples, or pins in place or any questionable skin condition should not use the volumeter. A tape measure can be used to measure parts of the hand or forearm. Common sites

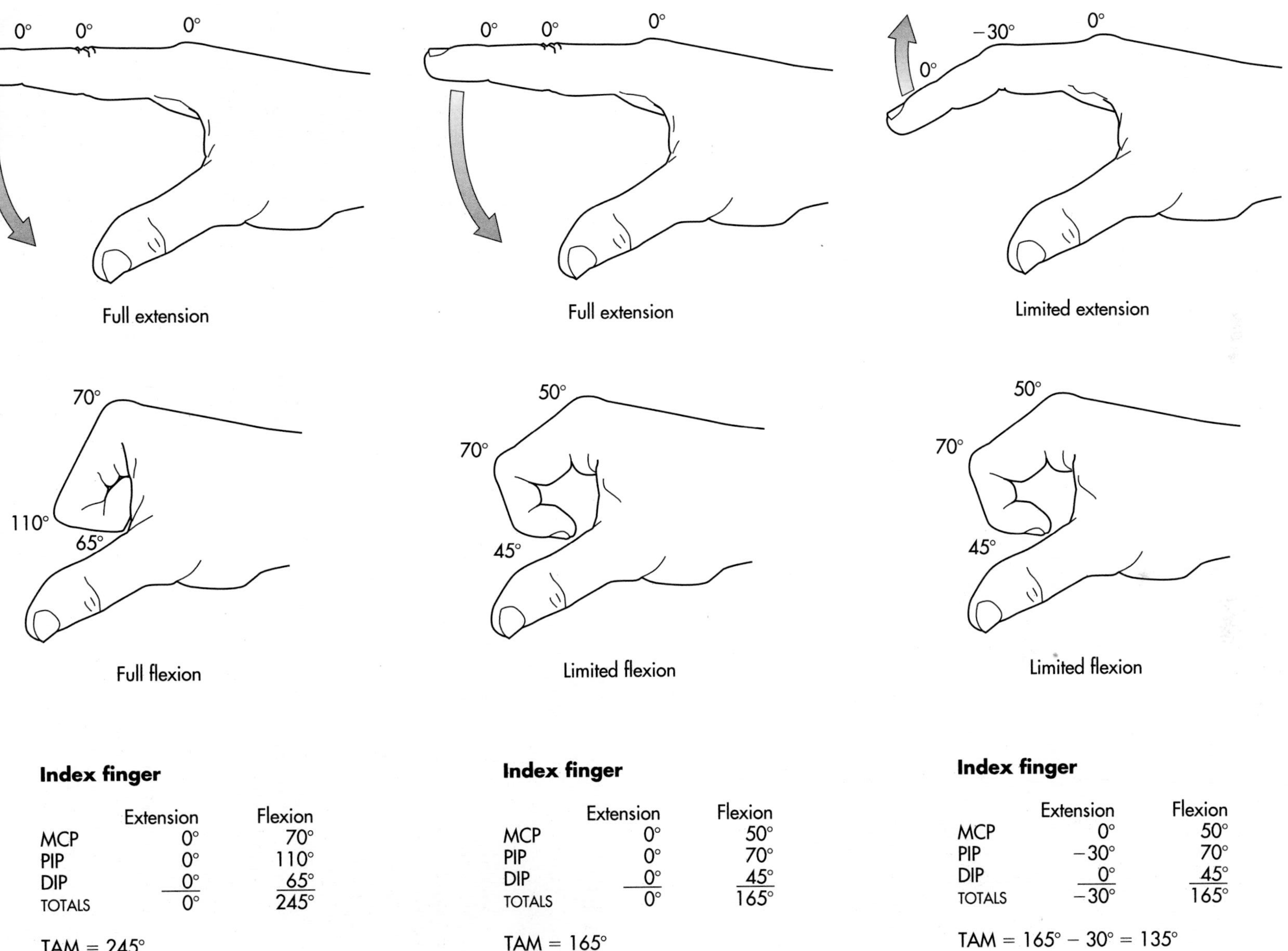


*Figure 35-1* Measurement of total active range of motion (TAM) in the hand.

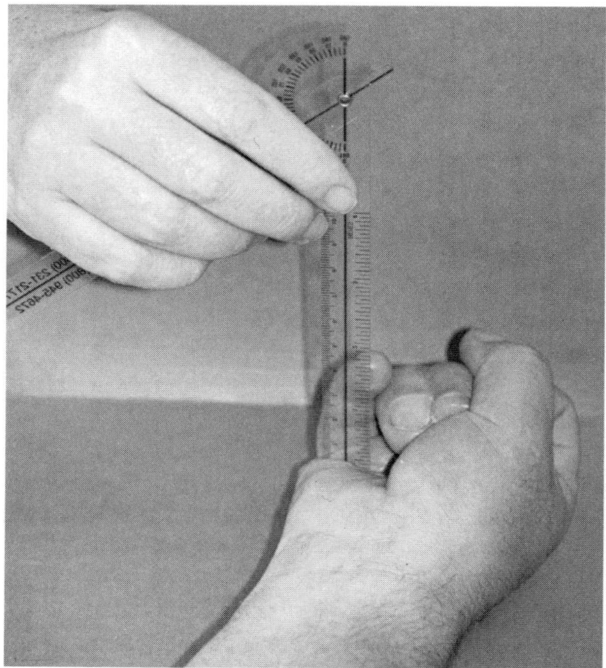

*Figure 35-2* Measuring distance between finger pulp and distal palmar crease.

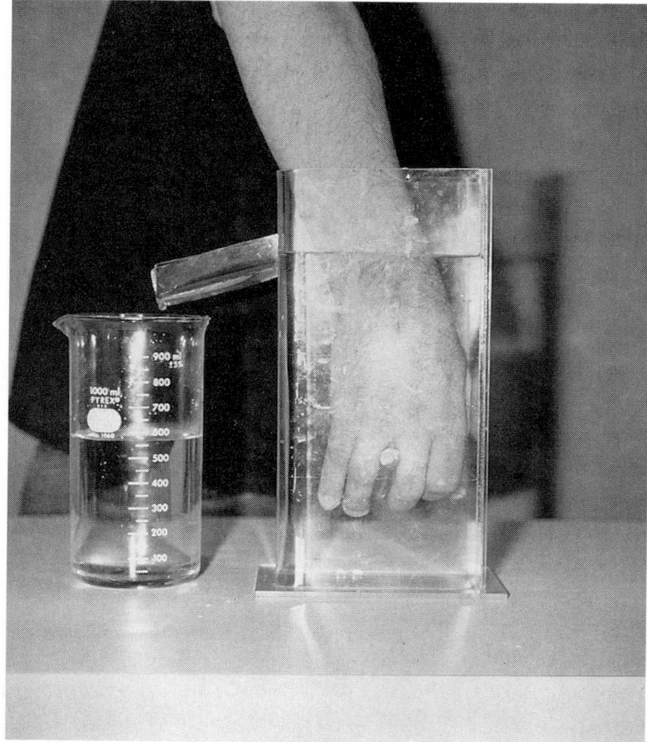

*Figure 35-3* Volumeter used to measure volume of both hands for comparison. Increased volume indicates edema.

are around the distal palmar crease, ulnar styloid of the wrist, or over the joints or phalanxes. When using a tape measure for the hand, it is important to note at what time of the day the measurements were taken so the assessment can be repeated.

To assess an individual finger (or when a volumeter is contraindicated), a tape measure or jeweler's ring-size standards can be used. Measurements should be made before and after treatment, especially after the application of thermal modalities or splinting. While patients often will have subjective complaints relating to swelling, objective data of circumference or volume will help the therapist to assess the response of the tissues to treatment and activity. Edema control techniques will be discussed later in this chapter.

### Strength Assessment

Upper extremity strength assessment should be performed after the healing phase of trauma. Strength testing is not performed after recent trauma or surgery and should be deferred until the patient has been cleared for full-resistive activities, usually 8 to 12 weeks after injury. Strength in the hand is measured in several ways: grip strength, pinch strength, and manual muscle testing.

#### *Grip Strength*

The dynamometer is recommended for assessing **grip strength** (Figure 35-4). The subject should be seated with the shoulder adducted and neutrally rotated, the elbow flexed at 90 degrees[46] forearm in the neutral position, and the wrist between 0 and 15 degrees of ulnar deviation. Three trials are taken of each hand with the dynamometer handle set at the second position.[44] The dynamometer should be lightly held by

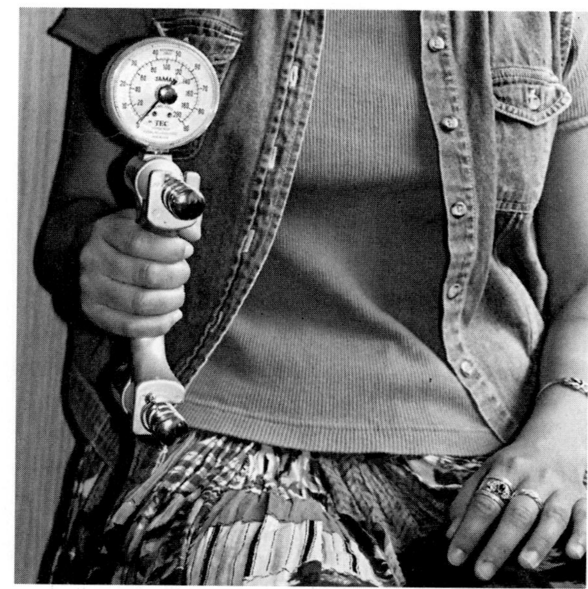

*Figure 35-4* Jamar dynamometer is used to measure grip strength.

the examiner to prevent accidental dropping of the instrument. A mean of the three trials should be reported. The noninjured hand is measured for comparison. Normative data may be used to compare strength scores.[35,45] Variables such as age will affect the strength measurements.

### *Pinch Strength*

**Pinch strength** should be tested with a pinch gauge. The pinch gauge (B & L Engineering) has been found to be the most accurate.[44] Two-point pinch (thumb tip to index fingertip), lateral or key pinch (thumb pulp to lateral aspect of the middle phalanx of the index finger), and three-point pinch (thumb tip to tips of index and long fingers) should be measured. As with the grip dynamometer, three successive trials should be obtained and compared bilaterally[35] (Figure 35-5).

### *Manual Muscle Testing*

Manual muscle testing is also used to evaluate upper extremity strength. Accurate assessment is especially important when preparing the patient for tendon transfers or other reconstructive surgery because it individuates each intrinsic and extrinsic muscle of the hand. It is not customary to perform a manual muscle test during a routine hand evaluation, except when a specific diagnosis (e.g., peripheral nerve injury or neuromuscular disease) warrants detailed investigation.

Additional information about manual muscle testing is referred to in the References at the end of this chapter.

Maximum voluntary effort during grip, pinch, or muscle testing will be affected by pain in the hand or extremity. Therefore subjective complaints should be noted if the patient's ability to exert true force is limited. Localization of the pain or symptoms and consistency of pain complaints will help the therapist to determine the role that pain is playing in the recovery from injury.

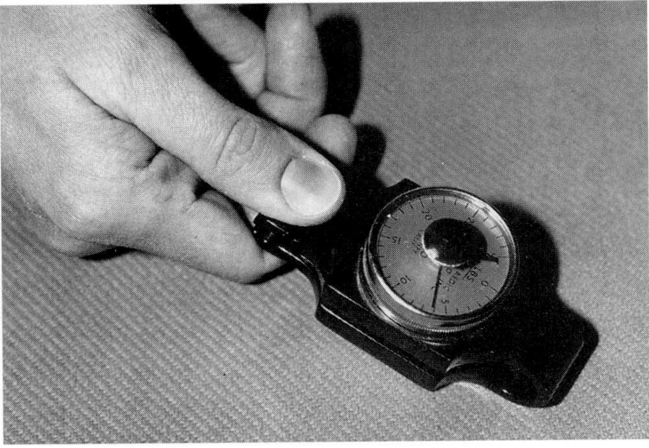

*Figure 35-5* Pinch gauge is used to measure pinch strength in a variety of prehension patterns.

## Soft Tissue Assessment

### *Joint Assessment*

Joints may develop dysfunction after trauma, immobilization, or disuse. Mennell[48] emphasizes the importance of the small, involuntary motions of the joint that he refers to as "joint play."[48] Others[51] describe these as "accessory motions." Joint play or accessory motions are those movements that are nonvoluntary and may be performed only by someone else.[34] One example of accessory motion is joint distraction, in which the OTR firmly but gently stretches the ligaments surrounding the joint. One name for this treatment is *joint mobilization.* It may be helpful to restore joint play with this technique before attempting passive or active ROM.[49]

Guidelines must be followed in applying joint mobilization techniques, and they should not be attempted by the untrained or inexperienced practitioner. Postgraduate courses are offered in joint mobilization of the extremities, and the therapist must be familiar with the arthokinematics (movements of joint surfaces) of each joint as well as with the techniques used.

### *Extrinsic and Intrinsic Assessment*

Limitations in joint motion may also be caused by tightness of the extrinsic or intrinsic muscles and tendons. Various injuries may cause adhesions or shortening (tightness) of the intrinsic hand muscles. For **joint assessment** the OTR must passively place the MCPs, PIPs, and DIPs in a series of recommended positions.[2]

## Sensibility Assessment

Any patient who has sustained a direct injury to a peripheral nerve or who is suspected of having a condition that may compress a peripheral nerve needs to be fully assessed in the area of **sensibility.** The ability of the hand to function, explore, and interact with the environment is dependent on sensibility.[3] Therefore the COTA must be familiar with all sensibility tests and how their results impact treatment and function. However, it is the OTR who performs the assessment.

### *Mapping*

Sensibility testing can begin with sensory mapping of the entire volar surface of the hand.[14] The areas are carefully marked and transferred to a permanent record. Mapping should be repeated at monthly intervals during nerve regeneration.

## Categories of Tests

A variety of evaluations may be required to adequately assess sensibility. These tests can be divided into three categories: (1) modality tests for pain, heat, cold, and touch pressure; (2) functional tests to assess the quality of sensibility or what Moberg described as "tactile gnosis," such as stationary and moving two-point discrimination and the Moberg Pick-up Test; and (3) objective tests that do not require active participation by the patient, including the wrinkle test, the ninhydrin sweat test, and nerve conduction studies.[50]

### *Sympathetic Function*

Recovery of the **sympathetic function** (sweating, pain, and temperature discrimination) may occur early but does not correlate with functional recovery.[23] O'Rain[62] observed that denervated skin does not wrinkle. Therefore nerve function may be tested by immersing the hand in water for 5 minutes and noting the presence or absence of skin wrinkling. This test may be especially helpful in diagnosing a nerve lesion in young children. The ability to sweat is also lost in a nerve lesion. A ninhydrin test[51] evaluates sweating of the finger.

The wrinkle test and the ninhydrin test are objective tests of sympathetic function. Recovery of sweating has not been shown to correlate with the recovery of sensation, but the absence of sweating correlates with the lack of discriminatory sensation. Other signs of sympathetic dysfunction are smooth, shiny skin; nail changes; and "pencil pointing," or tapering of the fingers.[62]

### *Nerve Compression and Nerve Regeneration*

Sensibility testing is done (1) to assess the recovery of a nerve after laceration and repair; (2) to determine the presence of a nerve compression syndrome and the return of nerve function after surgical decompression; and (3) to determine the efficacy of conservative treatment to reduce compression. Therefore tests such as vibratory tests may be interpreted differently depending on the mechanism of nerve dysfunction.

*Tinel's sign and Phalen's test* Although these tests are not considered to be tests of sensibility, they are used to assess the rate of nerve recovery (Tinel's) and are considered "provocative" tests in nerve compression syndromes because they will elicit the pathological response of the nerve when used. During the first 2 to 4 months after nerve suture, axons will regenerate and travel through the hand at a rate of about 1 mm per day or 1 inch per month (2.54 cm). Tinel's sign may be used to follow this regeneration.[38] The test is performed by tapping gently along the course of the nerve, starting distally and moving toward the nerve suture to elicit a tingling sensation in the fingertip. The point at which tapping begins to elicit a tingling sensation is noted and indicates the extent of sensory axon growth. As regeneration occurs, hypesthesias will develop. Although this hypersensitivity may be uncomfortable to the patient, it is a positive sign of nerve growth. A treatment program for desensitization of hypersensitive areas can be initiated as soon as the skin is healed and can tolerate gentle rubbing and immersion in textures. Desensitization is discussed further in the treatment section.

The examiner may attempt to elicit Tinel's sign in nerve compression by tapping the median nerve at the level of the wrist carpal tunnel.[48] Tinel's sign is positive if there is a tingling along the course of the nerve distally when tapped. Phalen's test will also produce the nerve parasthesias present in compression of the median nerve. The patient is asked to hold the wrist in a fully flexed position for 60 seconds. It is considered positive if tingling occurs within this time.[48]

### *Vibration*

Tuning forks are used for assessing the return of vibratory sensation after nerve repair as regeneration occurs and as a guideline for initiating a sensory reeducation program.[24,25] There are also commercially available vibrometers to detect abnormal sensation.

Vibration and the Semmes-Weinstein monofilament tests[9] are more sensitive in picking up a gradual decrease in nerve function in the presence of nerve compression where the nerve circuitry is intact. Therefore vibration, Semmes-Weinstein, and electrical testing are reliable and sensitive tests for early detection of carpal tunnel syndrome and other nerve compression syndromes. Vibration and Semmes-Weinstein tests can be performed in the clinic with no discomfort to the patient and are excellent screening tools when nerve compression is suspected.[8,30]

### *Touch Pressure*

Moving touch is tested with the eraser end of a pencil. The eraser is placed in an area of normal sensibility and, pressing lightly, is moved to the distal fingertip. The patient notes when the perception of the stimulus changes. Light and heavy stimuli may be applied and noted.[23] Constant touch is tested by pressing with the eraser end of the pencil, first in an area with normal sensibility and then moving distally. The patient responds when the stimulus is altered again; light and heavy stimulus may be applied.[23] The Semmes-Weinstein monofilaments are the most accurate instrument for assessing cutaneous pressure thresholds.[9] The test is composed of 20 nylon monofilaments housed in plastic hand-held rods. Markings on the probes range from 1.65 to 6.65. Normal fingertip sensibility has been found to correspond to the 2.44 and 2.83 probes.

The monofilaments must be applied perpendicularly to the skin and are applied just until the monofilament bends. Results can be graded from normal light touch (probes 2.83 and above) to loss of protective sensation (probes 4.56 and below).

### *Two-Point and Moving Two-Point Discrimination*

Discrimination, the second level of sensibility assessment, requires the subject to distinguish between two direct stimuli. A variety of devices have been used in measuring two-point discrimination. The bent paper clip is inexpensive but often has burrs on the metal tip. Other devices include industrial calipers and the Disk-Criminator.[41] A device with parallel prongs of variable distance and blunted ends should produce replicable results.

Moving two-point discrimination is slightly more sensitive than stationary two-point discrimination.[39] Two point values increase with age in both sexes, with the smallest values occurring between the ages of

10 and 30. Females tend to have smaller values than men, and there is no significant difference between dominant and nondominant hands.[39]

### *Modified Moberg Pick-Up Test*

Recognition of common objects is the final level of sensory function. Moberg used the phrase "tactile gnosis" to describe the ability of the hand to perform complex function by feel. Moberg described the Pick-Up Test in 1958,[59] which was later modified by Dellon.[23] This test is used with either a median nerve injury or a combination of median and ulnar nerves. Clinically, it has been observed that it takes twice as long to perform the tests with vision occluded than with vision not occluded. The test is performed as follows:

1. Nine or ten small objects (coins, paper clips etc.) are placed on a table, and the patient is asked to place them one at a time in a small container as quickly as possible while looking at them. The patient is timed.
2. The test is repeated for the opposite hand with vision.
3. The test is repeated for each hand with the vision occluded.
4. The patient is asked to identify each object one at a time with and then without vision.

It is important to observe any substitution patterns that may be used when the patient cannot see the objects.

## FUNCTIONAL EVALUATION

**Evaluation of hand function** or performance is important because the physical evaluation does not measure the patient's ingenuity and ability to compensate for the loss of strength, ROM, sensation, or for the presence of deformities.[17] The results of the physical evaluation will, however, increase the therapist's understanding of functional impairment and of why patients function the way they do.[47]

The occupational therapy practitioner should observe the effect of dysfunction on use of the hand during ADL. In addition, a standardized performance evaluation, such as the Jebsen Test of Hand Function[31] or the Carroll Quantitative Test of Upper Extremity Function,[17] should be administered. These tests can be within the scope of the COTA role.

### Jebsen Hand Function Test

This test was developed to provide objective measurements of standardized tasks with norms for patient comparison. It is a short test that is assembled by the administrator. It is easy to administer and inexpensive. The test consists of seven subtests: (1) writing a short sentence, (2) turning over 5-inch cards three times, (3) picking up small objects and placing them in a container, (4) stacking checkers, (5) eating (simulated), (6) moving large empty cans, and (7) moving large weighted cans. Norms are provided for dominant and nondominant hands for each subtest and are also divided by sex and age. Instruction for assembling the test, as well as specific instructions for administering it, are provided by the authors.[31] This has been found to be a good test for overall hand function.

### Quantitative Upper Extremity Function Test

Described by Carroll,[17] this test was designed to measure ability to perform general arm and hand activities used in daily living. It is based on the assumption that complex upper extremity movements used to perform ordinary ADL can be reduced to specific patterns of grasp and prehension of the hand, supination and pronation of the forearm, flexion and extension of the elbow, and elevation of the arm.

The test consists of the following six parts: (1) grasping and lifting four blocks of graduated sizes to assess grips; (2) grasping and lifting two pipes of graduated sizes from a peg to test cylindrical grip; (3) grasping and placing a ball to test spherical grasp; (4) picking up and placing four marbles of graduated sizes to test fingertip prehension or pinch; (5) putting a small washer over a nail and putting an iron on a shelf to test placing; and (6) pouring water from a pitcher to a glass and a glass to a glass; placing hand on top of head, behind head, and to mouth; and writing the name to assess pronation, supination, and elevation of the arm. The test uses simple, inexpensive, and easily acquired materials. Details of materials and their arrangement, test procedures, and scoring can be found in the original source.[18]

### Dexterity Tests

Other tests that have been found to be useful in the evaluation of hand dexterity are the Crawford Small Parts Dexterity Test,[19] the Bennett Hand Tool Dexterity Test,[11] the Purdue Pegboard Test,[60] and the Minnesota Manual Dexterity Test.[58] The Valpar Corporation has developed a number of standardized tests that measure an individual's ability to perform work-related tasks. They provide information about the test taker's results compared with industry performance standards. All of these tests include comparison with normal subjects working in a variety of industrial settings. This information can be used in predicting the likelihood of successful return to a specific job. These tests are especially useful when administering a work capacity evaluation. Tests may be purchased and come with standardized norms and instructions for administering the test. Melvin[47] lists additional hand function tests.

## GOAL-DIRECTED TREATMENT TECHNIQUES

### Edema Reduction

Edema is a normal consequence of trauma but must be quickly and aggressively treated to prevent permanent stiffness and disability. Within hours of trauma, vasodilation and local edema occur.

Early control of edema should be achieved through elevation, massage, compression, and active ROM. The patient is instructed at the time of injury to keep the hand elevated, and a compressive dressing is applied to reduce early swelling. Pitting edema is present early and can be recognized as a bloated swelling that "pits" when pressed. This may be more pronounced on the dorsal surface where the venous and lymphatic systems provide return of fluid to the heart. Active motion is especially important to produce retrograde venous and lymphatic flow; active ROM moves this fluid back into the general circulatory system.

If the swelling continues, a serofibrinous exudate invades the area. Fibrin is deposited in the spaces surrounding the joints, tendons, and ligaments, resulting in reduced mobility, flattening of the arches of the hand, tissue atrophy, and further disuse.[42] Normal gliding of the tissues is reduced, and a stiff, often painful hand will be the result. Scar adhesions will form and further limit tissue mobility. If untreated, these losses may become permanent.

Early recognition of persistent edema through volume and circumference measurement is important. It may be necessary to use several of the suggested edema control techniques.

### Elevation

Early elevation with the hand above the heart is essential. Slings tend to reduce blood flow and should be avoided. Resting the hand on pillows while seated or lying down is effective. Resting the hand on top of the head or using devices that elevate the hand with the elbow in extension have been suggested. Suspension slings may be purchased or fabricated.

The patient should use the injured hand for ADL within the limitations of resistance prescribed by the physician. Light ADL that can be accomplished while the hand is in the dressing are permitted.

### Contrast Baths

Alternating soaks of cold and warm water that is 66° and 96° F (18.9° and 35.6° C) have been recommended as a method preferred over warm water soaks or whirlpool baths. The contrast baths can be done for 20 minutes, alternating the hand between cool water for 1 minute and warm water for 1 minute. Start and end with cool water. A sponge can be placed in each tub so that the hand can be exercised during the soaking period. The tubs should be placed as high as possible to provide elevation of the extremity. The alternating warm and cool water will cause vasodilation and vasoconstriction, resulting in a pumping action on the edema. Contrast baths, along with elevation and active motion, may reduce edema and alleviate pain.

### Retrograde Massage

A retrograde massage may be done by the practitioner, but it should be taught to the patient so that it can be done frequently throughout the day. The massage assists in blood and lymph flow. It should be started distally and stroked proximally with the extremity in elevation.[22] Active motion should follow the massage but muscle fatigue should be avoided.

In more severe cases, when the hand and forearm are involved, retrograde massage is a two-stage procedure. First, begin proximally (i.e., midforearm to "empty" the proximal body part). Next, the hand, or distal part, is massaged so that this fluid may be emptied into an available space.

### Pressure Wraps

Wrapping with **Coban** elastic[26] may be used to reduce edema (Figure 35-6). Starting distally, the finger is wrapped snugly with Coban. Care must be taken not to pull the Coban too tightly as this may constrict circulation. Each involved finger should be wrapped distally to proximally until the wrap is proximal to the edema. The wrap remains in place for 5 minutes and then is removed. Active exercise may be done while the finger is wrapped or immediately after. Measurements should be taken before and after treatment to document an increase in ROM and a decrease in edema. The wrapping may be repeated three times a day.

Light compression may be applied throughout the day with a light Coban wrap, an Isotoner glove, or a

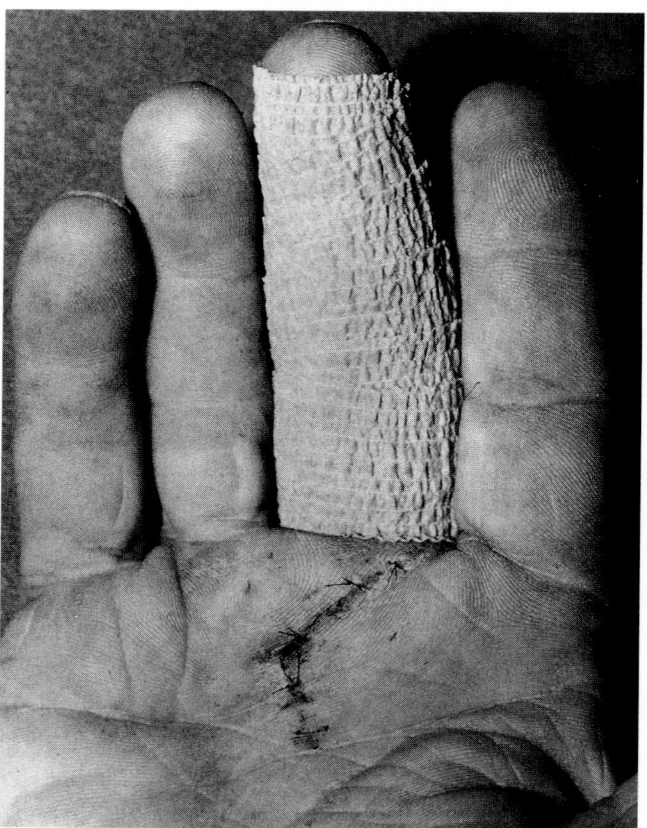

*Figure 35-6* One-inch Coban is wrapped with minimal pressure from distal to proximal.

custom-made garment by Bioconcepts or Jobst (Figure 35-7). The compression should not be constricting and should be discontinued if ischemia results. Elastic ace bandages may be used for larger areas. A 3- or 4-inch wide elastic bandage may be used when the entire hand and forearm require a gentle pressure wrap. A variety of pressure wraps are used by hand centers. Tubular gauze and Digisleeves[2] provide compression to a specific finger. No one method is superior to the other. A combination of techniques used at different stages of healing and according to patient comfort may be the most effective.

#### *Active Range of Motion*

Normal blood flow is dependent on muscle activity. Active motion does not mean wiggling the fingers, but rather maximum available ROM done firmly. Casts and splints must allow mobility of uninjured parts while protecting newly injured structures. The shoulder and elbow should be moved several times a day. The importance of active ROM for edema control, tendon gliding, and tissue nutrition cannot be overemphasized.

### Range of Motion Improvement

To improve ROM, the following questions must be answered:

1. What is the available passive ROM?
2. Is muscle strength available?
3. Can the tendons glide?

Passive ROM gives information about the noncontractile structures, such as ligaments surrounding the joint. Passive ROM is assessed by the therapist moving the joint throughout its available ROM. Active ROM gives information about the contractile units moving the joint. When there is more passive ROM than active ROM, there is a problem with the contracting unit (i.e., muscle weakness or tendon adherence). If PROM is limited, the specific cause of the limitation must be addressed by the therapist together with treatment strategies to improve AROM.

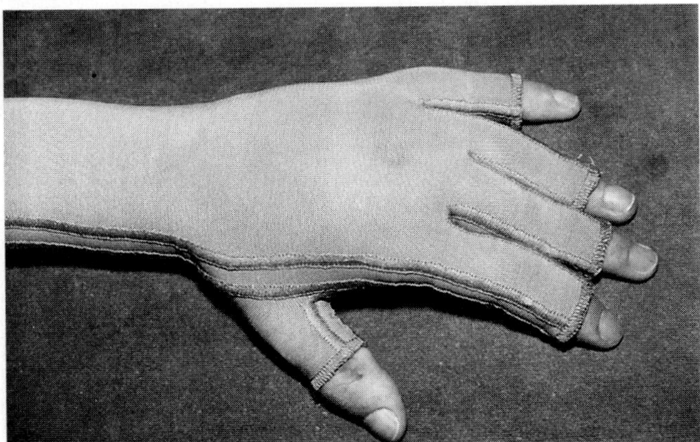

*Figure 35-7* Custom-fit Jobst garment may be used to reduce edema and to reduce or prevent hypertrophic scar formation after burns or trauma.

To improve passive ROM, the OTR may use a combination of the following: modalities to improve tissue elasticity, joint mobilization techniques to restore joint play, passive ROM to involved joint, and dynamic or static progressive splinting. The COTA may supplement these passive ROM treatment strategies with specific exercises or activities targeted to the involved structures. The clinician must be sensitive to the patient's age and interest when selecting activities. As with any rehabilitation program, the patient should be provided with a specific home exercise program that will supplement and reinforce the therapy.

### Soft Tissue Mobility Improvement

Many hand therapy patients have experienced an invasive event to the hand, be it through trauma or surgical intervention. Therefore the COTA must be familiar with wound healing theory to assist the OTR in managing the acute hand injury or surgery. All wounds lead to formation of scars, which are necessary for healing. It is the practitioner's responsibility to use techniques that will modify and remodel the scar to preserve soft tissue mobility.

Tissues that have restored gliding have different scar architecture from those that do not develop the ability to glide. With gliding, the scar resembles the state of the tissues before injury, whereas the nongliding scar remains fixed on surrounding structures. Controlled tension on a scar has been shown to facilitate remodeling. Scar formation is also influenced by the patient's age and the quantity of scar deposited.[42]

#### *Pressure*

A hypertrophic scar, or a scar that is randomly laid down and thickened, is unable to glide properly and therefore may restrict active ROM, contribute to deformity, or be cosmetically unacceptable. The principal technique used to modify a scar is the application of pressure, similar to the techniques used in burn rehabilitation.

There are several types of commercially available products that when used in combination enable the clinician to manage scars effectively. For example, the following products can be used as the contact medium with the skin: Otoform, Silastic Elastomer, and Prosthetic Foam. These products are generally held in place with pressure devices such as Coban wrap, Isotoner gloves, ace bandages, or pressure elastic garments. Pressure should be applied for most of the 24-hour period and removed for bathing and exercise. As the scar changes in response to the pressure, the contact medium needs to be replaced. For those patients with burns, the garment is worn 23 hours per day and may need to be worn for 6 months to 18 months, depending on the severity of the burn.

*Massage*

Gentle to firm massage of the scarred area with a thick ointment, such as lanolin or Corrective Concepts Cream will rapidly soften scar tissue and should be followed immediately with active hand use, so that tendons will glide against the softened scar.[22] Vibration to the area with a small, low intensity vibrator will have a similar effect.[32] Active exercise with facilitation techniques, exercise against resistance, or functional activity should follow vibration. Massage and vibration may be started 4 weeks after the injury.

Thermal heat in the form of paraffin dips, hot packs, or Fluidotherapy immediately followed by stretching while the tissue cools will provide stretch to the scar tissue. Wrapping the scarred or stiff digit into flexion with Coban during the application of heat will often increase mobility in the area. Heat should not be used with insensate areas or if swelling persists.[33] These techniques can be carried out by the COTA under close supervision of a registered therapist.

*Active Range of Motion and Physical Agent Modalities*

Active ROM provides an internal stretch against a resistant scar, and its use cannot be overemphasized. When the patient is unable to achieve active range because of scar adhesions or weakness, an OTR may use a battery-operated neuromuscular electrical stimulator (NMES) that assists the motion.[65] High-voltage, direct-current ultrasound and a continuous passive motion machine may be judiciously used by the registered therapist. These modalities help increase motor activity and help remodel the scar. The use of all physical agent modalities requires a prescription from a physician and must be administered by a qualified registered therapist.

## SENSATION NORMALIZATION

As an injury to the hand resolves, the hand or a portion of it may be either hypersensitive or hyposensitive. For example, after trauma to a peripheral or digital nerve, sensibility can be expected to return in a certain order.[24] To facilitate the return of function to the peripheral or digital nerve, a program of sensory reeducation may be used. Alternatively, a patient may have a hypersensitive area, one that is excessively sensitive to even the lightest touch, making it almost impossible for that person to manipulate ordinary items. In this case, a program of desensitization is indicated.

### Sensory Reeducation

Evaluation of sensibility has been described earlier in this chapter. The OTR would use this information to prepare a program of sensory reeducation after nerve repair.

When a nerve is repaired, regeneration is not perfect, resulting in fewer and smaller nerve fibers and receptors distal to the repair. The goal of sensory reeducation is to maximize the functional level of sensation. All programs emphasize a variety of stimuli used in a repetitive manner to bombard the sensory receptors. A sequence of eyes-closed, eyes-open, eyes-closed is used to provide feedback during the training process. Sessions are limited in length to avoid fatigue and frustration. Objects must not be potentially harmful to the insensate areas to avoid further trauma. A home program should be provided to reinforce learning that occurs in the clinical setting.

The authors[14,23,62] have found that sensory reeducation can result in improved functional sensibility in motivated patients. Objective measurement of sensation after reeducation must be performed and then compared with initial testing to accurately assess the success of the program.

### Sensory Desensitization

**Sensory desensitization** techniques are based on the theory that nerve fibers that carry pain sensation can be positively influenced through the use of pressure, rubbing, vibration, TENS, percussion, and active motion.

Yerxa et al[67] have described a desensitization program that "employs short periods of contact with three sensory modalities: dowel textures, immersion or contact particles, and vibration." This program allows the patient to rank 10 dowel textures and 10 immersion textures on the degree of irritation produced by the stimulus. Treatment begins with a stimulus that is irritating but tolerable. The stimulus is applied for 10 minutes 3 or 4 times a day. The vibration hierarchy is predetermined and is based on cycles per second (cps) of vibration, the placement of the vibrator, and the duration of the treatment. The Downey Hand Center hand sensitivity test can be used to establish a desensitization treatment program and to measure progress in decreasing hypersensitivity.[66]

### Strength Improvement

Acute care is followed by a gradual return of motion, sensibility, and preparation to return to normal ADL. Strengthening of the injured and neglected extremity is usually not accomplished by patients at home because they are often fearful of further injury and pain. Because every hand clinic has its own armamentarium of strengthening exercises and media, only a few suggestions are provided here.

*Computerized Evaluation and Exercise Equipment*

**Baltimore Therapeutic Equipment (BTE)** has made available the BTE work simulator[21] (Figure 35-8), an electromechanical device that has more than 20 interchangeable tool handles and can be used for both work evaluation and upper extremity strengthening. Resistance can vary from no resistance to complete static resistance; tool height and angle are also adjustable. When used for strengthening, the resistance is usually set low and gradually increased, with concurrent increases in length of exercise. The BTE work simulator

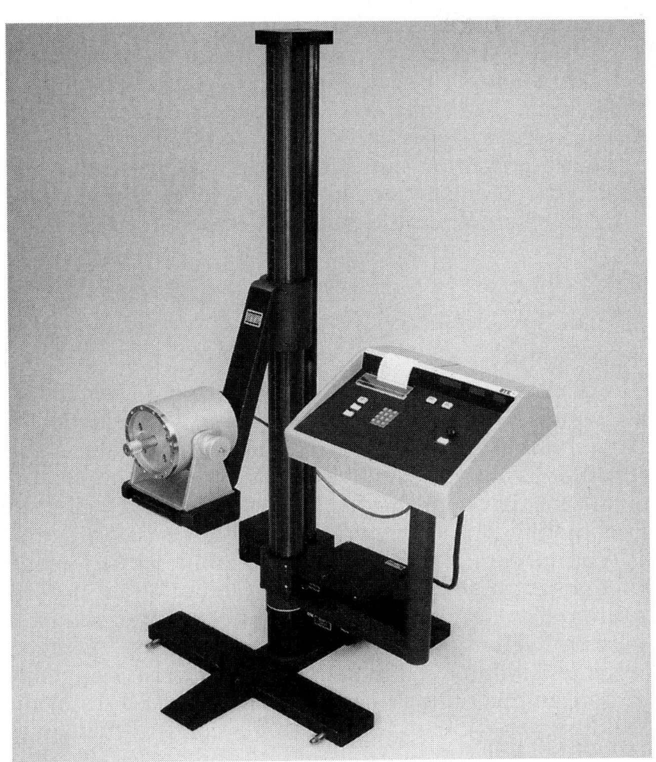

*Figure 35-8* The BTE Work Simulator is used to simulate real-life tasks. The patient's progress can be monitored through a computerized print-out, and the program can be modified to increase resistance and endurance.

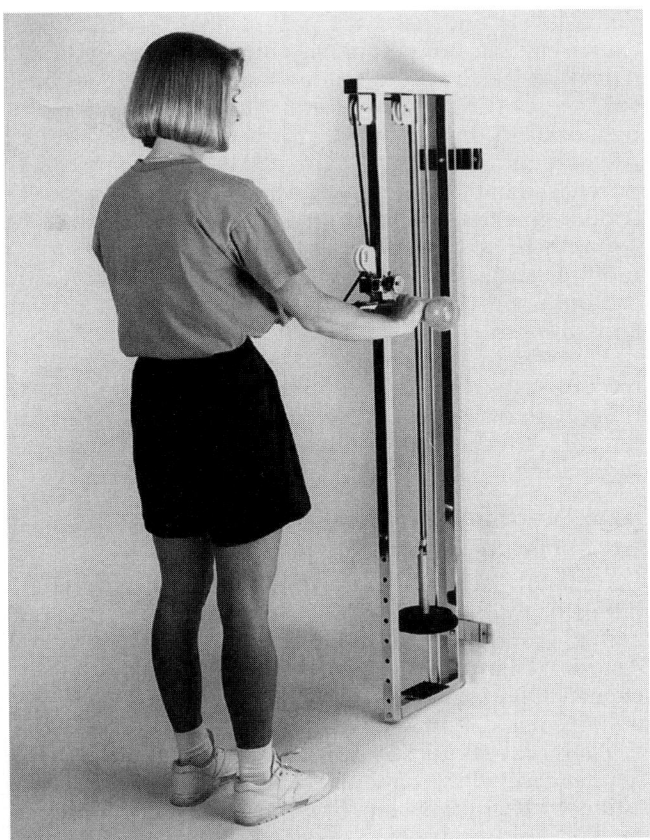

*Figure 35-9* Weight well used for upper extremity and pinch and grip strengthening. (Courtesy Karen Schultz Johnson.)

allows for close simulation of physical demands common to manual work in the real world.

Other computerized evaluation equipment includes the EVAL system, which allows the therapist to record the results of evaluation, to print a report, and to estimate the percentage of impairment. The Dexter Evaluation and Therapy System can be used to evaluate the patient, record and report the results of evaluation, establish an exercise program, record the results of each therapy session, and compare changes in the individual's strength or ROM. Portable systems are also being developed that will allow the therapist to record daily treatment and enter the information into a computerized network. Outcome data from many sources can then be compared. The advancement of technology in rehabilitation will allow greater efficiency of the therapist while capturing important information that is not available through traditional means.

### Weight Well

The **weight well**[5] (Figure 35-9) is available commercially. A variety of handle shapes are attached to rods with suspended weights. The rods are turned against resistance throughout the ROM to encourage full grasp and release of the injured hand, wrist flexion and wrist extension, pinch, and pronation and supination patterns. The weight well can be graded for resistance and repetitions and is an excellent tool for progressive resistive exercise.

### Theraband

**Theraband** is a 6-inch-wide (15.2 cm) rubber sheet that is available by the yard and is color coded by degrees of resistance. It can be cut into any length required and used for resistive exercise for the upper extremity. Use of Theraband is limited only by the therapist's imagination; it can be adapted to diagonal patterns of motion, wrist exercises, follow-up treatment of tennis elbow, and other uses. The Theraband can be combined with dowel rods and other equipment to provide resistance throughout the ROM. It is inexpensive and easy to incorporate into a home treatment program.

### Hand Strengthening Equipment

Hand grips of graded resistance are available from rehabilitation supply companies and sporting goods stores. They can be purchased with various resistance levels and used for progressive resistive hand exercises. The practitioner is cautioned against using overly resistive spring-loaded grippers such as those sold in sporting goods stores. These devices may be beneficial to the seasoned athlete but are usually too resistive for the recently injured. Therapy putty can be purchased in bulk and in grades of resistance. It is color coded to allow easy progression of the patient as strength improves. It can be adapted to most finger motions and is easily used as part of a home program; the amount given to the patient is adjusted to hand size and strength.

Household items such as spring-type clothespins have been used to increase strength of grasp and pinch. Imaginative use of common objects may originate with the clinician or the patient and is highly beneficial and motivating.

### ADL Function Improvement

#### *Functional Activities*

Functional activities are an integral part of rehabilitation of the hand. Functional activities may include crafts, games, dexterity activities, ADL, and work samples. Many of the treatment techniques described to this point are used to condition the hand for normal use.

Activities should be started as soon as possible at whatever level the patient can perform them, with adaptations to compensate for limited ROM and strength. They should be used in conjunction with other treatments. The OTR must continually assess the patient's functional capacities and initiate changes in the treatment program to introduce activities as soon as possible in the restorative phase.

Vocational and avocational goals should be noted at the time of initial evaluation and taken into account when planning treatment. The needs of a brick mason are likely to be quite different from those of a mother with small children—the environmental needs of the patient must not be neglected. Crafts should be graded from light to heavy resistance and from gross to fine dexterity. Crafts that have been found to work extremely well with hand injuries include macramé, Turkish knot weaving, clay, leather, and woodworking.

All of these crafts can be adapted and graded to the patient's capabilities and have been found to have a high level of patient acceptance. When integrated into a program of total hand rehabilitation, they are viewed as another milestone of achievement and not as a diversion to fill up empty hours. For example, the pride of accomplishment felt by a patient who sustained a Volkmann's contracture caused by ischemia and then completed the first project in nearly 4 years is evidence that crafts belong in hand rehabilitation.

Activities that do not have an end product but provide practice in dexterity and ADL skills also fit into the category of functional activities. Developmental games and activities that require pinch or grasp and release may be graded and timed to increase difficulty. ADL boards that have a variety of opening and closing devices provide practice for use of the hand at home and increase self-confidence. String and finger games are challenging and entertaining coordination activities that can be done in pairs. Many times a hobby can be adapted for use in the clinic. Fly-tying (making lures for trout from string and feathers) is a difficult dexterity activity but one that will be enjoyed by avid fishermen. Golf clubs and fishing poles can be adapted in the clinic to allow early return to a favorite form of relaxation. Humor and interaction with the therapists and other patients provide vital, but intangible benefits. Treatment should be planned to promote both.

## SPECIFIC INTERVENTIONS FOR SELECTED HAND INJURIES

### Amputations

A common injury among people using machinery such as saws and snow blowers, is a traumatically amputated finger tip or partial finger amputation. See Chapter 27 for information on upper extremity amputations, so the discussion here is concerned with partial finger and finger tip amputations.

The surgeon's goal is to ensure good skin coverage of the amputated part when replantation is not an option. This may be achieved in a variety of surgical methods. The goal of occupational therapy, however, remains essentially the same: wound care, desensitization, edema reduction, restoring ROM, and restoring full function. Edema reduction is a concern that must be addressed immediately. Elevation, massage, and gentle wraps can be initiated early postoperatively, possibly before ROM therapy is begun. However, all uninvolved joints must be ranged immediately.

Very often, patients with a partial finger or finger tip amputation are left with a hypersensitive residual finger tip. If left untreated, a patient would be unable to use that finger to touch or pick up most common objects. Once the wound is closed with satisfactory coverage (i.e., skin thick enough to act as a cushion to the underlying bone yet not so thin that skin breakdown is a constant concern) a program of desensitization can begin. Traditionally, this includes tapping on or near the finger tip, sensory stimulation with a variety of textures, vibration, and submerging the finger in a container of raw rice or other materials.[23]

ROM of the affected digit and adjacent fingers may be limited as a result of the patient's limited pain tolerance, edema, and fear of moving. This must be addressed immediately with an appropriate program in the clinic and then followed up with a home exercise program. Occasionally, a splint may be indicated to improve ROM in a stiff joint, usually the proximal interphalangeal (PIP) joint of the involved finger.

While these concerns are being addressed, the patient should be encouraged to use the hand in as many functional activities as possible, such as dressing, feeding, and other light activities. If the patient has a sedentary job, an early return to work is advised. People whose work demands heavy, bimanual activity may have to increase strength and endurance before returning to work. With appropriate rehabilitation, a single partial finger or finger tip amputation should have little impact on a person's ability to return to full employment.

### Flexor Tendon Injuries

Injuries to tendons may be isolated or occur in conjunction with other injuries, especially fractures or crushes. Both flexor (palmer) and extensor (dorsal) surfaces of the hand have been divided into distinct areas called *zones*. The way in which the injury is managed is dependent on the area or zone of the injury. **Flexor tendons** injured in the area between the distal palmar crease and the insertion of the flexor digitorum superficialis (zone 2) are considered to be the most difficult to treat, because the tendons lie in their sheaths in this area beneath the fibrous pulley system, and any scarring will cause adhesions. This area is often referred to as *no man's land*.

Primary repair of the flexor tendons within this zone is most frequently attempted after a clean laceration. Several methods of postoperative management have been proposed with the common goal to promote gliding of the tendons and to minimize the formation of scar adhesions. There are now three methods of postoperative management of lacerated flexor tendons: early active mobilization, controlled passive mobilization, and immobilization.

#### *Early Active Motion*

Dr. Harold Kleinert, a pioneer of flexor tendon surgery, was an early advocate of rubber band traction after repair of flexor tendons. This technique is often referred to as the *Klienert technique*. After surgical repair, rubber bands are attached to the nails of the involved fingers with a suture through the nail or with a hook held in place with cyanoacrylate glue. A dorsal blocking splint is fabricated from low-temperature thermoplastic material with the metacarpophalangeal (MCP) joints held in about 60 degrees of flexion and the PIPs in gentle flexion. The patient must be able to fully extend the IP joints actively within the splint or joint contractures will develop (Figure 35-10).

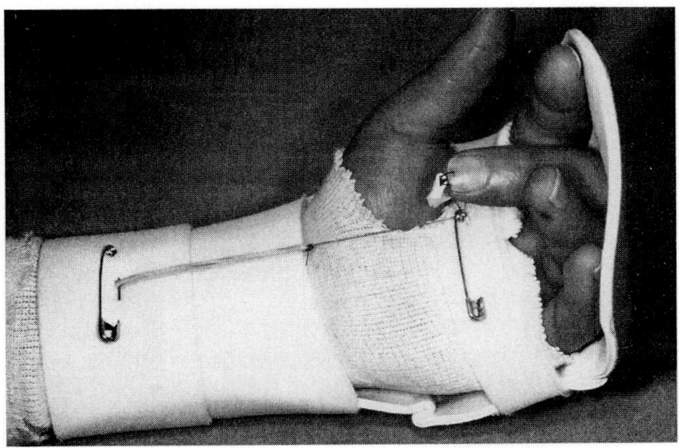

*Figure 35-10* The dorsal blocking splint allows for passive flexion of the digit(s) and full active extension at the PIP and DIP joints.

The patient wears this splint 24 hours a day for 3 weeks and is instructed to actively extend the fingers several times a day in the splint, allowing the rubber bands to pull the fingers into flexion. The movement of tendon through the tendon sheath and pulley system minimizes scar adhesions while enhancing tendon nutrition and blood flow. The dorsal blocking splint is removed at 3 weeks, and the rubber band is attached to a wrist band, which is worn for 1 to 5 additional weeks, depending on the judgment of the surgeon.

The primary disadvantage of this technique is that contractures of the PIP joints frequently occur as a result of too much tension on the rubber band or incomplete IP extension within the splint. Dynamic extension splinting of the PIP joint can be started at 5 to 6 weeks if a flexion contracture is present. To be successful, this technique requires a motivated patient who thoroughly understands the program. There are currently early active mobilization protocols that allow early active extension and flexion of the repaired tendons.[57] Only the most experienced OTR who is in close contact with the surgeon should attempt this protocol.

#### *Controlled Passive Motion: Duran and Houser Technique*

Duran and Houser[27] suggested the use of controlled passive motion to achieve optimal results after primary repair, allowing 3 to 5 mm of tendon excursion. They found this to be sufficient to prevent adherence of the repaired tendons. On the third postoperative day, the patient begins a twice daily exercise regimen of passive flexion and extension of 6 to 8 motions for each tendon. Care is taken to keep the wrist flexed and the MCPs in 70 degrees of flexion during passive exercise. Between exercise periods, the hand is wrapped in a stockinette. After 4½ weeks the protective dorsal splint is removed and the rubber band traction is attached to a wrist band. Active extension and passive flexion are done for 1 additional week and gradually increased over the next several weeks.

#### *Immobilization Technique*

A third postoperative protocol is complete immobilization for 3½ weeks after tendon repair. Immobilization may not result in consistently good results and may lead to a greater incidence of tendon rupture. However, if a patient appears to be unable to participate fully in treatment, a surgeon may elect this method.

#### *Postacute Flexor Tendon Rehabilitation*

When active flexion is begun out of the splint after any of the postoperative management techniques described previously, the patient should be instructed in exercises to facilitate differential tendon gliding.[63] Wehbe[64] recommends three positions: hook, straight fist, and fist, to maximize isolated gliding of the flexor digitorum superficialis and the flexor digitorum pro-

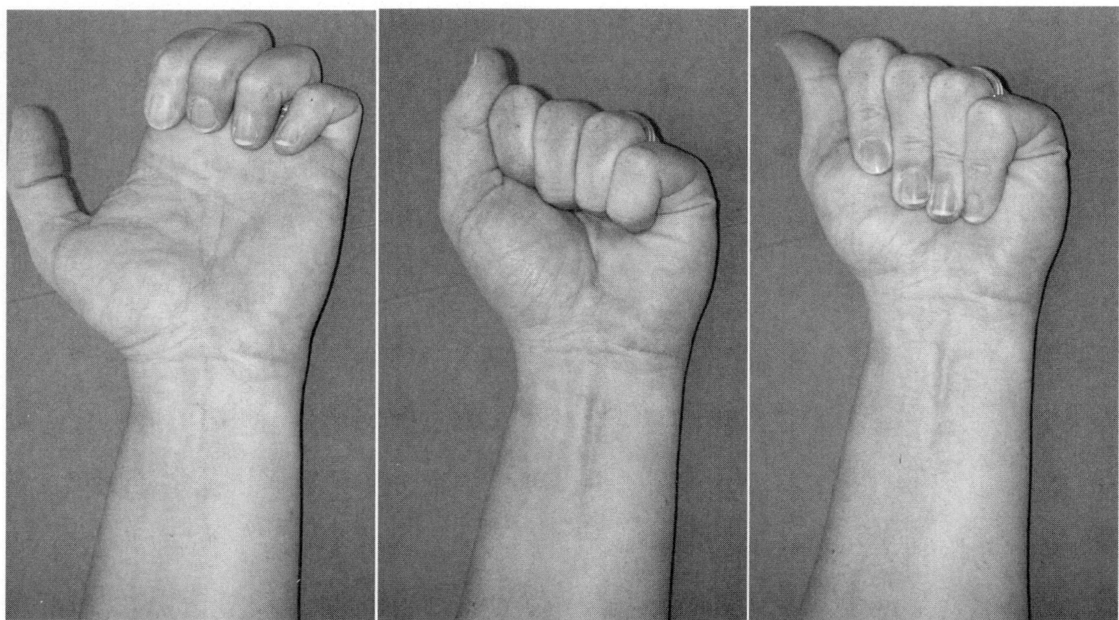

*Figure 35-11* Tendon gliding exercises. Patient starts with fingers in full extension and then makes each of these fist positions.

fundus tendons, as well as stretching of the intrinsic musculature and gliding of the extensor mechanism. Tendon gliding exercises should be done for 10 repetitions of each position, 2 to 3 times per day (Figure 35-11). Isolated exercises to assist tendon gliding may also be performed with a blocking splint[34] (Figure 35-12) or the opposite hand (Figure 35-13). The MCP joints should be held in extension during blocking so the intrinsic muscles that act on it cannot overcome the power of the repaired flexor tendons. Care should be taken not to hyperextend the PIP joint and overstretch the repaired tendons.

After 6 to 8 weeks, passive extension may be started, and a volar finger splint may be necessary to correct a flexion contracture at a PIP joint. A cylindrical plaster splint may be fabricated by the OTR to apply constant static pressure on the contracture as described by Bell-Krotoski [7](Figure 35-14).

After approximately 8 weeks the patient may begin light resistive exercises, light ADL, and other activities. The patient must avoid lifting with or applying excessive resistance to the affected hand. Sports activities should be discouraged. However, activities such as working with clay, woodworking, and macramé are excellent. Full resistance and normal work activities can be started at 3 months after surgery.

Although performance of ADL is generally not a problem, the therapist should ask patients about any problems they may have or anticipate. Disuse and neglect of a finger, especially the index finger, are common and should be prevented.

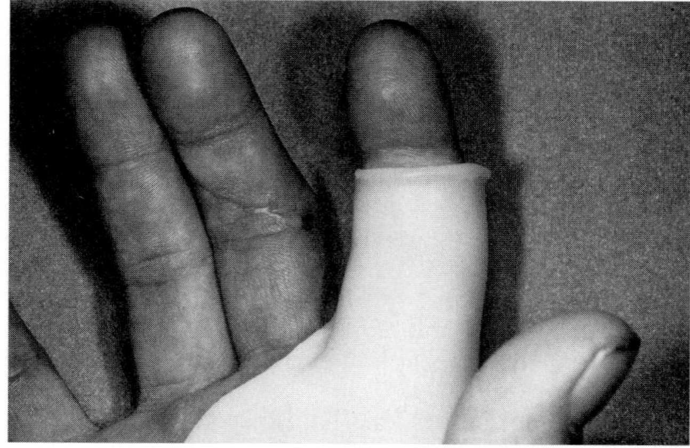

*Figure 35-12* A blocking splint can allow the patient to perform isolated tendon motion at a specified joint.

Gains in finger flexion and extension may continue to be recorded for 6 months postoperatively. A finger with limber joints and minimal scarring preoperatively will function better after repair than one that is stiff and scarred or has trophic skin changes.[16] A "functional" to "excellent" result is obtained when there is minimal extension lag at the PIP and distal interphalangeal (DIP) joints and the finger(s) can flex to the palm.[14]

### Extensor Tendon Injuries

Dorsal scar adherence is the most difficult problem after injury to the **extensor tendons,** because of the

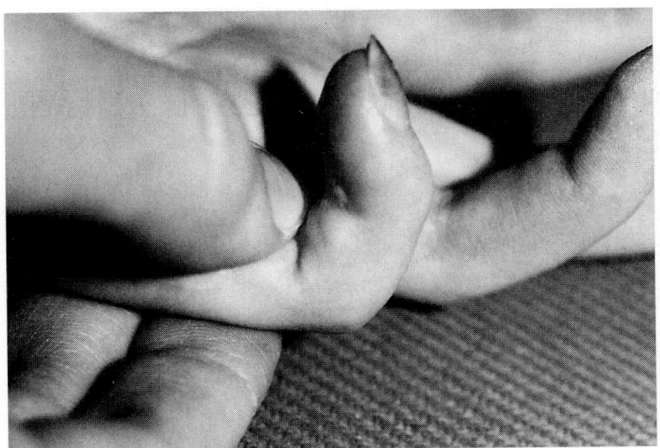

*Figure 35-13* Manual blocking of the MCP during active flexion of the PIP joint.

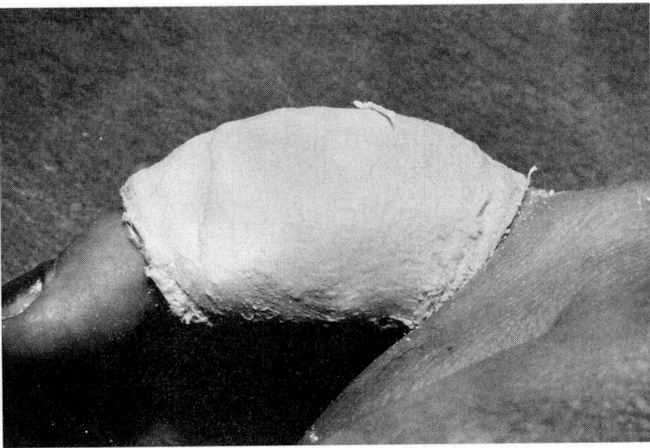

*Figure 35-14* Plaster cylindrical cast used to apply gentle static stretch to PIP joint.

tendency of the dorsal extensor hood to become adherent to the underlying structures and thus limit its normal excursion during flexion and extension. Extensor tendons proximal to the MCP joints frequently become adherent to the structures above and below them. This adherance results in either incomplete extension, also known as *extensor lag,* or incomplete flexion resulting from loss of gliding of the extensor tendon. Either of these conditions will require the OTR to begin a splinting program. The splint is worn for 3 weeks, with the initiation of active motion between the third and fourth weeks. A removable volar splint is used between exercise periods to protect the tendon for 2 additional weeks. Dynamic flexion splinting may be started 6 weeks after surgery to regain flexion if needed. Injuries to extensor tendons proximal to the MCP joint may be immobilized for 3 weeks. After this, the finger may be placed in a removable volar splint that is worn between exercise periods for an additional 2 weeks. Progressive ROM is begun after 3 weeks, and if full flexion is not regained rapidly, dynamic flexion may be started after 6 weeks.

Extensor tendon injuries that occur distal to the MCP joint require a longer period of immobilization (usually 6 weeks). A progressive exercise program is then initiated with dynamic splinting during the day and static splinting at night to maintain extension.

### Peripheral Nerve Injuries

Nerve injury may be classified into the following three categories:

1. Neurapraxia is contusion or bruise of the nerve. The nerve recovers function without treatment within a few days or weeks.
2. Axontmesis is an injury in which nerve fibers distal to the site of the injury degenerate, but the internal organization of the nerve remains intact. No surgical treatment is necessary, and recovery usually occurs within 6 months. The length of time may vary depending on the level of injury.
3. Neurotmesis is a complete laceration of the nerve. Microsurgical repair is required.

**Peripheral nerve injuries** may occur as a result of disruption of the nerve by a fractured bone, laceration, or crush injury. Symptoms of nerve injuries will include weakness or paralysis of muscles that are innervated by motor branches of the injured nerve and sensory loss to areas that are innervated by sensory branches of the injured nerve. Before assessing the patient for nerve loss, the therapist must be familiar with the muscles and areas that are innervated by the three major forearm nerves. A summary of upper extremity peripheral neuropathies can be found in Table 35-1.

#### *Peripheral Neuropathy*

The OTR may administer several quick clinical tests to detect dysfunction of peripheral nerves on the basis of the sensory and motor function of the individual nerve. The ulnar nerve may be tested by asking the patient to pinch with the thumb and index finger and palpating the first dorsal interrosseous muscles (Figure 35-15). The radial nerve may be tested by asking the patient to extend the wrist and fingers (Figure 35-16). Median nerve function is tested by asking the patient to oppose the thumb to the fingers [18] (Figure 35-17). Early signs of median nerve compression are sensory in nature and may be tested by performing Phalen's test and percussing over the median nerve at the wrist to elicit Tinel's sign as described earlier in this chapter.

Patients may also develop compression syndromes of the ulnar and radial nerves that will be indicated by parasthesias along the course of those nerves.

#### *Radial Nerve*

The radial nerve innervates the extensor-supinator group of muscles of the forearm. The sensory distribution of the radial nerve is a strip of the posterior

*Table 35-1*

## Nerve Injuries of the Upper Extremity

| *Nerve* | *Location* | *Affected* | *Test* |
|---|---|---|---|
| Radial nerve (posterior cord; fibers from C5, C6, C7, C8) | Upper arm | Triceps and all distal motors; sensory to SRN | MMT, sensory test |
| Radial nerve | Above elbow | Bracioradialis and all distal motors, sensory to SRN | MMT, sensory |
| Radial nerve | At elbow | Supinator, ECRL, ECRB, and all distal motors; sensory to SRN | MMT, sensory |
| Posterior interosseous nerve | Forearm | ECU, ED, EDM, APL, EPL, EPB, EIP; no sensory loss | Wrist extension—if present indicated PIN rather than high radial nerve |
| Radial nerve at ECRB, radial artery, arcade of Froshe, origin of supinator | Radial tunnel syndrome | Weakness of muscles innervated by PIN, no sensory loss | Palpation for pain over extensor mass; pain with wrist flexion and pronation, pain with wrist extension and supination; pain with resisted middle finger extension |
| Median nerve (lateral cord from C5, C6, C7; medial cord from C8, T1) | High lesions (elbow and above) | Paralysis/weakness of FCR, PL, all FDS, FDP, I and II; FPL, pronator teres and quadratus, opponens pollicis, APB, FPB (radial head), lumbricals I and II; sensory cutaneous branch of median nerve | MMT, sensory |
| Median nerve | Low (at wrist) | Weakness of thenars only | Inability to flex thumb tip and index finger tip to palm; inability to oppose thumb, poor dexterity |
| Median nerve under fibrous band in PT, beneath heads of pronator, arch of FDS, origin of FCR | Pronator syndrome | Weakness in thenars but *not* muscles innervated by AIN; sensory in median nerve distribution in hand | Provocative tests to isolate compression site |
| Median nerve under origin of PT, FDS to middle | Anterior interosseous nerve syndrome | Pure motor, no sensory; forearm pain preceding paralysis; weakness of FPL, FDP I and II, PQ | Inability to flex IP joint of thumb and DIP of index; increased pain with resisted pronation; pain with forearm pressure |
| Median nerve at wrist | Carpal tunnel syndrome | Weakness of median innervated intrinsics, sensory | Provocative tests, Tinel's, sensory |
| Ulnar nerve at elbow (branch of medial cord from C7, C8, T1) | Cubital tunnel syndrome | Weakness/paralysis of FCU, FDP III and IV, ulnar intrinsics; numbness in palmar cutaneous and dorsal cutaneous distribution; loss of grip and pinch strength | Pain with elbow flexion/extension |
| Ulnar nerve at wrist | Compression at Guyon's canal | Weakness and pain in ulnar intrinsics | Reproduced by pressure at site |

*SRN,* Superficial radial nerve; *MMT,* manual muscle test; *ECRL,* extensor carpi radialis longus; *ECRB,* extensor carpi radialis brevis; *ECU,* extensor carpi ulnaris; *ED,* extensor digitorum; *EDM,* extensor digiti minimi; *APL,* abductor pollicus longus; *EPL,* extensor pollicus longus; *EPB,* extensor pollicus brevis, *EIP,* extensor indicus proprius; *PIN,* posterior interosseus nerve; *FCR,* flexor carpi radialis; *PL,* palmaris longus; *FDS,* flexor digitorum superficialis; *FDP,* flexor digitorum profundus; *FPL,* flexor pollicus longus; *APB,* abductor pollicus brevis; *FPB,* flexor pollicus brevis; *AIN,* anterior interosseus nerve; *PT,* pronator teres; *FCR,* flexor carpi radialis; *PQ,* pronator quadratus; *IP,* interphalangeal; *DIP,* distal interphalangeal; *FCU,* flexor carpi ulnaris.

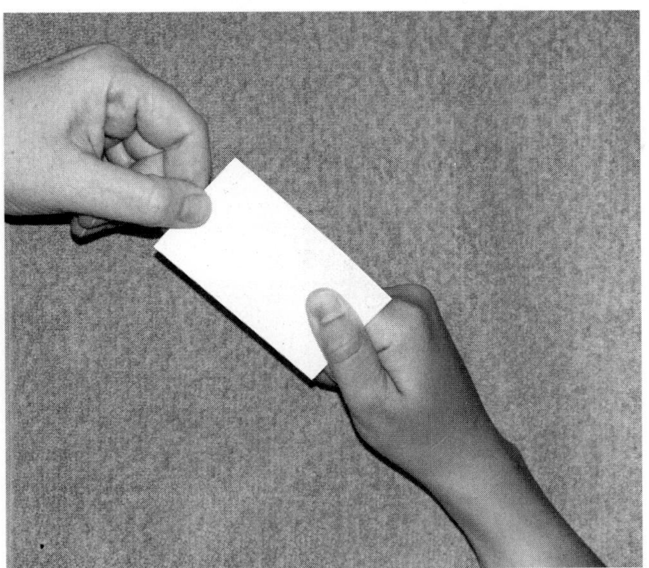

*Figure 35-15* Quick ulnar nerve function test.

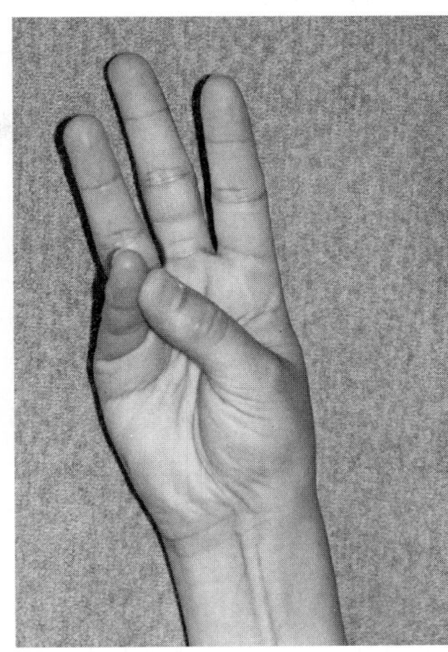

*Figure 35-17* Quick median nerve function test.

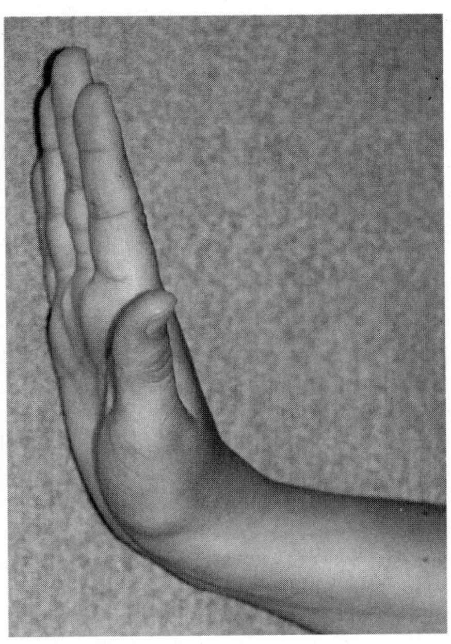

*Figure 35-16* Quick radial nerve function test.

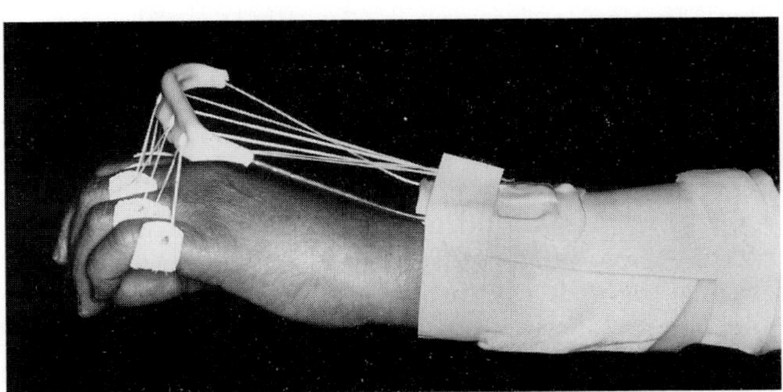

*Figure 35-18* Low profile radial nerve splint is carefully balanced to pull MCP joints into extension when wrist is flexed and allows the MCP joints to fall into slight flexion when wrist is extended, preserving normal balance between two joints and preventing joint contracture. (Courtesy Judy C. Colditz.)

upper arm and the forearm, dorsum of the thumb, as well as the index and middle fingers and radial half of the ring finger to the PIP joints. Sensory loss of the radial nerve does not usually result in dysfunction.

A dorsal splint that provides wrist extension, MCP extension, and thumb extension should be provided to protect the extensor tendons from overstretching during the healing phase and to position the hand for functional use (Figure 35-18). A dynamic splint is commonly provided.

### Median Nerve

The median nerve innervates the flexors of the forearm and hand and is often called the *eyes* of the hands because of its importance in sensory innervation of the volar surface of the hands. Median nerve loss may result from lacerations as well as from compression syndromes of the wrist, such as carpal tunnel syndrome.

Motor distribution of the median nerve is listed in Table 35-1. Sensory distribution of the median nerve is to the volar surface of the thumb, index, and middle

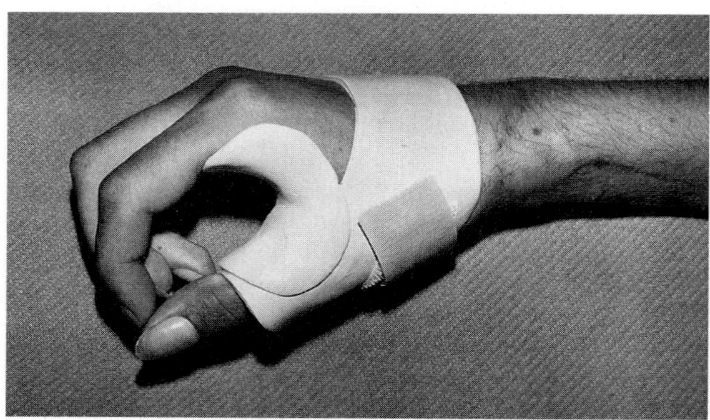

*Figure 35-19* A hand-based thumb positioning splint may be used with median nerve injury to preserve the web space and to position thumb for function.

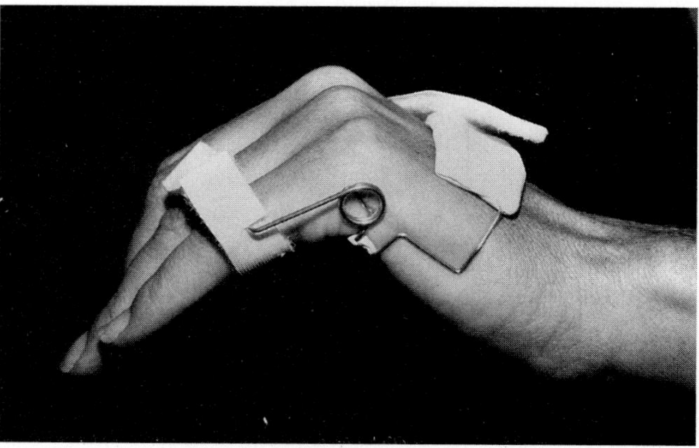

*Figure 35-20* A dynamic ulnar nerve splint blocks hyperextension of the MCP joints thus allowing extension of the PIP joints. (Splint courtesy Mary Dimick, University of California—San Diego Hand Rehabilitation Center, San Diego, Calif.)

fingers; radial half of the ring finger and dorsal surface of the index and middle fingers; and the radial half of the ring finger distal to the PIP joints. The sensory loss associated with median nerve injury is particularly disabling because there will be no sensation to the volar aspects of the thumb and index and long fingers and the radial side of the ring finger. When blindfolded, the patient will substitute pinch to the ring and small fingers to compensate for this loss.

Splints that position the thumb in palmar abduction and slight opposition will increase functional use of the hand (Figure 35-19). If clawing of the index and long fingers is present, a splint should be fabricated to prevent hyperextension of the MCP joints. Patients report that they avoid use of the hand with a median nerve injury because of lack of sensation rather than because of muscle paralysis. Despite this, the weakened or paralyzed muscles should be protected.

### *Ulnar Nerve*

The ulnar nerve in the forearm innervates only the flexor carpi ulnaris, the median half of the flexor digitorum profundus, and the intrinsic muscles of the hand (see Table 35-1). The sensory distribution of the ulnar nerve is the dorsal and volar surfaces of the little finger and the ulnar half of the dorsal and volar surface of the ring finger. An ulnar nerve injury results in hyperextension of the MCP joints of the ring and small fingers (*clawing*) caused by action of the extensor digitorum communis that is not held in check by the third and fourth lumbricals.[54]

Splints should block hyperextension of the MCP joints (Figure 35-20). The IP joints of the ring and small fingers will not demonstrate a great flexion deformity because of the paralysis of the flexor digitorum profundus. The hypothenar muscles and interossei will be absent. The wrist will assume a position of radial extension caused by the loss of the flexor carpi ulnaris.

Sensory loss of the ulnar nerve results in frequent injury (especially burns) to the ulnar side of the hand. Patients must be instructed in visual protection of the anesthetic area.

### *Postoperative Management After Nerve Repair*

After nerve repair the hand is placed in a position that will minimize tension on the nerve. For example, after the repair of the median nerve the wrist will be immobilized in a flexed position. Immobilization usually lasts 2 to 3 weeks, after which protective stretching of the joints may begin. The clinician must exercise great care not to put excessive traction on the newly repaired nerve.

Correction of a **contracture** (soft tissue shortening around a joint) may take 4 to 6 weeks. Active exercise is the preferred method of gaining full extension, although a light dynamic splint may be applied with the surgeon's supervision. Splinting to assist or substitute for weakened musculature may be necessary for an extended period during nerve regeneration. Splints should be removed as soon as possible to allow for active exercise of the weakened muscles. However, it is important to instruct the patient in correct patterns of motion so that substitution is minimized.

Initially, treatment is directed toward the prevention of deformity and correction of poor positioning during the acute and regenerative stages. Patients must be instructed in visual protection of the anesthetic area. ADL should be evaluated, and new methods or devices may be needed for independence. Use of the hand in the patient's work should be evaluated, and the patient should be returned to employment with any necessary job modifications or adaptations of equipment as soon as possible.

Careful muscle, sensory, and functional testing should be performed frequently. As the nerve regenerates, splints may be changed or eliminated. Exercises and activities should be revised to reflect the patient's new gains, and adaptive equipment should be discarded as soon as possible.

As motor function begins to return to the paralyzed muscles, a careful program of specific exercises should be devised to facilitate the return. Neuromuscular electrical stimulation (NMES)[10] may be used by the OTR to provide an external stimulus to help strengthen the newly innervated muscle. When the muscle receives a good rating, functional activities should be used to complete the return to normal strength.

### Fractures

In treating a hand or wrist **fracture** (broken bone), the surgeon will attempt to achieve good anatomical position through either a closed (nonsurgical) or open (surgical) reduction. Internal fixation with Kirschner wires, metallic plates, and screws may be used to maintain the desired position. External fixation may also be used with internal fixation. The hand is usually immobilized in wrist extension and MCP joint flexion with extension of the distal joints whenever the injury allows this position.[65] Trauma to bone may also involve trauma to tendons and nerves in the adjacent area. Treatment must be geared toward the recovery of all injured structures.

Occupational therapy may be initiated during the period of immobilization, which is usually 3 to 5 weeks. Uninvolved fingers of the hand must be kept mobile through the use of active motion. Edema should be carefully monitored, and elevation is required whenever edema is present.

As soon as there is sufficient bone stability, the surgeon will allow mobilization of the injured part. The surgeon should provide guidelines for the amount of resistance or force that may be applied to the fracture site. Activities that correct poor motor patterns and encourage use of the injured hand should be started as soon as the hand is pain free. Early motion will prevent the adherence of tendons and reduce edema through stimulation of the lymphatic and blood vessels.

When the brace or cast is removed, the patient's hand must be assessed. If edema is present, edema control techniques can be initiated with techniques described earlier in this chapter. A baseline ROM should be established, and the application of appropriate splints may begin. A splint may be used to correct a deformity that has resulted from immobilization or may be used to protect the finger from additional trauma to the fracture site. An example of this type of splinting is the Velcro "buddy" splint (Figure 35-21). A dorsal block splint that limits full extension of the finger may be used after a fracture or dislocation of the PIP joint. A dynamic splint may be used to achieve full ROM or prevent the development of further deformity at 6 to 8 weeks after fracture.

Intraarticular (inside the joint) fractures may result in injury to the cartilage of the joint, resulting in additional pain and stiffness. An x-ray examination will indicate if there has been damage to the joint surface that might limit the treatment of the joint. Joint pain and stiffness after fracture without the presence of joint damage should be alleviated by a combination of thermal modalities, restoration of joint play, or joint mobilization and corrective and dynamic splinting, followed by active use. Resistive exercises can be started when bony healing has been achieved.

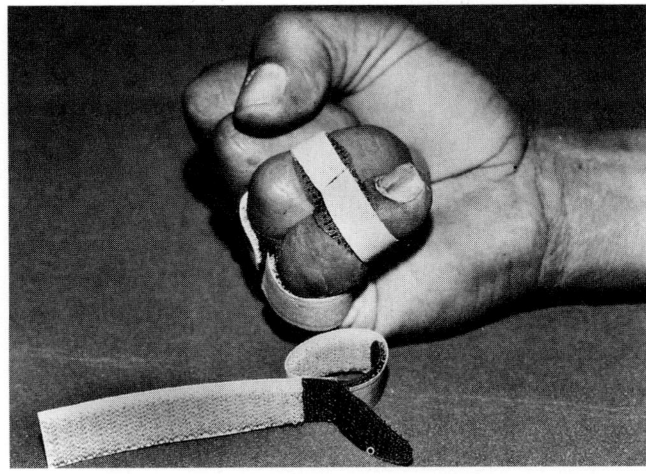

*Figure 35-21* Velcro "buddy" splint/strap may be used to protect a finger following a fracture or to encourage movement of a stiff finger.

Wrist fractures are common and may present special problems for the surgeon and therapist. Colle's fractures of the distal radius are the most common injury to the wrist[12] and may result in limitations in wrist flexion and extension, as well as in pronation and supination, resulting from the involvement of the distal radioulnar joint. Use of splints, active motion that emphasizes wrist movement, and joint mobilization may be beneficial. The weight well (see Figure 35-9) may be used to provide resistance to wrist motions.

The scaphoid is the second most commonly injured bone in the wrist[12] and is often fractured when the hand is dorsiflexed at the time of injury. Fractures to the proximal portion of the scaphoid may result in nonunion because of poor blood supply to this area. Scaphoid fractures will require a prolonged period of immobilization, sometimes up to several months in a cast, with resulting stiffness and pain. Care should be taken to mobilize noninvolved joints early.

Stiffness and pain are common complications of fractures, but the control of edema coupled with early motion and good patient instruction and support will minimize these complications.

### Reflex Sympathetic Dystrophy

**Reflex sympathetic dystrophy (RSD)** is a term used to describe a disabling reaction to pain that is "generated by an abnormal sympathetic reflex."[37,52] The hallmarks of RSD are pain; edema; blotchy-looking, shiny skin; and coolness of the hand. There may be excessive sweating or dryness. The degree of trauma does not correlate with the severity of the pain and may occur after any injury. It appears to be triggered by a cycle of vasospasm and vasodilation after an injury. Abnormal edema and constrictive dressings or casts may be a factor in initiating the vasospasm. A vasospasm "causes tissue anoxia and edema and therefore more pain, which continues the abnormal cycle."[10,55] Circulation is decreased, which causes the extremity to become cool and pale. Fibrosis after tissue anoxia and the production of protein-rich exudates results in joint stiffness. The patient may cradle the hand and prefer to keep it wrapped. There may be an exaggerated reaction to touch, especially light touch. Osteoporosis may be apparent on x-ray films by 8 weeks after trauma. Burning pain associated with causalgia is a symptom that is often alleviated by surgical interruption of the sympathetic nerve pathways.

There are three stages of RSD. Stage I may last up to 3 months. It is characterized by pain, pitting edema, and discoloration. Stage II may last an additional 6 months. Pain, brawny edema (hard and thick), stiffness, redness, heat and bony demineralization are usually found in this stage. The hand usually has a glossy appearance. Stage III may last up to several years or indefinitely. Pain usually peaks and decreases over time. Thickening around the joints occurs and fixed contractures may be present. If there is swelling, it is hard and not responsive to techniques such as elevation. The hand may be pale, dry, and cool. There may be significant dysfunction of the limb.

RSD is treated by decreasing sympathetic stimulation. It is most responsive in Stage I. The first goal of treatment is reduction of the pain and hypersensitivity to light touch. This may be accomplished with application of warm (not hot) moist heat, fluidotherapy, gentle handling of the hand, accupressure, desensitization, and TENS before AROM. Treatment that increases pain (such as passive ROM) should be avoided. Many patients respond well to gentle retrograde massage that reduces the edema and reintroduces touching of the hand. Stellate ganglion blocks to eliminate the pain are effective early. This procedure requires a surgeon to selectively anesthetize the stellate ganglion or nerve bundle. This usually results in a marked decrease in pain. This surgical treatment should be coordinated with therapy so the patient can perform AROM and functional activities during the period after the blocks. A variety of drugs may be used that reduce the vasoconstrictive action of the peripheral vessels. A stress-loading program that has been used effectively to reduce symptoms of RSD has been described.[61] It can easily be adapted for home use.

Edema control techniques should be started immediately. Biofeedback training for relaxation may help muscle spasming and ischemia, as well as reduce anxiety.

RSD will frequently trigger shoulder pain and stiffness, resulting in shoulder-hand syndrome or a "frozen" shoulder. Therefore active ROM and functional activities should include the entire upper quadrant. Skateboard exercises are helpful in the early stages for active-assistive exercise of the shoulder. Splints that reduce joint stiffness should be used as tolerated. A tendency to develop RSD should be suspected in any patient who seems to complain excessively about pain, appears anxious, and complains of profuse sweating and temperature changes in the hand. Patients will tend to overprotect the hand. Early intervention with a structured therapy program of functional activities, group interaction, and exercises that include the hand and shoulder may prevent the occurrence of a fully developed RSD. This is a problem that is best recognized early and treated with tempered aggressiveness and empathy.

### Cumulative Trauma Disorder

A number of terms are used to describe the conditions that occur when the musculoskeletal system is subjected to repeated stress. Some of the terms used are overuse syndromes, repetitive stress or strain injuries (RSIs), repetitive motion injuries, and **cumulative trauma disorders (CTDs).** In the United States, the term CTD is most commonly used. The incidence of CTD in the United States is on the rise, with 281,800 cases reported in private industry in 1992.[56] Between 1981 and 1992, CTD increased from 18% to 62% of all worker's compensation claims filed. The term cumulative trauma disorder should be considered descriptive in nature—it describes the mechanism of injury but is not a diagnosis. Today, many workers are required to perform the same repetitive motor task 6 or more hours a day. For example, a worker who is required to stand on an assembly line doing the same task repeatedly or type on a computer all day long may exemplify the type of person who could develop CTD. Work-related activities that are considered high-risk factors for CTD are repetition, high force, awkward joint posture, direct pressure, vibration, and prolonged static positioning.[4] The human body was not made to work this way, even though today's technology and need for productivity may encourage this type of behavior. In addition, it is not uncommon for many people to have second jobs or pursue rigorous leisure activities. It must be remembered that CTD may take many weeks, months, or years to develop and may take just as long to resolve.

Cumulative trauma occurs when force is repeatedly applied to the same muscle or muscle group, causing an inflammatory response in the tendon, muscle, or nerve.[55] Muscle fatigue is an important aspect of cumulative trauma and can be relieved by rest. However, chronic fatigue, the usual condition of these patients, cannot be relieved by rest alone. In these circumstances, it is important to examine the patient's job requirements and leisure activities.

Diagnoses associated with cumulative trauma usually fall within the following three categories: tendonitis, nerve compression syndromes, and myofascial pain. Common examples of CTD involving the tendons are lateral epicondylitis (tennis elbow), and DeQuervain's disease. A well-known nerve compression syndrome is carpal tunnel disease, which is a compression of the median nerve at the level of the wrist. Poor posture and positioning of the body out of normal alignment are often the cause of myofascial pain. This is a difficult diagnosis to make because the pain is often referred to a distal area. An accurate diagnosis of any of these conditions is difficult and should be done by a skilled physician, often with input from an experienced OTR.

When supervised the COTA may assist in the treatment of these patients. In the acute phase, the goal of treatment is to reduce inflammation through rest. Splints are used for immobilization, often in combination with physician-prescribed antiinflammatory medication. In this phase the patient may be placed on an active therapy program consisting of modalities to reduce pain and stretching of the affected musculature to prevent joint stiffness. The patient should be instructed not to engage in activities that cause pain.

As the acute symptoms decrease, the patient begins the exercise phase of treatment. This phase of treatment adds resistive exercise but only after the muscle has been warmed by slow stretching. Resistance should be increased slowly and should not result in increased pain. Patients are instructed to stretch at home, especially before activity, three times per day for an indefinite period of time.

To control symptoms in the long term, patients must become aware of what triggers their symptoms and learn early intervention if symptoms reappear. Modalities to reduce pain—splints, stretching, and modified activities—combined with proper body mechanics are usually effective. The key is that patients learn self-management techniques and take an active role in their treatment. When it has been established that the patient's job demands have caused the CTD, an evaluation of the job site, tools used, and body mechanics during work activities may be indicated. The job site evaluation is done by the OTR with permission from the patient and employer. The COTA may assist the therapist in gathering information from the patient about job requirements to help determine if a job site analysis is indicated.

## SUMMARY

The OTR usually carries out the assessment of the hand-injured patient with assistance from the COTA. The OTR establishes the intervention strategy for each patient. The COTA may assist in certain defined areas and in some areas may carry out the treatment independently. However, it is imperative that COTAs who work with this population be familiar with assessment and intervention concepts. COTAs who elect to work in this specialty area are encouraged to further develop service competency by participating in continuing education and on-site supervision.

## *Selected Reading Guide Questions*

1. Describe the various sensory tests and their appropriate uses.
2. What are two tools used to measure edema? Discuss the rationale for each.
3. Name two objective tests of sympathetic function.
4. What is the only technique that is always appropriate for acute hand injury?
5. Name the components of a hand evaluation.
6. What are the benefits for using the Jebsen Test of Hand Function?
7. If no goniometer is available, describe another method of evaluating gross finger flexion.
8. What are the goals of occupational therapy with a patient who has had a finger tip amputation?
9. Name the three types of pinch that are routinely assessed for strength. Name two functional activities for each of these pinch types.
10. Name the three levels of peripheral nerve injury.
11. Why is the median nerve sometimes referred to as the "eyes of the hand?"
12. Why do we see "clawing" in the small and ring fingers after ulnar nerve injury?
13. What splint position is indicated after a low-level median nerve injury that has resulted in paralysis?
14. Once a patient has been cleared for strengthening, name two clinic activities and two craft activities that will achieve this goal.
15. Describe two treatment strategies to reduce finger tip hypersensitivity.
16. Describe the appropriate splint immediately after flexor tendon repair. What is the rationale of the Kleinert protocol?
17. Name the surgical intervention to relieve the pain associated with RSD. Describe its implications for occupational therapy treatment.
18. Discuss the three categories of cumulative trauma disorders. What is the goal in the acute phase of cumulative trauma disorder?

### *REFERENCES*

1. American Occupational Therapy Association: Official AOTA statement on physical agent modalities, *AJOT* 45:1075, 1991.
2. American Society for Surgery of the Hand: *The hand examination and diagnosis,* ed 3, New York, 1990, Churchill Livingstone.
3. Anthony MS: Sensory evaluation. In Clark G et al, editors: *Hand rehabilitation: a practical guide,* New York, 1993, Churchill Livingstone.
4. Armstrong TJ: Cumulative trauma disorders of the upper limb and identification of work-related factors. In Millender LH, Louis DS, Simmons BP, editors: *Occupational disorders of the upper extremity,* New York, 1992, Churchill Livingstone.
5. Barber LM: Occupational therapy for the treatment of reflex sympathetic dystrophy and post-traumatic hypersensitivity of the injured hand. In Fredericks S, Brody GS, editors: *Symposium on the neurologic aspects of plastic surgery,* St Louis, 1978, Mosby.
6. Barber LM: Desensitization of the traumatized hand. In Hunter JM et al, editors: *Rehabilitation of the hand,* ed 3, St. Louis, 1990, Mosby.

7. Bell-Krotoski JA: Plaster cylinder casting for contractures of the interphalangeal joints. In Hunter JM et al, editors: *Rehabilitation of the hand,* ed 3, St Louis, 1990, Mosby.
8. Bell-Krotoski JA: Sensibility testing: state of the art. In Hunter JM et al, editors: *Rehabilitation of the hand,* ed 3, St Louis, 1990, Mosby.
9. Bell-Krotoski JA: Light touch-deep pressure testing using Semmes-Weinstein monofilaments. In Hunter JM et al, editors: *Rehabilitation of the hand,* ed 3, St Louis, 1990, Mosby.
10. Benton LA et al: *Functional electrical stimulation: a practical clinical guide,* ed 2, Downey, Calif, 1981, Rancho Los Amigos Hospital.
11. Bennett GK: *Hand-tool dexterity test,* New York, 1981, Harcourt, Brace, Jovanovich.
12. Boyes JH: *Bunnell's surgery of the hand,* ed 5, Philadelphia, 1970, JB Lippincott.
13. Boyes JH, Stark HH: Flexor-tendon grafts in the fingers and thumb, *J Bone Joint Surg* 53A:1332, 1971.
14. Callahan AD: Methods of compensation and reeducation for sensory dysfunction. In Hunter JM et al, editors: *Rehabilitation of the hand,* ed 3, St Louis, 1990, Mosby.
15. Cambridge CA: Range of motion measurements of the hand. In Hunter JM et al, editors: *Rehabilitation of the hand,* ed 3, St. Louis, 1990, Mosby.
16. Cannon NM et al: Control of immediate postoperative pain following tenolysis and capsulectomies of the hand with TENS, *J Hand Surg* 8:625, 1983.
17. Carroll D: A quantitative test of upper extremity function, *J Chronic Dis* 18:479, 1965.
18. Chusid JG: *Correlative neuroanatomy and functional neurology,* ed 19, Los Altos, Calif, 1985, Lange.
19. Crawford JE, Crawford DM: *Crawford small parts dexterity test manual,* New York, 1981, Harcourt, Brace, Jovanovich.
20. Creelman G: *Volumeters unlimited,* Idyllwild, Calif.
21. Curtis RM, Engalitcheff J: A work simulator for rehabilitating the upper extremity: preliminary report, *J Hand Surg* 6:499, 1981.
22. Cyriax JH: Clinical application of message. In Basmajian JV: *Manipulation, traction, and massage,* ed 3, Baltimore, 1985, Williams & Wilkins.
23. Dellon AL: *Evaluation of sensibility and reeducation of sensation in the hand,* Baltimore, 1981, Williams & Wilkins.
24. Dellon AL, Curtis RM, Edgerton MT: Reeducation of sensation in the hand after nerve injury and repair, *Plast Reconstr Surg* 53:297, 1974.
25. Dellon AL: The vibrometer, *Plast Reconstr Surg* 71:427, 1983.
26. Donatelli R, Owens-Burkhart H: Effects of immobilization on the extensibility of periarticular connective tissue, *J Orth Sports Phys Ther* 3:67, 1981.
27. Duran RJ et al: Management of flexor tendon lacerations in zone 2 using controlled passive motion postoperatively. In Hunter JM et al, editors: *Rehabilitation of the hand,* ed 3, St Louis, 1990, Mosby.
28. English CB, Rehm RA, Petzoldt RL: Blocking splints to assist finger exercise, *AJOT* 36:259, 1983.
29. Fee EE, Moran CA: *Clinical assessment recommendations,* Indianapolis, 1981, American Society of Hand Therapists.
30. Gelberman RH et al: Sensibility testing in peripheral nerve compression syndromes, *JBJS* 65A:632, 1983.
31. Jebsen RH et al: An objective and standardized test of hand function, *Arch Phys Med Rehabil* 50:311, 1969.
32. Kamentz HL: Mechanical devices of massage. In Basmajian JV: *Manipulation, traction and massage,* ed 3, Baltimore, 1985, Williams & Wilkins.
33. Kasch MC: Clinical management of scar tissue, *OT Health Care* 4(3/4):37, 1987.
34. Kessler RM, Hertling D: Joint mobilization techniques. In Kessler RM, Hertling D: *Management of common musculoskeletal disorders,* New York, 1983, Harper & Row.
35. Kellor M et al: *Technical manual of hand strength and dexterity test,* Minneapolis, 1971, Sister Kenny Rehabilitation Institute.
36. Kelsey JL et al: *Upper extremity disorders: a survey of their frequency and cost in the United States,* St Louis, 1980, Mosby.
37. Lankford LL: Reflex sympathetic dystrophy. In Hunter JM et al, editors: *Rehabilitation of the hand,* ed 3, St Louis, 1990, Mosby.
38. Lister GL: *The hand: diagnosis and indications,* ed 3, New York, 1993, Churchill Livingstone.
39. Louis DS et al: Evaluation of normal values for stationary and moving two-point discrimination in the hand, *J Hand Surgery* 99:552, 1984.
40. Lundborg G: *Nerve injury and repair,* New York, 1988, Churchill Livingstone.
41. Mackinnon SE, Dellon AL: Two-point discrimination tester, *J Hand Surg* 10A:906, 1985.
42. Madden JW: Wound healing: the biological basis of hand surgery. In Hunter JM et al, editors: *Rehabilitation of the hand,* ed 3, St Louis, 1990, Mosby.
43. Maitland GD: *Peripheral manipulation,* Boston, 1977, Butterworth.
44. Mathiowetz V et al: Reliability and validity of grip and pinch strength evaluations, *J Hand Surg* 9A:222, 1984.
45. Mathiowetz V et al: Grip and pinch strength: normative data for adults, *Arch Phys Rehabil* 66:69, 1985.
46. Mathiowetz V, Remmells C, Donoghue L: Effects of elbow position on grip and key pinch strengths, *J Hand Surg* 10A:694, 1985.
47. Melvin JL: *Rheumatic disease occupational therapy and rehabilitation,* ed 3, Philadelphia, 1989, FA Davis.
48. Mennell JM: *Joint pain,* Boston, 1964, Little, Brown.
49. Mennell JM, Zohn DA: *Musculoskeletal pain diagnosis and physical treatment,* Boston, 1976, Little, Brown.
50. Moberg E: Objective methods of determining functional value of sensibility in the hand, *J Bone Joint Surg* 40A:454, 1958.
51. Moberg E: Aspects of sensation in reconstructive surgery of the upper extremity, *J Bone Joint Surg* 46A:817, 1964.
52. Omer GE: Management of pain syndromes in the upper extremity. In Hunter JM, et al, editors: *Rehabilitation of the hand,* ed 3, St Louis, 1990, Mosby.
53. O'Rain S: New and simple test of nerve function in the hand, *Br Med J* 3:615, 1973.
54. Parry CBW: *Rehabilitation of the hand,* ed 4, London, 1984, Butterworth.
55. Rempel DM: Work-related cumulative trauma disorders of the upper extremity, *JAMA* 267:838-842, 1992.
56. Silverstein S: Preventive medicine standards on cumulative trauma would cover every employee in the state, *LA Times,* January 13, 1994.
57. Stewart KM, VanStrien G: Postoperative management of flexor tendon injuries. In Hunter JM et al, editors: *Rehabilitation of the hand,* ed 4, St Louis, 1995, Mosby.
58. Swanson AB, Swanson GD, Goran-Hagert C: Evaluation of impairment of hand function. In Hunter JM, et al, editors: *Rehabilitation of the hand,* ed 4, St Louis, 1990, Mosby.
59. Szabo RM et al: Vibratory sensory testing in acute peripheral nerve compression, *J Hand Surg* 9A:104, 1984.
60. Tiffin J: *Purdue pegboard examiner manual,* Chicago, 1968, Science Research Associates.
61. Watson HK, Carlson L: Treatment of reflex sympathetic dystrophy of the hand with an active "stress loading" program, *J Hand Surg* 12A:779, 1987.
62. Waylett-Rendall J: Sensibility evaluation and rehabilitation. In *Orthopedic Clinics of North America,* vol 19(1), Philadelphia, 1988, WB Saunders.
63. Wehbé MA, Hunter JM: Flexor tendon gliding in the hand, Pt II: differential gliding, *J Hand Surg* 10A:575, 1985.
64. Wehbé MA: Tendon gliding exercises, *Am J Occup Ther* 41:164, 1987.
65. Wilson RE, Carter MS: Management of hand fractures. In Hunter JM et al, editors: *Rehabilitation of the hand,* ed 3, St Louis, 1990, Mosby.
66. Wolf SL: *Electrotherapy,* New York, 1981, Churchill Livingstone.
67. Yerxa EJ et al: Development of hand sensitivity test for the hypersensitive hand, *Am J Occup Ther* 37:176, 1983.

No Power Point ✓
Handouts ✓
Questions - printed + in folder

# Chapter 36

# Spinal Cord Injuries

*Carole Adler*
*Diane D. Hardy*

## Chapter Objectives

*After studying this chapter, the student or practitioner will be able to:*

1. Define terminology relevant to spinal cord injury.
2. Identify key muscles for each level of spinal cord injury.
3. Describe functional expectations for each level of spinal cord injury.
4. Identify assistive devices commonly recommended for spinal cord injury.
5. Describe treatment precautions and treatment interventions for complications of spinal cord injury.
6. Explain the purpose and importance of a well-integrated exercise program for the patient with a spinal cord injury.
7. Describe the purpose of positioning as it relates to abnormal tone.
8. Describe the three areas that are important for successful self-care task completion.

## Key Terms

quadriplegia
paraplegia
vertebrae
spinal cord
complete injury
incomplete injury
Brown-Sèquard syndrome
spinal shock
decubitus ulcers
autonomic dysreflexia
tenodesis

Rehabilitation of the individual with a spinal cord injury is a lifelong process that requires readjustment in nearly every aspect of life. Occupational therapy plays a very important role in the total treatment program. The registered occupational therapist (OTR) must evaluate the patient to determine functional capabilities and then define realistic goals to improve function in activities of daily living (ADL).

The patient's self-esteem is critical in providing motivation for rehabilitation. Occupational therapy practitioners must be sensitive to the significant losses and psychological shock of a spinal cord injury as they guide the patient to cope with task performance dysfunction. As the patient confronts limitations and concentrates on capabilities, function can improve, and with it the patient's image of self as a competent performer in the world.

Spinal cord injuries have many causes. The most common are trauma from motor vehicle accidents, violent injuries such as gunshot and stab wounds, falls, sports accidents, and diving accidents.[4,10] Normal spinal cord function may also be disturbed by diseases such as tumors, myelomeningocele, syringomyelia, multiple sclerosis, and amyotrophic lateral sclerosis. This chapter will emphasize the rehabilitation of the individual with a traumatic spinal cord injury.

## RESULTS OF SPINAL CORD INJURY

Spinal cord injury results in quadriplegia or paraplegia. **Quadriplegia** is any degree of paralysis of the four limbs, trunk musculature, and pelvic organs. There may be partial upper extremity (UE) function, depending on the level of the cervical lesion. **Paraplegia** is paralysis of the lower extremities (LEs) with some involvement of the trunk and pelvic organs, depending on the level of the lesion.[4,10]

### Review of Normal Anatomy

The spine or vertebral column is a flexible, bony structure that provides support and protection (Figure 36-1). It consists of 33 individual bones called **vertebrae** that sit one on top of another and support the head, ribs, shoulders, and arms. Each vertebra is cushioned by an intervertebral disk (composed primarily of cartilage) that acts as a shock absorber for the weight of the body. The disks account for approximately one third of the length of the spinal column.

The vertebrae are stabilized by ligaments and muscles, which also allow the spine flexibility of movement. Torn ligaments and muscles cause instability. The primary sections of the vertebral column include the cervical spine (C1 to C7), thoracic spine (T1 to T12), and lumbar spine (L1 to L5). At the base of the vertebral column are five fused vertebrae that are collectively called the *sacrum* and a small bony tip called the *coccyx*.

The **spinal cord** extends from the base of the brain to the second lumbar vertebra and carries sensory and motor information to and from the brain. Nerve fibers from the spinal cord exit via spinal nerves that carry impulses to and from muscles, tendons, and body organs.

There are 31 pairs (right and left) of spinal nerves; each has two pathways—sensory and motor. Eight pairs of cervical nerves (C1 to C8) control the head, neck, arms, hands, and diaphragm. Twelve pairs of thoracic nerves (T1 to T12) control the chest, back, and abdomen. Five pairs of lumbar nerves (L1 to L5) control the legs and feet. Five pairs of sacral nerves (S1 to S5) control the bowels, bladder, and sexual functions.

The spinal cord also houses the autonomic nervous system, which is responsible for "fight or flight" responses. The spinal cord terminates at L1-L2, where it tapers off and is commonly referred to as the cauda equina or "horse's tail."

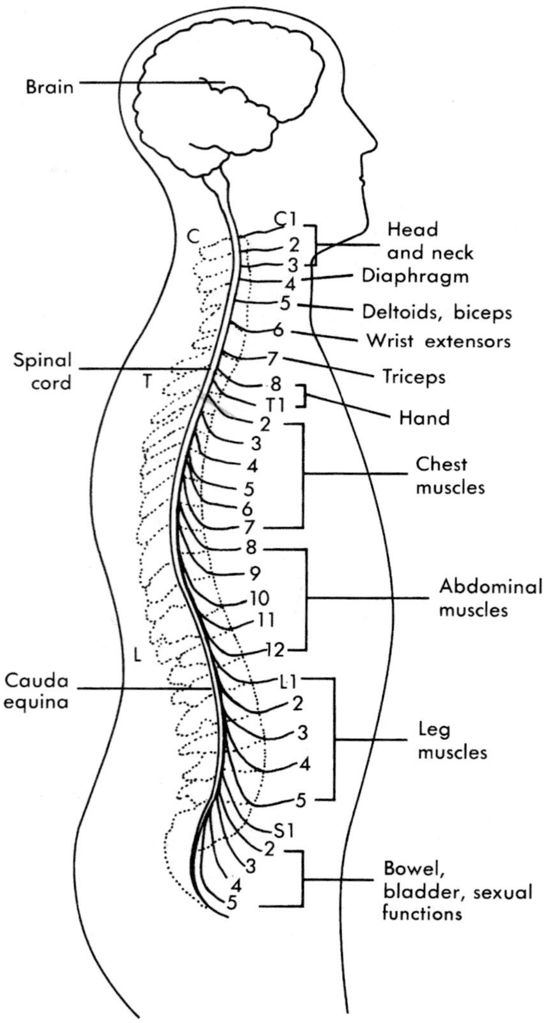


*Figure 36-1* Spinal nerves and the major areas of the body they supply. (From Paulson S, editor: *Santa Clara Valley Medical Center spinal cord injury home care manual,* ed 2, San Jose, Calif, 1994, Santa Clara Valley Medical Center.)

### Classification of Injuries

Spinal cord injuries are referred to in terms of the regions (cervical, thoracic, and lumbar) of the spinal cord in which they occur and the numerical order of the neurological segments. The level of spinal cord injury indicates the last fully functioning neurological segment of the cord; for example, C6 refers to the sixth neurological segment of the cervical region of the spinal cord as the last fully intact neurological segment.[4,9] Neurological segments correspond to the spinal nerves. Note that although there are only 7 cervical vertebrae, there are 8 cervical nerve roots and thus 8 cervical neurological segments.

Lesions may be complete or incomplete, indicating the severity of damage to the cord. Complete lesions result in absence of motor or sensory function of the spinal cord below the level of the injury. Incomplete lesions may involve several neurological segments and some spinal cord function may be partially or completely intact.[3,9] Table 36-1 lists the key muscles or groups innervated at each level. It is essential for the certified occupational therapy assistant (COTA) to know this information because it determines which functions will be intact and which will require compensatory techniques, adaptive equipment, or environmental modification. The information in Table 36-1 should be compared with that in Figure 36-1 for a fuller understanding.

### Complete and Incomplete Injuries

The extent of neurological damage depends on the location and severity of the injury (Fig. 36-1). A **complete injury** results in total paralysis and loss of sensation below the level of the lesion. In an **incom-**

Table 36-1

### Neurological Levels and Innervation of Key Muscles

| *Neurological level* | *Key muscles* |
|---|---|
| C4 | Diaphragm (for breathing) |
| C5 | Deltoid, biceps |
| C6 | Wrist extensors |
| C7 | Triceps |
| C8 | Flexor digitorum |
| T1 | Hand intrinsics |
| T2-L1 | Chest muscles and abdominals |
| L2 | Iliopsoas (hip flexor) |
| L3 | Quadriceps (knee extensor) |
| L4 | Anterior tibialis (ankle dorsiflexor) |
| L5 | Extensor hallicus longus (big toe extensor) |
| S1, S2 | Gastrocnemius (ankle plantar flexor) |

**plete injury** there is some degree of preservation of the sensory or motor nerves below the lesion. The American Spinal Injury (ASIA) Impairment Scale[1] is the current standard for classifying spinal cord injuries (Box 36-1).

Incomplete injuries are categorized according to the area of damage: central, lateral, anterior, or peripheral. These areas refer to the part of the cord that is affected.

### *Central Cord Syndrome*

Central cord syndrome results when there is more cellular destruction in the center of the cord than in its periphery. There is greater paralysis and sensory loss in the UEs because these nerve tracts are more centrally located than nerve tracts for the LEs.

### *Brown-Séquard Syndrome (Lateral Damage)*

**Brown-Séquard syndrome** results when only one side of the cord is damaged, as it often is in a stabbing or gunshot injury. Below the level of injury there is motor paralysis and loss of proprioception on the ipsilateral side and loss of pain, temperature, and touch sensation on the contralateral side.

### *Anterior Spinal Cord Syndrome*

Anterior spinal cord syndrome results from injury that damages the anterior spinal artery or the anterior aspect of the cord. There is paralysis and loss of pain, temperature, and touch sensation. Proprioception is preserved.

### *Cauda Equina (Peripheral)*

Cauda equina injuries involve peripheral nerves rather than the spinal cord directly. Because peripheral nerves possess a regenerating capacity that the cord does not, there is a better prognosis for recovery.[5]

Box 36-1

### Standard ASIA Neurological Classification of Spinal Cord Injury

**ASIA scale A**

Indicates a *complete* lesion with no motor or sensory function preserved in the sacral segments S4 to S5

**ASIA scale B**

Indicates an *incomplete* lesion in which only sensation is present below the neurological level, including the sacral segments S4 to S5

**ASIA scale C**

Indicates an *incomplete* lesion with motor function below the neurological level and the majority of key muscles below the level having strength grade of less than 3

**ASIA scale D**

Indicates an *incomplete* lesion with motor function preserved below the neurological level and the majority of key muscles below the level having a muscle grade of 3 or greater

**ASIA scale E**

Indicates that motor and sensory function are normal

From American Spinal Injury Association: *Standards for neurological and functional classification of spinal cord injury,* Chicago, Ill, 1992, The Association.

## Stages of Recovery

### *Spinal Shock*

Immediately after spinal cord injury the victim enters a stage of **spinal shock,** a sudden neurovascular shutdown that may last from hours to several weeks. The patient is prone to low blood pressure and hypothermia. Reflex activity ceases below the level of the injury.[9] The bladder and bowel are flaccid. Deep tendon reflexes are decreased. As spinal shock recedes, spasms may occur in both the UEs and LEs.

### *Recovery from Spinal Shock*

As spinal shock ends, sensory loss continues. In patients whose injuries are above T12 the bladder and bowel usually become spastic (which is referred to as an *upper motor neuron bladder*). In lesions at L1 and below, the bladder and bowel usually remain flaccid (which is referred to as a *lower motor neuron bladder*).

### Prognosis for Recovery

The extent of recovery depends first on whether the lesion is complete or incomplete. Motor return is unlikely in complete lesions that result in no sensation or return of motor function below the level of lesion between 24 to and 48 hours after the injury.

## MEDICAL AND SURGICAL MANAGEMENT OF THE PERSON WITH A SPINAL CORD INJURY

It is helpful for the COTA to have some awareness of the medical care of the spinal cord patient immediately after the injury. The main objectives at the early stages of spinal cord injury are stabilization of the spinal cord and the vertebral column and reduction of pressure on the cord and the nerve roots. Careful examination, stabilization, and transportation of the patient by emergency medical and rescue personnel may prevent a temporary or slight spinal cord injury from becoming more severe or permanent.

Initial care in the emergency room and hospital is directed toward preventing further damage to the spinal cord and reversing neurological damage if possible by stabilizing and reducing pressure on the injured neurological structures.[4,7,9] A catheter is usually placed in the patient's bladder for drainage of urine. Various radiological assessments (x-ray, magnetic resonance imaging [MRI]) are ordered.

The patient is placed on a rotating kinetic bed (Figure 36-2) that allows for skeletal traction and immobilization. The constant rotation of the bed provides continuous pressure relief, promotes mobilization of respiratory secretions, and gives easy access to the patient's entire body for bowel, bladder, and hygiene care.

Surgery may be needed to decompress the spinal cord and stabilize and align the spine.[4,9] In some cases the patient may be allowed to heal without surgery. As soon as possible a portable means of immobilization (usually a halo vest for cervical injuries and a thoracic brace or body jacket for thoracic injuries) is provided (Figure 36-3). This enables the patient to be transferred to a standard hospital bed and subsequently to be up in a wheelchair and involved in an active therapy program as soon as 1 to 2 weeks after injury. Being up in a wheelchair shortly after injury can significantly reduce risks from further medical complications such as deep venous thrombosis (DVT), joint contractures, and the general deconditioning that follows prolonged bed rest.

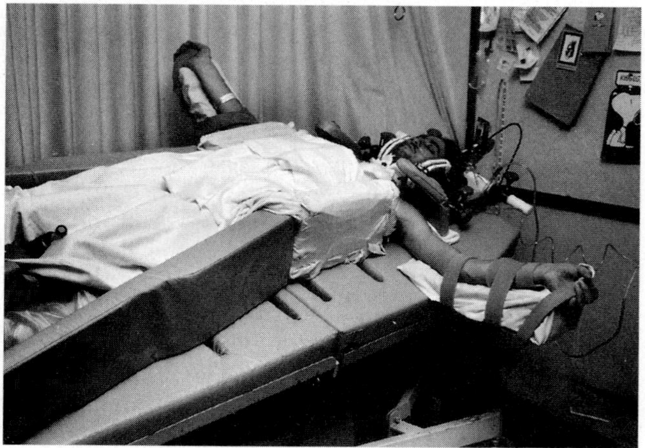

*Figure 36-2* Kinetic bed with arm positioner. (Occupational Therapy Department, Santa Clara Valley Medical Center, San Jose, Calif.)

### Complications of Spinal Cord Injury

#### *Skin Breakdown, Pressure Sores, or Decubitus Ulcers*

The spinal cord injury patient is at high risk of developing pressure sores or **decubitus ulcers.** The patient cannot feel the pressure and shearing of prolonged sitting or lying in one position or the presence of pain or heat against the body. (Shearing is pressure against the skin that causes the skin to slide in a direction opposite to that of the underlying tissues[2]). Pressure, heat, and shearing can destroy skin and underlying tissue. The areas most likely to develop skin breakdown are bony prominences over the sacrum, ischium, trochanters, elbows, and heels. Other bony prominences such as the iliac crest, scapula, knees, toes, and rib cage are also at risk.

It is important for all rehabilitation personnel to be aware of the signs of developing skin problems. At first the area reddens, yet it blanches (whitens) when pressed. Later the reddened or abraded area does not blanch. This indicates that necrosis has begun. Finally, a blister or ulceration appears in the area. If allowed to progress, a sore can become quite severe, destroying underlying tissues, and going as deep as the bone.

Skin breakdown can be prevented by relieving and eliminating pressure points and protecting vulnerable areas from excessive shearing, moisture, and heat. Turning schedules must be followed consistently. Patients should be taught how to inspect their own skin at regular intervals with a mirror or caregiver assistance. Skin should be inspected twice a day and any reddened areas reported to the OTR and nursing staff. Skin damage can develop within 30 minutes, so frequent weight shifting, repositioning, and constant attention are essential if skin breakdown is to be prevented.[9,12]

Occupational therapy practitioners can educate the patient to prevent pressure sores. The patient should be taught to make sure that clothing, shoes, and orthoses (body jackets, splints) fit properly, and to be wary of heavy seams, rear pockets, and rivets in clothing. Mattress overlays and padding of body prominences may also be used.

#### *Decreased Vital Capacity*

Decreased vital capacity will be a problem in people with cervical and high thoracic lesions as a result of weakness or paralysis of the diaphragm and the intercostal and latissimus dorsi muscles. Such patients will have limited chest expansion and decreased ability to cough with consequent increased risk for respiratory tract infections. Symptoms include a shallow cough, congestion, and low energy levels. It is important for the OTR and COTA to discuss treatment options and for the COTA to have a clear understanding of how to perform a manually assisted cough.

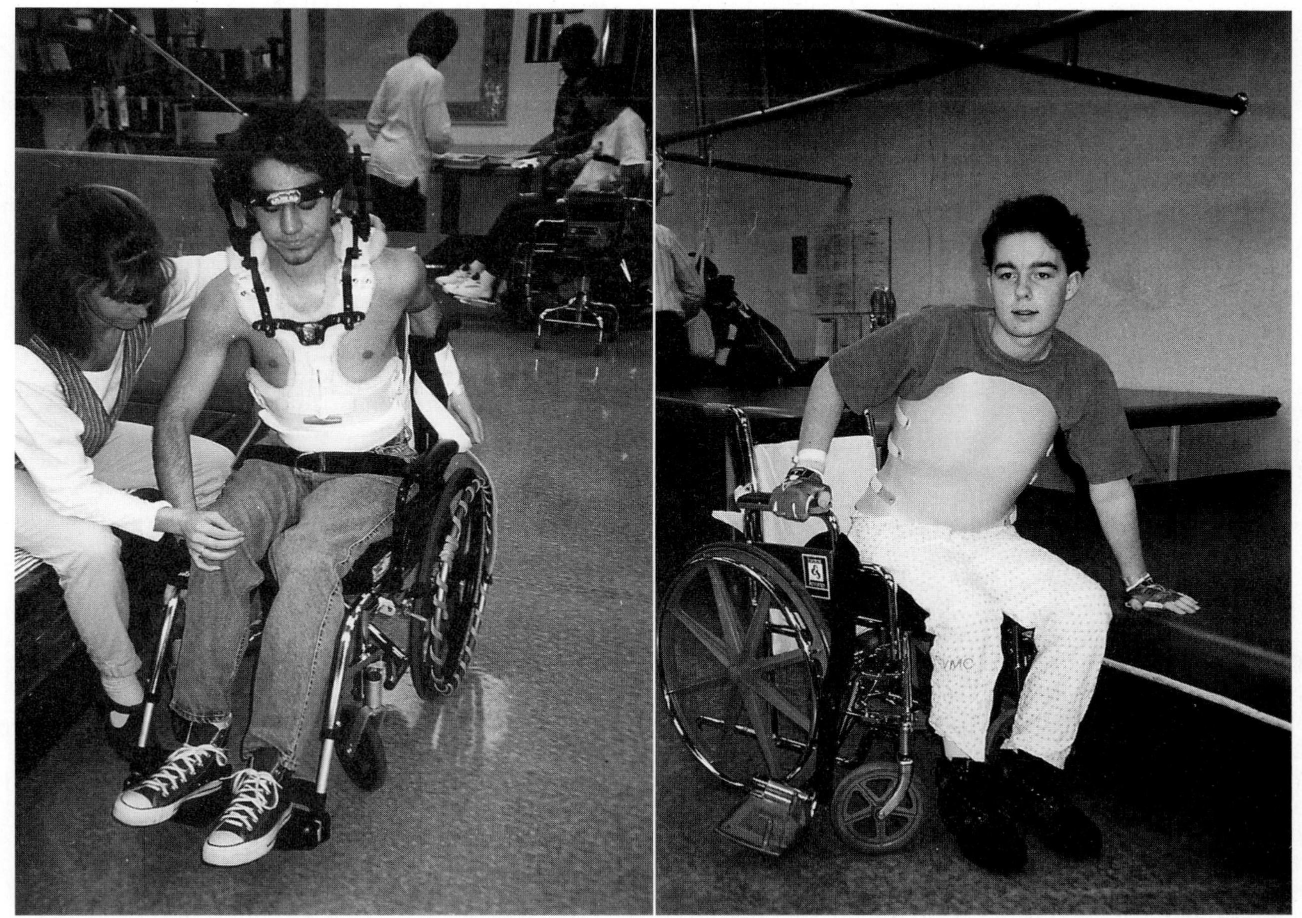


*Figure 36-3* **A,** Halo vest—neck immobilization device for quadriplegic and high level paraplegia. **B,** Body jacket—immobilization device for paraplegia.

### *Osteoporosis of Disuse*

Osteoporosis is likely to develop in patients with spinal cord injuries because of disuse of long bones, particularly of the LEs. A year after the injury the osteoporosis may be sufficiently advanced for pathological fractures to occur in any of several sites in the LEs. (Pathological fractures are usually not seen in UEs.) Daily standing on a tilt table or at a standing frame may slow the onset of osteoporosis[9,12]; however, a standing program must be ongoing if it is to be effective and therefore must fit into the patient's daily ADL routine after discharge. The COTA will need to observe and teach the patient precautions to avoid injury while bathing and performing LE dressing.

### *Orthostatic Hypotension*

Lack of muscle tone in the abdomen and LEs leads to pooling of blood in these areas with resultant decrease in blood pressure (hypotension). A sudden decrease in pressure occurs when the patient goes from a supine to an upright position or changes body position too quickly. Symptoms are dizziness, nausea, and loss of consciousness.[4] The patient must be reclined quickly, and if sitting in a wheelchair should be tipped back with legs elevated until symptoms subside. With time this problem can diminish as sitting tolerance and level of activity increases; however, some people continue to experience hypotensive episodes. Abdominal binders, leg wraps, antiembolism stockings, and medications can aid in reducing symptoms.

### *Autonomic Dysreflexia*

**Autonomic dysreflexia** is a medical emergency and is potentially life-threatening. Individuals with spinal cord injuries above the T6 level are more prone to this complication, which occurs more often in patients with complete lesions. It is caused by reflex action of the autonomic nervous system in response to some stimulus, such as a distended bladder, fecal mass, bladder irritation, rectal manipulation, extreme temperature, tight clothing, skin irritation, or an uncomfortable position.

The symptoms are pounding headache, anxiety, perspiration, flushing of the skin, chills, nasal congestion, hypertension (blood pressure elevated as high as 250/150), and bradycardia.

The patient should not be left alone.[4,9,12] Medical help must be summoned *immediately*. Autonomic dysreflexia is treated by placing the patient in an upright position and loosening anything restrictive such as abdominal binders or elastic stockings to reduce blood pressure. The legbag tubing should be checked for obstruction. Blood pressure and other symptoms should be monitored until back to normal. Dysreflexia can occur at any time after the injury.

### *Spasticity*

Spasticity is a result of most spinal cord injuries.[13] Muscles below the level of injury contract involuntarily. Patterns of spasticity change over the first year, gradually increasing in the first 6 months and reaching a plateau about 1 to 2 years after the injury. A small amount of spasticity is useful and can help to maintain muscle bulk, assist in joint range of motion (ROM), and assist during wheelchair and bed transfers and mobility. A sudden increase in spasticity can alert the patient to other medical problems, such as bladder infections, skin breakdown, or fever.

### *Heterotopic Ossification*

Heterotopic ossification (HO), also called *ectopic bone,* is bone that develops in abnormal locations.[13] It most often occurs in the muscles around the hip and knee but occasionally also at the elbow and shoulder. The first symptoms are swelling, warmth, and decreased joint ROM. The onset of HO is usually 1 to 4 months after injury. Treatment consists of medication and maintenance of joint ROM during the early stage of active bone formation. The objective is to preserve the functional ROM necessary for mobility and for good wheelchair positioning and neutral symmetrical placement of the pelvis. If HO progresses to the point of limiting hip flexion, the sitting position will be abnormal. This will contribute to trunk deformities such as scoliosis and kyphosis with subsequent skin breakdown at the ischial tuberosities and sacrum.[4,9]

### *Sexual Function*

The sexual drive and need for physical and emotional intimacy are not changed by spinal cord injury. There are, however, problems of mobility, dependency, and body image in addition to complicating medical problems and the attitudes of partners and society that affect social and sexual roles, access, and interest. Sexuality is an important part of life, and rehabilitation is not complete until people are comfortable with their sexual and social roles.

Sexual education and counseling must be geared to the needs of individual patients and their significant other. In some instances, social interaction skills will need improvement before sexual activity can be considered. Occupational therapy practitioners play an important role in providing information and a forum to deal with these issues (see Chapter 14).[8]

## OCCUPATIONAL THERAPY INTERVENTION

### Evaluation

During the assessment process the OTR will evaluate the following:

- UE ROM
- UE motor skills, strength, coordination, and endurance
- Need for splinting and positioning devices
- Anticipated adaptive and durable medical equipment
- Muscle tone
- Wrist and hand function
- Trunk control and posture
- Sensation
- ADL, self-care, household, community, and leisure interests

Supplemental evaluation may be required, depending on the initial evaluation. These assessments may include the following:

- Assistive technology
- Sensory integration
- Prevocational assessment
- Perception (especially for combined spinal cord injury/traumatic brain injury [TBI] diagnoses)
- Cognition (especially for combined spinal cord injury/TBI diagnoses)
- Adaptive driving
- Home, school, and work place evaluation

The COTA can assist the OTR by assessing the patient's self-care skills and needs and by determining or identifying structural concerns within the home.

Performing ADLs is an important part of the occupational therapy evaluation. The purpose is to determine present and potential levels of functional ability. If the patient is cleared of bedrest precautions, then evaluation and simultaneous treatment should begin as soon as possible after injury. Light activities such as feeding, light hygiene at the sink, and object manipulation may be appropriate depending on the level of injury. The COTA may be involved in this part of the evaluation.

Direct interaction with the patient's family and friends will provide valuable information regarding the patient's support systems while in the hospital and more importantly after discharge. Information gained informally can assist in later caregiver training in areas in which the patient may require the assistance of others to accomplish self-care and mobility tasks.

In addition to physical and functional assessments the occupational therapy practitioner has the opportunity to observe patients' psychosocial adjustment to the disability and life in general as evidenced by the activities in which they participate.[9] This is an important time to establish rapport and mutual trust that will facilitate participation and progress in later and more difficult phases of rehabilitation. An individual's motivation, determination, socioeconomic background, education, family support, acceptance of disability, problem-solving abilities, and financial resources can prove to be invaluable assets or limiting factors in determining the outcome of rehabilitation.[6]

### Establishing Treatment Objectives

The patient and the rehabilitation team should work together to establish treatment objectives because the primary objectives of the team may not be those of the patient. More participation can be expected if the patient's priorities are respected to the extent that they are achievable and realistic.

The general objectives of treatment for the person with spinal cord injury are the following:

1. To maintain or increase joint ROM and prevent deformity by means of active and passive ROM and splinting and positioning
2. To increase strength of all innervated and partially innervated muscles through the use of enabling and purposeful activities
3. To increase physical endurance by means of functional activities
4. To develop the patient's maximal independence in all aspects of self-care, mobility, homemaking, and parenting skills
5. To explore leisure interests and vocational potential
6. To aid in the psychosocial adjustment to disability
7. To evaluate, recommend, and train in the use and care of necessary durable medical and adaptive equipment
8. To ensure safe and independent home accessibility through home modification recommendations
9. To instruct the patient in communication skills necessary for training caregivers to provide safe assistance

The patient's length of stay in the inpatient rehabilitation program and ability to participate in outpatient therapy will determine the appropriateness and priority of the listed activities.

### Treatment Methods

#### *Acute Phase*

During the acute or immobilized phase of the rehabilitation program, the patient may be in traction or wearing a stabilization device such as a halo brace or body jacket. Good skin care and proper hygiene are imperative when using any device. COTAs have an important role in helping the patient deal with the need for these devices and in learning the appropriate use and precautions and adaptations as identified by the OTR.

Medical precautions must be in force during this period. Flexion, extension, and rotary movements of the spine and neck are contraindicated. It is essential that the COTA who interacts with a patient in the acute phase have a clear understanding of how to handle the medical equipment involved.

Splints may be designed and fabricated by occupational therapy practitioners to support the wrist and hands properly for function and appearance. Such splints are dorsal rather than ventral in design to allow maximal sensory feedback while the patient's hand is resting on any surface. The COTA should be aware of the correct positioning and strapping of the splint and of the need for skin inspection.

Active and active-assisted ROM of all joints within strength, ability, and tolerance levels should be performed. Progressive resistive exercises to wrists may be carried out. These interventions may be delegated to the COTA.

The patient should be encouraged to engage in self-care activities such as eating, writing, and hygiene if possible with the use of simple devices such as a universal cuff or a custom writing splint. Even though the patient may be immobilized in bed, discussion of anticipated durable medical equipment (DME), home modifications, and caregiver training should be initiated to allow sufficient time to prepare for discharge.

#### *Active Phase*

*Development of upright tolerance*

During the active or mobilization phase of the rehabilitation program, the patient can sit in a wheelchair and should begin developing upright tolerance. It is at this time that the patient should learn a method for relieving sitting pressure to prevent decubitus ulcers on the ischial, trochanteric, and sacral bony prominences. The patient with at least F+ (3+) shoulder and elbow strength bilaterally can relieve pressure on the buttocks by leaning forward over the feet. Simple cotton webbing loops are secured to the back frame of the wheelchair (Figure 36-4).

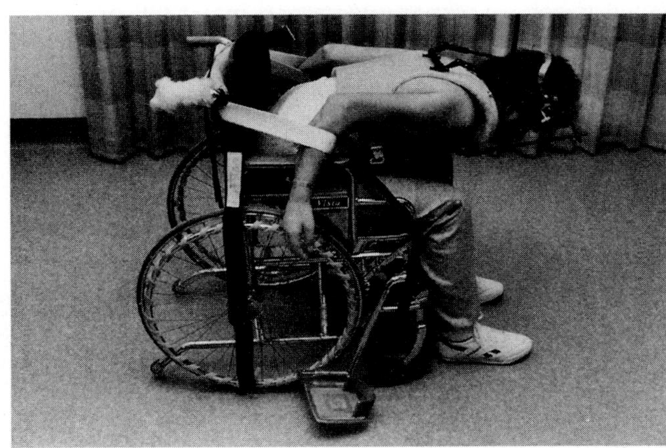

*Figure 36-4* Forward weight shift with loops attached to wheelchair frame. C6 quadriplegic with symmetrical grade 4 deltoids and biceps.

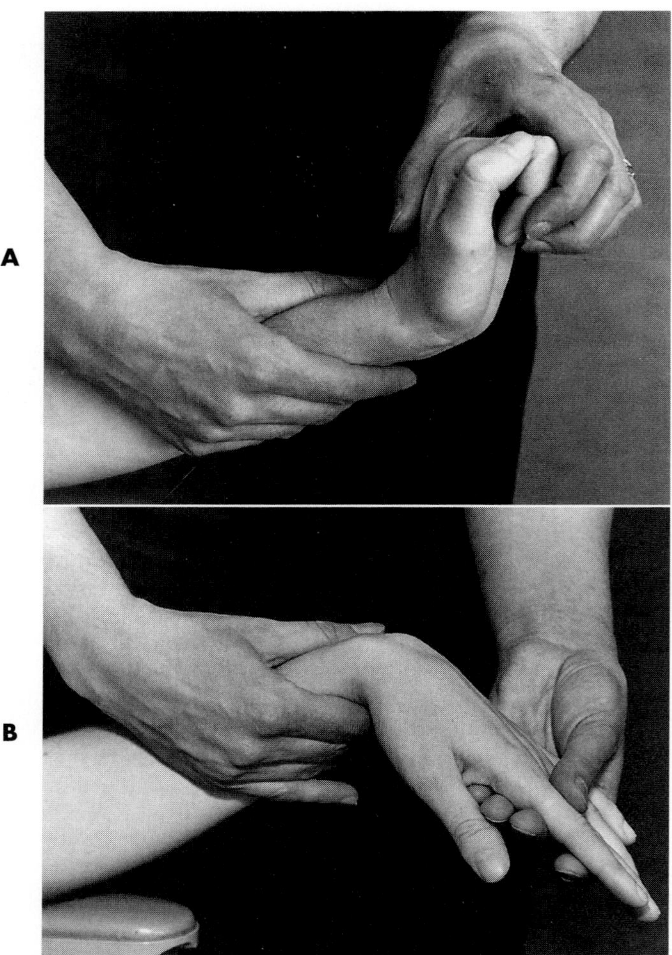


*Figure 36-5* **A,** Wrist is extended when fingers are passively flexed. **B,** Wrist is flexed when fingers are passively extended.

A person with low quadriplegia (C7 neurological level or below) or paraplegia and intact UE musculature can perform a full depression weight shift off the arms or wheels of the wheelchair. Weight shifts should be performed at least every 30 minutes until skin tolerance is determined.

*Maintenance of range of motion*

Active and passive ROM exercises should be continued regularly to prevent contractures. The elbows may be splinted or casted to correct contractures that are developing. In patients who have wrist extension that will be used to substitute for absent grasp through tenodesis action of the long finger flexors, it is desirable to develop some tightness in these tendons to give some additional tension to the tenodesis grasp. **Tenodesis** is the reciprocal motion of the wrist and fingers that occurs during active wrist flexion and extension. The desirable contracture is developed by ranging finger flexion with the wrist fully extended and finger extension with the wrist flexed, thus never allowing the flexors or extensors to be in full stretch over all of the joints that they cross[12] (Figure 36-5). See also Chapter 22 for further discussion of tenodesis.

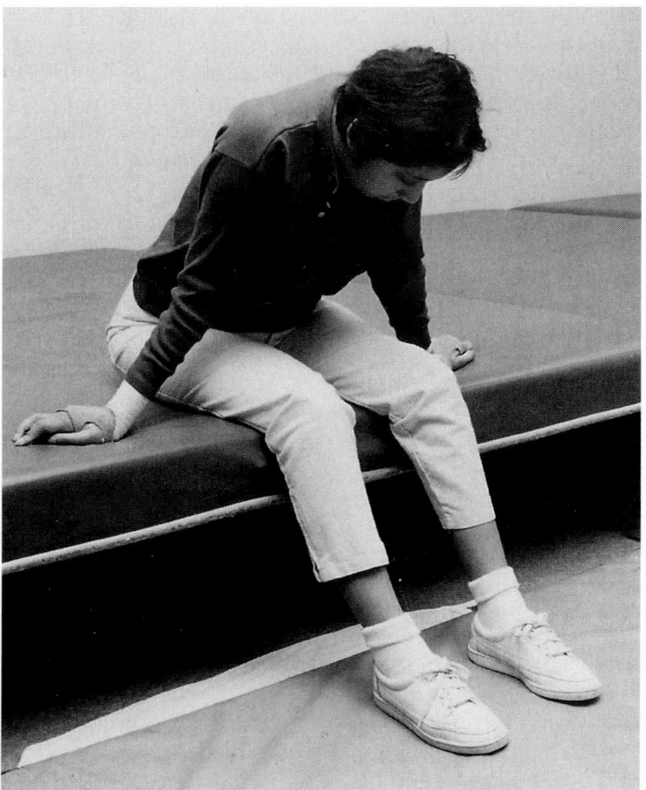

*Figure 36-6* C6 quadriplegic. Forward sitting balance is maintained (without triceps) by locking elbows—a valuable skill for bed mobility and transfers.

Elbow contractures should never be allowed to develop. Full elbow extension is essential to allow "propping" to maintain balance during static sitting and to assist in transfers. With zero triceps strength, a person with C6 quadriplegia can maintain forward sitting balance by shoulder depression and protraction, external rotation, and full wrist extension (Figure 36-6).

*Muscle strengthening*

For the spinal cord injury patient, exercise can mean the difference between independence and dependence. A well-integrated exercise program is initiated early in treatment to prevent atrophy in weakened muscles, to maximize upper body strength, and to increase endurance for self-care task follow-through. The COTA must work closely with the OTR to provide an exercise program to meet each patient's needs. It is also important to have a good understanding of how endurance and coordination affect overall functional performance.

1. *Head and neck:* Building strength, endurance, and coordination for head and neck musculature (C2 to C5 patient) are often achieved through

mouthstick activities. To engage in mouthstick activities in the upright position, the patient must have attained head and neck stability. Activities can then be introduced that demand more controlled head and neck movements. Examples can include page turning, typing (using an electric typewriter or computer keyboard), and painting. Patients who are unable to work against gravity may be able to perform mouthstick tasks in a semireclined position. Isometric exercises can also strengthen head and neck muscles.

2. *Endurance training:* Endurance and muscle strength have the same importance when it comes to functional performance outcome. The majority of ADL routines require repeated performance of motor patterns for task completion. For example, consider eating—the hand-to-mouth movements are repeated over an extended time.
3. *Coordination:* For the quadriplegic patient, tasks that are customarily done at a fine motor level will have to be performed by less refined gross motor patterns. For example, writing or typing is normally performed by muscles of the wrist and hand, which are stabilized by the steadiness of the rest of the UE and the trunk. The patient with a C5 to C6 quadriplegia must relearn how to achieve the distal control for writing or typing by relying solely on the proximal musculature of the upper extremities. If the patient has spasticity or altered sensory feedback, this will make the relearning process even more difficult.[6] It is important that the OTR and COTA frequently meet to coordinate training so that only essential motor patterns that will enhance function are developed.
4. *Upper body:* Progressive resistive exercise and resistive activities can be applied to innervated and partially innervated muscles. Shoulder musculature should be exercised with emphasis on the latissimus dorsi (shoulder depressors), deltoids (shoulder flexors, abductors, and extensors), and the remainder of the shoulder girdle and scapular muscles for proximal stability. The triceps, pectoralis, and latissimus dorsi muscles are needed for transfers and shifting weight when in the wheelchair. Wrist extensors should be strengthened to maximize natural tenodesis function, thereby maximizing the necessary prehension pattern in the hand for functional grasp and release. The treatment program should be graded to increase the amount of resistance that can be tolerated during activity.

There are a variety of exercises that a COTA can use when working with a spinal cord injury patient. The patient who is innervated at C6 has an imbalance in muscle function (between agonists and antagonists). It is important for the OTR and COTA to develop a strengthening program that will strengthen weaker muscles that are necessary for successful task performance. Patterns to emphasize include forward and overhead reach, hand-to-mouth-to-plate pattern, and wheelchair propulsion.

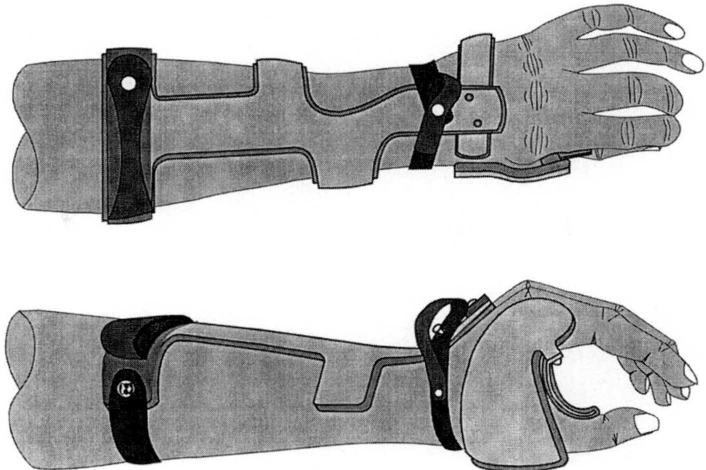

*Figure 36-7* Long opponens splint. (Courtesy Thomas R. Lunsford.)

*Orthoses*

Upper extremity orthotics help prevent deformities by positioning weak muscles and protecting joint structures from unnatural forces caused by weakened or absent musculature. Splints are used for proper positioning and should be incorporated into daily functional activities. Some splints enhance natural tenodesis action, enabling the C5-C6 or C6 patient to pinch and grasp objects. There are four types of wrist-hand orthoses for spinal cord injury patients:

1. *The short opponens* provides stabilization of carpometacarpal (CMC) and metacarpophalangeal (MCP) of thumb while in an opposed position. This splint is used with C6 patients during tenodesis grasp training.
2. *The long opponens* is also known as a *static wrist and hand orthosis.* This device is designed to provide the hand and wrist with the proper static functional position (Figure 36-7).
3. *The wrist driven wrist-hand orthosis (WDWHO)* is also known as the wrist-driven flexor hinge hand splint and is commonly used for the C6 quadriplegic with fair plus or better wrist extensors and poor or less finger flexion for grasp. The splint is wrist driven, providing the patient with a variety of pinch size options (Figure 36-8).
4. *The ratchet wrist-hand orthosis (WHO)* is primarily used with the C5 quadriplegic with absent to poor wrist extensor strength (Figure 36-9).

Lower extremity orthotic devices are used by complete paraplegics, T10 and below, incomplete quadriplegics, and paraplegics to allow the patient to stand or walk during functional activities. Patients are

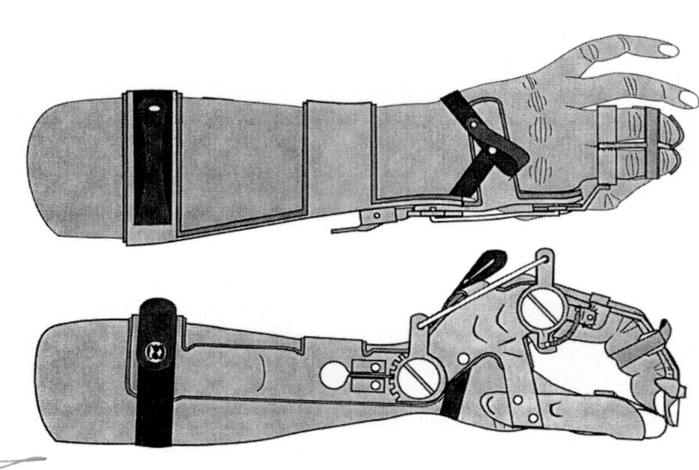

*Figure 36-8* Wrist-driven wrist-hand orthosis (WDWHO). (Courtesy Thomas R. Lunsford, The Woodlands, Tex.)

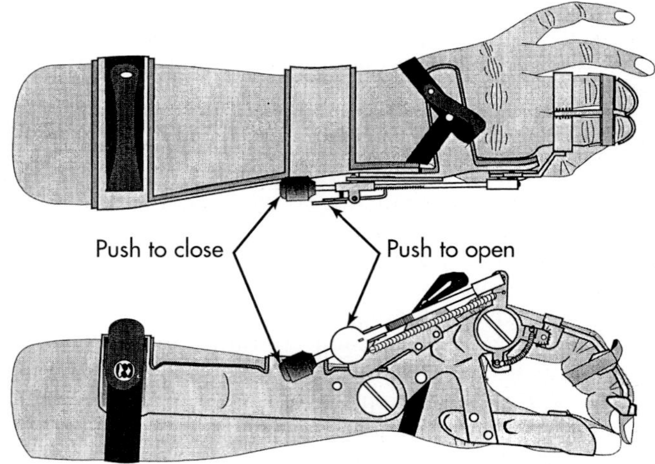


*Figure 36-9* Ratchet wrist-hand orthosis (WHO). (Courtesy Thomas R. Lunsford, The Woodlands, Tex.)

taught to independently don, doff, and care for these assistive devices.

It is important to combine passive ROM with orthosis use to prevent joint and muscle stiffness. The COTA is involved throughout the education and treatment process and can work with the patient to develop a wearing schedule that includes the following:

1. Monitoring the wear time of the orthosis, initially 30 to 45 minutes
2. Beginning a wearing schedule of 2 hours "on" (with assessment for pressure after the first hour) and 1 hour "off"
3. Wearing at night as tolerated, in keeping with the training schedule, to minimize interruption of sleep
4. Increasing wear to full night and day use as the patient's tolerance allows
5. Removing the orthosis one to two times daily for cleaning and ROM

*Assistive devices: provision and training*

There are many assistive devices and equipment items that can be useful to the person with a spinal cord injury. However, it is most desirable for the patient to perform the task with no equipment or as little as possible. Modified techniques can enable efficient performance without the need for costly or bulky equipment. When appropriate, the universal cuff for holding eating utensils, toothbrushes, pencils, and paintbrushes is a simple and versatile device that offers increased independence (see Figure 17-37).

A wrist cock-up splint to stabilize the wrist with attachment of the universal cuff can be useful for persons with little or no wrist extension. A plate guard, cup holder, extended straw with straw clip, and nonskid table mat can facilitate independent feeding (see Figure 17-37). The wash mitt and soap holder or soap-on-a-rope can make bathing easier; however, the added difficulty of donning and doffing such equipment must be considered. Many people with quadriplegia can use a button hook to fasten clothing (see Figure 17-8). A transfer board is an option for safe transfers. Muscle strength and coordination can be developed through treatment so much that the patient may grow out of equipment that was initially provided.

*Selection and measurement for durable medical equipment*

The assessment, ordering, and fitting of DME, such as wheelchairs, seating and positioning equipment, mechanical lifts, beds, and bathing equipment, is an extremely important part of the rehabilitation program. Such equipment should be specifically evaluated, however, and ordered only at the time when definite goals and expectations are known. Inappropriate equipment can impair function and cause further medical problems such as skin breakdown or trunk deformity.

The clinician must account for all functional, positioning, environmental, psychological, and financial considerations when evaluating the patient's equipment needs. The desired equipment (especially wheelchairs and positioning devices and bathing equipment) should be available for demonstration by the patient before final ordering. It is imperative that clinicians involved in the evaluation and ordering of this costly and highly individualized equipment be familiar with what is currently on the market and be knowledgeable in ordering equipment that will provide optimal function and body positioning on a short- and long-term basis to the patient. See Chapter 18 for a more in depth discussion of wheelchairs, seating, and positioning equipment.

An increasing number of individuals with high-level spinal cord injuries (C4 and above) are surviving and participating in active rehabilitation programs. Their treatment and equipment needs are unique and extremely specialized, ranging from mouthsticks and environmental control systems to ventilators and sophisticated electric wheelchairs and drive systems (Table 36-2). COTAs should expect and seek close supervision for all aspects of care for this unique patient population.

*Activities of daily living*

The COTA is likely to be most involved with the spinal cord injury patient in the area of ADL, in particular basic ADL such as eating, dressing, and grooming. Because of the complexities and differences from one spinal cord injury level to the next, it is not possible to provide details for all levels (see Table 36-2).

- *Positioning:* The aim of positioning is to minimize abnormal tone, accommodate deformities, and provide enough postural support to increase stability without reducing mobility or interfering with movements. The most appropriate position is dependent on the patient's physical ability, needs for task completion, and functional changes to come. When planning for ADL retraining, position must be kept in the forefront.
- *Eating:* Eating independently is often the first functional self-care task initiated with the spinal cord injury patient. There is a high level of motivation to eat independently as well as a sense of accomplishment for a task well done. The task of eating includes drinking from a cup or straw, eating with fingers, eating with utensils, and arranging the setup required to eat a meal, cut food, and open containers.
- *Hygiene and grooming:* With daily practice, creativity, problem solving, and the use of adaptive and orthotic equipment, independence in these areas can be attained.[6] Oral-facial hygiene tasks and grooming can include face washing, teeth brushing or denture care, shaving, and make-up application. Successful task completion is dependent on tenodesis function, appropriate assistive devices, available endurance, coordination, and muscle strength.
- *Dressing:* A patient's motivation to perform the task of dressing is very important. Without the motivation to succeed, the goals will be unattainable. The goal of dressing should be mutually agreed on by the patient, the family members, and the therapist. It takes hours of training, problem solving, and adapting to the proper use of equipment and compensatory techniques to achieve the desired goal.[6]

  Motivation and the ability to problem solve will directly affect the patient's ability to accomplish a task. Physical factors that may influence dressing skill performance include bed mobility (rolling and positioning lower extremities), body weight, age, spasticity, flexibility, arm and hand function, and endurance. When initiating dressing training, the COTA must be aware of patient precautions, restrictions, and limitations.

  **Upper body:** Two basic techniques are used for upper body dressing: over the head and around the back. Dressing training begins with the C6 quadriplegic; however, there are C5 and C5,C6 patients who have attained success with dressing tasks.[6] The option of participating in dressing training should always be offered to the patient. Details on specific sequences for dressing and other ADL can be found in Chapter 17.

  **Lower body:** There are several basic techniques for lower body dressing that can be used by the COTA. Initially, if upright tolerance has been achieved, begin teaching the patient to dress with the head of the bed in a full upright position. In this position the patient must be wearing the appropriate body stabilizer. If the body jacket is not in place the head of the bed may be elevated to no more than a 30 degree angle.

  **Equipment:** Assistive devices often used for lower and upper body dressing tasks include reachers, dressing sticks, leg pull-ups or ranging straps, dressing loops, sock-donning devices, zipper pullers, and buttonhooks. Rope ladders are used to assist the patient into a long-sit position, and aid in stabilization and positioning for lower body dressing. The techniques chosen for successful lower body dressing are determined by the patients upper extremity strength, endurance, and lower body ROM.
- *Bathing:* Before initiating bathing training it is important to assess the bathroom in the patient's home. Completion of a home evaluation early in the rehabilitation process is necessary to help determine equipment needs, available working space, and the need for possible structural modifications.

  Equipment suggestions include the following:
  1. Rolling shower-commode wheelchair
  2. Padded tub transfer bench (with or without cutout)
  3. Shower chair with back and suction cup feet
  4. Grab bars for support and stability
  5. Handheld shower nozzle with on and off device on the handle
  6. Wash mitts with a Velcro D-ring closure or elastic edge
  7. Long-handled bath brush with angled handle
  8. Soap-on-a-rope worn around the neck or attached to bath chair
  9. Towels adapted by adding loops to the ends or sewing eyelet holes across the ends.
- Bathing is an important aspect of self-care performance for the patient at C6 or lower level. The COTA needs to be aware of any physical restrictions and limitations. Those patients wearing Ky-

*Text continued on p. 604*

*Table 36-2*

## Functional Outcomes Based on Level of Injury*

| *Neurological level and muscles innervated†* | *Movements possible* | *Pattern of weakness* | *Functional capabilities and limitations* |
|---|---|---|---|
| **C1-C3** | | | |
| Sternocleidomastoids<br>Upper trapezius<br>Levator scapulae | Neck control | Total paralysis of trunk, UEs, and LEs<br>Dependence on respirator | Is totally ADL dependent<br>Instructs others in care<br>Propels power wheelchair equipped with portable respirator and chin or breath controls<br>Operates communcation devices and environmental control systems with mouthstick or pneumatic control<br>Requires full-time attendant care |
| **C3-C4** | | | |
| *Trapezius (superior, middle, and inferior)‡*<br>*Diaphragm (C3-C5)*<br>Cervical and paraspinal muscles | Neck movements, scapular elevation<br>Inspiration | Paralysis of trunk, UEs, and LEs<br>Difficulty in breathing and coughing | Uses wheelchair full time—can talk through all set-ups and train caregivers in care<br>May require respiratory assistance full time or part time<br>Requires maximum assistance for skin inspection (cannot position mirrors but should inspect self)<br>Accomplishes activities (e.g., typing, page turning, and manipulation of table top objects and games) through use of mouthstick<br>Operates power wheelchair with chin or breath<br>Requires full-time attendant care |
| **C5** | | | |
| All muscles of shoulder at least partially innervated except latissimus dorsi and coracobrachialis | Shoulder extension and horizontal abduction (weak) | Absence of elbow extension, pronation, and all wrist and hand movements | Unable to roll over or reach sitting position without hospital bed with rails<br>Needs assistance in transfers |
| *Partial deltoids* | Shoulder flexion, shoulder abduction to 90 degrees | Total paralysis of trunk and LEs | If good muscle power, may perform UE dressing with minimum assistance<br>Depends on others for skin inspection |

*These guidelines were developed primarily from experience. The outcomes reflect the highest level of independence that may be expected of a complete injury given optimum circumstances. Let the reader be aware that these are meant as guidelines only and not as outcomes to be expected in all cases.
†Each level includes the muscles and functions of the preceding levels.
‡Key muscles are in *italics*.

*Table 36-2*

## Functional Outcomes Based on Level of Injury*—cont'd

| *Neurological level and muscles innervated†* | *Movements possible* | *Pattern of weakness* | *Functional capabilities and limitations* |
|---|---|---|---|
| **C5—cont'd** | | | |
| *Biceps brachii*<br>Brachialis<br>Brachioradialis | Elbow flexion and supination | | Performs independent indoor activities in wheelchair with hand rim adaptations<br>Uses power wheelchair for long distance and outdoors |
| Levator scapulae, diaphragm, scleni—fully innervated<br>Rhomboids (major and minor)<br>Serratus anterior (C5-C7)<br>Teres major (C5, C6)<br>Subscapularis (C5, C6)<br>Pectoralis major (C5-C8, T1)<br>Infraspinatus<br>Supraspinatus<br>Teres minor (C5, C6) | Scapular adduction and downward rotation (weak)<br>Scapular abduction and upward rotation (weak)<br>Shoulder internal rotation (weak)<br>Shoulder horizontal adduction (weak)<br>Shoulder external rotation | Low endurance because of paralysis of intercostals and low respiratory reserve | With splints, adaptive equipment and attendant setup, performs eating, light hygiene, makeup, shaving, handwriting (sufficient for legal signature), telephoning, and typing activities<br>Requires at least part-time attendant care; instructs caregivers in all self-care mobility, and functional set-ups<br>Directs bowel and bladder management<br>May drive a van with significant adaptations |
| **C6** | | | |
| All partially innervated C5 muscles now fully innervated except serratus and pectoralis major | Full strength to shoulder flexion and extension, abduction and adduction, internal and external rotation, and elbow flexion | Absence of elbow extension and ulnar wrist extension | Performs many activities independently with equipment or natural tenodesis grasp<br>Uses tenodesis splint or universal cuff for eating with regular utensils; performs personal hygiene and grooming (oral and upper body) activities, UE dressing, hand-writing, typing, telephoning, and light kitchen activities<br>Rolls from side to side in bed with aid of bed rails<br>Moves from supine to sidelying to sit with minimum assistance |
| Partial but significant innervation to serratus anterior (C5-C7) | Scapular abduction and upward rotation | | Independently propels wheelchair on level terrain and minimum grade inclines with plastic or foam-coated rims |

Continued.

*Table 36-2*

## Functional Outcomes Based on Level of Injury*—cont'd

| *Neurological level and muscles innervated*† | *Movements possible* | *Pattern of weakness* | *Functional capabilities and limitations* |
|---|---|---|---|
| **C6—cont'd** | | | |
| Latissmus dorsi (C6-C8) | Shoulder extension and internal rotation | Possible low endurance because of reduced vital capacity | Relieves pressure independently when sitting, using loops, and during forward weight shift |
| *Pectoralis major (C5-C8, T1)* | Shoulder horizontal adduction and internal rotation | Absence of wrist flexion<br>Total paralysis of trunk and LEs | Independently manages communication devices with adapted equipment |
| Coracobrachialis (C6, C7) | Shoulder flexion | | Assists in transfers by substituting shoulder adduction and rotation for elbow extension and may be independent with aid of transfer board |
| Pronator teres (C6, C7) | Forearm pronation | | |
| Supinator | Complete innervation for forearm supination | | |
| *Extensor carpi radialis longus and brevis (C6, C7)* | Radial wrist extension | | Drives with adaptations |
| | | | Performs independent skin inspection with mirrors |
| | | | Assists caregiver in bladder care |
| | | | Requires adaptive equipment and assistance for bathing and bowel care |
| | | | May require part-time attendant care |
| | | | May participate in sports (quad rugby, swimming) |
| **C7-C8** | | | |
| Shoulder prime movers—fully innervated, as well as rest of partially innervated C6 muscles | Full strength of all shoulder movements, radial wrist flexors and extensors, and strong pronation | Lack of trunk muscles—compromised full shoulder stability | Performs transfers to and from bed and wheelchair independently |
| *Triceps brachii* | Elbow extension | | |
| Extensor carpi ulnaris (C6-C8) | Ulnar wrist extension | | Rolls over, sits up, and moves about in a standard bed |
| *Flexor carpi radialis* | Radial wrist flexion | | Dresses independently and performs personal hygiene activities |
| *Flexor digitorum superficialis and profundus (C7, C8, T1)* | Proximal interphalangeal (PIP) and distal interphalangeal (DIP) flexion | Limited grasp, release and dexterity because of incomplete innervation of hand intrinsics | Independently eats (usually with no assistive devices)<br>May use tenodesis splint because of weakness of grasp |
| *Extensor digitorum communis (C6-C8)* | Metacarpophalangeal extension | | Propels manual wheelchair (may need friction tape on handrims for long distances, may need assistance on rough terrain)<br>Drives with adaptations |

*These guidelines were developed primarily from experience. The outcomes reflect the highest level of independence that may be expected of a complete injury given optimum circumstances. Let the reader be aware that these are meant as guidelines only and not as outcomes to be expected in all cases.

†Each level includes the muscles and functions of the preceding levels.

‡Key muscles are in *italics*.

Table 36-2

## Functional Outcomes Based on Level of Injury*—cont'd

| *Neurological level and muscles innervated†* | *Movements possible* | *Pattern of weakness* | *Functional capabilities and limitations* |
|---|---|---|---|
| **C7-C8—cont'd** | | | |
| Extensor pollicis longus and brevis<br>Abductor pollicis longus | Thumb extension (metacarpophalangeal, and interphalangeal (IP)<br>Thumb abduction | Total paralysis of LEs<br>Weakness of trunk control<br>Limited endurance because of reduced respiratory reserve | Performs independent bladder and bowel care<br>Performs independent skin inspection<br>Performs light housework if possible<br>May participate in preparation for sexual activity (i.e. undressing, condom and diaphragm use) |
| **C8-T1** | | | |
| All muscles of UEs—fully innervated<br>Pronator quadratus | Forearm pronation | Paralysis of LEs | Independently performs bed activities, wheelchair transfers, and self-care and personal hygiene activities |
| Flexor carpi ulnaris | Ulnar wrist flexion | Weakness of trunk control | Manages manual wheelchair on all surfaces |
| *Lumbricales and interossei dorsales and palmares*<br>Palmar interrossei | Metacarpophalangeal flexion<br>Finger adduction | Reduced endurance because of low respiratory reserve | Transfers from wheelchair to floor and return with standby assistance<br>Gets up and down from standing frame independently<br>Performs independent bladder and bowel care and skin inspection |
| Flexor pollicis longus and brevis<br>Adductor pollicis<br>*Opponens digiti minimi*<br>*Opponens pollicis* | Thumb flexion (metacarpophalangeal, IP)<br>Thumb adduction<br>Opposition of fifth finger<br>Thumb opposition | | Independently manages communication devices<br>Drives with adaptations<br>Performs light housekeeping activities independently |
| **T4-T9** | | | |
| All muscles of upper extremities plus partial innervation of intercostal muscles and long muscles of the back (sacrospinalis and semispinalis) | All arm functions, partial trunk stability, endurance increased because of better respiration | Partial trunk paralysis and total paralysis of LEs | Independently performs all self-care activities<br>Independently manages manual wheelchair and transfers<br>May use standing frame independently<br>Drives car with adaptations<br>Independently performs light housekeeping activities |

*Continued.*

Table 36-2

Functional Outcomes Based on Level of Injury*—cont'd

| *Neurological level and muscles innervated*† | *Movements possible* | *Pattern of weakness* | *Functional capabilities and limitations* |
|---|---|---|---|
| **T10-L2** | | | |
| Intercostal muscles fully innervated<br>Abdominal muscles partially to fully innervated (recuts abdominis, internal and external obliques) | Partial to good trunk stability<br>Increased physical endurance | Paralysis of LEs<br>Possible flaccid bowel, bladder and decreased sexual function (e.g., no erection, sensation, or ejaculation) | Independently performs self-care, work, personal hygiene, sports, and housekeeping activities<br>Ambulates with difficulty using braces and crutches; however, wheelchair often chosen for speed, energy conservation, and sports<br>Drives car with hand controls |
| **L3-L4** | | | |
| Low back muscles<br>Hip flexors, adductors, quadriceps | Trunk control and stability<br>Hip flexion, hip adduction, knee extension | Partial paralysis of lower extremities—hip extension, knee flexion, and ankle and foot movements | Independently performs all activities previously outlined<br>Ambulates independently with short leg braces using crutches<br>May still use a wheelchair for convenience, energy conservation, and sports |
| **L5-S3** | | | |
| Hip extensors—gluteus maximus and hamstrings<br>Hip abductors—gluteus medius and gluteus minimus<br>Knee flexors—hamstrings, sartorius, and gracilis<br>Ankle muscles—tibilis anterior, gastrocnemius, soleus, and peroneus longus<br>Foot muscles | Partial to full control of LEs | Partial paralysis of LEs especially in distal segment | Independently performs all activities<br>May require limited bracing for ambulation<br>May have volitional bowel, bladder, and sexual function<br>May drive car without modifications |

*These guidelines were developed primarily from experience. The outcomes reflect the highest level of independence that may be expected of a complete injury given optimum circumstances. Let the reader be aware that these are meant as guidelines only and not as outcomes to be expected in all cases.
†Each level includes the muscles and functions of the preceding levels.
‡Key muscles are in *italics*.

dex and Jewett orthoses may shower with the braces in place.

*Psychological support*

The occupational therapy practitioner should continue to provide psychological support by allowing and encouraging the patient to express frustration, anger, fears, and concerns.[10] The occupational therapy clinic can provide an atmosphere of support with other inpatients and outpatients who can offer their experiences and problem-solving advice to those in earlier phases of their rehabilitation.

*Home management*

During the initial evaluation process, home management roles, responsibilities, goals, and options are discussed and addressed. Training for home management skills will continue on an outpatient or in-home basis. Roles will depend on the patient's functional status, living situations, and prioritization of time and energy management.

The ability to participate minimally, or with complete independence, in home management activities is important to the spinal cord injury patient. The COTA may enable this by providing instruction in techniques and use of adaptive equipment and orthotic devices. Modification to the home environment may be needed to increase independence and safety during performance of home management activities. In-home alterations may involve rearrangement of home furnishings and kitchen appliances to increase accessibility.

### *Community Reentry*

The reintegration experience should be provided before discharge. Skills are successfully learned through participation. Successful community living requires not only physical performance, but also psychosocial readiness, and the ability to seek assistance and verbally direct another person when assistance is required. Rehearsing potential situations and planning ahead through role play and simulation will help the patient prepare for community reentry.

#### *Leisure skills*

A COTA can expose patients to leisure and recreational activities individually and in a group setting. The exposure usually builds interests and a desire to participate in the activity. Occupational therapy's role includes providing equipment, training, enhancement of skills, encouragement, and support. Leisure skills participation should be viewed as part of a well-integrated lifestyle.

#### *Group programs*

Spinal cord injury patients are excellent candidates for group activities as an adjunct to individual therapy sessions. Possible group activities include the following:

1. Quadriplegic ADL communication group
2. Independent eating group
3. Community reentry group for paraplegics and quadriplegics
4. Meal preparation group
5. Vocational group
6. Upper body motor skills group

Group activities should be matched to the patient's goals and determined jointly by the OTR and the COTA. It is appropriate for the COTA to lead such groups.

#### *Patient, family, and caregiver education*

To make a successful transition to community living, the patient and family or other caregivers need to be able to follow through with and support the objectives of the treatment plan. The patient and any significant others should be involved in setting the short- and long-term goals. Training and education must begin early in the rehabilitation process and continue throughout the patient's stay and should focus on ROM and deformity control, positioning, skin protection and inspection, splint and orthosis use, self-care, and appropriate use of adaptive devices and equipment.

### *Discharge Planning*

Occupational therapy is involved with discharge planning as are the other disciplines and the patient and family. Among the many issues that the occupational therapy practitioner addresses are (1) additional training the family or caregiver will need, (2) carry over of learned self-care tasks into the home, (3) whether patients will be able to adequately communicate their needs to another person, and (4) whether patients' home environments are conducive to meeting self-care needs. Additional responsibilities for occupational therapy staff include the following:

1. Determining and ordering equipment needed for the home
2. Ensuring that the home and school evaluations are completed
3. Providing awareness and education for an adaptive driving program
4. Determining the need for outpatient therapy
5. Providing the patient with a home exercise program

#### *Home evaluation*

When place of discharge is determined and the patient can tolerate leaving the hospital for a few hours, a home evaluation should be performed. Although this evaluation is usually performed by a highly skilled OTR, the COTA may contribute as well. Clinicians should understand safety and accessibility options for a variety of environments.

### *Outpatient Rehabilitation*

Under current reimbursement pressures and practice restrictions, patients should anticipate extended rehabilitation on an outpatient basis or by means of home therapy. This may include assessment and progressive treatment in areas such as adaptive driving, home management, leisure activities, workshop skills, and vocational potential. Such activities can improve socialization skills and provide a milieu for assessing problem-solving skills and potential work habits as well.

#### *Paraplegic patients*

Outpatient rehabilitation should emphasize higher learning skills including the following:

1. Home management tasks
2. Enhancement of transfer skills with a slide board or depression transfer
3. Community reentry program
4. Ambulation training with or without braces
5. Reassessment of specific self-care tasks after the removal of the halo or jacket

6. Improvement of one- and two-handed activities in the standing position
7. Upper body strength and endurance program
8. Adaptive driving program assessment and training
9. Home program with emphasis on specific need areas

*Quadriplegic patients*

Outpatient rehabilitation should emphasize skills that will enhance independence:

1. Upper extremity strength, endurance, and coordination to facilitate follow-through with ADL
2. Refinement of self-care skills
3. Household management
4. Community reentry
5. Wrist and hand orthosis training
6. Technology assessment
7. Adaptive driving program assessment and training
8. Patient, family, and caregiver training

### *Vocational Assessment and Rehabilitation*

Vocational possibilities for persons with high levels of spinal cord injury are limited by the sheer magnitude of the physical disability. Many patients must change their vocation or alter former vocational goals. Low aptitude, poor motivation, and lack of interest and perseverance on the part of many patients make vocational rehabilitation challenging. The COTA, during the process of the treatment program and through the use of ADL, craft, and work simulation activities, can observe and help to assess the patient's level of motivation, functional intelligence, aptitudes, attitudes, interests, and personal vocational aspirations. The COTA can observe the patient's attention span, concentration, manual ability with splints and devices, accuracy, speed, perseverance, work habits, and work tolerance level. This information should be communicated to the OTR. Ultimately, the patient may be referred to a vocational rehabilitation specialist.

## AGING WITH SPINAL CORD INJURY

After survival of acute spinal cord injury, the primary goal of rehabilitation is defined in terms of independence. Independence has become the measure of quality of life for people with disabilities, an idea accepted and often perpetuated by professionals and survivors.[11]

Occupational therapy practitioners treating patients with spinal cord injuries have a considerable influence on the level of independence throughout the course of the patients' lives. The COTA who understands the aging process in both the able-bodied and the disabled individual will be more prepared to offer appropriate options and foster attitudes that will enhance the quality of the patient's life at any age.

Physical aging can occur at varying rates. In persons with spinal cord injuries, aging is usually accelerated by secondary effects of the disability such as the presence of muscle imbalance, infections (both urinary and respiratory), deconditioning, pain, and joint degeneration as a result of overuse. One of four spinal cord injury survivors has survived 20 years after the injury.[9] Persons who become quadriplegic in their twenties (which is when the majority of spinal cord injuries occur) develop the degenerating conditions of normal aging earlier than normal, usually before their forties.[4] When this occurs, someone who may have been independent in transfers at home and in loading a wheelchair in and out of the car may now require assistance getting in and out of bed and have to trade the car for a van requiring costly modifications.

It is important for the COTA to appreciate why good trunk alignment and seating is essential from the onset in preventing fixed trunk and pelvic deformities such as kyphosis and scoliosis that can lead to considerable skin problems and uncorrectable cosmetic deformities years later. In addition, the COTA should be aware that manual wheelchair propulsion may damage a weak shoulder even though it provides the advantage of cardiopulmonary conditioning. The increased fatigue and weakness often associated with normal aging may motivate the individual with a spinal cord injury to give up a manual wheelchair for a power model.

## SUMMARY

A spinal cord injury can result in significant paralysis of limbs and trunk. The degree of residual motor and sensory dysfunctions depends on the level and severity of the lesion. After a spinal cord injury, bony realignment and stabilization is established surgically or with braces. A spinal cord injury puts the patient at risk for many medical complications including skin breakdown, decreased vital capacity, and autonomic dysreflexia.

Occupational therapy focuses on helping the patient achieve optimum independence and functioning. The occupational therapy program includes measures for physical restoration; self-care, independent living skills; and educational, work, and leisure activities. The psychosocial adjustment of the patient is very important, and all clinicians should offer emotional support toward this end in every phase of the rehabilitation program.

The evaluation and establishment of the initial treatment plan by the OTR will provide the COTA with the direction for an effective occupational therapy program. It is important to remember that a patient's motivation is often related to emotional stability and to relationships with family and friends. Each patient must be treated individually. There is no generic, universal approach to the treatment of the spinal cord injury patient. Clinical reasoning skills, insight, and creativity on the part of staff will help the patient overcome fears of dependency and move toward a more positive self-image and successful performance of ADL.

It is important for the OTR and COTA to meet on a regular basis to discuss medical status, treatment gains, setbacks, program goals, equipment needs, and goal attainment. Clear and frequent communication and collaboration between the OTR and COTA will optimize the rate of progress and move the patient most rapidly toward successful rehabilitation.

## Selected Reading Guide Questions

1. Describe the difference between a C5 and C6 quadriplegic.
2. Describe the difference between a complete and an incomplete lesion.
3. What are the characteristics of autonomic dysreflexia?
4. How does postural hypotension affect function?
5. What is the purpose of a wrist-driven WHO?
6. What level of injury requires a wrist-driven WHO?
7. How is wrist extension used to affect grasp by the patient with quadriplegia?
8. Why is tightening of the long finger flexors an important goal to attain for the quadriplegic?
9. Describe four self-care activities that the patient with a C6 spinal cord injury may be expected to accomplish.
10. List four assistive devices commonly used by a person with quadriplegia and explain the purpose of each.

### REFERENCES


1. American Spinal Injury Association: *Standards for neurological and functional classification of spinal cord injury,* Chicago, Il, 1992, The Association.
2. Anderson KN, editor: *Mosby's medical, nursing, and allied health dictionary,* ed 4, St Louis, 1994, Mosby.
3. Bromley I: *Tetraplegia and paraplegia: a guide for physiotherapists,* ed 3, New York, 1985, Churchill Livingstone.
4. Freed MM: Traumatic and congenital lesions of the spinal cord. In Kottke FJ, Lehmann JF, editors: *Krusen's handbook of physical medicine and rehabilitation,* Philadelphia, 1990, WB Saunders.
5. Hanak M, Scott A: *An illustrated guide for health care professionals,* New York, 1983, Springer Verlag.
6. Hill JP, editor: *Spinal cord injury, A guide to functional outcomes in occupational therapy,* Rockville, Md, 1986, Aspen.
7. Malick MH, Meyer CMH: *Manual on the management of the quadriplegic upper extremity,* Pittsburgh, 1978, Harmarville Rehabilitation Center.
8. Paulson S, editor: *Santa Clara Valley Medical Center spinal cord injury home care manual,* ed 3, San Jose, Calif, 1994, Santa Clara Valley Medical Center.
9. Pierce DS, Nickel VH: *The total care of spinal cord injuries,* Boston, 1977, Little, Brown.
10. Spencer EA: Functional restoration. In Hopkins HL, Smith HD, editors: *Willard and Spackman's occupational therapy,* ed 8, Philadelphia, 1993, JB Lippincott.
11. Whiteneck et al, editors: *Aging with spinal cord injury,* New York, 1993, Demos.
12. Wilson DJ, McKenzie MW, Barber LM: *Spinal cord injury: a treatment guide for occupational therapists,* Thorofare, NJ, 1984, Slack.
13. Yarkony GM: *Spinal cord injury, medical management and rehabilitation,* Gaithersburg, Md, 1994, Aspen.


### RECOMMENDED READING


Ford JR, Duckworth B: *Physical management for the quadriplegic patient,* Philadelphia, FA Davis.

Green R: *Human sexuality: a health practitioners text,* ed 2, Baltimore, Williams & Wilkins.

Somers F: *Spinal cord injury functional rehabilitation,* Norwalk, Conn, 1992, Appleton and Lange.

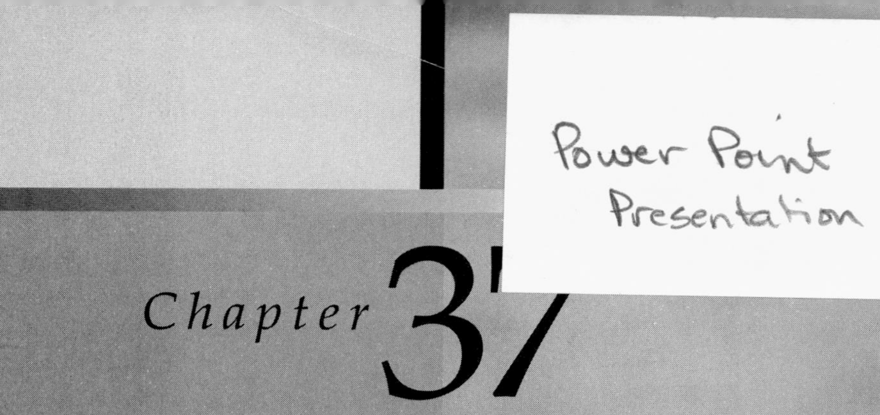


Chapter 37

# Traumatic Brain Injuries

*Katie Schlageter*
*Maureen Michele Matthews*
*Michelle Tipton-Burton*

## Chapter Objectives

*After studying this chapter, the student or practitioner will be able to:*

1. Define traumatic brain injury and identify its common causes.
2. Describe the range of clinical symptoms seen in the traumatic brain injury population.
3. Differentiate between treatment for a beginning level traumatic brain injury patient and an intermediate to advanced level traumatic brain injury patient.
4. Explain how cognitive and perceptual deficits impact ADL function.
5. Describe the principles of a seating program.
6. Explain the purpose of a behavior management program.
7. Describe sensory regulation treatment in the beginning level patient and its purpose.
8. Given specific patient problems, identify and describe appropriate adaptive and compensatory treatments.

## Key Terms

traumatic brain injury (TBI)
open brain injury
closed brain injury
primary damage
diffuse axonal injury (DAI)
secondary damage
posttraumatic amnesia
decorticate posturing
decerebrate posturing
postural deficits
impaired initiation
sensory regulation treatment
pelvic alignment

**Traumatic brain injury (TBI)** results from a penetrating (open) or nonpenetrating (closed) injury to the skull. No two brain injuries are identical. Some are significant enough to cause immediate death whereas others result in little if any measurable damage.

Survivors of TBI may show a variety of problems. No two patients have exactly the same symptoms. One TBI patient may be emerging from coma and respond inconsistently and nonpurposefully to painful stimuli. Another may be very confused and hit, grab, or strike out when overstimulated. A TBI patient may walk and be slightly uncoordinated but have problems in abstract reasoning and may act in ways that are socially inappropriate. The range of disability found in TBI patients is more diverse than in other central nervous system disorders.

This chapter will present an overview of TBI rehabilitation, emphasizing treatment areas in which the certified occupational therapy assistant (COTA) might be expected to participate, including contracture management related to spasticity, behavioral issues, visual deficits, and community reintegration. The incidence, pathophysiology, medical/surgical management, and evaluation of severity of injury will be introduced briefly. The patient's clinical picture (physical, cognitive, behavioral, visual, perceptual, functional, and psychosocial aspects) will be presented in more detail; this will differentiate patients functioning at a beginning level from those functioning at an intermediate to advanced level. Occupational therapy evaluation, which is primarily the responsibility of the registered occupational therapist (OTR), will be discussed briefly.

## BACKGROUND

### Incidence

The recent incidence of TBI in the United States is about 325,000 cases per year.[37] The number of TBIs has been declining, a trend that is attributed to a reduction in drunk driving; increased use of seat belts, airbags, motorcycle helmets; and increased public education on prevention of TBI.[35]

The leading causes of severe TBI are motor vehicle accidents (MVAs) and falls. TBI occurs three times more frequently in men than in women. The risk is greater among children 4 to 5 years old, males 15 to 24 years old, the elderly, and people who have had previous brain injuries. Mortality is higher in adults than in children. Most individuals who experience a TBI are from a lower socioeconomic status and are single. A high percentage of persons with TBI have a history of drug and alcohol abuse, or a psychiatric history.[20]

### Pathophysiology

An **open brain injury** typically is caused by a gunshot wound or fragments from exploding objects. A **closed brain injury** occurs when rotational acceleration and deceleration forces are applied to the head and cause brain tissue to shear (tear apart). Closed brain injuries often result from MVAs. Both primary and secondary damage may result from a closed brain injury.

#### *Primary Damage*

**Primary damage** occurs at the time of a closed brain injury. The damage is caused by localized contusions and **diffuse axonal injury (DAI).** Contusions (bruises) occur in the frontal and temporal regions when the brain slides and strikes the rough skull. They are usually bilateral but are asymmetrical in severity. Localized contusions may also be found under areas of depressed skull fracture.[6]

DAI results from shearing forces that occur between the different components of the brain. The corpus collosum and the brain stem are the most commonly affected areas.[1,2,6] DAI causes widespread brain damage. Damage may be severe enough to induce a coma or so mild that only a concussion, or brief loss of consciousness, results.[4]

#### *Secondary Damage*

**Secondary damage** may evolve over time. Secondary effects include intracranial hematomas, cerebral edema, raised intracerebral pressure, hydrocephalus, intracranial infection, and posttraumatic epilepsy. Widespread brain damage can result from secondary damage.[17] Diagnosis and treatment of these secondary changes during the acute phase of the injury will help to minimize neurological dysfunction and prevent further brain damage.

## MEDICAL AND SURGICAL MANAGEMENT

The priority in the management of the TBI adult is to minimize the primary impact damage and prevent or treat secondary insults.[27] The patient with a severe brain injury may experience many complications.[7,25] Suctioning, intubation, or tracheostomy may be needed for an impaired airway. The medical team will be concerned with shock, spinal and soft tissue injuries, and preventing further damage to the brain. The neurosurgeon may perform an emergency craniotomy to prevent bleeding or decrease rising intracranial pressure.[27]

Nutritional needs are usually treated initially with intravenous maintenance. For patients with impaired oral bulbar status a nasogastric tube is inserted through the nose or a gastrostomy tube is surgically placed in the stomach. The patient can receive nutrients through these tubes until able to consume sufficient calories orally.

An incontinent patient may require catheterization. Later in the rehabilitation phase, when functions start to return, a bowel and bladder program is initiated. After the initial evaluation and treatment (management in the emergency room and operating room), the patient is usually transferred to the intensive care unit (ICU). In the ICU the patient is monitored for secondary complications. The clinical neurological status is frequently reassessed.[33] The patient is transferred to the acute care service or to a rehabilitation unit when medically stabilized and having no symptoms of serious infection.

### Occupational Therapy in the ICU

Occupational therapy treatment in the ICU should be performed by an OTR because vigilant and constant evaluations are necessary. Occupational therapy goals in the ICU include increasing functional endurance, establishing a bed and wheelchair positioning program, preventing contractures, and establishing a baseline cognitive status.

Usually a patient with an open brain injury or craniectomy defect greater than 5 cm by 5 cm requires a helmet when out of bed to protect the open skull from further brain injury.[10]

If seizures occur the facility protocol is followed. The objective is to protect the patient from self-inflicted harm.

## SEVERITY OF INJURY

Management of TBI varies greatly depending on severity. No absolute measure of severity of brain injury exists; but duration and depth of coma and length of **posttraumatic amnesia** (PTA) (the amount of time it takes for continuous memory to return after an injury) are the most accepted criteria.[11,17] The most dramatic recovery usually occurs during the first 6 months, but neurological recovery can continue for years.

#### Posttraumatic Amnesia

After the patient has emerged from coma, the best guide to the severity of the diffuse damage is the duration of PTA. Longer PTAs are associated with worse cognitive and motor ability.[18]

#### Functional Assessment

A number of assessment scales are used and produce data for clinical research, clinical evaluation, program evaluation, and prediction of outcome.[14] The Glasgow Outcome Scale,[15] the Disability Rating Scale,[14,32] the Functional Independence Measure,[13] the Community Integration Questionnaire,[36] and the Rancho Los Amigos Scale of Cognitive Functioning[31] (Box 37-1) are standardized assessment scales used in evaluating persons with TBI. The OTR may participate in using an assessment scale; the COTA should be familiar with the scale used at the facility.

Persons recovering from a TBI evolve along a continuum from comatose (at one end of the spectrum) to fully functional in all situations. The Rancho Los Amigos Scale of Cognitive Functioning[31] divides recovery into eight stages. Being familiar with these stages will prove invaluable in recognizing the normal course of recovery.

#### Clinical Picture of Persons With Traumatic Brain Injury

The patient with a TBI may present in many different ways depending on the type, severity, and location of the injury. The patient may have severe limitations in most of the areas listed below or the patient may have very subtle deficits, evident only in high level, complex activities.

##### *Physical Status*

The physical deficits encountered in patients with TBI can vary from severe motor involvement (in one to four extremities) to full isolated control with minimally impaired coordination and muscle strength. Most patients who require occupational therapy will exhibit deficits in one or more of the following areas: primitive reflexes, muscle tone, motor control, strength, posture, range of motion (ROM), sensation, endurance, and total body function.

##### *Abnormal Reflexes*

Typical reflexes seen in the low level TBI adult include the asymmetrical tonic neck reflex and the symmetrical tonic neck reflex. Treatment is focused not only on inhibiting these brain stem reflexes but replacing them with new motor programs to facilitate improvement in function.[5]

##### *Abnormal Muscle Tone*

In the TBI adult, muscle tone varies from hypotonus (flaccidity) to hypertonus (spasticity). When muscles are flaccid, the resistance to passive movement is diminished and the stretch reflexes are dampened. When an entire upper extremity is hypotonic, such as in the days directly after the injury, the arm appears "floppy."

##### *Spasticity*

Spasticity may range from minimal to severe in any particular muscle or muscle group. The patient in coma may develop **decorticate posturing** (sustained contraction and posturing of both upper extremities [BUE] in flexion and the trunk and both lower extremities [BLE] in extension) or **decerebrate posturing** (sustained contraction and posturing of the trunk and extremities in extension) in the first days or weeks after injury. These postures generally diminish over time as the patient makes a neurological recovery.

Spasticity will fluctuate with changes in the patient's position, volitional movement, medication, any infections or illness, an increase in pain or discomfort, or a change in emotions. Long-term consequences of spasticity include compromised function in activities of daily living (ADL), difficulty with transfers, difficulty in positioning the patient in bed or in the wheelchair, gait deviations, poor speech and breath control, painful spasms, and contracture formation.[26]

##### *Muscle Weakness*

Muscle weakness is a decrease in muscle strength without the presence of spasticity. When muscle weakness is present in BUE, impaired coordination (both gross and fine motor control) will be evident.

##### *Ataxia*

Ataxia is an abnormality of movement and disordered muscle tone seen in patients with damage to the cerebellum or to the sensory pathways. The patient with ataxia has lost the ability to make small, minute adjustments that allow for smooth coordination of movement. Ataxia can be a significant impediment to achieving a functional goal.

##### *Impaired Motor Control*

Impairments in motor control in BUE as well as BLE may result from an imbalance in muscle tone and muscle weakness. Usually one side of the body is more involved. Motor control allows for smooth purposeful movements of body parts during functional tasks.

##### *Postural Deficits*

**Postural deficits** develop as a result of an imbalance in muscle tone throughout the body, impaired motor control, delayed or absent righting reactions, and impaired vision, cognition, and perception. Abnormal postures frequently exhibited in adults with moderate to severe TBI include the following:

Box 37-1

## Levels of Cognitive Functioning

**I No Response** Patient appears to be in a deep sleep and is completely unresponsive to any stimuli presented.

**II Generalized Response** Patient reacts inconsistently and nonpurposefully to stimuli in a nonspecific manner. Responses are limited in nature and are often the same regardless of stimulus presented. Responses may be physiological changes, gross body movements, and/or vocalization. Often the earliest response is to deep pain. Responses are likely to be delayed.

**III Localized Response** Patient reacts specifically but inconsistently to stimuli. Responses are directly related to the type of stimulus presented as in turning head toward a sound or focusing on an object presented. Patient may withdraw an extremity and/or vocalize when presented with a painful stimulus. Patient may follow simple commands in an inconsistent, delayed manner, such as closing eyes or squeezing or extending an extremity. After external stimulus is removed, patient may lie quietly and may also show a vague awareness of self and body by responding to discomfort by pulling at nasogastric tube or catheter or resisting restraints. Patient may show bias by responding to some persons (especially family, friends) but not to others.

**IV Confused-Agitated** Patient is in a heightened state of activity with severely decreased ability to process information. Patient is detached from the present and responds primarily to his own internal confusion. Behavior is frequently bizarre and nonpurposeful relative to immediate environment. Patient may cry out or scream out of proportion to stimuli even after removal, show aggressive behavior, attempt to remove restraints or tubes, or crawl out of bed in a purposeful manner. Patient does not, however, discriminate among persons or objects and is unable to cooperate directly with treatment effort. Verbalization is frequently incoherent and/or inappropriate to the environment. Confabulation may be present; patient may be euphoric or hostile. Thus gross attention is very short and selective attention is often nonexistent. Being unaware of present events, patient lacks short-term recall and may be reacting to past events. Patient is unable to perform self-care (feeding, dressing) without maximum assistance. If not disabled physically, patient may perform motor activities as in sitting, reaching, and ambulating as part of agitated state and not as a purposeful act or on request necessarily.

**V Confused, Inappropriate, Nonagitated** Patient appears alert and is able to respond to simple commands fairly consistently. However, with increased complexity of commands or lack of any external structure, responses are nonpurposeful, random, or at best fragmented toward any desired goal. Patient may show agitated behavior, not on an internal basis (as in Level IV), but rather as a result of external stimuli, and usually out of proportion to the stimulus. Patient has gross attention to the environment but is highly distractible and lacks ability to focus attention to a specific task without frequent redirection back to it. With structure, patient may be able to converse on a social, automatic level for short periods of time. Verbalization is often inappropriate; confabulation may be triggered by present events. Patient's memory is severely impaired, with confusion of past and present in reaction to ongoing activity. Patient lacks initiation of functional tasks and often shows inappropriate use of objects without external direction. Patient may be able to perform previously learned tasks when structured, but is unable to learn new information. Patient responds best to self, body, comfort—and often family members. Patient can usually perform self-care activities with assistance and may accomplish feeding with maximum supervision. Management on the ward is often a problem if the patient is physically mobile; patient may wander off either randomly or with vague intention of "going home."

**VI Confused-Appropriate** Patient shows goal-directed behavior but is dependent on external input for direction. Response to discomfort is appropriate and patient is able to tolerate unpleasant stimuli (as NG tube) when need is explained. Patient follows simple directions consistently and shows carry-over for such relearned tasks (such as self-care). Patient is at least supervised with old learning; unable to maximally assist for new learning with little or no carry-over. Responses may be incorrect due to memory problems, but they are appropriate to the situation. They may be delayed, and patient shows decreased ability to process information with little or no anticipation or prediction of events. Past memories show more depth and detail than recent memory. The patient may show beginning awareness of situation by realizing an answer isn't known. Patient no longer wanders and is inconsistently oriented to time and place. Selective attention to tasks may be impaired especially with difficult tasks and in unstructured settings but is now functional for common daily activities (30 minutes with structure). Patient shows at least vague recognition of some staff and has increased awareness of self, family, and basic needs (such as food), again in an appropriate manner as in contrast to Level V.

From Rancho Los Amigos Medical Center: *Original scale: levels of cognitive functioning,* Downey, Calif, 1980, Ranchos Los Amigos Medical Center, Adult Brain Injury Service.

Continued.

Box 37-1

## Levels of Cognitive Functioning—cont'd

**VII Automatic-Appropriate** Patient appears appropriate and oriented within hospital and home settings and goes through daily routine automatically but is frequently robotlike; minimal to absent confusion but has shallow recall of what has been done. Patient shows increased awareness of self, body, family, foods, people, and interaction in the environment. Patient has superficial awareness of but lacks insight into his condition, demonstrates decreased judgment and problem-solving, and lacks realistic planning for his future. Patient shows carry-over for new learning but at a decreased rate. Patient requires at least minimal supervision for learning and for safety purposes. Patient is independent in self-care activities and supervised in home and community skills for safety. With structure, patient is able to initiate tasks in social and recreational activities in which he now has interest. Judgment remains impaired, such that patient is unable to drive a car. Prevocational or avocational evaluation and counseling may be indicated.

**VIII Purposeful and Appropriate** Patient is alert and oriented, is able to recall and integrate past and recent events, and is aware of and responsive to his culture. Patient shows carryover for new learning if acceptable to and life role and needs no supervision after activities are learned. Within physical capabilities, patient is independent in home and community, activities including driving. Vocational rehabilitation, to determine ability to return as a contributor to society (perhaps in a new capacity), is indicated. Patient may continue to show a decreased ability, relative to premorbid abilities, reasoning, tolerance for stress, judgment in emergencies, or unusual circumstances. Patient's social, emotional, and intellectual capacities may continue to be at a decreased level but are functional for society.

- Head/neck: Forward flexion or hyperextension
- Scapula: Humeral depression with protraction, retraction, or downward rotation
- Upper extremities: Possible bilateral or unilateral involvement; typically have elbow flexion, humeral adduction and internal rotation, forearm pronation, and flexion of wrist and fingers
- Trunk: Kyphosis, scoliosis, loss of lordosis
- Pelvis: Posterior pelvic tilt and pelvic obliquity
- Lower extremities: Hip adduction, knee flexion, plantar flexion, and inversion; if in a persistent vegetative state, may have severe extensor spasms

### *Limitations of Joint Motion*

Loss of ROM is a common problem. Treatment for loss of ROM varies depending on the cause. Therefore it is essential that the OTR determine the cause of the loss of ROM before the COTA begins treatment.

### *Loss of Sensation*

TBI adults may present with loss of any of the following: light touch sensation, sharp or dull discrimination, proprioception, kinesthesia, or stereognosis in the extremities. Cranial nerve involvement may cause loss of pain and light touch sensation in the face and impaired senses of taste and smell.

### *Decreased Functional Endurance*

Decreased endurance and vital capacity are common in TBI persons. Medical complications such as pneumonia or infections and deconditioning from prolonged bed rest diminish the patient's ability to participate in therapy programs.

### *Loss of Total Body Function*

Total body function skills are head and trunk control, sitting and standing balance, reaching, bending, stooping, and functional ambulation. Total body function skills are necessary for performing both basic and advanced level ADL.

## Dysphagia

TBI patients may demonstrate dysphagia in any of the four stages of swallowing: oral preparatory, oral, pharyngeal, and esophageal. Typically, more than one abnormality in swallowing is observed.[21] In addition, the cognitive, behavioral, and linguistic problems evident in the TBI patient further complicate the ability to manage the intake of food and liquids.[23]

## Cognitive Status

Cognitive deficits, to varying degrees, are common in the TBI population and include decreased levels of attention, impaired memory, impaired initiation, diminished safety awareness, decreased ability to accurately process information, and difficulty with executive functions and abstract thinking.

### *Reduced Attention and Concentration*

The patient with a brain injury often loses not only the ability to concentrate for any length of time but also the ability to filter out distraction.

### *Impaired Memory*

There are several types of memory impairments, ranging from the inability to recall a few words just heard (immediate memory), to forgetting what happened in the last treatment session (short-term memory), to forgetting events that occurred 24 hours ago or years before the injury (long-term memory). Memory loss is manifested in the inability to learn and carry over new tasks and contributes to confusion.

#### *Impaired Initiation*

**Impaired initiation,** or difficulty in beginning the first actions, steps, or stages of a task, can significantly impact the ability to live independently.

#### *Decreased Safety Awareness*

Unsafe behaviors found in some persons with TBI may be a result of impulsiveness, decreased insight into the disability, impaired judgment, or a combination of all of these. Decreased insight, disorientation, and impaired memory can contribute to the patient's inability to recognize limitations for specific situations or analyze consequences of actions.

#### *Delayed Processing of Information*

Difficulty with processing visual and auditory information within a normal time frame is referred to as *delayed processing.* The delay may be a few seconds or minutes. The clinician must allow the patient sufficient time to respond during treatment.

#### *Impaired Executive Functions and Abstract Thinking*

Executive functions are needed to set goals and to plan and effectively complete tasks. This requires high-level problem solving, reasoning, and judgment. Patients with brain injuries tend to analyze problems in concrete terms, interpreting all information at the most literal level. Functional independence, including appropriate social skills, and successful return to work demands the mastering and manipulation of these executive functions.[22]

### Behavioral Status

Behavioral impairments are a natural part of the recovery from a TBI. Nonetheless, behavioral problems are disturbing for both the treatment team and the families. Behavioral management is a necessary component of TBI rehabilitation.

Working with someone with behavioral problems can be frustrating and at times frightening. Untrained staff frequently reinforce the patient's behavior through their own behavior.

Common behaviors observed in the TBI population include agitation, combativeness, disinhibition, and refusal to cooperate. The patient who is unable to filter distractions becomes agitated in a noisy environment, and a patient who is agitated may become combative and kick, bite, grab, or spit. The correct environment and an appropriate approach may reduce this problem. This type of behavior may occur in isolation; however, some patients go through a period of combativeness where they act this way for weeks or months during any interactions with others. When this occurs, a strict behavior management program must be immediately established and enforced by all team members.

A disinhibited patient may lack awareness of the external environment and consequently may remove clothes in the treatment gym or flirt with the doctor. Other examples of socially inappropriate and disinhibited behavior are shouting obscenities or making indiscriminate sexual advances to a stranger in the community. Patients who refuse to cooperate with the treatment team may do so because of a behavioral deficit.

The cognitive and behavioral aspects of a TBI are complex and interrelated. Behavior exhibited by the patient with a TBI correlates significantly with the level of cognitive function.

### Visual Status

TBI may significantly impact a previously intact visual system. Visual problems found after a traumatic brain injury include a "lazy eye" with double vision, blurring of vision, inability to smoothly adjust from near to far vision, jerky eye movements, poor tracking (inability to follow objects), field defects (ability to see only part of an image), reduced blink rate, and incomplete eyelid closure.[9] Visual impairments will impair ADL performance.

### Perceptual Motor Skills

The ability to accurately take in information and respond to people and objects within the environment is necessary for successful, independent function.[3] The TBI patient may have difficulty with perceptual-motor skills that previously were taken for granted. Depending on the nature and extent of damage, the impairment may involve visual, perceptual, or perceptual-motor skills. TBI patients may experience impairments in the following areas: praxis (action), body scheme (recognizing body parts), figure ground, position in space, size and shape discrimination, spatial attention (ability to notice items on one side, usually the left), part/whole integration (being able to recognize the whole object from some of its parts), or visual organization. If a person cannot differentiate between underpants and a shirt, recognize arms, or locate a sock on a patterned bedspread, dressing is indeed a challenge.

### Psychosocial Factors

Family and friends are an integral part of the rehabilitation process, especially in the beginning stages, because they may be able to elicit a response from the patient when no one else can.

Family role changes and the patient's coping mechanisms for dealing with these changes must be considered. The patient may go from being extremely independent to being totally dependent. It is often difficult for family members to understand the uncontrolled behavior that they observe in their loved one. No matter how cognizant the family and the patient are of the disability, it disrupts the family structure.

Previous education and values affect the patient's progress toward independence.

### Functional Status

Self-care deficits found in persons with TBI include difficulty with feeding, dressing, hygiene, grooming, bathing, and/or toileting. Impairments of mobility may be evident in moving in bed, a wheelchair, transferring, or walking. Housekeeping, cooking, and childcare abilities may be disturbed. Speech and symbolic language may be impaired. The patient may be unable to use public transportation, drive, shop, or work.

## OCCUPATIONAL THERAPY EVALUATION

Evaluations of a TBI adult will be performed by the OTR. A review of the therapist's findings and treatment plan are essential prerequisites to treatment. The therapist's findings establish a baseline for treatment. By being familiar with the findings the COTA will be introduced to the patient's unique clinical picture.

## GENERAL AIMS AND METHODS OF TREATMENT FOR THE BEGINNING-LEVEL PATIENT

The aims of treatment for the beginning level patient (levels I to III [see Box 37-1])[31] are to increase the patient's level of response and overall awareness. Input must be well structured and broken down into simple steps. Enough time must be allowed for a response, which often is delayed during this phase of treatment.

Treatment at this stage can be broken down into six areas: sensory regulation, wheelchair positioning, bed positioning, casting and splinting, dysphagia management, and family and caregiver training. The treatments occur simultaneously to optimize the patient's progress.

### Sensory Regulation Program

Should the patient present with no response to pain, touch, sound, or sight or exhibit only a generalized response to pain, the goal of treatment is to increase the patient's level of awareness by trying to arouse the patient with controlled sensory input.

**Sensory regulation treatment** incorporates visual, auditory, tactile and other stimuli into specific tasks such as rolling in bed. The patient is actively engaged in the activity as opposed to having the stimulus presented to the passive patient. The program is multisensory and meaningful, and the treatments are usually brief (initially about 10 minutes), incorporating both sides of the body. The modalities used are common, everyday tasks such as hygiene, bed mobility, and turning on the radio. The clinician continually observes the patient during the activity and documents any changes in behavior such as head turning in response to sounds, visual attention and tracking, vocalizations, and following commands.

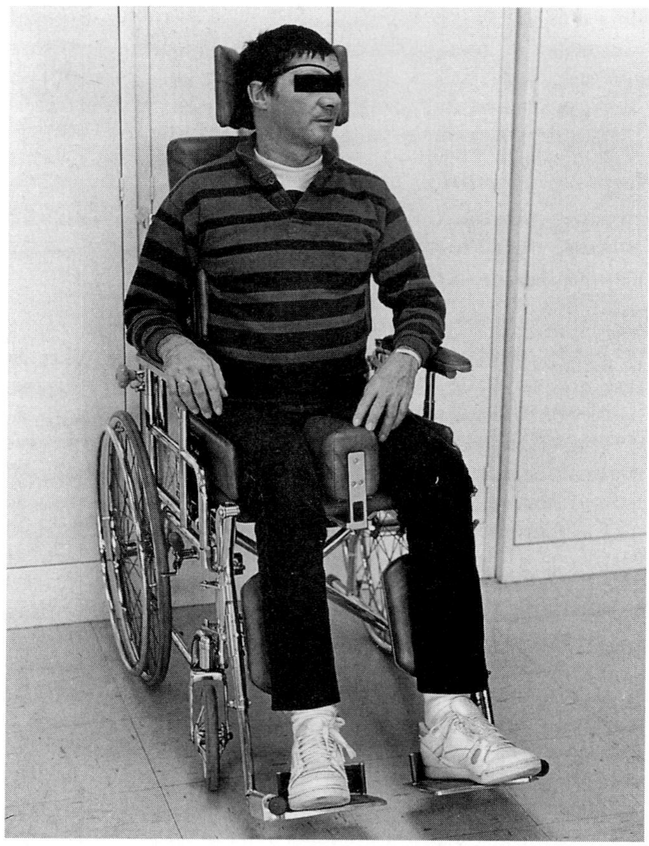

*Figure 37-1* Improved posture and trunk alignment is achieved with positioning devices.

### Wheelchair Positioning Program

Seating and positioning is often a challenging task. Proper positioning assists in the prevention of skin breakdown and joint contractures, facilitates normal tone, optimizes cognition, improves behavior, and promotes safety. Effective seating and positioning requires a stable base of support at the pelvis, maintaining the trunk in midline, and placing the head in an upright posture for functional upper extremity use (Figure 37-1). Positioning should alleviate postural deficits and place the patient in good postural alignment. Although the OTR may establish the initial seating and positioning program, daily follow-through is often deferred to the COTA. Familiarity with the principles of seating and positioning will help quickly identify and correct positioning problems.

#### *Pelvis*

Wheelchair positioning should begin with **pelvis alignment** because poor hip placement alters head and trunk alignment and influences tone in the extremities. A solid seat insert can be placed underneath the patient

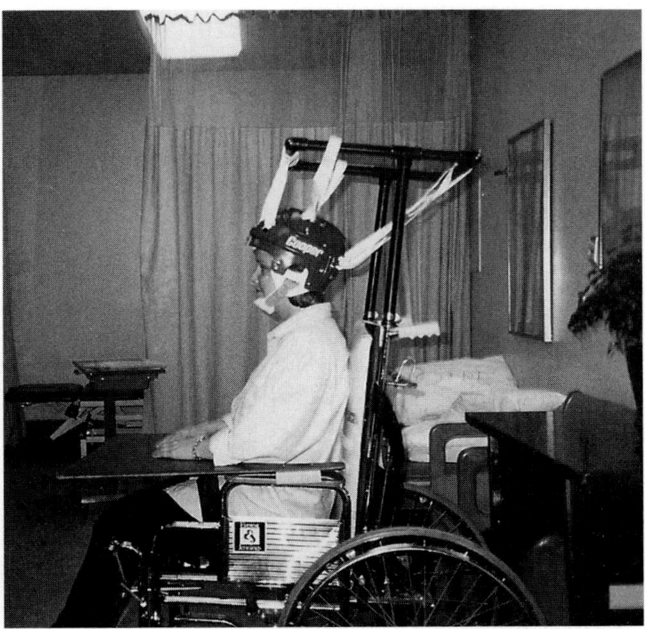

*Figure 37-2* Dynamic head control device.

to facilitate a neutral to slight anterior tilt of the pelvis. A lumbar support may maintain a natural curve in the spine. A seat insert that is slightly wedged (with the downward slope pointing toward the back of the wheelchair) can be used to flex the hips to help inhibit extensor tone in the hip and lower extremities. A seat belt angled across the pelvis will help to maintain the desired position.

#### *Trunk*

Positioning the trunk occurs after the pelvis is properly positioned. A solid back insert or solid contoured back is placed behind the patient's back to facilitate a more erect posture of the spine. Lateral trunk supports can be used to eliminate scoliosis; a chest strap or crossed chest straps will decrease kyphosis, retract the shoulders, and expand the upper chest. The pelvic position should be reevaluated if the clinician is having difficulty maintaining the patient's trunk in midline.

#### *Lower Extremities*

Thigh pads placed along the lateral aspect of the thigh may be used to decrease lower extremity (LE) abduction, or an abductor wedge may be placed between the LEs just proximal to the knees to eliminate LE adduction. A foot wedge is placed on top of the foot plate if plantar flexion contractures are present in one or both feet.

#### *Upper Extremities*

A lap tray is generally used to support the upper extremities (UEs). This maintains the UEs on the same height surface and does not disturb trunk alignment. The UEs should be positioned with the shoulders in slight flexion and external rotation, the elbows in slight flexion, the wrists and fingers in a functional position.

#### *Head*

Attaining a neutral, midline head position can be difficult when the patient has little to no active head control. Most head control devices are static positioning devices. The head is kept from falling forward by a forehead strap. Caution must always be taken to avoid overstressing the cervical area or giving excessive resistance to a spastic neck. It is often difficult to avoid this with static devices. Reclining the patient back will eliminate this problem but weight bearing through the trunk and pelvis and visual interaction with the environment will be reduced.

An alternative to static head positioning is dynamic head positioning. The advantages of such a device are that it places the head in good alignment on the trunk and distributes pressure equally. In addition, it allows the patient to begin initiating head movements actively (Figure 37-2).

Wheelchair positioning involves constantly reevaluating and adapting the equipment to meet the changing needs of the patient. It should be done by the COTA only under the close supervision of a registered therapist.

### Bed Positioning

Bed positioning is critical. The TBI patient generally has bilateral involvement, requiring a program for sidelying on both sides. A schedule for prone lying may also be used during the day to maintain ROM in hip and knee extension.

### Splinting and Casting

Splinting and casting may be used when tone interferes with functional movement and ADL independence, when passive range of motion (PROM) is limited, and when there is potential for contractures. If PROM and wheelchair and bed positioning are sufficient to maintain ROM in the UEs, splinting and casting are not indicated.

The goals of splinting and casting are to reduce abnormal tone or soft tissue tightness, increase or maintain PROM, increase the functional potential of the UE, prevent skin breakdown (e.g., in the palmar surface of the hand), and simplify management of care (e.g., bathing, dressing, and performing bowel and bladder care) for the beginning level patient.

The most commonly used splint for the beginning level patient is the stretch splint. This splint places the wrist and fingers in extension and abducts the thumb (Figure 37-3). The stretch splint is a resting splint and should not be worn during functional activities. A typical splint schedule begins with 2 hours on and 2 hours off. The goal is generally to increase the wearing time to about 8 continuous hours. This varies from patient to patient.

A casting program is implemented when other methods for managing spasticity are no longer effec-

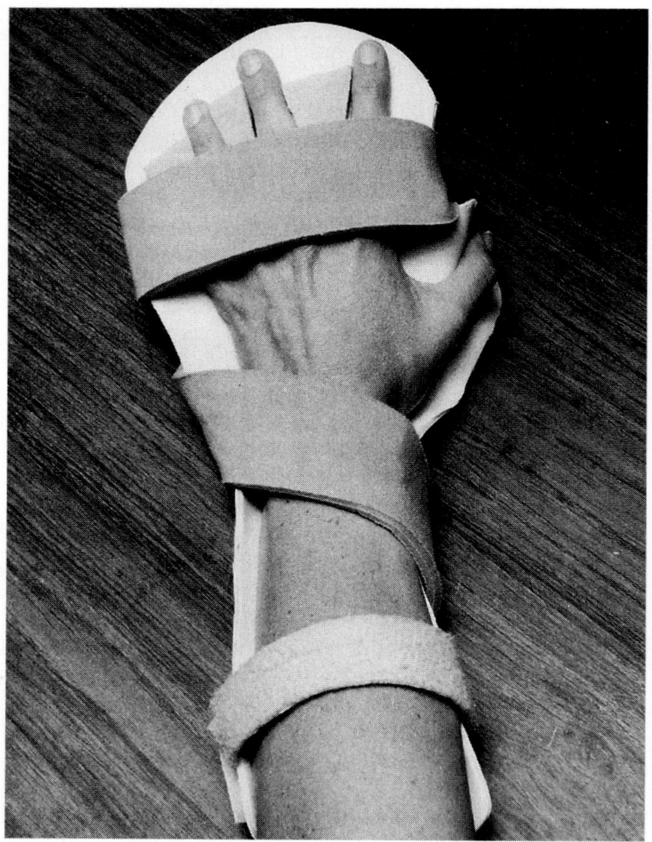

*Figure 37-3* Stretch splint.

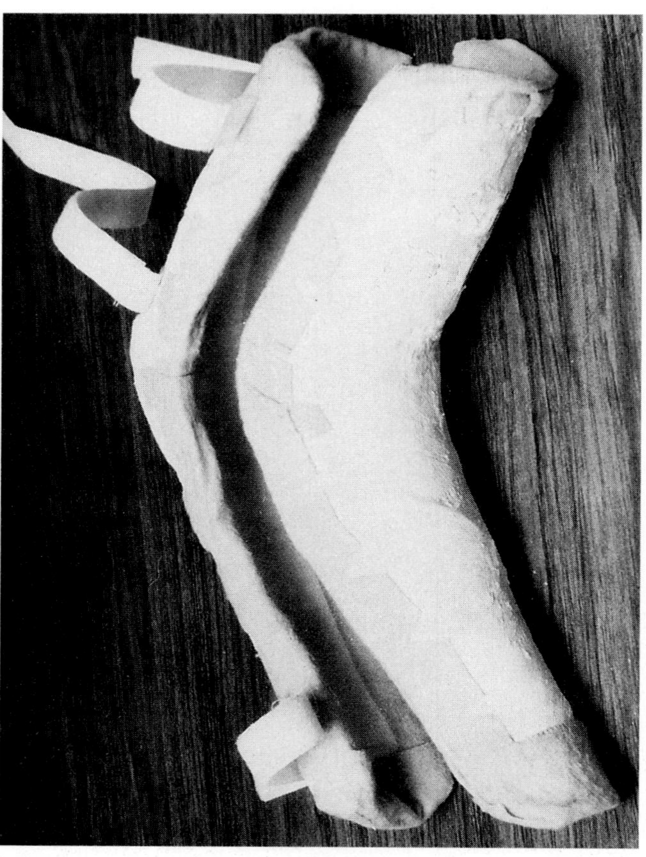

*Figure 37-4* Bivalved cast.

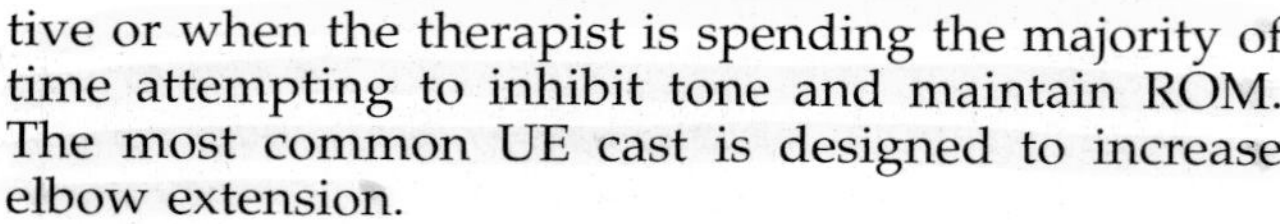

tive or when the therapist is spending the majority of time attempting to inhibit tone and maintain ROM. The most common UE cast is designed to increase elbow extension.

Casts can be fabricated out of fiberglass or plaster. Fiberglass is preferred because it is lighter in weight, sets (hardens) more quickly, and is easier to apply than plaster. As with splinting, training and practice in casting are required to attain proficiency.

Serial casting (as its name suggests) uses a series of casts that gradually stretch out the contracture, each new cast being slightly closer to the desired end position. Serial casting usually requires at least two clinicians, one to position and hold the extremity and one to apply the cast. Serial casts are generally left on the patient for several days and then removed. The patient's skin is examined for blistering and reddened marks. If skin integrity is good, a new cast (closer to the desired ROM) is applied.

Once the desired ROM has been attained, the last cast is removed and the edges of both halves of the cast are finished (Figure 37-4). The bivalved cast is then worn by the patient to maintain the ROM. COTAs are often called on to do the finishing work in bivalve casting.

### Dysphagia

The patient emerging from coma may have swallowing difficulty and require a feeding evaluation and intervention (see Chapter 19) for specifics.

### Caregiver Training

Education of the caregivers (which may or may not include family members) starts the first time the professional meets them. The clinician should provide information according to each person's ability to handle and process it. Caregivers play an essential part in eliciting the patient's responses and often play a large role in the programs for sensory regulation, bed positioning and ROM. Caregiver training is generally graded so that they learn to assist with complex patient handling, like transferring, after basic skills are mastered.

## TREATMENT OF THE INTERMEDIATE- AND ADVANCED-LEVEL PATIENTS

### Neuromuscular Impairments

The types of motor impairment present in the TBI patient are numerous. Weakness, spasticity, rigidity, soft tissue contractures, primitive reflexes, loss of postural reactions and impaired sensation affect the patient's ability to perform activities independently and with normal motor control.

The prerequisites for normal movement include normal postural tone, normal integration of flexor and extensor control (reciprocal innervation), normal proximal stability, and selective movement patterns.[16] Although the program for each patient with TBI is individualized, the common principles of treatment are (1) to progress proximal to distal, (2) to establish symmetrical posture, (3) to integrate both sides into activities, (4) to encourage bilateral weight bearing, and (5) to introduce a normal sensory experience. A variety of treatment approaches, including neurodevelopmental treatment (NDT), proprioceptive neuromuscular facilitation (PNF), myofascial release, Rood techniques, and physical agent modalities can be effective for this patient population. In fact, successful treatment will use more than one technique. Such techniques require specialized training including hands-on practice. Once competency has been attained in a technique, the COTA may use it during patient care under the guidance of an OTR.

The trunk is the foundation for limb movements. Treatment of the trunk should focus on achieving alignment and stimulating activity in the trunk muscles. Alignment will facilitate stability. Once trunk control improves, treatment should progress to the upper extremities.

Many patients with TBI present with fairly intact motor control. These patients ambulate independently and incorporate both upper extremities into functional activities. Closer observation, however, reveals subtle trunk and UE deficits related to coordination and speed of movement. The treatment program is aimed at improving dynamic standing balance for all activities. UE treatment programs are designed to increase scapular stability and improve fine motor control. Activities should focus on improving the patient's speed while maintaining good coordination.

Ataxia is a common and frustrating problem that often develops early, persists into the late rehabilitation phase, and may remain permanently. Various treatment methods have been tried. Weighting body parts and using resistive activities appear to improve control during performance of tasks but show inconsistent carryover of control when the weights are removed. Weighted eating utensils and cups may compensate for ataxia in the UEs. Weighted devices are limited in their effectiveness.

All treatment should be activity based. Any adjunctive techniques such as NDT mobilizations must be followed by an activity that is meaningful and requires the same movement.

### Cognitive Retraining

Cognitive retraining is generally accomplished through functional activities. Simulations may distress the patient; the confused patient may become agitated when given sequence cards to put in order. The same sequencing deficit may be addressed by having the patient assemble a foot stool. The TBI patient may automatically understand the task and may participate for a longer period of time because it is familiar and makes sense.

Planning, organizational, and money management strategies can be practiced in an activity such as planning a vacation. Another patient can work on attention span, frustration tolerance, delays in processing information by playing with a child for an hour. Sequencing, organization, and problem solving can be addressed within the task of changing a washer in a dripping faucet. The activity chosen for each patient should be age appropriate, challenging, and of interest to the person.

Computer use has become popular in cognitive-perceptual training programs. The computer uses visual and auditory stimulation and feedback. It does not provide adequate tactile and proprioceptive stimulation, which are vital for training. Computers may have a place in cognitive-perceptual training but should be used in conjunction with other approaches.

### Behavior Strategies

Intervention strategies used to decrease and eliminate problem behaviors can be divided into two categories: environmental and interactive.

Environmental interventions use alterations in the environment to facilitate appropriate behaviors, inhibit unwanted behaviors, and maintain the safety of the patient. The first step in altering the environment is often to place the patient in a quiet, isolated room without a roommate. The television and radio are turned off, and the door is closed. Extraneous information on the walls and excess furniture are removed from the room.

Further steps may be needed such as one to one nursing care and a cubicle bed. A cubicle bed may be used in place of a standard hospital bed when patients are extremely agitated and at risk for falling or crawling out of bed. A cubicle bed is comprised of a mattress that sits on the floor and four padded walls. The patient must be able to be transferred from the floor to and from a wheelchair with assistance. Alarm systems and walkie-talkies may also assist in maintaining patient and staff safety.

Interactive interventions are the approaches that the staff and caregivers use when working with the patient. These include speaking in a calm, soothing, and concise manner to an agitated patient. Detailed explanations only increase the patient's confusion. When the patient has difficulty initiating tasks, the practitioner should physically assist the patient through the beginning of the activity or verbally cue the patient to begin the activity.[34]

Another behavior management technique is diversion. Should patients become agitated during an activity or interaction and be unable to redirect themselves, the clinician creates a diversion. Diversions include changing the subject, introducing a caregiver, or creating a harmless physical distraction. A "new" face can often elicit cooperation from a resistive patient.

### Vision

Vision deficits are variable in the TBI population. Vision testing by an optometrist or ophthomologist and corrective lenses are a first step.

Vision exercises may also be indicated. A series of activities is designed to increase the patients' awareness of visual deficits, increase function while maximizing residual vision, and develop compensatory skills. Treatment programs may be designed by the OTR. A COTA who has attained service competency in this area may provide treatment.

Compensatory strategies for visual field deficits include outlining work before beginning a task and using a colored border along one side of a page of a book to facilitate efficient reading. Using large objects during treatment, increasing task lighting and using contrasting colors (e.g., marking the stove dials with red nail polish) are other adaptations.

### Perceptual Training

There are two classifications of perceptual training: adaptive and remedial. The adaptive approach is based on the theory that recovery results from the use of intact brain areas to perform functional activities in modified ways.[28] Training of perceptual deficits occurs through repetitive practice of one or more ADL. For example, the patient is taught to compensate for a perceptual deficit by practicing dressing on a daily basis. This functional approach includes making the patient aware of the problem, teaching the patient to work with the deficit and adapting the environment to compensate for deficits.

The remedial approach assumes that the adult brain is sufficiently plastic to repair and reorganize itself after injury.[29] Sensory integration,[3] NDT,[8] and transfer of training techniques are all examples of this approach.

Current research in motor learning and the neurobiology of learning suggests that both remedial and adaptive approaches are beneficial to the adult with a brain injury. Functional training (adaptive approach) is appropriate for patients who respond to their environment and situations at a very concrete level and are unable to transfer cognitive-perceptual learning to different situations.[29] A remedial approach works best with patients who function at a more abstract level. These patients will be able to carry over a new technique learned (e.g., one-handed dressing) to a new situation.

### Self-Care

ADL retraining improves the patient's functional independence and allows work on the patient's deficits within meaningful, routine, and familiar tasks. Hygiene or dressing activities must often be broken down into smaller segments to facilitate functional improvements because of the patient's cognitive, behavioral, and perceptual status. Backward chaining (having the patient complete the end of the task) and sequence cards are ways to grade the activity to a particular patient's abilities. A self-care program is usually fairly structured, with the patient following the same daily routine in the same environment. As the patient reaches a supervised level, more emphasis is placed on ability to complete the tasks when the routine is disrupted or altered in some way.

The clinician must beware of techniques that increase functional independence but reinforce abnormal motor patterns. The COTA should clarify with the OTR whether the goal is to facilitate normal movement during ADL or to allow for independence in ADL with poor technique. In general, NDT principles such as normalizing tone and using both sides of the body are incorporated into self-care activities. The emphasis in treatment is to improve the quality of the patient's movements while maximizing independent performance. Compromising normal movements to obtain independence in a task is not usually advisable.

However, in certain situations normal movement must be compromised for patient safety. For example, a patient who still requires hands-on assist for normalizing muscle tone during transfers but is returning to independent living within a few days may need to use a different technique. The independent and safe technique may cause an increase in abnormal tone.

### Eating

Patients with TBI also exhibit frequent problems in feeding themselves. An eating or dining program often begins in isolated areas such as the patient's bedroom or a quiet kitchen. Eating is graded to more social situations such as in the dining room with other patients or in the kitchen at home with the family. A rocker knife, plate guard, or commuter mug may be introduced if a patient has difficulty with strength, coordination, or perceptual deficits. Introducing one item at a time may help with decreased attention and left-side neglect. When a patient is impulsive, the COTA or OTR may teach the strategy of placing the fork down after each bite to ensure that the patient chews and swallows completely before initiating the next bite.

### Functional Mobility

Mobility training can be subdivided into bed mobility, transfer training, wheelchair mobility, and functional ambulation. The NDT principles of bilateral involvement, equal weight bearing, and tone normalization are used with these activities.

#### *Bed Mobility, Wheelchair Management, and Functional Ambulation*

The bed mobility skills typically taught to the patient with brain injury are scooting up and down in bed, rolling, bridging, moving from supine to a sitting position and back, and moving from sitting to standing and back. Wheelchair management includes the ability to manage wheelchair parts (e.g., removing a foot plate) and propel the wheelchair both indoors and outdoors on different surfaces. The techniques used for bed mobility and wheelchair management are similar to those used with the cardiovascular accident population but are adapted as needed for patients with bilateral involvement.

Functional ambulation refers to the patient's ability to walk during functional activities. Although physical therapists teach ambulation skills, the occupational therapy clinician facilitates carry over of ambulation into daily living tasks such as getting dressed, preparing a meal, and mopping a floor. During activity, the patient may be doing more than just walking (i.e., carrying a plate, holding a purse, sweeping with a broom, or carrying a baby).

#### *Transfers*

Cognitive, perceptual, and physical status affects the type of transfer used in training. Memory and limited carry over of information require the technique and sequence to be consistent among all staff members treating the patient. It is preferable that transfers be practiced moving to both sides if possible. Often a patient becomes proficient in a transfer with an approach to one side only and is dismayed in a public rest room to discover that this particular approach is not possible.

All family members and caregivers should be trained and cleared by the treating clinician before transferring a patient alone. The timing of this training depends on the patient's functional level, and the family and caregivers' abilities. Training alleviates many of the fears and decreases the chance of failure during the first week at home.

### Group Treatment

Most TBI programs use group treatment as a supplement to individual treatment, because it provides learning experiences not available in individual therapy. Group treatment provides structured socialization in which patients can develop more appropriate psychosocial skills. Psychosocial deficits are a major barrier to successful reintegration of the TBI individual into family and community.

Groups allow persons with brain injuries to get feedback from their peers. Often patients make changes in their behavior in response to peer feedback.[19,24,30] Groups tend to be functionally based. Goals include improving ability to monitor conversations and behavior, improving executive functioning, improving functional money management skills, increasing the frequency of age-appropriate behavior, improving posture and gait patterns, improving functional memory, and increasing socialization.[12] Groups may be facilitated by one discipline but are frequently multidisciplinary. A cooking group might be led by both an occupational therapy staff member and a speech therapy staff member. Cooking is the medium in which individual patients might address their own goals, such as reading and following directions, successfully preparing a meal, carrying food across a room, and safe use of a stove. In group treatment, the clinician must understand each patient's individual goals, so that the patient can attain optimum value from the experience.

### Home Management

As the patient gains increased skills and independence in dressing, feeding, and functional mobility, treatment is expanded to include kitchen and homemaking tasks. Homemaking activities are dusting, sweeping, mopping, vacuuming, making the bed, laundry, and cleaning the kitchen and bathroom. Other home management activities include money management activities (balancing the checkbook, paying bills, and budgeting), home repairs, yard work, simple car repairs, and maintenance such as washing the car and changing the oil. Examples of high-level activities include planning a vacation, organizing a file cabinet, ordering from a catalog, and filing income tax.

It is important to determine the patient's interests and previous level of function before initiating treatment. Some patients make only simple meals using, at most, a microwave oven, while others are gourmet cooks. Some patients do not perform any other household activities except making their own bed and possibly doing their personal laundry. Introducing activities patients did not perform prior to their injury is likely to increase agitation.

Training is graded to suit the patient's functional level. Beginning tasks might include simple sandwich or hot soup preparation. Depending on the patient's cognitive status, the clinician may place all food items on the table and have the patient verbally review the task before doing it for the first time. At the end of the session, the next day's activities can be discussed. A session such as this requires simple sequencing, organizing, and memory for the task. As the patient improves, more demands may be made until the patient reaches the established long-term goals.

### Community Reintegration

In the rehabilitation process the patient with a TBI often reaches a maximum level of independence in the protected and structured atmosphere of the hospital. This independence does not necessarily follow over into the community when the patient encounters unfamiliar people, situations, and problems. Community reintegration must be included in the occupational therapy program before discharge.

### Home Health

There are some important differences in occupational therapy services provided within the patient's home compared with other treatment settings. The relationship between the clinician, patient, and family changes. The clinician is a consultant as well as an invited guest.

Therapeutically, clinicians have less control in the home where the family unit is the key to successful treatment. If the family does not support or agree with the treatment goals, the goals will not be accomplished. It is important to establish patient-focused goals with the patient and family. It is also essential to integrate patients back into their community (i.e., school, church, work, friends).

## SUMMARY

Treatment of the brain-injured adult is challenging and requires flexibility, stamina, and a great deal of creativity. Behavioral deficits frequently have a significant impact on the treatment program. Most patients have a multitude of deficits. Goals should be interdisciplinary and established to meet the specific needs of each patient. Treatment of the TBI population should be functionally based. Treatment provided within the context of activities has meaning for these patients, allows documentation of functional changes, and provides concrete evidence of improvement to third party payors.

## *Selected Reading Guide Questions*

1. Define traumatic brain injury (TBI).
2. List some of the causes of TBI.
3. What is a diffuse axonal injury (DAI) and what kind of damage does it cause?
4. Describe the physical deficits that one might encounter in a beginning level TBI patient.
5. Describe the cognitive deficits that might be encountered in a person who has sustained a TBI.
6. Look at the Rancho Los Amigos Scale of Cognitive Functioning and imagine that you are working with a level VII patient. How might you grade the activity of ordering a pizza for a patient at this level?
7. If a TBI patient refused to work on a cooking activity, what might some of the causes be?
8. Describe why serial casting is used.
9. How might a figure ground deficit, a visual field cut, and size discrimination deficit impact an individual's ability to cook?
10. Why might a TBI patient hit, kick, or bite?
11. Explain why functional activities might work better than sequencing cards for the TBI patient.
12. Why might a family member of a person with TBI have difficulty accepting the patient's behavior?
13. Why is transfer training not a good choice for the first caregiver training session?
14. Should the COTA pursue an adaptive or remedial approach to perceptual-motor treatment when a TBI patient functions at a concrete level?
15. List two components of a behavior management program.

## *Exercises*

1. Cover the left side of each lens of a pair of sunglasses with masking tape and put the glasses on. Now try to read a book. Then try to tie your shoes with one hand.
2. Choose any ADL activity and explain how it might be graded during treatment for each of the eight stages on the Rancho Los Amigos Scale of Cognitive Functioning.

### *REFERENCES*


1. Adams JH et al: Brain damage in fatal non-missile head injury, *J Clin Pathol* 33:1132-1145, 1980.
2. Anderson L: *NeuroCare patient safety assessment,* Concord, Calif, 1989, NeuroCare Rehabilitation Without Walls.
3. Ayres AJ: *Sensory integration and learning disorders,* Los Angeles, 1972, Western Psychological Services.
4. Bakay L, Glasauer FE: *Head injury,* Boston, 1980, Little, Brown.
5. Bly L: *NDT and motor learning theory.* Paper presented at the Seventh Annual Interdisciplinary Bobath Symposium, San Francisco, April 1994.
6. Bontke CF: Medical advances in the treatment of brain injury. In Kreutzer JS, Wehman P: *Community integration following traumatic brain injury,* Baltimore, 1990, Brookes.
7. Chusid JG: *Correlative neuroanatomy and functional neurology,* ed 19, Los Altos, Calif, 1985, Lange.
8. Davies PM: *Starting again,* Berlin, 1994, Springer-Verlag.
9. Efferson L: *Early intervention in identification and remediation of visual problems in traumatic brain injury.* Paper presented at the Sixteenth Annual Santa Clara Valley Medical Center Head Trauma Conference, San Jose, Calif, April 1993.
10. Englander J: Personal communication, October 4, 1993.
11. Giles GM, Fussey I: Models of brain injury rehabilitation: from theory to practice. In Fussey I, Giles GM: *Rehabilitation of the severely brain-injured adult,* London, 1988, Croom Helm.
12. Goble L, Hier-Wellner S, Lee D: The role of community reintegration activities in a day treatment service, *Physical Disabilities Special Interest Section Newsletter* 12(3):7-8, 1989.
13. *Guide to the uniform data set for medical rehabilitation,* (Adult FIM), Version 4.0, Buffalo, NY 14214, 1993, Research Foundation, State University of New York at Buffalo.
14. Hall KM: Overview of functional assessment scales in brain injury rehabilitation, *NeuroRehabil* 2(4):98-113, 1992.
15. Hall KM, Cope DN, Rappaport M: Glasgow outcome scale and disability rating scale: comparative usefulness in following recovery in traumatic head injury, *Arch Phys Med Rehabil* 66:35-37, 1985.
16. Hulme JB: Advanced problem solving: the interrelationship of trunk and limb function in abnormal movement patterns. Paper presented at the Seventh Annual Interdisciplinary Bobath Symposium, San Francisco, Calif, April 1994.
17. Jennett B, Teasdale G: *Management of head injuries,* Philadelphia, 1981, FA Davis.
18. Katz DI: Neuropathology and neurobehavioral recovery from closed head injury, *J Head Trauma Rehabil* 7(2):1-15, 1992.
19. Klupt R, Baker E, Patsy D: The importance of functional activities on an inpatient brain injury unit, *Physical Disabilities Special Interest Section Newsletter* 12(3):6-7, 1989.
20. Kraus JF et al: The incidence of acute brain injury and serious impairment in a defined population, *Am J Epidemiol* 119:186-201, 1983.
21. Lazarus CL: Swallowing disorders after traumatic brain injury, *J Head Trauma Rehabil* 4(4):34-41, 1989.
22. Lezak M: The problem of assessing executive functions, *Int J Psychol1 17:281-297, 1982.*
23. Logemann JA: Evaluation and treatment planning for the head-injured patient with oral intake disorders, *J Head Trauma Rehabil* 4(4):24-33, 1989.

24. Lundgren CC, Persechino EL: Cognitive group: a treatment program for head injured adults, *Am J Occup Ther* 40(6):397-401, 1986.
25. MacKinnon JD: Personal communication, June 6, 1994.
26. Mann N: Spasticity in traumatic brain injury. Paper presented at the Fifteenth Annual Santa Clara Valley Medical Center Head Trauma Conference, San Jose, Calif, April 1992.
27. Miller JD: Early intervention and management. In Rosenthal M et al: *Rehabilitation of the head-injured adult,* Philadelphia, 1984, FA Davis.
28. Neistadt ME: A critical analysis of occupational therapy approaches for perceptual deficits in adults with brain injury, *Am J Occup Ther* 44(4):299-304, 1990.
29. Neistadt ME: Perceptual retraining for adults with diffuse brain injury, *Am J Occup Ther* 48(3):225-233, 1994.
30. Oblender MM: Cognition groups in the rehabilitation of head injured adults, *Physical Disabilities Special Interest Section Newsletter* 12(3):5-6, 1989.
31. Rancho Los Amigos Medical Center: *Levels of cognitive functioning,* Downey, Calif, Rancho Los Amigos Medical Center, Adult Brain Injury Service, 1980.
32. Rappaport M et al: Disability rating scale for severe head trauma: coma to community, *Arch Phys Med Rehabil* 63:118-123, 1982.
33. Rimel RW, Jane JA: Characteristics of the head-injured patient. In Rosenthal M et al: *Rehabilitation of the head-injured adult,* Philadelphia, 1984, FA Davis.
34. Santa Clara Valley Medical Center: *Behavior management program policy and procedure manual,* San Jose, Calif, 1993, Santa Clara Valley Medical Center.
35. Shilling M: A formula to estimate incidence, *Community Integration* 2(3):8-9, 1992.
36. Willer B et al: Assessment of community integration following rehabilitation for traumatic brain injury, *J Head Trauma Rehabil* 8(2):75-87, 1993.
37. Willer B, Abosh S, Dahmer E: Epidemiology of disability from traumatic brain injury. In Wood R: *Neurobehavioral sequelae of traumatic brain injury,* London, 1990, Taylor and Francis.

# Chapter 38

# Burns

*Elizabeth A. Rivers*

## Chapter Objectives

*After studying this chapter, the student or practitioner will be able to:*

1. List the functions of skin and identify changes caused by a burn injury.
2. List the treatment goals for the three phases of burn wound healing.
3. Discuss the value of elevated, antigravity positioning for the burn patient and give one example.
4. Discuss scar management and give one example of a technique used to prevent or minimize scarring.
5. Prioritize rehabilitation goals to achieve maximum recovery with least cost to patient.
6. List two ways the occupational therapy practitioner prevents infection transfer.
7. Prioritize adaptations for function and list two reasons why such adaptations are discontinued early for burned persons.

## Key Terms

skin
epidermis
dermis
burn
eschar
extent of burn
percentage of the total body surface area (%TBSA)
depth of burn
edema
autograft
split-thickness skin graft (STSG)
cultured epidermal autograft (CEA)
microvascular skin flap autograft
full-thickness skin graft
hypertrophic scar
contracture
psychological reactions
burn care multidisciplinary team
wound maturation
skin conditioning
support or pressure garments

The annual incidence of burn-related injuries in the United States is decreasing. Presently it is estimated at 1.25 million, of which over 51,000 require hospitalization and 5,500 die.[3] Improvements in comprehensive burn rehabilitation continue.[4,11] Recovery after a burn is a long and arduous process. Severely burned survivors experience a myriad of continuing medical, functional, and psychosocial problems. Nonetheless, those who want to return to their level of function they had before their injury can anticipate recovery very near that capacity.

Burn care professionals use advanced medical and surgical techniques and focus on pain-free motion, functional recovery, and quality of life as well as survival after a burn.

## THE SKIN

The **skin**[8,10,12,14,25] is the largest organ of the body and primarily serves as an environmental barrier. Skin is waterproof, protects from infection, controls body temperature, prevents fluid loss, provides vast sensory information and contributes to identity.

Skin has two basic layers: the epidermis and the dermis[8,10,25] (Figure 38-1). The skin growth cells (germinal keratinocytes) are in the **epidermis.** The melanocytes (pigment or color-producing cells) are found at the dermo-epidermal junction.

The **dermis** is composed of highly structured and organized collagen, wandering cells (white blood cells, macrophages, fibroblasts, endothelial cells), blood vessels, elastic fibers, and a glue-like substance of glycosaminoglycans (GAG), which is also known as "ground substance." The dermis does not regenerate and heals by scar formation.

A **burn** is a permanent destruction of tissue caused by release of energy from an external agent. **Eschar,** pronounced "es-kar," is the dead epidermis and necrotic dermis that remain attached to the wound bed. Most thermal burns are of varying depths (Table 38-1).

When the skin is damaged, innumerable systemic, physiological, and functional problems begin.[10,13,14,25,26] The basis for safe burn treatment is detailed knowledge and understanding of normal skin anatomy, physiology, wound healing, and infection control; this requires continuing study and research by all team members.

## MEASURES OF BURN INJURY SEVERITY

### Percentage of Total Body Surface Area Involved

The **extent of the burn** is classified as a **percentage of the total body surface area (%TBSA)** burned. Two methods used to estimate burn size are the "rule of nines" and the Lund and Browder chart.[21] The rule of nines, developed in the 1940s by Pulaski and Tennison and communicated by word of mouth, divides the body surface into areas of 9%, with the perineum making up 1%. Although simple, the rule of nines is relatively inaccurate, especially for children (Figure 38-2). The Lund and Browder chart[21] provides a more accurate estimate of %TBSA involved and is used in most burn centers.

### Burn Depth

An accurate **depth of burn** is difficult to estimate. It is based on experienced clinical observation of the appearance, sensitivity, and pliability of the wound.[10,14] The burn is described as a superficial-, partial-, or full-thickness injury (see Table 38-1). For treatment planning, the team should remember that the wound is dynamically changing.[14]

### Mechanism of Injury

Thermal injuries are caused by exposure to flames, steam, hot liquids, hot metals, or extreme cold. Heat injury accounts for most burns[30]; about 75% of these accidents are preventable.

## HOSPITAL MEDICAL MANAGEMENT

### Initial Care

Burn injury causes extensive shifts of body fluids.[14] Fluids and electrolytes are replaced intravenously to

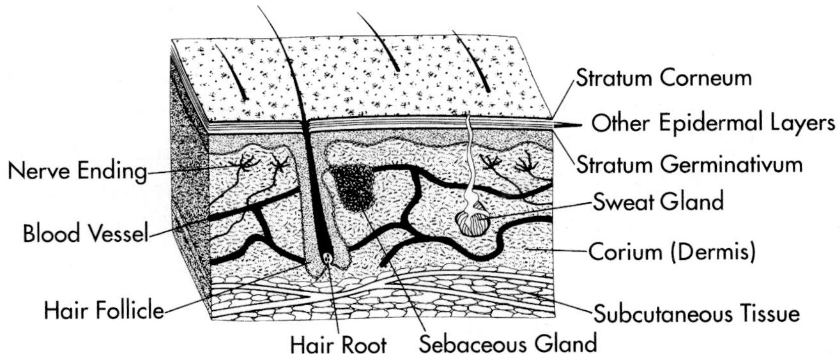


*Figure 38-1* Cross section of the skin. (From Iles RL: *Wound care: the skin,* 1988, Marion Laboratories.)

Table 38-1

## Depth of Injury Correlated With Anticipated Healing Time and Treatment Interventions

| *Injury depth* | *Healing time* | *Wound outcome* | *Therapy treatment modalities* |
|---|---|---|---|
| Superficial epidermis (first degree burn) | 1 to 5 days for spontaneous healing | No problems after healing | Elevation to decrease limb pain<br>Wound washing<br>On healed wound, aloe or other moisturizer to reduce dry skin and itching<br>Therapist consultation rare |
| Superficial dermis (superficial partial-thickness burn or second degree burn) | 14 days for spontaneous healing | Possible pigment (color) changes | Modalities listed above plus:<br>More careful wound care<br>Active elevated exercise<br>Protective garments<br>Sunscreen<br>Acknowledgment of patient's pain and inconvenience |
| Deep reticular dermis (deep partial-thickness burn or second degree) | 21 days* for spontaneous healing<br>(If grafted, see below) | Probable pigment changes<br>Reduced skin durability<br>Severe scarring<br>Sensory changes<br>Sweating changes<br>Edema in dependent limbs, usually temporary | Modalities listed above plus:<br>Therapists consultation by burn team<br>More frequent active elevated exercise<br>Elevated positioning, splints, or both<br>Vascular support garments†<br>Moisturization and lubrication of healed skin<br>Prolonged stretch to involved joints twice daily until contractures resolve<br>Daily living skills practice<br>Psychological therapy<br>Team collaboration to prevent stress disorder |
| Subcutaneous tissue (full-thickness burn or third degree burn) | Cannot heal spontaneously<br>Variable healing time<br>If small burn, approximated wound edges with primary closure; If very large burn, cultured epidermal autograft (CEA)‡ | Outcomes listed above plus:<br>Additional sweating loss<br>Possible loss of involved finger or toe nails<br>Possible additional sensory loss<br>No hair over grafts | Modalities listed above plus:<br>Postoperative positioning or immobilization<br>Initiation of exercise despite pain, very slow weaning from analgesics and medications for stress<br>Vibration for itching<br>Additional education for skin precautions<br>Support/pressure garments<br>Early return to recreation, work, school, family, and community responsibilities |
| Muscle, tendon, bone (fourth degree burn) [historic term—rarely used] | Variable healing time<br>Amputation or reconstructive surgery such as flaps needed§ | Variable | Modalities listed above plus:<br>Deep tendon massage to prevent tethered skin<br>Adapted equipment<br>Prosthetic fitting and training if indicated<br>Additional counseling for stress<br>Work retraining if unable to return to preburn employment safely |

*If surgeon grafts burn by 14 days, fewer scars form with improved functional outcome, less pain, and shortened hospital length of stay.[22]
†Gradient pressure progressively decreases the rate of pressure applied by an elastic bandage or cylindrical pressure sleeve, keeping the most pressure on the distal limb and the least pressure around the proximal area of the extremity.
‡Areas of CEA show permanent fragility; loss of temperature control; and dry, blister-prone skin with permanently changed sensation.
§Early amputation with closure using healthy tissue shortens hospital length of stay, decreases pain and wound breakdown, improves prosthesis fit, and simplifies prosthesis use. However, wounds are rarely of single depth through skin and muscle.

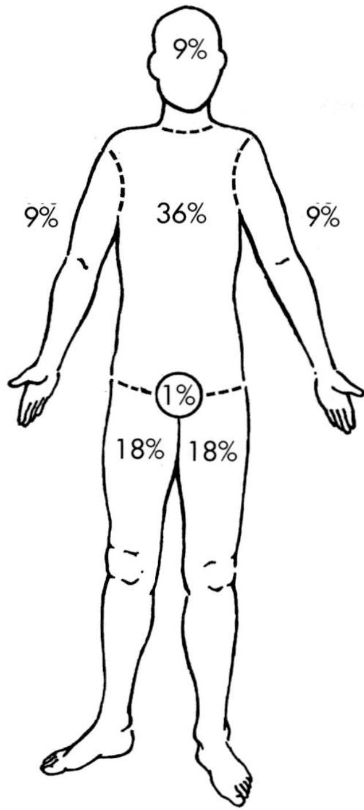


*Figure 38-2* Rule of nines.

prevent shock and death. **Edema** (swelling) is the first problem treated by the occupational therapy practitioner.

In circumferential full-thickness burns, the leathery eschar is inelastic, impairing normal circulation. Escharotomy (incision through destroyed skin) is performed by the surgeon to improve circulation[14] and is usually painless because the nerve endings are destroyed in a full-thickness burn (Figure 38-3).

### Wound Care

A shower or submersion cleansing of the wound and uninvolved areas is done on admission and daily. Various topical agents are applied to reduce bacterial counts in the wounds. All staff observe universal infection control precautions according to the hospital's rules (see Chapter 12). The occupational therapy practitioner decontaminates all equipment, materials, and surfaces between patient contacts.[14,36]

### Skin Grafting

When the depth and extent of the wound will require 3 or more weeks for healing, surgery will decrease hospital length of stay, pain, and scar or contracture complications.[10,14] With the patient anesthetized, the surgeon excises (removes) the eschar, controls bleeding in the recipient area and places an autograft. An **autograft** is a surgical transplantation of the person's own skin from an unburned area (donor site). The sheet or meshed (perforated evenly by machine) **split-thickness skin graft (STSG)** is applied to the

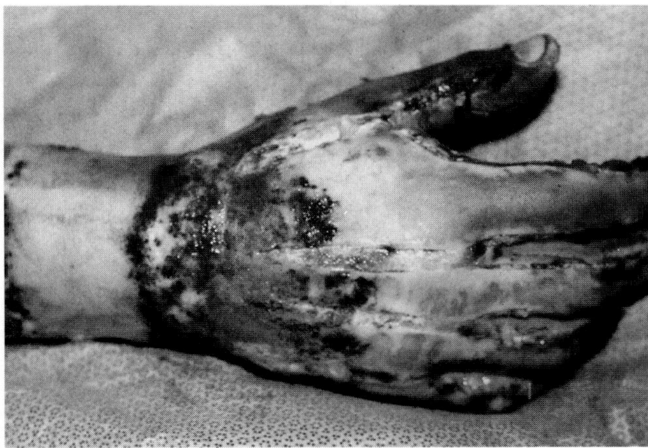

*Figure 38-3* Escharotomies on the dorsum of the hand with a full-thickness burn injury.

clean excised wound (graft recipient site). As the size of a survivable burn increases, available donor sites for autograft decrease. For this reason, alternatives to autografts such as the **cultured epidermal autograft (CEA)** are being explored.[9] When the wound is limited in size but the defect is so deep that tendon survival or graft adherence is extremely doubtful, a plastic surgeon covers the area with a **microvascular skin flap autograft.**[10] Because a **full-thickness skin graft** requires wound closure by an STSG or edge-to-edge sutures, it is usually reserved for reconstruction.

### Pain

Pain[24] is defined as an unpleasant sensory and emotional response to a stimulus associated with actual or potential tissue damage.[24] Burn pain severity cannot be predicted; it is influenced by burn depth and location, patient age, gender, ethnicity, education, occupation, history of drug or alcohol abuse, and psychiatric illness. A burn medication protocol includes long-acting narcotics for background pain, short-acting drugs for procedural pain, and medications to decrease anxiety. Procedural pain occurs when something is done to the patient such as wound cleansing, dressing changes, or therapy.[10,24,31] If possible, schedule exercise sessions when pain medications are at peak effectiveness. As the wound heals, a patient gradually decreases the dosage and frequency of drugs and usually requires minimal pain medications by discharge.

### Scar Formation

A **hypertrophic** scar is a hard, red, collagenous bundle of connective tissue raised above the surface of the burn wound.[26] Initially, healed burn wounds usually appear red and flat. Hypertrophic scars commonly become visible 6 to 8 weeks after wound closure. The functional or cosmetic significance of hypertrophic scars varies with the anatomical location of the wound. Race, age, the location, and depth of the burn wound have been reported to influence hypertrophic scarring.[10,22,25]

### Contracture Development

Normal wound healing occurs by contraction.[10,25] In addition, the burned patient often chooses to lie in a flexed, adducted, "fetal" position, the position of withdrawal from pain. If the patient does not actively stretch the healing wound to its original length, the new collagen fibers in the wound shorten.[14] A **contracture** is limited joint motion caused by shortened soft tissue, tendons, ligaments, blood vessels, and nerves or by calcium deposits surrounding the involved joint.

### Psychosocial Factors

During hospitalization, the patient experiences fear, isolation, dependency, and pain. Potential **psychological reactions** include depression; withdrawal reactions to disfigurement; regression; and anxiety and uncertainty about the ability to resume work, family, community, and leisure roles. During each contact, the COTA and OTR provide emotional support and education to facilitate adjustment, coping mechanisms, and self-direction.

## BURN REHABILITATION

### The Team

The **burn care multidisciplinary team** is composed of the patient and family, physicians, nurses, physical therapists (PTs) and physical therapist assistants (PTAs),[27] registered occupational therapists (OTRs), certified occupational therapy assistants (COTAs), dietitians, social workers, respiratory therapists, art and play therapists, recreational therapists, clergy, case managers, visiting caregivers, chaplains, and vocational counselors. Nationally, team members available to the burn patient vary widely.[4,7,11,33] Specific role delineation varies with state licensure or certification regulations and hospital or facility policies.[4,7,27]

### Phases of Recovery

Burn management can be divided into three overlapping phases: (1) acute care, (2) surgical and postoperative care, and (3) rehabilitation (inpatient and outpatient).[34]

The acute care phase occurs in the first 72 hours after a major burn injury. If the wound is superficial, a person experiences only this phase.

The surgical and postoperative phase follows the acute phase. Vulnerability to wound infection, sepsis, and septic shock predominate at this time.

The final phase is the postgrafting or wound maturation period when the patient is medically stable. Inpatient and outpatient treatments are provided during this phase, which the American Burn Association (ABA) calls *rehabilitation.*[34] Besides depth and %TBSA, other factors affecting outcome[33] are the quality of wound healing, scar formation, and effectiveness of team collaboration. This is the longest, most rigorous, and challenging phase. The COTA provides treatments at this time.

### Goals of Rehabilitation

Considering the functional, cosmetic, and psychosocial consequences of a severe burn injury, the team focuses on cost-effective, successful outcomes[15] (see Table 38-1 and Figure 38-4).

#### *Acute Care Phase*

During the acute care phase, medical management and patient survival predominate. For OT goals, see the short-term goals in Figure 38-4.

#### *Surgical and Postoperative Phase*

OT goals during the surgical and postoperative phase promote skin graft adherence while preserving or assisting function when possible. The graft recipient area is immobilized after surgery. The preferred position and length of immobilization vary by physician preference and burn center; however, the range is from 1 to 7 days.[10]

#### *Rehabilitation Phase*

The overlapping third phase of recovery is the postgrafting, **wound maturation** period. It begins as wound closure occurs. The patient becomes medically stable and external life support and monitoring tubes are discontinued. A wound is considered mature when it is soft, the proper color, flat, durable, and supple. Wound maturation time varies from less than a year to 2 years and in growing children up to 5 years.[30]

Care during the rehabilitation phase focuses on achieving independence while preventing deformity and contractures.[18] Patient and family prepare for discharge, and the COTA recommends practical program modifications. Once the individual is home, therapist and physician follow-up, psychological support, and intervention are provided to restore motivation, self-confidence, and social interaction.

At discharge or soon after, the patient will do the following:

1. Direct **skin conditioning** and wound care; bathe, moisturize skin, and perform self-care with minimal assistance; independently don and remove vascular supports; and preserve healed burn wounds, grafts, and donor areas while resuming preburn activity
2. Recover 80% of preburn active ROM, demonstrate prolonged stretching to decrease joint and skin contractures, and avoid joint deterioration
3. Recover 80% of preburn strength (as compared with norms for age) to return to preburn functional activities in home and community
4. Develop endurance to tolerate 2 hours of work equivalent activity and 8 hours of activities including safe homemaking or home chores
5. Recover coordination sufficient for work and daily living skills with minimal adaptive equipment and at preburn flexibility and speed

**Standing Burn Rehabilitation Orders**

Patient name: ______________________________ Diagnosis/onset: ______________________

Precautions: ________________________________________________________________

Duration of treatment: _________________________________________________________

Frequency of treatment: BID __________ Daily __________ 3×week __________ Other __________

**Long-term goals**

1. Patient recovers preburn status for active range of motion, strength, endurance, and coordination.
2. Edema is controlled by elevated positioning and external vascular supports.
3. Patient uses protective interventions for sensory, vascular, and pigment changes.
4. Burn wounds, grafts, and donor areas are healed, durable, soft, flat, proper color, pain-free, and itching is controlled.
5. Patient learns care of wound and healed skin.
6. Patient returns, as an outpatient, to preburn daily living, school, vocational, and avocational activities in home and community.
7. Patient copes constructively with stress symptoms and changed body appearance.

**Short-term goals**

*Routine burn rehabilitation protocol:*

1. Evaluate and treat deficits in range of motion of burned areas, and one joint proximal and one joint distal:
   A. Active range of motion with terminal stretch to contracted joints
   B. Prolonged stretch to all contractures that persist more than 1 day
   C. Ambulation with the use of a walker with an overhead bar as soon as medically stable
   D. Bicycle or equivalent aerobic exercise
   E. Gentle reciprocal pulleys if shoulders are involved
   F. Foam or rubberband gripper if no finger joint damage
2. Orthotics: Evaluate and obtain physician order as needed.
3. Evaluate and treat edema with extremity elevation, antigravity positioning, arm wedges, vascular support, or scar compression as appropriate. Patient learns figure-eight application of elastic bandages to legs—applied for 23 hours per day, including independent application and removal.
4. Evaluate and treat deficits or changes in sensation including itch management and applying lotion to healed dry areas.
5. Desensitization to healed areas with lotion and progressing.
6. Daily living skills: Evaluate and treat deficits as appropriate.
7. Teach home exercise program as soon as patient is alert.
8. Incorporate family (and patient as soon as alert) goals in plans.

*Figure 38-4* Short- and long-term burn rehabilitation goals.

6. Control limb edema with vascular supports 23 hours a day combined with elevated positioning to prevent wound breakdown, decrease scar formation, and prevent cellulitis
7. Demonstrate independent donning and doffing of splints to modify burn scars, remember to wear devices for the prescribed number of hours and be able to explain the purpose of these devices
8. Learn and use protective outdoor interventions such as flap hats or sunscreen clothing in the sun and layered winter clothing to avoid wound breakdown and hyperthermia or hypothermia
9. Demonstrate successful use of interventions such as cutting nails, applying lotion, and vibrating and desensitizing to control itching and avoid excoriation of wounds
10. Participate in appropriate, coordinated planning for discharge from burn care
11. Explore vocational issues with a vocational rehabilitation or school counselor to resume work or school
12. Explore and participate in recreational activities, leisure planning, and social and community reintegration while wearing external vascular supports and splints
13. If not consistently independent in hygiene, use of support garments, and homemaking, hire and supervise appropriate attendant help
14. Learn to cope constructively with stress symptoms, changed body appearance, intimacy issues, and adjustment to disability and seek assistance from psychologist or counselor as needed
15. Participate in a survey of home needs emphasizing independence and safety; use mobility aids and adaptive equipment in home if needed; determine the level of assistance required after discharge

## ROLE OF OCCUPATIONAL THERAPY

There is no substitute for early and consistent intervention by OTs. When burn team disciplines work closely together and communicate accurately and frequently, patients benefit from the skills and viewpoints of all. Then documentation and communication with third party payers, home care facilities, and families are consistent and coordinated.

Occupational therapy in burn care draws on specialized knowledge of environments, sexuality, cultural and family influences, anatomy, physiology, kinesiology, neurology, infection control, and psychosocial development. The OTR and COTA's skills, therapeutic approach, energy, and creativity become part of the strengths and resources that are available to the burned patient and the family.

Often a COTA is part of the team at a rehabilitation center to which grafted and stable burn patients are referred before returning home. After the patient is stable, and in collaboration with an OTR, a COTA may provide inpatient and outpatient daily living skills practice; follow up with exercise treatment such as Baltimore Therapeutic Equipment (BTE), Biodex programs, and adapted games; make adaptations for support garments and clothing; remeasure patients for custom-fitted garments as assigned; and teach homemaking. Depending on local practice regulations, exclusion criteria for COTA treatment includes patients with more than 20% TBSA burn, more than one joint involved, exposed tendons, hand or toe burns, face grafts, or inhalation injuries or who are medically unstable. In some hospitals, a qualified and experienced COTA reports and documents patient change, recommends or performs reevaluations, and collaborates with the patient and social worker to resolve transportation, shopping, and homemaking limitations.

### Assessment

If possible the OTR completes initial patient evaluation[28] within the first 24 to 48 hours, first obtaining data on burn etiology, medical history, any secondary diagnoses, and precautions from the medical chart. The OTR looks at the wounds to determine the extent and depth of injury, noting critical areas involved, and interviews the patient to establish rapport and obtain specific information such as hand dominance, pre-

*Table 38-2*

**Antideformity Positioning**

| *Body area* | *Antideformity position* | *Equipment/technique* |
|---|---|---|
| Mouth | Varied | Regular food (i.e., not cut into small pieces), straw for thick liquids, exercise, microstomia splint |
| Ears/face | Position that prevents pressure | No pillows, ear protection headgear, cut-out cushions in airbed, head of bed elevated to decrease edema and risk of aspiration |
| Neck | Neutral/slight extension | No pillow (or neck extended by foam wedge), elevation and head cut-out air flow or bead bed, foam neck splint conformer, Watusi collar, triple component neck splint |
| Chest/abdomen | Trunk extension, shoulder retraction | Head of bed lowered, towel roll beneath spine, clavicle straps |
| Axilla | Shoulder abducted 90 to 100 degrees | Arm boards, foam wedges, overhead traction slings, axillary total contact splint, clavicle straps, overhead wheeled walker |
| Elbow/forearm | 10 degrees short of full elbow extension, forearm neutral | Foam wedge pillows, arm boards, conformer splints, dynamic splints |
| Wrist/hand | Wrist extended 30 degrees, thumb abducted and extended, metacarpophalangeal (MCP) flexion 50 to 70 degrees, interphalangeal (IP) extension | Elevation above heart with pillows or foam wedges when lying down or sitting; suspension slings, deltoid aid, overhead bar on wheeled walker when walking |
| Hip/thigh | Neutral extension, hips abducted 10 to 15 degrees | Bed elevation changed for prone/sidelying positions, trochanter rolls, pillow between knees, wedges |
| Knee/lower leg | Knee extension for circumferential burn, slight flexion for anterior burn | Foot of bed positioned to elevate feet when sitting, knee conformer, casts, dynamic splints |
| Ankle/foot | Neutral or 0 to 5 degrees dorsiflexion | Cut-out heel cushions, airflow bed with foot cushion, custom splint, cast, ankle-foot orthosis (AFO) |

vious functional limitations, daily activities before the injury, psychological status, and spiritual and cultural values.[19]

### Acute Care Phase Treatments

#### *Exercise*

Acute care treatments[15,28,30] (see Table 38-1, Table 38-2, and Figure 38-4) include range of motion (ROM), which is a primary component in every burn treatment plan. Active, active-assisted, or prolonged stretch exercises are used depending on the patient's condition. Exercise in acute care preserves ROM and functional strength and decreases edema. Ambulation begins as soon as it is medically safe. The patient who has a lower extremity (LE) burn wears elastic wraps. These are applied in a figure-eight pattern—from the metatarsal heads, including the heel, to the groin. Avoid prolonged dangling of feet or static standing to prevent edema formation and unnecessary discomfort.

Strength and endurance activities are introduced early. Research and experience have shown that graded progressive exercise is not deleterious in acute burn recovery.[15,17,28,30]

If comatose or on a ventilator, the patient is dependent on nursing for self-care. As soon as the patient is medically cleared to eat, the OTR or experienced COTA assesses eating skills. Dressings, edema, and pain may impair self-feeding motions initially, and adaptive equipment may be used for a short time. Temporary adaptive equipment includes built-up and extended-handle utensils and a plate guard. Depending on amputations and the burn site, early simple grooming, toileting, and phone management are encouraged. All professional staff convey the expectation of early, independent, patient-initiated activities of daily living (ADL) with normal movement patterns within a normal time.

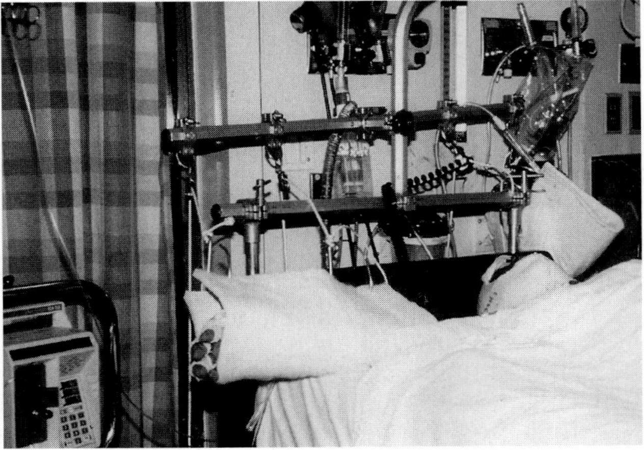

*Figure 38-5* Supine shoulder positioning with overhead traction and felt slings.

#### *Edema Management*

During acute care, elevated positioning limits edema formation.[14,26] The extremity or head is raised above heart level (Table 38-2, Figure 38-5). Vary positions to improve patient comfort and normal joint function. The OTR or experienced COTA makes the daily positioning program and changes clearly visible to all team members including the patient, family, nurses, and doctors.

#### *Splinting*

A splint used during the acute phase is usually applied during rest, with activity and exercise emphasized while the patient is awake. The volar burn hand splint is designed to provide approximately 30 degrees wrist extension, 50 to 70 degrees metacarpophalangeal (MCP) joint flexion, full interphalangeal (IP) extension, and the thumb abducted and extended[5] (Figure 38-6). It is secured in place with a figure eight wrap of gauze bandage. Straps are not used on acute burn splints because of the potential tourniquet effect and infection control concerns. Splints require daily assessment and alteration as edema and fit change.

### Surgical and Postoperative Phase Treatments

A period of postoperative immobilization assists graft adherence and vascularization. Bulky restrictive dressings with standard positioning equipment (see Figure 38-5) frequently are adequate. Splints may be ordered. Positioning procedures are checked by the team each day for graft and patient safety.

Exercises for adjacent body areas are discontinued until resumed by the physician. The average immobilization is 3 to 5 days, with 7 to 10 days for cultured epidermal grafts. The physician, OTR, and experienced COTA view the unbandaged graft and donor sites to determine graft integrity, exposed tendons, and bleeding areas before resuming exercises.

If permitted, temporary, simple techniques such as overhead mirrors, prism glasses for those supine in bed, or universal cuffs and extended-handle utensils for self-care to preserve feelings of self-worth and orientation are provided by the experienced COTA.

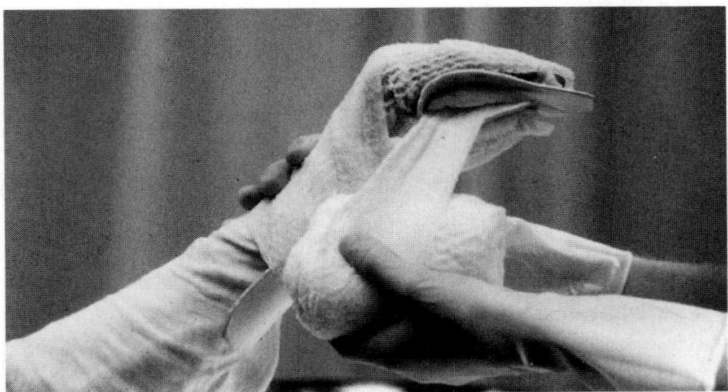

*Figure 38-6* Postburn hand splint. Note wrapping approach for the thumb.

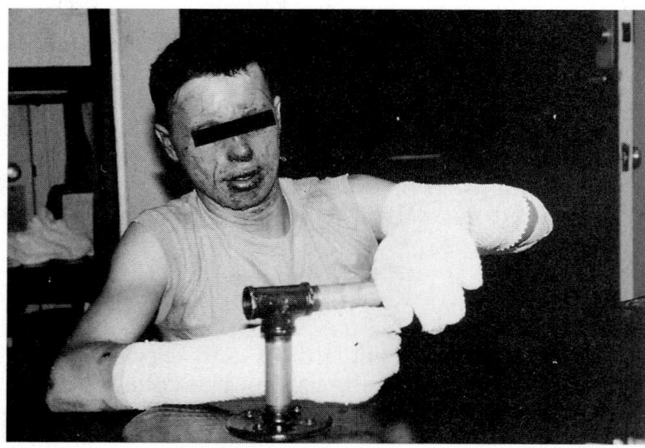

*Figure 38-7* Commonly used pipe tree is a good activity for hand exercise after a burn injury.

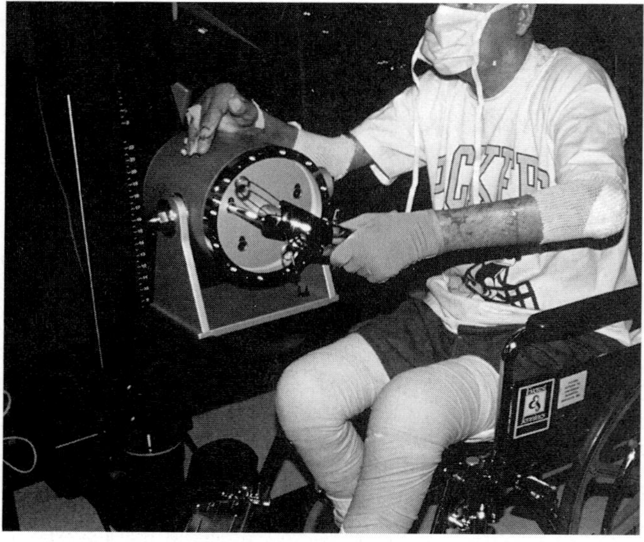

*Figure 38-8* A presized intermediate glove is worn all the time, including during exercise and activity, to condition the skin and control edema. BTE provides work simulation. Note elastic wraps to legs—toe to groin—bilaterally.

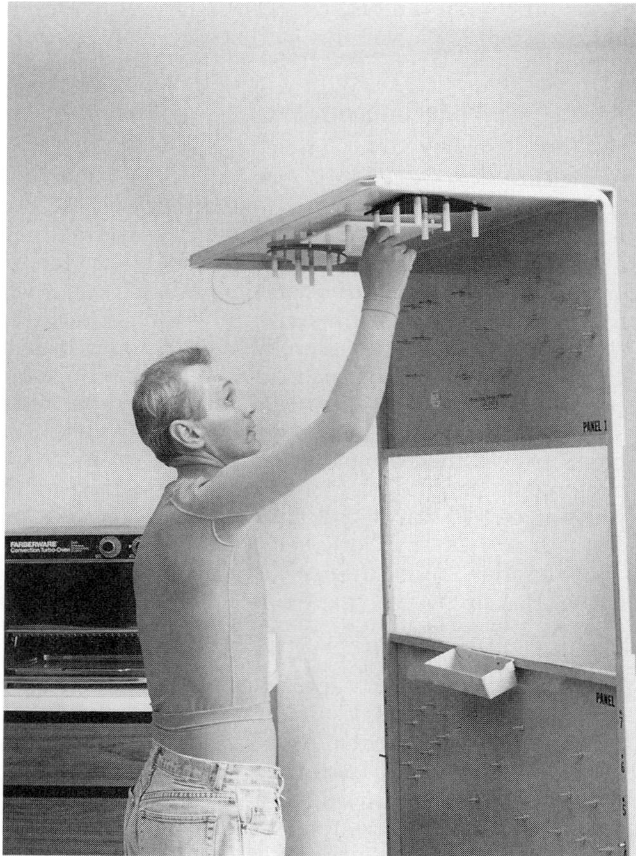

*Figure 38-9* A combined ROM and skin conditioning activity. Use of the Valpar whole body ROM for UE exercise while wearing compression garments.

### Rehabilitation Phase Treatments

Exercise is the most important treatment component in the rehabilitation phase (see Table 38-1, Table 38-2, and Figure 38-4) and is not unique for burn injuries (Figures 38-7 to 38-11). Depending on joints involved, every treatment during the intense rehabilitation phase overlaps with another treatment. For example, active exercise during ambulation includes stretching shoulders, elbows, and hands by grasping and releasing an overhead walker bar (see Figure 38-10) and increasing the number of laps the patient makes. Stair climbing and more vigorous patient-initiated exercise begin along with tub and car transfers. Rehabilitation equipment such as grippers, hand-manipulation boards, pipe trees, reciprocal pulleys, stationary bicycle, the BTE work simulator, Work Evaluation Systems Technology (WEST), the Valpar whole body exerciser (see Figure 38-9) musical or computer keyboards, homemaking, work simulation activity, or weighted pulleys may be used to increase range, strength, and endurance. Timers and written graph reminders give the person control of the duration and frequency of activity as well as providing objective documentation of improvement.

Stretching increases flexibility and fluidity of movement.[18] Perform a slow, sustained stretch with a full-length mirror to see and correct abnormal postures. Combine activities and do composite stretches such as using plastic syringe cases as mouth cones (Figure 38-12) while lying prone to stretch hips, shoulders, and elbows. Other possibilities include (1) stretching shoulders and elbows while vibrating an itching back or combing hair; (2) reaching overhead to punch a balloon after every 10 repetitions of stationary bicycling; (3) cutting foods independently, drinking from a cup without a straw or using straw with thickened liquids only, or opening the mouth to eat regular raw fruits or vegetables; (4) elevating arms while eating and tucking

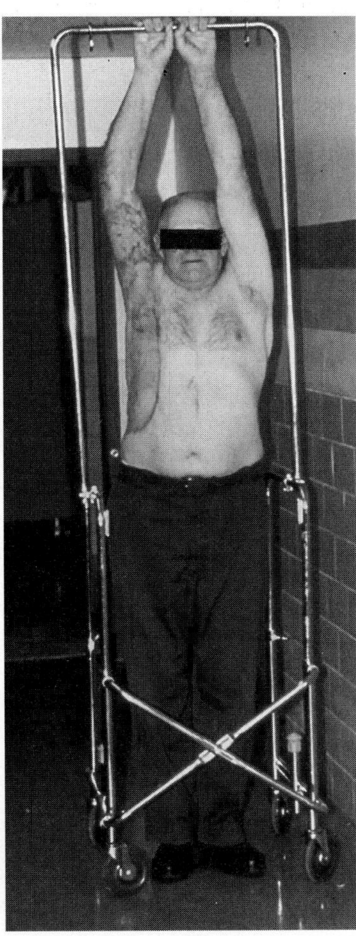

*Figure 38-10* Wheeled walker equipped with an overhead bar helps patient stretch axillary contracture during ambulation.

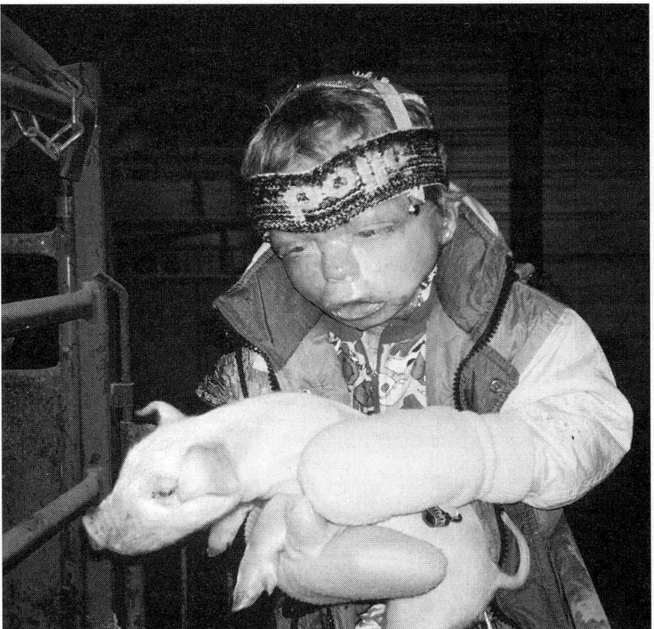

*Figure 38-11* Mittens, layered clothing, and scarves protect child doing winter chores from frostbite.

feet under a chair to stretch knee flexion and ankle dorsiflexion during a meal.

Control edema until there is no swelling.[13] In healed, severe burns of the hand, edema occurs because of decreased hand use, dependent positioning without adequate external support, and the tourniquet action of circumferential UE scarring. When edema is present, motion is limited and painful, the skin is prone to damage from shearing forces, and fibrosis may result. Often an Isotoner glove adequately controls hand swelling (see Figure 38-8).

In addition to controlling edema, **support or pressure garments** help to manage hypertrophic scars[35] but use must be supervised to avoid complications.[20,22,23,32] Custom-made support garments can be fitted once the patient's weight is stable, the healed skin does not stick to support, and skin is durable. Use of compression garments is controversial because there are no long-term, prospective, randomized, controlled studies that document whether they make a difference in time of wound maturity, quality of tissue, or comfort.[16] Based on anecdotal information, many surgeons

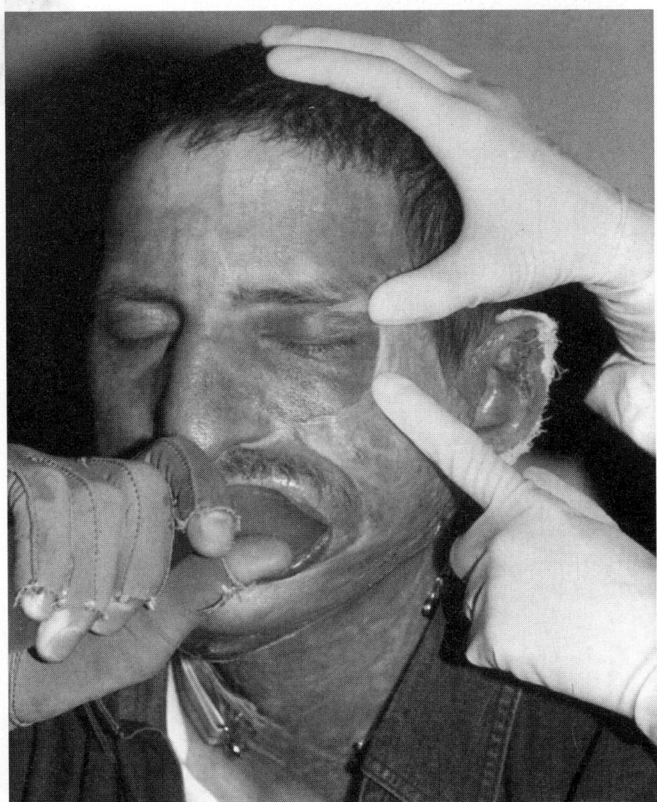

*Figure 38-12* Combined facial stretching with hand strengthening. Patient wearing Isotoner glove for hand edema uses syringe case to stretch left cheek pouch while COTA stretches facial contracture band. Note neck splint.

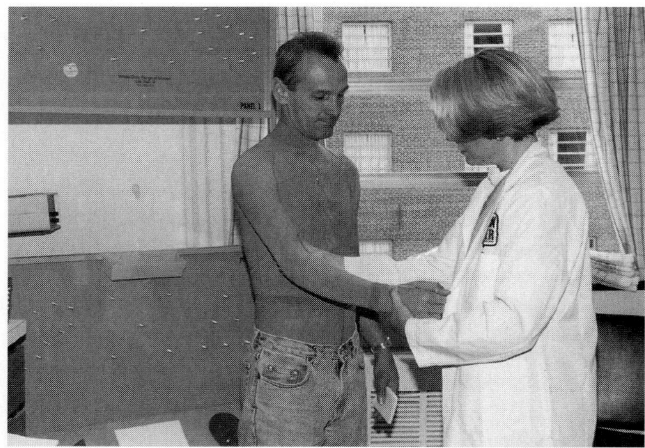

*Figure 38-13* Assess the fit of custom-made compression garments frequently to ensure adequate compression for scar management.

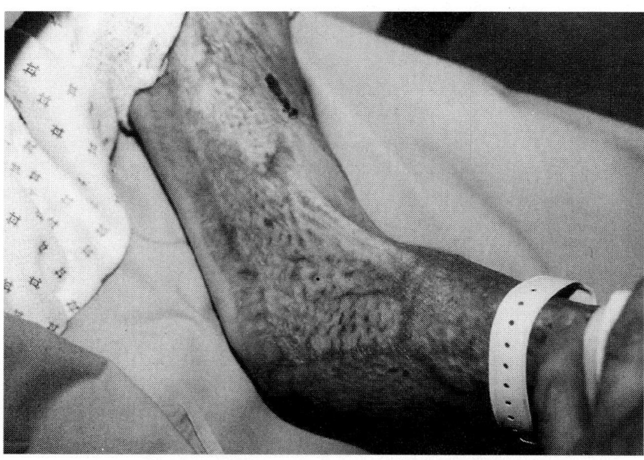

*Figure 38-14* Example of scar contracture of antecubital skin of elbow. Note taut, shortened skin when elbow is being extended.

A

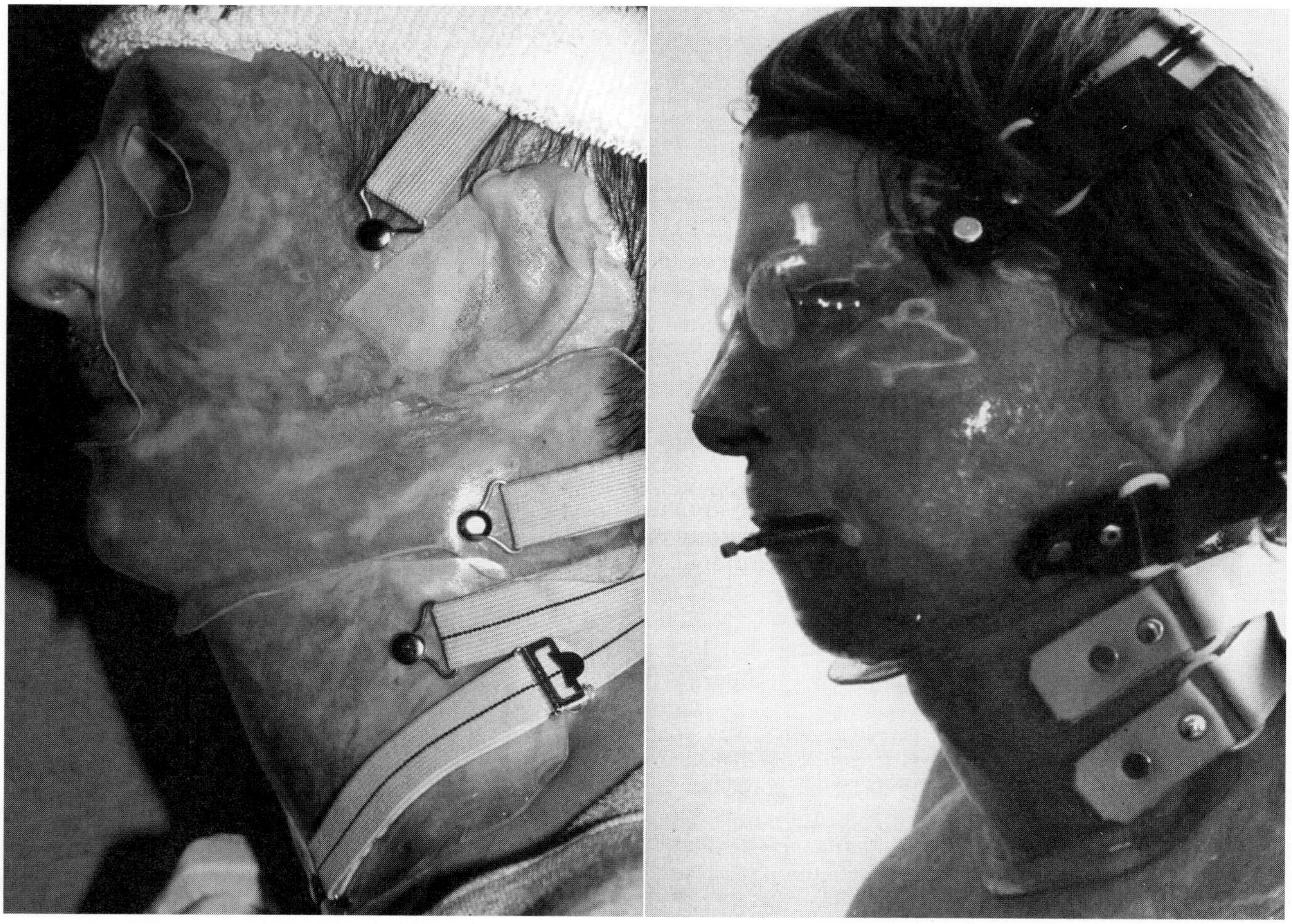

B

*Figure 38-15* Transparent facial orthosis and neck orthosis. **A,** Day facial and neck orthoses fitted to blanch or turn raised scar tissue white. **B,** Night face and neck orthoses with humidity domes for eyes and microstomia prevention appliance for mouth stretch.

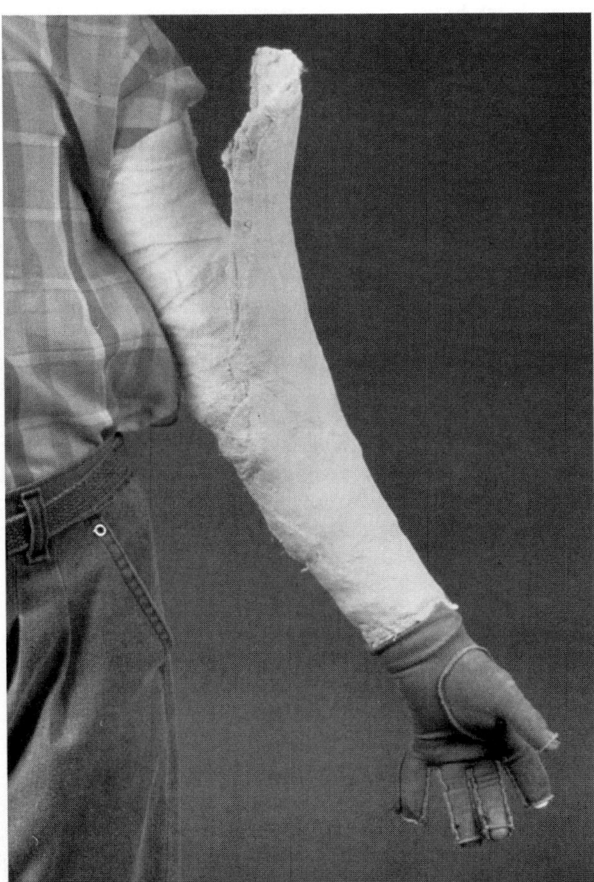

*Figure 38-16* Treatment of elbow scar contracture with a serial fall-out elbow cast applied at maximum elbow extension at night blocks flexion and allows full, painless extension by morning when cast is removed. After several weeks, contracture does not reform and cast is discontinued.

still recommend garments for all donor sites, graft sites, and burn wounds that take more than 2 to 3 weeks to heal.[9] The OTR or experienced COTA often measures, orders, and checks the fit (Figure 38-13) of the custom-made garments (see Resources at end of chapter).

All custom-made garments need to be measured and ordered following the special instructions of each company. To provide adequate scar compression, garments must be worn 23 hours a day; they are removed only for bathing, massage, or changing into a clean garment.

Scar contracture is often the primary cause of dysfunction (Figure 38-14). Splints at this stage (1) limit or reverse potentially disabling or disfiguring contracture formations (Figure 38-15), (2) increase ROM, (3) distribute pressure over problem hypertrophic scar areas, or (4) assist function. Serial drop-out casts[29] (Figure 38-16), used for progressive scar elongation, have the additional advantages of moisturizing and softening the scar, preventing orthotic slippage, and ensuring a consistent wearing schedule.

Before discharge, fears of heat sources such as hot water, the stove, or an iron are addressed during homemaking practice. The COTA teaches burn prevention techniques at this time and consults with the psychologist when behavioral desensitization procedures are indicated.

Physical tolerance and work skills assessment assists return to work. Vocational rehabilitation referrals are sometimes needed. Functional activities and work skills are assigned to improve work tolerances, strength, endurance, and flexibility. Lifting, stooping, pushing, pulling, handling, and manipulating are a few examples of common job activities incorporated by therapists. A job analysis interview, as part of the activity needs analysis, will provide a basis for beginning work conditioning. Outpatient OT is replaced as soon as possible by participation in health clubs, school swimming, gymnastic or sports programs, general home management, and work activity.

In the outdoor environment, special techniques are needed to protect the patient. The COTA gives the following suggestions to avoid injuries from sun exposure: wear light-colored, lightweight, nonrestrictive clothing, sandal shoes, and a cool flap hat or wide brimmed hat; use a battery fan and spray bottle to increase evaporative cooling; wear sunglasses; drink more fluids; avoid vasoconstricting drugs such as cigarettes; work in a shaded area; and apply sunscreen. Unprotected sun exposure results in blotchy, unpredictable tanning. If pigment is absent in the healed wound, severe tissue damage can result from sun exposure.

A healed wound has increased sensitivity to cold because of a changed ability to sweat and constrict or dilate capillaries in the scar tissue. If the patient lives in a cold climate, the COTA gives these general safety recommendations: keep vehicles well maintained; have a cell phone; keep blankets, extra mittens (not gloves), warm clothing/boots, candles, and snacks in the vehicle; wear insulated, waterproof boots; use safety shoes with fiberglass toe and shank if approved by employer; wear hats or an insulated hood and multiple-layer, nonrestrictive clothing made of wind-resistant fabric (see Figure 38-11); and avoid vasodilating drugs such as alcohol or vasoconstricting drugs such as cigarettes.

Many burn centers offer school reentry programs for children that educate teachers and students about burn injuries and explain the purpose of compression garments, splints, exercise, and care of the skin.[2,6] The program goals are to prevent unnecessary restrictions to the child's activities, decrease teasing, ensure splint and exercise assistance, remind schoolmates that the burned child is the same as before on the inside, and ease the transition back to school.[2,12,19]

Patient and family collaboration and motivation promote successful outcomes. For instance, Olympic achievement and the support of Fidel Castro were incentives for the 1996 Cuban 800-meter silver medalist Ana Quirot to recover full function after a 40% TBSA full-thickness burn of the face, neck, and upper torso from a cooking fire. Cliff Meidl is an inspiring American example of the triumph of the human spirit over burn injury. Three heart attacks, two toe amputations, loss of the use of both knees, and a severe burn from a 30,000 volt electrical injury during construction work sidelined the former soccer player. His doctor reconstructed his legs with a muscle transplant. Then he said, "Now you do your 50%. Go for it and try to prove us wrong. Try to walk." This was something Meidl and the doctors thought he'd never do. "Someone told me winners never quit and quitters never win, and that there's no such thing as an overachiever or underestimator," Meidl said. "I lived by that philosophy and used it a lot as a crutch because there's lots of dips and turns along the road." He was selected for the 1996 US Olympic team in the four-man flatwater kayak 1000 meter event.

## SUMMARY

Advances in burn care continue to improve burn injury outcomes. Today, most patients recovering from a burn injury can expect to return to a near-normal life, including early return to school or work.

The OTR and COTA provide exercise, ADL, skin-conditioning activities, positioning techniques, splints, patient education, vascular support, and compression garments. Reassessment of patient needs and function throughout recovery promotes effective economical treatment progression.

Burn scars last forever, although they can be modified slightly by surgery or camouflage make-up. Three fourths of burn injuries could have been prevented. Thoughtful COTAs incorporate burn prevention when they do therapy with the frail, the elderly, the socioeconomically burdened, or risk-taking youth who have immature judgment. The American Burn Association, and local fire fighting departments provide prevention materials.

## Sample Treatment Plan

**Case study**

***Personal data***

Name: Mr. J.
Age: 36
Religion: Native-American who uses healing stones
Diagnosis: Partial-thickness and full thickness burn; 20% TBSA involving right arm and hand, right anterior axillary fold, chest, neck, and face
Mechanism of injury: Carburetor backfired while he was examining it and clothing caught fire
Marital status: Recently married, planning to have children
Employer: Northwest Airlines
Job duties: Computer design, drafting, on-site management of building construction
Education: College degree
Wife's employer: Hospital—laboratory technician
Insurance: Both covered by Mr. J.'s insurance
Financial status: Both incomes needed for mortgage payments and remodeling of new home
Recreational hobbies: Spectator sports, motorcycle riding and repair, home renovations
Dominant hand: Right
Length of stay: 21 days
Grafts: STSG meshed to right hand, sheet STSG to face

See the OT Evaluation Summary that follows for details of the evaluation and treatment plan. Based on the summary of the acute care and OT treatment plan, assess OT treatment changes in surgical and rehabilitative stages of care.

**Follow-up care**

Mr. and Mrs. J., the COTA, and the OTR collaborate to update the treatment plan and revise the face mask fit every 2 weeks for a minimum of 2 months. If scar activity is stabilized and the patient independently evaluates scar control, therapy visits are reduced to once a month with the scheduled clinic time until the patient is discharged from all follow-up care.

### OT Evaluation Summary

| *Acute care phase* | *Current status* | *Short-term (1 week) goals (including education)* |
|---|---|---|
| UE, LE, face, trunk function<br>• ROM<br>• Strength<br>• Sensation<br>• Mobility | • ROM—eyelids do not close when asleep<br>• Mouth increased from small to medium size microstomia prevention appliance (MPA)<br>• Shoulder flexion and abduction limited to 0 to 150 degrees; elbow flexion limited to 10 to 90 degrees | • Close eyelids tightly 3 to 5 times each hour from 6 AM to 11 PM to elongate contracting upper and lower lids.<br>• Increase mouth stretches to 6 cc tube by next week.<br>• Improve wound healing by keeping right UE limber and participating more vigorously in active ROM in all joints burned within limits of pain, endotracheal tube, and intravenous lines. |

## Sample Treatment Plan—cont'd

### OT Evaluation Summary—cont'd

| *Acute care phase* | *Current status* | *Short-term (1 week) goals (including education)* |
|---|---|---|
| | • Right wrist extension decreased—unable to extend wrist actively past neutral, approximately 20 degree wrist extension after 20 minutes of prolonged stretch<br>• Supination limited 20 degrees actively and 60 degrees passively bilaterally<br>• Hand function—active ROM: MCPs 0 to 45 degrees PIPs 15 to 30 degrees DIP 0 degrees<br>• Unwilling to do prolonged stretch independently because of pain and medication sleepiness<br>• When cued, does relaxation breathing before exercise<br>• Increased sensitivity to touch and cocontraction from pain in past week<br>• Distraction from pain, irritation from nasogastric feeding tube, coughing up secretions<br>• Needs cueing for each exercise<br>• Since off ventilator, ambulates to chair independently and forgets tall walker<br>• Good functional strength | • Four times daily, reach for bed traction bar above head with both hands, hold stretch, count to 15.<br>• Use BTE in rehabilitation clinic and soft foam gripper increasing to rubber band exerciser when IPs closed.<br>• Remember to use overhead walker for ambulating.<br>• Learn quad sets and ankle pumps to use when grafted.<br>• Discuss pain and distraction with surgeon and psychologist, use recommendations and share with therapist. |
| Positioning and edema management<br>• Foam wedge<br>• Traction | • Positioning—no head pillow because of face and neck burns, elevated head of bed; shoulders at 90 degrees forward flexion in chair, at 90 degrees abduction in bed (using bedside table to support end of wedge); elbow extension; forearm in neutral; hands slightly elevated<br>• Pillow behind back when in chair to allow neck extension when sitting | • Keep injured areas elevated. Use wedges or airplane bed attachment at all times.<br>• Change position every 2 hours when awake by elevating head of bed, flexing knees, turning, dangling, sitting, standing, or walking.<br>• Learn importance of using tall walker for edema control when ambulating.<br>• Beginning middle of week, independently direct elevation and move furniture to achieve elevated positioning for arms and, if needed, legs.<br>• Review positioning with COTA each afternoon. |
| Orthotics<br>• Splints<br>• Casts<br>• Support garments | • Wears large or extra-large microstomia prevention appliance<br>• Uses Exudry pad or equivalent neck dressing to improve neck contours<br>• Wears wrist-hand-finger orthosis in IP extension, MP flexion, wrist 30 degrees extension, thumb abduction/flexion secured with Kerlix coarse mesh gauze wrap at bedtime<br>• Wears elastic wraps on legs during day | • Keep microstomia prevention appliance in mouth all night and loosen (not remove) to avoid discomfort of insertion and removal. Change to wearing 5 to 30 minutes of each waking hour as soon as tolerated.<br>• Remember to ask for wrist-hand-finger orthosis at bedtime.<br>• Remove leg elastic wraps at bedtime as soon as tolerated. |

*Continued.*

## Sample Treatment Plan—cont'd

### OT Evaluation Summary—cont'd

| *Acute care phase* | *Current status* | *Short-term (1 week) goals (including education)* |
|---|---|---|
| Daily living skills (evaluation done by COTA and OTR) | • Unable to pick up anything because of open fingertips<br>• Uses elastic wrap or tape on comb, toothbrush, fiber pen, spoon and fork for eating because of hand edema<br>• Needs assistance bathing<br>• Cannot apply lotion to dry lips before eating or moisturize healed areas yet<br>• Can remove elastic wraps with help<br>• Cannot don own clothing because of too much wound drainage, tube feeding supplements and gas pains causing clothing to be temporarily too tight around waist | • Operate nurse call button with foot or arm by middle of week<br>• Independently eat, brush teeth, comb hair, sign forms, and clean glasses by end of week using gross grasp<br>• Family will bring large jogging shorts and shirt. Slip on shoes after grafting. |
| Patient and family involvement with therapy | • Given outpatient instruction book for education in anticipated course of wound, graft, and donor healing<br>• Home therapy program and education reviewed with wife and parents on several occasions<br>• Written exercise program being followed by patient—still needs maximum help from therapist at this point, facial and hand edema interfere, groggy from medications and does not remember exercises from one session to the other<br>• Works with vigor and is cooperative during therapy sessions when analgesia effective<br>• Wears healing stones | • Family will begin to learn active ROM exercise program for face, neck, UEs and follow through in the evening with patient.<br>• Work on memory, negotiation, and team work during therapy. Take responsibility to inform others of desires and wishes.<br>• Family will follow through with patient's independent exercises and therapy program.<br>• Change velcro healing stone pocket as needed. |
| Equipment | — | • Use foam wedge, overhead walker, foam tape, and large handles temporarily for utensils. |

## Selected Reading Guide Questions

1. What are the two layers of the skin?
2. Name two factors considered in determining burn severity.
3. What is an escharotomy?
4. Describe two factors that can affect the quality of burn wound healing and lead to scar formation.
5. When ROM is evaluted during rehabilitation care, which factors may limit full ROM?
6. Why may a patient need temporary adaptations for self-care during acute care?
7. What is the primary objective for positioning during acute care?
8. Why are patients immobilized postoperatively?
9. How soon after grafting can gentle, active ROM be resumed?
10. How soon after surgery should an intermediate garment or support dressing be applied?
11. Why are skin conditioning activities used in burn rehabilitation? Provide examples of skin conditioning techniques.
12. When a splint is ordered in the acute phase, what is the preferred wearing schedule? Why?
13. When a splint for grafting is ordered, what is the preferred wearing schedule? Why?
14. What is the primary cause of dysfunction after a burn injury?

15. Which points should be covered in a home program?
16. What are possible causes of limitations in ADL during the rehabilitation phase?
17. How does a patient recover work skills?
18. Are splints always used during the rehabilitation care phase?
19. Name three interventions to prevent sunburn.
20. When should patient education about burn injury and rehabilitation begin?

## REFERENCES


1. American Burn Association: *Burn care services in North America.* 1995, The Association.
2. Blakeney P et al: Efficacy of school reentry programs, *J Burn Care Rehabil* 16:469-72, 1995.
3. Brigham PA, McLoughlin E: Burn incidence and medical care use in the United States: Estimates, trends, and data sources, *J Burn Care Rehabil* 17(2):95-107, 1996.
4. Cromes GF, Helm PA: The status of burn rehabilitation services in the United States: results of a national survey, *J Burn Care Rehabil* 13(6):656-662, 1993.
5. Daugherty MB, Carr-Collins JA: Splinting techniques for the burn patient. In Richard RL, Staley MJ, editors: *Burn care and rehabilitation principles and practice,* Philadelphia, 1994, FA Davis.
6. Doctor ME: Commentary, *J Burn Care Rehabil* 16(4):466-468, 1995.
7. Fakhry SM et al: Regional and institutional variation in burn care, *J Burn Care Rehabil* 16:86-90, 1995.
8. Falkel JE: Anatomy and physiology of the skin. In Richard RL, Staley MJ, editors: *Burn care and rehabilitation principles and practice,* Philadelphia, 1994, FA Davis.
9. Hansbrough JF: Current status of skin replacements for coverage of extensive burn wounds, *J Trauma* 30(suppl 12):155-162, 1990.
10. Heimbach DM, Engrav LH: Surgical management of the burn wound, New York, 1984, Raven.
11. Helm PA: Burn rehabilitation: Dimensions of the problem. In Salisbury RE: *Clinics in plastic surgery,* Philadelphia, 1992, WB Saunders.
12. Helm PA, Fisher SV: Rehabilitation of the patient with burns. In Delisa J, Currie D, Gans B, editors: *Rehabilitation medicine principles and practice,* ed 2, Philadelphia, 1988, JB Lippincott.
13. Hunter JM, Mackin EJ: Management of edema. In Hunter JM et al, editors: *Rehabilitation of the hand,* St Louis, 1990, Mosby.
14. Johnson C: Pathologic manifestations of burn injury. In Richard RL, Staley MJ, editors: *Burn care and rehabilitation principles and practice,* Philadelphia, 1994, FA Davis.
15. Jordan CL, Allely RA, Gallagher J: Self-care strategies following severe burns. In Christiansen C, editor: *Ways of living: self-care strategies for special needs,* Rockville, Md, 1994, American Occupational Therapy Association.
16. Laubenthal KN et al: Prospective randomized study of the effect of pressure garment therapy on pain and pruritus in the maturing burn wound, *Proc American Burn Association* 28:161, 1996.
17. Leman CJ et al: Exercise physiology in the acute burn patient: Do we really know what we're doing? *Proc American Burn Assoc* 24:91, 1992.
18. Leman CJ, Ricks N: Discharge planning and follow-up burn care. In Richard RL, Staley MJ, editors: *Burn care and rehabilitation principles and practice,* Philadelphia, 447-472, 1994, FA Davis.
19. Leslie G et al: Native Americans: a challenge for the pediatric burn team (poster), *Proc American Burn Assoc* 28:147, 1996.
20. Leung KS et al: Complications of pressure therapy for post-burn hypertrophic scars: biochemical analysis based on 5 patients, *Burns* 10:434-438, 1983.
21. Lund C, Browder N: The estimation of area of burns, *Surg Gynecol Obstet* 79:352-355, 1944.
22. Miles WK, Grigsby L: Remodeling of scar tissue in the burned hand. In Hunter JM et al, editors: *Rehabilitation of the hand,* ed 3, St Louis, 1990, Mosby.
23. Nahieli O et al: Oro-maxillofacial skeletal deformities resulting from burn scar contractures of the face and neck, *Burns* 21(1):65-69, 1995.
24. Pain management of the burn patient, *J Burn Care Rehabil* 16(3):343-376, 1995.
25. Peacock EE Jr: *Wound repair,* ed 3, Philadelphia, 1984, WB Saunders.
26. Price H: Connective tissue in wound healing. In Wolf SL et al, editor: *Wound healing: Alternatives in management: contemporary perspectives in rehabilitation,* Philadelphia, FA Davis.
27. Richard R et al: Algorithm to guide burn patient treatment by physical therapist assistants (PTAs), *Poster Proc American Burn Association* 28:160, 1996.
28. Richard RL, Staley MJ: Burn patient evaluation and treatment planning. In Richard RL, Staley MJ, editors: *Burn care and rehabilitation principles and practice,* Philadelphia, 1994, FA Davis.
29. Ricks N, Meager D: The benefits of plaster casting for lower extremity burns after grafting in children, *J Burn Care Rehabil* 13:465-468, 1992.
30. Rivers EA, Fisher SV: Burn rehabilitation. In O'Young BJ, Yong MA, Steins SA, editors: *Physical medicine and rehabilitation secrets,* Philadelphia, 1996, Hanley & Belfus.
31. Rivers EA, Fisher SV: Advances in burn rehabilitation. In Kottke JF, Amate EA, editors: *Clinical advances in physical medicine and rehabilitation,* Washington, DC: 334-357, 1991, Pan American Health Organization, Regional Office of the World Health Organization.
32. Robertson CF et al: Obstructive sleep apnea: A complication of burns to the head and neck in children, *J Burn Care Rehabil* 6:353-357, 1985.
33. Saffle JR, Davis B, Williams P: Recent outcomes in the treatment of burn injury in the United States: a report from the American Burn Association Patient Registry, *J Burn Care Rehabil* 16(3): 219-232; 288-289, 1995.
34. Upright J et al: American Burn Association Committee on the Organization and Delivery of Burn Care: Burn care outcomes and clinical indicators, *J Burn Care Rehabil* 17(3):17A-39A, 1996.
35. Ward RS: Pressure therapy for the control of hypertrophic scar formation after burn injury: A history and review, *J Burn Care Rehabil* 12(3):257-262, 1991.
36. Weber JM, Thompkins DM: Improving survival: Infection control and burns, *Am Assoc Crit Care Nurs* 4(3):414-423, 1993.


## RECOMMENDED READING


Campbell MK, Covey MH, editors: Topics in acute care and trauma rehabilitation, *Burn Trauma,* Vol 1, 1987.

Fisher SV, Helm PA, editors: *Comprehensive rehabilitation of burns,* Baltimore, 1984, Williams & Wilkins.

Richard RL, Staley MJ, editors: *Burn care and rehabilitation principles and practice,* Philadelphia, 1994, FA Davis.


## RESOURCES FOR CUSTOM-MADE GARMENTS

Barton Carey
Perrysburg, Ohio
(800) 421-0444

Bio-Concepts
Phoenix, AZ
(800) 421-5647

Beiersdorf-Jobst Institute
Toledo, Ohio
(800) 537-1063

# Index

**F**

## T

# Selected Abbreviations from Medicine and Rehabilitation*

| | |
|---|---|
| % TBSA | Percent of total body surface area (burns) |
| A-P, AP | Anteroposterior |
| a.c. | Before meals (ante cibum) |
| a.m.a. | Against medical advice |
| AAROM | Active assisted range of motion |
| ABA | American Burn Association |
| ACL | Allen Cognitive Level |
| ADHD | Attention deficit hyperactivity disorder |
| ADL | Activities of daily living |
| AI | Aortic insufficiency |
| AIDS | Acquired immune deficiency syndrome |
| ALS | Amyotrophic lateral sclerosis |
| AMA | American Medical Association |
| AML | Acute myelocytic leukemia |
| AOTA | American Occupational Therapy Association |
| ARDS | Acute respiratory distress syndrome |
| AROM | Active range of motion |
| ASD | Atrial septal defect |
| ASHD | Arteriosclerotic heart disease |
| BBB | Blood brain barrier, bundle branch block |
| b.i.d. | Twice a day (bis in die) |
| BM | Bowel movement |
| BMR | Basal metabolic rate |
| BP | Blood pressure |
| BPH | Benign prostatic hypertrophy |
| BSA | Body surface area |
| BTE | Baltimore Therapeutic Equipment (work simulator) |
| BUE | Both upper extremities |
| BUN | Blood urea nitrogen |
| c̄ | with (cum) |
| C1-C7 | Levels of cervical spine or spinal nerves |
| CA | Chronological age, cervicoaxial |
| CAD | Coronary artery disease |
| CARF | Commission on Accreditation of Rehabilitation |
| CAT, CT | Computerized axial tomography |
| CC | Chief complaint |
| cc | Cubic centimeter |
| CCU | Coronary care unit |
| CEA | Cultured epidermal autograft (burns) |
| CHAMPUS | Civilian Health and Medical Program of the Uniformed Services |
| CHD | Coronary heart disease |
| CHF | Congestive heart failure |
| CLD | Chronic liver disease |
| CMV | Cytomegalovirus |
| CNS | Central nervous system |
| COPD | Chronic obstructive pulmonary disease |
| COTA | Certified occupational therapy assistant |
| CPM | Continuous passive motion |
| CPR | Cardiopulmonary resuscitation |
| CSF | Cerebrospinal fluid |
| CTD | Cumulative trauma disorder |
| CVA | Cerebrovascular accident (stroke) |
| D/C | Discontinue, discharge |
| DAI | Diffuse axonal injury |
| DEG | Degeneration, degree |
| DIP | Distal interphalangeal |
| DOB | Date of birth |
| DRG | Diagnosis related group |
| DTR | Deep tendon reflex |
| DTs | Delirium tremens |
| DVT | Deep venous thrombosis |
| Dx | Diagnosis |
| ECG, EKG | Electrocardiogram, electrocardiograph |
| ECT | Electroconvulsive therapy |
| EEG | Electroencephalogram, electroencephalograph |
| EMG | Electromyogram |
| FBS | Fasting blood sugar |
| FH | Family history |
| FUO | Fever of unknown origin |
| FWB | Full weight bearing |
| GI | Gastrointestinal |
| GSW | Gunshot wound |
| GTT | Glucose tolerance test |
| h.d. | At bedtime (hora decubitus) |
| h.s. | At bedtime (hora somni) |
| HBV | Hepatitis B vaccine |
| HCFA | Health Care Financing Administration |
| HIV | Human immunodeficiency virus |
| HR | Heart rate |
| HVGS | High voltage galvanic stimulation |
| IBD | Inflammatory bowel disease |
| ICU | Intensive care unit |
| IH | Infectious hepatitis |

*Modified from Austrin MG, Austrin MR: *Learning medical terminology*, ed 8, St Louis, 1995, Mosby.